Thieme

Comprehensive Management of Vestibular Schwannoma

Editor

Matthew L. Carlson, MD
Professor of Otolaryngology and Neurosurgery
Program Director, Neurotology and Skull Base Surgery Fellowship
Department of Otolaryngology–Head and Neck Surgery
Mayo Clinic
Rochester, Minnesota

Associate Editors

Michael J. Link, MD
Professor of Neurosurgery and Otolaryngology
Program Director, Neurosurgical Skull Base Fellowship
Department of Neurologic Surgery
Mayo Clinic
Rochester, Minnesota

Colin L. W. Driscoll, MD
Professor and Chair
Department of Otolaryngology–Head and Neck Surgery
Mayo Clinic
Rochester, Minnesota

Brian A. Neff, MD
Associate Professor of Otolaryngology
Department of Otolaryngology–Head and Neck Surgery
Mayo Clinic
Rochester, Minnesota

Jamie J. Van Gompel, MD
Associate Professor of Neurosurgery and Otolaryngology
Program Director, Neurosurgery Residency Program
Department of Neurologic Surgery
Mayo Clinic
Rochester, Minnesota

Kelly D. Flemming, MD
Associate Professor of Neurology
Department of Neurology
Mayo Clinic
Rochester, Minnesota

John I. Lane, MD
Professor of Radiology
Department of Radiology
Mayo Clinic
Rochester, Minnesota

Neil T. Shepard, PhD
Professor of Audiology and Vestibular Medicine
Department of Otolaryngology–Head and Neck Surgery
Mayo Clinic
Rochester, Minnesota

Robert L. Foote, MD
Professor and Chair
Department of Radiation Oncology
Mayo Clinic
Rochester, Minnesota

Illustrated by:
Robert F. Morreale, MS, CMI, FAMI
Assistant Professor of Biomedical Communications
Division Chair, Biomedical and Scientific Visualization
Mayo Clinic
Rochester, Minnesota

Thieme
New York • Stuttgart • Delhi • Rio de Janeiro

Executive Editor: Timothy Y. Hiscock
Managing Editor: J. Owen Zurhellen IV
Director, Editorial Services: Mary Jo Casey
Editorial Assistant: Keith Palumbo
Production Editor: Sean Woznicki
International Production Director: Andreas Schabert
Editorial Director: Sue Hodgson
International Marketing Director: Fiona Henderson
International Sales Director: Louisa Turrell
Director of Institutional Sales: Adam Bernacki
Senior Vice President and Chief Operating Officer: Sarah Vanderbilt
President: Brian D. Scanlan

Library of Congress Cataloging-in-Publication Data

Names: Carlson, Matthew L. (Professor of Otolaryngology and Neurosurgery), editor. Title: Comprehensive management of vestibular schwannoma / [edited by] Matthew L. Carlson [and 8 others] ; illustrated by Robert F. Morreale.
Description: New York : Thieme, [2019] | Includes bibliographical references and index.
Identifiers: LCCN 2018061415| ISBN 9781626233317 (hardcover : alk. paper) | ISBN 9781626233324 (e-book)
Subjects: | MESH: Neuroma, Acoustic–diagnosis | Neuroma, Acoustic–therapy Classification: LCC RC280.E2 | NLM WV 250 | DDC 616.99/385–dc23 LC record available at https://lccn.loc.gov/2018061415

Thieme Publishers New York
333 Seventh Avenue, New York, NY 10001 USA
+1 800 782 3488, customerservice@thieme.com

Thieme Publishers Stuttgart
Rüdigerstrasse 14, 70469 Stuttgart, Germany
+49 [0]711 8931 421, customerservice@thieme.de

Thieme Publishers Delhi
A-12, Second Floor, Sector-2, Noida-201301
Uttar Pradesh, India
+91 120 45 566 00, customerservice@thieme.in

Thieme Publishers Rio de Janeiro, Thieme Publicações Ltda.
Edifício Rodolpho de Paoli, 25º andar
Av. Nilo Peçanha, 50 – Sala 2508,
Rio de Janeiro 20020-906 Brasil
+55 21 3172-2297 / +55 21 3172-1896
www.thiemerevinter.com.br

Cover design: Thieme Publishing Group
Typesetting by Thomson Digital, India

Printed in Germany by CPI books, Leck 5 4 3 2 1

ISBN 978-1-62623-331-7

Also available as an e-book:
eISBN 978-1-62623-332-4

Important note: Medicine is an ever-changing science undergoing continual development. Research and clinical experience are continually expanding our knowledge, in particular our knowledge of proper treatment and drug therapy. Insofar as this book mentions any dosage or application, readers may rest assured that the authors, editors, and publishers have made every effort to ensure that such references are in accordance with **the state of knowledge at the time of production of the book.**

Nevertheless, this does not involve, imply, or express any guarantee or responsibility on the part of the publishers in respect to any dosage instructions and forms of applications stated in the book. **Every user is requested to examine carefully** the manufacturers' leaflets accompanying each drug and to check, if necessary in consultation with a physician or specialist, whether the dosage schedules mentioned therein or the contraindications stated by the manufacturers differ from the statements made in the present book. Such examination is particularly important with drugs that are either rarely used or have been newly released on the market. Every dosage schedule or every form of application used is entirely at the user's own risk and responsibility. The authors and publishers request every user to report to the publishers any discrepancies or inaccuracies noticed. If errors in this work are found after publication, errata will be posted at www.thieme.com on the product description page.

Some of the product names, patents, and registered designs referred to in this book are in fact registered trademarks or proprietary names even though specific reference to this fact is not always made in the text. Therefore, the appearance of a name without designation as proprietary is not to be construed as a representation by the publisher that it is in the public domain.

Dedicated to Becky, Leif, Bryn, Soren, and Lars.

Contents

Preface

Despite being histologically benign and relatively uncommon, otolaryngologists and neurosurgeons have maintained a lasting and deep-rooted fascination with the management of vestibular schwannoma. The desire to improve the lives of patients with vestibular schwannoma drove refinements in middle and posterior fossa skull base approaches, the early adoption of the operating microscope, and intraoperative cranial nerve monitoring. Over the last century, vestibular schwannoma characteristically defined the subspecialties of neurotology and neurologic skull base surgery and cultivated the multidisciplinary collaboration that exists today.

Arising from the frequent collision between dogmatic views and innovative advances, the treatment of vestibular schwannoma bears a storied past of controversy. With the advent of minimally invasive methods of radiation delivery, in combination with an increased understanding of the natural history of the disease, the modern management of vestibular schwannoma has become considerably more complex. New advancements generate fresh controversies, yet many of the original debates between pioneering surgeons have once again emerged as the pendulum swings between conservatism and definitive cure.

The chief objective of this project was to create a comprehensive clinical textbook covering all aspects of vestibular schwannoma management. This book encompasses 84 focused chapters authored by a cadre of international experts based on specific topic expertise, with illustrations by Bob Morreale, a senior medical illustrator at the Mayo Clinic. Substantiated by an editorship comprised of microsurgeons, radiation oncologists, neurologists, neuroradiologists, and audiologists, an earnest attempt was made to place equal emphasis on all management modalities, with the goal of providing unbiased information about each aspect of care. Wherever possible, summary tables within various chapters were included to provide the reader with a rapid clinical reference based on evidence from the world literature rather than focusing solely on expert opinion.

This book will guide trainees and practicing physicians through the evaluation, surgical and non-surgical management, rehabilitation, salient controversies and long-term outcomes of sporadic and neurofibromatosis type 2-associated vestibular schwannoma. Each chapter covers fundamental principles directed toward residents, fellows and early attending physicians as well as more advanced concepts that will appeal to mid- and later-career physicians who care for patients with vestibular schwannoma. Indeed, we hope that this book uniquely guides the care of patients with vestibular schwannoma for years to come.

"*We are like dwarfs sitting on the shoulders of giants. We see more, and things that are more distant, than they did, not because our sight is superior or because we are taller than they, but because they raise us up, and by their great stature add to ours.*"

– John of Salisbury, 1159

Harvey Cushing, Walter Dandy, Lars Leksell, and William House will forever be remembered for their contributions to the advancement of the field. As this book was written, two extraordinary "giants" in our field passed away: Albert L. Rhoton Jr. and Michael E. Glasscock III. Dr. Rhoton was internationally recognized as the father of microscopic neurosurgery whose principal aim surrounded educating microsurgeons worldwide in an effort to "make surgery more accurate, gentle and safe". We are immensely fortunate to present one of Dr. Rhoton's final chapter submissions, "Anatomy of Vestibular Schwannoma Surgery", a topic about which he was particularly passionate. This contribution comes full circle as Dr. Rhoton began his neurosurgical career at Mayo Clinic in 1966, publishing several of his early landmark papers on cerebellopontine angle and temporal bone anatomy. After training with Dr. William House in Los Angeles, Dr. Glasscock founded The Otology Group in Nashville, Tennessee in 1970. As he recalls, being the only fellowship-trained neurotologist east of the Mississippi for over a decade provided an unparalleled clinical experience in vestibular schwannoma microsurgery. His legacy continues through his over 70 neurotology fellows, many of whom are prominent leaders in the field today. We will forever be indebted to our late mentors.

Matthew L. Carlson, MD

Acknowledgments

I sincerely thank my co-editors, the contributors, and artist Robert F. Morreale for their high-quality and detailed work on this project. In addition, I am indebted to Timothy Hiscock, J. Owen Zurhellen, and Keith Palumbo at Thieme Publishers for the commitment, guidance, and patience during the development of the book manuscript.

Contributors

Siviero Agazzi, MD, MBA, FACS
Professor and Vice Chairman
Department of Neurosurgery
Director, Division of Cranial Surgery
University of South Florida
Tampa, Florida

Yuri Agrawal, MD, MPH
Associate Professor
Division of Otology, Neurotology and Skull Base Surgery
Department of Otolaryngology–Head and Neck Surgery
The Johns Hopkins University School of Medicine
Baltimore, Maryland

Sameer Ahmed, MD
Neurotology Fellow
Department of Otolaryngology–Head and Neck Surgery
University of Michigan
Ann Arbor, Michigan

David W. Andrews, MD
Anthony Alfred Chiurco Professor of Neurological Surgery
Director, Division of Neuro-oncologic Neurosurgery and Stereotactic Radiosurgery
Director, Stereotactic Radiosurgery Units, Jefferson Hospital for Neuroscience
Thomas Jefferson University Hospital
Philadelphia, Pennsylvania

H. Alexander Arts, MD, FACS
Professor of Otolaryngology and Neurosurgery
Department of Otolaryngology-Head and Neck Surgery
University of Michigan Health System
Ann Arbor, Michigan

Ramsey Ashour, MD
Assistant Professor
Department of Neurosurgery
Dell Medical School
University of Texas
Austin, Texas

Albert Attia, MD
Associate Professor of Radiation Oncology and Neurosurgery
Program Director, Radiation Oncology Residency Program
Director of Radiosurgery Program
Vanderbilt University Medical Center
Nashville, Tennessee

Seilesh C. Babu, MD
Program Director and Clinical Professor
Ascension St John Macomb Otolaryngology Residency Program
Michigan State University College of Human Medicine
East Lansing, Michigan
Division of Otology/Neurotology/Skull Base Surgery
Michigan Ear Institute
Novi, Michigan

Daniele Bernardeschi, MD, PhD
Department of Otorhinolaryngology–Head and Neck Surgery
Hôpital Pitié-Salpêtrière, AP-HP
Sorbonne Université
Paris, France

Jaishri O. Blakeley, MD
Professor
Director, Johns Hopkins Comprehensive Neurofibromatosis Center
Department of Neurology
The Johns Hopkins University School of Medicine
Baltimore, Maryland

Nikolas H. Blevins, MD
Larry and Sharon Malcolmson Professor
Chief, Division of Otology and Neurotology
Medical Director, Stanford Cochlear Implant Center
Department of Otolaryngology–Head and Neck Surgery
Stanford University School of Medicine
Stanford, California

Kofi Boahene, MD, FACS
Professor
Division of Facial Plastic and Reconstructive Surgery
Department of Otolaryngology–Head and Neck Surgery
The Johns Hopkins University School of Medicine
Baltimore, Maryland

Christian A. Bowers, MD
Assistant Professor
Department of Neurosurgery
Westchester Medical Center
New York Medical College
Valhalla, New York

Derald E. Brackmann, MD
House Clinic
Los Angeles, California

Joseph T. Breen, MD
Assistant Professor
Department of Otolaryngology–Head and Neck Surgery
University of Cincinnati College of Medicine
Cincinnati, Ohio

Marc R. Bussiere, MSc
Medical Physics
Department of Radiation Oncology
Massachusetts General Hospital
Boston, Massachusetts

Matthew L. Carlson, MD
Professor of Otolaryngology and Neurosurgery
Program Director, Neurotology and Skull Base Surgery Fellowship
Department of Otolaryngology–Head and Neck Surgery
Mayo Clinic
Rochester, Minnesota

Lucas P. Carlstrom, MD, PhD
Resident Physician
Department of Neurologic Surgery
Mayo Clinic
Rochester, Minnesota

Stephen P. Cass, MD, MPH/MSPH
Professor
Department of Otolaryngology
University of Colorado School of Medicine
Aurora, Colorado

Per Caye-Thomasen, MD, DMSc
Professor and Consultant
Department of Oto-rhino-laryngology, Head and Neck Surgery
Copenhagen University Hospital Rigshospitalet
Copenhagen, Denmark

Steven D. Chang, MD
Robert C. and Jeannette Powell Professor of Neurosurgery
Department of Neurosurgery
Stanford University School of Medicine
Stanford, California

Navjot Chaudhary, MD
Clinical Associate Professor
Department of Neurosurgery
Stanford University School of Medicine
Stanford, California

Brian S. Chen, MD
Division of Otology and Neurotology
Department of Otolaryngology–Head and Neck Surgery
Tripler Army Medical Center
Honolulu, Hawaii
Assistant Professor of Surgery
Uniformed Services University of the Health Sciences
Bethesda, Maryland

William R. Copeland III, MD
Neurosurgeon
Tenwek Hospital
Bomet, Kenya

Roberto A. Cueva, MD, FACS
Regional Neurotologist/Skull Base Surgeon
Southern California Permanente Medical Group
Voluntary Clinical Professor
University of California San Diego School of Medicine
San Diego, California

Nicholas L. Deep, MD
Neurotology Fellow
Department of Otolaryngology–Head and Neck Surgery
New York University Langone Medical Center
New York, New York

Jacqueline Diels, OT
Division of Otolaryngology-Head and Neck Surgery
University of Wisconsin Hospital and Clinics
Facial Rehabilitation Specialist
Facial Retraining LLC
Madison, Wisconsin

Colin L. W. Driscoll, MD
Professor and Chair
Department of Otolaryngology–Head and Neck Surgery
Mayo Clinic
Rochester, Minnesota

Heidi A. Edmonson, PhD
Department of Radiology
Division of Medical Physics
Mayo Clinic
Rochester, Minnesota

D. Gareth Evans, MD, FRCP
Professor
Department of Genomic Medicine
Division of Evolution and Genomic Science
University of Manchester
St. Mary's Hospital
Manchester, England, United Kingdom

Christopher J. Farrell, MD
Assistant Professor
Department of Neurosurgery
Sidney Kimmel Medical College at Thomas Jefferson University
Philadelphia, Pennsylvania

Ugo P. Fisch, MD, FRCS, FACS(Hon)
Professor
ENT Center
Hirslanden Klinik
Zürich, Switzerland

Kelly D. Flemming, MD
Associate Professor
Department of Neurology
Mayo Clinic
Rochester, Minnesota

Robert L. Foote, MD
Hitachi Professor of Radiation Oncology
Chair, Department of Radiation Oncology
Mayo Clinic
Rochester, Minnesota

William A. Friedman, MD
Professor and Chair
Department of Neurosurgery
University of Florida
Gainesville, Florida

David R. Friedmann, MD
Assistant Professor
Division of Otology, Neurotology, and Skull Base Surgery
Department of Otolaryngology–Head and Neck Surgery
New York University School of Medicine
New York, New York

Francesco Galletti, MD
Professor of Otolaryngology
Department Director
University of Messina
Messina, Italy

Bruce J. Gantz, MD
Professor and Chair
Department of Otolaryngology–Head and Neck Surgery
University of Iowa Hospitals and Clinics
Iowa City, Iowa

Caterina Giannini, MD, PhD
Professor of Laboratory Medicine/Pathology and Neurosurgery
Department of Laboratory Medicine and Pathology
Mayo Clinic
Rochester, Minnesota

Michael B. Gluth, MD, FACS
Associate Professor
Section of Otolaryngology–Head and Neck Surgery
Director, Comprehensive Ear and Hearing Center
Director, Bloom Otopathology Lab
The University of Chicago Medicine & Biological Sciences
Chicago, Illinois

John G. Golfinos, MD
Chair, Department of Neurosurgery
Associate Professor of Neurosurgery and Otolaryngology
New York University School of Medicine
New York, New York

Christopher S. Graffeo, MD
Resident Physician
Department of Neurologic Surgery
Mayo Clinic
Rochester, Minnesota

Richard K. Gurgel, MD
Associate Professor
Department of Otolaryngology–Head and Neck Surgery
University of Utah School of Medicine
Salt Lake City, Utah

Marlan R. Hansen, MD, FACS
Marvin and Rose Lee Pomerantz Professor
Departments of Otolaryngology-Head and Neck Surgery and Neurosurgery
University of Iowa
Iowa City, Iowa

David S. Haynes, MD, MMHC, FACS
Vice Chair, Chief Academic Officer
Professor of Otolaryngology, Neurosurgery, and Hearing and Speech Sciences
Neurotology Division/Fellowship Program/Cochlear Implant Program Director
Skull Base Center Co-Director
Vanderbilt University Medical Center
Nashville, Tennessee

Douglas K. Henstrom, MD
Assistant Professor
Department of Otolaryngology–Head and Neck Surgery
University of Iowa
Iowa City, Iowa

Susan J. Herdman, PhD, PT, FAPTA
Professor of Rehabilitation Medicine
Director, Division of Physical Therapy
Director, Vestibular Rehabilitation
Department of Rehabilitation Medicine
Emory University School of Medicine
Atlanta, Georgia

Travis C. Hill, MD, PhD
Resident Physician
Department of Neurosurgery
New York University Langone Medical Center
New York, New York

Joshua D. Hughes, MD
Resident Physician
Department of Neurologic Surgery
Mayo Clinic
Rochester, Minnesota

Jacob B. Hunter, MD
Assistant Professor
Department of Otolaryngology–Head and Neck Surgery
University of Texas Southwestern Medical Center
Dallas, Texas

John Huston III, MD
Professor
Department of Radiology
Mayo Clinic
Rochester, Minnesota

Brandon Isaacson, MD, FACS
Professor
Co-Director, Comprehensive Skull Base Program
Chair, Otolaryngology Resident Selection Committee
Department of Otolaryngology–Head and Neck Surgery
University of Texas Southwestern Medical Center
Dallas, Texas

Robert K. Jackler, MD
Sewall Professor and Chair
Department of Otolaryngology–Head and Neck Surgery
Professor of Neurosurgery and Surgery
Stanford University School of Medicine
Stanford, California

Jeffrey T. Jacob, MD
Neurosurgeon
Michigan Head and Spine Institute
Novi, Michigan

Michael E. Johnson, MD, PhD
Assistant Professor
Department of Anesthesiology and Perioperative Medicine
Mayo Clinic
Rochester, Minnesota

Michel Kalamarides, MD, PhD
Professor
Department of Neurosurgery
Hopital Pitié-Salpêtrière, AP-HP
Sorbonne Université
Paris, France

Nickalus Khan, MD
Resident Physician
Department of Neurosurgery
University of Tennessee Health Science Center
Memphis, Tennessee

Matthew L. Kircher, MD
Assistant Professor
Department of Otolaryngology–Head and Neck Surgery
Loyola University Medical Center
Maywood, Illinois

Ruwan Kiringoda, MD
Director, Neurotology and Hearing Implants
Palo Alto Medical Foundation
Palo Alto, California

Narayan R. Kissoon, MD
Assistant Professor of Neurology and Anesthesiology
Division of Headache, Department of Neurology
Division of Pain Medicine
Department of Anesthesiology and Perioperative Medicine
Mayo Clinic
Rochester, Minnesota

Douglas Kondziolka, MD, MSc, FRCSC, FACS
Gray Family Professor of Neurosurgery
Vice-Chair, Clinical Research
Professor of Radiation Oncology
Director, Center for Advanced Radiosurgery
NYU Langone Medical Center
New York University
New York, New York

Jennifer Kosty, MD
Clinical Skull Base and Cerebrovascular Fellow
Department of Neurosurgery
Louisiana State University Health Sciences Center, Shreveport
Shreveport, Louisiana

J. Walter Kutz Jr., MD, FACS
Associate Professor
Department of Otolaryngology–Head and Neck Surgery
University of Texas Southwestern Medical Center
Dallas, Texas

John I. Lane, MD
Professor
Department of Radiology
Mayo Clinic
Rochester, Minnesota

Shannon Langmead, CRNP, CNRN
Senior Adult Nurse Practitioner, Neurology and Neuro-Oncology
Clinical Coordinator, Johns Hopkins Comprehensive Neurofibromatosis Center
The Johns Hopkins University School of Medicine
Baltimore, Maryland

Michael J. LaRouere, MD
Neurotology Fellowship Director
Michigan Ear Institute
Farmington Hills, Michigan

Gregory P. Lekovic, MD, PhD
Chief, Division of Neurosurgery
House Clinic
Clinician-Scientist
House Ear Institute
Los Angeles, California

Dan Leksell, MD
Chairman
Leksell Gamma Knife Society
Stockholm, Sweden

John P. Leonetti, MD
Professor
Director of Skull Base Surgery
Department of Otolaryngology–Head and Neck Surgery
Division of Cranial Base Surgery
Loyola University Health System
Maywood, Illinois

Michael J. Link, MD
Professor of Neurosurgery and Otolaryngology
Program Director, Neurosurgical Skull Base Fellowship
Department of Neurologic Surgery
Mayo Clinic
Rochester, Minnesota

Haisong Liu, PhD
Associate Professor
Department of Radiation Oncology
Sidney Kimmel Medical College
Thomas Jefferson University
Philadelphia, Pennsylvania

Simon K. W. Lloyd, MBBS, BSc(Hons), MPhil(Cantab), FRCS (ORL-HNS)
Professor of Neurotology and Skull Base Surgery
Salford Royal and Manchester University NHS Foundation Trusts
Manchester, England, United Kingdom

Jay S. Loeffler, MD
Herman and Joan Suit Professor of Radiation Oncology
Chief, Department of Radiation Oncology
Massachusetts General Hospital
Boston, Massachusetts

Morten Lund-Johansen, MD, PhD
Professor and Consultant Neurosurgeon
Department of Neurosurgery
Haukeland University Hospital
Professor I, Institute of Clinical Medicine
University of Bergen
Bergen, Norway

L. Dade Lunsford, MD, FACS
Lars Leksell Distinguished Professor
Director, Center for Image-Guided Neurosurgery
Director, Residency Training Program
Department of Neurological Surgery
UPMC Presbyterian Hospital
University of Pittsburgh
Pittsburgh, Pennsylvania

Daniele Marchioni, MD
Professor and Head
Department of Otorhinolaryngology
University of Verona
Verona, Italy

Samir Mardini, MD
Professor of Surgery
Chair, Division of Plastic Surgery
Department of Surgery
Mayo Clinic
Rochester, Minnesota

Sam J. Marzo, MD
Professor and Chairman
Department of Otolaryngology–Head and Neck Surgery
Loyola University Health System
Maywood, Illinois

Bill Mastrodimos, MD, JD
Voluntary Clinical Professor
University of California San Diego School of Medicine
Regional Skull Base Neurosurgeon
Southern California Permanente Medical Group
San Diego, California

Sean O. McMenomy, MD
Professor, Department of Otolaryngology and Neurosurgery
Director, Neurotology Fellowship Program
Department of Otolaryngology-Head and Neck Surgery
New York University School of Medicine
New York, New York

Beth N. McNulty, MD
Assistant Professor
Division of Otology, Neurotology, and Cranial Base Surgery
Department of Otolaryngology–Head and Neck Surgery
University of Kentucky College of Medicine
Lexington, Kentucky

Theodore R. McRackan, MD, MSCR
Assistant Professor
Director, Skull Base Center
Department of Otolaryngology–Head and Neck Surgery
Medical University of South Carolina
Charleston, South Carolina

Gautam U. Mehta, MD
Neurosurgeon
House Clinic
Los Angeles, California

Aaron Metrailer, MD
Neurotology Fellow
Michigan Ear Institute
Farmington Hills, Michigan

L. Madison Michael II, MD, FACS, FAANS
Associate Professor
Department of Neurosurgery
University of Tennessee Health Science Center
Semmes-Murphey Clinic
Memphis, Tennessee

David A. Moffat, BSc(Hons), MA(Hon), MBBS, PhD, FRCS
Department of Skull Base Surgery
Addenbrookes Hospital
Cambridge University Teaching Hospitals NHS Trust
Cambridge, England, United Kingdom

Ashkan Monfared, MD
Associate Professor
Departments of Surgery and Neurosurgery
George Washington University
Washington, DC

Edwin M. Monsell, MD, PhD
Professor
Department of Otolaryngology–Head and Neck Surgery
Wayne State University School of Medicine
Detroit, Michigan

Dennis M. Moore, MD
Assistant Professor
Department of Otolaryngology–Head and Neck Surgery
Loyola University Health System
Maywood, Illinois

Erling Myrseth, MD, PhD
Professor
Department of Neurosurgery
Haukeland University Hospital
Bergen, Norway

Brian A. Neff, MD
Associate Professor
Department of Otolaryngology–Head and Neck Surgery
Mayo Clinic
Rochester, Minnesota

Ajay Niranjan, MD, MBA
Professor of Neurosurgery
Director, UPMC Brain Mapping Center
Director of Radiosurgery Research, Center of Image-Guided Neurosurgery
Department of Neurological Surgery
UPMC Presbyterian
University of Pittsburgh
Pittsburgh, Pennsylvania

Georg Norén, MD, PhD
Professor Emeritus
Department of Neurosurgery
Warren Alpert Medical School of Brown University
Providence, Rhode Island

Brendan P. O'Connell, MD
Assistant Professor
Department of Otolaryngology–Head and Neck Surgery
University of North Carolina
Chapel Hill, North Carolina

Steven R. Otto, MA
House Clinic
Los Angeles, California

Scott R. Owen, MD
Director of Facial Plastic and Reconstructive Surgery
University of Iowa Hospitals and Clinics
Iowa City, Iowa

James A. Owusu, MD
Facial Plastic and Reconstructive Surgeon
Department of Head and Neck Surgery
MidAtlantic Permanente Medical Group
McLean, Virginia

Enrico Pasanisi, MD
Associate Professor of Otolaryngology
University of Parma
Parma, Italy

Neil S. Patel, MD
Neurotology Fellow
Department of Otolaryngology–Head and Neck Surgery
Mayo Clinic
Rochester, Minnesota

Stanley Pelosi, MD
Department of Otolaryngology
Long Island Jewish Medical Center
New Hyde Park, New York

Avital Perry, MD
Resident Physician
Department of Neurologic Surgery
Mayo Clinic
Rochester, Minnesota

Matthieu Peyre, MD, PhD
Department of Neurosurgery
Hopital Pitié-Salpêtrière, AP-HP
Sorbonne Université
Paris, France

Daniel R. Pieper, MD†
Department of Neurosurgery and Skull Base Surgery
Michigan Head and Spine Institute
Providence Park Hospital
Novi, Michigan

† *deceased*

Crystal Pitts, AuD
Department of Otolaryngology–Head and Neck Surgery
University of Michigan
Ann Arbor, Michigan

Scott R. Plotkin, MD, PhD
Professor
Department of Neurology
Harvard Medical School
Stephen E. and Catherine Pappas Center for Neuro-Oncology
Massachusetts General Hospital
Boston, Massachusetts

Bruce E. Pollock, MD
Professor of Neurosurgery and Radiation Oncology
Department of Neurologic Surgery
Mayo Clinic
Rochester, Minnesota

Sampath Chandra Prasad, MBBS, MS, DNB, FEB-ORLHNS
Consultant Otolaryngology-Head and Neck Surgery
Manipal Hospital
Bangalore, India

Livio Presutti, MD
Professor and Head
Department of Otolaryngology
University Hospital of Modena
Modena, Italy

Daniel L. Price, MD
Associate Professor
Program Director, Otolaryngology Residency Program
Department of Otolaryngology–Head and Neck Surgery
Mayo Clinic
Rochester, Minnesota

Aditya Raghunathan, MD, MPH
Assistant Professor
Department of Laboratory Medicine and Pathology
Mayo Clinic
Rochester, Minnesota

Richard T. Ramsden, MBE, FRCSEd, FRCSEng
Former Professor of Otolaryngology
Manchester Royal Infirmary and Salford Royal Hospital
Manchester, England, United Kingdom

Aaron K. Remenschneider, MD, MPH
Assistant Professor
University of Massachusetts Medical School
UMASS Memorial Medical Center
Worcester, Massachusetts

Albert L. Rhoton Jr., MD†
R. D. Keene Family Professor and Chairman Emeritus
Department of Neurosurgery
University of Florida College of Medicine
Gainesville, Florida

† *deceased*

Daniel S. Roberts, MD, PhD
Assistant Professor of Surgery
Division of Otolaryngology
University of Connecticut School of Medicine
Farmington, Connecticut

Jon Robertson, MD
Professor
Department of Neurosurgery
University of Tennessee Health Science Center
Semmes-Murphey Clinic
Memphis, Tennessee

Joseph P. Roche, MD
Assistant Professor
Division of Otolaryngology-Head and Neck Surgery
Department of Surgery
University of Wisconsin School of Medicine and Public Health
Madison, Wisconsin

J. Thomas Roland Jr., MD
Mendik Foundation Chairman of Otolaryngology-Head and Neck Surgery
Professor of Otolaryngology and Neurosurgery
New York University Langone Medical Center
New York, New York

Alessandra Russo, MD
Department of Otology and Skull Base Surgery
Gruppo Otologico
Piacenza-Rome, Italy

Raghuram Sampath, MD
Skull Base Fellow
Department of Neurosurgery
University of Colorado
Denver, Colorado

Ravi N. Samy, MD
Associate Professor
Chief, Division of Otology/Neurotology
Program Director, Neurotology Fellowship
Department of Otolaryngology
University of Cincinnati
Cincinnati, Ohio

Nina Niu Sanford, MD
Assistant Professor
Department of Radiation Oncology
University of Texas Southwestern Medical Center
Dallas, Texas

Mario Sanna, MD
Professor of Otolaryngology
Gruppo Otologico
Piacenza and Rome, Italy

Marc S. Schwartz, MD
Department of Neurosurgery
University of California San Diego
San Diego, California

Alexander Sevy, MD
Assistant Professor
Department of Otolaryngology–Head and Neck Surgery
Louisiana State University
Baton Rouge, Louisiana

Jeffrey D. Sharon, MD
Assistant Professor
Director of Balance and Falls Center
Division of Otology, Neurotology, and Skull Base Surgery
Department of Otolaryngology–Head and Neck Surgery
University of California San Francisco
San Francisco, California

Jason P. Sheehan, MD
Professor
Department of Neurological Surgery
University of Virginia
Charlottesville, Virginia

Neil T. Shepard, PhD
Professor Emeritus of Audiology and Vestibular Medicine
Department of Otolaryngology–Head and Neck Surgery
Mayo Clinic
Rochester, Minnesota

Wenyin Shi, MD, PhD
Associate Professor
Co-Director, Brain Tumor Center
Co-Director, Stereotactic Radiosurgery Program
Department of Radiation Oncology
Sidney Kimmel Medical College
Thomas Jefferson University
Philadelphia, Pennsylvania

Helen A. Shih, MD, MPH
Associate Professor
Chief, CNS & Eye Services
Department of Radiation Oncology
Medical Director, Proton Therapy Center
Massachusetts General Hospital
Boston, Massachusetts

Robert Smee, MBBS, MA, FRANZCR
Associate Professor
Department of Radiation Oncology
Prince of Wales Hospital
Sydney, Australia

Clayton A. Smith, MD, PhD
Assistant Professor
Department of Radiation Oncology
Ochsner Medical Center
New Orleans, Louisiana

Davide Soloperto, MD, PhD
ENT Department, AOUI Verona
University of Verona
Verona, Italy

Sven-Eric Stangerup, MD, DMSc
Associate Professor
ENT Department
Copenhagen University Hospital
Copenhagen, Denmark

Olivier Sterkers, MD, PhD
Professor
Department of Otorhinolaryngology–Head and Neck Surgery
Hôpital Pitié-Salpêtrière, AP-HP
Sorbonne Université
Paris, France

Marissa A. Suchyta, BA
Division of Plastic Surgery
Department of Surgery
Mayo Clinic
Rochester, Minnesota

Alex D. Sweeney, MD
Assistant Professor of Otolaryngology and Neurosurgery
Dorothy L. McGee Endowed Chair
Bobby R. Alford Department of Otolaryngology–Head and Neck Surgery
Baylor College of Medicine
Houston, Texas

Abdelkader Taibah, MD
Department of Otology & Skull Base Surgery
Gruppo Otologico
Piacenza-Rome, Italy

Steven A. Telian, MD
John L. Kemink Professor of Neurotology
Department of Otolaryngology–Head and Neck Surgery
University of Michigan
Ann Arbor, Michigan

Philip V. Theodosopoulos, MD
Professor and Vice Chair of Neurological Surgery
Reza and Georgianna Khatib Endowed Chair in Skull Base Surgery
Director, Skull Base Tumor Program
Department of Neurological Surgery
University of California San Francisco
San Francisco, California

Michael J. Torrens, MPhil, ChM, FRCS
Department of Neurosurgery
Hygeia Hospital
Athens, Greece

Øystein V. Tveiten, MD
Department of Neurosurgery
Haukeland University Hospital
Department of Clinical Medicine
University of Bergen
Bergen, Norway

Jamie J. Van Gompel, MD
Associate Professor of Neurosurgery and Otolaryngology
Program Director, Neurologic Surgery Residency Program
Department of Neurologic Surgery
Mayo Clinic
Rochester, Minnesota

Harry van Loveren, MD
David W. Cahill Professor and Chair
Department of Neurosurgery and Brain Repair
Vice-Dean of Clinical Affairs
CEO, Byrd Alzheimer's Center and Research Institute
Director, USF Health Neuroscience Institute
University of South Florida Morsani College of Medicine
Tampa, Florida

Judy B. Vitucci, BBA
Former Chief Executive Officer
Acoustic Neuroma Association
Cumming, Georgia

Jeffrey T. Vrabec, MD
Otology, Neurotology, and Skull Base Surgery
Houston Methodist ENT & Facial Plastic Surgery
Houston, Texas

David D. Walker, MD
Assistant Professor
Department of Otolaryngology–Head and Neck Surgery
University of Arkansas for Medical Sciences
Little Rock, Arkansas

George B. Wanna, MD, FACS
Professor of Otolaryngology and Neurosurgery
Icahn School of Medicine at Mount Sinai
Chair, Department of Otolaryngology
New York Eye and Ear Infirmary of Mount Sinai and Mount Sinai Beth Israel
New York, New York

Bryan K. Ward, MD
Assistant Professor
Department of Otolaryngology–Head and Neck Surgery
The Johns Hopkins University School of Medicine
Baltimore, Maryland

Robert E. Watson Jr., MD, PhD
Associate Professor
Chair, Division of Neuroradiology
Department of Radiology
Mayo Clinic
Rochester, Minnesota

D. Bradley Welling, MD, PhD, FACS
Walter Augustus Lecompte Professor and Chair
Department of Otolaryngology–Head and Neck Surgery
Harvard University Medical School
Chief of Otolaryngology Head and Neck Surgery
Massachusetts Eye and Ear Infirmary
Department of Otolaryngology–Head and Neck Surgery
Massachusetts General Hospital
Boston, Massachusetts

Cameron C. Wick, MD
Assistant Professor
Department of Otolaryngology–Head and Neck Surgery
Washington University School of Medicine
St. Louis, Missouri

Eric P. Wilkinson, MD, FACS
House Ear Institute
Los Angeles, California

Amparo Wolf, MD, PhD
Neurosurgeon
Department of Clinical Neurological Sciences
London Health Science Centre
University of Western Ontario
London, Ontario, Canada

Yin Xia, MD, PhD
Professor
Department of Otorhinolaryngology
Beijing Tiantan Hospital
Capital Medical University
Beijing, China

Kathleen J. Yost, PhD
Associate Professor
Department of Health Sciences Research
Mayo Clinic
Rochester, Minnesota

A. Samy Youssef, MD, PhD, MSc, FAANS
Professor of Clinical Neurosurgery and Otolaryngology
Director, Complex Cranial and Skull Base Surgery
Program Director, Skull Base Surgery Fellowship
Department of Neurosurgery
University of Colorado Hospital
Aurora, Colorado

Part I

Background

I

1 History of Vestibular Schwannoma Surgery

Richard T. Ramsden

1.1 Introduction

When we consider the current state of the art in many areas of surgery, it is instructive and humbling to glance occasionally in the rearview mirror of history. Where we are now has only been reached because of the achievements of those who went before. Bernard of Chartres in the 12th century pointed out "that we see more and further than our predecessors not because we have keener vision or greater height, but because we are lifted up and borne aloft on their gigantic stature." While it is true that we may look back on some of the ideas and misconceptions from the past with incredulity or even, at times, amusement, one has to put the efforts of our predecessors into the context of the state of knowledge and technology of the day. We may rest assured that future generations of surgeons will look back at our early 21st century efforts with the same emotions.

1.2 Presurgical "Diagnostic" Era

The first date in the vestibular schwannoma (VS) saga is 1777, when Eduard Sandifort of Leiden recorded the first postmortem description of such a tumor, in a paper entitled "De duro quodam corpusculo, nervo auditorio adherente" ("Regarding a certain hard body adherent to the auditory nerve"). It was "not only connected to the lower part of the said nerve, but also to the nearest part of the medulla oblongata from which the two seventh nerves emerge, penetrating as far the foramen in the inner part of the petrous section of the temporal bone." The tumor was externally hard like cartilage, but soft inside. He concluded that this cause of deafness was beyond the reach of medication or surgery and was thus incurable[1] (▶ Fig. 1.1).

The 18th century saw the dawn of the Age of the Enlightenment and can be seen as the start of the era of scientific medicine. Central to this was the abandonment of the belief that disease was a God-given punishment and was to be suffered as the price of redemption. Anatomy had been studied for several hundred years (e.g., the detailed dissection of the middle ear by Vesalius in the 16th century), but there was no serious attempt to understand physiology, until the groundbreaking work by William Harvey on the circulation of the blood. Galenic theories were gradually being challenged, and many of the great thinkers of the day presented their own concepts of the function of the human body and its relationship with the mind. Diagnostic medicine was fueled by the study of the relationship of disease to postmortem findings. In particular, neuroanatomy advanced through the outstanding contribution of Soemmerring on the origin and classification of the 12 cranial nerves and the doctrine of localization of the senses, notably through the work of Hughlings Jackson, Eduard Hitzig, and David Ferrier in the 19th century. Neurologists, like doctors in all specialties, were increasingly attempting to correlate pathological anatomy with clinical presentation—diseased structure with disorders of function. There are many elegant accounts of these efforts in the early literature on VS, and Leveque-Lasource, in 1810 in the French Literature, was one of the first who described a case of blindness and deafness with voice changes and partial paralysis.[2]

Cruveilhier's 1835 report cannot be bettered as an account of the progression of the symptomatology of VS, from deafness to postmortem, in a young woman. He describes "Complete amaurosis; no less complete loss of taste and smell; partial deafness. Violent headache, numbness of the skin of the face, and at times sharp pain in the left thigh, which seems to alternate with the cephalgia. Intelligence remained unimpaired to the last; passionate wish to die, as the sole means of ending her sufferings … for the last two weeks of life she refused nourishment, and for the first time there was practically continuous nausea; violent efforts to vomit, which raised phlegm; … the patient lost consciousness and died after 24 hours of agony. My diagnosis had been this: compression of the brain by an expanded tumor, either at the expense of the meninges or in the thickness of the brain itself; the probability of the seat of this tumor being at the base of the skull." Cruveilhier describes the application of 16 leeches to the mastoid, bloodletting from the feet, electropuncture, and the use of moxas–downy vegetable material used in Oriental medicine as a counterirritant by igniting it on the skin.[3] It is clear that at that time diagnostic skills were progressing at a greater rate than therapeutic remedies.

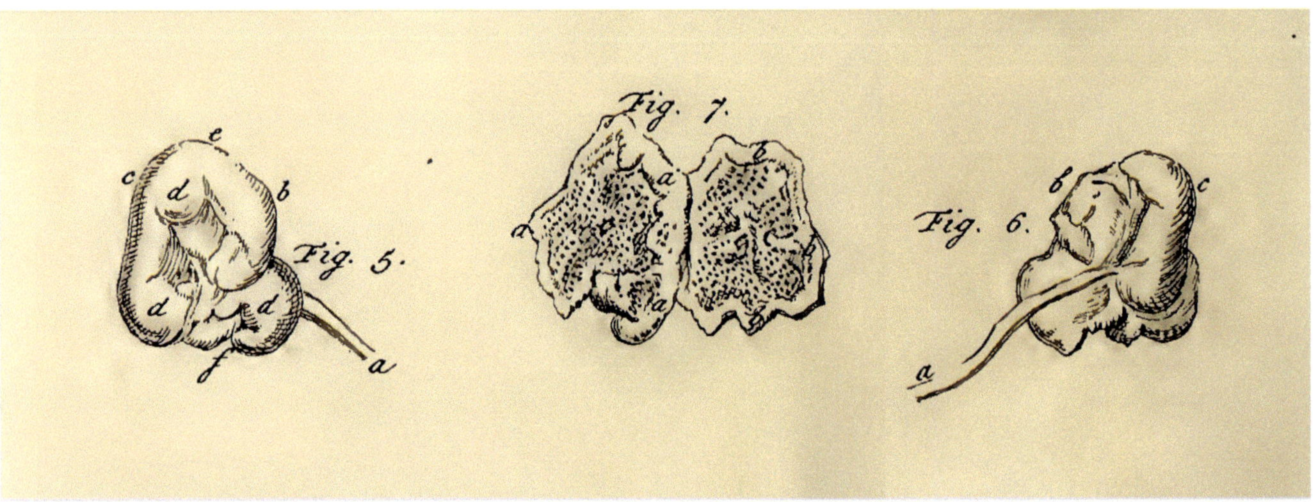

Fig. 1.1 The postmortem appearances of Sandifort's tumor.

Sir Charles Bell in Edinburgh provided one of the most detailed early accounts in the English language in his 1830 description of a young woman who presented to him with total anesthesia of the second and third divisions of the trigeminal nerve so that "the end of a feather passed three inches into the nostril gives her no sensation and does not produce sneezing." She went on to develop a hearing loss on the same side, giddiness, headache, and vomiting, and eventually died with brainstem failure, with clenching of her teeth, slurred speech, respiratory failure, and dysphagia. At postmortem, a tumor "the size of a pigeon's egg" was found occupying the cerebellopontine angle and indenting the pons and cerebellum. It was described as cystic and contained fluid the color of urine. The solid capsule resembled vitreous humor. The auditory nerve could not be identified and only the most medial quarter inch of the facial nerve and half inch of the trigeminal nerve could be seen to be free of tumor.[4] Throughout the 19th century, further important contributions to the localization of posterior fossa tumors and to cerebellar pathology were made by Hughlings Jackson,[5] Joseph Toynbee,[6] and William Gowers[7] in England; Ludwig Bruns[8] and Hermann Oppenheim[9] in Germany; and by Joseph Babinski[10] in France, eventually giving surgeons the confidence to locate and to attempt removal of posterior fossa lesions.

1.3 The Start of the Surgical Era and the Birth of Neurosurgery

The literature from the second half of the 19th century contains details, albeit somewhat scanty, of unsuccessful attempts at removal of what were most probably VSs. A patient was operated on by von Bergmann in Oppenheim's clinic in 1890, but the tumor was not actually found until after the patient's death.[11] Charles McBurney in New York unsuccessfully explored the posterior fossa of a patient of M. Allen Starr in 1891,[12] and Guldenarm operated for Winkler in Amsterdam in 1893, but the patient died soon after the operation.[13]

The literature has widely attributed the distinction of the first successful surgical removal of a VS in 1894 to the London-based neurosurgeon Sir Charles Ballance.[14] Harvey Cushing, however, disputes this, on the grounds that Ballance's tumor was broad based and attached to the posterior surface of the petrous bone and therefore more likely to be a meningioma. Furthermore, deafness was not mentioned as a symptom. ▶ Fig. 1.2 is taken from Ballance's own operative note and does indeed show the tumor to be broad based. The internal meatus is not widened and does not contain tumor and there is minimal compression of the brainstem. Ballance himself describes it as "a solid tumor found attached to dura over inner part of posterior surface of petrous – somewhat firmly fixed." Taken together, it does indeed seem to have been a meningioma, rather than a VS. In Cushing's view, the accolade should go to the Edinburgh surgeon, Thomas Annandale, in 1895: "a brilliant surgical result the first recorded."[15] Annandale studied medicine in Edinburgh, Scotland, where he eventually succeeded Joseph Lister as Regius Professor in 1877. Like all general surgeons of the day, he could turn his hand to anything, although most of his practice seems to have been orthopedic (▶ Fig. 1.3).

His famous case described by Gibson (1896)[16] and by Stewart (1895),[17] who was the resident physician at Edinburgh Royal Infirmary, was Isabella, aged 25 years and pregnant, with a 10-month history of frontal headache, giddiness, and difficulty walking. She was unable to hear the ticking of a watch in her right ear or a tuning fork placed on the vertex. Examination of the eyes revealed optic neuritis (papilledema) and both

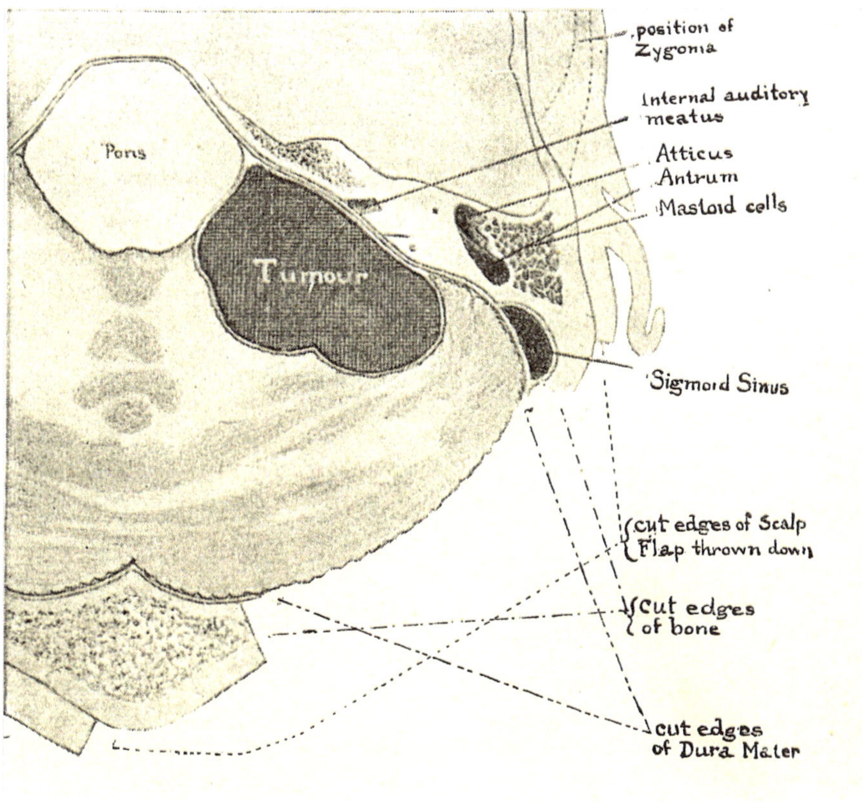

Fig. 1.2 Drawing taken from Ballance's operative note showing tumor attached to the petrous bone by a broad base, with minimal compression of the pons and an undilated internal meatus that appears free of tumor.

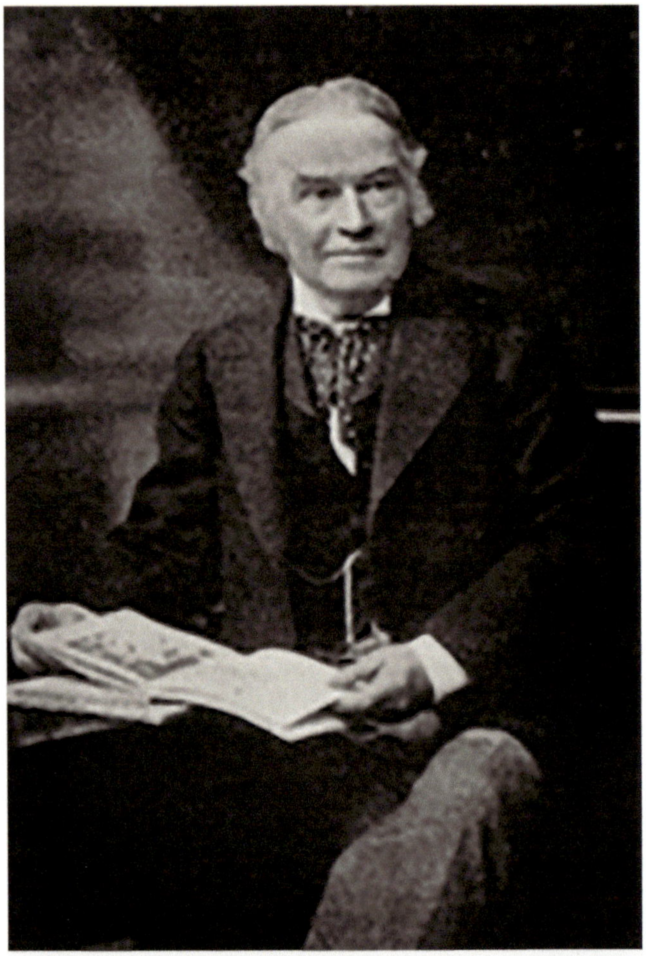

Fig. 1.3 Thomas Annandale of Edinburgh.

horizontal and vertical nystagmus. There was dilation of the contralateral pupil, palatal weakness with nasal regurgitation of fluids, and changes in her voice. She had exaggerated tendon reflexes on both sides and ankle clonus. Her gait was broad based and she had a tendency to fall to the right side especially when standing with the feet together and the eyes closed. There was therefore strong clinical evidence of a large posterior fossa lesion, and Stewart made the perspicacious observation "the labyrinthine deafness would be consistent with a lesion either of an auditory pathway in the cerebellum, or in the auditory nucleus or nerve itself." The differential diagnosis was tumor, gumma, or tuberculoma. Treatment with inunction of blue ointment and the antisyphilitic potassium iodide (her husband was a sailor "absent for protracted periods in distant parts of the world") proved ineffective and, on May 3rd 1895, Annandale trephined the skull over the right lobe of the cerebellum and removed a semicystic tumor the size of a pigeon's egg from "the lateral lobe of the cerebellum." Microscopic investigation showed it to be of the nature of a fibrosarcoma, at that time a rather imprecise term, but from the clinical description of the case it was most certainly a VS. Postoperatively, progress was "eminently satisfactory." Her headache was immediately better, her sickness ceased, and her nystagmus settled almost completely. The swallowing became perfect even for fluids. Her gait improved and her optic neuritis almost disappeared. Surprisingly, there is no mention in the clinical record of the postoperative function of the facial nerve. It is hard to imagine that it remained intact and it may just be that in 1895, a facial paralysis was not regarded as much of a price to pay for the successful removal of an intracranial tumor. Five months later, Isabella delivered a baby girl and the note from the general practitioner makes it clear that both mother and child were in excellent health. The author could find no reference in the literature to any further sorties into the cerebellopontine angle (CPA) by Annandale. It may well be that he decided to quit while he was ahead!

During the early decades of the 20th century, there were increasing numbers of attempts at tumor removal. The results were almost always apocalyptically dreadful. Krause reported an 84% operative mortality,[18] Borchardt reported 72%,[19] and Eiselsberg reported 75%.[20] Such statistics did nothing to encourage early intervention, and perpetuated the ominous outcome figures. Digital enucleation was common, with brain stem retraction and no understanding of the importance of the blood supply to the brainstem. Indeed, Ballance suggested that surgical outcomes could be improved if the anteroinferior cerebellar artery could be ligated prior to tumor removal. The need for speed driven by the still embryonic state of general anesthesia was a further contributing factor to the dire prognoses. At that time, the accepted approach to the tumor was via a large unilateral suboccipital craniotomy, often with resection of part of the cerebellum for access, and often as planned two- (or more) stage procedure. Furthermore, although localization was improving, it was still imperfect. Uncertainty as to the side of lesion would often mean that surgeons were obliged to remove all the bone from one lateral sinus to the other in search of the tumor.

Interestingly, the translabyrinthine approach to the tumor was first proposed in 1904 by Panse,[21] avoiding the need for brainstem retraction. He defined the limits of that approach as the lateral sinus, the jugular bulb, the internal carotid artery, and the temporal lobe, but felt that the facial nerve would usually have to be sacrificed, although he also suggested that it could be mobilized from the geniculate ganglion to the stylomastoid foramen, anticipating Ugo Fisch by several decades. It is unclear whether Panse ever used the approach himself, but operations were carried out by Kümmel in Heidelberg in 1909[22] and by Quix in Utrecht in 1911,[23] although Quix was not able to remove the tumor. Success was primarily limited because of the cramped access. The approach was cursorily dismissed by Ballance as "objectionable for obvious reasons" and for at least half a century was relegated to obscurity, although Cushing himself stated "it may in time become the operation of choice." Some surgeons did experiment with a combined suboccipital and transpetrosal approach removing bone as far as the internal meatus, but the results were just as disastrous.

1.4 The Era of Cushing and Dandy

Harvey Cushing was one of the medical greats and the father of the emerging specialty of neurosurgery. Most of the earlier surgeons were generalists who could turn their hands to almost anything. His name lives on in Cushing's disease, and he influenced the surgical practice of many fields. Working with the physicist William Bovie he introduced the use of electrocautery to surgical practice. After visiting Riva-Rocci, he introduced the sphygmomanometer to his practice and its use soon became commonplace in North America. He was the first to propose anesthetic monitoring during neurosurgery operations. It is, however, his contribution to the surgery of VS that concerns us here. His monograph "Tumors of the Nervus Acusticus and the Syndrome of the Cerebellopontile Angle" should be obligatory reading for all those working in this area.[15] He memorably compared the tumor with the bloody angle at the Battle of Gettysburg. Working at the Peter Bent Brigham Hospital in Boston, Cushing advocated a bilateral suboccipital approach through a cross-bow incision and, by performing an intracapsular subtotal debulking, reduced the perioperative mortality to 28% by 1915 and to 4% by 1931. Despite great strides in mortality reduction, facial nerve function was a secondary consideration, and its preservation was the exception rather than the rule. The bilateral craniectomy not only allowed wide decompression but also the possibility of exploring both sides in cases in which there was doubt as to the side of the tumor. His results were a spectacular improvement but did, of course, lead to recurrence, and his equally talented contemporary, one time pupil and eventual rival Walter E. Dandy of the Johns Hopkins Hospital in Baltimore, advocated total removal.[24] Dandy's contributions to neurosurgery were immense and included the introduction of pneumoencephalography, clipping of aneurysms, and the understanding of the mechanisms and the management of hydrocephalus. Despite these greatly improved results, there remained reluctance on the part of many neurosurgeons to advise surgery until the tumor was very large—thus continuing the "large tumor, poor outcome, avoid operating, large tumor" cycle.[25,26]

1.5 Concomitant Advances

Vestibular schwannoma surgery benefitted from advances in other fields of medicine, notably anesthesia, imaging, audiovestibular medicine, and microbiology. Blood transfusion was placed on a secure footing in the 1930s and 1940s, and neuroanesthesia became a specialty in its own right. The importance of the arterial blood supply to the brainstem was brought to surgeons' notice in 1949 by Atkinson, and the need to treat the anterior inferior artery in particular with respect was eventually realized.[27]

X-rays of the petrous bone became available in the 1920s, and tomography of the internal auditory canals was in routine use by the 1960s. The Technetium-99 scan was in use in the 1960s but was unable to reliably identify a CPA tumor of less than 3 cm in diameter. First generation CT scanners were introduced in the 1960s and MRI in the 1980s—the latter able to detect lesions of little more than a millimeter in diameter.[28]

Tests of hearing became more common in the 1940s and it was hoped that they would allow differentiation of neural lesions from those of the cochlea: Fowler's Alternate Loudness Balance test, Carhart's test for Tone Decay, Bekesy Audiometry, the Short Increase Sensitivity Index Test (SISI), the Loudness Discomfort Test, and Speech Audiometry. Shortly later came tests of the stapedial reflex, including threshold and decay. Individually and collectively, these tests were unreliable and as a result, undoubtedly, many tumors were missed. Many clinicians working in the 1970s were still using these tests as part of their routine workup given lack of diagnostic alternatives; however, these once ubiquitous tools have now been consigned to the dustbin of history. The audiological test that, for a time, held center stage was the auditory brainstem response (ABR) with a quoted sensitivity of 98%, which sounds impressive until one realizes that the specificity is very low.[28] Any sensorineural hearing loss greater than 70 dB, whether cochlear or retrocochlear, will be associated with an absent ABR response due to the severity of the deafness rather than the site of the lesion.

The caloric response was first described by Bárány in 1906 and the bithermal caloric test became an important tool in the diagnostic workup by the mid-20th century. Canal paresis on the side of the deafness was seen as a common feature of VS and was felt to be particularly indicative if there was no history of imbalance—findings that suggest slowly progressive pathology rather than an acute event.

During the 1970s, an algorithm was sought to rationalize the investigative protocol and a "rule of three" was adopted in many centers—if there were abnormalities on any two of ABR, caloric testing, and tomography of the internal auditory canals, one would then proceed to an "expensive" CT scan, or to myodil or air meatography. It seems a strange sequence of events looking back, as today any asymmetrical sensorineural hearing loss is routinely investigated with MRI, without any other diagnostic foreplay.

The first monocular otologic microscope was developed by a Swedish otologist, Carl Olof Nylen, in 1921. The following year, the illuminated binocular operative microscope was first adapted to otologic surgery by Gunnar Holmgren, while pioneering lateral canal fenestration surgery for otosclerosis.[29,30,31] Interestingly, despite the distinct advantages offered by the operating microscope in otologic surgery, many U.S. surgeons did not adopt its use for several decades secondary to significant limitations including narrow field of view, short working distance, poor illumination, large size, and poor maneuverability.[31] Following several key innovations of the commercial operating microscope, Bill House was the first American otologist to realize its full value. Neurosurgeons were initially slow to follow suit, but with time the operating microscope also became a standard part of the neurosurgical armamentarium. The development and refinement of electric and air-driven drills with cutting and diamond bur assortments occurred between the 1920s and 1940s.[29,30]

1.6 The House and Hitselberger Era: Modern Times

When Bill House entered the field of otolaryngology in the mid-1950s, VSs were rarely diagnosed until the patient had developed facial sensory changes or papilledema. House proposed the revolutionary idea of obtaining an X-ray of the internal auditory canals in all patients with unilateral sensorineural hearing loss, thus permitting earlier diagnosis in many patients. Following this strategy, House picked up a tumor in a young fireman with a unilateral hearing loss and a wide internal meatus and referred him to the neurosurgeon for, he assumed, excisional surgery. The neurosurgeon, however, advised against surgery on the grounds that the facial nerve could not be saved, the risk to life was too high, and he felt the tumor might not grow. Notably, at the time the California Tumor Registry recorded a 40% mortality rate for VS surgery. Within a year, however, the tumor had grown and the patient developed signs of increased intracranial pressure. House then observed “long and tedious surgery with the patient in the seated position.” The patient never regained consciousness.

The timing of House’s entry into the field was fortuitous, as many of the prerequisite innovations were available, including refined general anesthesia and antiseptic technique, the otologic drill, and the operating microscope. House recognized that the dilemma between early diagnosis and early tumor removal might be solved if the facial nerve could be saved. Using one of the first operating microscopes to be imported into the United States, he pioneered new temporal bone techniques on cadaver material in the Los Angeles County Morgue, initially the middle fossa approach and then the translabyrinthine approach. He teamed with a neurosurgeon, Bill Hitselberger, who was keen to work as a member of a team, but they met with considerable opposition from the general neurosurgical community who became very upset that an otologist should cross the sacred barrier of the dura. A standoff between the two sides at St Vincent’s Hospital in Los Angeles where they operated was resolved thanks to the negotiations of Bill’s brother Howard House, who threatened to remove his own considerable otological practice from the hospital if Bill House and Bill Hitselberger were not permitted to practice. They did get their way and the era of translabyrinthine surgery and the otoneurological team dawned (W.F. House, 1996, personal communication).[32] That is not to say that vitriolic arguments over the respective merits of the suboccipital and translabyrinthine approaches ceased, as they most certainly did not. Passionately held dogma was expounded from both sides, both in the literature and from the podium, and one was reminded of the observation of Sir William Osler that “the greater the ignorance the greater the dogmatism.” The truth of the matter, of course, is that the “best” approach is the one that works best for the individual surgical team, and the outcomes from experienced teams are often very similar, whichever approach is employed.

Following improvements in facial nerve functional outcomes with the adoption of microsurgical techniques and neuromonitoring, the next challenge for neurotological teams has been preservation of functional hearing, a feat that was realized early on in selected cases via the retrosigmoid or middle fossa approaches. Paralleling facial nerve outcomes, prospects of hearing preservation have been greatly facilitated by developments in cranial nerve monitoring.

Today, most developed skull base teams will be familiar with all approaches to the CPA and tailor the approach to the needs of the individual patient. Most large series report a perioperative mortality of well under 1%, a similar incidence of severe morbidity, a facial nerve preservation rate of 95%, with around 85% with House–Brackmann grade I or II function. By the early 1990s, in light of these improved results, microsurgical removal became the predominant VS management strategy. As reflected in the *National Institutes of Health 1991 Consensus Statement*,[33] the recommendation was surgery for all patients able and willing to undergo an operation, leaving observation and radiosurgery for those patients who were unwilling or deemed unable to tolerate surgery. Discussions regarding modern developments and trends in microsurgery, as well as nonoperative strategies including stereotactic radiation therapy and conservative observation, are reviewed in depth in later chapters.

References

[1] Sandifort E. De duram quodam corpusculo nervo auditorio adherente: observations anatomico-pathologicae. P v d Eyk & D Vygh. 1777;1:116–120
[2] Leveque-Lasource A. Observation sur un amaurosis et un cophosis, avec perte ou diminution de la voix, des mouvemens etc par suite de lesion organique apparente de plusieurs parties du cerveau. J Gen Med Chir Pharm. 1810; 37: 368–373
[3] Cruveilhier J. Tumours of the Nervus Acusticus and the Syndrome of the Cerebellopontile Angle. New York, NY: Haffner Publishing Company; 1917 (Reprinted 1963)
[4] Bell C. The Nervous System of the Human Body Embracing the Papers Delivered to the Royal Society on the Subject of Nerves. London: Longman Rees Orme Brown and Green; 1830;112–114
[5] Jackson H. Tumours at the base of the brain – death–autopsy–clinical remarks. Med Times Hosp Gazette. 1865:626–627
[6] Toynbee J. Neuroma of the auditory nerve. Tr Path Soc Lond. 1853; 4: 259–260
[7] Gowers W. A clinical lecture on a metastatic mystery. Lancet. 1905: 1593–1597
[8] Bruns L (1906) quoted by Cushing H (1917) Tumors of the Nervus Acusticus and the Syndrome of the Cerebello-pontile Angle Ch1 p4 reprinted 1963. Haffner Publishing Company New York
[9] Oppenheim H. Über mehrere Fälle von endocraniellem Tumor in welchem es gelang eine genaue Lokaldiagnose zu stellen. Berl klin Wochenschrift 1890:38–40
[10] Babinski R (1906) quoted by Cushing H (1917) Tumors of the Nervus Acusticus and the Syndrome of the Cerebello-pontile Angle Ch1 p4 reprinted 1963. Haffner Publishing Company New York
[11] Bergmann. quoted by Cushing H (1917) Tumors of the Nervus Acusticus and the Syndrome of the Cerebello-pontile Angle Ch10 p245 reprinted 1963. Haffner Publishing Company New York
[12] McBurney C, Starr M. A contribution to cerebral surgery: diagnosis, localization and operation for removal of three tumors of the brain: with some comments on the surgical treatment of brain tumors. Am J Med Sci 1893;361–387
[13] Cushing H. Tumors of the Nervus Acusticus and the Syndrome of the Cerebello-pontile Angle. New York, NY: Haffner Publishing Company; 1917 (reprinted 1963):245
[14] Ballance C. Some Points in the Surgery of the Brain and Its Membranes. London: McMillan and Co; 1907:276–282
[15] Cushing H. Tumors of the Nervus Acusticus and the Syndrome of the Cerebello-pontile Angle. New York, NY: Haffner Publishing Company; 1917 (reprinted 1963)
[16] Gibson GA. Remarks on the results of surgical measures in a series of cerebral cases. Trans Med Chir Soc Edinb. 1896; 15:27–46
[17] Stewart JP. A contribution to the localization of cerebellar lesions. Edinburgh Hospital Report.. 1895; 3:447–453
[18] Krause F. Zur Freilegung der hinteren Felsenbeinfläche and des Kleinhirns. Beitrage zur klinischen. Chirurgie. 1903; 37:728–764
[19] Borchardt M. Zur Operation der Tumoren des Kleinhirnbrückenwinkels. Berl klin Wchenschr 1905(xlii), 1033-1035
[20] Eiselsberg A Über die chirurgische Behandlung der Hirntumoren Tr Internat Cong Med Lond. 1913 Sect VII; 203-207
[21] Panse R. Klinische und pathologische Mitteilungen. IV Ein Gliom des Akustikus. Archiv Ohrenheilkunde.. 1904; 61:251–255
[22] Kümmel W. Otologische Gesichtspunkte bei der Diagnose und Therapie von Erkrankungen der hinteren Schädelgruppe. Deutsche Zeitschrift für Nervenheilkunde. 1909 xxxvi;132-142
[23] Quix F. Ein Fall von translabyrinthisch operiertem Tumor Akustikus. Ver Deutschen Otol Gselschaft.. 1912; 21:245–255
[24] Dandy WE. Results of removal of acoustic tumors by the unilateral approach. AMA Arch Surg. 1941; 42:1026–1033
[25] Pennybacker JB, Cairns H. Results in 130 cases of acoustic neurinoma. J Neurol Neurosurg Psychiatry. 1950; 13(4):272–277

[26] Northfield DWC. Acoustic neurinoma. J Neurol Neurosurg Psychiatry. 1950; 13(4):277–278

[27] Atkinson WJ. The anterior inferior cerebellar artery; its variations, pontine distribution, and significance in the surgery of cerebello-pontine angle tumours. J Neurol Neurosurg Psychiatry. 1949; 12(2): 137–151

[28] Selters WA, Brackmann DE. Acoustic tumor detection with brain stem electric response audiometry. Arch Otolaryngol. 1977; 103(4):181–187

[29] Mudry A. History of instruments used for mastoidectomy. J Laryngol Otol. 2009; 123(6):583–589

[30] Moberly AC, Fritsch MH. The evolution of mastoidectomy and tympanoplasty. Laryngoscope. 2010; 120 Suppl 4:S213

[31] Mudry A. The history of the microscope for use in ear surgery. Am J Otol. 2000; 21(6):877–886

[32] House WF. Transtemporal bone microsurgical removal of acoustic neuromas. Arch Otolaryngol. 1964; 80:731–742

[33] Acoustic neuroma. Consens Statement. 1991; 9(4):1–24

[34] Hinton AE, Ramsden RT, Lye RH, Dutton JEM. Criteria for hearing preservation in acoustic schwannoma surgery: the concept of useful hearing. J Laryngol Otol. 1992; 106(6):500–503

2 Historical Development of Radiation Modalities for Vestibular Schwannoma

L. Dade Lunsford, Ajay Niranjan, Georg Norén, and Dan Leksell

"The time to treat is when the tumor is no bigger than a grain of salt"

– Norman Dott[1]

2.1 Introduction

With earlier diagnosis of vestibular schwannoma (VS) related to the widespread availability of advanced imaging tools such as computed tomography (CT) and magnetic resonance imaging (MRI), the quandary of when and what treatment option to apply remains. Paralleling the advances in earlier detection based on more liberal indications for imaging—asymmetric hearing loss, tinnitus, or equilibrium disorders—the skill set required for surgical removal has advanced. The ability to excise a tumor while sparing existing cranial nerve function improved especially after the introduction of the operating microscope in the 1960s and the 1970s.

During the next 20 years, the consensus management for VS was surgical resection. While results improved with microsurgery, patients continued to be at risk for deafness, facial paralysis, and other cranial neuropathies, in addition to the less common risks of stroke, hemorrhage, and death. Various surgical approaches were refined by neurosurgeons and neurotologists, working alone or as a team, each with commendable rationales—improved facial function with expected deafness via the translabyrinthine approach or improved hearing preservation via the retrosigmoid or middle fossa approaches with somewhat higher risks of facial neuropathy. So what was the rationale and history behind the application of radiation modalities as an alternative to surgical resection?

2.2 The Development of Radiation Modalities

2.2.1 Early Efforts

The pioneering finding that conventional X-rays could detect disorders not apparent on physical examination led to the widespread use of cranial imaging. It was logical to expand the application of radiation to therapeutic needs, especially neoplasia. The energy delivered by orthovoltage X-ray devices quickly led to the finding that the therapeutic window (benefit vs. adverse effects) was relatively narrow. For targets not visible on the surface of the body, radiation delivery to the deeper target also meant that intervening tissues would receive the same dose of radiation. The consideration that faster dividing neoplastic cells would respond more to radiation doses than slow responding normal tissues led to the concept that the target dose needed to be divided into multiple treatment sessions. This so-called fractionation concept was designed to reduce collateral damage but produce preferential neoplastic tissue destruction by repeated hits to the same target.

The safer delivery of radiation to a deep-seated target in the body or skull required the development of higher energy X-ray devices called "linear accelerators." In addition to fractionation, use of multiple entry ports reduced the potential damage to intervening tissues between the radiation source and the target. In more recent years, the development of linear accelerators equipped with multileaf collimators dramatically improved the delivery of radiation while sparing regional normal tissue. Such devices are often guided by CT or MRI technologies. These developments have greatly improved the therapeutic window for delivery of radiation to deep-seated targets.

2.2.2 Particle Beams

Most radiation devices use gamma rays generated by decay of radioactive sources or X-rays generated by bombarding a tungsten plate with electrons. Alternatively, ionizing radiation can be produced by accelerated charged particles created by cyclotrons. Early pioneers in this effort included Lawrence who worked at the Lawrence Livermore Laboratories at Berkeley, California, in the late 1940s.[2] At that time, patients with pituitary tumors and even those with hormone-sensitive metastatic cancer were treated by pituitary ablation using protons. Work continued at Berkeley with both protons and helium ions in the treatment of both selected tumors and even arteriovenous malformations (AVMs).[3] Similar work was pursued at the Cambridge Cyclotron using protons. Kjellberg by the 1970s had treated a very large number of pituitary and AVM patients with Bragg peak stereotactic radiation done in a single procedure.[4,5] Despite relatively rudimentary methods to determine the target location and volume in the pre-CT era, the application of radiation modalities progressed.

2.3 The Early Work of Lars Leksell

Lars Leksell was one of the great pioneering neurosurgeons of the 20th century. Trained as a neurophysiologist and working in the lab of Ragnar Granit, Leksell was the first scientist to describe the gamma motor system for postural motor tone control. This work served as the base of his PhD degree. His neurosurgical education was obtained at the Serafimerlasarettet in Stockholm, Sweden, under the direction of Herbert Olivecrona, the pioneering Scandinavian neurosurgeon in the first half of the 20th century. During his training in the 1930s, Leksell immediately recognized the terrible risks that patients undertook, poor if any anesthesia, brain swelling, stroke, and a high risk of mortality. He was convinced there had to be a better way to access deep regions of the brain more safely.

Leksell completed a fellowship in stereotactic surgery in Philadelphia in 1947, studying with Temple University pioneers Ernest Spiegel and Henry Wycis. By 1949, he had published his first description of an arc-centered stereotactic guiding device.[6] This prototype device was further modified to link an orthovoltage X-ray device to the arc, generating photon beams that could be cross-fired on a cranial target. The term and field of stereotactic radiosurgery (SRS) was born[7] and the first patient with trigeminal neuralgia underwent irradiation of the gasserian ganglion using this prototype device.

Leksell was fascinated with the combination of better brain imaging and guiding devices. During his career, he evaluated conventional radiography, ultrasound, encephalography, CT, and finally MRI. His guiding devices were continually modified to facilitate higher quality imaging with the stereotactic frame in position. After target selection, both open stereotactic procedures and closed skull radiosurgical procedures were possible with the same guiding device.

During the late 1950s and early 1960s, Leksell collaborated with Swedish radiobiologist Börje Larsson to further study whether cross-fired radiation beams could be integrated with his stereotactic guiding devices. In 1951, Leksell published the article in which he described the potential methodology of SRS.[7] Larsson was working at the Gustav Werner Institute in Uppsala, Sweden, where a synchrocyclotron generated proton beams for physics studies. Together they performed an initial series of animal experiments. Goats were the preferred animal because they could thereafter live their natural lives at Larsson's farm. Following these studies, three patients underwent cross-fired proton radiation (not Bragg peak as performed at the Harvard Cyclotron Unit)[8,9].

The logistics were complex and Leksell and Larsson decided that a smaller more compact 179 source cobalt 60 unit cross-firing gamma rays made more sense. This self-contained technology allowed 4-mm beams to be focused on a small intracranial target. The unit itself could be placed in the local hospital environment. The first prototype Gamma Knife unit was installed in 1968 at the Sophiahemmet Hospital in Stockholm shortly after the first patient was treated in late 1967 just after loading the unit with sources at the nuclear reactor site Studsvik, Sweden. Thus, arrived the world's first noninvasive neurosurgical operating room. Despite Leksell's primary interest in functional neurosurgery, especially movement disorders and refractory severe obsessive compulsive and anxiety disorders, the first patient to undergo Gamma Knife radiosurgery had a craniopharyngioma.[10,11]

2.4 Application to Vestibular Schwannomas

Leksell himself had little interest in the potential commercial uses of his many inventions and was by nature cautious in the introduction of the new technologies he conceived. Various trainees or collaborators were tasked with individual application of both the prototype Gamma Knife and the second-generation device installed at the Radiumhemmet of the Karolinska Hospital in 1975 (▶ Fig. 2.1). Georg Norén was a disciple of Leksell and was in neurosurgical training at the Karolinska Institute, where Leksell served as professor for many years. After Leksell in 1969 had initiated the study by treating the first three patients, Dr. Norén gradually took over and was given the task of developing single session radiosurgical VS ablation using the prototype device.[12] At that time, the technologies to both diagnose and image the tumor target were rudimentary. In addition, the dose planning generally required that either a single or up to three overlapping isocenters were used to produce a complete and adequately precise dose distribution throughout the tumor. Jürgen Arndt, the first Gamma Knife medical physicist, was actively involved in this early development process. Dose planning initially was done based on partially computer-generated freehand-drawn tumor periphery and isodose configurations and the treatment time was calculated based on a nomogram. Starting in 1979, the display of the radiosurgical dose plan with the isodoses had to be printed at the appropriate magnification and then overlaid on hard copy CT images.

In addition to the imaging obstacles, the stereotactic frame itself did not fit into the aperture of the secondary and tertiary

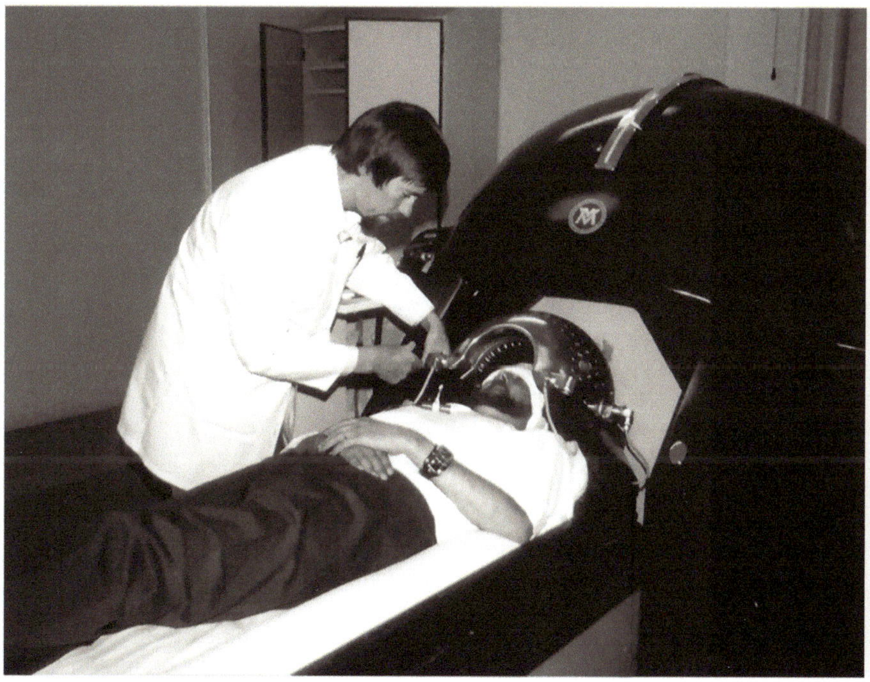

Fig. 2.1 Georg Norén positions a patient in the prototype Leksell Gamma Knife unit at the Sophiahemmet in Stockholm. The first vestibular schwannoma patients were treated with this first-generation device.

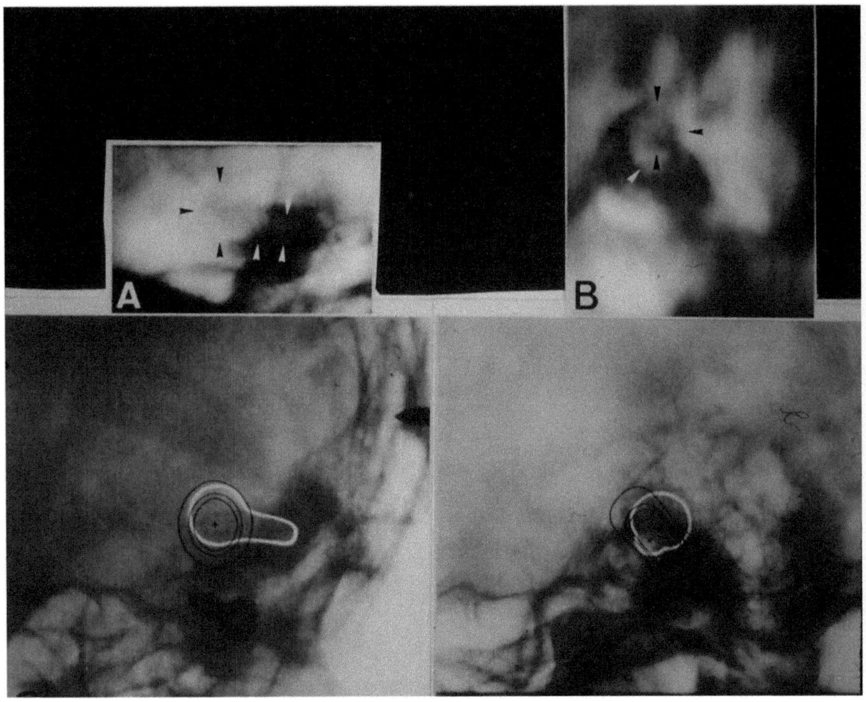

Fig. 2.2 Prior to the development of axial digital imaging technologies, the geometry of the vestibular schwannoma target was estimated using biplane air contrast encephalography.

collimators that focused the gamma rays through the slit-shaped collimators of the original prototype Gamma Knife. Innovative solutions included the use of a plaster of Paris and later thermoplastic cast wrapped around the patient's head (▶ Fig. 2.1). This strategy is strangely reminiscent of current-generation mask immobilization devices.

The first nine patients were imaged using air encephalography or positive contrast cisternography (▶ Fig. 2.2). In 1976, the first stereotactic CT for a VS patient was performed using an EMI scanner with water bag and a special interface without the frame attached during scanning.[13] The introduction of the first CT scanners without the water bag in 1979 facilitated the targeting of the tumor using thin slice axial imaging with the frame attached[14] (▶ Fig. 2.3). By 1987, more than 180 patients had been treated by radiosurgery.[15]

When the first nine VS patients were treated with the prototype Gamma Knife in the era between 1969 and 1974, nothing was known about optimal single radiation dose for these tumors. Leksell had come to the conclusion that a minimum dose to the tumor periphery of 25 to 35 Gy should be prescribed. There was evidence at the time that peripheral nerves would tolerate even higher doses. Remarkably, only one patient in this series had slight temporary facial hypesthesia and no one developed facial weakness. The tumor control overall was good. The size of the intracranial portion in this series in general was 1 to 2 cm. When the second Gamma Knife was installed in 1975, CT was available for the first time. The tumors actually were treated with a margin dose of 25 to 35 Gy. This resulted in a quite high incidence of trigeminal (18%) and facial (45%) neuropathy, as well as hearing loss. However, the tumor control was good. Starting in 1976, dose was reduced to 16 Gy, which reduced neuropathies other than hearing loss to a zero level. In this series, the size of the intracranial portion of the tumors was up to approximately 2.5 cm. For the first time, the 4-mm collimators were available, specifically designed to cover the intracanalicular portion of VSs.[16]

In 1988, a new Gamma Knife model B with freshly activated sources was installed at the Karolinska Hospital. Using identical dose planning and radiation dose levels, the incidence of facial weakness again increased to 27% (no facial hypesthesia documented).

Meanwhile, when the very first series of nine patients returned for follow-up, they underwent CT and later MRI. This imaging was meticulously compared to the earlier air and positive contrast studies. This revealed that these tumors had been treated with a peripheral dose in the range of 10 to 15 Gy. This explained the good tumor response paired with the almost nonexistent incidence of neuropathies. Based on these findings, Norén decided (Leksell had passed away in January 1986) to reduce the standard minimum peripheral tumor dose to 12 Gy prescribed to 50%. The 71 tumors treated between 1989 and 1990 demonstrated growth control (shrinkage or stable size) in 93% of cases.[16] Three tumors were retreated with Gamma Knife giving a total rate of growth control after radiosurgery of 97%.

Hearing levels were much harder to maintain and virtually all patients experienced hearing impairment over time. Overall, in this early experience, 20 of 180 patients had delayed tumor growth, 11 of who required delayed surgical removal and CSF diversion by shunting was required in 10%.[15] Norén's early work confirmed the potential future role that radiosurgery might achieve. He established new outcome benchmarks for VS management: life preservation, morbidity reduction, tumor growth prevention, and improved long-term cranial nerve outcomes.[17,18]

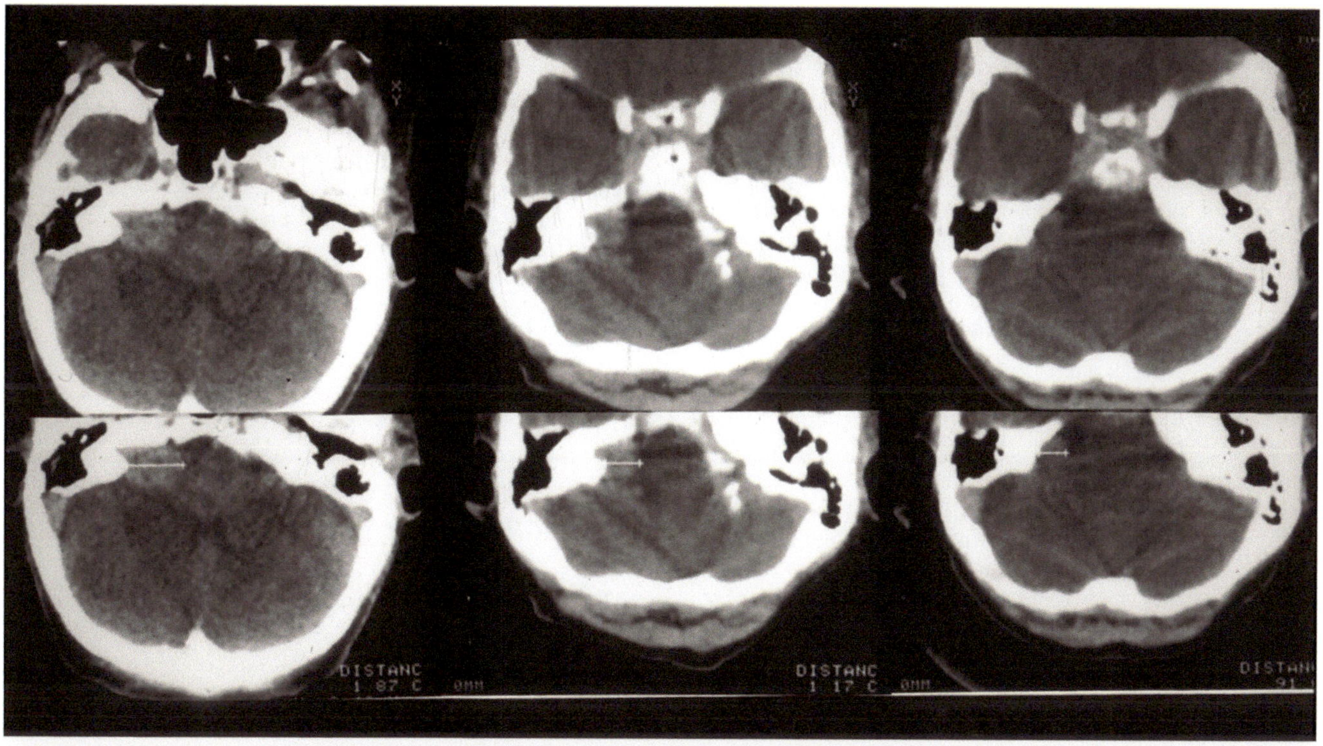

Fig. 2.3 An early Gamma Knife radiosurgery case using CT targeting, with follow-up at 1 and 2 years.

2.4.1 The Expansion of the Role of Gamma Knife Radiosurgery for Vestibular Schwannoma

In 1987, the first 201 source Gamma Knife (unit no. 5) was installed at Presbyterian University Hospital in Pittsburgh.[19] Among the earliest patients treated were those with VS. These patients wished to avoid the potential morbidity of microsurgical resection or had serious medical comorbidities precluding open surgery. All patients had enlarging symptomatic tumors confirmed by CT. It became clear in the first few years that the margin dose prescription suggested by the early Swedish experience resulted in too high a risk of new but usually transient facial and/or trigeminal neuropathy as well as inadequate hearing preservation rates. A margin dose de-escalation study commenced. Subsequent experience sought to define the therapeutic window—low cranial nerve complications plus long-term tumor control. During this dose optimizing era from 1987 to 1995, many other technological features emerged to further improve Gamma Knife SRS treatment. These advances included the first use of MRI to target the tumor (1991); improved multiple isocenter medical physics planning (first using KULA and then conversion to early generations of Leksell GammaPlan); and earlier detection and treatment of patients when tumor volumes were somewhat smaller. In addition, the installation of updated Gamma Knife technologies also contributed to ever improving outcomes. The U unit design gave way to the B unit, which facilitated reloading. The C unit incorporated true robotic positioning of the isocenters. The larger aperture, fully robotic Perfexion Gamma Knife was installed in Pittsburgh in 2006.

By 2017, almost 2,000 VS patients had undergone Gamma Knife SRS at the University of Pittsburgh Medical Center. Other worldwide centers reported large patient experience, including the Gamma Knife program at the Hôspital de la Timone in Marseille, France, where more than 3,000 VS patients underwent radiosurgery.[20] According to the tracking of patient volumes by the Leksell Gamma Knife Society, worldwide experience by 2016 had exceeded 100,000 VS patients. This experience was conducted using virtually the same paradigm at more than 300 worldwide centers: stereotactic frame application, high definition targeting most often with MRI, highly conformal and selective dose planning using advanced high-speed image-integrated computers (dose prescriptions typically of 11–13 Gy at the tumor margin), and single-session delivery of the therapeutic radiation—wheels-in to wheels-out in a single day.

Publications about outcomes after Gamma Knife SRS were produced at an impressive rate, so that by 2016 more than 300 publications related to outcomes of Gamma Knife radiosurgery for VS were available (▶ Fig. 2.4). Based on these scientific publications and many national and international forums, the value of radiosurgery as a primary management of VS was established. Long-term tumor control rates of more than 95%, facial neuropathy rates of less than 1%, and hearing preservation rates in 50 to 90% of patients (depending on preoperative tumor volume and hearing status) became an expected outcome for patients undergoing Gamma Knife SRS.[21]

2.5 Fractionated Radiation Therapy as an Alternative

Although fractionated radiation therapy quickly became a vital tool in the fight against malignant tumors of the brain, its application to slower growing benign skull base tumors such as VS was slow to develop. Fractionated radiation therapy delivered by linear accelerators was usually considered in patients who had growing residual tumors after attempted microsurgical resection or patients who were considered ineligible for initial surgery because of major medical comorbidities. Initial efforts were focused on safety (reduction of collateral damage to cranial nerve, brainstem, and temporal lobe). Similar to SRS, neither the cranial nerve tolerance nor the tumor control dose was known to early advocates of fractionated radiation therapy.[22] As linear accelerators improved using multileaf collimator systems and enhanced targeting using first CT data, and then eventually MRI data, the therapeutic window began to emerge.

Neither fractionation method nor the dose per fraction were known; so, many studies concentrated on the technology available (modified or commercially available Linacs) and the computer software dose planning (either homegrown or commercial). Both conventional fractionation methods such as 50 Gy at 1.8 Gy per fraction and hyperfractionated regimens in 3 to 10 sessions were reported in various publications.[23] In order to provide reasonable repeatable accuracy of dose delivery, most centers began to use relocatable mask fixation systems to immobilize the patient's head during the delivery of each radiation fraction.

As results accumulated, the same outcome analysis was applied to these fractionated radiation therapy paradigms: tumor control, cranial nerve response, detection of adverse radiation effects, and delayed hydrocephalus. Multileaf collimator radiation therapy devices, including cone beam CT target verification techniques, are widely commercially available across the world.

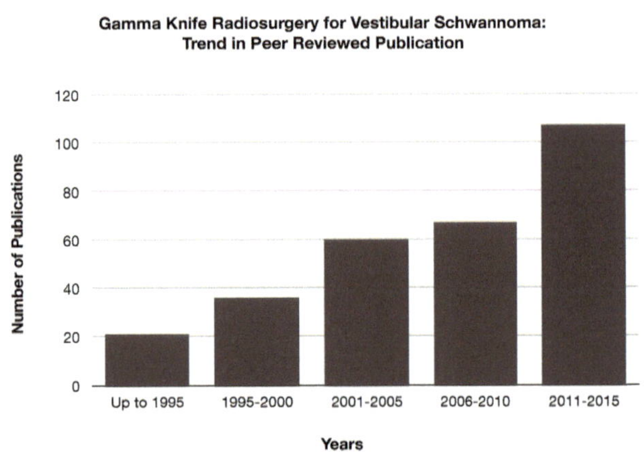

Fig. 2.4 The bar graph shows the trend of peer-reviewed publications using Gamma Knife radiosurgery for vestibular schwannomas.

2.5.1 The Development of CyberKnife Radiation Therapy

During the 1980s, Stanford neurosurgeon John Adler also spent time at the Karolinska Hospital observing the use of the Leksell Gamma Knife. Dr. Adler became convinced that photon radiation generated from a small light weight linear accelerator mounted on a commercial robot would allow similarly accurate and perhaps practical delivery of focused radiation to targets such as VS.[24] His prototype CyberKnife device also gradually evolved and was successfully marketed by Accuray. Scientific publications emerged to define its potential role as an alternative radiation delivery technique at selected centers across the world.[25,26,27,28]

2.5.2 Evolution of Particle Beam Delivery Techniques

Despite the early suggestion that radiation delivered either by cross-fired particle beams or Bragg peak technique might supplant other photon radiation techniques, accumulated data as to comparable effectiveness remain sparse. Centers involved in such efforts continue to advocate fractionation methods, and suggest that the radiobiological effectiveness of protons is superior to that of photon technologies. The data to support that contention seem very limited and largely accepted because of

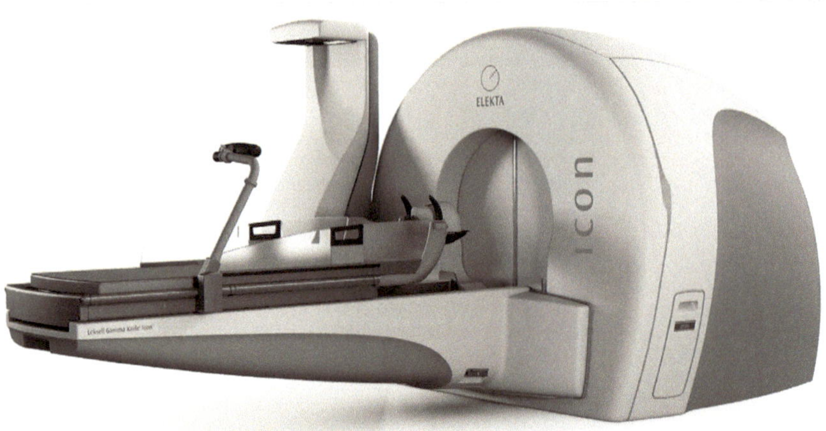

Fig. 2.5 The Leksell Gamma Knife icon: This model is equipped with on-board CT scanner and is capable of performing fractionation.

early experimental and clinical data that protons have an estimated 1.2 times greater radiobiological response compared to photons.[29,30] Because of the limited clinical application to VS, that contention remains largely unproven. The Bragg peak proton technique is often marketed to large hospitals as a method to reduce exit dose in a skull base tumor. However, the entrance dose of this technique within structures such as the temporal lobe often exceeds the dose delivered using stereotactic radiosurgical techniques.

Technologies to pinpoint the tumor target and safely deliver radiation to these tumors continue to evolve. Whether the target is immobilized using a stereotactic frame (where absolute submillimeter precision is needed) or a mask is under further study using both linear accelerator and newer Gamma Knife methodologies[31,32,33,34,35,36,37,38,39,40,41,42,43,44] (▶ Fig. 2.5).

References

[1] Dott NM. Chronic arachnoiditis and hydrocephalus in the surgical management of acoustic tumours; a plea for early operation. Proc R Soc Med. 1958; 51(11):897–899

[2] Lawrence JH. Proton irradiation of the pituitary. Cancer. 1957; 10(4): 795–798

[3] Fabrikant JI, Lyman JT, Hosobuchi Y. Stereotactic heavy-ion Bragg peak radiosurgery for intra-cranial vascular disorders: method for treatment of deep arteriovenous malformations. Br J Radiol. 1984; 57(678): 479–490

[4] Kjellberg RN. Stereotactic Bragg peak proton beam radiosurgery for cerebral arteriovenous malformations. Ann Clin Res. 1986; 18 Suppl 47:17–19

[5] Kjellberg RN, Shintani A, Frantz AG, Kliman B. Proton-beam therapy in acromegaly. N Engl J Med. 1968; 278(13):689–695

[6] Leksell L. A stereotaxic apparatus for intracerebral surgery. Acta Chir Scand. 1949; 99:229–233

[7] Leksell L. The stereotaxic method and radiosurgery of the brain. Acta Chir Scand. 1951; 102(4):316–319

[8] Leksell L, Larsson B, Andersson B, Rexed B, Sourander P, Mair W. Lesions in the depth of the brain produced by a beam of high energy protons. Acta Radiol. 1960; 54:251–264

[9] Andersson B, Larsson B, Leksell L, et al. Histopathology of late local radiolesions in the goat brain. Acta Radiol Ther Phys Biol. 1970; 9(5):385–394

[10] Backlund EO. The History and Development of Radiosurgery. New York, NY: Elsevier; 1992

[11] Ganz JC. Stockholm radiosurgery developing 1968–1982. Prog Brain Res. 2014; 215:85–94

[12] Norén G. Gamma knife radiosurgery of acoustic neurinomas. A historic perspective. Neurochirurgie. 2004; 50(2-3, Pt 2):253–256

[13] Bergström M, Greitz T. Stereotaxic computed tomography. AJR Am J Roentgenol. 1976; 127(1):167–170

[14] Leksell L, Jernberg B. Stereotaxis and tomography. A technical note. Acta Neurochir (Wien). 1980; 52(1-2):1–7

[15] Noren G, Arndt J, Hindmarsh T, Hirsch A. Modern Stereotactic Neurosurgery. Boston, MA: Martinus Nijhoff Publishing; 1988

[16] Norén G: Gamma Knife radiosurgery for acoustic neurinomas; in Gildenberg PL, Tasker RR (eds): Textbook of Stereotactic and Functional Neurosurgery. New York, McGraw-Hill, 1998, chap 90, pp 835844

[17] Hirsch A, Norén G, Anderson H. Audiologic findings after stereotactic radiosurgery in nine cases of acoustic neurinomas. Acta Otolaryngol. 1979; 88(3-4):155–160

[18] Norén G, Arndt J, Hindmarsh T. Stereotactic radiosurgery in cases of acoustic neurinoma: further experiences. Neurosurgery. 1983; 13(1):12–22

[19] Lunsford LD, Flickinger J, Lindner G, Maitz A. Stereotactic radiosurgery of the brain using the first United States 201 cobalt-60 source gamma knife. Neurosurgery. 1989; 24(2):151–159

[20] Régis J, Pellet W, Delsanti C, et al. Functional outcome after gamma knife surgery or microsurgery for vestibular schwannomas. J Neurosurg. 2013; 119 Suppl:1091–1100

[21] Lunsford LD, Niranjan A, Flickinger JC, Maitz A, Kondziolka D. Radiosurgery of vestibular schwannomas: summary of experience in 829 cases. J Neurosurg. 2005; 102 Suppl:195–199

[22] Newman H, Sheline GE, Boldrey EB. Proceedings: radiation therapy of tumors of the eighth nerve sheath. Am J Roentgenol Radium Ther Nucl Med. 1974; 120(3):562–567

[23] Andrews DW, Werner-Wasik M, Den RB, et al. Toward dose optimization for fractionated stereotactic radiotherapy for acoustic neuromas: comparison of two dose cohorts. Int J Radiat Oncol Biol Phys. 2009; 74(2):419–426

[24] Adler JR, Jr, Chang SD, Murphy MJ, Doty J, Geis P, Hancock SL. The Cyberknife: a frameless robotic system for radiosurgery. Stereotact Funct Neurosurg. 1997; 69(1–4, Pt 2):124–128

[25] Vivas EX, Wegner R, Conley G, et al. Treatment outcomes in patients treated with CyberKnife radiosurgery for vestibular schwannoma. Otol Neurotol. 2014; 35:162–170

[26] Sakamoto GT, Blevins N, Gibbs IC. Cyberknife radiotherapy for vestibular schwannoma. Otolaryngol Clin North Am. 2009; 42(4):665–675

[27] Chang SD, Gibbs IC, Sakamoto GT, Lee E, Oyelese A, Adler JR, Jr. Staged stereotactic irradiation for acoustic neuroma. Neurosurgery. 2005; 56(6): 1254–1261, discussion 1261–1263

[28] Ishihara H, Saito K, Nishizaki T, et al. CyberKnife radiosurgery for vestibular schwannoma. Minim Invasive Neurosurg. 2004; 47(5):290–293

[29] Kjellberg RN, Nguyen NC, Kliman B. [The Bragg Peak proton beam in stereotaxic neurosurgery]. Neurochirurgie. 1972; 18(3):235–265

[30] Kjellberg RN, Sweet WH, Preston WM, Koehler AM. The Bragg peak of a proton beam in intracranial therapy of tumors. Trans Am Neurol Assoc. 1962; 87:216–218

[31] Klijn S, Verheul JB, Beute GN, et al. Gamma Knife radiosurgery for vestibular schwannomas: evaluation of tumor control and its predictors in a large patient cohort in The Netherlands. J Neurosurg. 2015:1–8

[32] Boari N, Bailo M, Gagliardi F, et al. Gamma Knife radiosurgery for vestibular schwannoma: clinical results at long-term follow-up in a series of 379 patients. J Neurosurg. 2014; 121 Suppl:123–142

[33] Hasegawa T, Kida Y, Kato T, Iizuka H, Kuramitsu S, Yamamoto T. Long-term safety and efficacy of stereotactic radiosurgery for vestibular schwannomas: evaluation of 440 patients more than 10 years after treatment with Gamma Knife surgery. J Neurosurg. 2013; 118(3):557–565

[34] Kano H, Kondziolka D, Khan A, Flickinger JC, Lunsford LD. Predictors of hearing preservation after stereotactic radiosurgery for acoustic neuroma. J Neurosurg. 2009; 111(4):863–873

[35] Tamura M, Carron R, Yomo S, et al. Hearing preservation after gamma knife radiosurgery for vestibular schwannomas presenting with high-level hearing. Neurosurgery. 2009; 64(2):289–296, discussion 296

[36] Niranjan A, Mathieu D, Flickinger JC, Kondziolka D, Lunsford LD. Hearing preservation after intracanalicular vestibular schwannoma radiosurgery. Neurosurgery. 2008; 63(6):1054–1062, discussion 1062–1063

[37] Chopra R, Kondziolka D, Niranjan A, Lunsford LD, Flickinger JC. Long-term follow-up of acoustic schwannoma radiosurgery with marginal tumor doses of 12 to 13 Gy. Int J Radiat Oncol Biol Phys. 2007; 68(3):845–851

[38] Chung WY, Liu KD, Shiau CY, et al. Gamma knife surgery for vestibular schwannoma: 10-year experience of 195 cases. J Neurosurg. 2005; 102 Suppl:87–96

[39] Combs SE, Engelhard C, Kopp C, et al. Long-term outcome after highly advanced single-dose or fractionated radiotherapy in patients with vestibular schwannomas - pooled results from 3 large German centers. Radiother Oncol. 2015; 114(3):378–383

[40] Anderson BM, Khuntia D, Bentzen SM, et al. Single institution experience treating 104 vestibular schwannomas with fractionated stereotactic radiation therapy or stereotactic radiosurgery. J Neurooncol. 2014; 116(1):187–193

[41] Champ CE, Shen X, Shi W, et al. Reduced-dose fractionated stereotactic radiotherapy for acoustic neuromas: maintenance of tumor control with improved hearing preservation. Neurosurgery. 2013; 73(3):489–496

[42] Rasmussen R, Claesson M, Stangerup SE, et al. Fractionated stereotactic radiotherapy of vestibular schwannomas accelerates hearing loss. Int J Radiat Oncol Biol Phys. 2012; 83(5):e607–e611

[43] Kapoor S, Batra S, Carson K, et al. Long-term outcomes of vestibular schwannomas treated with fractionated stereotactic radiotherapy: an institutional experience. Int J Radiat Oncol Biol Phys. 2011; 81(3):647–653

[44] Collen C, Ampe B, Gevaert T, et al. Single fraction versus fractionated Linac-based stereotactic radiotherapy for vestibular schwannoma: a single-institution experience. Int J Radiat Oncol Biol Phys. 2011; 81(4):e503–e509

3 Epidemiology of Vestibular Schwannoma

Per Cayé-Thomasen and Sven-Eric Stangerup

3.1 Introduction

In a retrospective analysis from the Faroe islands[1] covering the period from 1962 to 1975, the incidence of primary intracranial neoplasms was found to be 9.9% in 50,000 inhabitants. In other series, vestibular schwannomas (VSs) were estimated to represent 8 to 10% of all intracranial tumors[2,3] and about 80% of all cerebellopontine tumors.[4]

In the period from January 1957 to July 1976, the incidence of VS in Denmark was estimated to be 5.4 VS per million persons per year based on publications from Danish neurosurgical departments.[5,6] In Aarhus County, Denmark, the incidence increased from 5.9 VS per million persons per year in the period from 1977 to 1981 to 18.3 VS per million persons per year in the period from 1992 to 1996.[7] In Manitoba, Canada, the incidence increased from 5 VS per million persons per year in the period[8] from 1980 to 1985 to 13 VS per million persons per year during the period[9] from 1987 to 1991. Other studies have found comparable incidences between 10 and 20 VS per million persons per year in the 1980s.[10,11,12,13,14] In a publication from the northwestern part of England, the incidence was found to be 10.4 VS per million persons per year during the period from 1990 to 1999.[15] In a recent publication from the United States,[16] the annual incidence in 2009 was found to be 11 VS per million persons per year.

In unselected autopsy series, the incidence of undiagnosed and "silent" VS was 0.8%[17] and 0.9%.[18] In Wittmaack's collection, gathered from 1908 to 1945, comprising 1,720 selected temporal bones, Eckermeier et al[19] found 30 neurinomas (1.7%), 8 of which were intrameatal with a diameter of 8 mm, whereas 22 had a diameter larger than 25 mm. In two histopathological studies on temporal bones, the incidence rates of undiagnosed and clinically silent VS were 2.4%[20] and 2.7%,[21] respectively.

Incidental findings of VS on brain magnetic resonance imaging (MRI) are reported to occur in 0.3, 0.5, and 1.6% of scans.[22,23,24] In two population-based incidence registries, the Central Brain Tumor Registry of the United States and the Los Angeles County Cancer Surveillance Program (1975–1998), the incidence of VS was similar: six VS per million persons per year and eight VS per million persons per year (1995–1998). Moreover, the incidence of primary nerve sheath tumors of the brain/central nervous system and of VS increased over time.[25]

3.2 Danish National Vestibular Schwannoma Database

Since 1976, patients diagnosed with VS in Denmark (population: 5.1 million in 1976 increasing to 5.6 million in 2013) have been referred to our tertiary referral center at Copenhagen University Hospital. Patient data such as sex, date of birth, zip code, day of diagnosis, tumor size, tumor location, pure-tone and speech audiometry, and other related data have been entered prospectively into the national database. In case of surgery, data were entered for the date of surgery, surgical approach, extent of resection, anatomical state of the facial nerve at the end of the operation, complications during and after surgery, as well as facial function at discharge from hospital and at 3, 6, 9, and 12 months after surgery. If the patient was allocated to "wait and scan" management, the intention was to perform annual MR scans as well as annual pure-tone and speech audiometry. These examinations were performed locally at the patient's home hospital and the MR images and the audiogram were sent to us for evaluation. After evaluation, the data were entered prospectively into the database.

3.3 Diagnosis

Since 1976, a total of 3,153 patients with a unilateral tumor of the internal auditory canal or cerebellopontine angle resembling VS have been diagnosed and registered in the database. The date of diagnosis was defined as the date of the first diagnostic computed tomography (CT) or MRI. Until 1985, the diagnosis of VS in Denmark was based on X-ray, X-ray tomography, and CT. The first MRI scanner became available in Denmark in 1985 and from 1990 onward, an increasing proportion of VS was diagnosed by MRI. Since 1995, MRI has made all such diagnoses, except in a few patients with metallic implants, extreme obesity, or claustrophobia.

3.3.1 Measurement of Tumor Size

According to the consensus meeting in Japan in 2003,[26] tumors were categorized as either purely intrameatal, with no size indication, or, in case the tumor extended into the cerebellopontine angle, as intra- and extrameatal, in which case the size of the tumor was measured by the largest extrameatal diameter. The intrameatal portion was not included in the assessment of tumor size for VS with cisternal growth.

3.3.2 Classification of Hearing

For the evaluation of hearing, the pure-tone average (PTA) was calculated as the mean of the hearing level (dB) at the frequencies 500, 1,000, 2,000, and 4,000 Hz. Speech discrimination (SD) audiometry had been performed in standardized quiet conditions, using word lists scoring by phonemes correctly repeated at the most comfortable hearing level, according to the masking rules.

For the classification of hearing, the modified Word Recognition Scoring classification[27] was used, with class 0: SD = 100%, class I: SD = 99 to 70%, class II: SD = 69 to 50%, class III: SD = 49 to 1%, and class IV: SD = 0%.

3.3.3 Patient Demographics and Tumor Characteristics

The median age of the 3,153 patients at diagnosis was 51.3 years (range: 15–93 years). The male:female ratio was 1,565:1,588. In 1,189 (38%) patients, the tumor was localized purely in the internal auditory canal (intrameatal) and in 1,964

(62%), the tumor extended into the cerebellopontine angle. The median size of the tumor at diagnosis was 14.3 mm, range intrameatal to 75 mm, extrameatally.

3.3.4 Incidence of Vestibular Schwannoma in Denmark

The annual number of diagnosed VS in Denmark has increased consistently from 15 tumors in 1976 to 178 tumors in 2012, corresponding to an increase in the annual incidence from 3.0 VS per million persons per year in 1976 to 32.0 VS per million persons per year in 2012 (▸ Fig. 3.1, ▸ Fig. 3.2).

The increase in the number of diagnosed VS has plausibly been caused by several factors, the most important being improved access to continuously evolving diagnostic equipment (i.e., MRI). Another cause may be heightened symptom awareness among the general population and especially among the elderly, as a longer and healthier lifetime may be expected in the developed countries. Also, better and more widespread audiological testing equipment has likely resulted in identification of more patients with asymmetric hearing loss. Enhanced testing and more frequent diagnosis of VS might in turn lead to increased awareness among general practitioners and otolaryngologists.

It is obvious, however, that the low incidence in the 1970s and early 1980s was due to poorer diagnostic means of that time (e.g., pneumatic cisternography and CT) with no or only a few MR scanners available. Furthermore, the diagnostic imaging of this period was by limited access reserved to patients of younger age, and small tumors in older patients were generally not diagnosed.[28]

3.4 Diagnosis of Intrameatal VS and Number of MR Scanners in Denmark

The increase in the number of MR scanners in Denmark is in accordance with the increase in the number of diagnosed intrameatal tumors (▸ Fig. 3.3). The first MR scanner in Denmark was installed in 1985. Since then, the continuously improved access to MR scanners and the introduction of gadolinium enhancement have had substantial influence on the diagnosis of small and purely intrameatal VS. Since 1980, the proportion of intrameatal VS has increased from 3 to 29% in 2001. Thus, the increase in the incidence can be attributed to an increasing number of diagnosed small and intrameatal VS. A major part of the small and intrameatal tumors occurs in elderly patients, who were not offered imaging in the earlier decades.[29]

As only a relatively small proportion of the small and purely intrameatal tumors grow following diagnosis, it has been proposed that the increase in incidence of diagnosed tumors may be explained by "fishing a pool" of previously undiagnosed tumors in elderly patients, rather than a factual increase in incidence. This has been strengthened by the fact that the smallest tumors were diagnosed in the oldest patients.

3.4.1 Size of Vestibular Schwannoma at Diagnosis

Throughout the period, the size of the tumors at the time of diagnosis has decreased considerably, from a mean size of 28 mm in the first 3-year period from 1976 to 1979 to 8.4 mm in the last 4-year period from 2009 to 2013 (▸ Fig. 3.4).

Looking at the eleven 3-year periods from 1976 to 2008, and the last 4-year period, it is seen that in the first periods, no purely intrameatal tumors was diagnosed, in contrast to the last

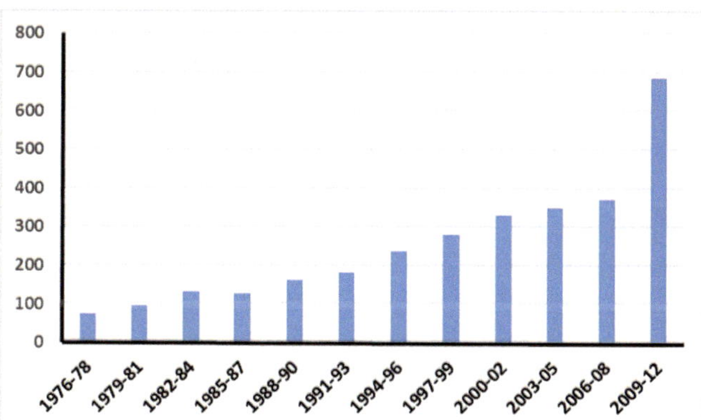

Fig. 3.1 Number of diagnosed vestibular schwannomas in Denmark, in 3-year periods from 1976 to 2008 and the 4-year period from 2009 to 2013.

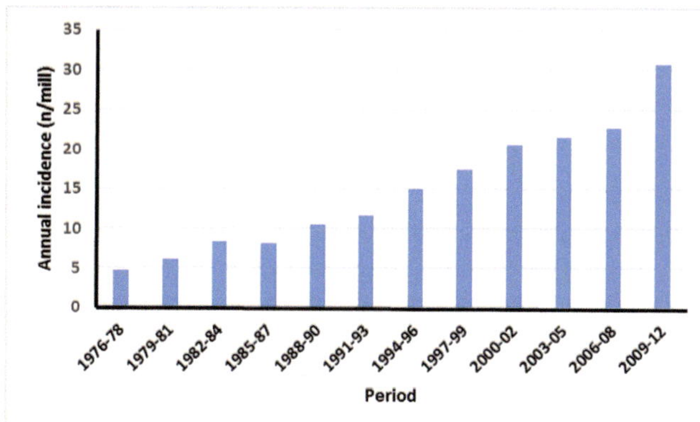

Fig. 3.2 Mean annual incidence (number/million/year) of vestibular schwannomas in Denmark, in 3-year periods from 1976 to 2008 and the 4-year period from 2009 to 2013.

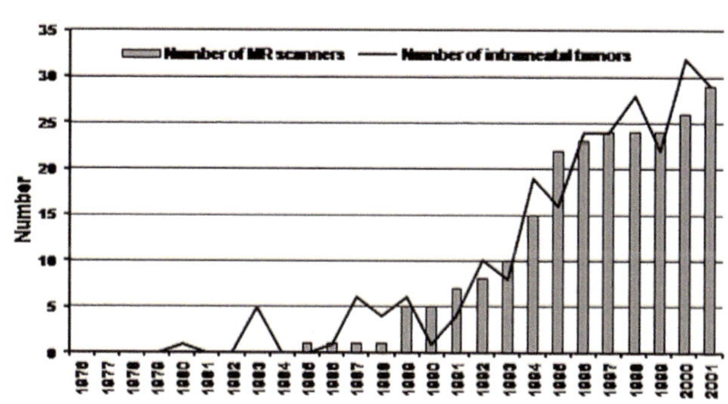

Fig. 3.3 Annual number of diagnosed intrameatal tumors and cumulated number of functioning MR scanners in Denmark.

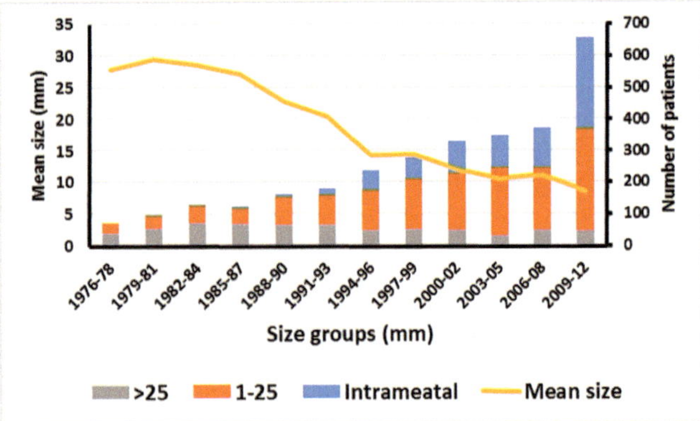

Fig. 3.4 Mean size and size groups of vestibular schwannomas in Denmark, in 3-year periods from 1976 to 2008 and the 4-year period from 2009 to 2013.

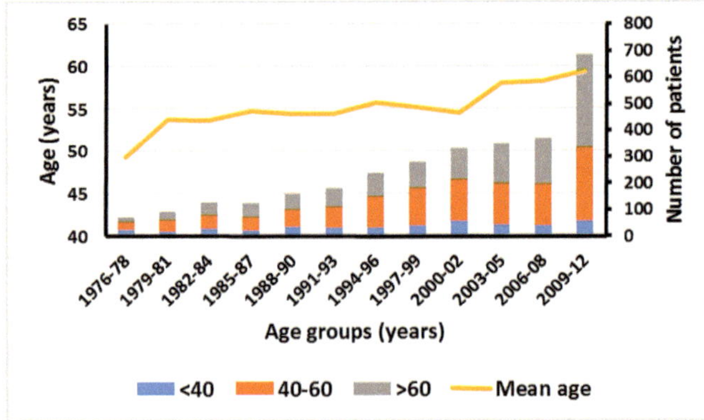

Fig. 3.5 Mean age and age groups of vestibular schwannomas in Denmark, in 3-year periods from 1976 to 2008 and the 4-year period from 2009 to 2013.

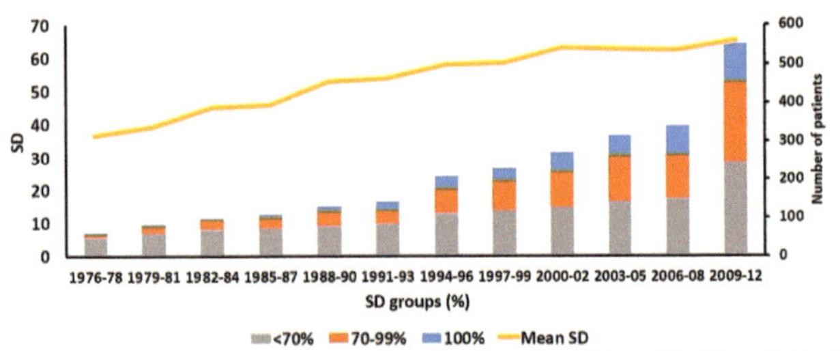

Fig. 3.6 Mean speech discrimination (SD) and SD groups of vestibular schwannomas in Denmark, in 3-year periods from 1976 to 2008 and the 4-year period from 2009 to 2013.

4-year period, where 44% of all diagnosed tumors was intrameatal. The percentage of medium sized tumors, 1 to 25 mm, was almost constant all through the periods. In contrast, the percentage of large tumors, larger than 25 mm, decreased from 54% in the first period to only 6% in the last period.

3.4.2 Age at Diagnosis

The age of the patients at the time of diagnosis of VS has been slowly increasing from 49 years in 1976 to 59 years in 2012 (▶ Fig. 3.5). The diagnostic age distribution during the 33-year period shows that the percentage of the middle-aged group between 40 and 60 years is almost constant at approximately half of patients. In contrast, the patient group younger than 40 years decreased from 30% of the patients in the first period to 8% of the patients diagnosed in the last period. The age group older than 60 years increased from 24% in the first period to more than half of the patients (51%) in the last period. Finally, the age group over 70 years increased from 3 to 14% during the same period.

3.4.3 Hearing at Diagnosis

In the earlier years, most (80%) patients diagnosed with VS had nonuseful hearing in the affected ear (▶ Fig. 3.6). However, in the last period, 56% of the patients had useful hearing with SD better than 70%. In fact, one-third of these patients had 100% SD at diagnosis.

3.5 Summary

In summary, the annual number of diagnosed VS is increasing. Only time can show if this reflects a true increase in incidence or if it is because of improved awareness and access to MR scanners. Considering the significant decrease in tumor size at diagnosis and better hearing, the increasing numbers are likely related to identification of previously unrecognized tumors. The increase in mean age at diagnosis in Denmark plausibly reflects the proliferation of MRI scanners and shift to offer older adults imaging.

References

[1] Joensen P. Incidence of primary intracranial neoplasms in an isolated population (the Faroese) during the period 1962–1975. Acta Neurol Scand. 1981; 64(1):74–78
[2] Walshe FMR. Intracranial tumors. A critical review. Q J Med. 1931; 24: 587–640
[3] Olivecrona H. Acoustic tumors. J Neurol Psychiatry. 1940; 3(2):141–146
[4] Lanser MJ, Sussman SA, Frazer K. Epidemiology, pathogenesis, and genetics of acoustic tumors. Otolaryngol Clin North Am. 1992; 25(3):499–520
[5] Overgaard J, Mosdal C. [Acoustic neurinoma. Neurosurgical treatment by suboccipital approach]. Ugeskr Laeger. 1981; 143(8):470–473
[6] Thomsen J, Tos M, Harmsen A, Riishede J, Thornval G. Surgery of acoustic neuromas. Preliminary experience with a translabyrinthine approach. Acta Neurol Scand. 1977; 56(4):277–290
[7] Mirz F, Pedersen CB, Fiirgaard B, Lundorf E. Incidence and growth pattern of vestibular schwannomas in a Danish county, 1977–98. Acta Otolaryngol Suppl. 2000; 543:30–33
[8] Sutherland GR, Florell R, Louw D, Choi NW, Sima AA. Epidemiology of primary intracranial neoplasms in Manitoba, Canada. Can J Neurol Sci. 1987; 14(4):586–592
[9] Frohlich AM, Sutherland GR. Epidemiology and clinical features of vestibular schwannoma in Manitoba, Canada. Can J Neurol Sci. 1993; 20(2):126–130
[10] Barker DJ, Weller RO, Garfield JS. Epidemiology of primary tumours of the brain and spinal cord: a regional survey in southern England. J Neurol Neurosurg Psychiatry. 1976; 39(3):290–296
[11] King TT. Tumours of eight cranial nerve. Br J Hosp Med. 1976; 16:259–272
[12] Nestor JJ, Korol HW, Nutik SL, Smith R. The incidence of acoustic neuromas. Arch Otolaryngol Head Neck Surg. 1988; 114(6):680

[13] Schoenberg BS, Christine BW, Whisnant JP. The descriptive epidemiology of primary intracranial neoplasms: the Connecticut experience. Am J Epidemiol. 1976; 104(5):499–510

[14] Moffat DA, Hardy DG, Irving RM, Viani L, Beynon GJ, Baguley DM. Referral patterns in vestibular schwannomas. Clin Otolaryngol Allied Sci. 1995; 20(1):80–83

[15] Evans DG, Moran A, King A, Saeed S, Gurusinghe N, Ramsden R. Incidence of vestibular schwannoma and neurofibromatosis 2 in the North West of England over a 10-year period: higher incidence than previously thought. Otol Neurotol. 2005; 26(1):93–97

[16] Kshettry VR, Hsieh JK, Ostrom QT, Kruchko C, Barnholtz-Sloan JS. Incidence of vestibular schwannomas in the United States. J Neurooncol. 2015; 124(2):223–228

[17] Leonard JR, Talbot ML. Asymptomatic acoustic neurilemoma. Arch Otolaryngol. 1970; 91(2):117–124

[18] Stewart TJ, Liland J, Schuknecht HF. Occult schwannomas of the vestibular nerve. Arch Otolaryngol. 1975; 101(2):91–95

[19] Eckermeier L, Pirsig W, Mueller D. Histopathology of 30 non-operated acoustic schwannomas. Arch Otorhinolaryngol. 1979; 222(1):1–9

[20] Hardy M, Crowe SJ. Early asymptomatic acoustic tumour. Arch Surg. 1936; 32:292–301

[21] Thomsen J, Jorgensen MB. Undiagnosed acoustic neurinomas. A presentation of 4 cases. Arch Klin Exp Ohren Nasen Kehlkopfheilkd. 1973; 204(3):175–182

[22] Onizuka M, Suyama K, Shibayama A, Hiura T, Horie N, Miyazaki H. Asymptomatic brain tumor detected at brain check-up. Neurol Med Chir (Tokyo). 2001; 41(9):431–434, discussion 435

[23] Vernooij MW, Ikram MA, Tanghe HL, et al. Incidental findings on brain MRI in the general population. N Engl J Med. 2007; 357(18):1821–1828

[24] Weber F, Knopf H. Incidental findings in magnetic resonance imaging of the brains of healthy young men. J Neurol Sci. 2006; 240(1–2):81–84

[25] Propp JM, McCarthy BJ, Davis FG, Preston-Martin S. Descriptive epidemiology of vestibular schwannomas. Neuro-oncol. 2006; 8(1):1–11

[26] Kanzaki J, Tos M, Sanna M, Moffat DA, Monsell EM, Berliner KI. New and modified reporting systems from the consensus meeting on systems for reporting results in vestibular schwannoma. Otol Neurotol. 2003; 24(4): 642–648, discussion 648–649

[27] Gardner G, Robertson JH. Hearing preservation in unilateral acoustic neuroma surgery. Ann Otol Rhinol Laryngol. 1988; 97(1):55–66

[28] Meyer TA, Canty PA, Wilkinson EP, Hansen MR, Rubinstein JT, Gantz BJ. Small acoustic neuromas: surgical outcomes versus observation or radiation. Otol Neurotol. 2006; 27(3):380–392

[29] Stangerup SE, Caye-Thomasen P, Tos M, Thomsen J. Change in hearing during 'wait and scan' management of patients with vestibular schwannoma. J Laryngol Otol. 2008; 122(7):673–681

4 Histopathology of Vestibular Schwannoma

Aditya Raghunathan and Caterina Giannini

4.1 Introduction

The eighth cranial nerve (vestibulocochlear nerve), which transmits auditory and vestibular input from the inner ear to the brainstem, represents the most common site of origin of intracranial schwannoma, followed at a distance by the fifth (trigeminal) nerve and other cranial nerves. Although the antiquated term "acoustic neurinoma/neuroma" is commonly used interchangeably with "vestibular schwannoma" (VS), the former is technically incorrect as the tumor is not a neuroma, nor does it typically arise from the cochlear nerve. Because these tumors arise from Schwann cells of the vestibular divisions of the eighth cranial nerve, the term VS is highly preferred. VSs are typically conventional schwannomas, benign nerve sheath tumors composed of well-differentiated Schwann cells at the histologic, immunophenotypic, and ultrastructural level. Uncommonly, cellular and epithelioid variants may occur.

4.2 Pathologic Features

4.2.1 Macroscopic Features

Vestibular schwannoma usually presents as a globular or lobulated mass on the surface of which the parent nerve is splayed. The cut surfaces are firm and often smooth, and sometimes may appear slightly lobulated. The color is usually homogenous light tan-pink to grey. Areas showing cystic change, dark red foci of hemorrhage, bright yellow foci corresponding to macrophage aggregates, and white areas corresponding to fibrosis may also be seen. The cystic and hemorrhagic changes may be extensive in fast growing or larger tumors.

Conventional Schwannoma

Most VSs have histopathological features of conventional schwannoma. Although frequently removed in a piecemeal fashion in multiple fragments, a well-formed fibrous pseudocapsule may be identified toward the periphery, and fascicles of the associated parent nerve may also be seen. The VS "capsule" has been shown to hold neoplastic cells, which carries implications with regard to tumor recurrence when "subcapsular dissection" is employed.[1] VSs characteristically show two intermingled, histologically distinct regions, designated Antoni A and Antoni B (▶ Fig. 4.1). Antoni A regions are composed of compact arrangements of elongated cells, arranged as sheets, intersecting fascicles, and, occasionally, palisades. The cells have eosinophilic cytoplasmic processes and indistinct cell membranes.

The nuclei are spindle shaped, tapering and wavy, with uniformly distributed chromatin and inconspicuous nucleoli. The most distinctive palisaded arrangements, termed "Verocay bodies," are composed of two parallel rows of nuclei separated by a relatively anuclear zone of eosinophilic fibrillary cytoplasmic processes (▶ Fig. 4.2). In contrast, Antoni B regions are relatively hypocellular, with a loose-textured pale-blue, myxoid stroma. The tumor cells in these regions have somewhat more ovoid to rounded nuclei and loosely knit cytoplasmic processes. These Antoni A and B regions can be present in variable relative proportions. Mitotic figures are rarely seen in conventional schwannomas.

Schwannomas are typically well vascularized, with blood vessels ranging from thick walled and hyalinized (▶ Fig. 4.1, *arrow*) to thin walled and dilated. Episodes of prior intratumoral bleeding may result in perivascular hemosiderin deposition. Aggregates of foamy macrophages may be seen, particularly adjacent to Antoni B regions. In long-standing tumors, scattered cells may show degenerative nuclear changes (the so-called ancient change/schwannoma), with markedly enlarged and hyperchromatic nuclei that have lost chromatin texture and may occasionally show intranuclear pseudoinclusions (▶ Fig. 4.3). Foci of bland, infarct-like necrosis, hyalinization, and calcification may

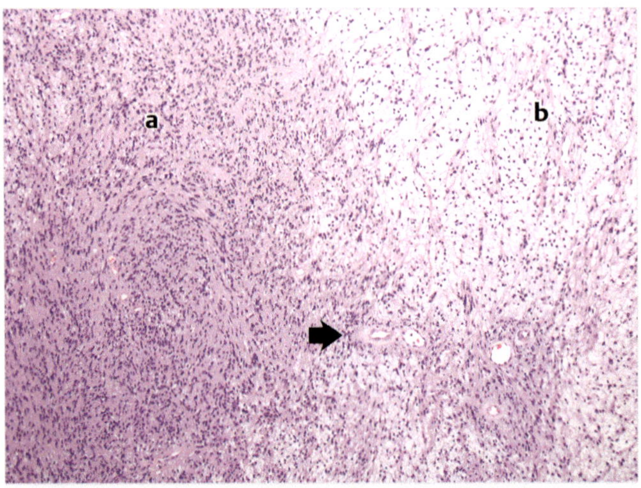

Fig. 4.1 Schwannomas are composed of intermingled regions of compact (Antoni A, **"A"**) and loose (Antoni B, **"B"**) cellularity. Hyalinized vessels are frequently seen (*arrow*).

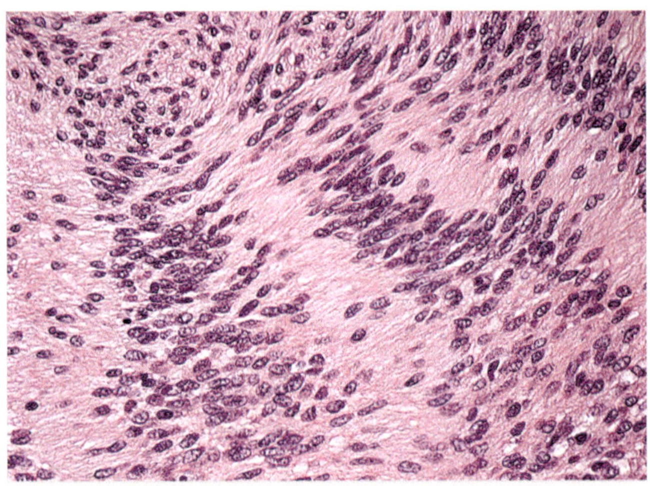

Fig. 4.2 Verocay bodies are a distinctive palisaded arrangement characteristic of schwannoma, composed of two parallel rows of nuclei separated by a relatively anuclear zone of eosinophilic fibrillary cytoplasmic processes.

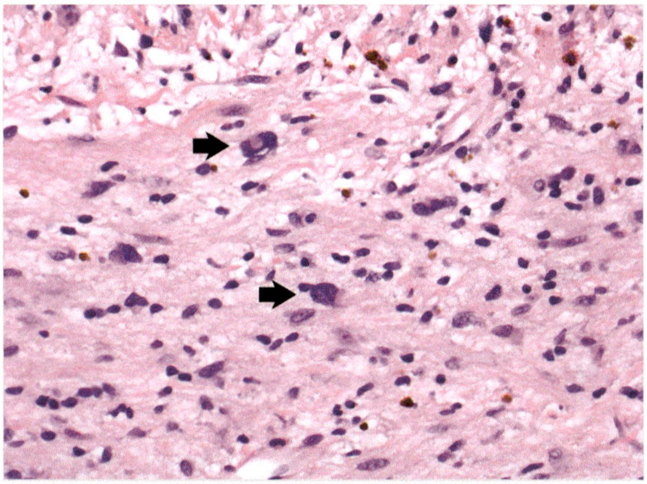

Fig. 4.3 Scattered cells may show degenerative nuclear changes (*arrows*), including enlargement, hyperchromasia, loss of chromatin texture, and, occasionally, intranuclear pseudoinclusions. However, these are of no prognostic significance.

also be present in long-standing cases. These findings are of no prognostic significance.

Epithelioid Schwannoma

In some schwannomas, the tumor cells may show epithelioid features, with more abundant cytoplasm, identifiable cell borders, and some degree of nuclear atypia.[2] These may be diagnosed as epithelioid schwannomas when such features are extensive. A recent series of 58 epithelioid schwannomas arising in various systemic sites did not identify any association with adverse outcomes, even in the presence of identifiable mitotic activity and moderate nuclear atypia.[3]

Cellular Schwannoma

Another variant that may rarely be seen in this region is the cellular schwannoma.[4,5] This tumor has high cellularity, is predominantly composed of Antoni A areas, and often has readily identifiable mitotic figures. However, even with elevated mitotic activity (generally no more than 4 mitoses per 10 high-power fields), these tumors have been well established to behave akin to conventional schwannoma. The significance of recognizing this variant lies in averting misdiagnosis as a malignancy and potential overtreatment.

Plexiform Schwannoma

This schwannoma variant is characterized by having a plexiform or multinodular manner of growth, and can be of the conventional or cellular type. Although some examples may have hypercellularity and increased mitotic activity, these behave as benign tumors. Plexiform schwannomas have been noted to have some association with the neurofibromatosis type 2 and with schwannomatosis.

Melanotic Schwannoma

The occurrence of melanotic schwannoma, a tumor characterized by advanced schwannian differentiation and extensive production of melanin pigment in the cerebellopontine angle (CPA), is exceptional. These tumors are composed of spindle and epithelioid cells, with moderate amounts of cytoplasm and intracytoplasmic brown to black pigment granules. The exceptionally rare occurrence of a pigmented tumor in the CPA should prompt consideration of primary melanocytic tumors of the central nervous system, which have malignant potential.[6]

As per the 2016 WHO Classification of Tumors of the Central Nervous System, conventional schwannomas correspond to WHO grade I tumors. Although epithelioid schwannomas are histologically distinct, plexiform schwannomas have a distinct growth pattern, and cellular schwannomas can harbor elevated mitotic activity, all of these variants also correspond to the WHO grade I designation. Melanotic schwannomas have not been assigned a grade, as experience with these rare tumors is limited.

4.3 Ancillary Studies

Ancillary studies may be used to confirm the diagnosis of schwannomas, and to distinguish these from histologically similar lesions. On immunohistochemical staining, schwannomas show characteristic widespread, strong cytoplasmic and nuclear staining of the S-100 protein and widespread nuclear expression of SOX10. The neurofilament immunostain may highlight rare intratumoral axonal filaments, but these are typically very sparse and may be seen in greater numbers toward the periphery. Few cases may also show patchy staining with glial fibrillary acid protein. Schwannomas are seen to have continuous basement membrane surrounding tumor cells on ultrastructural examination, particularly in Antoni A areas. This can also be demonstrated as pericellular deposition of reticulin by histochemistry, and pericellular collagen IV or laminin immunoreactivity. Although electron microscopy is not conventionally used for the diagnosis of schwannomas, ultrastructural features may be of value in the diagnosis of challenging cases. A characteristic, but nonspecific, ultrastructural finding is the presence of extracellular long-spacing collagen, termed "Luse bodies." Melanosomes in various stages of maturation can be seen by electron microscopy in melanotic schwannomas. Hereditary forms of schwannomas have been found to have constitutional and somatic mutations of the *INI1/SMARCB1* gene.[7] A mosaic pattern of loss of INI1 expression by immunohistochemistry is seen in tumors associated with schwannomatosis (about 90% of familial and 55% of sporadic cases) and neurofibromatosis type 2 (about 80% of cases), while being rare in solitary, sporadic schwannomas (about 5% of cases).[8] Mutations of the *NF2* tumor-suppressor gene and loss of expression of its product merlin have been identified in the majority of sporadic and NF2-associated VS, and the loss of merlin expression can be demonstrated by immunohistochemistry.[9,10]

4.4 Differential Diagnosis

4.4.1 Meningioma

Particularly the fibrous subtype may be composed of similar spindle-shaped cells, and pose a diagnostic challenge in this region. The presence of characteristic, tight meningothelial whorls or the presence of psammomatous calcifications may offer a diagnostic clue. Meningiomas are usually easily distinguished from schwannomas by immunohistochemical staining. Meningiomas show immunoreactivity with epithelial membrane antigen (EMA) and progesterone receptor (PR), which are not seen in schwannoma. On the other hand, S-100 protein expression is typically patchy when present, but may be more widespread among the fibrous and transitional subtypes of meningioma.[11] Meningiomas also lack pericellular basement membranes, which can be demonstrated by the absence of significant pericellular reticulin, collagen IV, or laminin staining.

Tumors of the ***solitary fibrous tumor (SFT)/hemangiopericytoma (HPC)*** family may also occur in the CPA region, albeit much less commonly. Tumors from this family show a morphological spectrum of high (HPC) to relatively low (SFT) cellularity, and extensive (SFT) to relatively sparse (HPC) collagen deposition. There is a chaotic or "patternless" arrangement of the constituent tumor cells, which have oval or elongated nuclei with finely distributed chromatin. In HPC, dilated thin-walled blood vessels showing few acute angle branching may also be seen. As with the soft-tissue counterparts, meningeal tumors of the SFT/HPC family have been shown to harbor *NAB2-STAT6* gene fusions, which can be detected by the nuclear expression of the STAT6 immunostain.[12]

Cellular schwannoma needs to be distinguished from ***malignant peripheral nerve sheath tumor (MPNST)***, which carries a dismal prognosis.[13,14,15] MPNST may arise de novo or they may develop secondarily within conventional type VS, either spontaneously or following radiation treatment. Concomitant MPNST cells in a background of conventional benign VS suggests secondary degeneration. The term ***malignant triton tumor*** historically has been used to describe MPNST with rhabdomyoblastic differentiation. This form of MPNST has been associated with prior irradiation in some cases and constitutes only approximately 5% of all MPNST cases. A history of extremely rapid tumor growth on serial imaging or fast deterioration of symptoms including facial paralysis should raise the suspicion for a malignant process, compared to the more indolent clinical course seen in most conventional VS. Thus, one theoretical advantage of microsurgery includes early histological confirmation of benign schwannoma, compared to conservative observation or stereotactic radiation where the diagnosis is only presumed based on history and imaging. The topic of radiation-induced tumorigenesis in the context of VS is discussed further in Chapter 24.

Unlike schwannoma, MPNST may show invasion of adjacent structures with a pseudocapsule formed by reactive fibrosis, and also lack distinct Antoni A and B areas and hyalinized blood vessels. The malignant cells in MPNST typically have somewhat monotonous hyperchromatic nuclei, and enlarged pleomorphic cells show viable chromatin, which can be distinguished from degenerative atypia seen in some schwannomas. Areas of tumor necrosis in MPNST are often geographic and may be surrounded by a palisaded rim of tumor cells. Mitotic activity is usually brisk, and atypical mitotic figures may also be identified. On immunohistochemical staining, MPNST typically shows a lesser extent of immunoreactivity for S-100 protein and neurofibromin, with the staining frequently appearing nonuniform, focal, and weak, and SOX10 expression may be absent or focal at best.[13] The elevated proliferative activity within MPNST can also be highlighted by Ki-67, which shows labeling indices of greater than 20%, a level which is not seen in cellular schwannoma.

Primary Melanocytic Tumors of the Central Nervous System

Primary melanocytic tumors of the central nervous system may also arise in the CPA region, and may need to be distinguished from melanotic schwannoma.[6] Melanocytic neoplasms typically lack the pericellular basement membranes seen in schwannomas, which can be demonstrated by the absence of the pericellular staining with reticulin and collagen IV. This can also be confirmed by electron microscopy if optimally preserved tissue is available. Of note, primary central nervous system melanocytic tumors frequently harbor *GNAQ*, *GNA11*, and *N-RAS* mutations, and rarely show *BRAF* and *KIT* mutations, which also helps distinguish these from systemic melanoma.[16,17]

4.5 Conclusion

Among tumors arising in the CPA, by far the most common is VS. The histological diagnosis of VS is relatively straightforward in a majority of cases, wherein classic features are readily identified. Schwannoma variants have been well described, and identification of these serves to avoid misdiagnosis as other more aggressive entities and overtreatment. Ancillary tests, including immunohistochemistry and electron microscopy, might be utilized in challenging cases, and usually serve to distinguish these tumors from histological mimics.

References

[1] Kuo TC, Jackler RK, Wong K, Blevins NH, Pitts LH. Are acoustic neuromas encapsulated tumors? Otolaryngol Head Neck Surg. 1997; 117(6):606–609

[2] Tan TC, Lam PW. Epithelioid schwannoma of the vestibular nerve. Singapore Med J. 2004; 45(8):393–396

[3] Hart J, Gardner JM, Edgar M, Weiss SW. Epithelioid schwannomas: an analysis of 58 cases including atypical variants. Am J Surg Pathol. 2016; 40(5):704–713

[4] Erlich SA, Tymianski M, Kiehl TR. Cellular schwannoma of the abducens nerve: case report and review of the literature. Clin Neurol Neurosurg. 2009; 111(5):467–471

[5] Ishii N, Sawamura Y, Tada M, Abe H. Acoustic cellular schwannoma invading the petrous bone: case report. Neurosurgery. 1996; 38(3):576–578, discussion 578

[6] Piedra MP, Scheithauer BW, Driscoll CL, Link MJ. Primary melanocytic tumor of the cerebellopontine angle mimicking a vestibular schwannoma: case report. Neurosurgery. 2006; 59(1):E206–, discussion E206

[7] Hulsebos TJ, Plomp AS, Wolterman RA, Robanus-Maandag EC, Baas F, Wesseling P. Germline mutation of INI1/SMARCB1 in familial schwannomatosis. Am J Hum Genet. 2007; 80(4):805–810

[8] Patil S, Perry A, Maccollin M, et al. Immunohistochemical analysis supports a role for INI1/SMARCB1 in hereditary forms of schwannomas, but not in solitary, sporadic schwannomas. Brain Pathol. 2008; 18(4):517–519

[9] Stemmer-Rachamimov AO, Xu L, Gonzalez-Agosti C, et al. Universal absence of merlin, but not other ERM family members, in schwannomas. Am J Pathol. 1997; 151(6):1649–1654

[10] Gutmann DH, Giordano MJ, Fishback AS, Guha A. Loss of merlin expression in sporadic meningiomas, ependymomas and schwannomas. Neurology. 1997; 49(1):267–270

[11] Artlich A, Schmidt D. Immunohistochemical profile of meningiomas and their histological subtypes. Hum Pathol. 1990; 21(8):843–849

[12] Fritchie K, Jensch K, Moskalev EA, Caron A, Jenkins S, Link M, Brown PD, Rodriguez FJ, Guajardo A, Brat D, Velázquez Vega JE, Perry A, Wu A, Raleigh DR, Santagata S, Louis DN, Brastianos PK, Kaplan A, Alexander BM, Rossi S, Ferrarese F, Haller F, Giannini C. HYPERLINK "https://www.ncbi.nlm.nih.gov/

pubmed/30584643" The impact of histopathology and NAB2-STAT6 fusion subtype in classification and grading of meningeal solitary fibrous tumor/hemangiopericytoma. Acta Neuropathol. 2018 Dec 24. doi: 10.1007/s00401-018-1952-6

[13] Pekmezci M, Reuss DE, Hirbe AC, et al. Morphologic and immunohistochemical features of malignant peripheral nerve sheath tumors and cellular schwannomas. Mod Pathol. 2015; 28(2):187–200

[14] Scheithauer BW, Erdogan S, Rodriguez FJ, et al. Malignant peripheral nerve sheath tumors of cranial nerves and intracranial contents: a clinicopathologic study of 17 cases. Am J Surg Pathol. 2009; 33(3):325–338

[15] Carlson ML, Jacob JT, Habermann EB, Glasgow AE, Raghunathan A, Link MJ. Malignant peripheral nerve sheath tumors of the eighth cranial nerve arising without prior irradiation. J Neurosurg. 2016; 125(5):1120–1129

[16] Gessi M, Hammes J, Lauriola L, et al. GNA11 and N-RAS mutations: alternatives for MAPK pathway activating GNAQ mutations in primary melanocytic tumours of the central nervous system. Neuropathol Appl Neurobiol. 2013; 39(4):417–425

[17] Küsters-Vandevelde HV, Klaasen A, Küsters B, et al. Activating mutations of the GNAQ gene: a frequent event in primary melanocytic neoplasms of the central nervous system. Acta Neuropathol. 2010; 119(3):317–323

5 Molecular Biology of Sporadic and NF2-Associated Vestibular Schwannoma

Aaron K. Remenschneider, Ruwan Kiringoda, and D. Bradley Welling

5.1 Introduction

The field of molecular research in vestibular schwannomas (VSs) began when mutations in the neurofibromatosis type 2 (*NF2*) tumor suppressor gene were identified in surgically removed specimens. Since then, a significant amount of new knowledge about the *NF2* gene and its protein product, Merlin, has been attained. Advances over the last 30 years in molecular biology have led to greater insight into the etiology and pathogenesis of VS. The underlying purpose of molecular research in VS is to identify potential targets and therapies for successful medical treatment; however, such options have yet to be firmly established.

This chapter will focus on the structure and function of the *NF2* gene, its protein product, Merlin, and will review associated, known molecular biologic pathways. This field of research is constantly evolving with new pathways and protein interactions emerging on a regular basis. For a more in-depth understanding of the myriad molecular pathways in VS tumorigenesis, the reader is referred to two recent articles published on the topic by Petrilli and Fernández-Valle[5] and Cooper and Giancotti (Cooper J, Giancotti FG. Molecular insights into *NF2*/Merlin tumor suppressor function. FEBS Lett. 2014 Aug 19;588 (16):2743-52). In light of described pathways, available and potential medical treatment options will also be discussed.

5.2 *NF2* Gene

VSs harbor mutations in the tumor-suppressor gene, *NF2*, resulting in abnormal Merlin production. The first studies to localize the gene responsible for Merlin production were performed in 1982 on meningioma samples and pointed toward chromosome 22.[1] In 1987, linkage analysis was used to confirm this location.[2] Genetic linkage analysis and tumor deletion mapping provided precise localization of the *NF2* gene to 22q12.2 in 1993.[3,4] Recently, mutations in *NF2* have also been discovered in several other tumors including the following malignancies: melanoma, mesothelioma, breast, colorectal, hepatic, prostate, and clear cell renal cell carcinoma.[5]

5.2.1 Merlin

In the 1990s, early characterizations of Merlin described a novel moesin-, ezrin-, radixin-like protein, taking its name from its structure.[3,4] Merlin is a 595-amino acid protein composed of an N-terminal domain, a coil–coil domain, and a carboxyl terminal domain. It can be regarded as a scaffold protein most commonly found at the plasma membrane. Merlin functions as a tumor suppressor that also plays an important role in schwannoma cell motility, cell adhesion, and cell proliferation.[6,7]

Merlin has structural similarity to the protein 4.1 superfamily known as the "ERM family," and functions in linking plasma membrane receptors to cytoskeletal components.[5] Relative conservation of the N-terminus domain known as the FERM region (*F* for 4.1 protein, *E* for ezrin, *R* for radixin, and *M* for moesin) characterizes the gene family, and sequence alignment demonstrates 64% similarity for Merlin at the conserved FERM domain.[4] The FERM domain in Merlin differs from the ERM proteins in that Merlin possesses a unique actin-binding motif at the N-terminal domain, in lieu of the conventional C-terminal actin binding site.[8,9] Moreover, while all ERM proteins form inter- and intramolecular associations, Merlin's associations are relatively weaker and more dynamic.[5] Nevertheless, these interactions appear critical for tumor-suppressor function.

Merlin's activity is controlled via phosphorylation. The process of dephosphorylation has been thought to activate Merlin by changing its structure from an unfolded, open state to its folded, active form as a tumor suppressor.[10,11] Recent work has suggested that while phosphorylation inactivates Merlin's role as a tumor suppressor, the protein remains in the closed configuration, without significant conformation change (▶ Fig. 5.1).[12] Activated Merlin appears to play critical roles in multiple molecular pathways that regulate cell cycle, which will be described later in this chapter.

5.2.2 *NF2*/Merlin Inactivation in Tumor Biology

Inactivation of both alleles of the *NF2* tumor-suppressor gene is necessary for the development of both spontaneous and NF2-associated VS.[3,4] Patients with inherited NF2 syndrome obtain one mutated copy of the *NF2* gene through autosomal dominant transmission. But unlike most autosomal dominant conditions, in which one copy of the altered gene is sufficient to result in phenotypic disease, both copies of the *NF2* gene must be altered to result in tumor formation. Somatic mutations in the *NF2* gene then occur during the patient's life, resulting in schwannomas or other tumors of the nervous system. Given the high probability of intergenerational transmission, selected at-risk populations should pursue genetic testing for the *NF2* mutation.[13]

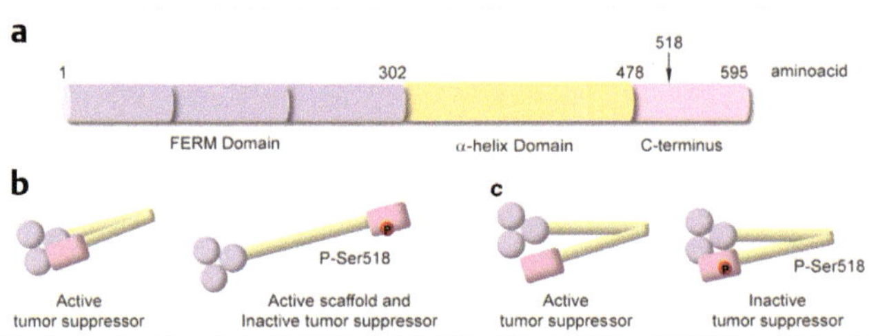

Fig. 5.1 Merlin's domain organization and molecular conformation. (**a**) Diagram of Merlin's structural domains. (**b**) Diagram or Merlin's molecular conformation based on ERM analogy. (**c**) Diagram of Merlin's molecular conformation based on the experimental data. (Used with permission from Petrilli and Fernández-Valle.[5])

In sporadic VS, spontaneous mutations of *NF2* within Schwann cells of the vestibular nerve are thought to be responsible for tumor formation. Isolated, unilateral VSs frequently harbor identifiable mutations in both copies of the *NF2* gene.[14,15,16]

5.2.3 *NF2* Mutation Type May Predict Severity of Disease

While mutations in the *NF2* gene are responsible for both sporadic and NF2-associated VS, there is significant variability in clinical presentation of both sets of patients.[17,18] Differences in disease severity may be related to the mutation type, as a wide range of mutations have been found in genetic studies of NF2 patients.[19] Approximately 65% of mutations seen in NF2 patients result in a truncated gene product (nonsense or frameshift mutations).[18] Studies evaluating genotype–phenotype relationships have determined that truncated *NF2* products lead to more severe clinical disease. Patients with milder disease tend to harbor missense mutations or DNA alterations that are not found by conventional mutation detection strategies.[18] Merlin proteins containing missense mutations may be stably expressed but defective in their ability to suppress cell division.[15,20,21] Today, it is known that one risk for a poorer prognosis in NF2 patients is related to the type of mutation—specifically the presence of a truncating mutation.

Patients with sporadic VS tend to have different types of *NF2* mutations than patients with NF2 syndrome.[15] Between 76 and 89% of sporadic VS cases have been found to harbor small deletions,[14,15,22] whereas only 42% of NF2-associated tumors harbor small deletions.[15] More common in NF2-associated tumors were single base pair point mutations.[15] Differences in mutation types likely result in varied presence and composition of the defective Merlin protein. However, the downstream effects on intracellular signaling pathways may represent an additional source of differential tumor growth patterns between patients.

5.3 Molecular Roles of Merlin

As a member of the FERM gene family, it is known that Merlin's main molecular role is to link plasma membrane receptors to the cortical actin cytoskeleton.[4] As such, Merlin modulates receptor-mediated signaling pathways that control cell proliferation and survival. These downstream pathways include contact inhibition/suppression of cell proliferation, ras-related C3 botulinum toxin substrate 1 (RAC1)-mediated cytoskeletal pathways, receptor tyrosine kinase (RTK), phosphatidylinositol 3-kinase (PI3K)/AKT serine/threonine kinase (AKT)/mammalian target of rapamycin (mTOR), and hippo pathways.[5,23] Loss of Merlin production or loss of normal Merlin function results in increased activation of these signaling pathways, leading to cellular growth, division, and tumorigenesis. Merlin tumor suppression acts via numerous pathways, and, thus, normally prevents unchecked growth in a number of distinct fashions. Currently, there is no clear indication which pathway is most important for tumorigenesis.

5.3.1 Contact Inhibition/Suppression of Cell Proliferation

Merlin is activated in conditions of increased cell density, and the resultant CD4-mediated interactions suppress cell proliferation. Merlin has been found to co-localize with the plasma membrane protein CD44.[24] Merlin and CD44 form a "molecular switch" whereby at low cell density, Merlin exists in a phosphorylated complex with ezrin, moesin, and CD44 that is growth permissive; at high cell density, Merlin becomes hypophosphorylated and inhibits cell growth through signals from the extracellular matrix (ECM; ▶ Fig. 5.2).[25] Cell–cell contact, in particular, plays a role in Merlin activity; loss of cell adhesion results a near-complete dephosphorylation of Merlin, while replating cells reverses this process.[25] In a murine model, Bai et al showed that increased expression of wild-type Merlin in Tr6BC1 schwannoma cells inhibits hyaluronic acid binding to CD44, supporting the idea that the interaction between CD44

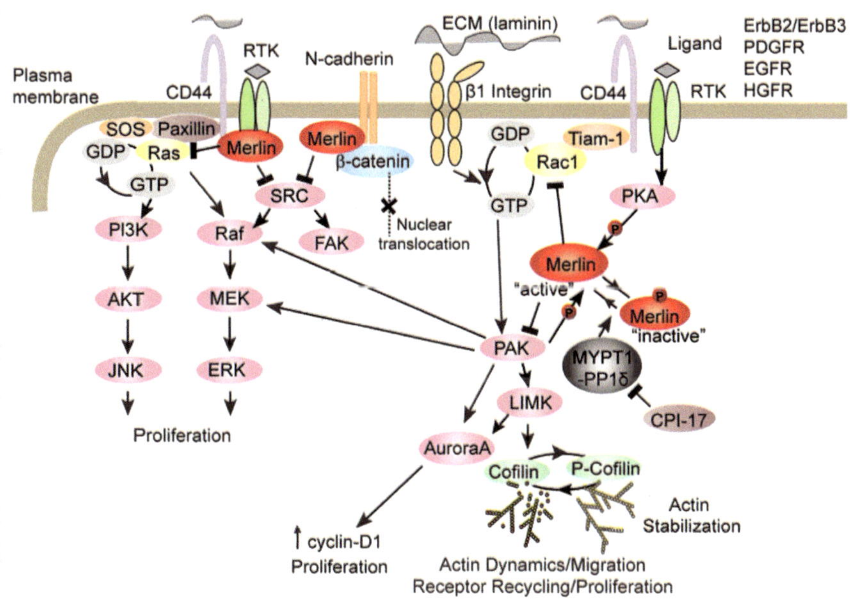

Fig. 5.2 Merlin inhabits membrane receptors and Rho GTPase family signaling cascade. (Used with permission from Petrilli and Fernández-Valle.[5])

and Merlin is at least partially responsible for tumor growth suppression.[26]

5.3.2 RAC11-Mediated Cytoskeletal Pathway

Merlin localizes predominantly to the membrane–cytoskeleton interface. Similar to the ERM proteins, Merlin most likely acts as a linker between plasma membrane molecules and the cytoskeleton, functioning in membrane organization.[24] Loss of Merlin results in deregulation of the actin cytoskeleton. Acting via CD44, Merlin triggers RAC1-dependent cytoskeleton-associated processes that modulate growth factor and ECM signals (▶ Fig. 5.2).[11] Expression of the activated GTPase RAC1 decreases the association of Merlin with the cytoskeleton via dephosphorylation. Furthermore, increased expression of Merlin inhibits RAC-induced signaling via phosphorylation.[10] Merlin inhibits the activation of the kinase Pak1, preventing cell cycle progression. Studies have shown that p21 (RAC1) activated kinase 1 (PAK1) substrates as well as the associated LIM domain kinases 1 and 2 (LIMK1, LIMK2) modulate actin dynamics and translocate into the nucleus to regulate cell cycle progression.[27]

5.3.3 The Mammalian Target of Rapamycin Pathway

Merlin has also been found to serve a tumor-suppressor function via the pro-proliferative mTOR pathway. Constitutive activation of this signaling pathway has been demonstrated in NF2-schwannomas and meningiomas.[5] The loss of Merlin has been shown to activate PI3K, which starts a signaling cascade resulting in activation of mTOR and cell proliferation (▶ Fig. 5.3). Inhibitors of PI3K have been tested in an *in vivo* Merlin-deficient mouse, with resultant strong antiproliferative activity.[28] Further downstream, PI3K activates AKT via phosphorylation in a manner that is regulated by two histone deacetylases (HDAC) and protein phosphatase 1 (PP1) (▶ Fig. 5.3). HDAC may provide another potential target for therapy along the mTOR pathway as HDAC inhibitors have been shown to decrease human schwannoma cell proliferation in an allograft model.[29,30] Finally, new studies relate the potential for Merlin to directly inhibit mTOR signaling, independent of PI3K or AKT activation, although the particular mechanism of action remains unclear.[31] These findings reiterate the potential need for multiple, simultaneous therapeutic approaches.

5.3.4 Mammalian Hippo Pathway

Recent studies have implicated Merlin within the mammalian hippo pathway, where it appears that Merlin negatively regulates cell division at two cellular locations: the nucleus and cell cortex. Normally, the mammalian hippo pathway works through a series of protein kinases to eventually phosphorylate and inactivate the Yes-associated protein/tafazzin (YAP/TAZ) complex, blocking their role in the nucleus as transcription factor coactivators (▶ Fig. 5.4).[32] While Merlin is commonly thought to exist as a plasma membrane protein, it can also be transported throughout the cell by microtubule motors, facilitating intranuclear localization and direct inhibition of transcriptional factors.[33] Merlin loss in human meningioma specimens is associated with increased intranuclear YAP, leading to activation of proliferative transcription factors.[34] Interestingly, YAP/TAZ has recently been identified as having mechanosensor properties that appear to be modulated by Merlin.[27] Stretching, rigidity, and cell density affect YAP/TAZ activity, but activation appears to be modulated through a Merlin-dependent mechanism.[35] Lastly, cellular cortex components such as angiomotins (AMOT) appear to complex with YAP/TAZ and prevent their intranuclear localization.[36] Normal AMOT function may depend on Merlin, as studies have identified colocalization of AMOT and Merlin,[37] but this part of the mammalian hippo pathway requires further exploration.

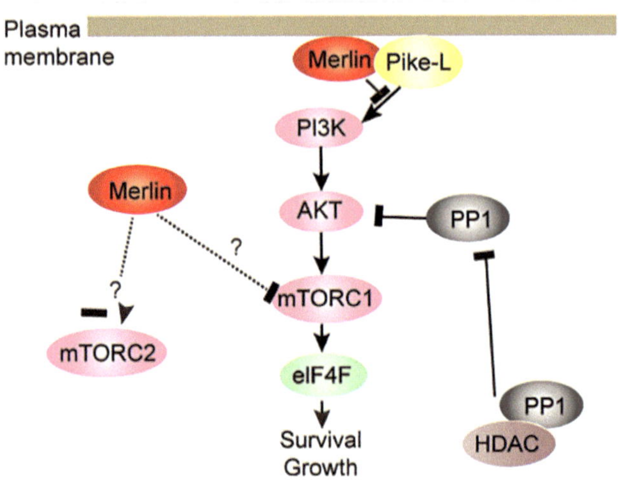

Fig. 5.3 Merlin inhibits PI3K/mTORC1/AKT signaling pathways. (Used with permission from Petrilli and Fernández-Valle.[5])

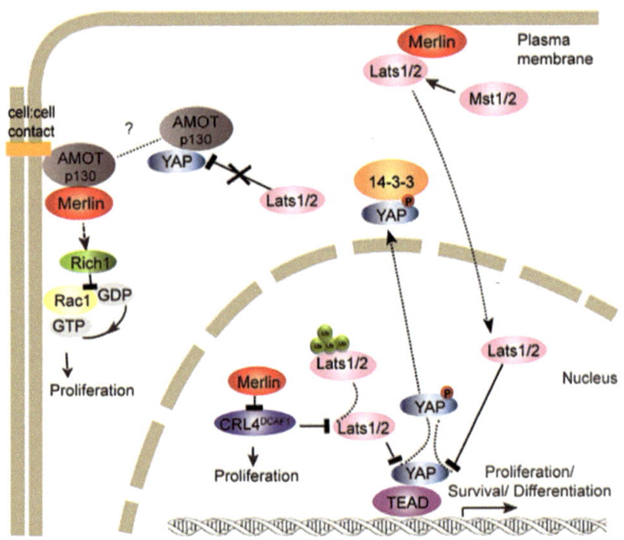

Fig. 5.4 Role of Merlin in the activation of the mammalian hippo pathway. (Used with permission from Petrilli and Fernández-Valle.[5])

5.3.5 Additional Merlin Pathways

Beyond the discrete signaling cascades described earlier, Merlin has also been found to be important in cell signaling along a variety of other pathways.[5] Recent work on the RAS pathway,[38] the signal transducer and activator of transcription 3 and 5 (STAT3, STAT5) signaling cascades,[39] and mitogen activated protein (MAP) kinase pathway[40] have added further complexity to the role Merlin plays in tumor suppression. These findings suggest a near-ubiquitous role for Merlin in proliferative cell signaling.

5.4 Epigenetic Pathways of Vestibular Schwannoma Tumorigenesis

Several studies genotyping VS tumor samples found rates of wild-type *NF2* genes as high as 47 to 70%[41,42] raising the suspicion of an alternate tumorigenic pathway. Several studies have evaluated mRNA transcription levels in schwannomas from patients without identified *NF2* mutations and found significantly decreased transcript levels.[43] Epigenetic changes including DNA methylation and histone deacetylation are known to decrease gene transcription and could account for reduced or absent Merlin production in patients with sporadic VS.

5.4.1 DNA Methylation

Early studies suggested that between 20 and 40% of sporadic VS demonstrated methylated *NF2*,[44,45] resulting in silencing of the gene and a downstream absence of Merlin. It was hypothesized that hypermethylation of *NF2* may be one explanation for tumorigenesis in patients with wild-type alleles or no loss of *NF2* heterozygosity. Recent work using updated, more precise techniques has suggested that, in fact, promoter regions and the *NF2* gene itself are actually hypomethylated, casting doubts upon the previous work.[41,42,46]

5.4.2 Histone Deacetylation

Changes in the acetylation or deacetylation of histones associated with the *NF2* gene affect gene transcription and subsequent Merlin production. Specifically, histone deacetylation results in tighter histone binding of DNA with resultant silencing of the associated genes. As a tumor suppressor, the *NF2* gene may be inactivated with resultant tumorigenesis if the associated histones are deacetylated. Perhaps the greatest evidence for a potential role of overactive histone deacetylases in schwannomas has been from several studies evaluating AR-42, a histone deacetylase inhibitor. VS xenografts exposed to AR-42 showed arrest of proliferation in cell culture, and volumetric reductions in size in a mouse model.[29,30] These data suggest that normal Merlin function may be partially restorable through activation of a silenced, but functional *NF2* gene. Clinical trials in humans using AR-42 for VS and meningioma are currently underway.[47]

5.5 Non-Merlin Molecular Pathways in Vestibular Schwannoma Tumorigenesis

5.5.1 Vascular Endothelial Growth Factor

Tumors growing larger than 2 mm within the central nervous system require a structured blood supply for delivery of nutrients and oxygen,[48] and prior studies have demonstrated that such growth is highly dependent on vascular endothelial growth factor (VEGF).[49] This glycoprotein binds to either VEGFR-1 or VEGFR-2 receptors, initiating vascular proliferation. In one series, 100% of VS expressed VEGF,[50] while in two different studies, VEGFR-1 was found in VS tumors at high levels.[51,52] In VS, a relationship has been observed between the growth rate/size of tumor and the number of feeding blood vessels. Because VEGF expression has also been correlated to the growth rate of the tumors,[53] clinical trials in patients with NF2 using bevacizumab, an anti-VEGF antibody, have been performed.[50] Early results from this study suggest that bevacizumab reduces tumor burden by up to 26% and offers hearing stability or improvement over the short term. Bevacizumab does carry side effects including hypertension and proteinuria, which must be carefully monitored.[54]

5.5.2 P53

Given its important role in cell cycle regulation, p53 has been evaluated in VS. Like Merlin, p53 functions as a tumor suppressor and is involved in cellular apoptosis along with the Fas cell surface death receptor (FAS)/Fas ligand (FASL), BCL2, apoptosis regulator (Bcl-2) and BCL2-associated X, and apoptosis regulator (BAX) pathways.[55] Early work evaluated mutations within p53 in 21 cases of VS and neither mutations nor deletions were found, suggesting p53 is likely not involved with tumorigenesis or cell proliferation in VS.[56] However, recent work using newer immunoblot techniques and evaluating downstream elements suggests that MDM2 protooncogene (MDM2)/p53 pathway may be upregulated in some sporadic VS.[57] Likewise recent unpublished work has found p53 upregulation in recurrent VS specimens. Further investigation of this pathway is likely forthcoming.

5.6 Drug Targets and Treatment

Consideration of therapeutic targets is only possible within the context of a thorough understanding of the molecular pathways that drive VS formation and growth. The *NF2* gene and its protein product, Merlin, have been the focus of significant research given their now defined role in tumor pathogenesis. With an increased understanding of Merlin's role in contact inhibition/suppression of cell proliferation, RAC1-mediated cytoskeletal pathways, receptor tyrosine kinase (RTK), PI3K/AKT/mTOR, and hippo pathways, multiple potential targets are emerging.[58,59] New low-toxicity biologic therapies developed for other tumors also mean that previously unconsidered targets in VS can now be explored. Please see Chapter 83 for an in-depth review

Table 5.1

Drug	Target	Author (ref no.)	Main results
Bevacizumab	VEGF	Plotkin et al[50]	Tumor shrinkage and mild hearing improvement in 9 of 10 patients
		Plotkin et al[60]	Tumor shrinkage in > 50% of 31 analyzed patients
		Mautner et al[61]	> 40% tumor shrinkage in 2 of 2 patients
		Wong et al[62]	Mouse model showing decrease of tumor vasculature after bevacizumab. Tumor growth decreased and the survival of treated mice extended by 50%
		Farschtschi et al[63]	Reduced dose of drug can decrease side effects while also stabilizing tumor growth and hearing
Erlotinib	EGFR	Plotkin et al[64]	No radiographic or hearing response in 11 patients
Imatinib	PDGF	Altuna et al[65]	In vitro study demonstrating apoptosis and inhibition of cell proliferation
		Yener et al[66]	In vitro study demonstrating reduction of angiogenesis in tissue specimens of NF2 related as well as sporadic tumors
Lapatinib	EGFR/ErbB2	Ahmad et al[67]	In vitro study demonstrating decrease of cell growth and proliferation in VS cell cultures
		Ammoun et al[68]	In vitro study demonstrating decrease proliferation in a human schwannoma model
		Karajannis et al[69]	Phase II trial demonstrating hearing and tumor volume responses in lapatinib-treated NF2 patients
Ponatinib	PDGFRα/β, AKT, MEK1/2-ERK1/2, STAT3		Early results from in vitro study demonstrating block of G1 cell cycle progression in Merlin/*NF2*-deficient Schwann cells
Nilotinib	PDGFR, c-kit	Sabha et al[70]	In vitro study showing dose-dependent inhibition of cell proliferation in human *NF2*-null schwannoma cell line
Sorafenib	VEGFR-2, PDGFRβ, c-kit	Subbiah et al[71]	Used in combination with histone deacetylase inhibitor without clear effects
Axitinib	VEGFR, c-kit, PDGFRβ		Potential drug with targets and presumed activity similar to sorafenib
AR42	PI3K/AKT	Bush et al[29]	Growth inhibition of schwannoma cells
FRAX597	PAK	Licciulli et al[72]	In vitro study displaying reduced schwannoma cell proliferation and an in vivo experiment indicating impairment in tumor development
Rapamycin	MTORc1	Giovannini et al[73]	Tumor growth arrest in 1 NF2 patient
Aspirin	COX-2	Kandathil et al[74]	Inverse association between aspirin use and tumor growth

Abbreviations: VEGF, vascular endothelial growth factor; EGFR, epidermal growth factor receptor; PDGF, platelet-derived growth factor; NF2, neurofibromatosis type 2; VS, vestibular schwannoma.
Vestibular Schwannoma Therapeutics, Targets and Main Results from Clinical and In Vitro Studies. Table Updated and modified from Devries et al, Otology and Neurotology 2015;36(7), now including additional studies since November 2015.

of medical therapies in VS and NF2 such as VEGF, (bevacizumab), ERBB2 receptor (trastuzumab), EGFR tyrosine kinase (erlotinib), HER2 (lapatinib), and PAK1 (IPA-3; ▶ Table 5.1). The interested reader may also review Chapter 78 for an in depth discussion on the genetics in NF2.

5.7 Conclusion

A better understanding of the molecular mechanisms of tumorigenesis in VS is still needed. Only after a thorough description of molecular pathways can appropriate molecular targets for therapy be considered. The loss of function of Merlin in humans most commonly affects Schwann, meningeal, or ependymal cells, whereas other mutated cell types, where typically Merlin is ubiquitous, are not tumorigenic. This implies a tissue-specific microenvironment that remains unclear. The recent discovery of Merlin inactivation in common human malignancies merits further investigation, as there may be potential for therapeutics with efficacy across diagnoses. Given the realization of Merlin's complex signaling pathways, successful treatment strategies may require combinatorial molecular therapies. Recent therapeutics demonstrating success, such as VEGF inhibitors, imply non-Merlin targets should also be pursued. Additionally, gene therapy replacement of the defective *NF2* gene is a future goal as hurdles to gene therapy are resolved.

References

[1] Zang KD. Cytological and cytogenetical studies on human meningioma. Cancer Genet Cytogenet. 1982; 6(3):249–274

[2] Rouleau GA, Wertelecki W, Haines JL, et al. Genetic linkage of bilateral acoustic neurofibromatosis to a DNA marker on chromosome 22. Nature. 1987; 329(6136):246–248

[3] Rouleau GA, Merel P, Lutchman M, et al. Alteration in a new gene encoding a putative membrane-organizing protein causes neuro-fibromatosis type 2. Nature. 1993; 363(6429):515–521

[4] Trofatter JA, MacCollin MM, Rutter JL, et al. A novel moesin-, ezrin-, radixin-like gene is a candidate for the neurofibromatosis 2 tumor suppressor. Cell. 1993; 72(5):791–800

[5] Petrilli AM, Fernández-Valle C. Role of Merlin/NF2 inactivation in tumor biology. Oncogene. 2016; 35(5):537–548

[6] McClatchey AI, Giovannini M. Membrane organization and tumorigenesis–the NF2 tumor suppressor, Merlin. Genes Dev. 2005; 19(19):2265–2277

[7] Okada T, You L, Giancotti FG. Shedding light on Merlin's wizardry. Trends Cell Biol. 2007; 17(5):222–229

[8] Sivakumar KC, Thomas B, Karunagaran D. Three dimensional structure of the closed conformation (active) of human merlin reveals masking of actin binding site in the FERM domain. Int J Bioinform Res Appl. 2009; 5 (5):516–524

[9] Xu HM, Gutmann DH. Merlin differentially associates with the microtubule and actin cytoskeleton. J Neurosci Res. 1998; 51(3):403–415

[10] Shaw RJ, Paez JG, Curto M, et al. The Nf2 tumor suppressor, merlin, functions in Rac-dependent signaling. Dev Cell. 2001; 1(1):63–72

[11] Sherman LS, Gutmann DH. Merlin: hanging tumor suppression on the Rac. Trends Cell Biol. 2001; 11(11):442–444

[12] Sher I, Hanemann CO, Karplus PA, Bretscher A. The tumor suppressor merlin controls growth in its open state, and phosphorylation converts it to a less-active more-closed state. Dev Cell. 2012; 22(4):703–705

[13] Welling DB, Packer MD, Chang LS. Molecular studies of vestibular schwannomas: a review. Curr Opin Otolaryngol Head Neck Surg. 2007; 15(5):341–346

[14] Jacoby LB, MacCollin M, Louis DN, et al. Exon scanning for mutation of the NF2 gene in schwannomas. Hum Mol Genet. 1994; 3(3):413–419

[15] Welling DB, Guida M, Goll F, et al. Mutational spectrum in the neurofibromatosis type 2 gene in sporadic and familial schwannomas. Hum Genet. 1996; 98(2):189–193

[16] Welling DB, Lasak JM, Akhmametyeva E, Ghaheri B, Chang LS. cDNA microarray analysis of vestibular schwannomas. Otol Neurotol. 2002; 23(5):736–748

[17] Bikhazi PH, Lalwani AK, Kim EJ, et al. Germline screening of the NF-2 gene in families with unilateral vestibular schwannoma. Otolaryngol Head Neck Surg. 1998; 119(1):1–6

[18] Ferner RE, O'Doherty MJ. Neurofibroma and schwannoma. Curr Opin Neurol. 2002; 15(6):679–684

[19] Sughrue ME, Yeung AH, Rutkowski MJ, Cheung SW, Parsa AT. Molecular biology of familial and sporadic vestibular schwannomas: implications for novel therapeutics. J Neurosurg. 2011; 114(2):359–366

[20] Gutmann DH, Giordano MJ, Fishback AS, Guha A. Loss of merlin expression in sporadic meningiomas, ependymomas and schwannomas. Neurology. 1997; 49(1):267–270

[21] MacCollin M, Braverman N, Viskochil D, et al. A point mutation associated with a severe phenotype of neurofibromatosis 2. Ann Neurol. 1996; 40(3): 440–445

[22] Sainz J, Huynh DP, Figueroa K, Ragge NK, Baser ME, Pulst SM. Mutations of the neurofibromatosis type 2 gene and lack of the gene product in vestibular schwannomas. Hum Mol Genet. 1994; 3(6):885–891

[23] Stamenkovic I, Yu Q. Merlin, a "magic" linker between extracellular cues and intracellular signaling pathways that regulate cell motility, proliferation, and survival. Curr Protein Pept Sci. 2010; 11(6):471–484

[24] Sainio M, Zhao F, Heiska L, et al. Neurofibromatosis 2 tumor suppressor protein colocalizes with ezrin and CD44 and associates with actin-containing cytoskeleton. J Cell Sci. 1997; 110(Pt 18):2249–2260

[25] Morrison H, Sherman LS, Legg J, et al. The NF2 tumor suppressor gene product, merlin, mediates contact inhibition of growth through interactions with CD44. Genes Dev. 2001; 15(8):968–980

[26] Bai Y, Liu YJ, Wang H, Xu Y, Stamenkovic I, Yu Q. Inhibition of the hyaluronan-CD44 interaction by merlin contributes to the tumor-suppressor activity of merlin. Oncogene. 2007; 26(6):836–850

[27] Petrilli A, Copik A, Posadas M, et al. LIM domain kinases as potential therapeutic targets for neurofibromatosis type 2. Oncogene. 2014; 33(27): 3571–3582

[28] Petrilli AM, Fuse MA, Donnan MS, et al. A chemical biology approach identified PI3K as a potential therapeutic target for neurofibromatosis type 2. Am J Transl Res. 2014; 6(5):471–493

[29] Bush ML, Oblinger J, Brendel V, et al. AR42, a novel histone deacetylase inhibitor, as a potential therapy for vestibular schwannomas and meningiomas. Neuro-oncol. 2011; 13(9):983–999

[30] Jacob A, Oblinger J, Bush ML, et al. Preclinical validation of AR42, a novel histone deacetylase inhibitor, as treatment for vestibular schwannomas. Laryngoscope. 2012; 122(1):174–189

[31] James MF, Han S, Polizzano C, et al. NF2/merlin is a novel negative regulator of mTOR complex 1, and activation of mTORC1 is associated with meningioma and schwannoma growth. Mol Cell Biol. 2009; 29(15):4250–4261

[32] Piccolo S, Dupont S, Cordenonsi M. The biology of YAP/TAZ: hippo signaling and beyond. Physiol Rev. 2014; 94(4):1287–1312

[33] Benseñor LB, Barlan K, Rice SE, Fehon RG, Gelfand VI. Microtubule-mediated transport of the tumor-suppressor protein Merlin and its mutants. Proc Natl Acad Sci U S A. 2010; 107(16):7311–7316

[34] Striedinger K, VandenBerg SR, Baia GS, McDermott MW, Gutmann DH, Lal A. The neurofibromatosis 2 tumor suppressor gene product, merlin, regulates human meningioma cell growth by signaling through YAP. Neoplasia. 2008; 10(11):1204–1212

[35] Dupont S, Morsut L, Aragona M, et al. Role of YAP/TAZ in mechanotransduction. Nature. 2011; 474(7350):179–183

[36] Robinson BS, Moberg KH. Cell-cell junctions: α-catenin and E-cadherin help fence in Yap1. Curr Biol. 2011; 21(21):R890–R892

[37] Yi C, Troutman S, Fera D, et al. A tight junction-associated Merlin-angiomotin complex mediates Merlin's regulation of mitogenic signaling and tumor suppressive functions. Cancer Cell. 2011; 19(4):527–540

[38] Jin H, Sperka T, Herrlich P, Morrison H. Tumorigenic transformation by CPI-17 through inhibition of a merlin phosphatase. Nature. 2006; 442(7102):576–579

[39] Scoles DR, Nguyen VD, Qin Y, et al. Neurofibromatosis 2 (NF2) tumor suppressor schwannomin and its interacting protein HRS regulate STAT signaling. Hum Mol Genet. 2002; 11(25):3179–3189

[40] Lim JY, Kim H, Jeun SS, Kang SG, Lee KJ. Merlin inhibits growth hormone-regulated Raf-ERKs pathways by binding to Grb2 protein. Biochem Biophys Res Commun. 2006; 340(4):1151–1157

[41] Kullar PJ, Pearson DM, Malley DS, Collins VP, Ichimura K. CpG island hypermethylation of the neurofibromatosis type 2 (NF2) gene is rare in sporadic vestibular schwannomas. Neuropathol Appl Neurobiol. 2010; 36(6):505–514

[42] Lee JD, Kwon TJ, Kim UK, Lee WS. Genetic and epigenetic alterations of the NF2 gene in sporadic vestibular schwannomas. PLoS One. 2012; 7(1):e30418

[43] Zhang Z, Wang Z, Sun L, et al. Mutation spectrum and differential gene expression in cystic and solid vestibular schwannoma. Genet Med. 2014; 16 (3):264–270

[44] Kino T, Takeshima H, Nakao M, et al. Identification of the cis-acting region in the NF2 gene promoter as a potential target for mutation and methylation-dependent silencing in schwannoma. Genes Cells. 2001; 6(5):441–454

[45] Gonzalez-Gomez P, Bello MJ, Alonso ME, et al. CpG island methylation in sporadic and neurofibromatis type 2-associated schwannomas. Clin Cancer Res. 2003; 9(15):5601–5606

[46] Torres-Martín M, Lassaletta L, de Campos JM, et al. Genome-wide methylation analysis in vestibular schwannomas shows putative mechanisms of gene expression modulation and global hypomethylation at the HOX gene cluster. Genes Chromosomes Cancer. 2015; 54(4):197–209

[47] Welling B. Exploratory Evaluation of AR-42 Histone Deacetylase Inhibitor in the Treatment of Vestibular Schwannoma and Meningioma. ClinicalTrials.gov 2016; Available at: https://clinicaltrials.gov/ct2/show/NCT02282917. Accessed December 12, 2018

[48] Folkman J. Seminars in Medicine of the Beth Israel Hospital, Boston. Clinical applications of research on angiogenesis. N Engl J Med. 1995; 333(26):1757–1763

[49] Ferrara N, Gerber HP, LeCouter J. The biology of VEGF and its receptors. Nat Med. 2003; 9(6):669–676

[50] Plotkin SR, Stemmer-Rachamimov AO, Barker FG, II, et al. Hearing improvement after bevacizumab in patients with neurofibromatosis type 2. N Engl J Med. 2009; 361(4):358–367

[51] Cayé-Thomasen P, Werther K, Nalla A, et al. VEGF and VEGF receptor-1 concentration in vestibular schwannoma homogenates correlates to tumor growth rate. Otol Neurotol. 2005; 26(1):98–101

[52] Uesaka T, Shono T, Suzuki SO, et al. Expression of VEGF and its receptor genes in intracranial schwannomas. J Neurooncol. 2007; 83(3):259–266

[53] Cayé-Thomasen P, Baandrup L, Jacobsen GK, Thomsen J, Stangerup SE. Immunohistochemical demonstration of vascular endothelial growth factor in vestibular schwannomas correlates to tumor growth rate. Laryngoscope. 2003; 113(12):2129–2134

[54] Slusarz KM, Merker VL, Muzikansky A, Francis SA, Plotkin SR. Long-term toxicity of bevacizumab therapy in neurofibromatosis 2 patients. Cancer Chemother Pharmacol. 2014; 73(6):1197–1204

[55] Mawrin C, Kirches E, Dietzmann K, Roessner A, Boltze C. Expression pattern of apoptotic markers in vestibular schwannomas. Pathol Res Pract. 2002; 198 (12):813–819

[56] Monoh K, Ishikawa K, Yasui N, Mineura K, Andoh H, Togawa K. p53 tumor suppressor gene in acoustic neuromas. Acta Otolaryngol Suppl. 1998; 537:11–15
[57] Chen Y, Wang ZY, Wu H. P14ARF deficiency and its correlation with overexpression of p53/MDM2 in sporadic vestibular schwannomas. Eur Arch Otorhinolaryngol. 2015; 272(9):2227–2234
[58] Ammoun S, Hanemann CO. Emerging therapeutic targets in schwannomas and other merlin-deficient tumors. Nat Rev Neurol. 2011; 7(7):392–399
[59] Blakeley JO, Plotkin SR. Therapeutic advances for the tumors associated with neurofibromatosis type 1, type 2, and schwannomatosis. Neuro-oncol. 2016; 18(5):624–638
[60] Plotkin SR, Merker VL, Halpin C, et al. Bevacizumab for progressive vestibular schwannoma in neurofibromatosis type 2: a retrospective review of 31 patients. Otol Neurotol. 2012; 33(6):1046–1052
[61] Mautner VF, Nguyen R, Kutta H, et al. Bevacizumab induces regression of vestibular schwannomas in patients with neurofibromatosis type 2. Neuro-oncol. 2010; 12(1):14–18
[62] Wong HK, Lahdenranta J, Kamoun WS, et al. Anti-vascular endothelial growth factor therapies as a novel therapeutic approach to treating neurofibromatosis-related tumors. Cancer Res. 2010; 70(9):3483–3493
[63] Farschtschi S, Kollmann P, Dalchow C, Stein A, Mautner VF. Reduced dosage of bevacizumab in treatment of vestibular schwannomas in patients with neurofibromatosis type 2. Eur Arch Otorhinolaryngol. 2015; 272(12):3857–3860
[64] Plotkin SR, Halpin C, McKenna MJ, Loeffler JS, Batchelor TT, Barker FG, II. Erlotinib for progressive vestibular schwannoma in neurofibromatosis 2 patients. Otol Neurotol. 2010; 31(7):1135–1143
[65] Altuna X, Lopez JP, Yu MA, et al. Potential role of imatinib mesylate (Gleevec, STI-571) in the treatment of vestibular schwannoma. Otol Neurotol. 2011; 32 (1):163–170
[66] Yener U, Avsar T, Akgün E, Şeker A, Bayri Y, Kılıç T. Assessment of antiangiogenic effect of imatinib mesylate on vestibular schwannoma tumors using in vivo corneal angiogenesis assay. J Neurosurg. 2012; 117(4):697–704
[67] Ahmad ZK, Brown CM, Cueva RA, Ryan AF, Doherty JK. ErbB expression, activation, and inhibition with lapatinib and tyrphostin (AG825) in human vestibular schwannomas. Otol Neurotol. 2011; 32(5):841–847
[68] Ammoun S, Cunliffe CH, Allen JC, et al. ErbB/HER receptor activation and preclinical efficacy of lapatinib in vestibular schwannoma. Neuro-oncol. 2010; 12(8):834–843
[69] Karajannis MA, Legault G, Hagiwara M, et al. Phase II trial of lapatinib in adult and pediatric patients with neurofibromatosis type 2 and progressive vestibular schwannomas. Neuro-oncol. 2012; 14(9):1163–1170
[70] Sabha N, Au K, Agnihotri S, et al. Investigation of the in vitro therapeutic efficacy of nilotinib in immortalized human NF2-null vestibular schwannoma cells. PLoS One. 2012; 7(6):e39412
[71] Subbiah V, Slopis J, Hong DS, et al. Treatment of patients with advanced neurofibromatosis type 2 with novel molecularly targeted therapies: from bench to bedside. J Clin Oncol. 2012; 30(5):e64–e68
[72] Licciulli S, Maksimoska J, Zhou C, et al. FRAX597, a small molecule inhibitor of the p21-activated kinases, inhibits tumorigenesis of neurofibromatosis type 2 (NF2)-associated Schwannomas. J Biol Chem. 2013; 288(40):29105–29114
[73] Giovannini M, Bonne NX, Vitte J, et al. mTORC1 inhibition delays growth of neurofibromatosis type 2 schwannoma. Neuro-oncol. 2014; 16(4): 493–504
[74] Kandathil CK, Dilwali S, Wu CC, et al. Aspirin intake correlates with halted growth of sporadic vestibular schwannoma in vivo. Otol Neurotol. 2014; 35 (2):353–357

Part II

Disease Presentation and Diagnostic Evaluation

II

6 Disease Presentation of Sporadic Vestibular Schwannoma

Christopher S. Graffeo, William R. Copeland III, and Michael J. Link

6.1 Introduction

The clinical presentation of sporadic vestibular schwannoma (VS)—a spontaneous disease without the evidence of an underlying genetic syndrome, in particular neurofibromatosis type 2—is relatively homogenous, with a small number of dominant symptomatologies accompanied by several uncommon variants or anecdotal exceptions. Symptoms of VS occur either as a direct result of their involvement of the vestibulocochlear system or from compression of adjacent structures—including the facial nerve, trigeminal nerve, cerebellum, brainstem, or fourth ventricle. Notably, the fraction of diagnoses made incidentally has grown markedly in recent history, attributable to the growing availability of high-resolution magnetic resonance imaging (MRI) technology, and the rise in the use of this imaging modality for surveillance in unrelated disease such as headache.

6.2 Vestibulocochlear Presentations

Overwhelmingly, unilateral sensorineural hearing loss dominates the landscape of VS clinical presentation, most often occurring with a characteristic high-frequency loss (▶ Fig. 6.1). In several large cohorts documenting the natural history of these tumors, subjective hearing deficits have been reported from 26 up to 95% of patients—with equal or higher rates detected on audiometric testing.[1,2,3,4] Unilateral tinnitus represents the second most common cochlear symptom, occurring in 12 to 60% of patients, and frequently accompanied by a nonspecific sense of aural fullness.[1,2,3,4,5,6] In spite of this, delay in identification of an underlying VS in patients with auditory symptoms is common, with mean time to diagnosis averaging 3.7 to 7.6 years after symptom onset in these same series.

By contrast, sudden hearing loss is an uncommon presentation of VS, accounting for 2 to 7% of patients, with waxing and waning symptoms indicating intermittent cochlear dysfunction occurring less frequently still.[1,2,7,8,9] When approached from the perspective of clinical assessment in sudden sensorineural hearing loss, discovery of an underlying VS is rare, accounting for less than 5% of all patients.[10] Nevertheless, where present, sudden hearing loss may benefit from corticosteroid therapy—either via a short oral course or intratympanic injection—although the results of relevant clinical trials have been equivocal, and not specifically designed or powered to look at the VS subpopulation.[11,12]

As with cochlear nerve symptoms, vestibular dysfunction is prominent in the clinical presentation of VS, typically precipitating symptoms of dizziness, imbalance, or gait unsteadiness, whereas spells of true vertigo are less common. Clinical complaints invoking the vestibular system arise in 14 to 61% of VS patients; as with hearing loss, formal testing on asymptomatic individuals often discloses a degree of dysfunction that is either clinically insignificant or that the patient is able to unconsciously compensate.[1,2,3,4,5,13] Where vestibulopathies were parsed in detail and reported independently, gait disturbance was noted in approximately 40%, although the fraction attributable to concomitant brainstem compression is difficult to establish definitively.[1,4,8] Frequently, vestibulopathy in VS is complex, with one in three patients reporting multiple concomitant symptoms.[1]

6.3 Trigeminal Facial Presentations

After hearing loss and vestibulopathy, craniofacial sensory changes localizing to the trigeminal nerve represent the next most common group of presenting symptoms. Numbness predominates, affecting 7 to 49% of all patients in at least one distribution, with a preponderance of V2 symptoms.[1,2,3,4] Less commonly, involvement of the ipsilateral nerve may induce trigeminal neuralgia or paresthesia, which occur in approximately 1 to 3% of patients and share the same preference for a V2 distribution.[1,4,8] In these patients, tumors can present with classic trigeminal neuralgia symptoms, a specific unrelated complaint such as otalgia, or a nonspecific facial pain syndrome.[4,14] Very rarely, contralateral facial pain has been documented, with symptomatic resolution following removal of the tumor.[15] In the vast majority of cases involving trigeminal symptoms, diagnostic delays are less significant than in the setting of hearing loss, with most patients reporting symptoms over 0.6 to 1.3 years prior to diagnosis.[1,2,3,4,5] Motor trigeminal symptoms are infrequently reported, but in one large study, mastication

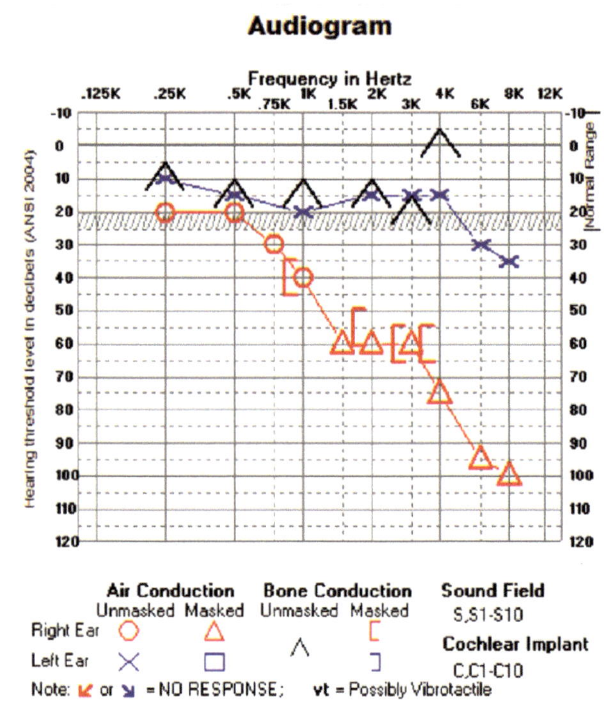

Fig. 6.1 Audiogram demonstrating unilateral high-frequency sensorineural hearing loss, characteristic of vestibular schwannoma.

disorders were observed in 3% of patients, and the ipsilateral corneal reflex was noted to be absent in 15%.[4]

Facial nerve symptoms are uncommon but by no means unheard of; however, the presence of a facial nerve paresis at diagnosis should significantly raise the index of suspicion for a primary facial nerve tumor or malignancy. Notwithstanding, several large series report a limited incidence of facial weakness or hemifacial spasm in patients with confirmed eighth nerve tumors, with an overall incidence of 1 to 4%.[1,2,3,4] Hemifacial spasm and taste disturbance are less common still, occurring in less than 1 to 4% of patients at primary presentation in larger series, with rare case reports documenting hemifacial spasm as the primary presenting symptom—including one instance of ipsilateral hearing loss and contralateral hemifacial spasm, which resolved following tumor resection.[1,3,4,16,17] Diagnostic delays in patients with isolated facial nerve symptoms are slightly more pronounced than those with trigeminal symptoms, typically leading to the identification of a VS within 2 years. Of note, although the majority of these symptoms occurred in patients with simultaneous hearing loss, the observed results are preserved in cohorts with normal hearing—studies in patients without a hearing deficit revealed that most patients presented with vestibular, trigeminal, and facial neuropathies, in that order.[18]

6.4 Headache and Incidental Diagnosis

The relationship between headache symptoms and VS presentation is nuanced, and very much intertwined with changing patterns in imaging referrals. In particular, headache as a component of a clinical syndrome precipitated by the tumor—typically one that also involves some combination of hearing loss, vestibulopathy, and trigeminal dysfunction—should be distinguished from chronic headache as an isolated symptom, the evaluation of which ultimately led to an MRI of the brain and the incidental discovery of a VS. When surveyed, more than 60% of VS patients endorsed a history of chronic headaches prior to treatment, a third of which were classified as severe.[19] By contrast, headache as the only presenting symptom at the time of diagnosis is rare, accounting for 1 to 12% of patients.[1,2,19] Of note, this fraction of VS patients has grown in an approximately linear fashion over several decades, in close parallel to the ready availability of MRI scanners and their increasing role in the workup of routine neurologic issues such as chronic headache.[1,2,5,19,20,21,22]

Closely related to this phenomenon is the increasing prevalence of incidental VS diagnosis in asymptomatic individuals who underwent surveillance imaging for unrelated pathology. With the rise in availability of high-resolution MRI technology, a range of neurologic diagnoses including multiple sclerosis, benign intracranial tumors, and others are routinely followed with serial imaging studies, which has dramatically increased the likelihood of capturing a tumor that would previously have gone undiagnosed for years—if not the patient's entire life.[5,20,21,22,23] Even in the absence of regular imaging, the chances of identifying an incidental VS on a one-time imaging study has been reported as 0.2% in the general population—a small but significant contributor to the rising tumor incidence, as routine MRI studies become increasingly common in a broad range of neurologic workups.[23] For a more detailed discussion of the epidemiology of VS, including changing trends in incidence, please refer to Chapter 3.

6.5 Mass Effect and Hydrocephalus

In the absence of obstructive hydrocephalus, compression of the brainstem by a large VS is most likely to precipitate symptoms related to the spectrum of cranial neuropathies described earlier—alone or in combination. Upper motor neuron signs are very uncommon, but have also been reported.[4] As one would intuit, the propensity for brainstem compression is strongly associated with increasing tumor size.[1,2,3,4] Cerebellar compression can be challenging to discriminate from vestibulopathy, and the symptoms are frequently comorbid—particularly in the gait domain. Nevertheless, studies that have explicitly included cerebellar tests such as ataxia, intention tremor, or dysdiadochokinesis have identified specific signs in up to 14 to 20% of patients.[1,2] Similarly, diplopia is a rarely reported presenting feature of VS presentation, attributable either to atypical superomedial tumor extension compressing the brainstem or fourth or sixth nerve, or to a feature of slowly progressive hydrocephalus.[24] Lower cranial nerve deficits are an even less common manifestation of mass effect in large tumors, observed in 1 to 3% of patients—typically as hoarseness or dysphagia.[1,4]

The development of symptomatic hydrocephalus requires a large tumor causing significant compression of the fourth ventricle and obstruction of the physiologic pathways for CSF egress. Correspondingly, the signs and symptoms of intracranial hypertension almost never occur in the absence of other neurologic deficits—although one case report does describe the diagnosis of VS after incidental discovery of papilledema in an otherwise asymptomatic patient without ventriculomegaly.[25] By contrast, radiographic ventriculomegaly is frequently identified in the setting of VS, and explicit evaluation discloses a much higher prevalence of clinical symptoms among these patients. Most frequently, findings are consistent with the chronic picture classically associated with normal pressure hydrocephalus—cognitive decline, urinary incontinence, and gait abnormalities—but more precipitous mental status changes attributable to acute intracranial hypertension may occur, as can visual disturbances including diplopia and blurred vision, which have been reported in 1 to 3% of patients.[1,2,25,26]

In one large series of cerebellopontine angle masses—the vast majority of which were VS—ventriculomegaly was observed in 14% of patients, of whom 12% demonstrated frank obstruction.[27] Further clinical evaluation of patients with obstructive hydrocephalus revealed at least one symptom of normal pressure hydrocephalus in 92%, and four patients from this subgroup presented with symptoms of acute intracranial hypertension, including two examples each of papilledema and mental status changes, requiring intervention in all cases. Another study of 400 VS patients identified ventriculomegaly in 13% (of which 21% were obstructive) with five patients demonstrating signs of acute intracranial hypertension.[28] Still other studies have demonstrated radiographic ventriculomegaly in up to 18% of patients, with the prevalence of obstruction reaching 39%; in most cases, a significant association was observed between tumor size and degree of fourth ventricular compression, extent of ventriculomegaly, and the prevalence of hydrocephalus symptoms.[5,27,28,29] For further details regarding recommendations for perioperative management of hydrocephalus, please refer to Chapter 46.

6.6 Conclusion

Although the most common presenting symptoms of sporadic VS are quite characteristic—unilateral sensorineural hearing loss, tinnitus, and dizziness—the broader clinical picture can be somewhat more variable, particularly in terms of how symptoms are subjectively experienced by patients and what ultimately brings them to medical attention. That these symptoms tend to develop indolently complicates things further, as do the rarities of VS presentation—the full swath of which encompasses symptoms ranging from sudden-onset hearing loss to altered mental status, facial paresis, visual changes, dysphagia, headache, and many others. In parallel, the ongoing expansion of access to MRI technology has markedly increased the fraction of incidental diagnoses, demanding a shift in overarching clinical management paradigms. Taken together, these features outline the broad landscape of VS, the diagnosis of which presents only the first of many key management challenges.

References

[1] Matthies C, Samii M. Management of 1000 vestibular schwannomas (acoustic neuromas): clinical presentation. Neurosurgery. 1997; 40(1):1–9, discussion 9–10

[2] Tos M, Charabi S, Thomsen J. Clinical experience with vestibular schwannomas: epidemiology, symptomatology, diagnosis, and surgical results. Eur Arch Otorhinolaryngol. 1998; 255(1):1–6

[3] Rosenberg SI. Natural history of acoustic neuromas. Laryngoscope. 2000; 110 (4):497–508

[4] Huang X, Xu J, Xu M, et al. Clinical features of intracranial vestibular schwannomas. Oncol Lett. 2013; 5(1):57–62

[5] Babu R, Sharma R, Bagley JH, Hatef J, Friedman AH, Adamson C. Vestibular schwannomas in the modern era: epidemiology, treatment trends, and disparities in management. J Neurosurg. 2013; 119(1):121–130

[6] Samii M, Matthies C. Management of 1000 vestibular schwannomas (acoustic neuromas): the facial nerve-preservation and restitution of function. Neurosurgery. 1997; 40(4):684–694, discussion 694–695

[7] Mathew GD, Facer GW, Suh KW, Houser OW, O'Brien PC. Symptoms, findings, and methods of diagnosis in patients with acoustic neuroma. Laryngoscope. 1978; 88(12):1893–1903, 1921

[8] Berrettini S, Ravecca F, Russo F, Bruschini P, Sellari-Franceschini S. Some uncharacteristic clinical signs and symptoms of acoustic neuroma. J Otolaryngol. 1997; 26(2):97–103

[9] Yanagihara N, Asai M. Sudden hearing loss induced by acoustic neuroma: significance of small tumors. Laryngoscope. 1993; 103(3):308–311

[10] Sauvaget E, Kici S, Kania R, Herman P, Tran Ba Huy P. Sudden sensorineural hearing loss as a revealing symptom of vestibular schwannoma. Acta Otolaryngol. 2005; 125(6):592–595

[11] Wei BP, Stathopoulos D, O'Leary S. Steroids for idiopathic sudden sensorineural hearing loss. Cochrane Database Syst Rev. 2013(7):CD003998

[12] Schreiber BE, Agrup C, Haskard DO, Luxon LM. Sudden sensorineural hearing loss. Lancet. 2010; 375(9721):1203–1211

[13] Samii M, Matthies C. Management of 1000 vestibular schwannomas (acoustic neuromas): hearing function in 1000 tumor resections. Neurosurgery. 1997; 40(2):248–260, discussion 260–262

[14] Matsuka Y, Fort ET, Merrill RL. Trigeminal neuralgia due to an acoustic neuroma in the cerebellopontine angle. J Orofac Pain. 2000; 14(2):147–151

[15] Eftekhar B, Gheini M, Ghodsi M, Ketabchi E. Vestibular schwannoma with contralateral facial pain - case report. BMC Neurol. 2003; 3:2

[16] Han I-B, Chang JH, Chang JW, Huh R, Chung SS. Unusual causes and presentations of hemifacial spasm. Neurosurgery. 2009; 65(1):130–137, discussion 137

[17] Nishi T, Matsukado Y, Nagahiro S, Fukushima M, Koga K. Hemifacial spasm due to contralateral acoustic neuroma: case report. Neurology. 1987; 37(2): 339–342

[18] Lustig LR, Rifkin S, Jackler RK, Pitts LH. Acoustic neuromas presenting with normal or symmetrical hearing: factors associated with diagnosis and outcome. Am J Otol. 1998; 19(2):212–218

[19] Carlson ML, Tveiten OV, Driscoll CL, et al. Risk factors and analysis of long-term headache in sporadic vestibular schwannoma: a multicenter cross-sectional study. J Neurosurg. 2015; 123(5):1276–1286

[20] Stangerup SE, Tos M, Caye-Thomasen P, Tos T, Klokker M, Thomsen J. Increasing annual incidence of vestibular schwannoma and age at diagnosis. J Laryngol Otol. 2004; 118(8):622–627

[21] Stangerup SE, Tos M, Thomsen J, Caye-Thomasen P. True incidence of vestibular schwannoma? Neurosurgery. 2010; 67(5):1335–1340, discussion 1340

[22] Stangerup SE, Caye-Thomasen P. Epidemiology and natural history of vestibular schwannomas. Otolaryngol Clin North Am. 2012; 45(2):257–268, vii

[23] Vernooij MW, Ikram MA, Tanghe HL, et al. Incidental findings on brain MRI in the general population. N Engl J Med. 2007; 357(18):1821–1828

[24] Morrison GA, Sterkers JM. Unusual presentations of acoustic tumours. Clin Otolaryngol Allied Sci. 1996; 21(1):80–83

[25] Grainger J, Dias PS. Case report: optic disc edema without hydrocephalus in acoustic neuroma. Skull Base. 2005; 15(1):83–86, discussion 86–88

[26] van Meter WS, Younge BR, Harner SG. Ophthalmic manifestations of acoustic neurinoma. Ophthalmology. 1983; 90(8):917–922

[27] Pirouzmand F, Tator CH, Rutka J. Management of hydrocephalus associated with vestibular schwannoma and other cerebellopontine angle tumors. Neurosurgery. 2001; 48(6):1246–1253, discussion 1253–1254

[28] Gerganov VM, Pirayesh A, Nouri M, et al. Hydrocephalus associated with vestibular schwannomas: management options and factors predicting the outcome. J Neurosurg. 2011; 114(5):1209–1215

[29] Rogg JM, Ahn SH, Tung GA, Reinert SE, Norén G. Prevalence of hydrocephalus in 157 patients with vestibular schwannoma. Neuroradiology. 2005; 47(5): 344–351

7 Auditory and Vestibular Testing Relevant to Vestibular Schwannoma

Crystal Pitts and Steven A. Telian

7.1 Introduction

In the same way that the identification and management of vestibular schwannoma (VS) has developed, so has there been an evolution of audiologic and vestibular testing methods. This has led to earlier identification of tumors, particularly those of smaller size at the time of diagnosis, which is often associated with improved outcomes related to hearing preservation and facial nerve function following surgical intervention. Most often, the patient initially presents with auditory and/or vestibular system complaints that require investigation and lead to the diagnosis. The purpose of this chapter is to provide an overview of current testing measures available to assess the integrity of the auditory and vestibular systems in patients with VS.

7.2 Audiometric Testing

Basic audiometric testing is typically performed when a patient complains of hearing loss, tinnitus, or difficulty understanding conversational speech, all rather common in patients with VS. The various portions of the audiometric testing battery can highlight abnormalities that are suspicious for retrocochlear pathology.

7.2.1 Pure-Tone Air and Bone Conduction

The audiogram is a graphic representation of a person's hearing sensitivity across a range of frequencies important for speech understanding, and provides information about the integrity of the entire auditory system from the peripheral end organ to the level of the auditory cortex in the brain. Behavioral threshold search is performed utilizing earphones (insert or circumaural) and a bone conduction oscillator. Patients with VS will often demonstrate asymmetrical hearing thresholds that are poorer in the affected ear, though hearing may be completely normal with no significant asymmetry noted. The type of hearing loss typically associated with a VS is sensorineural, with a potential sensory component due to changes in the cochlea itself or a strictly neural hearing loss from isolated auditory nerve impact. The pure-tone audiogram itself does not provide site-of-lesion information but can be used in conjunction with other testing measures to determine the status of the cochlea versus the auditory nerve, as described later. In 1977, Johnson classified a large cohort of patients with VS according to the patterns of hearing loss configuration: high frequency (66%), flat (13%), trough shape or mid frequency (12%), and low frequency (9%).[1] At least one subsequent large study confirmed similar percentages.[2]

7.2.2 Word Recognition Testing

Speech reception thresholds (SRT) are determined by having the patient repeat a familiar list of two-syllable words called spondees. The SRT is identified as the presentation level at which the subject correctly identifies 50% of the spondees presented. Word recognition testing is then performed at a "comfortable" listening level (usually between 35 and 50 dB above the SRT) using monosyllabic words. This test assesses the patient's ability to recognize and repeat an unfamiliar list of words utilizing audition alone (without lip reading). Patients with retrocochlear pathology often have poorer word recognition scores (WRS) than might be expected given the pure-tone thresholds and SRT in the affected ear.

7.2.3 Rollover

Patients with VS often demonstrate a positive rollover test, as defined by a decline in WRS as a function of increasingly louder presentation levels. A rollover index of 0.42 to 0.45 has been found to be suspicious for a retrocochlear lesion.[3,4] However, the sensitivity of the rollover test is generally regarded to be poor, considering that normal results can be obtained on a significant number of patients with confirmed VS. Still, a positive rollover test in conjunction with other abnormal findings (asymmetrical hearing loss and/or absent acoustic reflexes) strongly suggests that retrocochlear pathology may be present.

7.2.4 Acoustic Reflex Thresholds/Decay

Acoustic reflex thresholds are tested by recording the lowest level that a change in tympanic membrane (TM) compliance can be observed as the stapedius muscle contracts in response to a loud sound stimulus. A small contribution to the acoustic reflex threshold also comes from the tensor tympani muscle.[5,6] The afferent limb of the ipsilateral acoustic reflex travels via the auditory nerve to the cochlear nucleus and then to the superior olivary complex and the facial nerve nucleus in the pons, where the efferent limb via the facial nerve on the same side activates the stapedius muscle. This contracts, reducing mobility of the stapes and thus the entire ossicular chain, causing a measurable reduction in TM compliance recorded in the same ear. The contralateral acoustic reflex crosses to the superior olivary complex and facial nerve nucleus in the contralateral brainstem before traveling via the facial nerve to activate the stapedius muscle in the opposite ear. When a VS is present along the auditory nerve pathway, normal transmission of the afferent auditory signal to the brainstem is altered, either by compression or vascular disruption, often resulting in an elevated or absent acoustic reflex when the sound stimulus is presented to the affected ear even if there is excellent residual hearing. The ipsilateral reflex in the unaffected ear should not be impacted. Patients with VS may also demonstrate positive reflex decay, which means that the reflex cannot be sustained while a continuous tone is presented to the affected ear (typically 10 dB above the acoustic reflex threshold). When reflex decay is present, the reflex measured in the contralateral ear will rapidly decline to at least half of the initial compliance value. Studies have shown that abnormal acoustic reflexes have a sensitivity of only 75 to 82% for confirmed cases of VS, but a low specificity of only 11 to 30%.[1,7] The low sensitivity rate is due primarily to the very small prevalence of acoustic tumors in the population undergoing audiometric testing for hearing complaints. Thus, the significance of abnormal acoustic reflex testing should be interpreted only in conjunction with other auditory test measures.

7.3 Electrophysiology

7.3.1 Auditory Brainstem Response

Auditory brainstem response (ABR) evaluations can provide information about the integrity of the auditory pathway as afferent signals travel to the brainstem. Studies have shown that the sensitivity of the ABR in diagnosing VS is between 85 and 95%. The sensitivity rate for small tumors remains somewhat controversial, with reported values ranging from 58 to 92% for tumors measuring less than 1 cm.[8,9,10] For tumors less than 1 cm, Don et al advocated use of the stacked ABR, which utilizes a derived-band technique by recording click responses in the presence of high-pass masking filters of various cutoff frequencies and then subtracting each response from subsequent runs. Their study showed a sensitivity of 95% and a specificity of 88% for small VS. Though not widely adopted, additional studies replicating this work may lead to more widespread use of the stacked ABR technique for screening purposes.[11]

During a diagnostic evaluation for asymmetrical auditory symptoms such as hearing loss, tinnitus, perceived distortion of sound, or aural fullness, an ABR may be requested to screen for retrocochlear pathology. The neurodiagnostic ABR is performed while the patient lies quietly with eyes closed, or even more optimally, in a state of natural sleep. It is a far-field recording, with surface electrodes positioned on either the forehead or the vertex and at the level of the ear (either on the mastoid, earlobe, or anterior to the tragus). A loud click stimulus is delivered to the ears monaurally via insert earphones at 80 to 95 dB HL at a moderate rate of 20 to 30 clicks per second. This stimulus represents information mainly from the basilar (high-frequency) portion of the cochlea. Free-running EEG and EMG are monitored throughout the recording, which is ideally paused whenever large muscle artifact is present due to patient movement, swallowing, or tensing of the jaw. These artifactual EMG signals can obliterate the much smaller EEG response from the auditory pathway. Averaged EEG information collected within the first 10 ms after the onset of each stimulus is analyzed for delays in the evoked waves related to the auditory pathway and/or gross deviation from the anticipated response morphology. Five peaks are identified in a normal ABR waveform and are currently believed to originate from the following neural generators:

- Wave I—compound auditory nerve action potential in the distal portion of cranial nerve VIII.
- Wave II—proximal portion of cranial nerve VIII.
- Wave III—cochlear nucleus.
- Wave IV—superior olivary complex.
- Wave V—lateral lemniscus/inferior colliculus; the most robust wave of the ABR.

The morphology of the ABR is qualitatively analyzed for the presence or absence of waveform components, as well as for their reproducibility. Timing characteristics, such as absolute and interpeak wave latencies, are analyzed within and between ears. Significant findings include prolonged Wave I–III, III–V, or I–V interpeak latencies, delayed absolute latency of Wave V, or a significant interaural difference between ears for any of these parameters. The presence of a tumor within the internal auditory canal or cerebellopontine angle can affect the timing relationship of the ABR in the affected ear or cause a complete absence of synchronized neural activity. See ▶ Fig. 7.1 for an example of an ABR recording.

The person's hearing status as measured via conventional pure-tone audiometry may not correlate with the ABR response in the predicted fashion. For example, a person may have completely normal hearing thresholds but demonstrate an abnormal or even absent ABR. Likewise, a person with moderate hearing loss and a tumor of large size may still have a measurable ABR. When discussing management options for tumors, knowing the ABR status of the patient is sometimes helpful. When surgical intervention for hearing preservation is considered, patients with normal ABRs are likely to have better outcomes.[9] The ABR also provides a baseline for intraoperative neurophysiologic monitoring of auditory nerve function during resection of cerebellopontine angle tumors via a middle cranial fossa or retrosigmoid approach. Currently, given the widespread access and very high sensitivity and specificity of

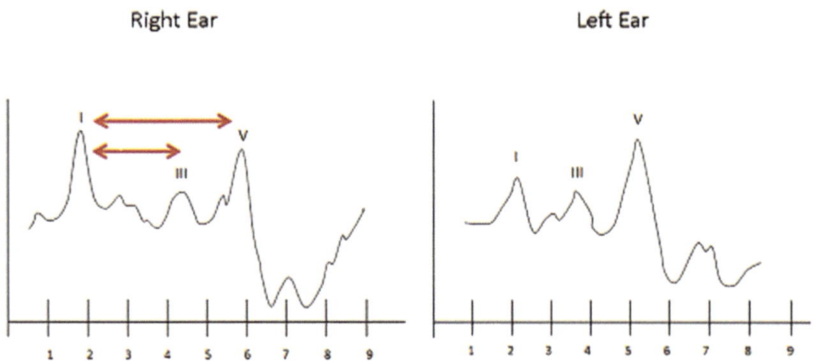

Fig. 7.1 Example of an auditory brainstem response (ABR) of a patient with a right vestibular schwannoma. Waveform morphology is excellent bilaterally; however, prolonged Wave I–III and I–V interpeak latencies are noted for the right ear. The left ABR is within normal limits.

gadolinium-enhanced MRI for detecting VS, ABR is no longer used at most centers in the United States as a diagnostic screening tool for VS. However, many centers still utilize preoperative and/or intraoperative ABR testing for cases where VS hearing preservation surgery is a consideration.

7.3.2 Electrocochleography

Electrocochleography (ECoG) may be performed if enhanced resolution of Wave I of the ABR is desired, as this wave corresponds to the action potential of the ECoG response. To measure ECoG, a TM surface electrode is placed deep within the patient's ear canal under microscopic visualization, with a soft tip positioned against the TM. An insert earphone is then placed into the ear canal to deliver click stimuli, and the responses are averaged in the same fashion as an ABR recording. ECoG is beneficial when there is some degree of cochlear hearing loss present because the TM electrode will detect a larger amplitude for Wave I (whole nerve action potential) due to its close proximity to the cochlear promontory. This modality may also enhance intraoperative monitoring of auditory nerve function in hearing preservation cases. If Wave I is not present or reliably repeatable on the far-field ABR recording, the enhanced resolution of the action potential measured with ECoG will allow feedback regarding cochlear function throughout tumor dissection and may help determine whether observed changes in the ABR are related to vascular versus neural injury.

7.3.3 Otoacoustic Emissions

Evoked otoacoustic emissions (OAEs) are often measured in conjunction with a neurodiagnostic ABR evaluation. OAEs originate from the outer hair cells and provide information regarding cochlear function. A probe tip, hermetically sealed in the patient's lateral ear canal, delivers sound stimuli (two tones of different frequency for distortion product OAEs, or a click stimulus for transient evoked OAEs). The probe includes a microphone that, in a normally conducting ear, records sound waves that result from the oscillatory movement of the TM driven by the cochlea through the middle ear.[12] If a patient with a VS has significant hearing loss that is purely neural due to brainstem and/or cochlear nerve compression, OAEs may be intact, reflecting healthy cochlear function with good vascular supply to the cochlea. This has been shown to be a favorable prognostic indicator for hearing preservation when surgical intervention is considered.[13]

7.4 Vestibular Testing

Patients with VS rarely experience intense vertigo, but may complain of imbalance, motion-provoked dizziness, or oscillopsia (the inability to maintain clear vision with head movement) due to an impairment of the vestibulo-ocular reflex (VOR). Various portions of the balance function testing battery can identify abnormalities associated with VS. These tests may be performed prior to diagnosis if a patient reports dizziness or balance system complaints, or as part of a preoperative evaluation to establish baseline vestibular function.

7.4.1 Vestibular Evoked Myogenic Potentials

Vestibular evoked myogenic potential (VEMP) testing is an electrophysiological measure that can determine function of either the inferior or superior division of the vestibular nerve. VEMP responses may be elicited by a loud air-conduction acoustic stimulus, bone-conduction clicks, or mechanical taps to the patient's forehead. The cervical VEMP (cVEMP) is generated by the saccule, which is primarily innervated by the inferior division of the vestibular nerve. Responses can be recorded even if the audiogram demonstrates a profound hearing loss. The cVEMP is an inhibitory response that is typically measured by a recording electrode on the ipsilateral sternocleidomastoid muscle. The patient is instructed to maintain tonic muscle contraction while the stimulus is delivered. The threshold and amplitude of the evoked relaxation potential in the muscle is measured and compared with the opposite side. See ▶ Fig. 7.2 for an example of a cVEMP. The ocular VEMP (oVEMP) gives information about the status of the utricle and related afferents in the superior division of the vestibular nerve. It is measured by recording electrodes placed under the eyes of the patient, who is instructed to gaze upward during stimulus delivery. The response is measured from the inferior rectus muscle contralateral to the ear of stimulation. Abnormal oVEMP findings include responses that are significantly reduced in amplitude relative to the healthy ear or absent if the utricle is completely unresponsive. See ▶ Fig. 7.3 for an example of an oVEMP.

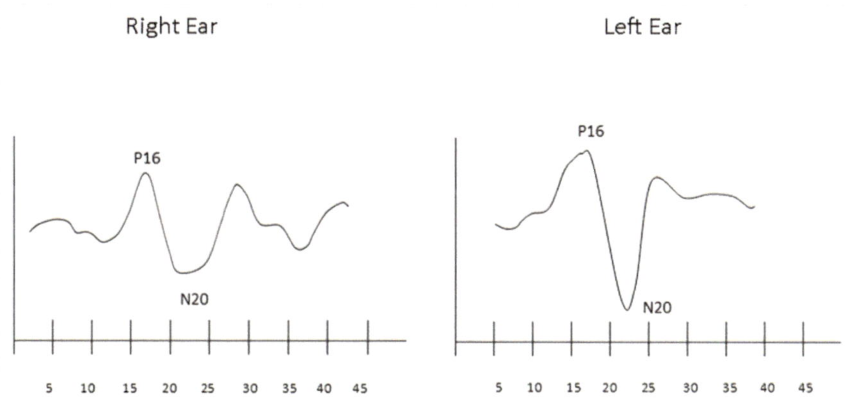

Fig. 7.2 Example of a cervical vestibular evoked myogenic potential (cVEMP) of a patient with a right vestibular schwannoma. Responses are obtained bilaterally; however, the amplitude of response obtained with right ear stimulation is significantly smaller than with left ear stimulation.

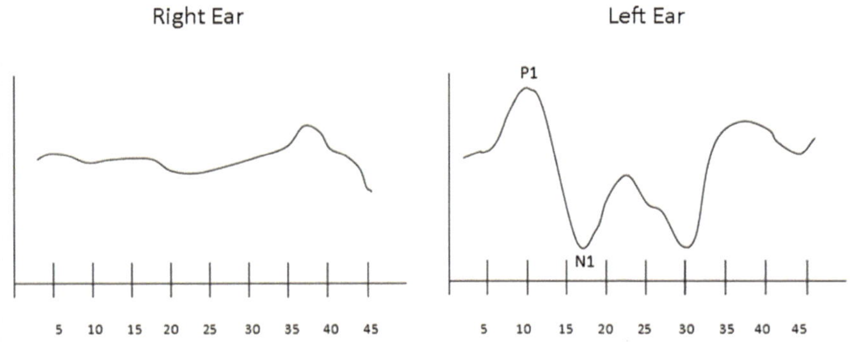

Fig. 7.3 Example of an ocular vestibular evoked myogenic potential (oVEMP) from a patient with a right vestibular schwannoma. A robust response is obtained with stimulation of the left ear, but the oVEMP is absent when the right ear is stimulated.

Several studies have demonstrated that VEMP responses may be absent or abnormal in patients with confirmed VS.[14,15,16] A study of 170 patients with VS demonstrated that 80% showed an abnormal cVEMP in the affected ear, which was consistent with other smaller studies.[14] VEMP is a useful part of the diagnostic battery, but detection of VS is difficult based on VEMP testing alone.[15] Preoperatively, patients may undergo cVEMP and oVEMP testing in an effort to separately evaluate the function of the inferior and superior vestibular nerves, though correlation of VEMP results with nerve of tumor origin remains controversial. One small study showed that cVEMP results coupled with the caloric test accurately predicted when the tumor either involved both branches of the nerve or the inferior branch only.[16] Another study showed no correlation between oVEMP, cVEMP, and caloric results relative to nerve of origin.[17] A third study showed inconsistent prediction of the nerve of origin, rendering predictions impossible based on preoperative VEMP studies alone.[18] To date, there is no consensus regarding the role of VEMP as a preoperative tool for identifying the nerve of tumor origin.

7.4.2 Videonystagmography

Videonystagmography (VNG) testing is performed utilizing video-oculography goggles and recording the corresponding eye movement tracings in both the horizontal and vertical planes. Abnormal eye movements (nystagmus) may be observed in patients with VS in several portions of the VNG test battery. Spontaneous and positional nystagmus may be present when the patient's eyes are observed in darkness in various positions while sitting and lying down. Typically, when it is present in patients with VS, the observed nystagmus is significantly suppressed with visual fixation, indicating peripheral vestibular system involvement. Transient evoked nystagmus might be observed immediately following a passive head shake in either the horizontal or vertical plane as the examiner stresses the VOR. When VOR impairment is present, the direction of the fast phase of the nystagmus during spontaneous and/or post head shake testing indicates whether the lesion is in a paretic (fast phase beating away from the affected ear) or irritative status (fast phase beating toward the affected ear). Gaze testing is performed by having the patient fixate on a target centered in front of them or offset in the horizontal or vertical plane. Patients with large VS greater than 3.5 cm may exhibit Bruns' gaze nystagmus, where fine, low-grade nystagmus is seen when gaze is directed to the side of the healthy ear (vestibular origin) and large amplitude nystagmus is seen when gaze is directed to the side of the affected ear (central origin due to cerebellar compression).[19] Hyperventilation-induced nystagmus may be observed in patients with VS. This is believed to be due to a transient improvement in the axonal conduction along a partially demyelinated vestibular afferent pathway due to the reduction of extracellular calcium resulting from hyperventilation.[20] Studies have shown that 58 to 82% of patients with confirmed VS demonstrate hyperventilation-induced nystagmus compared with 18 to 34% of patients with unilateral vestibular system involvement of other causes.[20,21] The bithermal caloric test evaluates function of the horizontal semicircular canal and the corresponding vestibular afferent fibers within the superior vestibular nerve in response to warm (44 °C) and cool (30 °C) stimulation. Irrigations may be performed utilizing air or water as the caloric stimulus. The peak slow component eye velocity is recorded for each irrigation and an inter-ear calculation is performed to determine whether a significant asymmetry is present. Several studies have evaluated the prevalence of caloric weakness in VS patients, with results ranging from 66 to 94% in this population.[22,23,24,25] Dynamic visual acuity testing can evaluate for oscillopsia by comparing the patient's ability to read from a Snellen eye chart, comparing acuity measured both at rest and during passive head rotation. Since the VOR is responsible for stabilizing the eyes during head movement, visual blurring may occur during head rotation as a result of retinal slip when a deficit is present. This is more common in the setting of bilateral vestibulopathy, but can be seen in unilateral pathology on occasion. If dynamic vision deteriorates to more than a two-line difference compared to static testing, the test is considered positive for oscillopsia.

When a patient with a VS demonstrates a unilateral weakness on caloric testing, the remainder of the VNG evaluation can give information about the compensation status of the lesion. For example, if abnormal eye movements are noted in the form of spontaneous, positional, and/or post–head shaking nystagmus, the lesion is considered to be uncompensated from a physiological perspective. As VSs are typically slow growing, many patients with normal central nervous system function are able to compensate for the weakening peripheral input as the tumor grows, and consequently few will report dizziness or balance difficulties. The amount of caloric asymmetry that is present preoperatively is an important point to discuss with the patient, as those that retain normal or only mildly asymmetrical function will most likely experience severe vertigo immediately following surgical resection of the tumor. Regardless of their preoperative status, most patients will benefit from evaluation and treatment by a physical therapist or other professional experienced in vestibular rehabilitation. Preoperative counseling and postoperative supervision will assist them in learning and implementing postoperative gaze stabilization and balance exercises, optimizing their eventual recovery.

7.4.3 Rotary Chair

Rotational testing may be performed in addition to VNG to assess a wider frequency range of VOR function and will help determine the level of physiological compensation. During sinusoidal testing, the patient sits upright with their head tilted slightly forward to place the horizontal semicircular canal at a 90-degree angle relative to the earth–vertical axis of rotation. Both horizontal semicircular canals are simultaneously stimulated as the chair rotates in a sinusoidal pattern with a peak velocity of 50 to 60 degrees per second, generating physiologic nystagmus. Various parameters of the nystagmus are analyzed across the frequency range including VOR gain, phase, and symmetry. When a unilateral weakness is measured on caloric testing (assuming normal function in the healthy ear), patients will typically demonstrate evidence of increased phase leads with normal VOR gain. If the lesion appears in a physiologically uncompensated state, slow component eye velocity asymmetries may be measured with slower eye speeds noted during rotation to the affected side, although symmetry values may be normal if the person is adequately compensated. The rotational step test is performed by rapidly accelerating the patient, which deflects the cupula and generates a brisk nystagmus, and then maintaining a constant rotational velocity to allow the nystagmus to decay as the cupula returns to its resting position. The patient is then abruptly decelerated to a stop, causing a reversal of endolymph flow and another burst of nystagmus that beats in the opposite direction. Rotational steps are performed for both clockwise and counter-clockwise rotations. The amount of time it takes for the nystagmus to exponentially decay during each step is used to calculate the vestibular time constant. Patients with VS may demonstrate asymmetrically short time constants on the rotational step test.

7.4.4 Computerized Dynamic Posturography

The sensory organization test (SOT) is performed by measuring the patient's postural sway in the anteroposterior plane throughout various conditions utilizing visual, vestibular, and somatosensory inputs in various combinations. The six test conditions evaluate the three input domains with reference to the patient's postural sway and can isolate performance dysfunction patterns. For example, a person with a unilateral weakness will typically demonstrate increased sway or fall reactions when forced to rely on vestibular system inputs alone. This indicates that the patient's vestibular paresis is uncompensated from a functional perspective. The SOT demonstrates high test–retest reliability[26] and may be used to identify patients who would particularly benefit from an evaluation by a vestibular physical therapist.

7.5 Conclusion

The completion of various audiometric, electrophysiologic, and vestibular evaluations can highlight abnormalities that may be associated with the diagnosis of VS. It is not possible for any single test of auditory or vestibular function to definitively predict the presence of a VS. Rather, a combination of abnormal results in the audiovestibular test battery has greater reliability in raising suspicion for retrocochlear pathology. Evaluation of baseline function can be beneficial not only to offer an explanation of symptoms but also to help guide discussions regarding management options for treating the tumor, preoperative counseling, and to identify patients who are candidates for auditory and vestibular rehabilitation.

References

[1] Johnson EW. Auditory test results in 500 cases of acoustic neuroma. Arch Otolaryngol. 1977; 103(3):152–158

[2] Gordon ML, Cohen NL. Efficacy of auditory brainstem response as a screening test for small acoustic neuromas. Am J Otol. 1995; 16(2):136–139

[3] Jerger J, Jerger S. Diagnostic significance of PB word functions. Arch Otolaryngol. 1971; 93(6):573–580

[4] Dirks DD, Kamm C, Bower D, Betsworth A. Use of performance-intensity functions for diagnosis. J Speech Hear Disord. 1977; 42(3):408–415

[5] Ochi K, Ohashi T, Kinoshita H. Acoustic tensor tympani response and vestibular-evoked myogenic potential. Laryngoscope. 2002; 112(12):2225–2229

[6] Mukerji S, Windsor AM, Lee DJ. Auditory brainstem circuits that mediate the middle ear muscle reflex. Trends Amplif. 2010; 14(3):170–191

[7] Kotlarz JP, Eby TL, Borton TE. Analysis of the efficiency of retrocochlear screening. Laryngoscope. 1992; 102(10):1108–1112

[8] El-Kashlan HK, Eisenmann D, Kileny PR. Auditory brain stem response in small acoustic neuromas. Ear Hear. 2000; 21(3):257–262

[9] Wilson DF, Hodgson RS, Gustafson MF, Hogue S, Mills L. The sensitivity of auditory brainstem response testing in small acoustic neuromas. Laryngoscope. 1992; 102(9):961–964

[10] Schmidt RJ, Sataloff RT, Newman J, Spiegel JR, Myers DL. The sensitivity of auditory brainstem response testing for the diagnosis of acoustic neuromas. Arch Otolaryngol Head Neck Surg. 2001; 127(1):19–22

[11] Don M, Kwong B, Tanaka C, Brackmann D, Nelson R. The stacked ABR: a sensitive and specific screening tool for detecting small acoustic tumors. Audiol Neurootol. 2005; 10(5):274–290

[12] Kemp DT, Brown AM. An integrated view of the cochlear mechanical nonlinearities observable in the ear canal. In: DeBoer E, Viergever MA, eds. Mechanics of Hearing. The Netherlands: The Hague; 1983:75–82

[13] Kim AH, Edwards BM, Telian SA, Kileny PR, Arts HA. Transient evoked otoacoustic emissions pattern as a prognostic indicator for hearing preservation in acoustic neuroma surgery. Otol Neurotol. 2006; 27(3):372–379

[14] Patko T, Vidal PP, Vibert N, Tran Ba Huy P, de Waele C, de Waele C. Vestibular evoked myogenic potentials in patients suffering from an unilateral acoustic neuroma: a study of 170 patients. Clin Neurophysiol. 2003; 114(7):1344–1350

[15] Takeichi N, Sakamoto T, Fukuda S, Inuyama Y. Vestibular evoked myogenic potential (VEMP) in patients with acoustic neuromas. Auris Nasus Larynx. 2001; 28(1) Suppl:S39–S41

[16] Chen CW, Young YH, Tseng HM. Preoperative versus postoperative role of vestibular-evoked myogenic potentials in cerebellopontine angle tumor. Laryngoscope. 2002; 112(2):267–271

[17] Iwasaki S, Murofushi T, Chihara Y, et al. Ocular vestibular evoked myogenic potentials to bone-conducted vibration in vestibular schwannomas. Otol Neurotol. 2010; 31(1):147–152

[18] Tsutsumi T, Tsunoda A, Noguchi Y, Komatsuzaki A. Prediction of the nerves of origin of vestibular schwannomas with vestibular evoked myogenic potentials. Am J Otol. 2000; 21(5):712–715

[19] Lloyd SK, Baguley DM, Butler K, Donnelly N, Moffat DA. Bruns' nystagmus in patients with vestibular schwannoma. Otol Neurotol. 2009; 30(5):625–628

[20] Choi KD, Kim JS, Kim HJ, et al. Hyperventilation-induced nystagmus in peripheral vestibulopathy and cerebellopontine angle tumor. Neurology. 2007; 69(10):1050–1059

[21] Robichaud J, DesRoches H, Bance M. Is hyperventilation-induced nystagmus more common in retrocochlear vestibular disease than in end-organ vestibular disease? J Otolaryngol. 2002; 31(3):140–143
[22] Tringali S, Charpiot A, Ould MB, Dubreuil C, Ferber-Viart C. Characteristics of 629 vestibular schwannomas according to preoperative caloric responses. Otol Neurotol. 2010; 31(3):467–472
[23] Fisch U, Wegmüller A. Early diagnosis of acoustic neuromas. ORL J Otorhinolaryngol Relat Spec. 1974; 36(3):129–140
[24] Okada Y, Takahashi M, Saito A, Kanzaki J. Electronystagmographic findings in 147 patients with acoustic neuroma. Acta Otolaryngol Suppl. 1991; 487 (487):150–156
[25] Kentala E, Pyykkö I. Clinical picture of vestibular schwannoma. Auris Nasus Larynx. 2001; 28(1):15–22
[26] Ford-Smith CD, Wyman JF, Elswick RK, Jr, Fernandez T, Newton RA. Test-retest reliability of the sensory organization test in noninstitutionalized older adults. Arch Phys Med Rehabil. 1995; 76(1):77–81

8 Diagnostic Imaging of Sporadic Vestibular Schwannoma and Other CPA Lesions

John I. Lane

8.1 Imaging Technique

Imaging of the internal auditory canal (IAC), cerebellopontine angle (CPA), and labyrinthine structures is most often performed as a screening study to exclude vestibular schwannoma (VS) in the patient presenting with asymmetric sensorineural hearing loss (SNHL) or as part of a "watch and wait" strategy in following up patients with previously diagnosed schwannomas. Magnetic resonance (MR) has replaced computed tomography (CT) as the primary imaging modality of choice. Diagnostic examinations can be obtained at either 3T or 1.5T. The higher field strength available at 3T offers the ability to achieve higher resolution images at shorter acquisition times. Disadvantages of 3T including increased susceptibility artifact at air–bone interfaces and increased banding artifact with use of 3D gradient echo (GRE) sequences (Fast Imaging Employing Steady-state Acquisition [FIESTA], Constructive Interference in the Steady State [CISS]) should be considered when deciding between these two commonly available MR platforms. The current preference at our institution is to scan at 3T using imaging sequences that eliminate or significantly reduce higher field strength artifacts (e.g., replacing the more commonly employed 3D GRE sequence with 3D fast spin echo [FSE] sequence). Improved image resolution can also be maximized with the use of multichannel coils, such as a 32- or 64-channel head coil depending on the available 3T platform.

Selection of imaging sequences is critical in achieving maximal image resolution. At the author's center, the current protocol utilizes higher resolution submillimeter 3D acquisitions with isotropic voxel sizes (Table 8-1). These sequences permit multiplanar reconstructions (▶ Fig. 8.1A–F), replacing the previously employed 3- to 4-mm 2D sequences that required separate planes of acquisition.

T2-weighted MR cisternography performed at small fields of view (FOV) to include 3D FSE T2 or 3D GRE (or T2*) acquisitions have become the standard of care when imaging the IAC. At 3T, 3D FSE offers distinct advantages over 3D GRE. Specifically, 3D FSE produces less susceptibility artifact at the skull base compared to 3D GRE and has the added advantage of eliminating problems with banding artifact inherent to 3D GRE imaging[1] (▶ Fig. 8.2). Image blurring, a consequence of the long-echo trains employed with high-resolution 3D FSE techniques, can be minimized by employing variable flip angle acquisitions.[2] Our protocol also includes a 3D fluid-attenuated inversion recovery (FLAIR) sequence to assess for any change in labyrinthine fluid signal not detectible on the T2 cisternogram sequences (▶ Fig. 8.1D).

To date, utilization of T1-weighted 3D sequences when imaging the IAC has not been as widely accepted compared to their 2D counterparts but are gaining in popularity because of the superior image resolution and multiplanar reformatting capability available with 3D acquisitions. 3D T1-weighted images can be produced using FSE or GRE sequencing. T1-weighted 3D GRE images differ slightly in appearance from T1-weighted 3D FSE in that flow-related enhancement is noted within the major vascular structures (i.e., adjacent internal carotid arteries) on 3D GRE (▶ Fig. 8.3A). 3D T1 FSE also provides better resolution of the fluid-filled labyrinthine structures against the background of dense labyrinthine bone than 3D T1 GRE (▶ Fig. 8.3B).

All 3D sequences, if acquired at isometric voxel size, allow for multiplanar reconstructions obviating the need for additional planes of acquisition. 3D sequences are more sensitive to motion artifact due to longer imaging times when compared to 2D sequences and therefore the patient's ability to remain still during image acquisition needs to be taken into account when protocoling the study.

The use of contrast in the imaging evaluation of VS has been considered standard practice and continues to be part of the routine examination in most centers. We routinely employ fat saturation on the postcontrast sequences to increase the conspicuity of pathologic contrast enhancement, particularly following fat graft placement, and eliminate the possibility of confusing enhancement with hyperintense marrow fat around the porus acusticus and within the petrous apex. Because of the

Table 8.1 3T protocol for IAC/CPA MR imaging

	Sag T1 FLAIR	Ax T2 FLAIR FS	Ax T2 FS	Ax SPACE T2	Ax SPACE T1	Gad Ax T1 FS SPACE	Gad Ax SPACE T2 FLAIR
TR (ms)	1,900	9,000	4,010	1,500	700	700	5,000
TE (ms)	9	135	99	202	32	32	358
FOV (mm)	240	220	220	150	150	150	150
Data matrix	224 × 320	224 × 320	269 × 384	320 × 320	192 × 192	192 × 192	192 × 256
Number of averages	1	1	2	1.4	1.7	1.7	2
Flip angle (degree)	–	180	150	140	–	–	–
Bandwidth (Hz)	260	289	260	651	651	651	488
Voxel size (mm^3)	00.8 × 0.8 × 5.0	0.7 × 0.7 × 4.0	0.6 × 0.6 × 4.0	0.2 × 0.2 × 0.5	0.4 × 0.4 × 0.8	0.4 × 0.4 × 0.8	0.3 × 0.3 × 1.2
Scan duration (min)	1:58	4:32	2:34	6:33	5:33	5:33	6:27

Abbreviations: TR, time to refocusing pulse; TE, time to echo; FOV, field of view; SPACE, sampling perfection with application optimized contrasts using different flip angle evolution; FLAIR, fluid-attenuated inversion recovery.

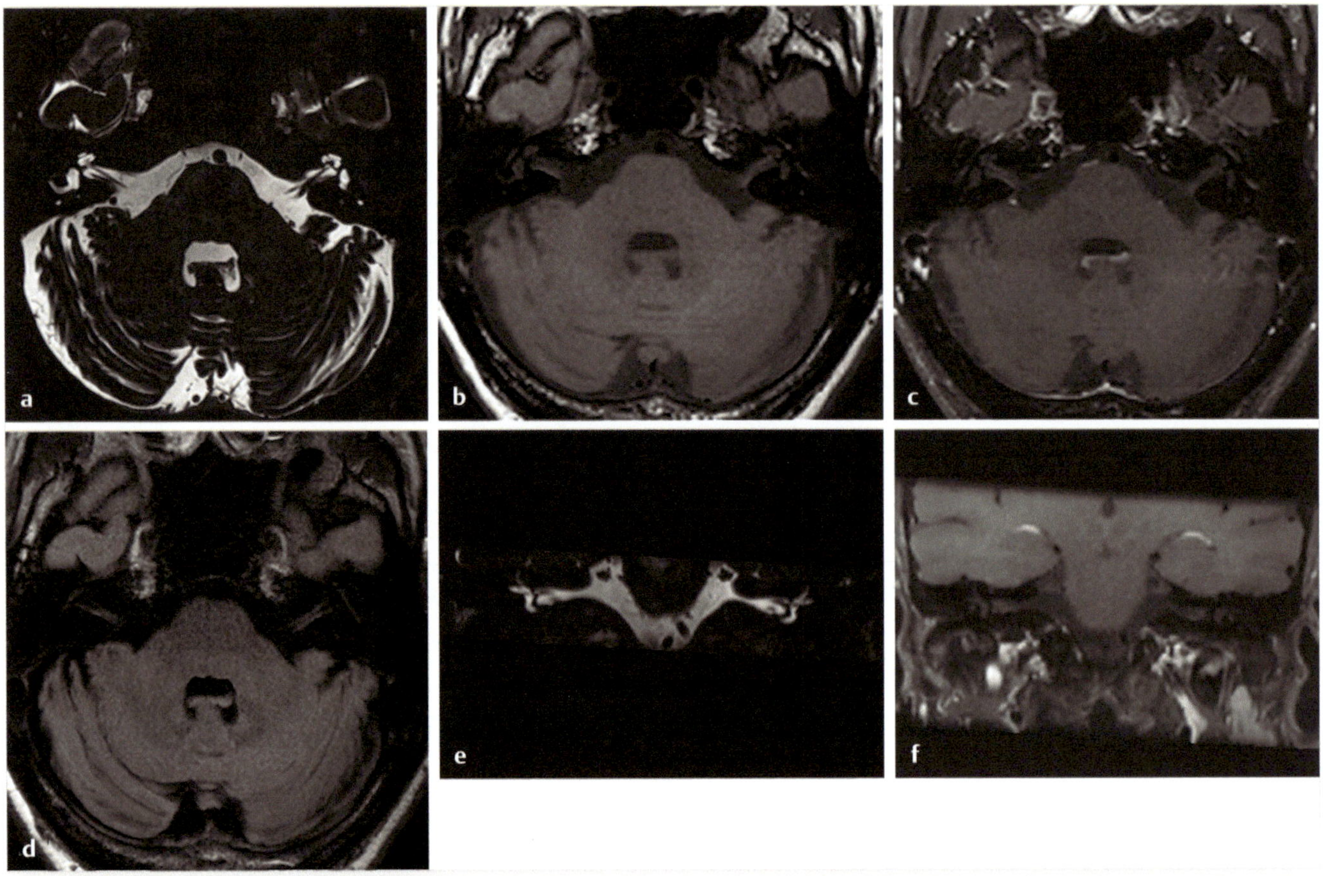

Fig. 8.1 Normal 3T IAC MR examination using 3D technique. (**a**) Axial T2-weighted 3D fast spin echo (FSE), (**b**) T1-weighted 3D FSE, (**c**) axial contrast-enhanced, fat-saturated T1-weighted 3D FSE, (**d**) axial 3D FLAIR. (**e** and **f**) Coronal reconstructions from axial T2- and T1-weighted FSE acquisitions, respectively.

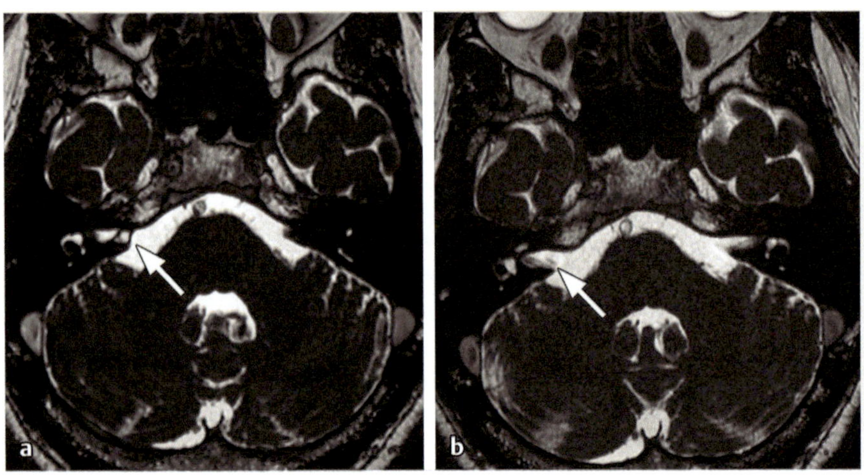

Fig. 8.2 3D T2-weighted MR imaging of the IAC. (**a**) 3D gradient echo (GRE) and (**b**) 3D fast spin echo (FSE) sequences at 3T employed to rule out IAC or CPA angle masses. Note banding artifact obscuring the right porus acusticus (*arrow*) which is widely patent on FSE sequence (*arrow*).

low diagnostic yield of adding contrast to the screening exam, some authors have advocated the use of noncontrast MR examinations, in an effort to reduce scan time and cost.[3,4] Recent studies have demonstrated that certain gadolinium chelate products are deposited in body tissues.[5,6,7] As a result of these studies and those demonstrating the low diagnostic yield of adding contrast to the examination, we may anticipate a future demand for noncontrast MR evaluations at least until more pharmacologically stable contrast agents become available. MR angiography and MR venography can be added to the imaging protocol to exclude vascular lesions of the IAC and CPA.

8.2 Anatomic Variants

Variations in the anatomy of the temporal bone may have important implications for avoiding surgical complications

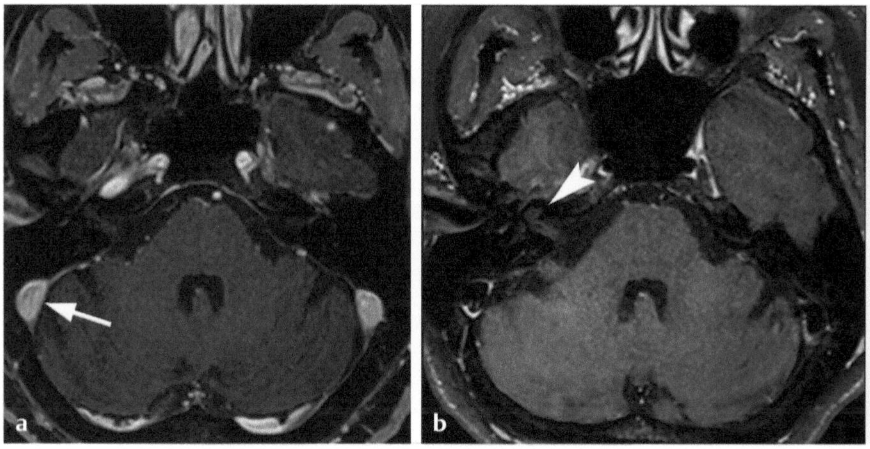

Fig. 8.3 3D T2-weighted MR imaging of the IAC. (**a**) Axial 3D GRE-based and (**b**) axial 3D FSE-based fat-saturated contrast-enhanced imaging. Note potentially distracting flow-related enhancement within adjacent vascular structures with 3D GRE technique (*arrow*) and improved conspicuity of labyrinthine structures on 3D FSE image (*arrowhead*).

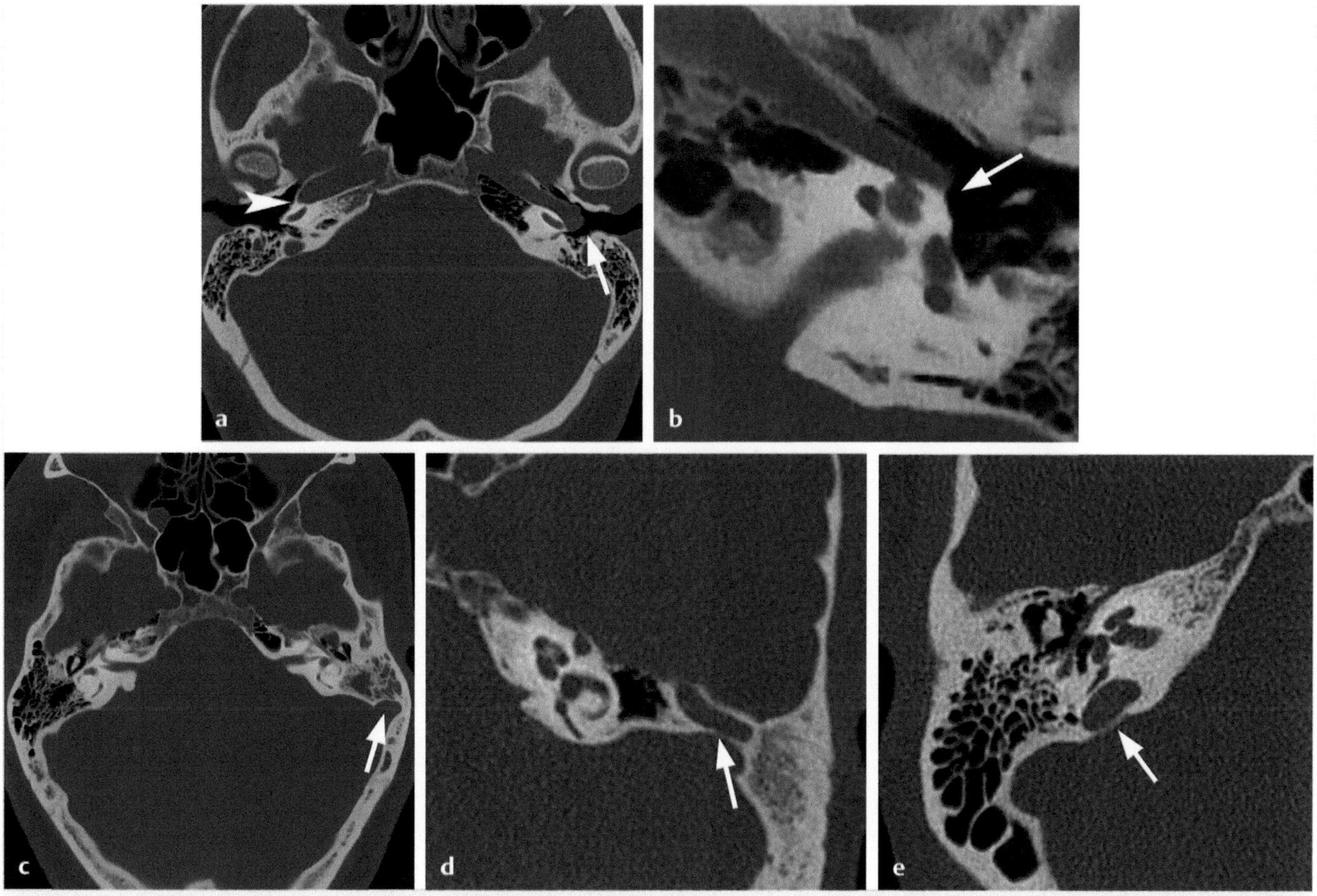

Fig. 8.4 Vascular anatomic variants of the temporal bone. Axial CTs of the temporal bone. (**a**) Aberrant ICA on the left (*arrow*). Note the position of normal contralateral carotid canal relative to cochlear promontory (*arrowhead*). (**b**) Lateralized ICA on the left (*arrow*). (**c**) Left anterior sigmoid sinus (*arrow*). (**d**) Prominent emissary vein adjacent to the tegmen. (**e**) High-riding jugular bulb on right (*arrow*).

during VS resection. Most of these variants are best delineated with high-resolution multidetector or cone beam CT. Vascular variants would include anterior sigmoid sinus, high jugular bulb, unusual emissary veins of the temporal bone, and aberrant or lateralized internal carotid artery (▶ Fig. 8.4). An anterior sigmoid sinus can be recognized when this structure is anteriorly displaced into the mastoid cavity, thereby restricting transmastoid access even with extensive decompression and placing it at risk for injury.[8] Variable pneumatization of the petrous portion of the temporal bone to include the margins of the IAC may predispose to postoperative cerebrospinal fluid (CSF) leaks if care is not taken to recognize these variants preoperatively and carefully seal off these air cells during surgery. Retained secretion within these air cells may produce the appearance of enhancing "pseudolesions" on MR and, if necessary, may be confirmed with temporal bone CT (▶ Fig. 8.5).

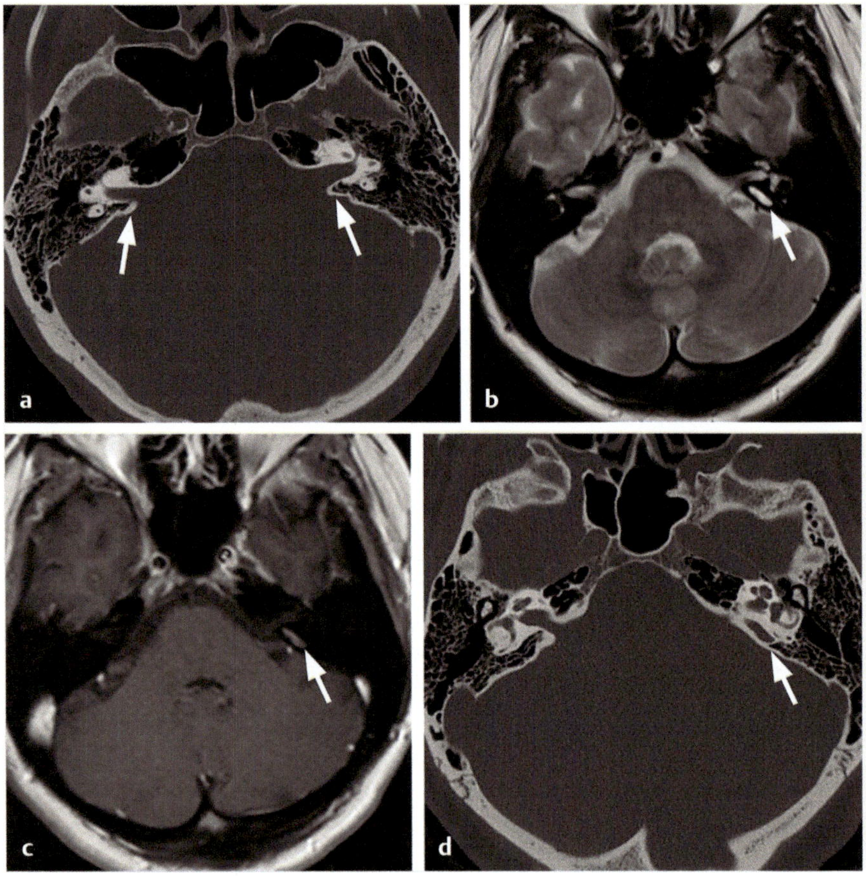

Fig. 8.5 Variations in temporal bone pneumatization. (**a**) Axial CT demonstrating pneumatization adjacent to the porus acusticus (*arrows*). (**a–c**) Axial T2 and postcontrast T1-weighted images, respectively, demonstrated T2 hyperintense, contrast-enhancing "pseudolesion" easily recognized as a fluid-filled air cell on **d**, axial CT (*arrow*).

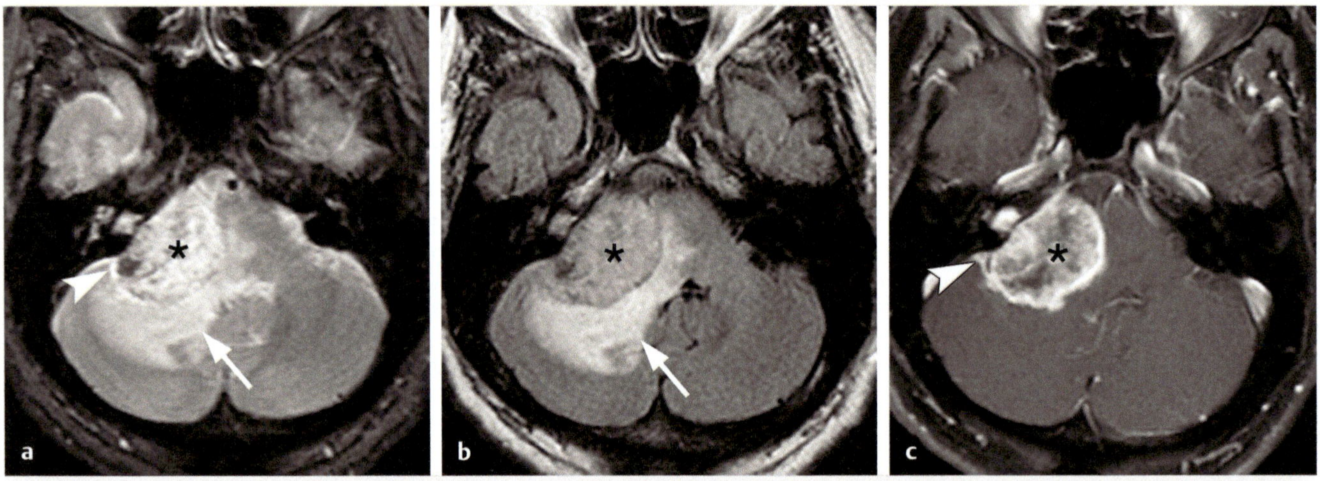

Fig. 8.6 Large vestibular schwannoma. (**a, b**) Axial T2 and FLAIR images, respectively, demonstrating characteristic inhomogeneous signal within the large CPA mass (*asterisk*) with brainstem compression and intra-axial edema (*arrow*). (**c**) Axial T1 demonstrating inhomogeneous pattern of enhancement (*asterisk*). Note CPA component of the tumor centered on the IAC and acute dural angles typical of vestibular schwannoma (*arrowhead*).

8.3 Differential Diagnosis of Cerebellopontine Angle and Internal Auditory Canal Lesions

Vestibular schwannoma is the most commonly encountered mass within the CPA cistern. When small, these lesions are isolated to the IAC but as they increase in size, they will protrude into the adjacent CPA cistern. The CPA component is centered at the porus acusticus and will usually form acute angles with the adjacent dural surface (▶ Fig. 8.6), a useful feature when considering meningioma in the differential diagnosis as CPA meningioma will typically be located eccentric to the porus and form obtuse dural angles. It is important to note the degree

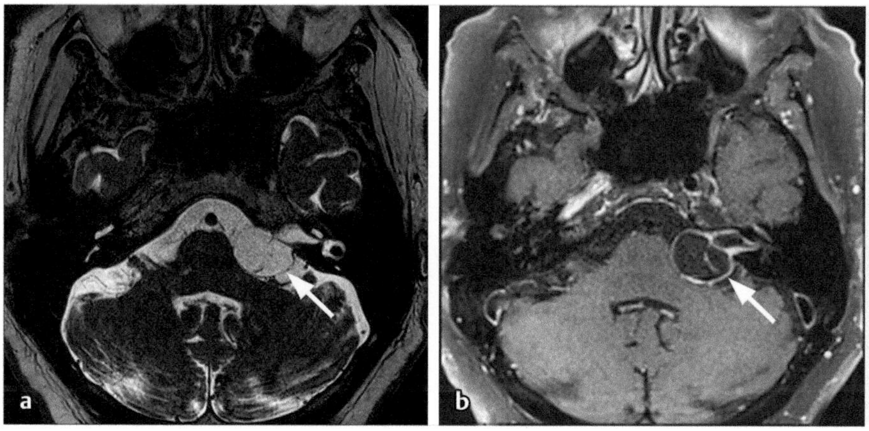

Fig. 8.7 Cystic vestibular schwannoma. (**a**) T2 axial image demonstrating predominately cystic schwannoma in the left CPA cistern with intracanalicular extension (*arrow*). (**b**) Fat-saturated contrast-enhanced T1 image demonstrates peripheral enhancement of peripheral soft-tissue capsule and internal septa (*arrow*).

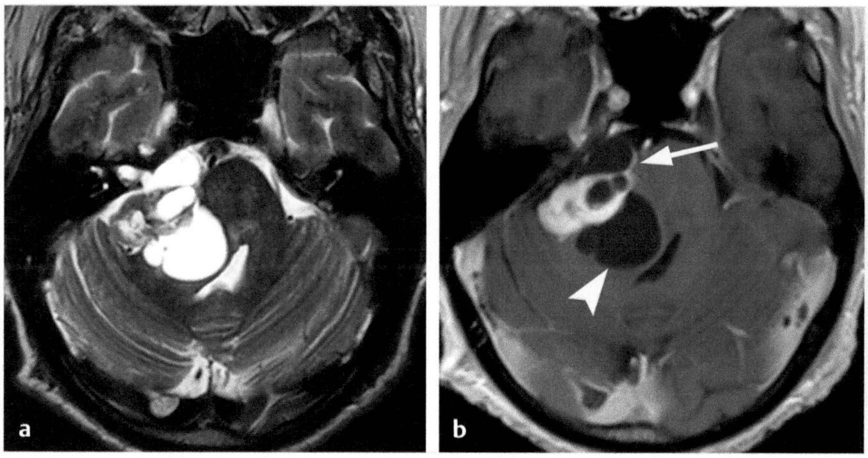

Fig. 8.8 Cystic vestibular schwannoma with dominant peritumoral arachnoid cyst. (**a**) T2-weighted axial image demonstrates cystic schwannoma occupying the right CPA cistern. (**b**) Contrast-enhanced T1-weighted axial image distinguishes peripherally enhancing intratumoral cysts (*arrow*) from nonenhancing peritumoral arachnoid cyst (*arrowhead*).

of lateral extension of the lesion into the fundus as this may have implications for the choice of surgical approach and probability of successful hearing preservation. Large lesions will usually demonstrate inhomogeneous T2 signal and enhancement (▶ Fig. 8.6), in contradistinction to meningiomas, characterized by their homogenous features. VS characterized by increased T2 signal has been correlated with softer, more easily "suckable" tumors with a tendency toward better facial nerve outcomes when compared to T2 hypointense tumors.[9] VS also typically enhances in an inhomogeneous fashion compared to meningiomas, which are characterized by a homogenous pattern of enhancement.

VSs are more often solid but cystic components are not uncommon particularly with larger lesions. The presence of intratumoral cysts within a large tumor may portend faster growth, and more difficult surgical resection with regard to facial nerve outcome.[10,11] Rarely, these tumors may be predominately cystic (▶ Fig. 8.7). Occasionally, VS may incite an inflammatory response within the adjacent arachnoid with the development of peritumoral cysts (▶ Fig. 8.8). The peripheral location and lack of enhancement of the cyst wall are features that can be useful in differentiating a peritumoral cyst from a cystic component of the primary tumor.

Demonstrating the nerve of origin may be possible with smaller intracanalicular lesions, an observation that may have prognostic significance if surgery is considered. Likewise, the presence of fluid within the fundus of the IAC ("fundal cap") lateral to the tumor may portend a better outcome regarding hearing preservation following a middle cranial fossa or retrosigmoid resection.[12,13] Alteration of the normal fluid signal within the ipsilateral labyrinth and fundus on T2 and FLAIR sequences is often associated with tumors obstructing the IAC (decreased signal on 3D GRE and increased signal on 3D FLAIR; ▶ Fig. 8.9). This finding has been ascribed to pathologically increased levels of protein related to the IAC obstruction. These signal changes have been correlated with increased SNHL compared to tumors of similar size without labyrinthine/fundal fluid signal changes.[14]

Large tumors which compress the brainstem and cerebellum may demonstrate peritumoral intra-axial edema (▶ Fig. 8.6), a finding usually indicative of increased tumor vascularity and associated with an increased risk of brainstem adherence and hemorrhagic complications at surgery.[15]

Intralabyrinthine extension of tumor can rarely be associated with intracanalicular tumors and is more often seen in patients with neurofibromatosis type II. Extension may be observed into the cochlea through the modiolus (transmodiolar extension) or into the vestibular (transmacular extension) and can be appreciated as filling defects within the labyrinthine fluid on T2 cisternogram images or as focal intralabyrinthine enhancement on the postcontrast images (▶ Fig. 8.10). Intralabyrinthine tumors may also rarely occur as primary inner ear schwannomas without intracanalicular components (▶ Fig. 8.11). Use of higher resolution techniques has led to an increase in diagnosis

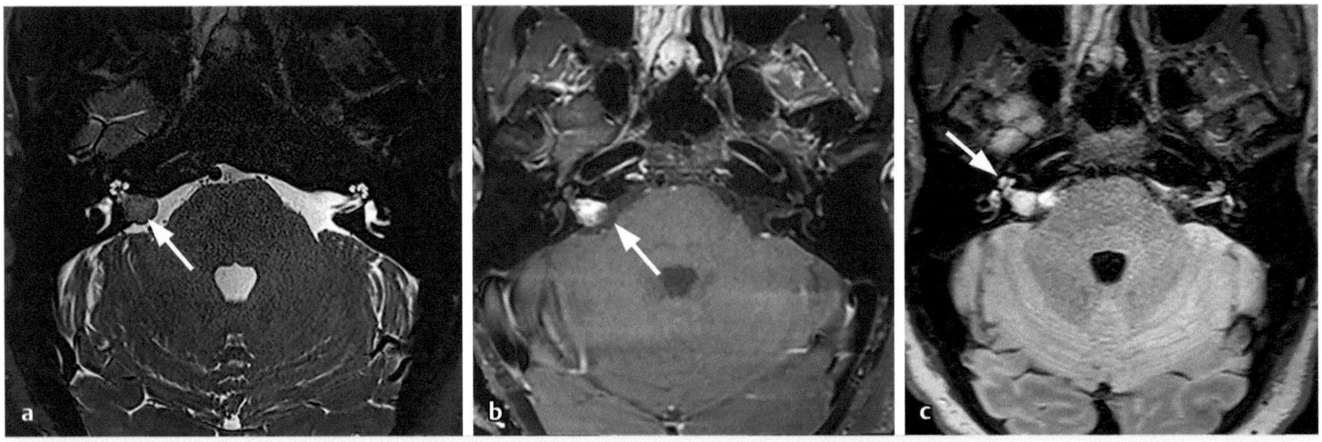

Fig. 8.9 Vestibular schwannoma with altered labyrinthine fluid signal. (**a**) 3D T2-weighted and (**b**) fat-saturated contrast-enhanced 3D T1-weighted axial images demonstrating intracanalicular schwannoma in the right internal auditory canal with slight protrusion into the cerebellopontine angle cistern (*arrow*). Note moderately inhomogeneous pattern of contrast enhancement. (**c**) 3D FLAIR demonstrates increased signal within the right cochlea and vestibule compared to contralateral inner ear indicative of increased protein content within the labyrinthine fluid (*arrow*).

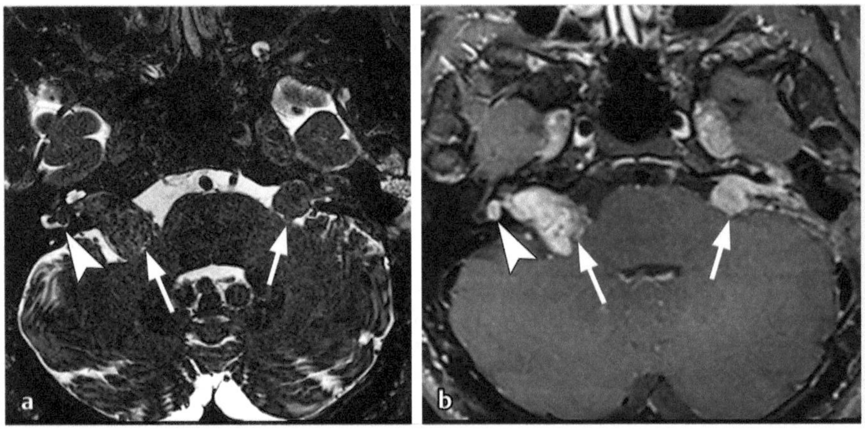

Fig. 8.10 Bilateral vestibular schwannomas in NF2 with intralabyrinthine extension on the right. (**a**) Axial T2-weighted image demonstrates bilateral CPA tumors (*arrows*) with replacement of normal fluid signal in the vestibule of the inner ear on the right. (**b**) Axial fat-saturated contrast-enhanced T1 image demonstrating bilateral CPA (*arrows*) and right intralabyrinthine schwannomas (*arrowhead*).

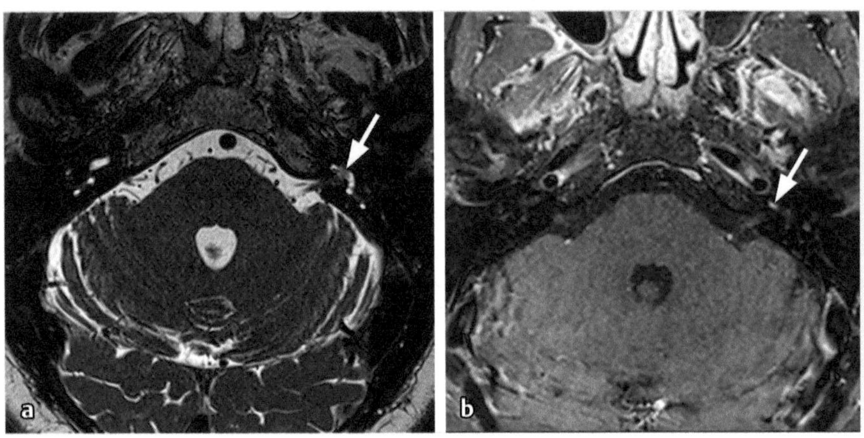

Fig. 8.11 Intralabyrinthine Schwannoma. (**a**) Axial T2-weighted image demonstrates a filling defect in the normal fluid signal with the basal turn on the left (*arrow*). (**b**) Axial contrast-enhanced, fat-saturated T1-weighted image demonstrates a corresponding focus of contrast enhancement consistent with intracochlear schwannoma (*arrow*).

of these lesions which often have identical clinical presentations compared to the more common IAC or CPA tumors. Classifications of these inner ear tumors according to location and extension have been proposed by Kennedy et al with further refinements suggested by Van Abel et al.[16,17]

CPA meningiomas as previously mentioned are characteristically eccentric to the porus, have obtuse rather than acute margins with adjacent dura, often have limited or no IAC extension, and classically have homogenous signal (isointense to adjacent brain) and enhancement characteristics (▶ Fig. 8.12). Thickening of enhancing dura adjacent to the tumor is characteristic ("dural tail") but not pathognomonic of meningioma. Calcifications may be seen in 10% and hyperostosis of adjacent cortical bone is not uncommon. Calcification will alter the

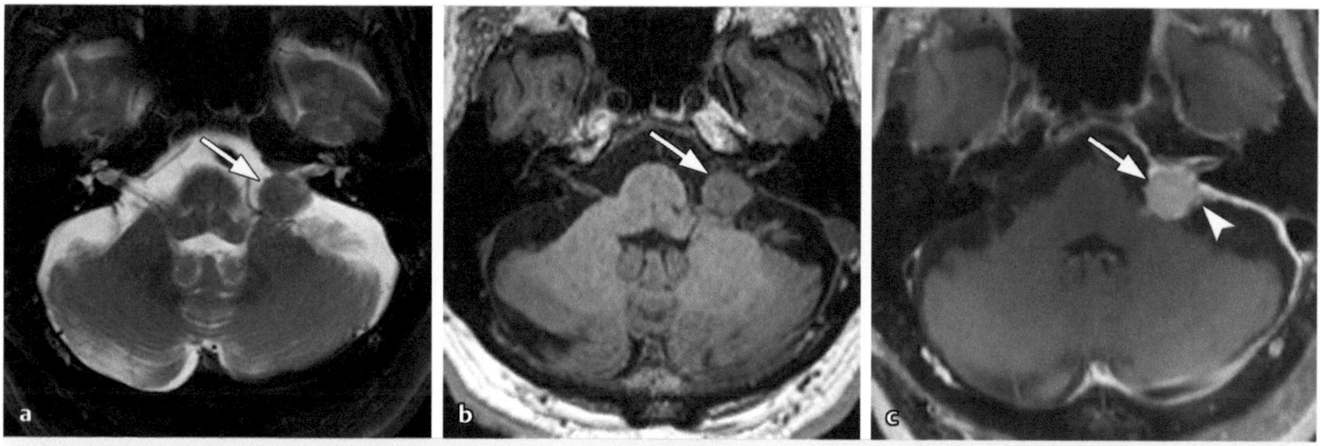

Fig. 8.12 Left CPA meningioma. **(a–c)** Homogenous signal and enhancement slightly eccentric to the porus acusticus of the IAC (*arrows*). Signal is isointense to brain on all sequences. Note the obtuse margin of tumor with adjacent dura and prominent "dural tail" (*arrowhead*).

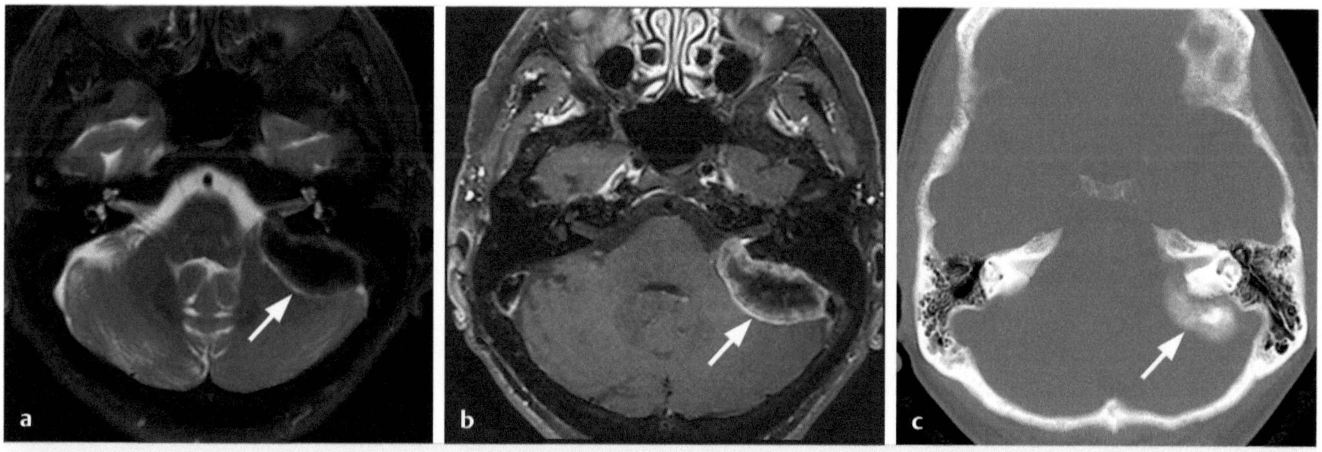

Fig. 8.13 Calcified CPA meningioma. **(a)** Axial T2-weighted image demonstrates extra-axial mass eccentric to the left IAC marked T2 hypointensity (*arrow*). **(b)** Axial contrast-enhanced fat-saturated T1 image demonstrates atypical peripheral enhancement with central T1 hypointensity (*arrow*). **(c)** Axial CT demonstrates central calcification (*arrow*) correlating with T2 and T1 hypointensity seen in **a** and **b**.

typical isointense homogenous T1 and T2 signal producing areas of marked hypointensity (▶ Fig. 8.13).

Epidermoids are congenital lesions arising from inclusion of epithelium during neural tube closure. They represent around 2% of intracranial masses and are most commonly encountered in the CPA.[18] These lesions are relatively isointense to CSF on T1- and T2-weighted sequences and usually appear slightly hyperintense to CSF on FLAIR sequences. They do not enhance on postcontrast sequences and characteristically demonstrate diffusion restriction on diffusion-weighted imaging, which helps further distinguish them from arachnoid cyst[19] (▶ Fig. 8.14).

Other nerve sheath tumors can occasionally mimic VS in the CPA. Facial nerve schwannomas can be indistinguishable on imaging from VS if isolated to the IAC and/or CPA without a labyrinth tail. Extension into the bony facial canal will often provide a clue as to the nerve of origin in these cases (▶ Fig. 8.15). Likewise, schwannomas of trigeminal origin involving the cisternal segment of the nerve may present in the superior CPA, but evidence of extension into Meckel's cave is often diagnostic[20] (▶ Fig. 8.16). Lower CPA schwannomas with extension into the jugular foramen (cranial nerves IX, X, XI) or hypoglossal canal (cranial nerve XII) may rarely mimic the more common CPA VS.[21]

Lipomas are most commonly encountered in the subarachnoid spaces of the basal cisterns or pericallosal regions.[22] They arise from meninx primitiva, the embryologic precursor to the arachnoid membrane.[23] In the CPA, the neurovascular bundle will commonly course through these lesions without evidence of mass effect or displacement, which explains why resection carries a higher risk of cranial nerve injury compared to other lesions that displace the neurovascular bundle over the capsule (▶ Fig. 8.17).

CPA arachnoid cysts have well-circumscribed margins, do not enhance, and will often displace adjacent neurovascular structures. They are isointense on all pulse sequences, and, unlike epidermoids, will not demonstrate restriction on diffusion-weighted images (▶ Fig. 8.18).

On occasion, cavernous hemangiomas may be encountered in the IAC and be indistinguishable on MR imaging from VS (▶ Fig. 8.19). They may demonstrate erosion of the bony cortex

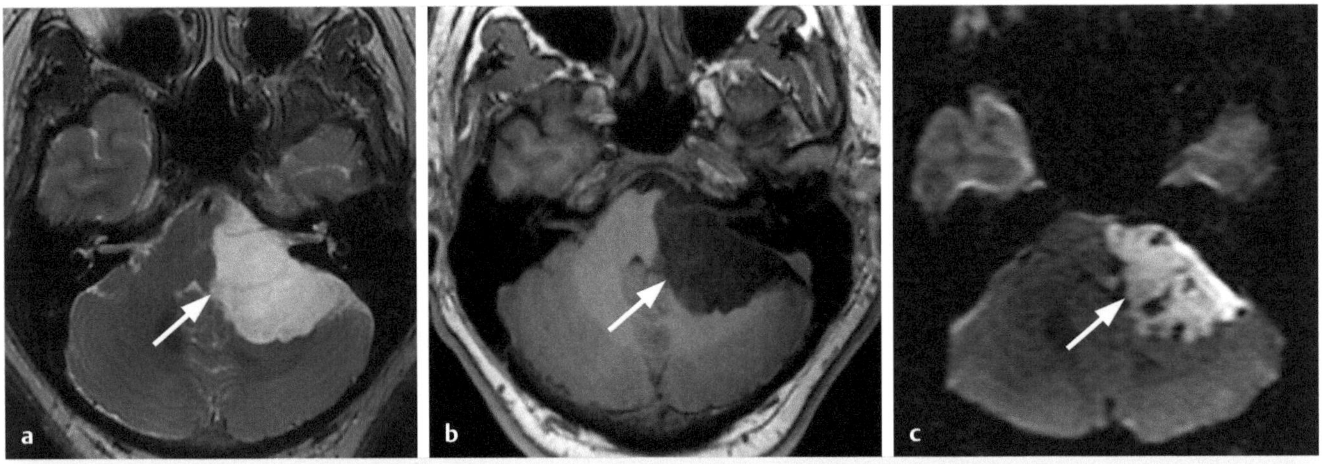

Fig. 8.14 CPA epidermoid. (**a, b**) Axial T2- and T1-weighted images, respectively, demonstrate extra-axial CPA angle mass with signal intensity relatively isointense to CSF (*arrows*). No enhancement was noted on the postcontrast sequences (not shown). (**c**) Diffusion-weighted image demonstrates markedly restricted diffusion (*arrow*). Combination of imaging characteristics are pathognomonic for epidermoid.

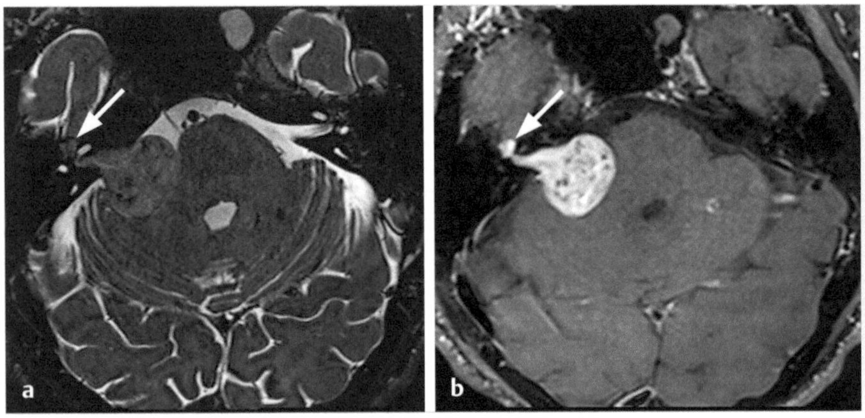

Fig. 8.15 Facial nerve schwannoma. (**a, b**) Axial T2 and fat-saturated contrast-enhanced T1-weighted images, respectively, demonstrate right CPA and IAC lesion which extends into labyrinthine segment of the facial nerve canal and geniculate ganglion identifying the facial nerve origin of this surgically proven facial nerve schwannoma.

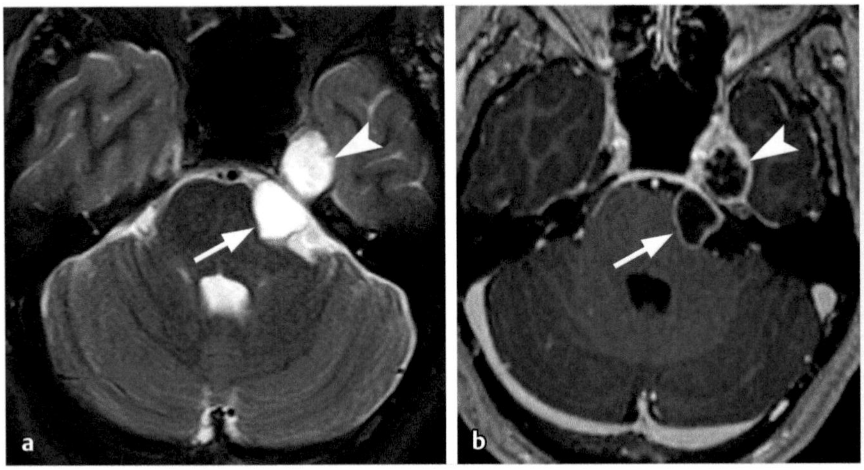

Fig. 8.16 CPA cystic trigeminal schwannoma. (**a**) Axial T2-weighted image demonstrates hyperintense left CPA mass (*arrow*) with anterior extension into Meckel's cave (*arrowhead*) indicative of trigeminal origin. (**b**) Axial contrast-enhanced fat-saturated T1-weighted images demonstrate peripheral pattern of enhancement consistent with a cystic tumor (*arrow*) and Meckel's cave extension (*arrowhead*).

of the IAC and intralesional calcification, best demonstrated on CT, which would allow differentiation from VS.[24] Other vascular lesions that may present as an IAC or CPA mass would include posterior circulation aneurysms, usually arising from the basilar artery or anterior inferior cerebellar artery. These lesions are characterized by signal voids on MR and, when large, peripheral thrombus surrounding a patent aneurysm lumen (▶ Fig. 8.20). Multiple signal voids in the CPA should raise concerns for central venous shunting in the setting of a dural arteriovenous fistula (▶ Fig. 8.21) and should warrant a diagnostic cerebral

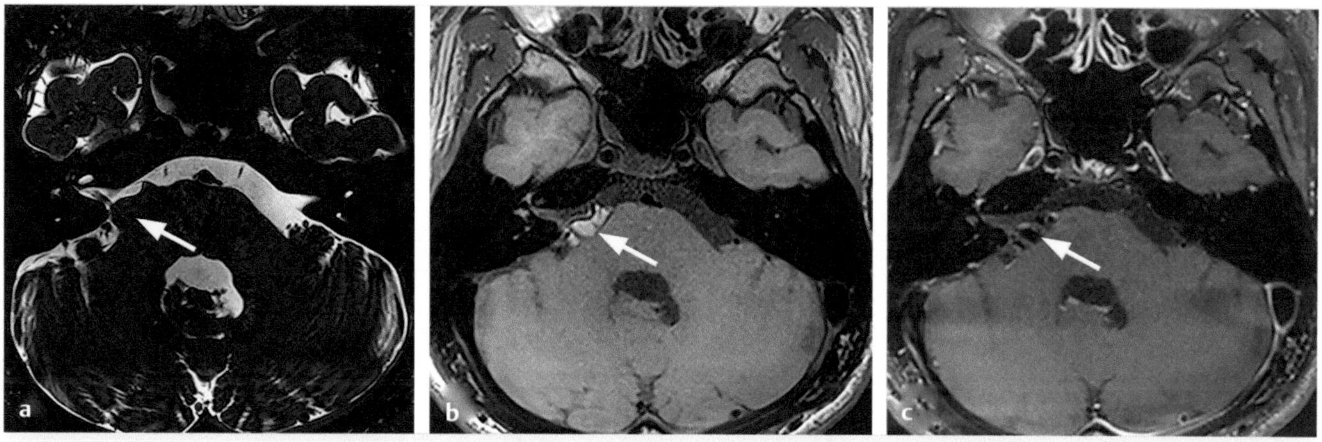

Fig. 8.17 CPA lipoma. (**a**) Axial T2-weighted image demonstrates lobulated right CPA hypointense mass (*arrow*). (**b**) Axial T1-weighted image without contrast characterizes mass as hyperintense consistent with fat (*arrow*). (**c**) Axial contrast-enhanced fat-saturated image demonstrates suppression of hyperintense fat signal (*arrow*) with minimal peripheral enhancement of adjacent venous structures.

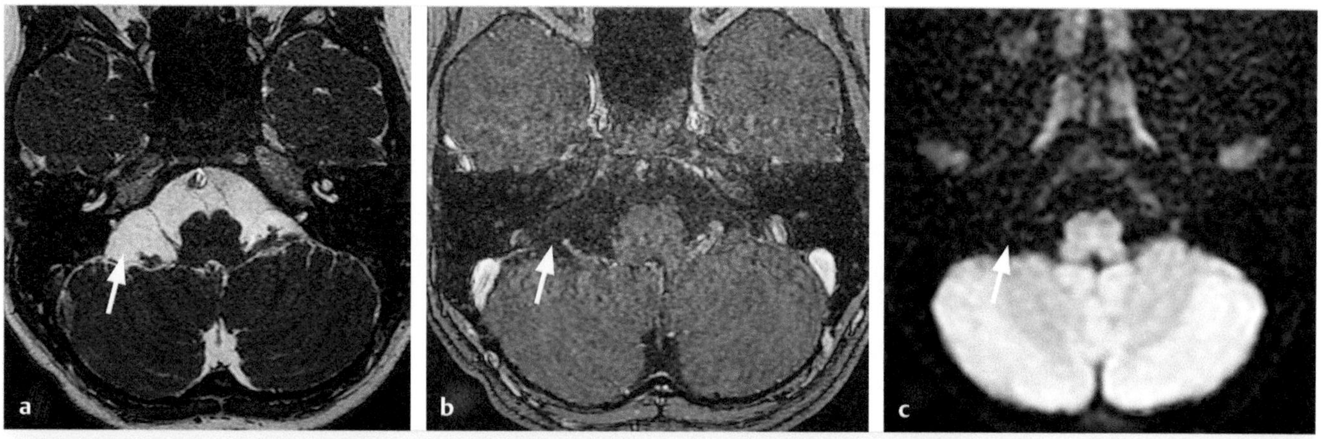

Fig. 8.18 CPA arachnoid cyst. (**a**) Axial T2 and (**b**) contrast-enhanced fat-saturated T1 sequences demonstrating cystic lesion in the inferolateral CPA which is isointense to CSF on all sequences (*arrows*). (**c**) Diffusion sequence demonstrating lack of diffusion restriction (*arrow*) distinguishes this lesion from an epidermoid.

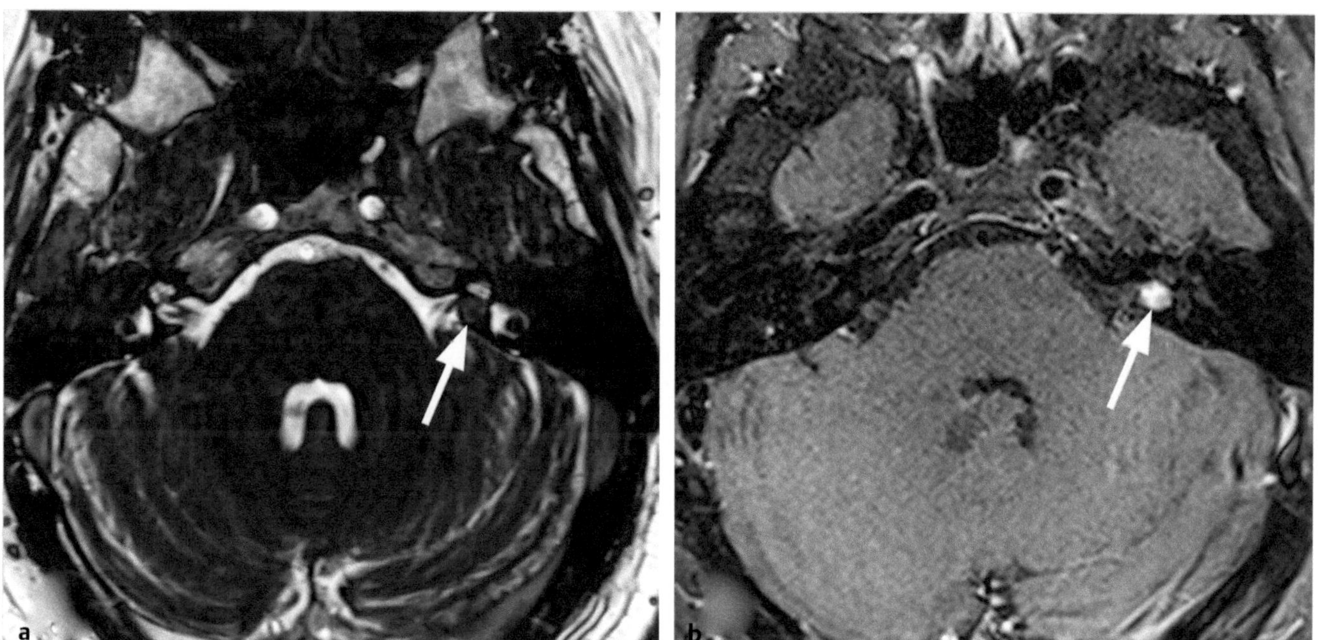

Fig. 8.19 IAC hemangioma. (**a**) Axial 3D GRE (FIESTA, CISS) image demonstrates filling defect in the left IAC (*arrow*). (**b**) Axial contrast-enhanced fat-saturated T1-weighted image demonstrates inhomogeneous enhancement of the lesion (*arrow*). Imaging features are indistinguishable from more common vestibular schwannoma. Cavernous hemangioma found at surgery.

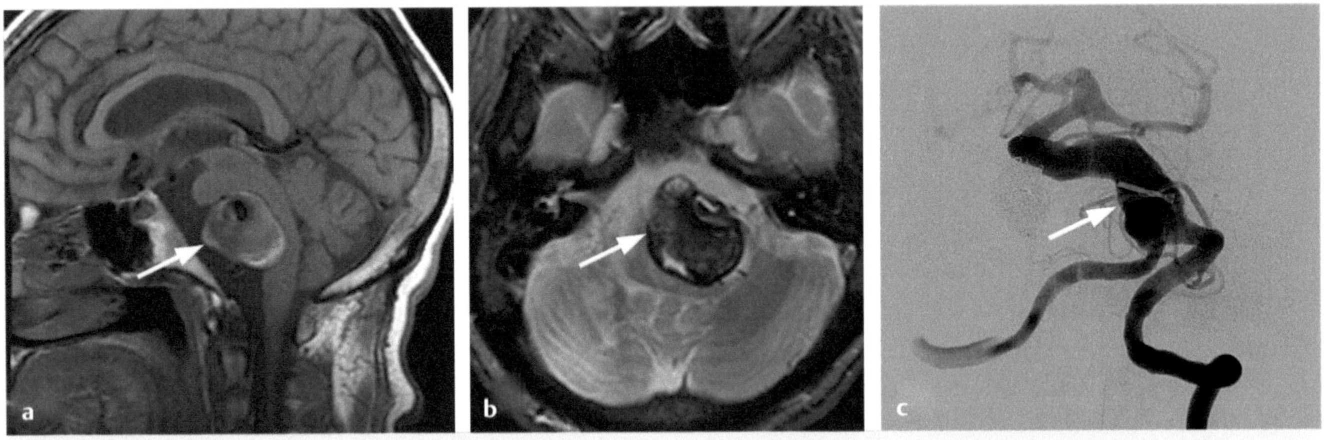

Fig. 8.20 Basilar artery fusiform aneurysm. (**a**) Sagittal T1-weighted and (**b**) axial T2-weighted images demonstrate peripheral T1 hyperintensity and T2 hypointensity consistent with thrombus (*arrows*) surrounding a central signal void consistent with partially thrombosed aneurysm. (**c**) Anterior projection from left vertebral artery angiogram demonstrates patent central lumen of large fusiform aneurysm of the basilar artery (*arrow*).

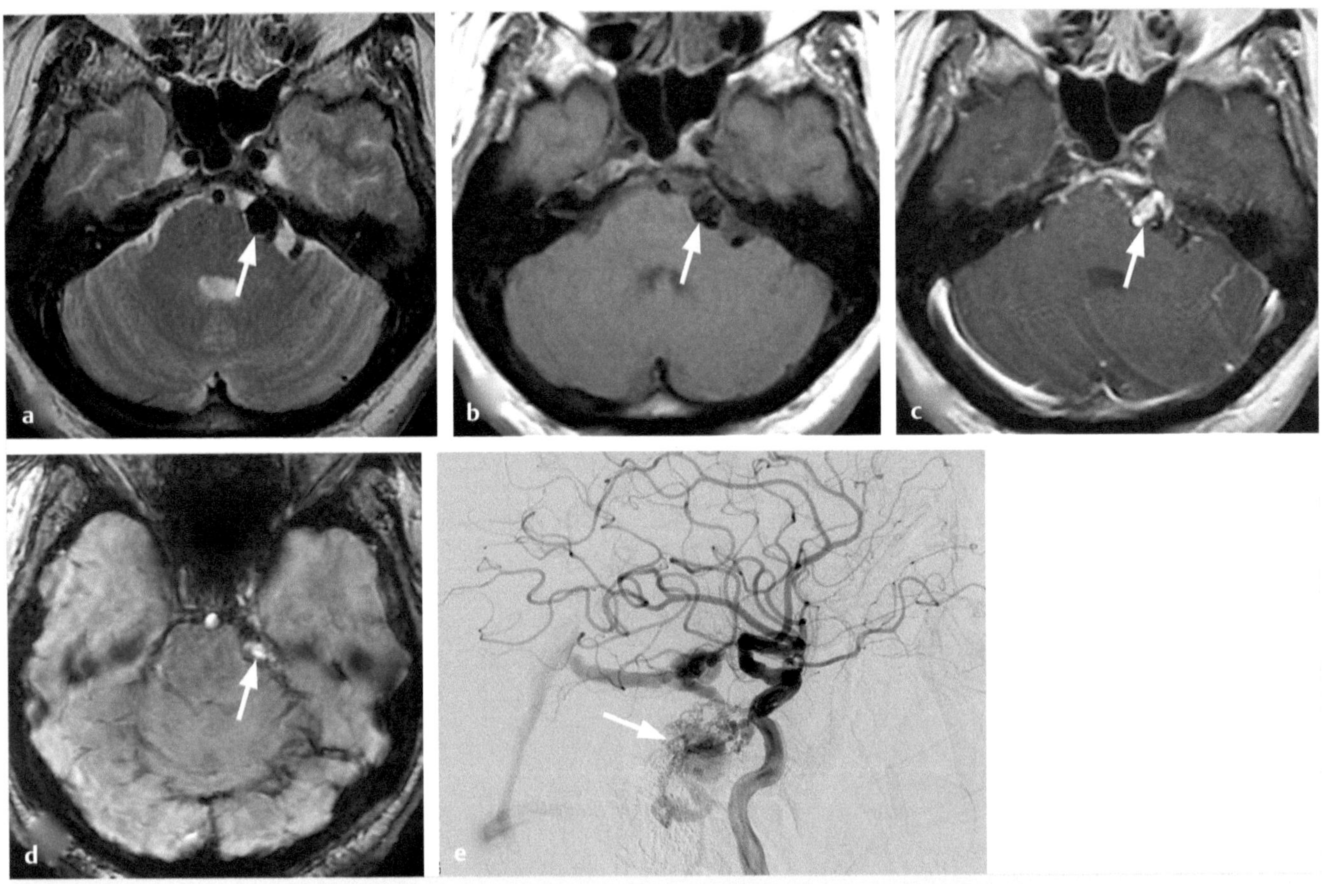

Fig. 8.21 CPA dural arteriovenous fistula. (**a**) Axial T2-weighted and (**b**) T1-weighted images demonstrating large signal void in the left CPA (*arrows*) consistent with venous shunting from a prominent dural arteriovenous fistula. (**c**) Axial postcontrast T1-weighed image demonstrates partial enhancement of the dilated, arterialized vein (*arrow*) and (**d**) susceptibility-weighted image demonstrates hyperintense flow-related enhancement (*arrow*) consistent with arterialization of central venous drainage. (**e**) Lateral projection from selective left internal carotid artery angiogram demonstrates dural fistula filling from the meningo-hypophyseal trunk with central venous shunting (*arrow*).

arteriogram. If central venous drainage is documented on angiography, embolization should be considered secondary to the high rate of cerebral hemorrhage.[25]

References

[1] Lane JI, Ward H, Witte RJ, Bernstein MA, Driscoll CL. 3-T imaging of the cochlear nerve and labyrinth in cochlear-implant candidates: 3D fast recovery fast spin-echo versus 3D constructive interference in the steady state techniques. AJNR Am J Neuroradiol. 2004; 25(4):618–622

[2] Lane JI, Witte RJ, Bolster B, Bernstein MA, Johnson K, Morris J. State of the art: 3 T imaging of the membranous labyrinth. AJNR Am J Neuroradiol. 2008; 29 (8):1436–1440

[3] Allen RW, Harnsberger HR, Shelton C, et al. Low-cost high-resolution fast spin-echo MR of acoustic schwannoma: an alternative to enhanced conventional spin-echo MR? AJNR Am J Neuroradiol. 1996; 17(7):1205–1210

[4] Abele TA, Besachio DA, Quigley EP, et al. Diagnostic accuracy of screening MR imaging using unenhanced axial CISS and coronal T2WI for detection of small internal auditory canal lesions. AJNR Am J Neuroradiol. 2014; 35(12): 2366–2370

[5] McDonald RJ, McDonald JS, Kallmes DF, et al. Intracranial gadolinium deposition after contrast-enhanced MR imaging. Radiology. 2015; 275(3):772–782

[6] Radbruch A, Weberling LD, Kieslich PJ, et al. Gadolinium retention in the dentate nucleus and globus pallidus is dependent on the class of contrast agent. Radiology. 2015; 275(3):783–791

[7] Kanda T, Ishii K, Kawaguchi H, Kitajima K, Takenaka D. High signal intensity in the dentate nucleus and globus pallidus on unenhanced T1-weighted MR images: relationship with increasing cumulative dose of a gadolinium-based contrast material. Radiology. 2014; 270(3):834–841

[8] Slattery WH. Neurofibromatosis. In: Brackmann DE, Shelton C, Arriaga M, eds. Otologic Surgery. 4th ed. Philadelphia, PA: Elsevier; 2016

[9] Copeland WR, Hoover JM, Morris JM, Driscoll CL, Link MJ. Use of preoperative MRI to predict vestibular schwannoma intraoperative consistency and facial nerve outcome. J Neurol Surg B Skull Base. 2013; 74(6):347–350

[10] Metwali H, Samii M, Samii A, Gerganov V. The peculiar cystic vestibular schwannoma: a single-center experience. World Neurosurg. 2014; 82(6): 1271–1275

[11] Zhu W, Mao Y. Cystic vestibular schwannomas: surgical considerations and outcomes. World Neurosurg. 2015; 83(5):742–743

[12] Goddard JC, Schwartz MS, Friedman RA. Fundal fluid as a predictor of hearing preservation in the middle cranial fossa approach for vestibular schwannoma. Otol Neurotol. 2010; 31(7):1128–1134

[13] Tringali S, Ferber-Viart C, Fuchsmann C, Buiret G, Zaouche S, Dubreuil C. Hearing preservation in retrosigmoid approach of small vestibular schwannomas: prognostic value of the degree of internal auditory canal filling. Otol Neurotol. 2010; 31(9):1469–1472

[14] Somers T, Casselman J, de Ceulaer G, Govaerts P, Offeciers E. Prognostic value of magnetic resonance imaging findings in hearing preservation surgery for vestibular schwannoma. Otol Neurotol. 2001; 22(1):87–94

[15] Samii M, Giordano M, Metwali H, Almarzooq O, Samii A, Gerganov VM. Prognostic significance of peritumoral edema in patients with vestibular schwannomas. Neurosurgery. 2015; 77(1):81–85, discussion 85–86

[16] Kennedy RJ, Shelton C, Salzman KL, Davidson HC, Harnsberger HR. Intralabyrinthine schwannomas: diagnosis, management, and a new classification system. Otol Neurotol. 2004; 25(2):160–167

[17] Van Abel KM, Carlson ML, Link MJ, et al. Primary inner ear schwannomas: a case series and systematic review of the literature. Laryngoscope. 2013; 123 (8):1957–1966

[18] Liu P, Saida Y, Yoshioka H, Itai Y. MR imaging of epidermoids at the cerebellopontine angle. Magn Reson Med Sci. 2003; 2(3):109–115

[19] Tsuruda JS, Chew WM, Moseley ME, Norman D. Diffusion-weighted MR imaging of the brain: value of differentiating between extraaxial cysts and epidermoid tumors. AJNR Am J Neuroradiol. 1990; 11(5):925–931, discussion 932–934

[20] Majoie CB, Hulsmans FJ, Castelijns JA, et al. Primary nerve-sheath tumours of the trigeminal nerve: clinical and MRI findings. Neuroradiology. 1999; 41(2): 100–108

[21] Bonneville F, Sarrazin JL, Marsot-Dupuch K, et al. Unusual lesions of the cerebellopontine angle: a segmental approach. Radiographics. 2001; 21(2): 419–438

[22] Bacciu A, Di Lella F, Ventura E, Pasanisi E, Russo A, Sanna M. Lipomas of the internal auditory canal and cerebellopontine angle. Ann Otol Rhinol Laryngol. 2014; 123(1):58–64

[23] Truwit, CL and Barkovich AJ Pathogenesis of Intracranial Lipoma: An MR Study in 42 Patients AJNR 11:665-674, July/August 1990

[24] Zhu WD, Huang Q, Li XY, Chen HS, Wang ZY, Wu H. Diagnosis and treatment of cavernous hemangioma of the internal auditory canal. J Neurosurg. 2016; 124(3):639–646

[25] Gandhi D, Chen J, Pearl M, Huang J, Gemmete JJ, Kathuria S. Intracranial dural arteriovenous fistulas: classification, imaging findings, and treatment. AJNR Am J Neuroradiol. 2012; 33(6):1007–1013

9 Emerging Imaging Techniques in Vestibular Schwannoma

Joshua D. Hughes, John Huston III, and John I. Lane

9.1 Introduction

Recently developed magnetic resonance imaging (MRI) techniques with potential applications for the evaluation of vestibular schwannoma (VS) include MR elastography (MRE) and diffusion tensor tractography. Although these techniques remain investigational, recently published work using both techniques in the preoperative evaluation of VS appears promising.

9.2 Magnetic Resonance Elastography

MRE is an emerging MR-based imaging sequence first described by Muthupillai et al[1] in 1995 that utilizes mechanical waves to quantify the shear modulus, or stiffness, of a substance in kilopascal (kPa). The three elements are (1) an external vibrating driver that transmits shear waves in adjacent tissue, (2) imaging the tissue of interest with a phase contrast MRI sequence, and (3) performing mathematical inversions of the wave images to create quantitative maps of tissue stiffness (▶ Fig. 9.1).[2] Essentially, MRE is a means of "palpating" a tissue with imaging and has been developed for liver, breast, skeletal muscle, heart, and brain.[3,4] The technology is most mature in hepatic applications and is replacing biopsy in many centers.[5]

In the brain, MRE is being used to evaluate stiffness in both global disease such as Alzheimer's,[6,7] multiple sclerosis,[8] and normal pressure hydrocephalus[9] and focal lesions such as meningioma,[10,11,12] glioblastoma,[12,13] pituitary macroadenoma,[12,14] and VS.[12] More recently, a form of MRE has been developed called slip-interface imaging (SII) to evaluate the surgical plane between extra-axial brain tumors and adjacent normal neural structures.[15] SII uses the wave images of MRE to create two images, shear line and octahedral shear strain (OSS) images (▶ Fig. 9.2). Shear-line imaging works by intravoxel phase dispersion and a low signal line indicates tissue separation, while lack of this line indicates adhesion. OSS works by the maximum change in shear displacement across all possible planes and is a measurable value, though on imaging it is typically indicated by an increasing orange-to-yellow color scale. Thus, MRE has the potential to provide preoperative evaluation of both tumor stiffness and tumor-brain adhesion. These are factors previously unreliably measured that may influence surgical difficulty, extent of resection, and complications such as facial nerve outcomes in VS resection.

Lee et al[16] speculated that VS consistency might impact facial nerve outcome after microsurgical resection, with firm, avascular tumors being more easily removed leading to less injury. In a prospective study, Esquia-Medina et al[17] have shown that tumor adhesion affects facial nerve outcomes; tumors with strong adhesion had poorer House-Brackmann scores.

However, no study has evaluated MRI characteristics for adhesion and only one study has evaluated for consistency in VS. Copeland et al[18] found that soft tumors tended to be T2 hyperintense, while firm tumors tended to be T2 hypointense. There was no correlation with tumor consistency and extent of resection or facial nerve outcomes. However, they preselected tumors that were very soft or hard at surgery; thus, the MRI findings may not apply for tumors that fall between those extremes.

Since MRE investigations have only recently been available to evaluate focal intracranial lesions, experience for evaluating consistency in VS is limited. In a mixed series including pituitary macroadenoma, meningioma, and glioblastoma, Sakai et al[12] reported on MRE stiffness in six patients with VS finding a mean shear stiffness range of 1.7 to 2.5 kPa and a maximum shear stiffness range of 1.7 to 3.7 kPa. They speculate MRE measurements might correlate with Antoni patterns on pathologic analysis.

At our institution, we have evaluated 11 VS and correlated MRE measurements for both consistency and adhesion[15] with surgical findings, extent of resection, and facial nerve outcome. Regarding consistency (▶ Fig. 9.3), surgeons categorized five VSs as soft, four as intermediate, and two as firm. For each category, mean MRE measurements increased (3.09 ± 0.58 [2.39–3.95], 3.17 ± 0.48 [2.58–3.74], and 3.5 ± 0.39 [3.26, 3.80] kPa, respectively), but the increases were not statistical significant (ANOVA, $p = 0.633$). Two soft tumors had MRE values greater than 3.0 kPa, but were vascular, a characteristic that may generate misleading MRE values in meningioma[10] and liver.[5]

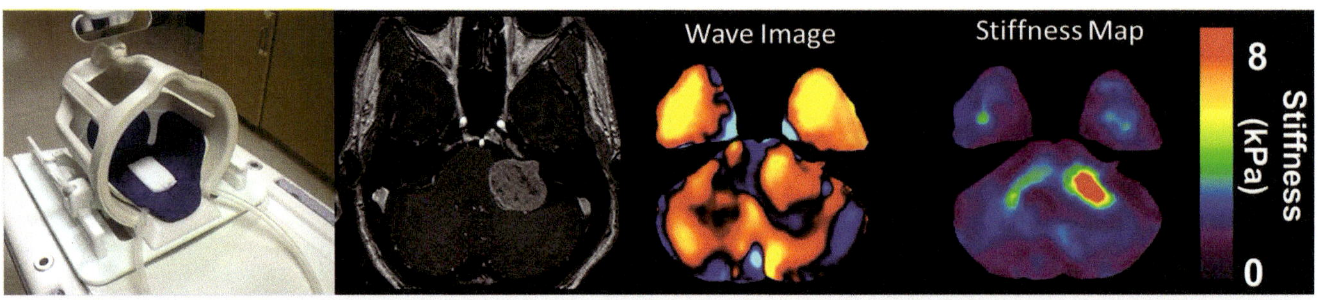

Fig. 9.1 Different components of MRE from left to right. A picture of the head driver that introduces waves into the brain during an MRI to obtain MRE images. A T1-weighted MRI shows a left-sided vestibular schwannoma that underwent MRE. An analysis of wave movement through the tissues by an algorithm creates a stiffness map.

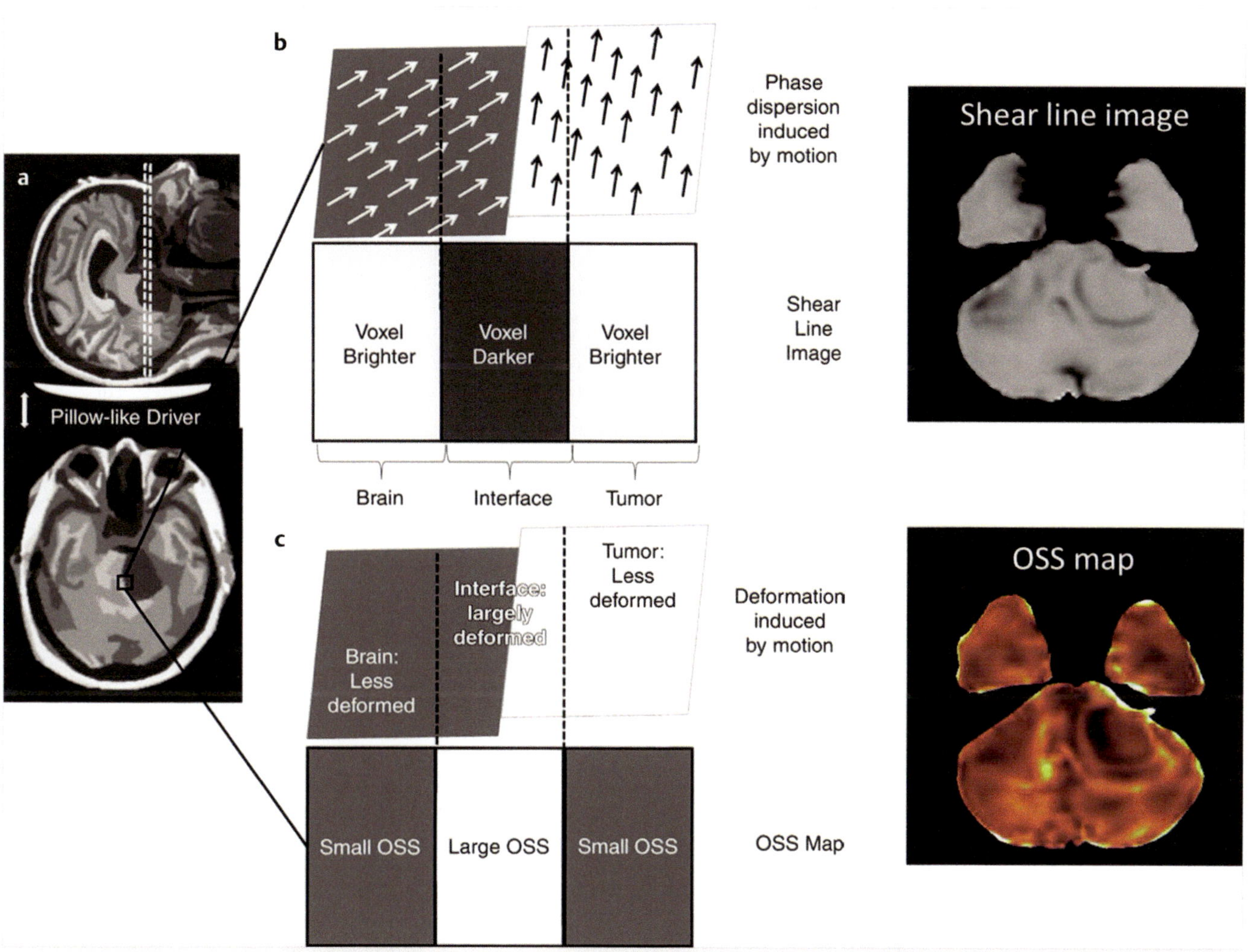

Fig. 9.2 Concept of slip interface imaging. (**a**) Shear waves are introduced into the brain by using a soft, pillow-like driver placed under the patient's head, with vibration direction indicated by *double-headed arrow*. The *dotted vertical lines* indicate the image plane. (**b**) Assuming a nonadhesive tumor, low-intensity shear lines can be made visible because of the intravoxel phase dispersion effect. The large differential motion between the tumor and the adjacent brain can create phase variations across the interface, which leads to magnitude signal loss. (**c**) Because of the independent motion of the tumor and the brain, differential motion between the tissues at the interface can be detected, which leads to large octahedral shear strain. Both images show tumors with no adhesion. Used with permission from: Yin Z, Glaser K J, Manduca A, et al. Slip interface imaging predicts tumor-brain adhesion in vestibular schwannomas. Radiology 2015;277:507-517.

Regarding tumor adherence, surgeons categorized five tumors as having complete, three as partial, and three as no separation. SII, using OSS as it correlates better than shear-line imaging,[15] categorized seven tumors as complete, three as partial, and one as no separation ($\kappa = 0.70$; 95% CI: 0.35–1.00; ▶ Fig. 9.4). Both tumors with discrepancy between SII and surgical findings had a cyst in the posterior portion of the tumor, a feature that may lead to poor correlation due to intratumoral motion in a heterogeneous lesion.[15] There was no correlation with MRE values or SII analysis with regard to extent of resection or facial nerve outcomes.

Currently, MRE is the only noninvasive imaging technique consistently able to evaluate tumor stiffness and tumor-brain adhesion. While more study is needed to determine the clinical utility of MRE for VS, it has demonstrated potential to allow better preoperative assessment of surgical difficulty, risk, and outcome.

9.3 Diffusion Tensor Imaging and Tractography

Diffusion-weighted imaging (DWI) was originally employed to identify areas of acute cerebral infarction characterized by restriction of normal Brownian motion of water molecules within the magnetic field. Diffusion tensor imaging (DTI) incorporates directionality into the DWI measurement. DTI is sensitive to motion that is in alignment with the applied MR gradients. Maximal anisotropic motion is detected when the gradients are parallel to existing white matter tracts. Color-coded anisotropy maps can be generated as a 3D model to depict the exact course and caliber of the white matter tracts or cranial nerves[19,20] (▶ Fig. 9.5).

This technique has recently been employed to define the course of the facial nerve within the cerebellopontine angle and

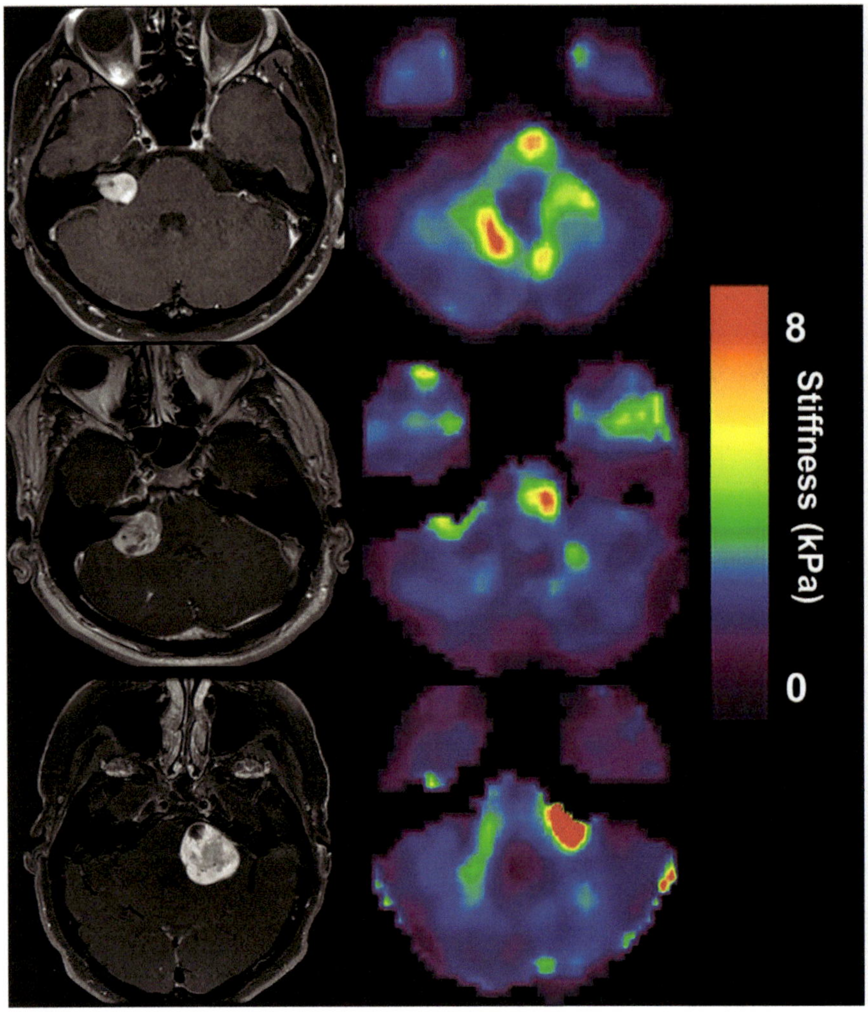

Fig. 9.3 T1 MRI with contrast images (*left*) showing three vestibular schwannomas with corresponding MRE stiffness maps (*right*) showing a soft, intermediate, and firm tumor (*top to bottom*).

internal auditory canal in proximity to VSs.[21,22,23,24,25,26] These studies have demonstrated that preoperative DTI with tractography has reliably predicted the position of the facial nerve in relation to the VS in approximately 80 to 90% of cases when correlated with intraoperative findings. However, the published surgical cohorts to date have been small and not all of these studies have included postoperative facial nerve outcome measures. Prospective controlled trials will be needed to determine if acquiring preoperative DTI tractography improves facial nerve functional outcomes after VS resection. In addition, the reliability and reproducibility of tractography data generated during the postprocessing may be highly dependent on the experience and knowledge of the operator and care must be taken to avoid variations in fractional anisotropy thresholding and fiber-tracking seed placement that could produce spurious tractography maps, particularly while attempting to track small cranial nerves.

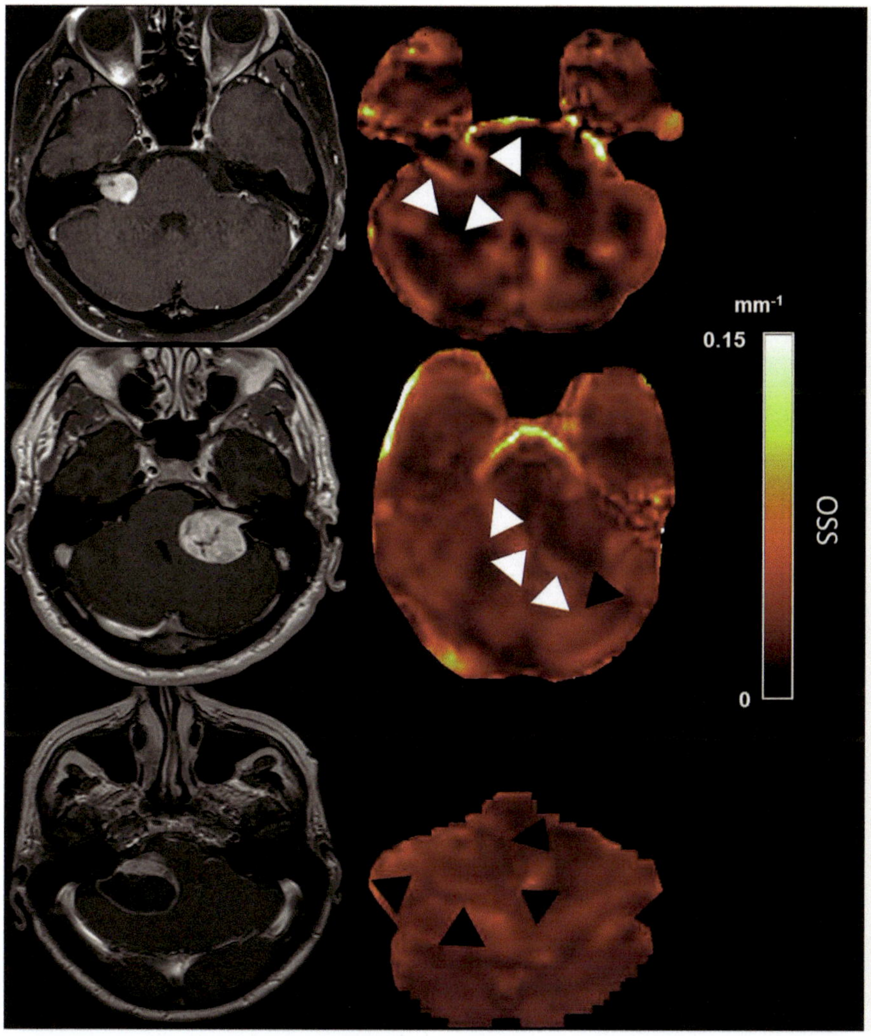

Fig. 9.4 T1 MRI with contrast images (*left*) showing three vestibular schwannomas with corresponding OSS maps (*right*) showing tumors with no, partial, and complete adhesion (*top to bottom*, *white arrows* show areas of no adhesion and *black arrows* show areas of adhesion).

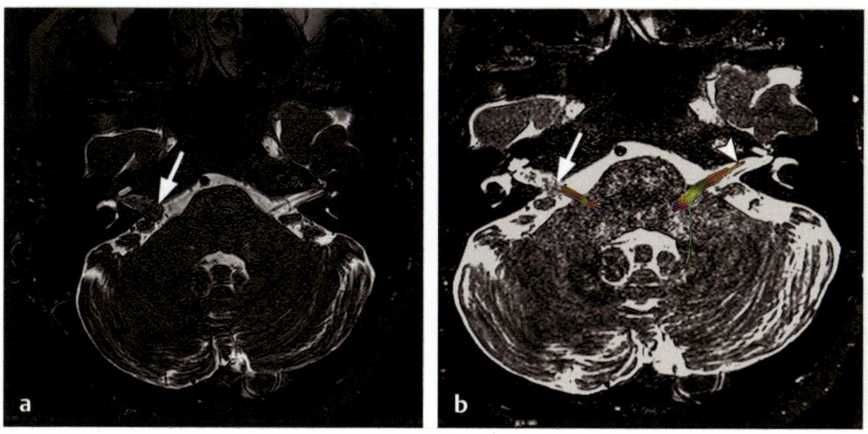

Fig. 9.5 (**a**) T2 SPACE axial image demonstrating right intracanalicular vestibular schwannoma (*arrow*). (**b**) Color-coded diffusion tensor fractional anisotropy map demonstrates abrupt attenuation of the fiber tracking at the interface between the tumor and the cochleovestibular trunk (*arrow*). The facial nerve was not reliably identified. Normal fiber tracking on the left (*arrow head*).

References

[1] Muthupillai R, Lomas DJ, Rossman PJ, Greenleaf JF, Manduca A, Ehman RL. Magnetic resonance elastography by direct visualization of propagating acoustic strain waves. Science. 1995; 269(5232):1854–1857

[2] Kruse SA, Rose GH, Glaser KJ, et al. Magnetic resonance elastography of the brain. Neuroimage. 2008; 39(1):231–237

[3] Glaser KJ, Manduca A, Ehman RL. Review of MR elastography applications and recent developments. J Magn Reson Imaging. 2012; 36(4):757–774

[4] Mariappan YK, Glaser KJ, Ehman RL. Magnetic resonance elastography: a review. Clin Anat. 2010; 23(5):497–511

[5] Venkatesh SK, Yin M, Ehman RL. Magnetic resonance elastography of liver: clinical applications. J Comput Assist Tomogr. 2013; 37(6):887–896

[6] Murphy MC, Curran GL, Glaser KJ, et al. Magnetic resonance elastography of the brain in a mouse model of Alzheimer's disease: initial results. Magn Reson Imaging. 2012; 30(4):535–539

[7] Murphy MC, Huston J, III, Jack CR, Jr, et al. Decreased brain stiffness in Alzheimer's disease determined by magnetic resonance elastography. J Magn Reson Imaging. 2011; 34(3):494–498

[8] Wuerfel J, Paul F, Beierbach B, et al. MR-elastography reveals degradation of tissue integrity in multiple sclerosis. Neuroimage. 2010; 49(3):2520–2525
[9] Freimann FB, Streitberger KJ, Klatt D, et al. Alteration of brain viscoelasticity after shunt treatment in normal pressure hydrocephalus. Neuroradiology. 2012; 54(3):189–196
[10] Hughes JD, Fattahi N, Van Gompel J, et al. Higher-resolution magnetic resonance elastography in meningiomas to determine intratumoral consistency. Neurosurgery. 2015; 77(4):653–658, discussion 658–659
[11] Murphy MC, Huston J, III, Glaser KJ, et al. Preoperative assessment of meningioma stiffness using magnetic resonance elastography. J Neurosurg. 2013; 118(3):643–648
[12] Sakai N, Takehara Y, Yamashita S, et al. Shear stiffness of 4 common intracranial tumors measured using MR elastography: comparison with intraoperative consistency grading. AJNR Am J Neuroradiol. 2016; 37(10):1851–1859
[13] Streitberger KJ, Reiss-Zimmermann M, Freimann FB, et al. High-resolution mechanical imaging of glioblastoma by multifrequency magnetic resonance elastography. PLoS One. 2014; 9(10):e110588
[14] Hughes JD, Fattahi N, Van Gompel J, Arani A, Ehman R, Huston J, III. Magnetic resonance elastography detects tumoral consistency in pituitary macroadenomas. Pituitary. 2016; 19(3):286–292
[15] Yin Z, Glaser KJ, Manduca A, et al. Slip interface imaging predicts tumor-brain adhesion in vestibular schwannomas. Radiology. 2015; 277(2):507–517
[16] Lee TK, Lund WS, Adams CB. Factors influencing the preservation of the facial nerve during acoustic surgery. Br J Neurosurg. 1990; 4(1):5–8
[17] Esquia-Medina GN, Grayeli AB, Ferrary E, et al. Do facial nerve displacement pattern and tumor adhesion influence the facial nerve outcome in vestibular schwannoma surgery? Otol Neurotol. 2009; 30(3):392–397
[18] Copeland WR, Hoover JM, Morris JM, Driscoll CL, Link MJ. Use of preoperative MRI to predict vestibular schwannoma intraoperative consistency and facial nerve outcome. J Neurol Surg B Skull Base. 2013; 74(6):347–350
[19] Hodaie M, Quan J, Chen DQ. In vivo visualization of cranial nerve pathways in humans using diffusion-based tractography. Neurosurgery. 2010; 66(4): 788–795, discussion 795–796
[20] Nucifora PG, Verma R, Lee SK, Melhem ER. Diffusion-tensor MR imaging and tractography: exploring brain microstructure and connectivity. Radiology. 2007; 245(2):367–384
[21] Chen DQ, Quan J, Guha A, Tymianski M, Mikulis D, Hodaie M. Three-dimensional in vivo modeling of vestibular schwannomas and surrounding cranial nerves with diffusion imaging tractography. Neurosurgery. 2011; 68(4):1077–1083
[22] Choi KS, Kim MS, Kwon HG, Jang SH, Kim OL. Preoperative identification of facial nerve in vestibular schwannomas surgery using diffusion tensor tractography. J Korean Neurosurg Soc. 2014; 56(1):11–15
[23] Gerganov VM, Samii M. Giant vestibular schwannomas. World Neurosurg. 2012; 77(5–6):627–628
[24] Ung N, Mathur M, Chung LK, et al. A systematic analysis of the reliability of diffusion tensor imaging tractography for facial nerve imaging in patients with vestibular schwannoma. J Neurol Surg B Skull Base. 2016; 77(4):314–318
[25] Yoshino M, Kin T, Ito A, et al. Combined use of diffusion tensor tractography and multifused contrast-enhanced FIESTA for predicting facial and cochlear nerve positions in relation to vestibular schwannoma. J Neurosurg. 2015; 123 (6):1480–1488
[26] Zhang Y, Chen Y, Zou Y, et al. Facial nerve preservation with preoperative identification and intraoperative monitoring in large vestibular schwannoma surgery. Acta Neurochir (Wien). 2013; 155(10):1857–1862

10 MRI Safety and Imaging Quality in Patients with Cochlear Implants or Auditory Brainstem Implants with Retained Internal Magnets

Robert E. Watson Jr., Matthew L. Carlson, and Heidi A. Edmonson

10.1 Introduction

Cochlear implantation (CI) is currently a standard intervention for rehabilitation of severe to profound sensorineural hearing loss, with over 300,000 implant recipients worldwide.[1] In addition, auditory brainstem implants (ABIs) have become increasingly used for rehabilitation of hearing loss in patients with neurofibromatosis type 2 (NF2). CIs are commonly used when an anatomically intact cochlear nerve exists, while ABI is generally reserved for NF2 patients where the continuity of the cochlear nerve has been compromised.[2] Concurrent with this, advanced medical imaging with MRI has become the gold standard for evaluation of many clinical conditions given its unparalleled soft-tissue contrast capabilities. NF2 patients with CIs or ABIs represent a specific population for which MRI is particularly important given their propensity for tumor development and long-term need for serial cranial and spine imaging.

In cases where a CI or ABI is performed, several options exist with regard to managing the internal magnet during MRI. Historically, it has been common practice to implant the patient with a nonferrous spacer and the patient would then have to use toupee tape or other inconvenient means to couple the internal and external device coils. More recently, many patients have simply been implanted with the expectation that internal magnet removal will be performed if/when head or body MRI is required in the future. Of course, magnet removal is not without risks, including device infection, period of non-use, silicone flange fatigue, and requirement of two local or general anesthetics. Only in the last decade have select centers begun scanning patients with retained internal magnets, under specific safety protocols.

Previously, most patients with implanted active electronic devices, including CIs and ABIs, and other devices, such as pacemakers and neurostimulators, could not be scanned due to patient safety concerns related to the unique conditions in MRI, as well as the possibility of damaging the device. More recently, procedures have been developed permitting some CI and ABI patients to be scanned, and manufacturers have increasingly been developing devices that are "MRI conditional"—that is, devices that are designed to withstand the MRI environment without injury to the patient while adhering to specific MRI scanning conditions.

It is important to understand that the term "MRI conditional" is not synonymous with "MRI compatible." In 2005, American Society for Testing and Materials (ASTM) International released terminology that was to be used in describing MRI safety, and these designations have been adopted by the United States Food and Drug Administration (FDA). These include "MRI safe," "MRI unsafe," and "MRI conditional" (▶ Fig. 10.1). MRI safe devices are considered safe under all MRI scanning scenarios, MRI unsafe devices are considered unsafe under all scenarios, and MRI conditional devices are those that minimize risk when the MRI exam is carefully tailored to permit this. Thus, an MRI conditional device may be within the MRI environment only when specific scanning conditions are adhered to; conversely, under certain inappropriate scanning conditions, these devices can be unsafe.

As CIs and ABIs contain electronic components as well as an internal magnet, they are particularly sensitive to MRI safety-related issues. To better understand these, it is valuable to have a basic appreciation of the three primary components of an MRI that work collectively to produce an image, and their related factors and forces that can pose safety issues due to the presence of implanted devices. These three components are the (1) main magnet; (2) gradient systems; and (3) radiofrequency (RF) coils (▶ Fig. 10.2).

The main magnetic field in contemporary clinical MRIs ranges from 1.0 to 3.0 tesla (1 tesla = 10,000 gauss; the earth's

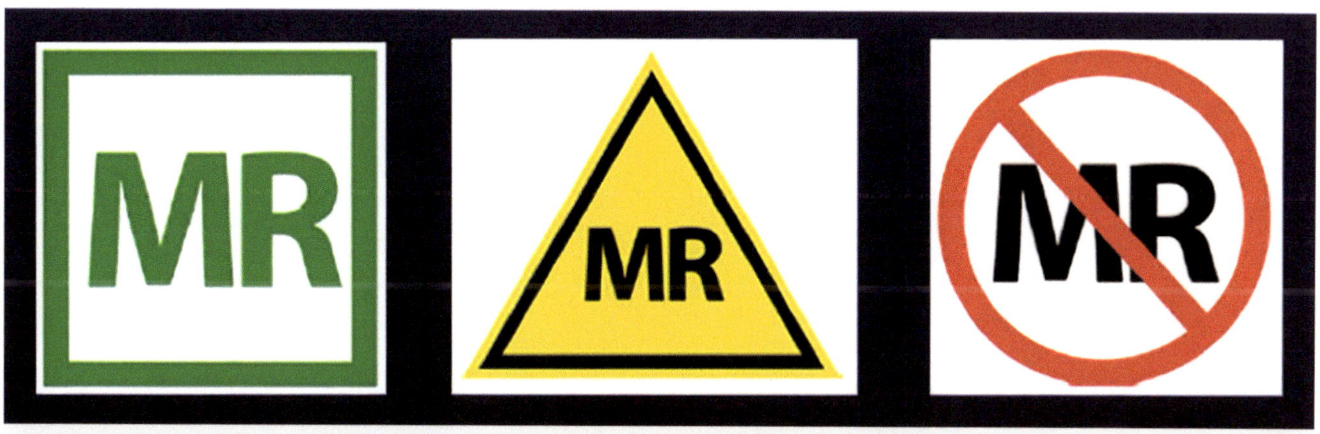

Fig. 10.1 2005 ASTM labeling for MRI safety. Labels used to indicate device compatibility with MRI: green square = MRI safe, yellow triangle = MRI conditional, red circle/slash = MRI unsafe. MRI conditional devices may only undergo MRI under specified conditions.

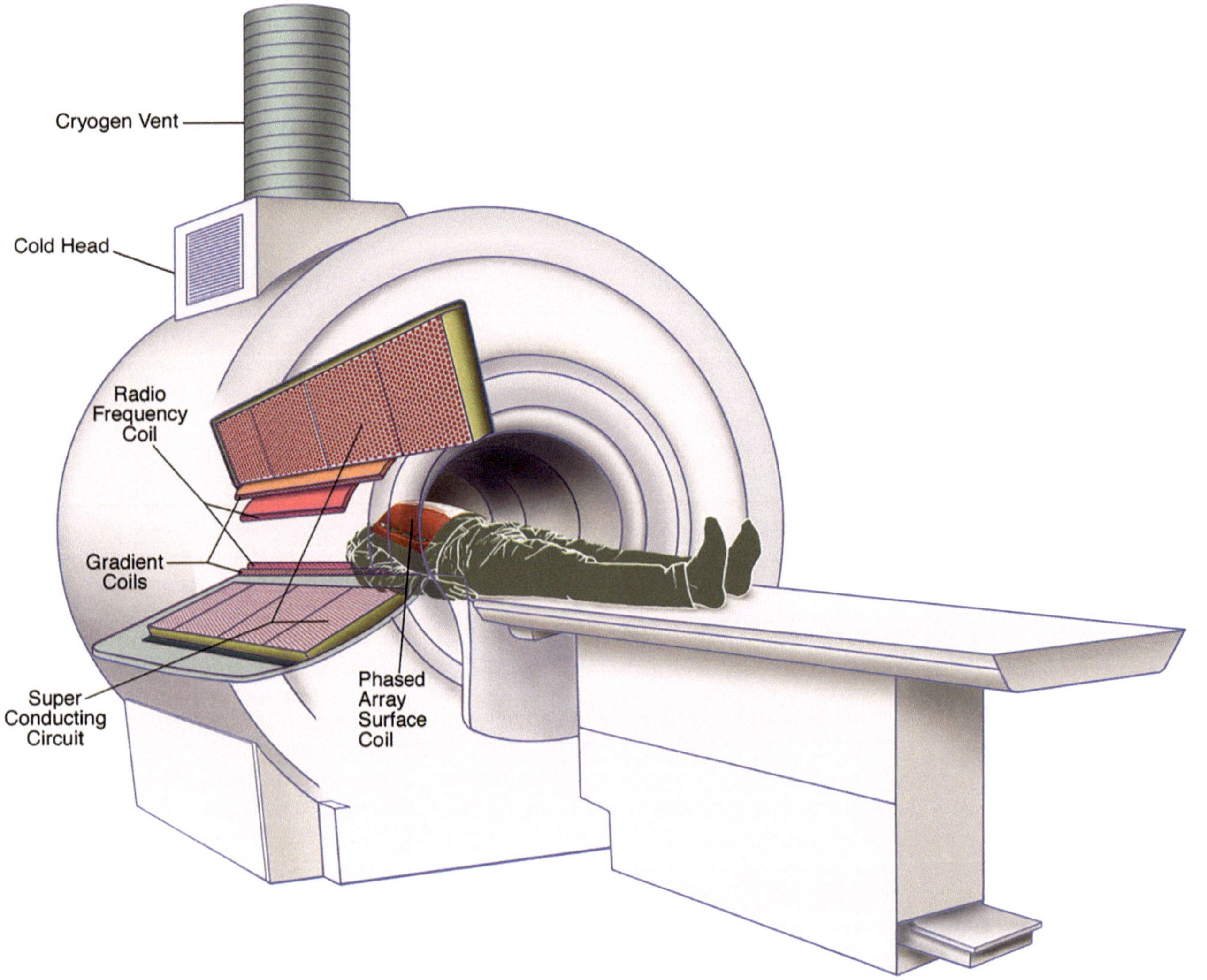

Fig. 10.2 Several components of an MRI are associated with the unique risks that can be encountered in CI and ABI patients while undergoing MRI examinations. The superconducting electromagnetic circuit imparts the main magnetic field. Adjacent to this are gradient coils, which permit spatial localization. Radiofrequency coils are adjacent to the bore of the magnet.

magnetic field is approximately 0.3–0.7 gauss). It is produced by coiling wire about the bore of the magnet, through which a current is passed, creating an electromagnet. By cooling the wires to temperatures approaching absolute zero with liquid helium, passage of very high currents (hundreds of amperes) is possible, producing superconducting magnets. The main magnetic field, B0, serves to align the proton magnetic moments.

Gradient systems (dB/dt), in an MR system, spatially locate the signal in three-dimensional space. Gradient coils alter the strength of the original main magnetic field allowing this. These gradient systems involve very rapidly fluctuating currents, producing the characteristic "knocking" and "banging" sounds in MRI. Given the electronic circuitry within CIs and ABIs, the changing magnetic field may induce signals that the patient perceives as clicking or other noises while the scanner is actively imaging.

The third component, RF coils, B1, deposits RF energy into the patient at the proton resonance frequency appropriate for the field strength of the magnet in order to elicit nuclear magnetization (i.e., it tips the magnetization into the transverse plane). Following this transmission, receiver coils detect the new emitting MRI signal.

10.2 MRI Safety Risks of Scanning Patients with Cochlear Implants and Auditory Brainstem Implants

10.2.1 Magnetic Translational Force and Torque

An object containing ferromagnetic components is subject to the extremely powerful magnetic attractive forces found in clinical MRIs. Ferromagnetic objects inadvertently brought into the scan room may become dangerous projectiles, which can result in injury or death.[3] Implanted devices containing ferromagnetic

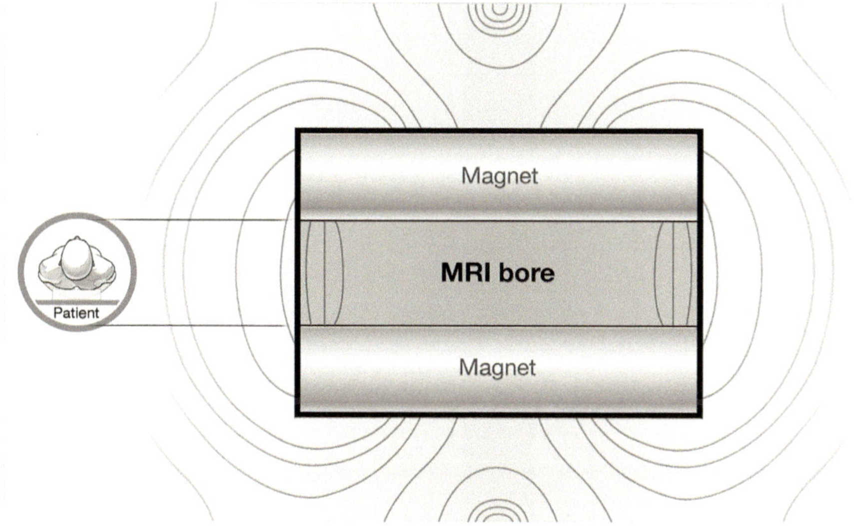

Fig. 10.3 Field lines of the static magnetic field. The magnetic field becomes increasingly strong as one approaches the mouth of the magnet.

components are subject to these same forces, including CIs and ABIs, especially those with an associated implanted magnet. The major effects exerted by the main magnetic field on ferromagnetic objects are translational forces and torque.

Translational force on a ferromagnetic object increases as a function of the field strength of the magnet, the amount of ferromagnetic material, the object's dimensions, and the gradient of the magnetic field strength at its position relative to the magnet. While the magnetic field is most powerful at isocenter within the magnet bore, it is the magnetic gradient, the difference in magnetic force per unit distance (known as spatial gradient magnetic field) that imparts the forces leading to translational force.[4] The spatial gradient magnetic field is different from the time-varying, gradient magnetic fields that are produced by gradient coils used to encode the position of the MRI signals. The largest magnetic spatial gradients are typically near the bore opening, and passing through this region imparts the greatest relative change in force on an object with ferromagnetic components as the distance changes (▶ Fig. 10.3). As a result, a patient with a ferromagnetic implant is at greatest risk for dislodgement of an object as they enter into and exit from a magnet bore. Hence, it is important to use a slow table speed as a patient with a ferromagnetic implant is put into and removed from the MRI. Contemporary MRIs in clinical use are electrically shielded, which minimizes the magnetic field outside the magnet. As a result, the magnetic field does not increase linearly as a patient approaches the magnet; it increases rapidly over a short distance, contributing to a high spatial gradient magnetic field. It is also valuable to recognize that Lenz's forces are also exerted when a *conductive* metal, including nonferromagnetic metals such as aluminum, develops magnetic field eddy currents when in powerful magnetic fields. Lenz's forces are greatest at the mouth of the magnet, where the spatial magnetic field gradient is highest, and tend to produce resistance opposite to the direction of motion. Patients with CIs and ABIs should avoid changing position while near the mouth of the magnet to reduce additional forces of the implant.

Torque, or the tendency for the magnetic moment of an object to align with the MRI magnetic field, is dependent on the square of the MRI magnetic field. Thus, the torque on the small internal magnet of the CI or ABI will be highest when at the center of the scanner bore.

10.2.2 Gradient Effects

Gradient systems tend to be relatively minor as they relate to CIs and ABIs. Generated eddy currents can contribute to heating of the device case (generally minor) as well as Lenz's effects, and current loops in device internal circuitry can have signals induced by the changing magnetic field, altering device output. In some situations in which an implanted electronic device is still functional in the MRI, as with cardiac pacemakers when a specific pacing rate is desired in a patient, the electronic circuitry can rarely become confused by unexpected signals, resulting in its returning to a baseline default mode ("power-on-reset").[5] As the external processors of CIs and ABIs are removed prior to entering the MRI suite and the device is not on, situations such as power-on-resets are not a factor.

10.2.3 Radiofrequency Effects and Risks of Possible Thermal Injuries and Burns

Patients can be burned by skin contacting or being in close apposition to the magnet bore, or coming too close to the body transmit coil. Currents within the body are induced by RF fields, and in a patient lying in the bore, skin to skin contact such as when inner thighs touch can result in burns if a conductive loop is formed. Similarly, in electronic implanted devices such as CIs and ABIs, RF induced currents could produce localized significant heating particularly in their lead systems due to their length and its relationship with RF wavelength and deposited energy by the antenna effect. As part of the MR conditions, the manufacturer typically provides a description of anticipated heating with the particular device, and may impose limits on the RF deposition used for the MRI study.

10.3 MRI Protocols and Safety Guidelines for CI Imaging

10.3.1 Current Food and Drug Administration Guidelines

United States FDA guidelines for conditional MR imaging in CI recipients is model-specific and continues to evolve with time.

Table 10.1 U.S. FDA approval for MRI conditional scanning of cochlear implants

Advanced Bionics (HiRes Ultra 3D)	Cochlear (Nucleus Profile and Freedom)	MED-EL (Synchrony)
United States FDA approved for 1.5 or 3.0 tesla with magnet in place	United States 1.5 tesla with internal magnet **in place**[a] 3.0 tesla with internal magnet **removed**	United States FDA approved for 1.5 or 3.0 tesla with magnet **in place**

[a]Requires specific bandaging protocol by manufacturer.
Note: MR conditions are model specific, and each model should be verified with the manufacturer for the associated MR conditions for safe scanning.

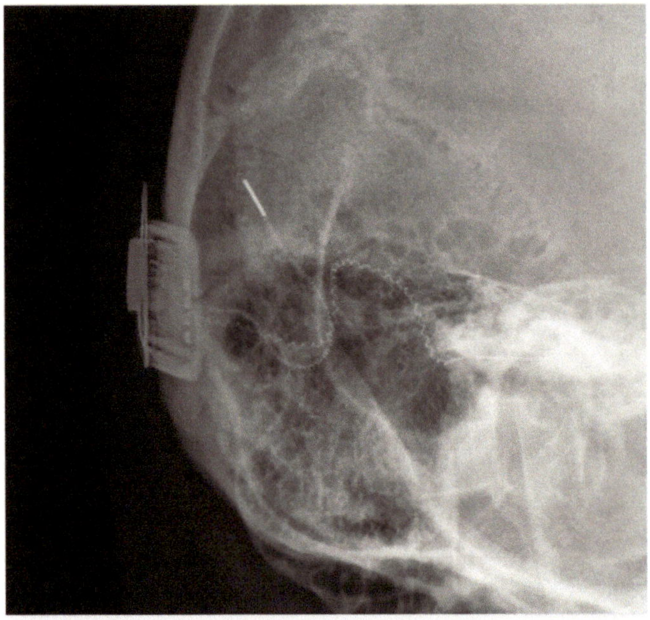

Fig. 10.4 Oblique plain film X-ray demonstrating the internal magnet in parallel with the internal RF coil wires, suggesting that the magnet is seated properly.

A summary of current FDA labeling for static magnetic field strength for modern CI devices is provided in ▶ Table 10.1. Additional MR conditions for gradient and RF effects may be periodically updated with the FDA; the most current MRI conditions from the manufacturer should always be consulted prior to any MRI exam. Beyond the static magnetic field strength guidelines, several notable differences between recent models and device manufacturers deserve mention. All three FDA-approved CI manufacturers currently employ a removable disc magnet system. The advantage of this arrangement is the flexibility to remove the internal magnet if needed to reduce, but not resolve, MR image degradation. As discussed earlier, magnet removal with replacement after imaging has some notable drawbacks and is not without risks including device contamination and infection, requirement for additional local or general anesthetics, and a period of non-use while the surgical site heals. Additionally, repetitive removal may result in material fatigue of the magnet flange, leading to an increased risk of spontaneous or MRI-associated displacement. Historically, all MED-EL devices have utilized a nonremovable internal magnet. This system does not permit magnet removal for artifact reduction; however, since the magnet is more firmly fixed within the receiver-stimulator housing, the risk of magnet displacement is reduced. In 2014, the SYNCHRONY CI system was released by MED-EL that contains an internal rotatable, self-aligning removable magnet designed to effectively reduce torque and associated discomfort. This new system includes a conical disc magnet that is removed from the underside of the implant, in order to reduce the probability of implant movement or displacement. Subsequently, in 2018, Advanced Bionics introduced the HiRes Ultra 3D implant that also contains a rotating, self-aligning magnet in order to reduce artifact, discomfort with scanning, and minimize risk of MRI-associated complications. Since these new systems were only released recently, there is little published data regarding the benefit over conventional magnet systems. Anecdotally, the authors have noticed a significant improvement in patient tolerance and comfort with these new systems.

10.3.2 Technique and Clinical Considerations

At the authors' center, a safety protocol has been established for performing MRI in patients with CIs or ABIs when a magnet is in place. All imaging studies are performed under the supervision of a radiologist, medical physicist, and otolaryngologist in order to improve patient tolerance, reduce procedural risks, and maximize imaging quality. Patients are routinely counseled regarding the potential for discomfort at the implant site, magnet migration, the very low risk of device malfunction, as well as the alternative of magnet removal before MRI. After informed consent and depending on the type of implanted magnet, an otolaryngologist applies a snug headwrap prior to MRI. We have found that a rigid unmolded 2 × 2 inch Aquaplast (Patterson Medical, Warrenville, IL) sheet with a single layer of Microfoam Surgical Tape (3 M Health Care, St. Paul, MN) placed directly over the receiver-stimulator followed by several layers of Kerlix Gauze (Covidien, Mansfield, MA) and a Coban Self-Adherent dressing provides an optimal balance of magnet immobilization and padding. Other groups have used similar card-like substrates or putty with good success. The primary goal of the headwrap is not to prevent device migration; rather it is mainly to counteract magnet canting or dislodgement. Thus, any bit of additional padding over the receiver-stimulator device results in undesirable "play," and greater risk of magnet movement.

Depending on patient tolerance, a local anesthetic block of the greater and lesser occipital nerves can be performed to reduce discomfort, utilizing a subcutaneous injection of 2% lidocaine several centimeters posteroinferior to the device. Injection directly over the device may create a potential space for magnet movement to occur and may risk bacterial seeding of the device, and therefore should be avoided. Additionally, an oral benzodiazepine is offered to patients with excessive anxiety or claustrophobia. After the MRI study is complete, the headwrap is removed and the scalp is examined to ensure no overlying pressure injury has occurred and that the magnet is flush with the CI receiver coil housing. Finally, the external coil is coupled to the device to ensure proper magnet alignment and functionality. In most cases, a dislodged magnet can be

Table 10.2 Studies including a minimum of 10 cochlear implant recipients undergoing 1.5–3 T MRI with internal cochlear implant magnet in place

Author (year)	CI ± ABI	No. of patients	No. of cases	MRI strength	No. of intolerant	Magnet canter or flip	CI malfunction	Inadequate head imaging from artifact
Crane et al (2010)	CI	16	22	1.5 T	1 of 16 (6%)	1 of 22[a] (5%)	0	1 of 16
Walton et al (2014)	CI + ABI	13	76	1.5 T	2 of 13 (15%)	1 of 76 (1%)	0	1 of 40
Kim et al (2015)	CI	18	30	1.5 T + 3 T	5 of 18 (28%)	2 of 30 (7%)	0	NR
Carlson et al (2015)	CI	16	34	1.5 T	2 of 16 (13%)	5 of 34 (15%)	0	1 of 18
Young et al (2016)	CI	11	13	1.5 T	NA[b]	4 of 13 (31%)	0	"All but 1 useful"

Abbreviations: ABI, auditory brainstem implant; CI, cochlear implant; NA, not available.
[a]Bilateral implants, both implants, implants with polarity reversal.
[b]All but one patient underwent sedation or general anesthesia from outset.

detected on physical exam, but in patients with thick subcutaneous tissue or bulky temporalis muscle it may be difficult to immediately identify. If there is suspicion for magnet rotation or canter, plain film X-ray should be obtained to further investigate position (▶ Fig. 10.4).

10.3.3 Surgical Considerations

While a detailed outline of surgical technique for CI is beyond the scope of this chapter, there are several considerations worth discussion. If repeat MR imaging is anticipated, for example in the case of tumor surveillance for NF2, it may be advantageous to position the internal receiver-stimulator device away from the region of interest to reduce problematic imaging artifact. In the authors' practice, we have found that placing the internal device more posterosuperior than what is typical draws the artifact away from the internal auditory canal. In a recent study, Todt et al analyzed optimal receiver-stimulator device position with respect to minimizing artifact at the internal auditory canal and labyrinth with 3-tesla MRI.[6] They found that a more posterior and horizontal position was advantageous. More recently, Sharon et al demonstrated that distance from the external auditory canal was significantly correlated with average image grade of view, while the angle between the nasion, external auditory canal, and magnet was not.[7] The second consideration is the theoretical risk of catastrophic injury in cases where the internal device is recessed in a bony well to the level of the dura, particularly in children. The authors are not aware of any cases to date where dura or parenchymal brain injury has occurred from device movement during MRI; however, delayed cerebrospinal fluid collection has been reported in children after standard CI utilizing a bony well.[8] Notably, thickness of adjacent bony skull is included in the MR conditions for certain CI models. A final consideration is the use of tight subperiosteal pocket technique, and the concern for whole device migration. It is feasible that early postoperative MR scanning may increase the risk of device migration, where a scar capsule has not yet healed around the device. In cases where a well and suture fixation is not performed, we commonly wait 2 or 3 months before obtaining the first MRI, unless there are strong clinical indications to undertake earlier imaging.

10.4 Adverse Events and Management

Fortunately, the prevalence of adverse events with MR imaging in CI recipients is low when performed by an experienced team in a controlled setting. The great majority of complications are associated with patient intolerance or discomfort, while less commonly, magnet canter, flip, or magnet polarity reversal may occur. While device malfunction and heating are theoretical risks, these events are evidently very rare based on published accounts in the literature. The risk of magnet displacement may be higher in patients who have had their magnet repeatedly removed and replaced for imaging, as this may cause fatigue and small tears in the silicone flange.[1] A summary of adverse events from previous published series having a minimum of 10 cases is reported in ▶ Table 10.2.

In many cases, patient anxiety, discomfort, and pain can be minimized through simple measures such as careful counseling prior to imaging, use of local anesthetic block, a snug but not overly tight headwrap, and use of an anxiolytic as outlined earlier. Additionally, providing a short break between studies for patients requiring several sequential scans, of the spine and head for example, may improve overall tolerance. For patients who require MR imaging but cannot tolerate the study with the magnet in place, traditional magnet removal can be considered. Alternatively, careful MR imaging of the patient while under general anesthesia is another option. Of course in the latter scenario, the patient will be unable to provide potentially important feedback regarding discomfort —a symptom that may indicate an impending or evolving adverse event.[9]

Several studies have demonstrated that use of a snug headwrap after placing a flat rigid platform directly over the magnet reduces internal magnet movement and risk of displacement. Different device manufactures provide various recommendations for headwrap application before MRI. Following the MRI study, if the magnet site appears proud or associated with raised somewhat inflamed appearing tissue, or if there is overlying redness, discomfort, or poor coupling with the external magnet, then internal magnet canter or displacement should be suspected. If clinical examination findings are inconclusive,

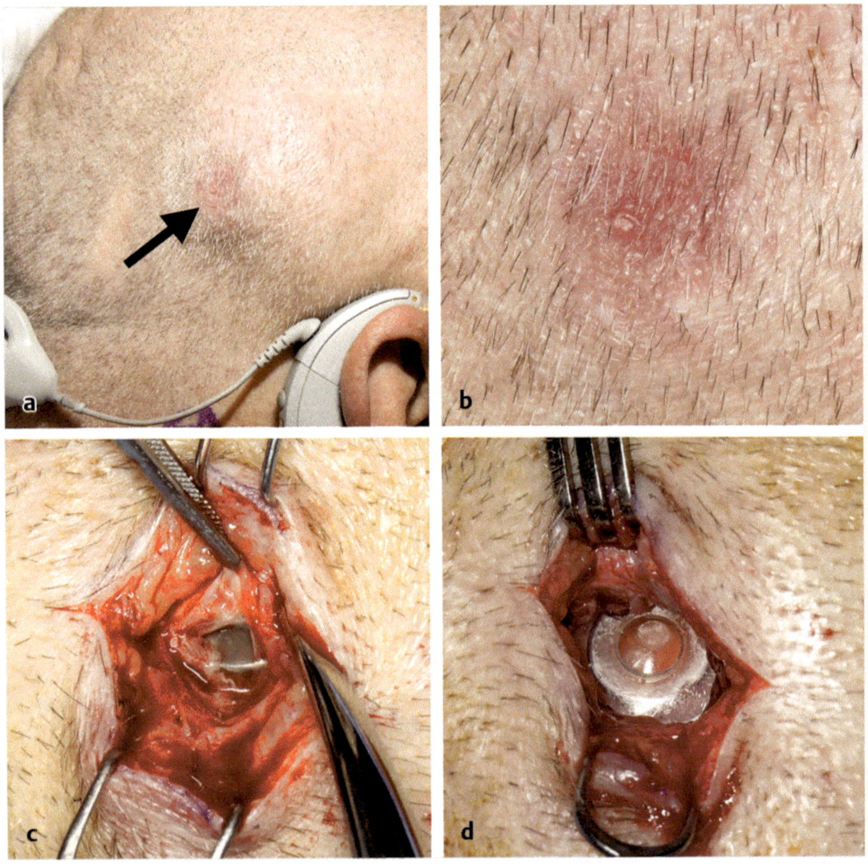

Fig. 10.5 (**a, b**), Adult man with NF2 and bilateral CIs who underwent 1.5-T MRI 5 months earlier and presented with focal discomfort and erythema (*arrow* in **a**) over the right CI site. **(c)** Under local anesthesia, a small linear incision was made and the implanted magnet was found adjacent to the silicone housing and flipped nearly 180 degrees; note the absence of a "star" on the face of the magnet used to mark correct orientation. **(d)** The magnet flange of the implanted device was found intact. (Used with permission from Carlson et al.[1])

secondary to thick subcutaneous tissue or temporalis muscle, then plain film X-ray can be used to further interrogate magnet seating. If the polarity of the internal magnet is completely reversed, the external magnet polarity can be flipped to restore device coupling.[10,11] However, if the internal magnet is not properly seated, there is a risk for soft-tissue complications over time[1] (▶ Fig. 10.5). While rare, loss of magnet strength has also been reported.[1] These cases can often be managed by simply increasing the magnet strength of the external magnet to improve coupling. If magnet canter is identified, it is possible that one edge of the magnet remains seated under the silicone flange and gentle manual pressure may "externally reduce" the magnet back into the silicone sleeve. We have successfully employed this technique in several patients. However, if this maneuver is unsuccessful, a default to surgical reseating of the magnet is required to reduce risk of later soft-tissue complications.[1]

10.5 MRI Scanning Protocol and Artifact Reduction Techniques

When an MRI exam is ordered, the radiologist and ordering clinician should consider alternate non-MRI imaging modalities that may answer the clinical question without the effort, inconvenience, and expense of conducting an MRI exam with the CI or ABI in place. For instance, musculoskeletal injuries may best be initially evaluated with ultrasound. In some settings, CT could serve as a viable alternative to MRI.

When MRI is required, the clinician and radiologist should expect significant artifact for intracranial exams. Artifacts manifest from the implanted magnet, causing off-resonance distortion and signal loss, as well as signal loss from implants that do not have a magnet in place (▶ Fig. 10.6). The artifact extends a greater distance from an implant with an internal magnet than one without. Pathology near the magnet may not be completely visualized, depending on the severity of the artifact and proximity to the device. It is notable that different planar views and different sequences will often exhibit varying degrees of artifact severity. In many cases, the radiologist and the clinician may be able to evaluate the area of interest simply by switching to coronal images, rather than axial images (▶ Fig. 10.7), or from contrast-enhanced T1-weighted images to FSE T2-weighted sequences, for example (▶ Fig. 10.8). As mentioned earlier, it is also advantageous to strategically place the receiver-stimulator further away from the area of interest in cases where serial imaging is anticipated (▶ Fig. 10.9).

Depending on the imaging technique used, there are various techniques to reduce the location or extent of the artifact. In general, special prescan tuning of the MRI scanner can be used to reduce the artifact, using the signal away from the implant to tune specifically to the tissue.[12] Adjusting the tuning may also shift the artifact away from the region of interest. Advanced scanning techniques, such as those used to image tissue near metallic implants, may also be helpful. Metal artifact reduction

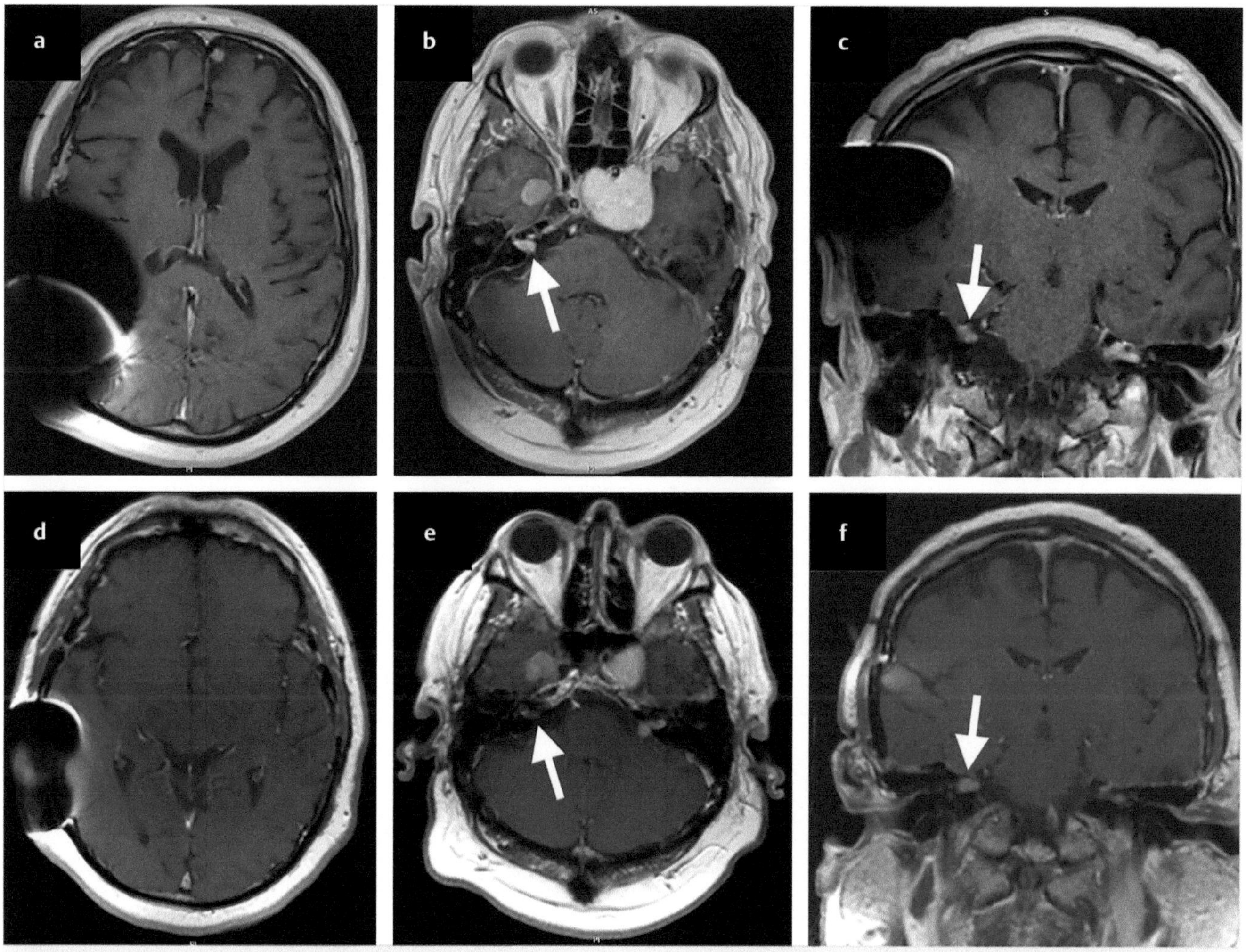

Fig. 10.6 Comparison of MRI imaging artifact with (ABC) and without (DEF) the internal magnet in place. Contrast-enhanced T1-weighted axial images (**a** and **d**) at the level of maximum image distortion demonstrate less ferromagnetic artifact with the internal magnet removed. Contrast-enhanced T1-weighted axial (**b** and **e**) and coronal (**c** and **f**) images demonstrate adequate visualization of the ipsilateral IAC (*arrows*) in both cases despite adjacent ferromagnetic artifact from the CI. Figures **b** and **e** are far enough from the magnet that both do not demonstrate significant artifact. (Used with permission from Carlson et al.[1])

scan techniques (e.g., MAVRIC or SEMAC) are commercially available[13] (▶ Fig. 10.10). Alternate data acquisition strategies such as PROPELLER or BLADE are more robust than echo planar imaging techniques that are typically used for diffusion-weighted imaging and can prove advantageous in the presence of the CI or ABI (▶ Fig. 10.11). Fat saturation techniques are extremely useful in identifying enhancing lesions near the skull base, particularly after placement of an abdominal fat graft. Improved visualization can sometimes be achieved with three-point Dixon techniques (▶ Fig. 10.12).

Artifacts may also originate from image-processing routines that rely on a calibration scan, such as parallel imaging. The calibration scan is typically a very fast measurement of the relative signal specific to each coil element within a particular imaging coil to help with encoding the position of the MR signal. The short, gradient echo scan will be very degraded by the presence of the implant. Thus, accelerated/parallel imaging and surface coil intensity corrections such as PURE, CLEAR, or Prescan Normalization should be avoided during the exam.

For implants that have MR conditions limiting the RF deposition below the normal mode operation of the MRI scanner, many of the techniques to reduce magnetic field artifacts tend to be RF intensive. The scanning technologist and associated personnel should be diligent in monitoring the RF deposition while making any significant changes to the typical scan protocol.

Given the artifacts induced by the device and the necessity for a properly trained MRI technologist to understand the required MR conditions, a facility should have a protocol and

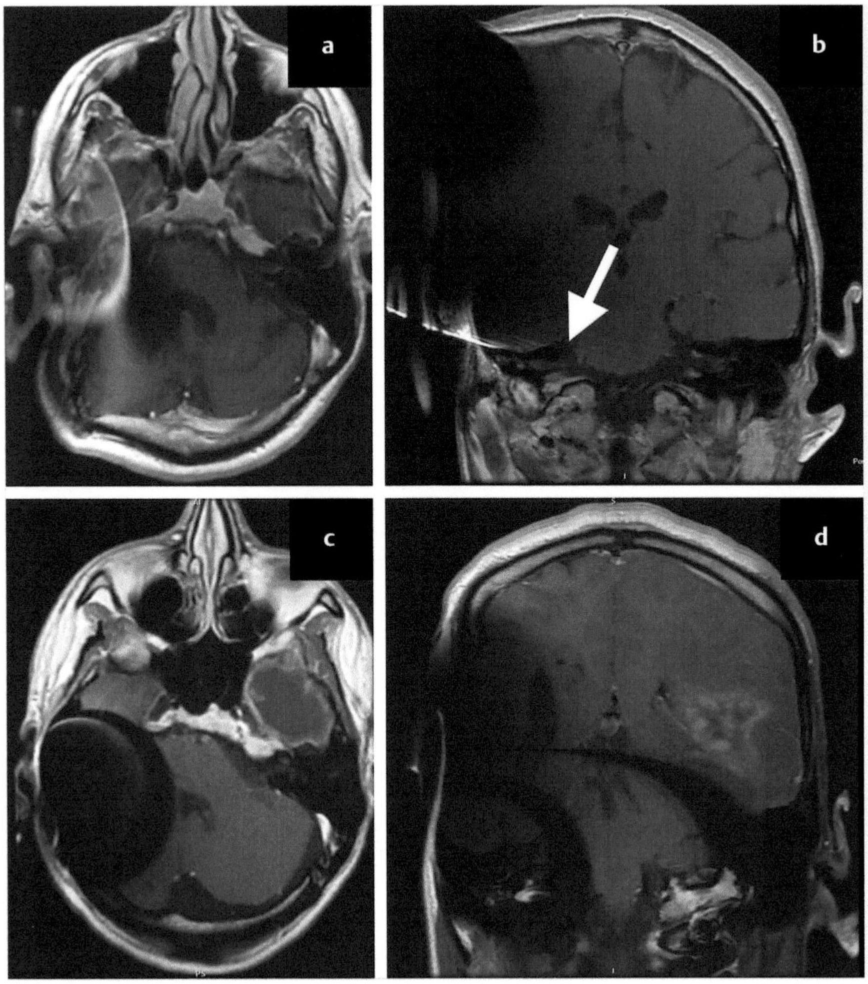

Fig. 10.7 Contrast-enhanced T1-weighted axial (a) and coronal (b) images in a patient with a right internal CI magnet in place, illustrating moderate distortion of the right skull base. It is difficult to delineate the right IAC on the axial view; however, coronal orientation offers improved visualization (*arrow*). Axial (c) and coronal (d) T1-weighted images illustrating a case of severe imaging artifact. In this case, the ipsilateral IAC could not be fully visualized, regardless of imaging sequence. (Used with permission from Carlson et al.[1])

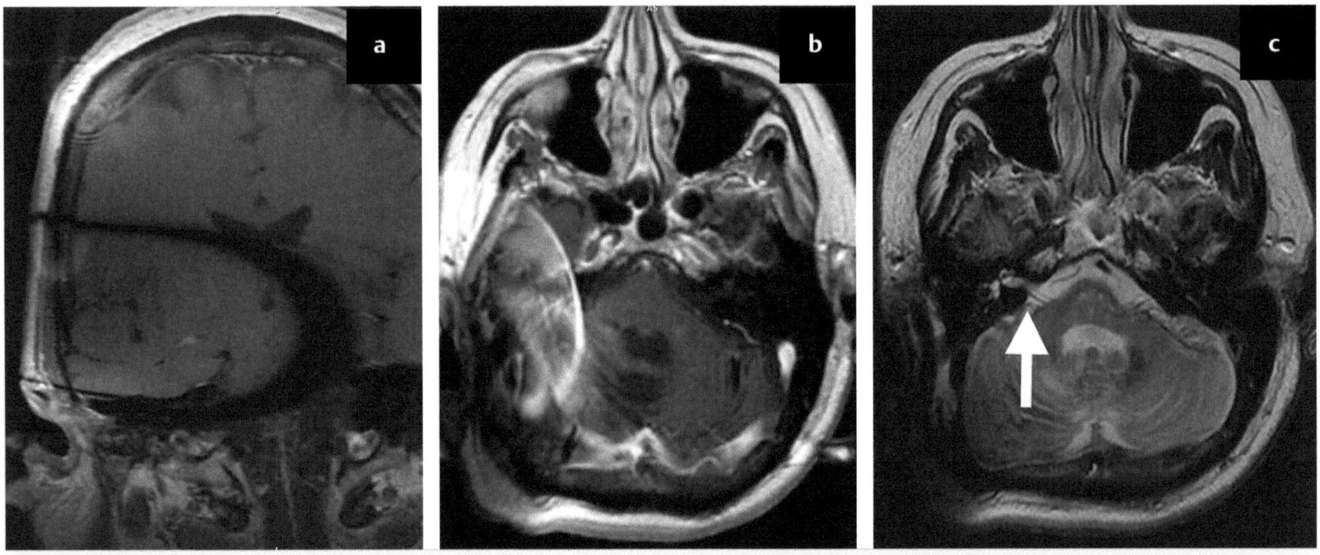

Fig. 10.8 Contrast-enhanced T1-weighted coronal (a) and axial (b) images demonstrating significant degradation of the right IAC by internal magnet artifact. (c) Axial FSE T2-weighted MRI in the same patient provided an unimpeded view of the ipsilateral IAC and CPA (*arrow*). (Used with permission from Carlson et al.[1])

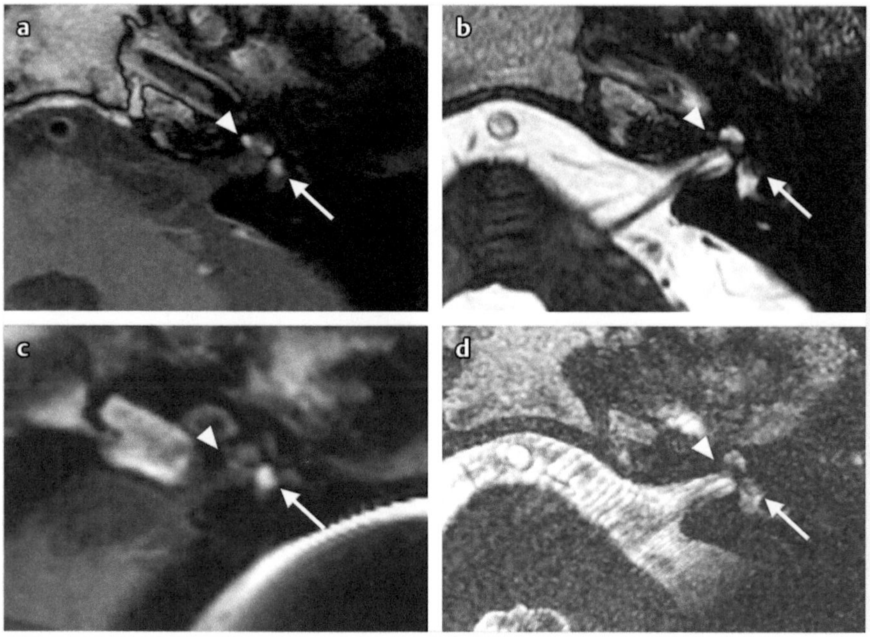

Fig. 10.9 Gadolinium-enhanced axial T1-weighted (**a**) and T2-weighted MRI (**b**) demonstrating a left-sided intralabyrinthine schwannoma. (**c** and **d**) Similar sequences after left-sided cochlear implantation. Note that despite imaging artifact, the ipsilateral inner ear and skull base can be adequately visualized (*white arrowhead* = intracochlear tumor component, *white arrow* = intravestibular tumor component). (Used with permission from Carlson et al.[1])

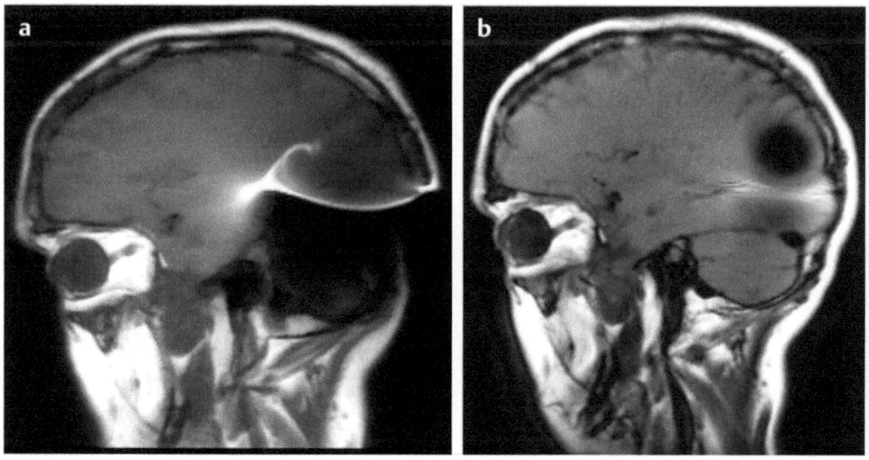

Fig. 10.10 Comparison of MRI imaging artifact without (**a**) and with (**b**) a metal artifact reduction scan technique (MAVRIC). ▶ Fig. 10.10**a** is a standard sagittal T1 spin echo image; ▶ Fig. 10.10**b**, with MAVRIC, demonstrates greater visualization of brain anatomy and substantially less artifact.

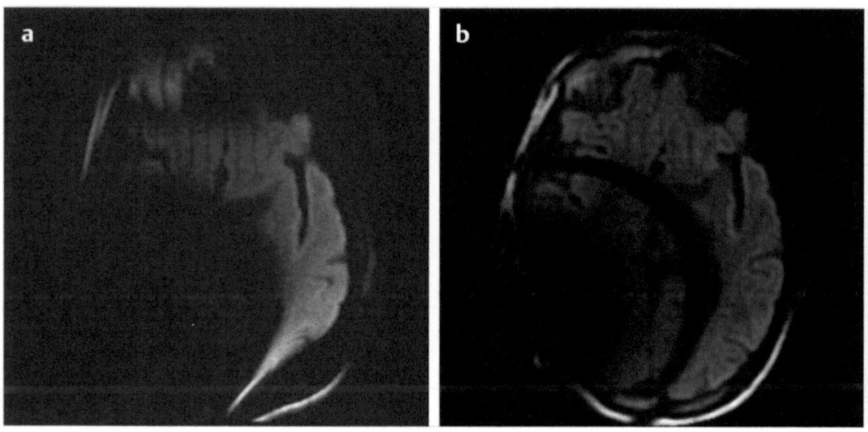

Fig. 10.11 Comparison of MRI imaging artifact with echo planar (**a**) and PROPELLER (**b**) technique in diffusion-weighted imaging (trace diffusion image). Note the significantly improved visualization of brain anatomy using PROPELLER technique.

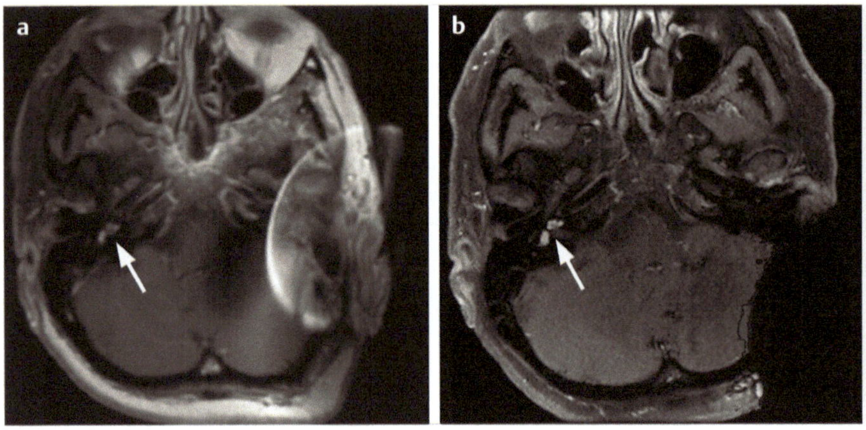

Fig. 10.12 Comparison of MRI imaging artifact with conventional fat saturation (**a**) and with three-point Dixon technique and localized shimming (**b**). Note the decreased artifact and conspicuity of enhancing right inner ear structures (*arrows*) with the Dixon technique.

plan to provide MR imaging services for patients with CIs and ABIs, and be prepared to refer to an alternate facility if unprepared for the technical challenges associated with these exams. Specifically, the MR facility should be familiar with imaging protocol modifications necessary to limit RF deposition, and also be prepared to address image artifacts for intracranial exams.

10.6 Conclusion

When performed under controlled conditions by an experienced team, 1.5-T MRI can be successfully carried out in most patients without the need for CI or ABI magnet removal. With scan sequence optimization, device-related artifact does not usually impede successful clinical imaging. Patients should be counseled regarding the risk of internal magnet movement that may occur in up to 15% of cases, even with headwrap application. If mild displacement of the internal magnet occurs, an attempt at reseating can be made by applying gentle firm pressure to the scalp over the internal magnet. If conservative measures fail, the magnet should be surgically repositioned to prevent scalp complications.

References

[1] Carlson ML, Neff BA, Link MJ, et al. Magnetic resonance imaging with cochlear implant magnet in place: safety and imaging quality. Otol Neurotol. 2015; 36 (6):965–971

[2] Carlson ML, Breen JT, Driscoll CL, et al. Cochlear implantation in patients with neurofibromatosis type 2: variables affecting auditory performance. Otol Neurotol. 2012; 33(5):853–862

[3] Landrigan C. Preventable deaths and injuries during magnetic resonance imaging. N Engl J Med. 2001; 345(13):1000–1001

[4] Shellock FG, Kanal E, Gilk TB. Regarding the value reported for the term "spatial gradient magnetic field" and how this information is applied to labeling of medical implants and devices. AJR Am J Roentgenol. 2011; 196(1): 142–145

[5] Higgins JV, Sheldon SH, Watson RE, Jr, et al. "Power-on resets" in cardiac implantable electronic devices during magnetic resonance imaging. Heart Rhythm. 2015; 12(3):540–544

[6] Todt I, Rademacher G, Mittmann P, Wagner J, Mutze S, Ernst A. MRI artifacts and cochlear implant positioning at 3 T in vivo. Otol Neurotol. 2015; 36(6): 972–976

[7] Sharon JD, Northcutt BG, Aygun N, Francis HW. Magnetic resonance imaging at 1.5 tesla with a cochlear implant magnet in place: image quality and usability. Otol Neurotol. 2016; 37(9):1284–1290

[8] Horton JD, Friedmann DR, Roland JT, Jr. Delayed extradural CSF collection following pediatric cochlear implantation: report of two cases. Otol Neurotol. 2016; 37(6):654–657

[9] Kim BG, Kim JW, Park JJ, Kim SH, Kim HN, Choi JY. Adverse events and discomfort during magnetic resonance imaging in cochlear implant recipients. JAMA Otolaryngol Head Neck Surg. 2015; 141(1):45–52

[10] Young NM, Rojas C, Deng J, Burrowes D, Ryan M. Magnetic resonance imaging of cochlear implant recipients. Otol Neurotol. 2016; 37(6):665–671

[11] Crane BT, Gottschalk B, Kraut M, Aygun N, Niparko JK. Magnetic resonance imaging at 1.5 T after cochlear implantation. Otol Neurotol. 2010; 31(8): 1215–1220

[12] Holz D, Jensen D, Proksa R, Tochtrop M, Vollmann W. Automatic shimming for localized spectroscopy. Med Phys. 1988; 15(6):898–903

[13] Edmonson HA, Carlson ML, Patton AC, Watson RE. MR Imaging and Cochlear Implants with Retained Internal Magnets: Reducing Artifacts near Highly Inhomogeneous Magnetic Fields. Radiographics 2018, 38(1): 94-106

Part III

Management: Overview

III

11 Current Trends in Vestibular Schwannoma Management

Ramsey Ashour, Harry van Loveren, and Siviero Agazzi

11.1 Introduction

Vestibular schwannoma (VS) management has evolved considerably since the first postmortem descriptions of this tumor in the late 18th century. Contemporary management options include observation, stereotactic radiosurgery or radiotherapy, and microsurgical removal. For each case, a variety of important factors influence the management strategy, including patient age and medical condition, tumor size, extent of hearing loss, patient preference, treating provider bias, and others. Overall trends have been driven by technological advances (i.e., operating microscope, magnetic resonance imaging [MRI], radiosurgery) that allow for safer and more effective treatment, improved disease detection resulting in smaller tumor size at the time of diagnosis, recent data on natural history demonstrating relatively low rates of tumor growth over time without treatment, and reduced tolerance of posttreatment morbidity. In this chapter, we review the evolution of VS management. Further discussion regarding the early developments and refinement of VS surgery and stereotactic radiation delivery are described in Chapters 1 and 2, respectively.

11.2 Microsurgery

The introduction of the operating room microscope and microsurgical techniques in the second half of the 20th century revolutionized intracranial and skull base surgery, and VS surgery in particular. The pioneering work of William House and William Hitselberger led to the popularization of the middle fossa and translabyrinthine microsurgical approaches and eventually to the development of the combined neurotology/neurosurgery skull base team that persists today.[1,2] Improvements in imaging (i.e., computed tomography [CT] and later MRI), audiologic testing, and neuromonitoring (e.g., facial and cochlear) facilitated timely and precise diagnosis, improved the safety of surgery, and allowed curative tumor resection to become a realistic treatment goal in most cases. Facial nerve preservation became the rule rather than the exception, and serious perioperative morbidity and mortality were dramatically reduced. By the early 1990s, in light of these improved results, microsurgical removal became the predominant VS management strategy. As reflected in the *National Institutes of Health 1991 Consensus Statement*,[3] the recommendation was surgery for all patients able and willing to undergo an operation, leaving observation and radiosurgery for those patients who were unwilling or deemed unable to tolerate surgery.

While scattered reports of successful hearing preservation were reported decades earlier, proactive microsurgery for attempted hearing preservation has arguably only been mainstream since the 1990s. Early detection in the MRI era has resulted in smaller tumor size at the time of diagnosis, which has further encouraged focus on the development of hearing preservation surgery techniques and monitoring technologies. This trend is clearly demonstrated by the increased use of the middle fossa and retrosigmoid approaches and decreased use of the translabyrinthine approach, comparing Acoustic Neuroma Association (ANA) surveys published in 1983 and 1998.[4] Furthermore, at the House Ear Clinic between 1992 and 1998, 45% of all surgical cases for VS were performed via the middle fossa approach,[5] whereas only 3.4% of cases were treated via middle fossa approach between 1968 and 1975 at the same institution.[6] More recently, similar comparison between the 1998 and 2008 ANA surveys again demonstrated a trend toward increased use of the middle fossa approach for small and medium size tumors, reflecting continued enthusiasm for hearing preservation surgery.[7]

11.3 Radiosurgery

As with microsurgical techniques, stereotactic radiosurgery similarly arose in the second half of the 20th century, in part, from a need to reduce the high rates of morbidity and mortality seen with surgical resection. In 1969, Lars Leksell first performed radiosurgery for VS at the Karolinska Institute in Sweden.[8] The early radiosurgery experience of the Karolinska group, performed on the basis of CT, metrizamide cisternography, or pneumoencephalography, demonstrated tumor control in 12 (86%) of 14 consecutive patients, with facial weakness in 5 (36%) and facial numbness in 2 (14%) patients.[9] Further advances in radiosurgery included the introduction of MRI, improvements in dose planning software, and reduction in the radiation dose to the margin of the tumor. By the early 1990s, these developments led to better tumor growth control results (> 95%) and lower rates of facial (< 10%) and trigeminal (< 10%) neuropathies.[10] With an increasing priority placed on hearing preservation, we have witnessed a shift toward continued marginal dose reduction and employment of cochlear shielding strategies. Currently, many centers utilize a marginal dose of 12 Gy in patients with pretreatment serviceable hearing. Additionally, the concept of limiting cochlear dose has become popular, since there are data to support that patients who receive greater than approximately 4 Gy to the modiolus are at increased risk for progression to nonserviceable hearing. This trend in dose reduction will likely continue in effort to elucidate the perfect balance between reliable tumor control and optimal long-term hearing outcomes.

As the availability of radiosurgical units was increasing, more data were emerging to support its safety and effectiveness, thus providing a rationale for its exponential increase. In 1998, Pollock et al predicted that equal numbers of VS patients in the United States would undergo radiosurgery and surgical resection between 2005 and 2010, and that more than two-thirds of patients would undergo radiosurgery by 2020.[11] While these predictions were not ultimately realized secondary to an apparent recent plateau in use, radiosurgery's increasing popularity since the time of its inception marks a notable paradigm shift in VS management. Specifically, radiosurgery has emerged as a viable and accepted alternative to surgery, even in young healthy patients, and is no longer considered merely a second option for elderly or unhealthy patients.

11.4 Observation and Natural History

During the 1990s and early 2000s, the vast majority of VS patients were offered some form of active treatment, either surgery or radiosurgery, whereas observation was generally reserved for elderly patients with small tumors. However, with a growing number of younger patients being diagnosed with smaller VSs and good hearing, the issue of tumor behavior and growth became increasingly relevant in terms of management strategy. Specifically, patients and clinicians alike began questioning the need for upfront treatment of small, asymptomatic or minimally symptomatic tumors, since intervention was unlikely to improve symptoms or quality of life.

Early studies evaluating the natural history of untreated VSs were generally limited by selection biases and short follow-up time, but some evidence encouraged treatment rather than observation. For example, in one study, a "wait and scan" approach revealed tumor growth in 90 (73%) of 123 observed patients at an average rate of 3.2 mm per year; notably, 21 (75%) of 28 patients initially considered candidates for hearing preservation surgery lost their candidacy during the observation period due to tumor growth or hearing loss.[12] Nevertheless, others reported unpredictable growth patterns, including continuous growth, growth followed by regression, regression followed by growth, saltatory growth, and so forth.[13]

In the largest natural history study published to date, Stangerup et al prospectively followed 1,818 consecutive patients with sporadic unilateral VSs diagnosed between 1976 and 2004 in Denmark.[14] In a country where all VSs are referred to and managed by a single center in Copenhagen, 729 patients were allocated to observation, 552 of these having at least two scans at the time of data analysis. During an observation period of up to 15 years (mean: 3.6 years), evidence of growth was observed in only 17% of the intrameatal tumors and 29% of the extrameatal tumors. This 2006 landmark study led many providers to reconsider management of smaller tumors, resulting in renewed enthusiasm for the wait-and-scan approach and an overall trend toward observation that persists today.[15]

11.5 Future Directions in Vestibular Schwannoma Management

Contemporary studies on VS management trends continue to document the fact that microsurgery remains the most common treatment modality across all tumor size categories (▶ Table 11.1).[7,15,16,17,18,19,20,21,22] However, surgery continues to decline as radiosurgery and observation are increasingly utilized, particularly for small- to medium-sized tumors (▶ Fig. 11.1, ▶ Fig. 11.2).

Hearing preservation remains of great interest to microsurgeons and radiosurgeons alike; however, optimal management of small VS in patients with good hearing remains a fiercely debated topic with growing evidence that observation not only offers the best chance to preserve good hearing for the longest possible time but also carries the lowest risk of facial neuropathy.[23] Furthermore, recent analyses suggest that quality of life is most significantly driven by the diagnosis and patient-specific factors rather than treatment modality.[24] In most cases, the observation cohort fairs best when long-term outcomes are compared.[23,25] Therefore, based on these data, one can expect that the trend toward increasing use of observation for small- to medium-sized VS will continue into the foreseeable future.[11]

Although large tumors with brainstem compression still require surgery, an increasing number of surgeons are exploring the strategy of subtotal resection to decompress the brainstem and minimize the risk of postoperative facial neuropathy, followed by radiation to the residual (▶ Fig. 11.3).[26,27] While this particular management strategy requires further study, it reflects an emphasis on quality of life and an associated reduction in tolerance for posttreatment facial neuropathy. Both of these trends are also expected to continue in the future.

11.6 Conclusion

Vestibular schwannoma management continues to evolve. Microsurgery remains the most common treatment modality across all tumor sizes; however, its use continues to decline slowly with greater acceptance of conservative observation and stereotactic radiosurgery. Radiosurgery has increased steadily over the past two decades, but not at the exponential rate that was once predicted. Recent trends suggest that its use has plateaued in the United States. Earlier disease detection, natural history data demonstrating high rates of radiographic stability without treatment for small tumors, and reduced tolerance for posttreatment morbidity have combined to result in an increased rate of observation for small- to medium-sized tumors. Reflecting a contemporary emphasis on quality of life and avoidance of posttreatment facial neuropathy, surgeons are exploring the strategy of subtotal resection followed by radiation for large tumors with brainstem compression. These trends in conservative management can be expected to continue in the future.

Table 11.1 Contemporary management trends for vestibular schwannoma

Year	Author	Time frame	Study detail	Surgery trend	Radiosurgery trend	Observation trend	Comment
2015	Carlson et al[15]	2004–2011	SEER database retrospective analysis of 8,330 patients	Decreased	No change	Increased	Surgery correlated with younger age and larger tumor size, trend toward decreased tumor size at the time of diagnosis
2014	Ahmed et al[16]	1996–2010	CHIDD database retrospective analysis of 6,545 patients	Decreased	N/A	N/A	Annual volume of surgical cases decreased by 28.5% in spite of increasing population growth. Presumed increased use of radiosurgery/observation during the study period
2014	Patel et al[7]	1966–2008	ANA 1998 and 2008 survey responses—3,305 patients analyzed	Decreased	Increased	Increased	Trend toward decreased tumor size at the time of diagnosis
2013	Babu et al[17]	2004–2009	SEER database retrospective analysis of 6,225 patients	Decreased	Increased	Increased	African Americans significantly less likely to receive surgery than whites despite larger tumors at diagnosis
2013	Patel et al[18]	2000–2007	NIS database retrospective analysis of 14,928 patients	Decreased	N/A	N/A	41% reduction in annual rate of surgical excisions, presumably increased use of radiosurgery/observation during this period
2013	Mackeith et al[19]	1990–2010	Single-center (Oxford) retrospective analysis of 714 patients	Decreased	Increased	Unchanged	Study center was found to treat much higher percentage of patients with radiosurgery (and less with surgery) compared with rest of UK
2012	Lau et al[20]	2004–2007	SEER database retrospective analysis of 2,448 patients	Decreased	Increased	Unchanged	Significant trends toward decreased surgery and increased radiosurgery noted for tumors < 2 cm: surgery correlated with younger age and larger tumor size
2010	Tan et al[21]	1997–2007	Single-center (Johns Hopkins) retrospective analysis of 835 patients	Decreased	Increased	Increased	Surgery correlated with younger age and larger tumor size, trend of decreased tumor size at the time of diagnosis
2007	Chen[22]	1990–2005	Single-center (private) retrospective analysis of 614 patients	Decreased	Increased	Increased	Trend toward increasing age and smaller tumor size at the time of diagnosis

Abbreviations: ANA, Acoustic Neuroma Association; CHIDD, California Hospital Inpatient Discharge Database; NIS, nationwide inpatient sample; SEER, surveillance epidemiology and end results.

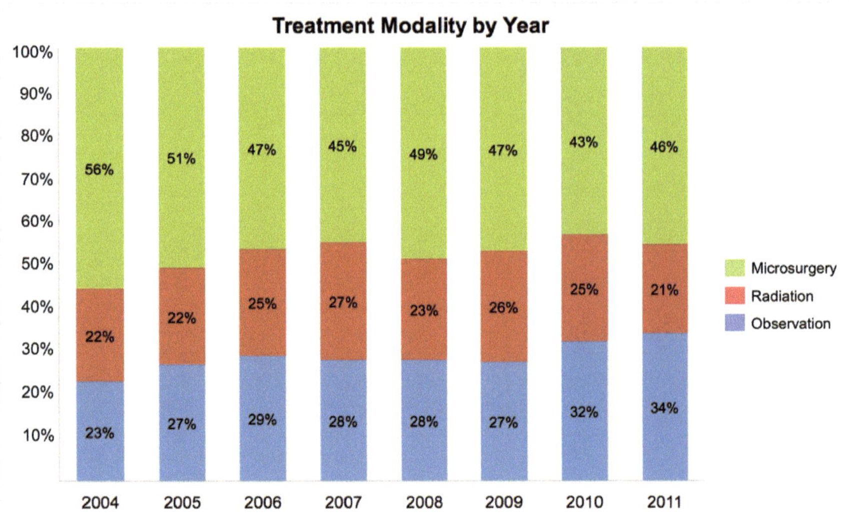

Fig. 11.1 Treatment modality by year among 8,330 patients with vestibular schwannoma (SEER Analysis, 2004–2011). (Carlson et al.[15])

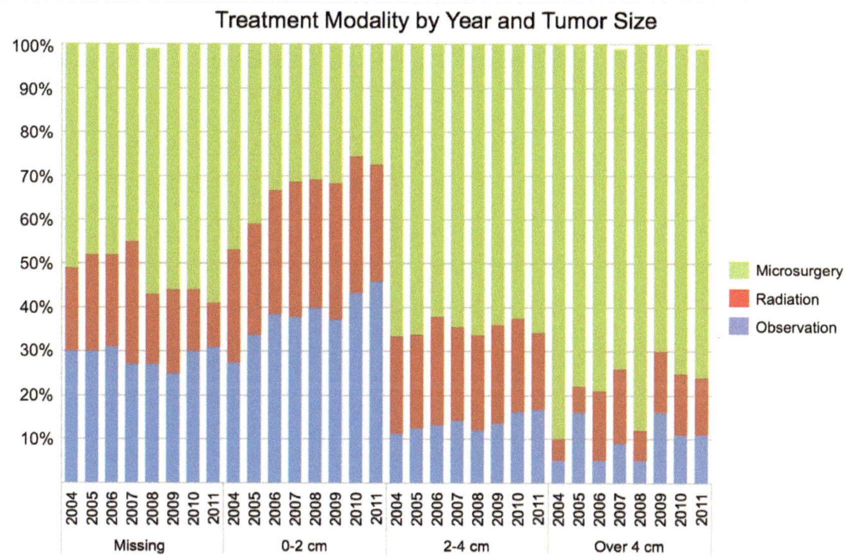

Fig. 11.2 Treatment modality by year and tumor size among 8,330 patients with vestibular schwannoma (SEER Analysis, 2004–2011). (Carlson et al.[15])

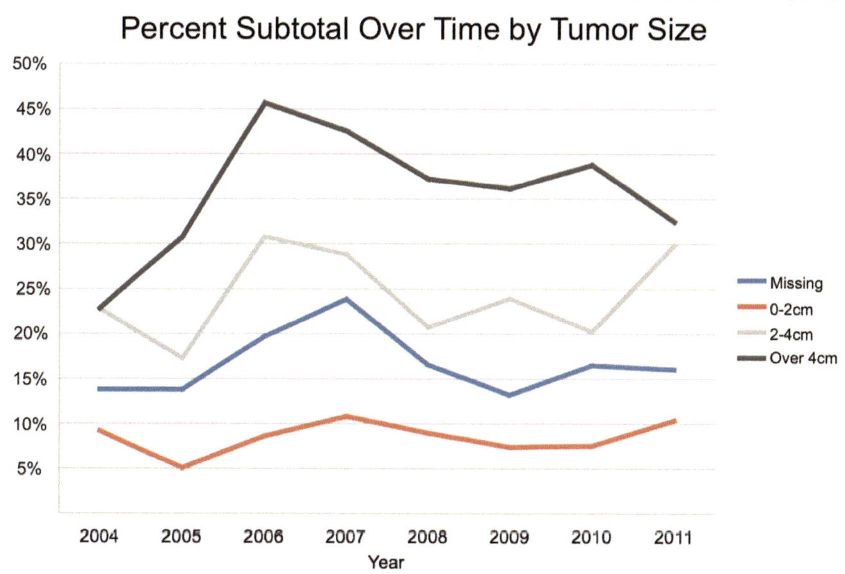

Fig. 11.3 Percentage of cases of vestibular schwannoma that received subtotal resection by year and tumor size (SEER Analysis, 2004–2011). (Carlson et al.[15])

References

[1] House WF. Surgical exposure of the internal auditory canal and its contents through the middle, cranial fossa. Laryngoscope. 1961; 71:1363–1385

[2] House WF. Transtemporal bone microsurgical removal of acoustic neuromas. Evolution of transtemporal bone removal of acoustic tumors. Arch Otolaryngol. 1964; 80:731–742

[3] Acoustic neuroma. Consensus Statement. 1991

[4] Cumming G. The Acoustic Neuroma Experience 1998. Member Survey (Patient Brochure). Acoustic Neuroma Association; 1998

[5] Brackmann DE, Owens RM, Friedman RA, et al. Prognostic factors for hearing preservation in vestibular schwannoma surgery. Am J Otol. 2000; 21(3):417–424

[6] Luetje C. Preface. In: House W, Luetje C, eds. Acoustic Tumors. Vol 1. Baltimore, MD: University Park Press; 1979:XIII–XIV

[7] Patel J, Vasan R, van Loveren H, Downes K, Agazzi S. The changing face of acoustic neuroma management in the USA: analysis of the 1998 and 2008 patient surveys from the acoustic neuroma association. Br J Neurosurg. 2014; 28(1):20–24

[8] Leksell L. A note on the treatment of acoustic tumours. Acta Chir Scand. 1971; 137(8):763–765

[9] Norén G, Arndt J, Hindmarsh T. Stereotactic radiosurgery in cases of acoustic neurinoma: further experiences. Neurosurgery. 1983; 13(1):12–22

[10] Flickinger JC, Kondziolka D, Pollock BE, Lunsford LD. Evolution in technique for vestibular schwannoma radiosurgery and effect on outcome. Int J Radiat Oncol Biol Phys. 1996; 36(2):275–280

[11] Pollock BE, Lunsford LD, Norén G. Vestibular schwannoma management in the next century: a radiosurgical perspective. Neurosurgery. 1998; 43(3): 475–481, discussion 481–483

[12] Charabi S, Thomsen J, Mantoni M, et al. Acoustic neuroma (vestibular schwannoma): growth and surgical and nonsurgical consequences of the wait-and-see policy. Otolaryngol Head Neck Surg. 1995; 113(1):5–14

[13] Shin YJ, Fraysse B, Cognard C, et al. Effectiveness of conservative management of acoustic neuromas. Am J Otol. 2000; 21(6):857–862

[14] Stangerup SE, Caye-Thomasen P, Tos M, Thomsen J. The natural history of vestibular schwannoma. Otol Neurotol. 2006; 27(4):547–552

[15] Carlson ML, Habermann EB, Wagie AE, et al. The changing landscape of vestibular schwannoma management in the United States–a shift toward conservatism. Otolaryngol Head Neck Surg. 2015; 153(3):440–446

[16] Ahmed OH, Mahboubi H, Lahham S, Pham C, Djalilian HR. Trends in demographics, charges, and outcomes of patients undergoing excision of sporadic vestibular schwannoma. Otolaryngol Head Neck Surg. 2014; 150(2):266–274

[17] Babu R, Sharma R, Bagley JH, Hatef J, Friedman AH, Adamson C. Vestibular schwannomas in the modern era: epidemiology, treatment trends, and disparities in management. J Neurosurg. 2013; 119(1):121–130

[18] Patel S, Nuño M, Mukherjee D, et al. Trends in surgical use and associated patient outcomes in the treatment of acoustic neuroma. World Neurosurg. 2013; 80(1–2):142–147

[19] Mackeith SA, Kerr RS, Milford CA. Trends in acoustic neuroma management: a 20-year review of the oxford skull base clinic. J Neurol Surg B Skull Base. 2013; 74(4):194–200

[20] Lau T, Olivera R, Miller T, Jr, et al. Paradoxical trends in the management of vestibular schwannoma in the United States. J Neurosurg. 2012; 117(3):514–519

[21] Tan M, Myrie OA, Lin FR, et al. Trends in the management of vestibular schwannomas at Johns Hopkins 1997–2007. Laryngoscope. 2010; 120(1):144–149

[22] Chen DA. Acoustic neuroma in a private neurotology practice: trends in demographics and practice patterns. Laryngoscope. 2007; 117(11): 2003–2012

[23] Carlson ML, Tveiten OV, Driscoll CL, et al. Long-term quality of life in patients with vestibular schwannoma: an international multicenter cross-sectional study comparing microsurgery, stereotactic radiosurgery, observation, and nontumor controls. J Neurosurg. 2015; 122(4):833–842

[24] Myrseth E, Møller P, Pedersen PH, Lund-Johansen M. Vestibular schwannoma: surgery or gamma knife radiosurgery? A prospective, nonrandomized study. Neurosurgery. 2009; 64(4):654–661, discussion 661–663

[25] Robinett ZN, Walz PC, Miles-Markley B, Moberly AC, Welling DB. Comparison of long-term quality-of-life outcomes in vestibular schwannoma patients. Otolaryngol Head Neck Surg. 2014; 150(6):1024–1032

[26] Monfared A, Corrales E, Theodosopoulos P, et al. Facial nerve outcome and tumor control rate as a function of degree of resection in treatment of large acoustic neuromas: preliminary report of the Acoustic Neuroma Subtotal Resection Study (ANSRS). Neurosurgery. 2016(2):194–203

[27] Schwartz MS, Kari E, Strickland BM, et al. Evaluation of the increased use of partial resection of large vestibular schwanommas: facial nerve outcomes and recurrence/regrowth rates. Otol Neurotol. 2013; 34(8): 1456–1464

12 Multidisciplinary Care of the Vestibular Schwannoma Patient: Building a Skull Base Team

Jeffrey T. Jacob, Matthew L. Carlson, Colin L. W. Driscoll, and Michael J. Link

12.1 Introduction

A strong multidisciplinary team, who shares a similar mindset in their approach to patient management, is a central component in providing optimal, comprehensive care for vestibular schwannoma (VS) patients. Establishing a multidisciplinary network of specialists within an established neurosurgical, otorhinological, and oncologic environment can present unique challenges. The ability to offer the complete spectrum of options available to treat VS in addition to other complex lateral skull base pathologies involves building a highly subspecialized team that successfully integrates all the available strategies and tailors treatment to what is most appropriate for each individual patient.

Counseling patients who are diagnosed with VS can be challenging. Given the variety of treatment options, presenting patients with an unbiased review of the advantages and disadvantages of various modalities is important for shared-decision making and supports true informed consent. It has been shown that patients themselves can be biased and committed toward a particular treatment strategy based on their initial consultations, the Internet, and other factors.[1,2] Furthermore, providers can be biased toward a certain modality depending on their comfort level, availability of radiation treatment platforms, or personal bias toward treatment strategies.

12.2 What Constitutes a Vestibular Schwannoma Team?

Undoubtedly, the most important aspect in building a successful skull base program is the people. The team itself can be led or co-managed by a variety of experienced practitioners, inclusive of a primary surgical team (e.g., neurosurgeon + neurotologist) or a combination of providers (e.g., neurosurgeon + neurotologist + radiation oncologist). There are excellent examples of providers in each of these specialties who have jointly contributed to the management of VS patients at many high-volume centers. While the titles are not important, whoever is seeing the patient should have experience with all forms of treatment, or be able and willing to bring in members of the team who do if they are not versed in one particular aspect of care.

12.2.1 Building an Effective Skull Base Team

Collectively, the team should have a unified vision in the general approach and management of patients. Important and often overlooked, the team must share mutual respect for all members. Respect for one another is likely the single most important trait for a successful team, both anecdotally and even as identified in systematic analyses defining healthcare teamwork competencies.[3] In addition, a cooperative and positive attitude, courage to disagree with each other, and even a sense of humor encompass almost equally important traits for the members of an effective healthcare team.[3]

Practicing as part of a team has very unique benefits to both the patient and the provider. A team approach brings in more perspective regarding the most appropriate management and may enlighten other members to options or issues they did not individually consider. Furthermore, it reduces fatigue both in the consultation aspect of seeing patients and among surgical colleagues during particularly long procedures and tedious dissections. Experienced input from a second set of eyes at critical decision-making points may improve the outcome. Often understated, the reduced psychological burden that comes from group decision making is invaluable. Moreover, collaboration also emphasizes the importance of being intellectually honest regarding the evaluation of complications and outcome.

The tireless multispecialty teamwork must occur seamlessly at all levels: from leadership to midlevel providers, schedulers, support staff, nursing, and even among billing staff. All personnel must understand the team approach. We have found that allowing the members of the team to interact with each other, by way of in-service education, joint conferences, multidisciplinary rounds, and joint clinics, has helped foster this relationship. Furthermore, the members of the team frequently have joint appointments to one another's department, which serves both to facilitate the relationship and to further reinforce the close partnership of the skull base team throughout the institution.

There is increasing evidence that overall outcomes are improved when VS surgeries are performed at high-volume centers and by high-volume providers through a team-based approach. This approach has demonstrated superior short- and long-term outcome, with shorter lengths of stay and reduced hospital cost.[4] Nonetheless, it is also the case that high-volume centers and high-volume surgeons tend to take on higher risk surgeries and perform more complete resection, as compared to lower-volume centers, which can artificially skew the risks and complications of treatment.[5] While it is difficult to categorically make the case for centralizing VS and other complex skull base surgery to a select few centers and providers, there are clear data to suggest that higher case volume may be a proxy of better access and outcomes that benefit patients due to refinement and standardization of clinical protocols, surgical technique, and streamlined postoperative care.[6]

12.3 The Initial Consult

When a patient is referred to our institution with a VS or other skull base pathology, they are jointly evaluated by both the neurosurgeon and neurotologist during their initial visit. This further emphasizes to the patient the team approach to care and allows the patient to complete his or her evaluation in a single setting. An unbiased approach to patients with VS, as well as flexibility and expertise in all management modalities, can facilitate clinical decisions based on the needs of a particular patient. Building a team with a diverse skill set and flexibility in approach helps deliver all available information to the patient in a balanced unbiased way to ensure that he or she understands the options for treatment leading to appropriate informed consent.

12.4 Operative Planning

Given the specialized equipment, monitoring, and positioning involved in joint cases, it is imperative that a highly specialized and knowledgeable operating room staff including the circulators, first assistants, and certified surgical technicians be trained specific to skull base surgery. Furthermore, it is vital that the surgeons jointly communicate with the operating room staff well in advance how the general flow of the operation will be conducted.

A collaborative investment in purchasing the necessary instruments and equipment that is frequently checked and stocked at all times prior to surgery is essential. In institutions that are just beginning their programs, the neurosurgical and otology teams need to discuss together each operation from start to finish to anticipate the commonly used "must-have" instruments and any other instruments that need to be ordered preoperatively, including necessary sutures, non-stick bipolars, microsurgical dissection instruments, drills, endoscopic sets, positioning tools, and navigational tools. Particularly important for any skull base practice is to think carefully about closure and reconstruction and anticipate the need for free tissue transfers, microvascular surgery, dural reconstruction, plating systems, and so on, prior to any planned procedure.

12.4.1 Neurophysiologic Monitoring

Neuromonitoring is an essential part of VS and lateral skull base surgery. The monitoring team needs to work closely with the surgical team to understand the monitoring needs for each individual case. Most importantly, a clear understanding of the intraoperative communication that will occur during the operation to assure proper monitoring and functional outcome is paramount. We have worked closely with our neurophysiology team and have tailored our facial nerve monitoring over time based on our clinical outcomes. We now encompass calculations based on interrogating facial nerve function intraoperatively through the neurophysiology team, and this information has proven useful to guide our resection for each individual case.[7]

12.4.2 Postoperative Care

The after-care of patients following skull base surgery is an extremely important and often overlooked aspect of care that can make or break an otherwise well-conducted operation. A surgical intensive care unit that is familiar with all aspects of postoperative VS patient care is essential. The care team and nursing staff need to be educated about appropriate hemodynamic monitoring, cranial nerve deficits and their appropriate management, and signs and symptoms of cerebrospinal fluid leak—such that when new changes occur, the surgical team is notified. Furthermore, the nursing staff needs to be aware that both the neurosurgical and neurotology teams are jointly involved in the care and management of VS patients.

12.4.3 Rehabilitation

A dedicated neurorehabilitation program specifically trained to address issues relevant to lateral skull base surgery such as cranial nerve deficits, vestibular rehabilitation, and speech/swallowing therapy is essential. It is important to make the rehabilitation team aware of the specific type of therapy patients require, as the rehabilitation needs are quite different from more common forms of neurorehabilitation such as stroke therapy for example. Furthermore, issues such as long-term postoperative dizziness and headache can be from other causes beyond having a tumor (vestibular migraine, etc.), and the expertise from specialized neurologists with specific expertise in headache management can be invaluable.

12.5 Neurofibromatosis Type 2

The care of the NF2 patient highlights the importance of close collaborative multidisciplinary care, where the neurosurgeon, neurotologist, and medical and radiation oncologists work diligently to provide comprehensive management. Given the complexity and evolving management in NF2, a joint clinic facilitates optimal communication and careful clinical, radiologic, and audiologic review that must be done to tailor the treatment for each individual patient. Furthermore, communication with the radiology department to assure that imaging for NF2 patients, in particular, is uniform from year to year to assure proper radiographic comparison can be very helpful. Lastly, it is essential that the audiology program is well versed in the management of patients with cochlear implants and auditory brainstem implants.

12.6 Research and Education

Given the complexity of lateral skull base surgery, the optimal center should be involved in the training and education of residents, fellows, and nurses. Additionally, the center should be actively involved in continuing medical education and patient education symposia or support groups. Equally important is the mission to help advance the field of VS management and lateral skull base surgery as a whole by participation in research, which may include basic or translational research, epidemiological, or clinical studies. While basic or translational research may be difficult for some institutions, all high-volume centers should perform retrospective or prospective outcome studies to assess the efficacy and safety of microsurgical and radiosurgical interventions. Maintaining a clinical database of all patients that have been evaluated in the joint practice, their treatment, outcomes, complications, and follow-up can be useful to facilitate intensive outcomes analysis to help improve the overall practice as well us to help develop standards of care and best practice guidelines.

12.6.1 Multidisciplinary Skull Base Conference

A specific multidisciplinary skull base conference, separate from the general neuro-oncology conference can be an important resource to optimize the management of select patients. In this forum, specialists with an identified interest and/or expertise in skull base tumors from neuropathology, neuroradiology, medical and radiation oncology, neurosurgery, neurotology, head and neck surgery, and rhinology meet and present the more unusual presentations or management dilemmas. In addition to the direct benefits toward patient care, this style of conference often fosters cross-specialty research collaboration and educational opportunities.

12.7 Conclusion

An abundance of data suggest that optimal management of VS requires a coordinated team-based multidisciplinary approach by experienced specialists, not only to deliver the chosen therapy but also to assist in the complex decision-making process. The most effective team has the greatest impact when they demonstrate a commitment to working collaboratively, commitment to the team members and organization, and a commitment to a quality outcome.[3] The mission of the skull base team should be to provide comprehensive care and support for all patients with complex cranial base disorders, provide education and training opportunities for team members and trainees at all levels, and to contribute to clinical and basic science research in VS and other lateral skull base disorders.

References

[1] Pogodzinski MS, Harner SG, Link MJ. Patient choice in treatment of vestibular schwannoma. Otolaryngol Head Neck Surg. 2004; 130(5):611–616

[2] Backous DD, Pham HT. Guiding patients through the choices for treating vestibular schwannomas: balancing options and ensuring informed consent. Otolaryngol Clin North Am. 2007; 40(3):521–540, viii–ix

[3] Leggat SG. Effective healthcare teams require effective team members: defining teamwork competencies. BMC Health Serv Res. 2007; 7:17

[4] Barker FG, II, Carter BS, Ojemann RG, Jyung RW, Poe DS, McKenna MJ. Surgical excision of acoustic neuroma: patient outcome and provider caseload. Laryngoscope. 2003; 113(8):1332–1343

[5] Curry WT, McDermott MW, Carter BS, Barker FG, II. Craniotomy for meningioma in the United States between 1988 and 2000: decreasing rate of mortality and the effect of provider caseload. J Neurosurg. 2005; 102(6):977–986

[6] Ward BK, Gourin CG, Francis HW. Vestibular schwannoma surgical volume and short-term outcomes in Maryland. Arch Otolaryngol Head Neck Surg. 2012; 138(6):577–583

[7] Schmitt WR, Daube JR, Carlson ML, et al. Use of supramaximal stimulation to predict facial nerve outcomes following vestibular schwannoma microsurgery: results from a decade of experience. J Neurosurg. 2013; 118(1):206–212

13 Patient Counseling Following Diagnosis of Sporadic Vestibular Schwannoma

Marc S. Schwartz

13.1 Introduction

In general, it is safe to say that patients newly diagnosed with a brain tumor face a period of anxiety and uncertainty. Obviously, there are different implications among various types of tumors. Many malignant tumors carry very grim prognoses, while for other types of tumors, including vestibular schwannomas (VS), prognoses are much more favorable. This generally good prognosis, however, does not imply that the decision-making process for VS patients is less complicated. Indeed, given the various endpoints of treatment, many of which have major implications regarding quality of life and well-being, there is a very high level of complexity.

It is rare for the skull base surgeon or other subspecialist to make the initial diagnosis of VS. Patients usually arrive already having received opinions from initial diagnosing physicians, family, and friends, as well as from the expanding resources available from the internet, social media, and patient advocacy groups. The information obtained in the course of diagnosis may be useful, confusing, misleading, or some combination of all three.

Despite the fact that VSs are all benign schwannomas originating from the vestibulocochlear nerve in the internal auditory canal and cerebellopontine angle, each tumor displays unique characteristics and each patient presents with a particular clinical picture. There are a number of very distinct but generally successful management options available. Treatment must therefore be individualized, taking into consideration the particulars of both tumors and patients.

13.2 Measuring Outcomes in Vestibular Schwannoma Treatment

In some types of disease, outcomes can be measured and described simply. Examples include measured decrease in blood pressure following administration of an antihypertensive medication and 5-year mortality following treatment of cancer. For VSs, measuring results is considerably more complicated.

The traditional outcomes of VS treatment are complication rate, facial nerve function, and hearing status. Although there may be interobserver variability, these are all factors that can be objectively measured and quantified.[1] Certainly, however, there are different tolerances for poor outcomes among different groups of VS patients. For instance, higher complication rates and worse facial nerve function are more acceptable in patients with giant VSs than in patients with intracanalicular tumors.

More recently, the importance of other, less readily quantified, outcome measures has come to light. Quality-of-life studies have shown that the importance of dizziness and headaches may meet or even exceed that of facial nerve and hearing function.[2] Yet more indistinct are the questions of patient satisfaction and socioeconomic effects.[3,4] These are measures that may be influenced by any number of controllable or noncontrollable factors. It is critical to understand that despite the increasing nebulousness of various measures, each of these retains some validity in determining how patients end up doing.

13.3 Vestibular Schwannoma Data and Treatment Options

In the most basic terms, VS patients face the options of observation, microsurgical resection, and stereotactic radiation. Of course, in some situations, the correct course of action is wholly apparent, such as in the patient with a giant tumor who requires microsurgical resection or the elderly, infirm patient with a small but growing tumor who would best be treated with stereotactic radiation. A majority of patients, however, lie somewhere between the extremes, and in these patients several options remain reasonable.

In the middle is the situation of *clinical equipoise*, in which more than one treatment option can be considered equally valid. Thus, a Venn diagram can be created outlining the options available to patients in various clinical situations (▶ Fig. 13.1). It is important to understand, however, that borders between different areas are not distinct lines. Rather, a continuum of states exists, ranging from situations in which there is only one good option to situations of true equipoise. An intermediate state in which one option can be generally recommended over another but in which either option is ultimately reasonable exists.

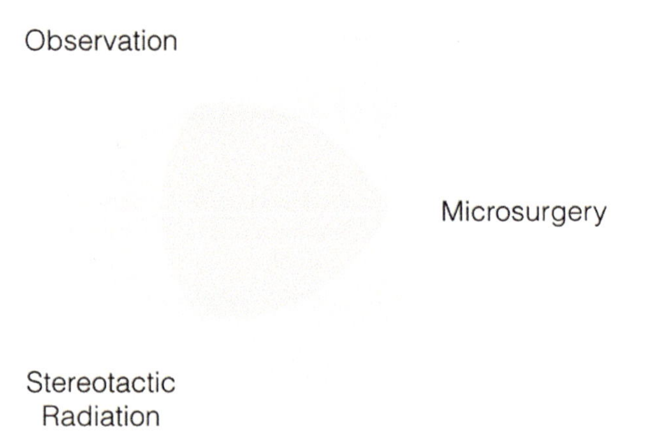

Fig. 13.1 Venn diagram detailing treatment options for patients with vestibular schwannomas. It should be understood that the delineation of intersections is not precise. Counseling of patients should differ significantly based on the location of the clinical situation in relation to this diagram. Location on the diagram can be influenced both by tumor factors and by patient factors.

As is evident to anyone in the field of VS treatment, there are clear differences of opinion from one practitioner to another in terms of the merits of the various treatment options. This is an unavoidable situation made possible by limitations in the measurability of the data regarding VS treatment. Most basically, there is no simple, binary treatment outcome measure. Various factors, including complication avoidance, facial nerve function, hearing, balance, ease of treatment, and other less well-defined aspects of quality of life are important, and the relative value of any one versus another is purely subjective.

Even for outcomes that can be measured, it is important to understand limitations of the data regarding VS treatment. Even most quantifiable outcome measures, such as facial nerve function, are subject to interobserver variability. As factors become more subjective, additional questions regarding reliability and validity become progressively more problematic. Furthermore, the quality of the data is in many regards not unassailable. Long-term follow-up of patients is only done with difficulty, and most series suffer from significant proportions of patients being lost to follow-up.[5] The endpoints of studies are also often less than ideal when considering a diagnosis of VS. The utility of short-term studies is limited when considering treatment of a benign process with the goal of long-term survival, often many decades, with the best possible function and quality of life. It is essentially inherently impossible to answer some of the most important questions.

13.4 The Psychology of Decision Making

Given the multiplicity of treatment options and the need to make a decision based on numerous factors, the possible outcomes of which can generally only be described imprecisely, it is important to understand the ways in which people actually make decisions. Being primarily a social science question, academic analysis of this process lies outside the field of VSs or skull base surgery.

In his book, "Thinking Fast and Slow," Kahneman has summarized the research in this area and proposed the "two-system" theory of decision making.[6] As described by this theory, people use two competing cognitive systems to make decisions. System I allows people to unconsciously and automatically make decisions based on impressions and associations. An example is 2 + 2 = 4. System II allows people to consciously and effortfully analyze information in a focused and rational manner. System II is used to compute the answer to more complex mathematical problems.

In the course of daily life, the human mind utilizes both systems organically in order to reach conclusions and make decisions as appropriately as possible. It is easy to understand how system II takes over from system I when people face complicated questions that cannot be easily answered. As may be counterintuitive, however, when problems become even more increasingly complex, system II cannot adequately analyze information, especially if much of that information is conflicting. When system II is overwhelmed, people make decisions using the impressions generated by system I, and they use system II to justify these impressions. The best and most obvious example of this is politics. Few of us would argue that, most basically, people's political views are derived from anything other than automatic, instinctual impressions.

Thus, in the treatment of VSs, it is important to understand that patients make decisions using a combination of both rational, thoughtful analysis and automatic, instinctual, subconscious thought. In the end, and probably in those cases in which the decision is closest to clinical equipoise and most complicated, it is usually system I which is ultimately dominant.

It is therefore important to understand that system I does not understand statistics or complex data. System I deals in impressions and is prone to various biases. For instance, a strong argument delivered confidently and forcefully will carry disproportionate weight, even if the data do not support any sort of strong position. Patients are also likely to assign disproportionate weight to the first opinion that they hear, even if this is from someone with little actual understanding or experience with VS care. System I also utilizes heuristics, or the substitution of a complex problem with an easier one. So, a patient may decide that microsurgical treatment is bad because a close relative deteriorated after craniotomy for a malignant brain tumor or that radiosurgery is bad because "radiation causes cancer." To system I, a single anecdote may carry greater weight than all published data combined.

Of course, it is tempting to argue that all effort should be made to bolster system II against system I for these types of difficult decisions. The problem with this, however, is that social science research has shown that people who rely on system I or gut instinct to make important decisions with multiple reasonable options generally end up happier than those who attempt to overanalyze with system II.[6,7]

In order to maximize outcomes and patient satisfaction, those treating patients with VS should therefore understand two important points. First, is it easy to mislead patients by manipulating their underlying biases; second, in situations at or near equipoise, patients are likely to end up more satisfied if they are allowed to follow their own instincts in deciding the best course of treatment.

13.4.1 Bias in Caregivers

While the preceding section is framed in terms of the process patients' decision making, it is important to understand that physicians and other caregivers are bound by the same psychological realities. Certainly, experts in the field of VS have a greater understanding of the literature and greater experience dealing with tumors than nearly any patient. Thus, they can claim a better ability to synthesize all of the complex information pertaining to the treatment of a particular case. It has been shown, however, that experts are not less dependent on biased, irrational decision-making processes than members of the general population.

13.5 Framing Options

The key question of patient counseling is how to help the patient best understand the options appropriate or inappropriate for the treatment of his or her VS. Options are realistically innumerable, including observation with serial MRIs, microsurgical resection via at least three surgical routes, stereotactic radiation via single- or multifraction treatment using various devices, strategies of tumor resection, treatment dosages, and combinations of treatments. Clearly, this can be overwhelming.

Psychological studies have shown that choice is good. People placed in situations without the ability to choose are generally less happy than those provided a choice. For most VS patients, this would seem to be a factor likely to lead to more satisfaction. It does not hold, however, that even more choice is better. This is thought to be in large part due to increasing effects of regret. While two or three options are better than none, progressively more choices actually decrease satisfaction, and even one or two additional ones may be worse than none at all.[7]

Thus, given the complexity of the decision-making process, it would seem best to counsel patients about the options available to them within a framework of a series of more manageable choices. Patients should be led through the process, discussing options, and detailing why any specific option may or may not be reasonable in their particular case.

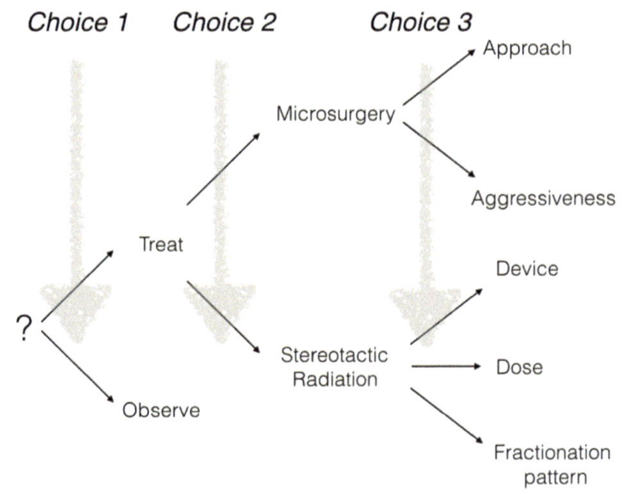

Fig. 13.2 Steps in the decision-making process regarding treatment of vestibular schwannomas. If not presented in an orderly fashion, the plethora of options can be overwhelming, and more important questions should be answered prior to considering the details.

13.5.1 Important Decisions

Patients should be counseled to make the important decisions about treatment first, before considering the details, which are likely to be confusing or even overwhelming. The important decisions are basically two choices each of which has two options. The first decision to be made is "does this tumor need to be treated now or can it be observed." If the tumor does need to be treated, the second decision is "should this tumor be treated by microsurgical resection or by stereotactic radiation."

These important decisions should be discussed comprehensively. Even if it is very clear that there is only one reasonable course of action, such as in the case of a young patient presenting with a giant tumor, the goal should be for the patient to understand why both observation and stereotactic radiation are not reasonable options. In other, less clear-cut cases, options should be framed in terms such as recommended, reasonable, and possible but not recommended.

It is also mandatory for physicians to discuss with patients the options for treatment in terms of both personal recommendations and the standard of care. It is unwise not to provide alternatives that may be interpreted as lying within the standard of care not only from a good practice perspective but for medicolegal reasons as well.[8]

13.5.2 The Details

Patients should be counseled that further decisions about treatment should be considered only after the important questions described in the previous section have been answered. These details are innumerable and opinions about them are likely to vary from center to center and from physician to physician. For patients electing to observe, options include the timing of the following scan and the criteria for determining growth. For patients electing microsurgical resection, options include surgical approach, aggressiveness of resection, and use of endoscopes. For those electing stereotactic radiation, details include single- or multifraction, which device to use, and prescribed dose (▶ Fig. 13.2).

In the end and within reason, there is little if any evidence that clearly supports any one of these options over the others. At the level of details, recommendations are generally based on specific surgeon comfort levels, availability of devices, academic interests, and other factors that reflect bias more than anything else. Of course, this does not preclude physicians from advocating what they think is best for their patients in their own hands (or in the hands of someone else). It is critical to help patients understand their choices and to help lead them toward a reasonable decision.

13.6 Managing Expectations

Happiness = Reality − Expectations

Although perhaps self-evident, social science research has shown this equation actually is true.[9] It is important for physicians treating patients with VSs to understand that when counseling, their tone of conversation may influence eventual outcome and patient satisfaction.

Especially given the competitive nature of VS practice, we must understand the implications of optimism versus realism. Patients seeking opinions for the treatment of their tumors may initially be buoyed by displays of certainty and optimism, justified or not. Indeed, research has shown that many people respond with trust and belief to forcefully stated, positive arguments.[6] This may be true even in situations in which the data do not support any strong, definitive assertions. On the other hand, introduction of uncertainty into the counseling process is likely not to be favorable for retention of patients and for business in general.

Caregivers should, however, clearly understand the potential costs of overoptimism in terms of eventual patient satisfaction. Patients with less than ideal outcomes who do not understand the implications of the various challenges often faced by VS patients over time or who do not understand the risks of treatment are likely to be left particularly bitter and unhappy.

13.7 Multiple Opinions

It is the nature of VS treatment that many patients will obtain multiple opinions regarding their care. This is yet another type of option that patients face, further adding to the complexity of the decision-making process. With many opinions, the point of diminishing returns is likely to be reached. In many cases, however, there is clear value in patients obtaining opinions from more than one physician or team. When opinions concur, patients may be more satisfied that they are receiving sound advice. When opinions differ, there is even greater value to new information. Within reason, patients should not be dissuaded from seeking additional opinions.

13.8 Conclusions

The decision-making process for VS treatment is complex. In counseling, patients should be guided toward treatment options appropriate for their specific cases on an individualized basis. In cases of clinical equipoise, patients are likely to be most satisfied with results if they are encouraged to decide on the course of action that is ultimately most aligned not only with their specific tumor and clinical issues but also with their own psychological factors. All physicians and other caregivers have biases, and this must be recognized in order to avoid the worst errors of decision making, including potential ethical lapses. The numerous choices for treatment can be overwhelming to patients, and options should be presented in a coherent manner which encourages understanding of important issues. Expectations should be appropriately managed. Except in emergency situations, which are very rare, patients should not be dissuaded from seeking further opinions.

References

[1] Fattah AY, Gurusinghe AD, Gavilan J, et al. Sir Charles Bell Society. Facial nerve grading instruments: systematic review of the literature and suggestion for uniformity. Plast Reconstr Surg. 2015; 135(2):569–579

[2] Carlson ML, Tveiten OV, Driscoll CL, et al. Long-term quality of life in patients with vestibular schwannoma: an international multicenter cross-sectional study comparing microsurgery, stereotactic radiosurgery, observation, and nontumor controls. J Neurosurg. 2015; 122(4):833–842

[3] Tos T, Cayé-Thomasen P, Stangerup SE, Tos M, Thomsen J. Patients' fears, expectations and satisfaction in relation to management of vestibular schwannoma: a comparison of surgery and observation. Acta Otolaryngol. 2003; 123(5):600–605

[4] Pritchard C, Clapham L, Davis A, Lang DA, Neil-Dwyer G. Psycho-socio-economic outcomes in acoustic neuroma patients and their carers related to tumour size. Clin Otolaryngol Allied Sci. 2004; 29(4):324–330

[5] Carlson ML, Jacob JT, Pollock BE, et al. Long-term hearing outcomes following stereotactic radiosurgery for vestibular schwannoma: patterns of hearing loss and variables influencing audiometric decline. J Neurosurg. 2013; 118 (3):579–587

[6] Kahneman D. Thinking Fast and Slow. New York, NY: Farrar, Straus and Giroux;2011

[7] Schwartz B. The Paradox of Choice: Why More is Less. New York, NY: Harper Perennial; 2004

[8] Ruhl DS, Hong SS, Littlefield PD. Lessons learned in otologic surgery: 30 years of malpractice cases in the United States. Otol Neurotol. 2013; 34(7):1173–1179

[9] Rutledge RB, Skandali N, Dayan P, Dolan RJ. A computational and neural model of momentary subjective well-being. Proc Natl Acad Sci U S A. 2014; 111(33):12252–12257

Part IV

Management: Conservative Observation

IV

14 Natural History of Tumor Growth in Sporadic Vestibular Schwannoma

Per Cayé-Thomasen, David A. Moffat, Simon K. W. Lloyd, and Sven-Eric Stangerup

14.1 Introduction

Sandifort was the first to describe a vestibular schwannoma (VS) in 1777 following a postmortem autopsy. Since the first attempts at surgical tumor removal at the end of the 19th century, it was assumed for almost a century that, if left untreated, these tumors would invariably continue to grow over time. Upon diagnosis, surgical treatment was therefore considered mandatory for decades, irrespective of tumor size. Approaching the end of the 20th century, some patients were, however, treated conservatively and observed for tumor growth by interval imaging, as surgery was considered too risky due to severe patient comorbidities and/or advanced age. In 1985, Silverstein et al were among the first to report on conservative management[1] and since then, a number of studies have documented that tumor growth following diagnosis was not inevitable and that some tumors do not grow for extended periods of time.

A large cerebellopontine angle tumor may be associated with serious complications and become life threatening due to brainstem compression. Thus, surgery is definitively advocated in patients with large VS. In patients with small- or medium-sized tumors, however, there are currently three management options: observation with interval imaging, surgery, or radiotherapy. Success of treatment is usually perceived to be control of tumor growth. Preservation of serviceable hearing in patients presenting with socially useful speech discrimination scores together with no or minimal treatment side effects are also regarded as important secondary outcomes. In order to justify invasive treatment by either surgery or radiotherapy for small- to medium-sized tumors, the outcome should be superior to that resulting from the natural history of the disease and should also be balanced against the need for intervention in order to avoid or minimize subsequent problems. Only a detailed knowledge of the natural history of these tumors will allow valid, evidence-based comparison of the outcome of observational management compared with active treatment. Accordingly, this chapter reviews the existing evidence on the natural history of tumor growth in patients observed with small- or medium-sized unilateral sporadic VS, whereas the natural history of hearing and vestibular function is addressed in Chapter 51. These issues are increasingly relevant for the patients and clinicians involved, as a steadily increasing number of patients are diagnosed with small- and medium-sized tumors, as reported in Chapter 3 on the epidemiology of VS.

14.2 Measurement of Tumor Size and Determination of Tumor Growth

According to the international consensus meeting in Japan in 2003,[2] a tumor should be defined as either intrameatal or extrameatal, the latter designating a tumor with growth into the cerebellopontine angle. The size of a tumor with cerebellopontine angle extension should be determined by measuring the largest extrameatal tumor diameter, excluding the intrameatal portion.

It should be emphasized that determined tumor size and growth rate may depend on the diagnostic tool (computed tomography [CT] vs. magnetic resonance imaging [MRI]), the method of measurement (e.g., plane of dimensions assessed), and the definition of growth (e.g., number of millimeter enlargement). The largest diameter measurement is considered adequate when merely questioning absolute growth,[3] which is the parameter relevant for clinical assessment and decision making, as it is the absolute size that determines the risk of brainstem or adjacent cranial nerve compression. Using contemporary MRI, diameter measurement error is up to 2 mm.[4] Thus, tumor growth should be defined as an increase of 2 mm or more when measuring any diameter.

14.3 Natural History of Vestibular Schwannoma Growth

The evidence for the natural history of VS growth presented in this chapter is based on a review of the literature using the databases PubMed and Embase, including studies published during the period 1984 to 2014. Clinical articles reporting original data (thus excluding reviews and meta-analyses) from observational studies based on case series/cohorts and with more than 30 patients were considered. In total, there were 53 studies identified in the VS literature that reported on sporadic unilateral VS growth using serial predominantly MR imaging, which offered a definition of tumor growth (directly or indirectly) and reported mean/median follow-up. Collectively, these 53 studies contain data on tumor growth from almost 6,000 patients[5,6,7,8,9,10,11,12,13,14,15,16,17,18,19,20,21,22,23,24,25,26,27,28,29,30,31,32,33,34,35,36,37,38,39,40,41,42,43,44,45,46,47,48,49,50,51,52,53,54,55,56,57] (▶ Table 14.1).

Weighted calculation based on the number of included patients in each publication produces an overall mean follow-up of 3.3 years, ranging from 0.5 to 10 years. Only three papers, representing 170 patients, have a mean follow-up of more than 5 years (5.5, 6.7, and 10 years, respectively).[35,42,54] Weighted calculation on the occurrence of growth showed that a mean of 33% of tumors grow within a mean observation period of 3.3 years (▶ Table 14.1). Growth after diagnosis is unpredictable in rate and time and does not appear to be related to age, sex, tumor size at diagnosis, symptoms, or any other recognized factor of relevance, although cystic tumors may display sudden and dramatic growth.[7] In addition, the risk of growth appears to be higher for tumors with extrameatal extension at diagnosis compared with tumors located exclusively within the internal auditory canal, although this may depend on the definition of growth (see later).

Table 14.1

Author	Year	Study design	Patients (number)	Mean follow-up (y)	Growth definition	Growth (%)
Stangerup et al[5]	2006	Pro	552 322 EM 230 IM	3.6	>2 mm Growth to CPA	29 17
Moffat et al[7]	2012	Pro	381	4.2	>2 mm	33
Bakkouri et al[8]	2009	Retro	325	1.0	≥3 mm	12
Martin et al[9]	2009	Pro	276	3.6	>2 mm	22
Suryanarayanan et al[10]	2010	Pro	240	3.6	≥1 mm	32
Al Sanosi et al[11]	2006	Retro	197	3.4	>0 mm	28
Caye-Thomasen et al[6]	2006	Pro	196 IM	4.4	Growth to CPA	19
Breivik et al[12]	2012	Pro	186	3.6	>2 mm	40
Agrawal et al[13]	2010	Retro	180	2.7	≥1 mm/y	37
Varughese et al[14]	2012	Pro	178 (88% IM)	3.6	≥1 mm/y	29
Ferri et al[15]	2013	Pro	161	0.5	≥2 mm	36
Ferri et al[16]	2008	Pro	123	4.8	≥2 mm	35
Quaranta et al[17]	2003	Retro	122	3.5	>2 mm	40
Fucci et al[18]	1999	Retro	119	2.5	>2 mm	30
Roehm and Gantz[19]	2007	Pro	114 (>65 y)	3.0	>0 mm	50
Fayad et al[20]	2014	Retro	114	4.8	≥2 mm	38
Battaglia et al[21]	2006	Retro	111	3.2	>0 mm	50
Bozorg Grayeli et al[22]	2005	Retro	111	2.8	>0 mm	47
Solares and Panizza[23]	2008	Retro	110	2.6	>2 mm	21
Hoistad et al[24]	2001	Retro	102	2.4	>1 mm	44
Kishore et al[25]	2003	Retro	100	3.2	>1 mm	29
Flint et al[26]	2005	Retro	100	2.2	>0 mm	36
Remenyi et al[27]	2009	Retro	95	3.7	>2 mm	23
Whitehouse et al[28]	2010	Retro	88	3.7	>1 mm	51
Shin et al[29]	2000	Retro	87	2.6	>0 mm	53
Moller et al[30]	2003	Pro	82	3.0	>0 mm	43
Rosenberg et al[31]	2000	Retro	80	4.4	>0 mm	58
Nutik and Babb[32]	2001	Retro	75	4.1	>0 mm	41
Tschudi et al[33]	2000	Retro	74	2.9	>0 mm	31
González-Orús Álvarez-Morujo et al[34]	2014	Retro	73	3.0	≥2 mm	12
Hajioff et al[35]	2008	Pro	72	10.0	>1 mm	35
Walsh et al[36]	2000	Retro	72	3.2	>0 mm	36
Bederson et al[37]	1991	Retro	70	2.2	>0 mm	53
Quaranta et al[38]	2007	Retro	70	2.8	>2 mm	40
Godefroy et al[39]	2009	Pro	70	3.6	≥2 mm	36
Deen et al[40]	1996	Retro	68	3.4	>0 mm	29
Mirz et al[41]	2000	Pro	64	3.6	>1 mm/y	23
Raut et al[42]	2004	Pro	61	6.7	>1 mm/y	50
Wiet et al[43]	1995	Retro	53	2.2	>0 mm	40
Strasnick et al[44]	1994	Retro	50	2.3	>0 mm	68
Herwadker et al[45]	2005	Pro	50	1.5	>3 × error, Bayesian	42
Nedzelski et al[46]	2008	Retro	50	3.5	≥1 mm	48
Pennings et al[47]	2010	Retro	47 IM	3.6	Growth to CPA	38
Régis et al[48]	2010	Pro	47 IM	3.7	>0 mm	74
Modugno et al[49]	1999	Retro	47	3.0	>0 mm	36
Stipkovits et al[50]	2001	Pro	44	3.5	>0 mm	18
O'Reilly et al[51]	2000	Retro	43	2.6	>0 mm	30
Perry et al[52]	2001	Retro	41 (>65 y)	3.5	>0 mm	51

Table 14.1 (*Continued*)

Author	Year	Study design	Patients (number)	Mean follow-up (y)	Growth definition	Growth (%)
Vokurka et al[53]	2002	Pro	38	1.0	> 3 × error, Bayesian	32
Martin et al[54]	1994	Retro	37	5.5	> 2 mm/y	30
Glasscock et al[55]	1997	Retro	34	2.4	> 2 mm/y	55
Lee et al[56]	2014	Retro	31 IM	2.6	≥ 2 mm	23
Sakamoto et al[57]	2001	Retro	31	2.8	> 1 mm/y	45
All studies	**-**	**-**	**5942**	**3.32**	**-**	**33.3**

Abbreviations: Pro, prospective; Retro, retrospective; CPA, cerebellopontine angle; EM, extrameatal tumors; IM, intrameatal tumors.
Notes: Studies on the natural history of vestibular schwannoma growth, listed by the number of observed patients (largest to smallest study size).

Although long-term data are scarce, it appears that tumor growth occurs almost exclusively within 5 years of diagnosis, and only rarely at a later stage. Growth may be continuous, but may also occur after a dormant period.[7] Similarly, approximately 20% of tumors stop growing following a period of growth demonstrable on MRI.[7] Notably, tumor shrinkage is also seen in approximately 5% of patients.[58] For those tumors that demonstrate growth, the growth rate varies from 2 to 16 mm per annum with a mean annual growth rate varying between 1.6 and 4.7 mm.[5,6,7,8,9,10,11,12,13,14,15,16,17,18,19,20,21,22,23,24,25,26,27,28,29,30,31,32,33,34,35,36,37,38,39,40,41,42,43,44,45,46,47,48,49,50,51,52,53,54,55,56,57,58]

14.4 Data Interpretation and Issues of Bias

When assessing available data on VS growth in observed patients, there are a number of issues to be considered. Although a significant amount of data has been gathered, a cautious interpretation of data robustness and the various actual and potential biases associated with the individual studies and the overall body of evidence is prudent and warranted.

14.4.1 Referral Bias

All but two studies[5,6] involved referral bias where patients may not be representative of the general population. The two papers not involving referral bias are both from the largest database on VS patients in the world, including all patients diagnosed in Denmark since 1976. This national database includes data on approximately 3,500 patients as of 2015, and 748 of the 5,942 patients included in this review are from the Danish database[5,6] (▶ Table 14.1). Applying a global perspective, the majority of the published data derives from a relatively limited number of countries and parts of the world, which also inevitably introduces inherent biases.

14.4.2 Selection Bias

All papers are subject to selection bias concerning tumor size, as larger tumors were excluded (and usually surgically excised) and the majority of papers involved some degree of patient selection bias concerning age and comorbidity. Large tumors are found more often in young patients and as surgery is performed in most of these cases, data on observation and growth are elusive for this population, which may disguise a potential correlation between age and the occurrence and rate of tumor growth. In addition, selection bias related to symptoms, typically hearing loss and vertigo/dizziness, also exists in a number of the studies.

14.4.3 Long-Term Follow-up

Loss to follow-up and incomplete data acquisition are yet other potential sources of bias, often but not solely depending on the study design, as these problems are more likely to occur in retrospective, compared with prospective studies (▶ Table 14.1).

14.4.4 Determination of Tumor Size and Growth

Most studies do not distinguish between purely intrameatal tumors and tumors with extrameatal extension, although some do. As the risk of growth appears to be smaller in purely intrameatal tumors, an uncertain degree of bias is likely to exist in studies pooling all tumors.

Most, but not all, studies define small- to medium-sized tumors as those having a maximal extrameatal diameter of less than 20 mm, not including the intrameatal portion of the tumor. Linear measurement of the largest extrameatal tumor diameter for tumor size determination has been used by most authors, although some have used linear measurement of the total tumor diameter, including the portion within the internal auditory canal, and have not, therefore, followed the recommendations of the international consensus document.[2] Yet others have used volume rendering or Bayesian methods for the evaluation of both tumor size and growth (▶ Table 14.1).

The definition of tumor growth varies between papers, introducing additional bias, either under- or overestimating the occurrence of growth. Most of the early studies did not take into consideration interobserver variability and errors of measurement, using greater than 0 mm tumor enlargement as a definition of growth. As knowledge of error of measurement was recognized by the research community and taken into account in the literature, more recent studies have used greater than 1 mm, greater than 2 mm, or even greater than 3 mm enlargement to define growth (see ▶ Table 14.1). The partial use of CT in some of the early studies is also a source of potential bias, as

CT is less accurate than MRI when estimating tumor size and growth.

14.4.5 Other Sources of Bias

Finally, some of the reporting centers have published more than one paper on their institutional experience with overlapping patient populations. Serial publications are common as updates on the original cohort become available or new additional cases are added. Thus, an unspecified number of patients have been tallied more than once in ▶ Table 14.1.

14.5 A Treatment Strategy Based on the Natural History of Tumor Growth

As an increasing number of small- and medium-sized VSs are diagnosed (see Chapter 3), the medical community is in need of a treatment strategy based on a thorough knowledge on the natural history of tumor growth and the natural history of audiovestibular function (see Chapter 51). Based on the data presented herein, the authors have adopted the following observational strategy for sporadic, noncystic VS with a maximal extrameatal diameter less than 15 to 20 mm:

1. Follow-up MRI 6 months after diagnosis for tumors with extrameatal extension and 12 months after diagnosis for purely intracanalicular tumors.
2. In case of no growth, yearly MRI for 4 years.
3. Followed by MRI every other year for 4 years.
4. Followed by MRI after a further 5 years.

Cystic tumors may display sudden and dramatic growth necessitating shorter MRI follow-up intervals (e.g., every 6 months for 2 years, followed by yearly scans). If significant growth occurs, active treatment with surgery or radiotherapy may be considered, but continuance of observational management may be reasonable depending on a number of other factors such as patient age, comorbidities, existing tumor-related deficits, tumor size, and growth rate. Both surgery and radiotherapy are associated with risks, and patients' quality of life may be better when their disease is observed rather than actively treated (see Chapter 60).

Some argue that follow-up can be safely terminated after 15 years of no tumor growth. Although anecdotally the risk of growth after 15 years appears to be negligible, very little data exist to support this. Thus, in order to clarify long-term risk and identify late growth, a follow-up MRI every 5 to 10 years for an indefinite and even life-long period may be appropriate.

14.6 Future Perspectives

Long-term observational studies on tumor growth and audiovestibular function are ongoing and will be essential in the design of future observational and treatment strategies. Quality-of-life studies are important and likely to influence recommendations for patients and clinicians.[59] Basic science and identification of genes, molecular pathways, and networks related to tumor growth are likely to change our approach to treatment including conservative management.[60] Medical treatment predicated on basic science is already an option in the treatment of VSs associated with neurofibromatosis type 2 (NF2), in the form of anti-vascular endothelial growth factor (anti-VEGF) antibody therapy. Tumor expression of VEGF is correlated positively with tumor growth[61,62] and anti-VEGF antibody treatment has been shown to stabilize growth or even reduce tumor size as well as improve hearing in some patients with NF2.[63,64] In addition, tumor expression of VEGF as determined by imaging has been shown to correlate with subsequent tumor growth, thus providing the first ever-prognostic instrument for these patients.[65] Recommended treatment and follow-up strategy may accordingly be individualized with primary active treatment or short interval follow-up MRI performed in patients with a high expression of tumor VEGF and longer interval follow-up MRI in patients with a low expression of VEGF. Although NF2-associated tumors are usually more aggressive, prognostic imaging modalities and pharmacological therapies developed for the treatment of NF2 will likely be applied to sporadic tumors in the future.

14.7 Conclusion

The literature review included in this chapter demonstrates that 33% of small- or medium-sized unilateral sporadic VSs will grow within 3.3 years of observation. Based on this evidence, it can be argued that active treatment of small- and medium-sized VS should await documented tumor growth in order to avoid overtreatment or treatment-related side effects that may be worse than the natural history and spontaneous course of the disease. It should be noted that only three papers on conservative management, representing 170 patients, have more than 5 years of follow-up (5.5, 6.7, and 10 years, respectively). Most studies show that if tumor growth occurs, it is usually detected within the first few years of diagnosis. However, long-term observational studies are desperately needed to guide the development of evidence-based surveillance algorithms designed to detect late tumor progression.

References

[1] Silverstein H, McDaniel A, Norrell H, Wazen J. Conservative management of acoustic neuroma in the elderly patient. Laryngoscope. 1985; 95(7)(,)(Pt 1): 766–770

[2] Kanzaki J, Tos M, Sanna M, Moffat DA, Monsell EM, Berliner KI. New and modified reporting systems from the consensus meeting on systems for reporting results in vestibular schwannoma. Otol Neurotol. 2003; 24(4):642–648, discussion 648–649

[3] Walsh RM, Bath AP, Bance ML, Keller A, Rutka JA. Comparison of two radiologic methods for measuring the size and growth rate of extracanalicular vestibular schwannomas. Am J Otol. 2000; 21(5):716–721

[4] Hougaard D, Norgaard A, Pedersen T, Bibby BM, Ovesen T. Is a redefinition of the growth criteria of vestibular schwannomas needed? Am J Otolaryngol. 2014; 35(2):192–197

[5] Stangerup SE, Caye-Thomasen P, Tos M, Thomsen J. The natural history of vestibular schwannoma. Otol Neurotol. 2006; 27(4):547–552

[6] Caye-Thomasen P, Hansen S, Dethloff T, Stangerup SE, Thomsen J. Sublocalization and volumetric growth pattern of intracanalicular vestibular schwannomas. Laryngoscope. 2006; 116(7):1131–1135

[7] Moffat DA, Kasbekar A, Axon PR, Lloyd SK. Growth characteristics of vestibular schwannomas. Otol Neurotol. 2012; 33(6):1053–1058

[8] Bakkouri WE, Kania RE, Guichard JP, Lot G, Herman P, Huy PT. Conservative management of 386 cases of unilateral vestibular schwannoma: tumor growth and consequences for treatment. J Neurosurg. 2009; 110(4):662–669

[9] Martin TP, Senthil L, Chavda SV, Walsh R, Irving RM. A protocol for the conservative management of vestibular schwannomas. Otol Neurotol. 2009; 30(3):381–385

[10] Suryanarayanan R, Ramsden RT, Saeed SR, et al. Vestibular schwannoma: role of conservative management. J Laryngol Otol. 2010; 124(3):251–257

[11] Al Sanosi A, Fagan PA, Biggs ND. Conservative management of acoustic neuroma. Skull Base. 2006; 16(2):95–100

[12] Breivik CN, Varughese JK, Wentzel-Larsen T, Vassbotn F, Lund-Johansen M. Conservative management of vestibular schwannoma-a prospective cohort study: treatment, symptoms, and quality of life. Neurosurgery. 2012; 70(5): 1072–1080, discussion 1080

[13] Agrawal Y, Clark JH, Limb CJ, Niparko JK, Francis HW. Predictors of vestibular schwannoma growth and clinical implications. Otol Neurotol. 2010; 31(5): 807–812

[14] Varughese JK, Breivik CN, Wentzel-Larsen T, Lund-Johansen M. Growth of untreated vestibular schwannoma: a prospective study. J Neurosurg. 2012; 116(4):706–712

[15] Ferri GG, Pirodda A, Ceroni AR, Fioravanti A, Calbucci F, Modugno GC. Management of growing vestibular schwannomas. Eur Arch Otorhinolaryngol. 2013; 270(7):2013–2019

[16] Ferri GG, Modugno GC, Pirodda A, Fioravanti A, Calbucci F, Ceroni AR. Conservative management of vestibular schwannomas: an effective strategy. Laryngoscope. 2008; 118(6):951–957

[17] Quaranta N, Baguley DM, Axon PR, et al. Conservative management of vestibular schwannomas. In: Baguley D, Ramsden R, Moffat D, eds. The Proceedings of the Fourth International Conference on Vestibular Schwannoma and Other CPA Lesions; 2003; Cambridge, UK; 2003:256–257

[18] Fucci MJ, Buchman CA, Brackmann DE, Berliner KI. Acoustic tumor growth: implications for treatment choices. Am J Otol. 1999; 20(4):495–499

[19] Roehm PC, Gantz BJ. Management of acoustic neuromas in patients 65 years or older. Otol Neurotol. 2007; 28(5):708–714

[20] Fayad JN, Semaan MT, Lin J, Berliner KI, Brackmann DE. Conservative management of vestibular schwannoma: expectations based on the length of the observation period. Otol Neurotol. 2014; 35(7):1258–1265

[21] Battaglia A, Mastrodimos B, Cueva R. Comparison of growth patterns of acoustic neuromas with and without radiosurgery. Otol Neurotol. 2006; 27 (5):705–712

[22] Bozorg Grayeli A, Kalamarides M, Ferrary E, et al. Conservative management versus surgery for small vestibular schwannomas. Acta Otolaryngol. 2005; 125(10):1063–1068

[23] Solares CA, Panizza B. Vestibular schwannoma: an understanding of growth should influence management decisions. Otol Neurotol. 2008; 29(6):829–834

[24] Hoistad DL, Melnik G, Mamikoglu B, Battista R, O'Connor CA, Wiet RJ. Update on conservative management of acoustic neuroma. Otol Neurotol. 2001; 22 (5):682–685

[25] Kishore A, Handoura L, O'Reilly BF, et al. Outcome of 100 vestibular schwannomas managed conservatively: a 10 year follow up study. In: Baguley D, Ramsden R, Moffat D, eds. The Proceedings of the Fourth International on Vestibular Schwannoma and other CPA Lesions; 2003; Cambridge, UK; 2003:58

[26] Flint D, Fagan P, Panarese A. Conservative management of sporadic unilateral acoustic neuromas. J Laryngol Otol. 2005; 119(6):424–428

[27] Remenyi J, Marshall A, Enticott JC, Briggs RJ. The prognostic value of speech recognition scores at diagnosis of vestibular schwannoma. J Clin Neurosci. 2009; 16(11):1460–1463

[28] Whitehouse K, Foroughi M, Shone G, Hatfield R. Vestibular schwannomas - when should conservative management be reconsidered? Br J Neurosurg. 2010; 24(2):185–190

[29] Shin YJ, Fraysse B, Cognard C, et al. Effectiveness of conservative management of acoustic neuromas. Am J Otol. 2000; 21(6):857–862

[30] Moller P, Myrseth E, Pedersen P-H, et al. Small vestibular schwannoma: results with observation, surgery and gamma-knife. In: Baguley D, Ramsden R, Moffat D, eds. Fourth International Conference on Vestibular Schwannoma and Other CPA Lesions; 2003; Cambridge, UK; 2003:39–40

[31] Rosenberg SI. Natural history of acoustic neuromas. Laryngoscope. 2000; 110 (4):497–508

[32] Nutik SL, Babb MJ. Determinants of tumor size and growth in vestibular schwannomas. J Neurosurg. 2001; 94(6):922–926

[33] Tschudi DC, Linder TE, Fisch U. Conservative management of unilateral acoustic neuromas. Am J Otol. 2000; 21(5):722–728

[34] González-Orús Álvarez-Morujo RJ, Alvarez-Palacios I, Martin-Oviedo C, Scola-Yurrita B, Arístegui-Ruiz MÁ. Conservative management of vestibular schwannoma. Acta Otorrinolaringol Esp. 2014; 65(5):275–282

[35] Hajioff D, Raut VV, Walsh RM, et al. Conservative management of vestibular schwannomas: third review of a 10-year prospective study. Clin Otolaryngol. 2008; 33(3):255–259

[36] Walsh RM, Bath AP, Bance ML, Keller A, Tator CH, Rutka JA. The role of conservative management of vestibular schwannomas. Clin Otolaryngol Allied Sci. 2000; 25(1):28–39

[37] Bederson JB, von Ammon K, Wichmann WW, Yasargil MG. Conservative treatment of patients with acoustic tumors. Neurosurgery. 1991; 28(5):646–650, discussion 650–651

[38] Quaranta N, Baguley DM, Moffat DA. Change in hearing and tinnitus in conservatively managed vestibular schwannomas. Skull Base. 2007; 17(4):223–228

[39] Godefroy WP, Kaptein AA, Vogel JJ, van der Mey AG. Conservative treatment of vestibular schwannoma: a follow-up study on clinical and quality-of-life outcome. Otol Neurotol. 2009; 30(7):968–974

[40] Deen HG, Ebersold MJ, Harner SG, et al. Conservative management of acoustic neuroma: an outcome study. Neurosurgery. 1996; 39(2):260–264, discussion 264–266

[41] Mirz F, Pedersen CB, Fiirgaard B, et al. Incidence and growth pattern of vestibular schwannomas in a Danish county, 1977Y98. Acta Otolaryngol Suppl. 2000; 543:30–33

[42] Raut VV, Walsh RM, Bath AP, et al. Conservative management of vestibular schwannomas - second review of a prospective longitudinal study. Clin Otolaryngol Allied Sci. 2004; 29(5):505–514

[43] Wiet RJ, Zappia JJ, Hecht CS, O'Connor CA. Conservative management of patients with small acoustic tumors. Laryngoscope. 1995; 105(8, Pt 1):795–800

[44] Strasnick B, Glasscock ME, III, Haynes D, McMenomey SO, Minor LB. The natural history of untreated acoustic neuromas. Laryngoscope. 1994; 104(9): 1115–1119

[45] Herwadker A, Vokurka EA, Evans DG, Ramsden RT, Jackson A. Size and growth rate of sporadic vestibular schwannoma: predictive value of information available at presentation. Otol Neurotol. 2005; 26(1):86–92

[46] Nedzelski JM, Schessel DA, Pfleiderer A, Kassel EE, Rowed DW. Conservative management of acoustic neuromas. Neurosurg Clin N Am. 2008; 19(2):207–216

[47] Pennings RJ, Morris DP, Clarke L, Allen S, Walling S, Bance ML. Natural history of hearing deterioration in intracanalicular vestibular schwannoma. Neurosurgery. 2011; 68(1):68–77

[48] Régis J, Carron R, Park MC, et al. Wait-and-see strategy compared with proactive Gamma Knife surgery in patients with intracanalicular vestibular schwannomas. J Neurosurg. 2010; 113 Suppl:105–111

[49] Modugno GC, Pirodda A, Ferri GG, et al. Small acoustic neuromas: monitoring the growth rate by MRI. Acta Neurochir (Wien). 1999; 141(10):1063–1067

[50] Stipkovits EM, Graamans K, Vasbinder GB, Van Dijk JE, Beek FJ. Assessment of vestibular schwannoma growth: application of a new measuring protocol to the results of a longitudinal study. Ann Otol Rhinol Laryngol. 2001; 110(4): 326–330

[51] O'Reilly B, Murray CD, Hadley DM. The conservative management of acoustic neuroma: a review of forty-four patients with magnetic resonance imaging. Clin Otolaryngol Allied Sci. 2000; 25(2):93–97

[52] Perry BP, Gantz BJ, Rubinstein JT. Acoustic neuromas in the elderly. Otol Neurotol. 2001; 22(3):389–391

[53] Vokurka EA, Herwadkar A, Thacker NA, Ramsden RT, Jackson A. Using Bayesian tissue classification to improve the accuracy of vestibular schwannoma volume and growth measurement. AJNR Am J Neuroradiol. 2002; 23 (3):459–467

[54] Martin CH, Fraysse B, Chelikh L, et al. Acoustic neuroma natural growth in older patients. J Fr Otorhinolaryngol. 1994; 43:392–397

[55] Glasscock ME, III, Pappas DG, Jr, Manolidis S, Von Doersten PG, Jackson CG, Storper IS. Management of acoustic neuroma in the elderly population. Am J Otol. 1997; 18(2):236–241, discussion 241–242

[56] Lee JD, Park MK, Kim JS, Cho YS. The factors associated with tumor stability observed with conservative management of intracanalicular vestibular schwannoma. Otol Neurotol. 2014; 35(5):918–921

[57] Sakamoto T, Fukuda S, Inuyama Y. Hearing loss and growth rate of acoustic neuromas in follow-up observation policy. Auris Nasus Larynx. 2001; 28 Suppl:S23–S27

[58] Huang X, Caye-Thomasen P, Stangerup SE. Spontaneous tumour shrinkage in 1261 observed patients with sporadic vestibular schwannoma. J Laryngol Otol. 2013; 127(8):739–743

[59] Irving RM, Beynon GJ, Viani L, Hardy DG, Baguley DM, Moffat DA. The patient's perspective after vestibular schwannoma removal: quality of life and implications for management. Am J Otol. 1995; 16(3):331–337

[60] Miller C, Sudhoff H, Jacob A. Vestibular schwannoma drug development: current state-of-the art. Curr Otorhinolaryngol Rep. 2014; 2:217–225

[61] Cayé-Thomasen P, Baandrup L, Jacobsen GK, Thomsen J, Stangerup SE. Immunohistochemical demonstration of vascular endothelial growth factor in vestibular schwannomas correlates to tumor growth rate. Laryngoscope. 2003; 113(12):2129–2134

[62] Cayé-Thomasen P, Werther K, Nalla A, et al. VEGF and VEGF receptor-1 concentration in vestibular schwannoma homogenates correlates to tumor growth rate. Otol Neurotol. 2005; 26(1):98–101

[63] Plotkin SR, Stemmer-Rachamimov AO, Barker FG, II, et al. Hearing improvement after bevacizumab in patients with neurofibromatosis type 2. N Engl J Med. 2009; 361(4):358–367

[64] Alanin MC, Klausen C, Caye-Thomasen P, et al. The effect of bevacizumab on vestibular schwannoma tumour size and hearing in patients with neurofibromatosis type 2. Eur Arch Otorhinolaryngol. 2015; 272(12):3627–3633

[65] Li KL, Djoukhadar I, Zhu X, et al. Vascular biomarkers derived from dynamic contrast-enhanced MRI predict response of vestibular schwannoma to antiangiogenic therapy in type 2 neurofibromatosis. Neuro-oncol. 2016; 18 (2):275–282

Part V

Management: Radiation

V

15 Principles of Radiobiology Relevant to Radiosurgery and Radiotherapy of Sporadic Vestibular Schwannoma

Robert Smee and Robert L. Foote

15.1 Introduction

With over 100 years of clinical practice and scientific evaluation, much is known about the application of radiotherapy to address malignancies. Important in this perspective is the relationship of cell kill versus cell survival. Simplistically, the former relates to eradicating cancer and the latter to preservation of adjacent normal tissue. The scientific endeavor to demonstrate and explain this is radiobiology. By this means, the clinical practice of radiotherapy is explained, and methods of modifying the standard approach explored. The basic component of the science is the cell-survival curve whereby in vitro a population of cells are irradiated, and the proportion of surviving cells, after varying doses and fractions over time, is evaluated. From this, the most valid demonstration of what is achieved is modeled by the linear quadratic (LQ) equation.[1,2] There are two components to the graphical demonstration of this equation: the alpha (α) component (single-hit/linear kinetics) and the beta (β) component (double-hit/quadratic kinetics).[2,3] Both malignant lesions and normal tissue can then be qualitatively described as being of early or late responding nature.[2]

There are significant challenges, however, in using this approach to describe what happens clinically when any form of radiotherapy is utilized to treat benign tumors, such as vestibular schwannomas.[4,5,6,7] Cell kill, while it can occur, at least with vestibular schwannoma, is much more difficult to demonstrate clinically and experimentally. Upward of 40% of treated vestibular schwannomas can demonstrate "central necrosis" radiologically in short-term follow-up, associated with a small component of volume expansion, subsequently settling down, and not regarded as true increase in size.[8] On magnetic resonance (MR), this central component has the imaging characteristics of necrosis (an implosion effect), demonstrated in the few publications where resected cases post–stereotactic radiosurgery have (SRS; ≥ 12 Gy single session) enlargement and are pathologically evaluated.[9] In a series where single-digit patient numbers were reported, ischemic infarction is evident, but with viable cells present on the periphery of the resected tumor.[10] This feature was evident in all four surgically resected cases in this series.[11]

The difficulty in extrapolating this circumstance is that, as stated earlier, only 40% of vestibular schwannomas treated demonstrate this central necrosis radiographically, there is still a minimum of another 50% of treated cases (given that > 90% are locally controlled) that do not demonstrate this feature but are still "controlled," with long-term follow-up. In addition, those operated upon post-SRS where enlargement is evident, that form part of the typically less than 10% of patients treated, may not be biologically the same as those who remain controlled.[12] An experimental model has been developed with a subrenal capsule xenograph in mice that may provide an answer.[4] Histological review indicates decreased tumor size with cytotoxic and vascular effect, at higher SRS doses than are used in the clinical situation.

Comparable control figures are reported for meningiomas, when treated by the same means, presumably with the same biological effect, but with a much lower circumstance of "central necrosis" demonstrated in follow-up. Conti et al, in describing the outcomes of CyberKnife management of perioptic meningiomas, discussed the radiobiology of hypofractionated multisession radiotherapy.[13] This is in the context of the optic nerve being the dose critical structure. This study graphically demonstrates using the LQ model, and an α/β of 2 for the tumor and 0.55 for the optic nerve, a means of creating a total dose and fraction number relationship for meningiomas, a tumor comparable to vestibular schwannomas. Others have reported, however, that the LQ model does not predict for optic neuropathy.[2,3,4]

Classical radiobiology, in demonstrating an effect, relies descriptively upon the four "Rs" (*r*e-oxygenation, *r*edistribution, *r*epopulation, and *r*epair) with intrinsic radiosensitivity added as a fifth in more recent years.[14] A concern is how applicable this methodology is to single session (≥ 12 Gy) SRS or multisession hypofractionated radiotherapy.[2,3,6] To date, it has not been evident whether there is a good alternative model, although the linear quadratic debate continues.[14] Radiobiological effects have been reported to impact upon the outcomes of treatment. In the early 1990s, long-term cranial nerve deficit rates post-SRS were regarded as being high, even in the context of high tumor control. Since then, there was a reduction in the utilized dose, with minor perceptible change in local control, but with improvement in cranial nerve preservation rates.[15] This dose change, associated with significant technological advances, accompanies many biological events.

15.2 Important Topics

15.2.1 The Biological Target

The question then is what is the biological target resulting in a clinical effect to which the LQ formula may be applicable. Is it the Schwann cells (with an answer potentially possible from the subrenal capsule xenograph model) or the endothelial cells that provide a vascular supply to the tumor?[11,16,17] Endothelial growth promoters are important with a demonstrated increased number of vessels, faster growth rate, and thus increased size with associated increase in vascular endothelial growth factor (VEGF) receptors in many NF2-related vestibular schwannoma, as well as in a number of sporadic cases.[11] This explains the benefit reported to VEGF inhibitors in the NF2-related vestibular schwannomas. There are very few clinical trials reported demonstrating a benefit in sporadic vestibular schwannoma for these drugs.

Apoptosis of schwannoma cells has been described with alterations in the absolute amount of Merlin detected as well as altering the schwannomin/Merlin ratio.[18] In one report, 60% of unilateral sporadic vestibular schwannomas were reported to have this feature.[18] Endothelial cell apoptosis has been reported at higher SRS doses than are utilized in the treatment of vestibular schwannoma.

Although not relevant initially, this phenomenon may explain the long-term hearing decline now being reported in follow-up, without any accompanying imaging change.[4]

15.2.2 Dose Rate Effect

Is there any importance of the treatment time?[19] The model B Gamma Knife treatment paradigm used limited number of isocenters with movement between each isocenter being manual not computerized. Hence, treatment times were long. Now with automated couch position movement, as in the Perfexion model, a greater number of isocenters are used but in a shorter treatment time. For both machinery types, there is a change in treatment times as the cobalt source ages. It is projected that this treatment time effect with comparable source strength may have resulted in an effective Gamma Knife model B dose of 14.41 to 15.43 Gy compared to a Perfexion model dose of 13 Gy, a 10 to 18% difference.[6] This may have partially explained or contributed to the higher complication rate seen at that time.[15] This dose-rate effect with different Gamma Knife devices is not apparent for the outcomes of treatment for arteriovenous malformations (AVMs).[19] For most linear accelerator-based approaches, dose rates are comparable as it would be unusual to treat in high dose rate physics/research mode.

15.2.3 Dose Inhomogeneity

The Gamma Knife approach uses a variable number of isocenters and prescribes dose to the 50% isodose line encompassing the entire tumor (margin dose). This results in dose inhomogeneity, certainly more than the usual single-isocenter linear accelerator-based treatment.[15] This is reported to result in better tumor control.[3] However, multiple linear accelerator-based series do not confirm this.

It should be noted that the majority of radiobiological models were developed for homogeneous dose distributions.[13] This is in contrast to most SRS series, where the SRS dose delivery, particularly where the Gamma Knife is used, is typically inhomogeneous. This further complicates the use of the LQ model to explain how SRS for vestibular schwannomas conceptually works.[20]

15.2.4 Single Fraction Effect

Vestibular schwannomas are regarded as a slow growing, late responding tissue. It could be considered that vestibular schwannomas are "relatively resistant" to the lower dose per fraction used in conventionally fractionated (1.8–2.0 Gy per fraction) courses of treatment. Hence, long-term tumor control is more likely to be higher with single session ≥ 12 Gy SRS treatment than where cumulative smaller fraction doses are used (1.8–2.0 Gy).[21] The literature does not verify this stance.

15.2.5 Multiple Fraction Effect

As per the aforementioned reports, long-term tumor control is equivalent; however, Andrews et al reported higher hearing preservation rates where 2.0 Gy fractions are used to administer a total dose of 50 Gy versus that outcome for single-session 12 Gy SRS.[22] This phenomenon is not explained well radiobiologically.

15.2.6 Volume Effect

As vestibular schwannomas enlarge, there is not only extension along the petrous ridge to involve more of the cerebellopontine angle (CPA), but there is also expansion and indentation into the adjacent brainstem. This indentation needs to be considered in a 3D sense, not as per single-slice transverse MR. Hence, the brainstem becomes a dose-limiting structure.[23] For many, this serves as a distinguishing point between single session ≥ 12 Gy SRS and conventionally or hypofractionated radiotherapy. Some Gamma Knife centers will still consider SRS, be it for selected patients, with reported low-morbidity rates.[24,25] The significance of the brainstem is that necrosis within that structure will have greater clinical effect than, say, the superiorly adjacent temporal lobe.[26]

Any tumor indenting into the brainstem is going to be of large volume. Do the large-volume vestibular schwannomas respond in the same way, to the same or lower dose, as small-volume tumors? Typically NF2-related tumors coming to SRS are larger than sporadic tumors, with lower likelihood of local control. Is this difference something inherently related to NF2 vestibular schwannomas, or is it that any type of large tumor does not do as well, and thus warrant a different treatment approach?[24] More clinical data are required to address this issue.

15.3 Complications

15.3.1 Cranial Nerves

Given the high tumor control rates, radiobiological attention has turned to examining complication rates, predominantly with hearing loss, although other cranial nerve effects are also noted. The LQ model does not represent well the risks of optic neuropathy, or other cranial nerve deficits, and hence can it be reliably used to define the risks of hearing loss, facial numbness, or facial weakness?[2,3] Other factors have been considered, such as the length of cranial nerve VIII within the treatment volume, and the specific dose to the cochlear apparatus.[19] As indicated earlier, the LQ model was developed for homogeneously treated targets, whereas for all Gamma Knife approaches, where multiple isocenters are treated and dose is prescribed to the 50% isodose line, there will be, more likely, considerable dose inhomogeneity with higher dose along the nerve. Yet there is, on average, comparability of hearing preservation rates between most Gamma Knife and linear accelerator-based series, the latter with more dose homogeneity and lower dose along the nerve.[27]

15.3.2 Malignancy

The consequences of treatment are important in addressing the appropriateness of any treatment method. While there are reported cases of malignancies arising in a presumed/known benign vestibular schwannoma, the Sheffield series of 5,000 patients with benign tumors treated by Gamma Knife SRS with 98% of patients accounted for contributing to the minimum 20-year follow-up documented no increased incidence of malignancy (compared to a matched population). This gives considerable confidence in continuing with this approach.[28] A further discussion regarding risk of malignancy following SRS or fractionated radiotherapy can be found in Chapter 24.

15.4 Protectors

There has been some work on developing radioprotectors for normal tissues, where high-dose conventionally fractionated radiotherapy is used in the treatment of malignancies. There is similar experimental work in developing pharmacological protectors to be used during the treatment of vestibular schwannomas.[19] Tumor tissue protection is obviously of concern in this circumstance.

15.5 Conclusion

Classical radiobiology has yet to fully explain what is happening in the radiotherapeutic management of vestibular schwannomas. While the LQ model is useful in explaining the treatment of cancers where cell kill and survival can be easily demonstrated clinically and radiographically, these concepts are not as applicable for benign tumors as cell kill does not have the same meaning. Central necrosis is evident post-SRS in a minority of treated vestibular schwannoma patients; however, for comparable tumors (meningiomas, other schwannomas, and pituitary tumors) the same change is not seen. Is there a difference in the radiobiology of vestibular schwannomas versus other benign tumors? Do vestibular schwannomas decrease in volume by cell kill or a reduction in cell size? Is there a major biological difference in what is happening in those vestibular schwannomas that remain stable in size for many years versus those in which volume reduction occurs? Considerable work still needs to be done to explain what is happening; simplistically accepting the LQ model to explain events will not help the science to advance.

Coincidently, using the LQ model to define normal tissue, specifically cranial nerve, tolerance in selecting a dose to be given to an adjacent benign tumor is fraught with concern. Fortunately, most tumors are controlled by modest SRS doses that historically have low prospect of creating harm. However, are we as confident about the tolerance of a damaged or compressed nerve as we are of that of a normal nerve? SRS has been shown to work in the great majority of tumors and to be reasonably safe in that same majority of patients. How it works needs further evaluation.

References

[1] Kirkpatrick JP, Meyer JJ, Marks LB. The linear-quadratic model is inappropriate to model high dose per fraction effects in radiosurgery. Semin Radiat Oncol. 2008; 18(4):240–243

[2] Niranjan A, Flickinger J. Radiobiology, principle and technique of radiosurgery. In: Regis J, Roche P, eds. Modern Management of Acoustic Neuroma. Vol 21. Basel, Switzerland: Karger; 2008:39

[3] Flickinger J. Radiobiological and dosimetric considerations in stereotactic radiosurgery. In: Pollock B, ed. Contemporary Stereotactic Radiosurgery. New York, NY: Futura; 2002:40

[4] Kondziolka D, Shin SM, Brunswick A, Kim I, Silverman JS. The biology of radiosurgery and its clinical applications for brain tumors. Neuro-oncol. 2015; 17(1):29–44

[5] Casentini L, Fornezza U, Perini Z, Perissinotto E, Colombo F. Multisession stereotactic radiosurgery for large vestibular schwannomas. J Neurosurg. 2015; 122(4):818–824

[6] Hopewell J, Millbar W, Lindquist C. Radiobiological principles: their application to gamma knife therapy. In: Kim D, Lunsford L, eds. Current and Future Management of Brain Metastasis. Vol 25. Pittsburg, PA: Karger; 2012:44

[7] Balagamwala EH, Chao ST, Suh JH. Principles of radiobiology of stereotactic radiosurgery and clinical applications in the central nervous system. Technol Cancer Res Treat. 2012; 11(1):3–13

[8] Delsanti C, Roche P, Thomassin J, Regis J. Morphological changes of vestibular schwannomas after radiosurgical treatment: pitfalls and diagnosis of failure. In: Regis J, Roche P, eds. Modern Management of Acoustic Neuroma. Vol 21. Basel, Switzerland: Karger; 2008:94

[9] Levivier M. Tissue changes after radiosurgery for vestibular schwannomas. In: Regis J, Roche P, eds. Modern Management of Acoustic Neuroma. Vol 21. Basel, Switzerland: Karger; 2008:101

[10] Kaye A, Briggs R, Morokoff A. Acoustic neurinoma (vestibular schwannoma). In: Kaye A, Laws E, eds. Brain Tumors. 3rd ed. Philadelphia, PA: Saunders Elsevier; 2012:532

[11] Yeung AH, Sughrue ME, Kane AJ, Tihan T, Cheung SW, Parsa AT. Radiobiology of vestibular schwannomas: mechanisms of radioresistance and potential targets for therapeutic sensitization. Neurosurg Focus. 2009; 27(6) E2:E2

[12] Pollock BE, Lunsford LD, Kondziolka D, et al. Vestibular schwannoma management: Part II. Failed radiosurgery and the role of delayed microsurgery. J Neurosurg. 2013; 119 Suppl:949–955

[13] Conti A, Pontoriero A, Midili F, et al. CyberKnife multisession stereotactic radiosurgery and hypofractionated stereotactic radiotherapy for perioptic meningiomas: intermediate-term results and radiobiological considerations. Springerplus. 2015; 4(37):37

[14] Brown JM, Carlson DJ, Brenner DJ. The tumor radiobiology of SRS and SBRT: are more than the 5 Rs involved? Int J Radiat Oncol Biol Phys. 2014; 88(2): 254–262

[15] Niranjan A, Lunsford L, Flickinger J, Kondziolka D. Acoustic neuroma radiosurgery: lessons learned. In: McDermott M, ed. Radiosurgery. Vol 7. Basel, Switzerland: Karger; 2010:143

[16] Song CW, Kim MS, Cho LC, Dusenbery K, Sperduto PW. Radiobiological basis of SBRT and SRS. Int J Clin Oncol. 2014; 19(4):570–578

[17] Karam SD, Bhatia S. The radiobiological targets of SBRT: tumor cells or endothelial cells? Ann Transl Med. 2015; 3(19):290–294

[18] Roche P, Bouvier C, Chinot O, Figarella-Branger D. Genesis and biology of vestibular schwannomas. In: Regis J, Roche P, eds. Modern Management of Acoustic Neuroma. Vol 21. Basel, Switzerland: Karger; 2008:24

[19] Flickinger J, Kondziolka D, Niranjan A, Lunsford L. Dose selection in stereotactic radiosurgery. In: Szeifert G, Kondziolka D, Levivier M, Lunsford L, eds. Radiosurgery and Pathological Fundamentals. Vol 20. Basel, Switzerland: Karger; 2007:29

[20] Anker C, Shrieve D. Basic principles of radiobiology applied to radiosurgery and radiotherapy of benign skull base tumours. In: Battista R, ed. Radiosurgery and Radiotherapy for Benign Skull Base Tumours. Vol 42. Philadelphia, PA: Elsevier; 2009:608

[21] Regis J, Roche P, Delsanti C, Soumare O, Thomassin J, Pellet W. Stereotactic radiosurgery for vestibular schwannoma. In: Pollock B, ed. Contemporary Stereotactic Radiosurgery. New York, NY: Futura; 2002:185

[22] Andrews DW, Suarez O, Goldman HW, et al. Stereotactic radiosurgery and fractionated stereotactic radiotherapy for the treatment of acoustic schwannomas: comparative observations of 125 patients treated at one institution. Int J Radiat Oncol Biol Phys. 2001; 50(5):1265–1278

[23] Ogunrinde O, Lunsford D, Kondziolka D, Bissonette D, Flickinger J. Cranial nerve preservation after stereotactic radiosurgery of intracanalicular acoustic tumors. In: Gildenberg P, ed. Stereotactic and Functional Neurosurgery. Basel, Switzerland: Karger; 1995:87–97

[24] Yang HC, Kano H, Awan NR, et al. Gamma Knife radiosurgery for larger-volume vestibular schwannomas: clinical article. J Neurosurg. 2013; 119 Suppl:801–807

[25] Inoue H, Nishi H, Shibazaki T, Ono N. Hearing preservation after radiosurgery combined with or without microsurgery for large vestibular schwannomas: preliminary results. In: Kondziolka D, ed. Radiosurgery. Vol 5. Basel, Switzerland: Karger; 2004:107–114

[26] Leith J, Cook S, Chougule P, et al. Intrinsic and extrinsic characteristics of human tumors relevant to radiosurgery: comparative cellular radiosensitivity and hypoxic percentages. In: Lindquist C, Kondziolka D, Loeffler, eds. Advances in Radiosurgery. New York, NY: Springer-Verlag; 1994:19

[27] Kim C-H, Chung KW, Kong D-S, et al. Prognostic factors of hearing preservation after gamma knife radiosurgery for vestibular schwannoma. J Clin Neurosci. 2010; 17(2):214–218

[28] Rowe J, Grainger A, Walton L, Silcocks P, Radatz M, Kemeny A. Risk of malignancy after gamma knife stereotactic radiosurgery. Neurosurgery. 2007; 60(1):60–65, discussion 65–66

16 Gamma Knife Radiosurgery for Treatment of Sporadic Vestibular Schwannoma

Michael J. Link, Bruce E. Pollock, Matthew L. Carlson, and Robert L. Foote

16.1 Introduction

Gamma Knife radiosurgery (GKRS) was developed by Lars Leksell, a Swedish neurosurgeon, in the 1950s as reviewed in Chapter 2.[1] Over the past more than 60 years, and especially in the past 30 years, GKRS has become a well-established, safe, and effective treatment for vestibular schwannomas (VSs) worldwide. According to the international treatment registry kept by the Leksell Gamma Knife Society, a total of 100,609 VSs were treated with GKRS between 1968, when the registry began, and 2016, the most recent year with complete data.[2] There is a clear worldwide trend over the past 15 years for an increasing number of VS patients per year being treated with GKRS (▶ Fig. 16.1). By 1995, a total of 4,810 patients, by 2005, 32,610 patients, and by 2016 more than 100,000 VS patients had been treated with GKRS. In 2016 alone, there were 7,709 VSs treated worldwide with GKRS, 1,160 of which were treated in North America. There are currently 116 Gamma Knife centers in the United States, and as of February 1, 2017, a total of 325 gamma units have been installed worldwide.

The general principle of GKRS involves application of a stereotactic head frame, which allows for rigid head fixation during treatment, and also allows for the establishment of a coordinate system. Next, a fiducial system attaches to the head frame during imaging, allowing a computer dose-planning system to reference the fiducials with the desired images, creating a stereotactic space. The dose-planning system then calculates summated isodose curves of individual "shots of radiation" taking into account the cumulative effect of isocenter placement, collimator size, weighting, and head angulation to create a highly conformal prescription isodose to cover the tumor.

We installed our first gamma unit (Model U) at the Mayo Clinic in 1990 and then subsequently upgraded to the Model B, Model C, 4C, and since 2007 have used the model Perfexion (▶ Fig. 16.2). The previous units used 201 Co^{60} radiation sources arranged more or less concentrically to provide an ovoid isocenter of radiation. The radiation beams could be collimated to 4, 8, 14, or 18 mm. Some of the 201 channels could be blocked in order to protect radiosensitive structures such as the lens of the eye, or to slightly "shape" the isocenter. Admittedly, the process of blocking more than a few beams was very labor intensive, and rarely employed. Thus, multiple differentially weighted isocenters were each assigned a unique x (right/left), y (anterior/posterior), and z (superior/inferior) coordinates in the stereotactic space. When the radiation contribution of each isocenter is summed, this then results in a very conformal radiation plan that highly matches the shape of the VS. The Perfexion unit, instead, uses 192 Co^{60} sources also arranged concentrically. The isocenters are further subdivided into eight sections of 24 sources. Each section can be automatically collimated to 4, 8, or 16 mm, or completely blocked. Thus, with this latest version of the gamma unit, there are thousands of different possible isocenters one could create. This allows for more flexibility when shaping each individual isocenter, which at times proves helpful to avoid radiation to critical structures. Also, a very conformal plan can be created with fewer individual isocenters or "shots," making treatment more efficient.

The purpose of this chapter is to review the technique and results of GKRS for VS, using contemporary techniques and dose. Primary endpoints of interest include tumor control, facial nerve, hearing and other cranial nerve morbidity, and other treatment-related side effects.

16.2 Technique

16.2.1 Patient Consultation

At our institution, all patients with sporadic VS are initially evaluated by a neurosurgeon and a neurotologist, and counseled regarding the options available for treatment of their tumor. Currently, we offer GKRS as a treatment option to all patients with tumors that have a maximum posterior fossa diameter of less than 2.5 cm. We have occasionally treated larger tumors and it is highly dependent on patient comorbidities, history of prior

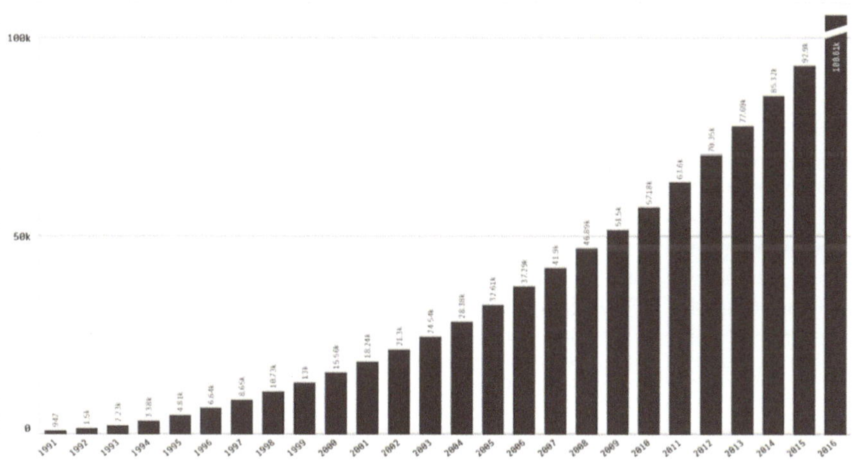

Fig. 16.1 Cumulative number of vestibular schwannoma patients treated with Gamma Knife radiosurgery worldwide by year. The percentage of centers submitting their numbers each year has varied between 68 and 100% from 1968 to 2016. The year 1991 reflects cumulative numbers since 1968 when the registry was begun. Data courtesy of the Leksell Gamma Knife Society.

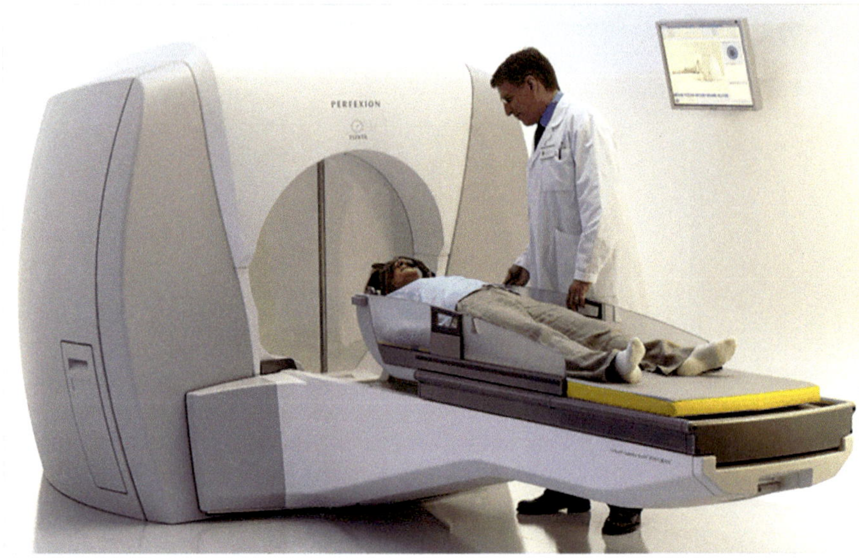

Fig. 16.2 The Perfexion unit, utilizing 192 Co^{60} sources. (Used with permission from Elekta AB, Stockholm, Sweden).

treatment, and preferences.[3] Patients who select GKRS are then also seen by a radiation oncologist the day prior to undertaking treatment, and the goals, risks, benefits, and alternatives of VS GKRS are reviewed yet again. An updated audiogram including pure-tone average (PTA) and speech discrimination scores (SDS) is obtained. Patients are instructed not to eat or drink anything after midnight the evening before the procedure. They are allowed to take any daily medications with a sip of water the morning of treatment and then are instructed to report to the hospital the morning of the outpatient treatment of their tumor. Patients are given 1 mg of oral midazolam for mild sedation and then transported to the gamma unit.

16.2.2 Head Frame Application

With the patient in the seated position, the head and hair are cleaned with 70% isopropyl alcohol and the Leksell model G stereotactic head frame is applied using local anesthesia (2:1 mixture of 1% lidocaine with 1:100,000 epinephrine and 0.25% Marcaine including 10% $NaHCO_3$) and four-point pin fixation. The head frame is positioned slightly eccentric to the side of the tumor with the ear bars resting in the ear canals. It is optimal to keep the base ring of the head frame as low as possible to minimize distortion artifact on the planning imaging. Five to 6 milliliters of local anesthetic are injected at the expected location of each of the pins, and after allowing ample time for the sites to become appropriately anesthetized, the pins are inserted through the skin to the outer table of the skull. We simultaneously tighten opposing pins (right anterior and left posterior; left anterior and right posterior) using hand tools only. We prefer that these be tightened to finger pressure tightness only. It is obviously critically important that the head frame does not move during imaging or treatment, but if the pins are over torqued it can bow the upright supports that can then warp the base ring and potentially alter how the fiducial boxes sit on the frame during imaging. This can introduce additional error into the stereotactic accuracy of the imaging. Most patients find the head frame application mildly uncomfortable and are left with a sense of head pressure for several minutes to an hour after application that then becomes minimally bothersome.

16.2.3 Imaging

The patient is then transported to the magnetic resonance imaging (MRI) suite where they undergo postgadolinium axial imaging with a standard fiducial box in place. The protocols we use to scan our patients are listed in ▶ Table 16.1. One-millimeter-thick axial postgadolinium images are used for planning. Sagittal and coronal reconstructions are performed by the Gamma Plan software (Elekta AB, Stockholm, Sweden) to also aid in dose planning. These sequences usually result in a mean stereotactic error of 0.1 to 0.3 mm and a maximum error of 0.3 to 0.7 mm. We will accept a mean error up to 0.3 mm, but we will rescan or repeat imaging on a different MR scanner for anything greater, until satisfied. A thin-slice noncontrast stereotactic computed tomographic (CT) scan of the temporal bones is then obtained to better define the bony margins of the internal auditory canal (IAC) and the inner ear structures such as the cochlea and vestibule (▶ Table 16.1). The MRI and CT imaging can be fused as well to allow a hybrid-type image to visualize the tumor optimally (MRI), as well as the surrounding inner ear structures (CT). In addition, nonstereotactic imaging such as FIESTA (Fast Imaging Employing Steady-state Acquisition), heavily T2-weighted, thin-slice axial imaging, obtained prior to GKRS for diagnostic purposes, can be coregistered with the stereotactic images on the day of GKRS in some cases for more definite estimation of the degree of fundal extension, for instance. Of note, all the stereotactic imaging must have a large enough field of view (FOV) to incorporate the fiducial markers to allow stereotactic registration. In our experience, it is difficult to acquire FIESTA imaging, for example, with a sufficiently large FOV without a bothersome amount of distortion while the patient is in the stereotactic head frame. All the imaging is transferred via the Ethernet to the planning computer workstation.

Skull and frame measurements are taken per a standardized protocol, and likewise entered into the workstation. These measurements provide an estimation of the size and shape of

Table 16.1 Imaging protocols for Gamma Knife radiosurgery dose planning using both Siemens Medical Solutions (Malvern, PA) and GE Healthcare (Chicago, IL), 1.5 or 3.0 Tesla magnet strength

Imaging options for Siemens Medical Solutions MRI scanners								
Sequence	**Plane**	**2D or 3D**	**Frequency**	**Phase**	**Slices**	**Field of view (cm)**	**Slice thickness (mm)**	**Signal averages**
Localizer	3-plane	2D	256	224	11	30	5	1
T1 FLASH	Axial	3D	256	256	60	25	1	2
T1 FLASH	Axial	3D	256	256	30	25	1	2
T1 Spin Echo	Axial	2D	256	256	30	24	3	2
T1 Spin Echo	Coronal	2D	256	256	30	24	3	2
T2 CISS	Axial	3D	256	256	64	25	0.5	2
MPRAGE	Axial	3D	256	256	144	25	1	1
Imaging options for GE medical solutions MRI scanners								
Sequence	**Plane**	**2D or 3D**	**Frequency**	**Phase**	**Slicers**	**Field of view (cm)**	**Slice thickness (mm)**	**Signal averages**
Localizer	3-plane	2D	256	128	11	30	10	1
MPRANGE	Axial	3D	256	224	80	24	1	1
T1 Spin Echo	Axial	2D	256	256	60	24	1.4	1
T2 Spin Echo	Axial	2D	256	320	25	25	1.8	1
GE Localizer	3-plane	2D	256	128	50	30	2.5	1
Brovo	Axial	3D	256	256	200	24	1	1
SPGR	Axial	3D	256	254	60	24	1	1
T1 Spin Echo-Flow Comp	Axial	2D	256	256	48	24	3	1
T1 Spin Echo-sat	Axial	2D	256	256	48	24	3	1
T1 Spin Echo	Axial	2D	256	256	24	24	1.1	1
SPGR	Axial	3D	256	256	74	30	4	1
Imaging options for CT scanner (Siemens F-128 scanner) for imaging temporal bones								
Siemens				**F-128**				
Scan type				Spiral				
Rotation time (s)				1				
Collimation				128x.6				
Pitch				0.6				
kVp				120				
Effective mA				350				
CARE dose 4D				Off				
Scan field (mm)				*300*				
Prep delay				Min allowable				
Min. Retro (mm)				*0.6*				
CTDI-vol (mGy)				*53.55*				
Base protocol				*Head routine*				

Note: Scan is acquired from top of C1 to top of petrous temporal bones (0-degree gantry tilt, no tilt).

the patient's head, which assists in the computerized calculation of the dose contribution of each individual beam of radiation to the total dose. They also serve as a check to make sure there will not be any collisions between the head frame or the patient's head and the treatment unit.

16.2.4 Dose Planning and Treatment

Treatment planning has been greatly facilitated by progressive improvements in the Gamma Plan software over the past 20 years. As detailed earlier, a combination of isocenters is selected, placed, and differentially weighted to create a highly conformal dose plan primarily based on the post-gadolinium axial SPGR (Spoiled Gradient Recalled Acquisition in the Steady State) imaging dataset (▶ Fig. 16.3). There has been a trend toward more isocenters per plan over the past two decades, but the plan may be rarely as simple as a single isocenter to more than 20, depending on size and shape of the VS. From 1990 to 1997, a total of 88 VS patients were treated at Mayo Clinic with a mean number of 5.3 isocenters per case, and between 1997 and 2004, the mean number of isocenters increased to 7.9 per case ($n = 205$ patients).[4] The evolution of dose planning, dose selection, and subsequent reduction in morbidity from the first decade of our practice is outlined in ▶ Table 16.2. During the last decade, there has been significant interest in cochlea dose as a possible risk factor for hearing loss following GKRS, and therefore blocking of certain sections of the isocenter can be employed to try and limit dose extending in the direction of the cochlea.

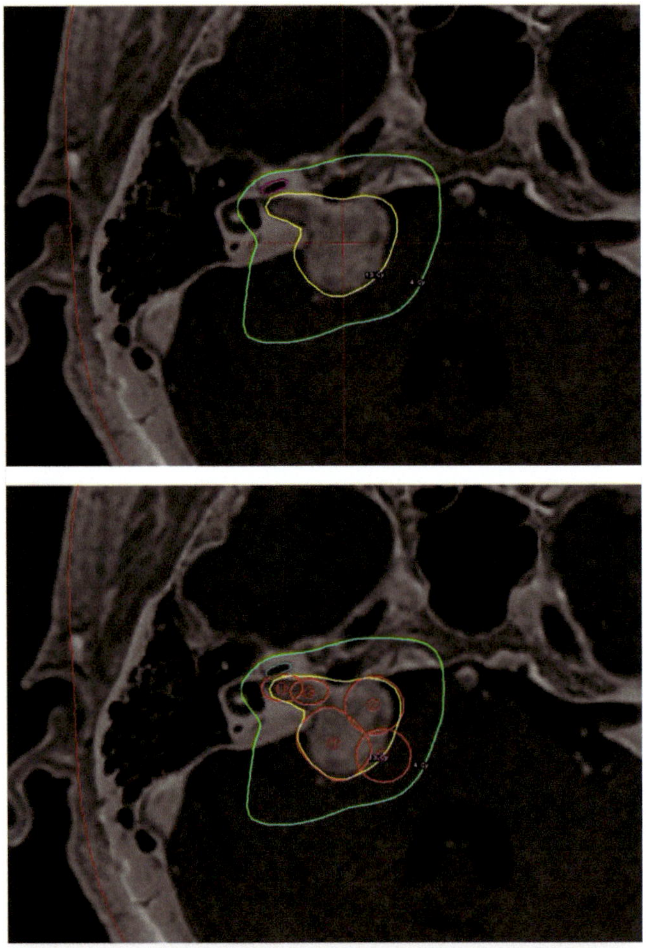

Fig. 16.3 Fused axial CT–MRI image demonstrating a typical treatment plan for a right-sided vestibular schwannoma utilizing a marginal dose of 13 Gy to the 50% isodose line (*yellow*). Multiple isocenters or "shots" (*red spheres*, bottom image) are arranged to cover the entire tumor volume, while limiting radiation to adjacent radiosensitive structures such as the brainstem and cochlea. For illustrative purposes, the 4-Gy isodose line is shown in *green*. Despite optimal planning, the cochlear volume receives more than 4 Gy given the significant fundal extension of the tumor.

Almost all tumors are treated at the 50% isodose line, by convention, as this allows for the steepest dose fall off. The great majority of VSs are now treated with 12.5 Gy to the 50% isodose line. A few years ago, the physicists at Elekta AB calculated a new tissue maximum ratio (TMR), thus effectively changing the calculated dose delivered; and therefore to stay consistent with our dose practice from the first 25 years of our experience, we increased the prescribed dose by an additional 0.5 to 1 Gy to deliver the same amount of radiation as had been previously used for VS. The latest version of Gamma Plan will provide the calculated dose for both the old and new TMR; so, the dose can be precisely adjusted if desired.[5] For patients with useful ipsilateral hearing (i.e., > 50% SDS), we most commonly prescribe 12.5 to 13 Gy, and for patients who are already functionally deaf in their tumor ear, we use 13.5 to 14.5 Gy to the 50% isodose line. For larger tumors (i.e., volume > 10 cm^3), we usually limit the prescription dose to 12 Gy in order to reduce the risk of treatment-associated edema and hydrocephalus. While other centers have published series using very low-dose GKRS for VS, we have been reluctant to use less than 12 Gy for any indication as we worry about a possible decreased efficacy below this dose.

There has been much discussion in the radiosurgical literature regarding the influence of cochlea dose on hearing outcomes for VS.[6,7,8,9,10,11,12] As a result, we routinely contour the cochlea on the planning of thin-slice CT of the temporal bones, and Gamma Plan allows determination of a mean, minimum, and maximum dose to the cochlea. However, we have not found cochlea dose to be an independent factor in predicting hearing outcome when accounting for other confounding factors.[13] Likely, the cause for hearing deterioration after GKRS is multifactorial and is most heavily impacted by hearing status at the time of treatment, volume treated, and marginal dose. To a lesser degree, loss of serviceable hearing may also be impacted by radiation dose to the cochlear nuclei in the brainstem, the cochlear nerve, and various aspects of the cochlea such as the stria vascularis—a structure that is thought to be particularly sensitive to the effects of ionizing radiation.[10] Based on current evidence in the literature, we attempt to limit the dose to the cochlea as much as feasible, but never at the expense of whole tumor coverage. That is, we always fully treat the lateral extent of the tumor as dictated by the detailed imaging at the time of radiosurgical planning, and we do not reduce the tumor marginal dose below 12 or 12.5 Gy to specifically reduce cochlea

Table 16.2 Evolution of dose planning, dose selection, and morbidity during the first decade of GKRS for VS at the Mayo Clinic

	1/1990–12/1993 (*N* = 44)	1/1994–5/1997 (*N* = 57)	6/1997–12/2000 (*N* = 84)
Tumor volume (cm^3)	3.2 (0.3–8.7)	4.6 (0.4–20.4)	2.4 (0.06–12.8)
Marginal dose (Gy)	18 (16–20)	15 (12–16)	13 (12–16)
Maximum dose (Gy)	36 (25–40)	30 (24–32)	27 (19–32)
No. of isocenters	5 (1–12)	6 (1–14)	8 (2–20)
Temporary VII deficit	11%	5%	1%
Permanent VII deficit	20.5%	10.5%	0%
Hemifacial spasm	7%	7%	3.6%
V paresthesias	36%	17.5%	3.6%
Hearing loss	75%	19%	22.6%

dose. Therefore, in our experience, if the tumor extends to the fundus of the IAC, there is no possibility of keeping the mean dose to the cochlea below 6 Gy for instance, and in some cases the cochlea dose may be as high as 10 Gy.[6,14] We do not routinely calculate dose to any other structures such as brainstem or trigeminal nerve, for instance, during dose planning.

During treatment, the head frame is locked into the treatment couch with the patient in a comfortable supine position. The patient's head can be elevated or lowered to maximize comfort. The machine then moves the patient automatically, in turn to each x, y, and z for each individual shot for the prescribed time until the treatment is complete. Depending on the number and size of isocenters used, dose prescribed, age of the Co^{60}, and to a lesser extent size of the patient's head, treatment times may vary from as little as approximately 20 minutes to as long as 2 hours. Once treatment is complete, the patient is removed from the gamma unit, the stereotactic head frame is removed, a light head dressing is applied, and the patient returns to the outpatient observation area. We administer 4 mg of intravenous dexamethasone after completion of the treatment, and after approximately 2 hours the patient is discharged. A minority of patients will develop significant scalp, periorbital, or facial edema related to the moderately large volume of local anesthetic used during head frame placement and occasionally some will report experiencing complete unilateral eye closure related to swelling; however, this edema always resolves within 48 to 72 hours with head elevation and application of cold compresses. Pin site infection requiring oral antibiotics has occurred in less than a dozen cases in more than 6,000 head frame placements at our institution. There have been no cases of osteomyelitis or need for intravenous antibiotic treatment.

16.3 Results

Since Georg Norén first performed GKRS to treat a VS at Karolinska Institute in Stockholm, in 1969, we have learned a great deal about the functional and radiographic outcomes of this modality. Various large-volume radiosurgical centers have reported hearing, facial nerve, other cranial nerve, and tumor control outcomes. Despite nearly 50 years of experience and more than 100,000 patients treated worldwide, there still remains some controversy regarding GKRS outcomes and how they should be reported. ▶ Table 16.3 summarizes select recent publications reporting clinical outcomes following low-dose (≤ 14 Gy marginal dose) Gamma Knife radiosurgery for sporadic VS.

16.3.1 Facial Nerve Outcomes

In the late 1980s and early 1990s, there was very limited information to guide dose selection for GKRS for VS. Subsequently, most centers, including ours, used 18 to 20 Gy to the 50% isodose line covering the tumor. At Mayo Clinic, between 1990 and 1993, 44 VSs were treated with a mean marginal dose of 18 Gy (range, 16–20 Gy) and a mean number of five isocenters (range, 1–12). Twenty-one percent of patients developed new permanent facial nerve weakness. The marginal dose was subsequently reduced in 1994 to a mean of 16 Gy, and then to a mean marginal dose of 13 Gy in 1996. Since then we have only had two cases of permanent facial paresis, one House-Brackmann (HB) grade III and one grade V, following GKRS for more than 600 presumed sporadic VS.[15] Rarely, patients will develop transient hemifacial spasm (HFS) approximately 4 to 12 months after treatment that consistently resolves within 3 to 6 months of onset. This usually correlates to fairly dramatic transient tumor swelling and loss of central enhancement, suggesting a robust inflammatory response in the tumor to the radiation. If the patient is disturbed by this symptom, we commonly prescribe a short course of dexamethasone and gabapentin or baclofen. In our prospective study comparing GKRS and microsurgical resection of VS, the only cases in the GKRS cohort ($n = 46$) to develop facial paresis were two patients who required microsurgical salvage after their tumors did not respond to radiation treatment.[16] There have been rare reports of acute facial paresis occurring immediately following GKRS for VS, but this is indeed extremely rare.[17,18,19]

Other centers report equally excellent early facial nerve outcomes using marginal doses of 12 to 13 Gy. In 2001, Flickinger et al, from the University of Pittsburgh, reported 99% HB grade I to II function following treatment of 192 patients with a median follow-up of 30 months.[19] Similarly, Régis et al, in 2002, reported no new facial nerve paralysis (100% HB grades I–II) among 104 patients with a minimum follow-up of 3 years, although two patients had transient weakness that resolved.[20] A more recent report from Régis et al reported a new facial nerve paresis rate of 0.5% among 2,336 VSs treated with GKRS, receiving a marginal dose of either 11 or 12 Gy at La Timone University Hospital in Marseille, France.[21] When higher marginal doses are used, as in our early experience, a higher incidence of facial nerve paralysis is reported. Hasegawa et al reported long-term follow-up on 73 sporadic VSs treated with marginal doses ranging from 10 to 18 Gy, with 7% developing permanent facial nerve palsy at 6 to 15 months following GKRS.[22] Boari et al reported long-term follow-up on 379 patients treated with marginal doses of 11 to 15 Gy, and 4 patients (1.1%) experienced new permanent facial nerve weakness.[23] Using contemporary imaging, dose planning software, and marginal doses of 12 to 14 Gy, we counsel patients that they have less than a 1% risk of permanent facial nerve weakness or HFS following GKRS to treat a VS under 2.5 cm in maximum posterior fossa diameter.[24]

16.3.2 Hearing Outcomes

One of the most fascinating questions in all of VS management is what is the true long-term hearing preservation rate following GKRS? The literature is often difficult to interpret when some authors only report PTA, for instance, a notoriously poor estimation of functional hearing.[25,26] When considering preservation of serviceable hearing to be a PTA less than 50 dB HL and an SDS greater than 50% (i.e., AAO–HNS class A and B or Gardner Robertson grade I and II), hearing preservation rates following GKRS range from 32 to 71% with variable lengths of follow-up extending from 3.5 to 9 years.[27,28,29,30,31,32] In a prospective, nonrandomized study comparing GKRS and microsurgery at Mayo Clinic, we obtained a serviceable hearing preservation rate of 61% in 46 patients treated with GKRS at a median follow-up of 42 months (range, 12–62 months).[16] A very similar prospective study undertaken by Myrseth et al, in Bergen,

Table 16.3 Recent publications reporting clinical outcomes following low-dose (≤ 14 Gy marginal dose) Gamma Knife radiosurgery for sporadic vestibular schwannoma

Author	Year of publication	No. of patients	Tumor size	Follow-up	Dose strategy	Tumor control	New facial nerve dysfunction	New trigeminal nerve dysfunction	Hydrocephalus	Hearing
Prospective studies										
Régis et al[20]	2002	97	Mean or median: NR	NR	12–14 Gy	97% no surgery	0% paresis, 3% hemispasm	4%	3% hydrocephalus	50% retained SH
Paek et al[62]	2005	25	Median: 3.0 cm^3	Median: 45 mo	12 Gy	92% no growth, 100% no surgery	0%	0%	0%	52% (13/25) retained SH
Pollock et al[15]	2006	46	Mean: 1.5 cm^3	Mean: 42 mo	Mean: 12.2 Gy	96% no surgery	0%	2%	4%	63% retained SH
Myrseth et al[32]	2009	60	Mean: 1.6 cm	All patients 2 y	12 Gy	98% no surgery	0%	NR	0%	76% and 68% retained SH at 1 and 2 y, respectively
Regis et al[37]	2010	34	Mean: 112.5 mm^3	Mean: 46 mo	Median: 12 Gy	97%	NR	NR	NR	At 3, 4, and 5 y, SH was retained in 77, 70, and 64%, respectively
Kim et al[64]	2011	41	Mean: 1.5 cm^3	Median: 30 mo	Median: 12 Gy	88% no growth, 98% no surgery	0%	0%	NR	61% (25/41) retained SH
Breivik et al[69]	2013	113	Mean: 3.9 cm^3	Mean: 55 mo	12 Gy	94% no additional treatment	0%	0%	NR	36% retained SH
Retrospective studies										
Prasad et al[57]	2000	96*	Mean: 2.7 cm^3	Mean: 4.3 y	Median: 13 Gy	94% no growth	2%	4%	0% hydrocephalus	58% (21/36) retained SH
Flickinger et al[19]	2001	190	Median: 2.7 cm^3	Median: 30 mo	Median: 13 Gy	5-y 97% no surgery	Actuarial 5-y 1%	Actuarial 5-y 3%	NR	81% (61/75) retained SH with a 5-y actuarial preservation rate of 74%
Petit et al[58]	2001	35*	Median: 1.8 cm	Median: 3.5 y	Median: 12 Gy	100% no growth and no surgery	4% transient, no permanent	0%	NR	100% with GR grade I or II at baseline retained GR grades I–III at follow-up
Iwai et al[59]	2003	51	Median: 3.6 cm^3	Median: 60 mo	≤ 12 Gy	96% no surgery	0% paresis, 6% hemispasm	0%	6%	56% (10/18) retained SH
Litvack et al[60]	2003	134	Median or mean: NR	Mean: 32 mo	12 Gy	97% no surgery	2% transient paresis, 6% transient spasm	6% transient	3%	62% (29/47) retained SH
Flickinger et al[61]	2004	313	Median: 1.1 cm^3	Median: 24 mo	Median: 13 Gy	6-y 99% no surgery	0%	4%		79% (218/246) retained SH
Hasegawa et al[40]	2005	317	Median or mean: NR	Median: 7.8 y	Mean: 13.2 Gy	91% no surgery	6% high-dose group, 1% transient in low-dose group	4% high-dose group, 2% low-dose group	7%	68% (50/74) retained SH with marginal dose ≤ 13 Gy
Massager et al[6]	2007	82	NR	Median: 2 y	12 Gy	99% no growth	NR	NR	NR	65% (39/60) retained SH

Table 16.3 (*Continued*)

Author	Year of publication	No. of patients	Tumor size	Follow-up	Dose strategy	Tumor control	New facial nerve dysfunction	New trigeminal nerve dysfunction	Hydrocephalus	Hearing
Chopra et al[26]	2007	216	Median: 1.3 cm^3	Median: 5.7 y	Median: 13 Gy	10-y 98% no surgery	0% paresis, 1% hemispasm	5%	NR	56.6% (60/106) retained SH. The 10-y actuarial preservation rate was 44.5%
Lasak et al[7]	2008	33	Mean: 1.48 cm^3	Median: 24 mo	12–13 Gy	94% no growth, 100% no surgery	3% transient hemispasm	3%	NR	90% (9/10) retained SH
Tamura et al[63]	2009	74	Median or mean: NR	Median: 48 mo	Median: 12 Gy	93% no additional treatment	1%	10%	NR	70% of patients with GR I at baseline retained SH at 8 y and beyond
Hasegawa et al[12]	2011	117	Median: 1.9 cm^3	Median: 74 mo	Median: 12 Gy	98% no growth	NR	NR	NR	At 3, 5, and 8 years, SH was retained in 55, 43, and 34%, respectively
Han et al[65]	2012	119	Mean: 1.95 cm^3	Mean: 55 mo	Median: 12 Gy	NR	NR	NR	NR	At 12, 24, 36, and 60 mo, SH was retained in 68.5, 62.5, 59.9, and 56.2%, respectively
Sun et al[66]	2012	190	Median: 3.6 cm^3	Median: 109 mo	≤14 Gy	90% no growth	14% transient paresis, 1% permanent	21% transient, 3% permanent	3%	86% (19/22) retained SH
Yomo et al[25]	2012	154	Mean: 0.73 mL	Mean: 60 mo	Mean: 12.1 Gy	95% no additional treatment	1%	1%	1%	58% retained SH
Baschnagel et al[67]	2013	40	Median: 0.23 cm^3	Median: 25 mo	Median: 12.5 Gy	100%	0%	0%		At 1, 3, and 5 y, SH was retained in 93, 77, and 74%, respectively
Carlson et al[35]	2013	44	Median: 715 mm^3	Median: 9.3 y	12–13 Gy	NA	NR	NR	NR	At 1, 3, 5, and 10 y, SH was retained in 80, 55, 48, and 23%, respectively
Kim et al[64]	2013	60	Mean: 0.34 cm^3	Median: 42 mo	Mean: 12.2 Gy	88% no growth, 100% no additional treatment	NR	NR	NR	At 1, 2, and 5 y, SH was retained in 70, 63, and 55%, respectively
Lunsford et al[41]	2013	829	Mean: 2.5 cm^3	NR	Median: 13 Gy	10-y 97% no additional treatment	0%	0.20%	0.80%	79% retained SH with marginal dose 12–13 Gy

Abbreviations: Mo, month; NA, not applicable; NR, not reported; SH, serviceable hearing.

Norway, reported hearing preservation in 68% of cases at 24 months of follow-up in 60 patients.[32,33] A more recent study including patients from both Mayo Clinic and Bergen, evaluating long-term quality of life in VS patients, included 114 patients with serviceable hearing who underwent GKRS.[34] At a mean follow-up of 7.3 years, 39 (34%) patients maintained serviceable hearing.[34] Since most patients diagnosed with a sporadic VS have three or four more decades of life, the issue of true long-term hearing preservation is keenly important. Yang et al performed a comprehensive analysis of the English-language literature in 2010, analyzing hearing preservation after radiosurgery.[34] The overall hearing preservation rate for 4,234 patients included in their analysis was 51% at a mean follow-up of 44.4 ± 32 months.[35] Unfortunately, most studies have mean follow-up of only approximately 5 years or less.

Hasegawa et al published one of the first studies reporting hearing outcomes with longer-term follow-up.[22] In 2005, they reported on 73 of 80 patients treated between 1991 and 2003. After a mean follow-up of 11.25 years, 7 of 19 (37%) patients who started with serviceable hearing retained functional hearing.[23] A later publication by the same authors, specifically analyzing hearing outcomes, found in the analysis of 117 patients with serviceable hearing at the time of GKRS, the actuarial 3-, 5-, and 8-year hearing preservation rates were 55, 43, and 34%, respectively—remarkably similar to Tveiten et al.[12,33]

In order to determine long-term hearing outcomes after GKRS at the Mayo Clinic, in 2013 we asked patients treated with GKRS between 1997 and 2002 to obtain a follow-up audiogram. Forty-four patients who started with serviceable hearing were assessed with a median duration of audiometric follow-up of 9.3 years. The Kaplan–Meier estimated rates of serviceable hearing at 1, 3, 5, 7, and 10 years following GKRS were 80, 55, 48, 38, and 23%, respectively.[36] The only factors on multivariate analysis associated with maintenance of serviceable hearing were pretreatment PTA and smaller tumor size (< 1 cm).[36]

Most notably, in the past few years, the groups from Marseille and Pittsburgh have separately reported that proactive GKRS treatment of VS is hearing protective.[25,37] For instance, Akpinar et al, compared patients with "normal hearing" (SDS > 70%) treated with GKRS either within 2 years ($n = 57$) of diagnosis or in a delayed fashion, after 2 years from diagnosis ($n = 31$).[36] The 1-, 3-, 5-, and 10-year estimated rates of retaining excellent hearing were 95, 89, 77, and 51%, respectively, in the cohort treated within 2 years of diagnosis. Alternatively, the 1-, 3-, 5-, and 10-year estimated rates of maintaining greater than 70% SDS hearing in the later-treated group were 84, 65, 33, and 29%, respectively.[37] However, there is also equally compelling data that GKRS may actually accelerate hearing loss following treatment. Yomo et al, working with the Marseille group, found that patients with good hearing (SDS > 70%) were experiencing hearing loss at a rate of −0.57 dB/year after initial diagnosis and at a rate of 3.59 dB/year after GKRS ($p = 0.007$).[38]

Primarily based on our and other publications looking at longer-term follow-up analysis of hearing outcomes following GKRS for VS, we counsel patients that overall there is a 50% chance of maintaining useful hearing at 5 years and a 25% probability of maintaining useful hearing at 10 years following treatment.[36] Patients who start with excellent hearing and have small tumors have the highest chance of maintaining hearing long term. Furthermore, although some authors have found cochlea dose to predict risk of hearing loss, we do not recommend undertreating the lateral fundal margin of a VS, for instance, in order to reduce the dose to the cochlea as we have not found it to be an important factor.[13] A more detailed discussion regarding the impact of radiation on hearing outcomes is reviewed in Chapter 52.

16.3.3 Tumor Control

Perhaps even more controversial than hearing preservation rates is the issue of what truly constitutes tumor control (▶ Fig. 16.4). Various definitions of GKRS treatment failure have been used by authors over the years including any tumor enlargement following treatment, tumor enlargement on at least two serial follow-up imaging studies, symptomatic tumor enlargement, the need for any additional treatment following GKRS, or even the need for any additional nonradiation treatment after GKRS (i.e., repeat GKRS does not constitute failure). In order to avoid overtreatment of cases that develop early transient post-GKRS tumor swell and subsequent volumetric stability or regression, we have consistently used serial growth seen on at least two, and often three or more, consecutive follow-up MRI scans following GKRS as a definition of failure as we feel the primary goal of GKRS is to prevent tumor growth. In 2009, we published a retrospective review of all sporadic VSs treated between 1990 and 2004 with GKRS at the Mayo Clinic, 293 cases in total. The median tumor margin dose was 13 Gy and 90% of cases had at least 2 years of imaging follow-up, with a mean follow-up of 60.9 ± 32.5 months. Clinical tumor control was 96% at 3 years and 91% at 7 years for patients treated with marginal doses ≤ 13 Gy, reflecting contemporary treatment techniques.[4] Hasegawa et al noted an actuarial 10-year progression-free survival rate of 93% in 57 patients with tumor volumes less than 10 cm^3, with a median duration of follow-up of 135 months.[22] Most series in the last decade report tumor control rates from 92 to 98%, with follow-up between 3 and 10 years.[8,9,26,39,40,41,42]

Once again depending on definition, tumor control rates have been reported as high as 98%, at a median follow-up of 5.7 years, using marginal doses of 12 or 13 Gy if the definition of tumor control is limited to lack of subsequent tumor resection.[21] Similarly, Boari et al reported a "retreatment-free" survival rate of 97.1% for 379 patients followed up for a median of 69.5 months after GKRS.[23] Régis et al likewise reported a tumor control rate of 97.5% for 2,336 patients that had a minimum of 3 years follow-up after GKRS using the definition of not receiving a second treatment for their VS as success.[43,44]

One of the most common criticisms regarding the reporting of results of GKRS to treat VS is that many tumors may not have been growing prior to radiosurgery, and therefore with follow-up of 3 to 5 years in many clinical series, perhaps GKRS is merely taking credit for a benign natural history. To further explore this possibility, we recently reported our analysis examining pretreatment growth rate as a predictor of tumor control following GKRS. We analyzed 68 patients who had documented tumor growth of at least 2 mm in maximum diameter and were subsequently treated at Mayo Clinic with GKRS between 2004 and 2014. Among 59 extracanalicular (EC) tumors, the combined pretreatment growth rate for VS that

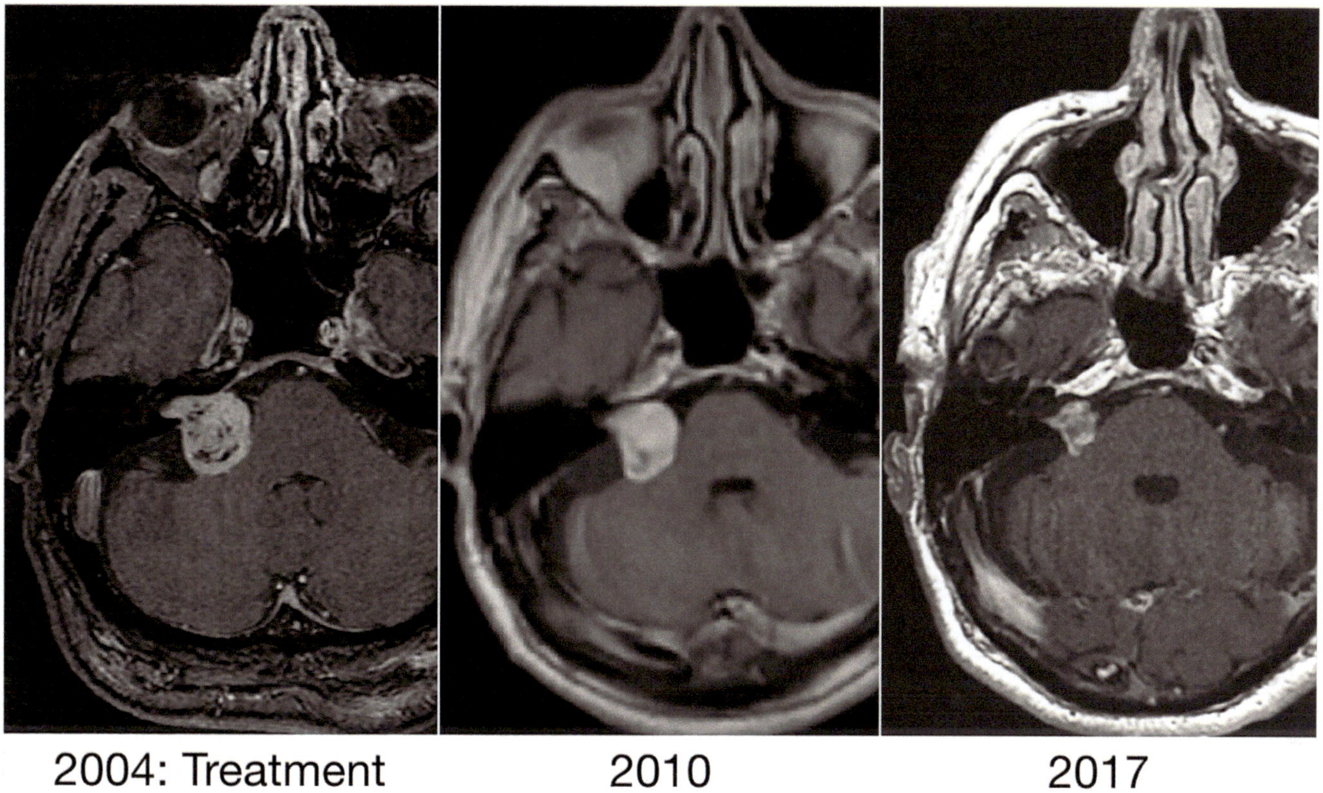

Fig. 16.4 Axial contrast-enhanced MRI demonstrating progressive volumetric tumor regression following Gamma Knife radiosurgery.

achieved tumor control was 2.08 mm/year prior to treatment, whereas the pretreatment growth rate for EC tumors that continued to increase in size following GKRS was 3.26 mm/year ($p = 0.009$). To simplify the analysis, a pretreatment growth rate of less than 2.5 mm/year was associated with a 97% (32 of 33 patients) tumor control rate. Conversely, if the tumor was growing ≥ 2.5 mm/year, only 69.2% (18 of 26 patients) achieved tumor control ($p = 0.007$).[45]

Of course, one wants to avoid subjecting a patient to an unnecessary second treatment, and the dynamic imaging changes that can occur early following GKRS are well reviewed in Chapter 25. Indeed, many VSs exhibit swelling or transient tumor enlargement before achieving radiographic stability or regression following GKRS and do not require additional treatment.[43,44,46] Therefore, we insist on progressive tumor growth on at least two consecutive scans following GKRS. For a good discussion of this controversy, we would encourage the reader to review the editorial by Régis et al and our reply recently published in *Journal of Neurosurgery*.[44]

If treatment failure is determined following GKRS, then typically surgical resection is recommended. Most centers with significant experience report that salvage surgery is more difficult following prior radiation, with worse facial nerve outcomes and a greater chance of not being able to achieve gross total resection (GTR).[48,49,50,51,52] We, along with our colleagues from Bergen, Norway, recently reviewed our experience with salvage microsurgery for VS after failed radiation treatment. Collectively, 37 patients underwent surgery following prior GKRS between 2003 and 2015, and the median time from radiation to surgical salvage was 36 months (range: 9.6–153 months). Compared to a cohort of radiation naive controls, matched for tumor size and patient age, we were much less likely to achieve GTR in the previously radiated tumors. The GTR rate was only 49% in the radiated group; however, there was not a significant difference in satisfactory postoperative facial nerve function between the radiated and nonirradiated patients.[52] Repeat GKRS has also been reported as an alternative to microsurgical salvage if the initial treatment is unsuccessful. Of course, several theoretical concerns regarding this strategy must be considered, including (1) the risk of a higher cumulative dose to adjacent structures; (2) the realistic probability of tumor control in a case that has already proved to be radioresistant, at least at low dose; (3) a concern for initial misdiagnosis of a benign VS or possible biological transformation to a more aggressive entity (e.g., sarcoma) resulting in delay of appropriate treatment; and (4) the presumed escalated surgical risks inherent to operating on a twice-radiated tumor, should radiation fail a second time. Despite these reservations, the preliminary results of repeat GKRS seem to indicate that this strategy is quite safe and has good efficacy in select cases.[53]

16.3.4 Other Complications

Other complications following GKRS for small- and medium-size VS using current dose planning and dose selection are fortunately extremely rare. Most series report less than a 5% risk of trigeminal dysfunction and secondary hydrocephalus following treatment. Both of these side effects are much more common in larger tumors.[23,24,43]

16.4 Conclusion

GKRS is safe and effective for the great majority of small- and medium-sized VS treated using contemporary dose planning and dose selection. For patients with serviceable hearing, a marginal dose of 12.5 Gy to the 50% isodose line is usually selected. Multiple isocenter plans designed to keep the cochlea dose as low as possible but still covering the entire tumor volume with the prescription isodose is recommended. Stereotactic MRI and CT are useful to maximize stereotactic accuracy, and reduce the risk of MR distortion interfering with the submillimeter accuracy of the gamma unit. When utilizing contemporary dose-planning strategies, the risk of permanent facial nerve paralysis following GKRS is ≤ 1%. Overall, approximately 50% of patients with serviceable hearing prior to GKRS (> 50% SDS and < 50 dB PTA) will retain useful hearing 5 years following treatment, with 25% still having useful hearing by 10 years after GKRS. Long-term tumor control can be expected in approximately 93% of VSs treated with GKRS; however, fast growing VS (> 2.5 mm/year) may respond less well to GKRS. Both repeat GKRS and salvage microsurgery are options if the initial treatment is not successful in halting tumor growth, determined by continuous volumetric progression on serial post-GKRS imaging studies.[54,55,56]

References

[1] Leksell L. The stereotaxic method and radiosurgery of the brain. Acta Chir Scand. 1951; 102(4):316–319

[2] Annual Treatment Statistics. Available at: https://www.lgksociety.com/library/annual-treatment-statistics/. Accessed September 20, 2018

[3] Milligan BD, Pollock BE, Foote RL, Link MJ. Long-term tumor control and cranial nerve outcomes following γ knife surgery for larger-volume vestibular schwannomas. J Neurosurg. 2012; 116(3):598–604

[4] Pollock BE, Link MJ, Foote RL. Failure rate of contemporary low-dose radiosurgical technique for vestibular schwannoma. J Neurosurg. 2009; 111(4):840–844

[5] Rojas-Villabona A, Kitchen N, Paddick I. Investigation of dosimetric differences between the TMR 10 and convolution algorithm for Gamma Knife stereotactic radiosurgery. J Appl Clin Med Phys. 2016; 17(6):217–229

[6] Massager N, Nissim O, Delbrouck C, et al. Irradiation of cochlear structures during vestibular schwannoma radiosurgery and associated hearing outcome. J Neurosurg. 2007; 107(4):733–739

[7] Lasak JM, Klish D, Kryzer TC, Hearn C, Gorecki JP, Rine GP. Gamma knife radiosurgery for vestibular schwannoma: early hearing outcomes and evaluation of the cochlear dose. Otol Neurotol. 2008; 29(8):1179–1186

[8] Kano H, Kondziolka D, Khan A, Flickinger JC, Lunsford LD. Predictors of hearing preservation after stereotactic radiosurgery for acoustic neuroma. J Neurosurg. 2009; 111(4):863–873

[9] Timmer FC, Hanssens PE, van Haren AE, et al. Gamma knife radiosurgery for vestibular schwannomas: results of hearing preservation in relation to the cochlear radiation dose. Laryngoscope. 2009; 119(6):1076–1081

[10] Wackym PA, Runge-Samuelson CL, Nash JJ, et al. Gamma knife surgery of vestibular schwannomas: volumetric dosimetry correlations to hearing loss suggest stria vascularis devascularization as the mechanism of early hearing loss. Otol Neurotol. 2010; 31(9):1480–1487

[11] Brown M, Ruckenstein M, Bigelow D, et al. Predictors of hearing loss after gamma knife radiosurgery for vestibular schwannomas: age, cochlear dose, and tumor coverage. Neurosurgery. 2011; 69(3):605–613, discussion 613–614

[12] Hasegawa T, Kida Y, Kato T, Iizuka H, Yamamoto T. Factors associated with hearing preservation after Gamma Knife surgery for vestibular schwannomas in patients who retain serviceable hearing. J Neurosurg. 2011; 115(6):1078–1086

[13] Jacob JT, Carlson ML, Schiefer TK, Pollock BE, Driscoll CL, Link MJ. Significance of cochlear dose in the radiosurgical treatment of vestibular schwannoma: controversies and unanswered questions. Neurosurgery. 2014; 74(5):466–474, discussion 474

[14] Linskey ME, Johnstone PA. Radiation tolerance of normal temporal bone structures: implications for gamma knife stereotactic radiosurgery. Int J Radiat Oncol Biol Phys. 2003; 57(1):196–200

[15] Pollock BE, Driscoll CL, Foote RL, et al. Patient outcomes after vestibular schwannoma management: a prospective comparison of microsurgical resection and stereotactic radiosurgery. Neurosurgery. 2006; 59(1):77–85, discussion 77–85

[16] Tago M, Terahara A, Nakagawa K, et al. Immediate neurological deterioration after gamma knife radiosurgery for acoustic neuroma. Case report. J Neurosurg. 2000; 93 Suppl 3:78–81

[17] Ogunrinde OK, Lunsford LD, Flickinger JC, Kondziolka DS. Cranial nerve preservation after stereotactic radiosurgery for small acoustic tumors. Arch Neurol. 1995; 52(1):73–79

[18] Pollack AG, Marymont MH, Kalapurakal JA, Kepka A, Sathiaseelan V, Chandler JP. Acute neurological complications following gamma knife surgery for vestibular schwannoma. Case report. J Neurosurg. 2005; 103(3):546–551

[19] Flickinger JC, Kondziolka D, Niranjan A, Lunsford LD. Results of acoustic neuroma radiosurgery: an analysis of 5 years' experience using current methods. J Neurosurg. 2001; 94(1):1–6

[20] Régis J, Pellet W, Delsanti C, et al. Functional outcome after gamma knife surgery or microsurgery for vestibular schwannomas. J Neurosurg. 2002; 97(5):1091–1100

[21] Régis J, Carron R, Delsanti C, et al. Radiosurgery for vestibular schwannomas. Neurosurg Clin N Am. 2013; 24(4):521–530

[22] Hasegawa T, Kida Y, Kobayashi T, Yoshimoto M, Mori Y, Yoshida J. Long-term outcomes in patients with vestibular schwannomas treated using gamma knife surgery: 10-year follow up. J Neurosurg. 2005; 102(1):10–16

[23] Boari N, Bailo M, Gagliardi F, et al. Gamma Knife radiosurgery for vestibular schwannoma: clinical results at long-term follow-up in a series of 379 patients. J Neurosurg. 2014; 121 Suppl:123–142

[24] Iwai Y, Yamanaka K, Kubo T, Aiba T. Gamma knife radiosurgery for intracanalicular acoustic neuromas. J Clin Neurosci. 2008; 15(9):993–997

[25] Yomo S, Carron R, Thomassin JM, Roche PH, Régis J. Longitudinal analysis of hearing before and after radiosurgery for vestibular schwannoma. J Neurosurg. 2012; 117(5):877–885

[26] Chopra R, Kondziolka D, Niranjan A, Lunsford LD, Flickinger JC. Long-term follow-up of acoustic schwannoma radiosurgery with marginal tumor doses of 12 to 13 Gy. Int J Radiat Oncol Biol Phys. 2007; 68(3):845–851

[27] Combs SE, Thilmann C, Debus J, Schulz-Ertner D. Long-term outcome of stereotactic radiosurgery (SRS) in patients with acoustic neuromas. Int J Radiat Oncol Biol Phys. 2006; 64(5):1341–1347

[28] Fukuoka S, Takanashi M, Hojyo A, Konishi M, Tanaka C, Nakamura H. Gamma knife radiosurgery for vestibular schwannomas. Prog Neurol Surg. 2009; 22: 45–62

[29] Kim KM, Park CK, Chung HT, Paek SH, Jung HW, Kim DG. Long-term outcomes of gamma knife stereotactic radiosurgery of vestibular schwannomas. J Korean Neurosurg Soc. 2007; 42(4):286–292

[30] Myrseth E, Møller P, Pedersen PH, Vassbotn FS, Wentzel-Larsen T, Lund-Johansen M. Vestibular schwannomas: clinical results and quality of life after microsurgery or gamma knife radiosurgery. Neurosurgery. 2005; 56(5):927–935, discussion 927–935

[31] Niranjan A, Mathieu D, Flickinger JC, Kondziolka D, Lunsford LD. Hearing preservation after intracanalicular vestibular schwannoma radiosurgery. Neurosurgery. 2008; 63(6):1054–1062, discussion 1062–1063

[32] Myrseth E, Møller P, Pedersen PH, Lund-Johansen M. Vestibular schwannoma: surgery or gamma knife radiosurgery? A prospective, nonrandomized study. Neurosurgery. 2009; 64(4):654–661, discussion 661–663

[33] Tveiten OV, Carlson ML, Goplen F, Vassbotn F, Link MJ, Lund-Johansen M. Long-term auditory symptoms in patients with sporadic vestibular schwannoma: An international cross-sectional study. Neurosurgery. 2015; 77(2): 218–227, discussion 227

[34] Yang I, Sughrue ME, Han SJ, et al. A comprehensive analysis of hearing preservation after radiosurgery for vestibular schwannoma. J Neurosurg. 2010; 112(4):851–859

[35] Carlson ML, Jacob JT, Pollock BE, et al. Long-term hearing outcomes following stereotactic radiosurgery for vestibular schwannoma: patterns of hearing loss and variables influencing audiometric decline. J Neurosurg. 2013; 118(3):579–587

[36] Akpinar B, Mousavi SH, McDowell MM, et al. Early radiosurgery improves hearing preservation in vestibular schwannoma patients with normal hearing at the time of diagnosis. Int J Radiat Oncol Biol Phys. 2016; 95(2):729–734

[37] Régis J, Carron R, Park MC, et al. Wait-and-see strategy compared with proactive Gamma Knife surgery in patients with intracanalicular vestibular schwannomas: clinical article. J Neurosurg. 2013; 119 Suppl:105–111
[38] Wowra B, Muacevic A, Jess-Hempen A, Hempel JM, Müller-Schunk S, Tonn JC. Outpatient gamma knife surgery for vestibular schwannoma: definition of the therapeutic profile based on a 10-year experience. J Neurosurg. 2013; 119 Suppl:114–118
[39] Chung WY, Liu KD, Shiau CY, et al. Gamma knife surgery for vestibular schwannoma: 10-year experience of 195 cases. J Neurosurg. 2013; 119 Suppl:87–97
[40] Hasegawa T, Fujitani S, Katsumata S, Kida Y, Yoshimoto M, Koike J. Stereotactic radiosurgery for vestibular schwannomas: analysis of 317 patients followed more than 5 years. Neurosurgery. 2005; 57(2):257–265, discussion 257–265
[41] Lunsford LD, Niranjan A, Flickinger JC, Maitz A, Kondziolka D. Radiosurgery of vestibular schwannomas: summary of experience in 829 cases. J Neurosurg. 2005; 102 Suppl:195–199
[42] Liu D, Xu D, Zhang Z, Zhang Y, Zheng L. Long-term outcomes after Gamma Knife surgery for vestibular schwannomas: a 10-year experience. J Neurosurg. 2006; 105 Suppl:149–153
[43] Marston AP, Jacob JT, Carlson ML, Pollock BE, Driscoll CLW, Link MJ. Pretreatment growth rate as a predictor of tumor control following Gamma Knife radiosurgery for sporadic vestibular schwannoma. J Neurosurg. 2017; 127(2): 380–387
[44] Régis J, Delsanti C, Roche PH. Editorial: Vestibular schwannoma radiosurgery: progression or pseudoprogression? J Neurosurg. 2017; 127(2):374–379
[45] Pollock BE. Management of vestibular schwannomas that enlarge after stereotactic radiosurgery: treatment recommendations based on a 15 year experience. Neurosurgery. 2006; 58(2):241–248, discussion 241–248
[46] Mindermann T, Schlegel I. How to distinguish tumor growth from transient expansion of vestibular schwannomas following Gamma Knife radiosurgery. Acta Neurochir (Wien). 2014; 156(6):1121–1123
[47] Friedman RA, Brackmann DE, Hitselberger WE, Schwartz MS, Iqbal Z, Berliner KI. Surgical salvage after failed irradiation for vestibular schwannoma. Laryngoscope. 2005; 115(10):1827–1832
[48] Friedman RA, Berliner KI, Bassim M, et al. A paradigm shift in salvage surgery for radiated vestibular schwannoma. Otol Neurotol. 2011; 32(8): 1322–1328
[49] Gerganov VM, Giordano M, Samii A, Samii M. Surgical treatment of patients with vestibular schwannomas after failed previous radiosurgery. J Neurosurg. 2012; 116(4):713–720
[50] Husseini ST, Piccirillo E, Taibah A, Almutair T, Sequino G, Sanna M. Salvage surgery of vestibular schwannoma after failed radiotherapy: the Gruppo Otologico experience and review of the literature. Am J Otolaryngol. 2013; 34 (2):107–114
[51] Wise SC, Carlson ML, Tveiten OV, et al. Surgical salvage of recurrent vestibular schwannoma following prior stereotactic radiosurgery. Laryngoscope. 2016; 126(11):2580–2586
[52] Fu VX, Verheul JB, Beute GN, et al. Retreatment of vestibular schwannoma with Gamma Knife radiosurgery: clinical outcome, tumor control, and review of literature. J Neurosurg. 2001; 6:1–9
[53] Lonneville S, Delbrouck C, Renier C, Devriendt D, Massager N. Repeat Gamma Knife surgery for vestibular schwannomas. Surg Neurol Int. 2015; 6:153
[54] Kano H, Kondziolka D, Niranjan A, Flannery TJ, Flickinger JC, Lunsford LD. Repeat stereotactic radiosurgery for acoustic neuromas. Int J Radiat Oncol Biol Phys. 2010; 76(2):520–527
[55] Liscak R, Vladyka V, Urgosik D, Simonova G, Vymazal J. Repeated treatment of vestibular schwannomas after gamma knife radiosurgery. Acta Neurochir (Wien). 2009; 151(4):317–324, discussion 324
[56] Yomo S, Arkha Y, Delsanti C, Roche PH, Thomassin JM, Régis J. Repeat gamma knife surgery for regrowth of vestibular schwannomas. Neurosurgery. 2009; 64(1):48–54, discussion 54–55
[57] Prasad D, Steiner M, Steiner L. Gamma surgery for vestibular schwannoma. J Neurosurg 2000; 92:745-759
[58] Petit JH, Hudes RS, Chen TT, Eisenberg HM, Simard JM, Chin LS. Reduced-dose radiosurgery for vestibular schwannomas. Neurosurgery 2001; 49:1299-1306; discussion 1306-1297
[59] Iwai Y, Yamanaka K, Shiotani M, Uyama T. Radiosurgery for acoustic neuromas: results of low-dose treatment. Neurosurgery 2003; 53:282-287; discussion 287-288
[60] Litvack ZN, Noren G, Chougule PB, Zheng Z. Preservation of functional hearing after gamma knife surgery for vestibular schwannoma. Neurosurg Focus 2003; 14:e3
[61] Flickinger JC, Kondziolka D, Niranjan A, Maitz A, Voynov G, Lunsford LD. Acoustic neuroma radiosurgery with marginal tumor doses of 12 to 13 Gy. Int J Radiat Oncol Biol Phys 2004; 60:225-230
[62] Paek SH, Chung HT, Jeong SS, et al. Hearing preservation after gamma knife stereotactic radiosurgery of vestibular schwannoma. Cancer 2005; 104:580-590
[63] Tamura M, Carron R, Yomo S, et al. Hearing preservation after gamma knife radiosurgery for vestibular schwannomas presenting with high-level hearing. Neurosurgery 2009; 64:289-296; discussion 296
[64] Kim JW, Kim DG, Paek SH, et al. Efficacy of corticosteroids in hearing preservation after radiosurgery for vestibular schwannoma: a prospective study. Stereotact Funct Neurosurg 2011; 89:25-33
[65] Han JH, Kim DG, Chung HT, et al. Hearing preservation in patients with unilateral vestibular schwannoma who undergo stereotactic radiosurgery: Reinterpretation of the auditory brainstem response. Cancer 2012; 118:5441-5447
[66] Sun S, Liu A. Long-term follow-up studies of Gamma Knife surgery with a low margin dose for vestibular schwannoma. J Neurosurg 2012; 117 Suppl:57-62
[67] Baschnagel AM, Chen PY, Bojrab D, et al. Hearing preservation in patients with vestibular schwannoma treated with Gamma Knife surgery. J Neurosurg 2013; 118:571-578
[68] Kim YH, Kim DG, Han JH, et al. Hearing outcomes after stereotactic radiosurgery for unilateral intracanalicular vestibular schwannomas: implication of transient volume expansion. Int J Radiat Oncol Biol Phys 2013; 85:61-67
[69] Breivik CN, Nilsen RM, Myrseth E, et al. Conservative management or gamma knife radiosurgery for vestibular schwannoma: tumor growth, symptoms, and quality of life. Neurosurgery 2013; 73:48-56; discussion 56-47

17 Linear Accelerator Radiosurgery for Treatment of Vestibular Schwannoma (Non-CyberKnife)

William A. Friedman

17.1 Introduction

Stereotactic radiosurgery (SRS) is a minimally invasive treatment modality that delivers a single session of radiation to a specific target while sparing surrounding tissue. Unlike conventionally fractionated radiotherapy, SRS does not maximally exploit the presumed higher radiosensitivity of brain lesions relative to normal brain (i.e., therapeutic ratio). Its selective destruction is dependent mainly on sharply focused high-dose radiation and a steep-dose gradient away from the defined target. The biological effect is irreparable cellular damage, presumably via irreparable DNA double-strand breaks, and delayed vascular occlusion within the high-dose target volume. Because a therapeutic ratio is not required, traditionally radioresistant lesions can be treated. Since ablative doses are used, however, any normal structure included in the target volume is subject to injury.

The basis for SRS was conceived over 60 years ago by Lars Leksell.[1] He proposed the technique of focusing multiple beams of external Cobalt-60 gamma ray radiation on a stereotactically defined intracranial target. The confluence of these intersecting beams results in very high doses of radiation to the target volume, but low doses to nontarget tissues along the path of any given beam. His team's implementation of this concept culminated in the development of the Gamma Knife. The modern Gamma Knife (Perfexion or Icon model) employs 192 Cobalt-60 radiation sources with a fixed circumferential array of collimators of varying size, such that all 192 gamma ray photon beams are focused on a single point or isocenter. The patient is stereotactically positioned in the Gamma Knife unit using a robotic treatment couch so that the intracranial target coincides with the isocenter of radiation. Using variable collimation, beam blocking, differential weighting of dose to each isocenter, and multiple isocenters, the radiation target volume is shaped to conform to the intracranial target. Further discussion regarding the Gamma Knife SRS platform can be found in Chapter 16.

An alternate radiosurgical solution using a linear accelerator (LINAC) was first described in 1984 by Betti and Derechinsky.[2] Colombo et al described such a system in 1985,[3] and LINACs have subsequently been modified in various ways to achieve the precision and accuracy required for radiosurgical applications.[4,5,6,7] In 1986, a team composed of neurosurgeons, medical physicists, and software engineers began development of the University of Florida LINAC-based radiosurgery system.[8] This system has been used to treat over 4,500 patients at the University of Florida since May 1988, and is in use at multiple sites worldwide. Many other commercial versions of radiosurgical systems are currently available, including the Brain Lab system (Novalis), the Radionics (X-knife) system, the Accuray (CyberKnife) system, among others.

Most LINAC radiosurgical systems rely on the same basic paradigm: A collimated X-ray beam is focused on a stereotactically identified intracranial target. The gantry of the LINAC rotates around the patient, producing an arc of radiation focused on the target (▶ Fig. 17.1). The patient couch is then rotated in the horizontal plane and another arc performed. In this manner, multiple non-coplanar arcs of radiation intersect at the target volume and produce a high target dose, with

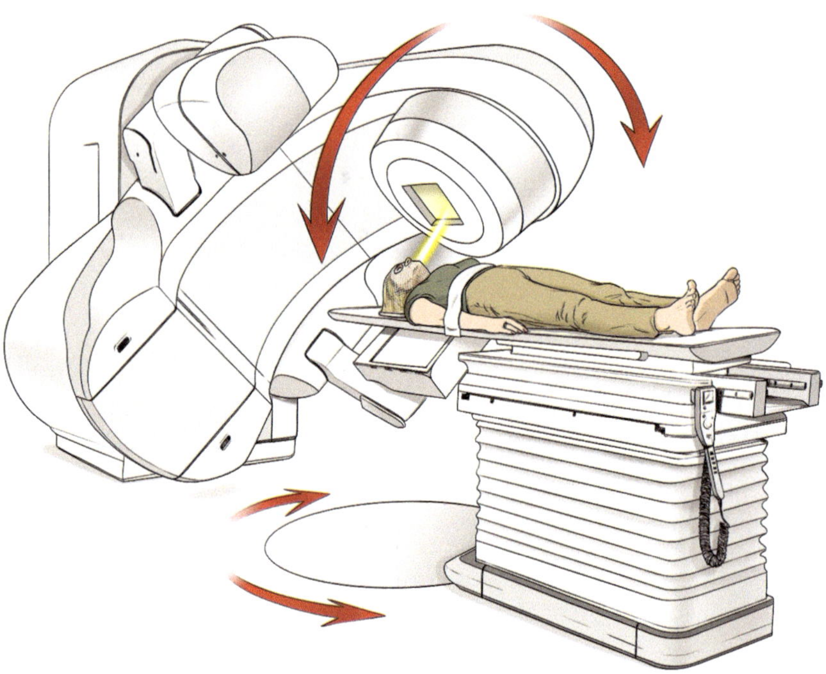

Fig. 17.1 Linear accelerators are the preferred device, worldwide, for conventional radiotherapy. They accelerate electrons to near light speed, then collide them with a heavy metal (like tungsten) in the head of the machine. The collision mainly produces heat, but a small percentage of the energy is converted into highly energized photons. These photons, because they are electronically produced, are called "X-rays." The X-ray radiation is collimated and focused on the target.

minimal radiation to surrounding brain. This dose concentration method is exactly analogous to the multiple intersecting beams of Cobalt-60 gamma ray radiation in the Gamma Knife.

The target dose distribution can be tailored by varying collimator sizes, eliminating undesirable arcs, manipulating arc angles, using multiple isocenters, and differentially weighting the dose to each isocenter.[9] In our center, multiple isocenters are used to achieve highly conformal dose distributions, analogous to the Gamma Knife technique. Some LINAC systems use an alternative approach that relies upon a computer-driven multileaf collimator to generate nonspherical beam shapes, which are conformal to the beam's eye view of the tumor. The multileaf collimator can be adjusted statically or dynamically as the LINAC gantry rotates. Intensity modulation can be used to achieve dose distributions that are close to those seen with multiple isocenters and treatment time can be reduced.

Achievable dose distributions are similar for LINAC-based and Gamma Knife–based systems. With both systems, it is possible to achieve dose distributions that conform closely to the shape of the intracranial target, thus sparing the maximum amount of normal brain. Recent advances in stereotactic imaging and computer technology for dose calculation and treatment planning, as well as refinements in radiation delivery systems, have led to improved efficacy, fewer complications, and a remarkable amount of interest in the various applications of SRS. Perhaps of equal importance is the fact that increasing amounts of scientific evidence have persuaded the majority of the international neurosurgical community that radiosurgery is a viable treatment option for selected patients suffering from a variety of challenging neurosurgical disorders. This chapter will present a brief description of LINAC radiosurgical technique, followed by a detailed review of the experience with vestibular schwannoma (VS) treatment. The interested reader can find an in-depth review of the CyberKnife system in Chapter 19.

17.2 LINAC Radiosurgery Technique

Although the details of radiosurgical treatment techniques differ somewhat from system to system, the basic paradigm is quite similar everywhere. The following is a detailed description of a typical radiosurgical treatment at the University of Florida.

Almost all radiosurgical procedures in adults are performed on an outpatient basis. The patient reports to the neurosurgical clinic the day before treatment for a detailed history and physical, as well as an in-depth review of images and treatment options. If radiosurgery is deemed appropriate, the patient is sent to the radiology department for a volumetric MRI scan. A radiosurgical plan can be generated, in advance, using this MRI study. The next morning, the patient arrives at 7:00 AM. A stereotactic head ring is applied under local anesthesia. No skin shaving or preparation is required. Subsequently, stereotactic CT scanning is performed. One millimeter slices are obtained throughout the entire head. The patient is then transported to an outpatient holding area where they wait until the treatment planning process is complete.

The stereotactic CT scan and the nonstereotactic volumetric MRI scan are transferred via Ethernet to the treatment-planning computer. The CT images are quickly processed so that each pixel has an anteroposterior, lateral, and vertical stereotactic coordinate, all related to the head ring previously applied to the patient's head. Using image fusion software, the nonstereotactic MRI is fused, pixel for pixel, with the stereotactic CT. The "pre-plan" performed the day before is, likewise, fused to the stereotactic CT. Final treatment planning then begins and continues until the neurosurgeon, radiation oncologist, and medical physicist are satisfied that an optimal dose plan has been developed. A variety of options are available for optimizing the dosimetry. The fundamental goal is to deliver a radiation in high-dose volume that is precisely conformal to the lesion shape (▶ Fig. 17.2) while delivering a minimal dose of radiation to all surrounding neural structures.

When dose planning is complete, the radiosurgical device is attached to the LINAC. The patient then is attached to the device and treated. The head ring is removed and, after a short observation period, the patient is discharged. The radiosurgical device is disconnected from the LINAC, which is then ready for conventional radiotherapy utilization. Close clinical and radiologic follow-up is arranged at appropriate intervals depending on the lesion treated and the condition of the patient.

17.3 Radiosurgery for Vestibular Schwannomas

Among benign intracranial tumors, VS has been one of the most frequent targets for SRS. Leksell first used SRS to treat a VS in 1969.[10] SRS is a logical alternative treatment modality for this tumor for several reasons. A VS is typically well demarcated from surrounding tissues on neuroimaging studies. The sharp borders of this noninvasive tumor make it a convenient match for the characteristically steep dose gradient produced at the

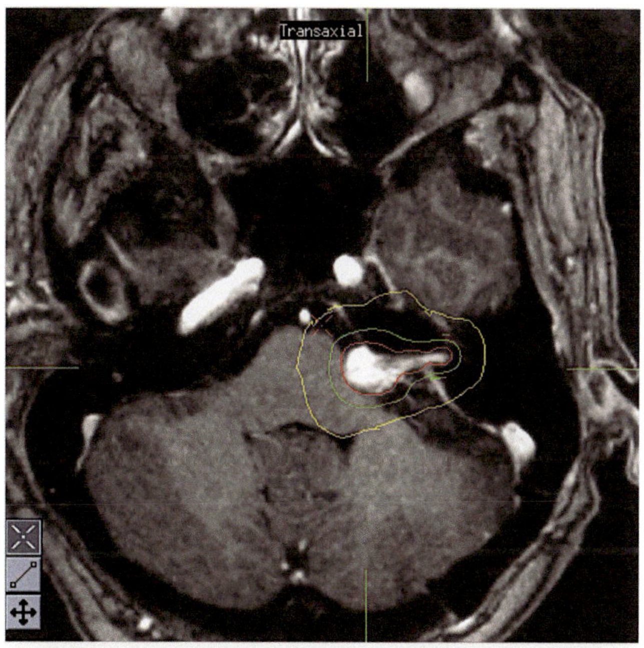

Fig. 17.2 In general, multiple isocenters are used to produce highly conformal dosimetry. Here, the *red line* is the prescription isodose line, the *green line* is 50% of the maximum dose, and the *yellow line* is 20% of the maximum dose.

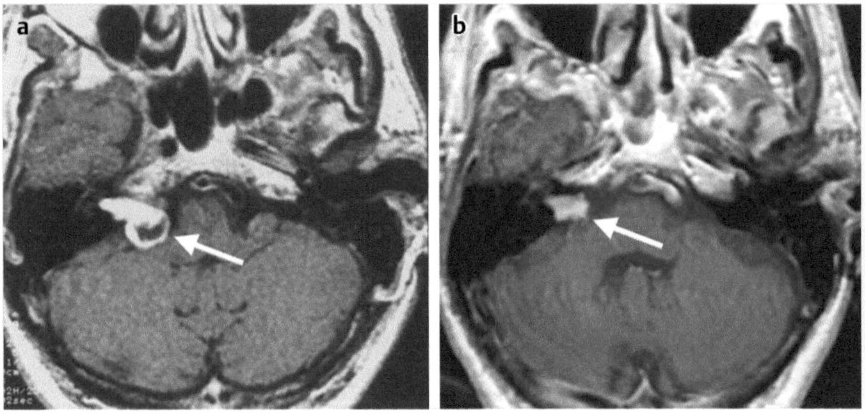

Fig. 17.3 (**a**) Contrast-enhanced axial MRI of the head shows a medium-sized right-sided sporadic vestibular schwannoma. (**b**) Four years posttreatment, the vestibular schwannoma has reduced in size.

boundary of a radiosurgical target. This allows the radiosurgeon to minimize radiation dose to normal tissue. Excellent spatial resolution on gadolinium-enhanced MRI facilitates radiosurgical dose planning. These tumors commonly occur in an older population that may be less fit for microsurgical resection under general anesthesia. Finally, the location of these tumors at the skull base in close proximity to multiple critical neurologic structures (i.e., cranial nerves, brainstem) can lead to appreciable surgical morbidity and very rare mortality even in expert hands. This makes the concept an effective, less invasive, less morbid alternative treatment that can be performed in a single day under local anesthesia attractive.

Certainly, the role of radiosurgery is limited by its inability to expeditiously relieve mass effect in patients for whom this is necessary. The radiobiology of SRS also requires lower, potentially less effective doses for larger target volumes in order to avoid complications. This limits the use of SRS to the treatment of smaller tumors (generally < 25 mm in diameter). Despite these limitations, there is a growing body of literature that substantiates the claim that radiosurgery is a safe and effective alternative therapy for VSs.

The published experience using LINAC-based SRS for the treatment of VS is relatively limited compared to the Gamma Knife literature. Foote et al[11] performed an analysis of risk factors associated with SRS for VS at the University of Florida. The aim of this study was to identify factors associated with cranial neuropathy following SRS for VS and to determine how such factors may be manipulated to minimize the incidence of SRS complications while maintaining high rates of tumor control. From July 1988 to June 1998, a total of 149 cases of VS were treated using LINAC SRS at the University of Florida. In each of these cases, the patient's tumor and brainstem were contoured in 1-mm slices on the original SRS targeting images. Resulting tumor and brainstem volumes were coupled with the original SRS plans to generate dose-volume histograms. Various tumor dimensions were also measured to estimate the length of cranial nerve that would be irradiated. Patient follow-up data, including evidence of cranial neuropathy and radiographic tumor control, were obtained from a prospectively maintained, computerized database. The authors performed statistical analyses to compare the incidence of posttreatment cranial neuropathies or tumor growth between patient strata defined by risk factors of interest. One hundred thirty-nine of the 149 patients were included in the analysis of complications. The median duration of clinical follow-up for this group was 36 months (range: 18–94 months). The tumor control analysis included 133 patients. The median duration of radiological follow-up in this group was 34 months (range: 6–94 months). The overall 2-year actuarial incidences of facial and trigeminal neuropathies were 11.8 and 9.5%, respectively. In 41 patients treated before 1994, the incidence rate of both facial and trigeminal neuropathies was 29%, but in the 108 patients treated since January 1994, these rates declined to 5 and 2%, respectively. An evaluation of multiple risk factor models showed that maximum radiation doses to the brainstem, treatment era (pre-1994 compared with 1994 or later), and prior surgical resection were all simultaneously informative predictors of cranial neuropathy risk. The radiation dose prescribed to the tumor margin could be substituted for the maximum dose to the brainstem with a small loss in predictive strength (▶ Fig. 17.2). The overall radiological tumor control rate was 93% (59% tumors regressed, 34% remained stable, and 7.5% enlarged), and the 5-year actuarial tumor control rate was 87% (95% confidence interval [CI]: 76–98%; ▶ Fig. 17.3). Based on this study, the authors currently recommend a peripheral dose of 12.5 Gy for almost all VSs, as this dose is most likely to yield long-term tumor control without causing cranial neuropathy. Since 1994, when the treatment dose was reduced to 12.5 Gy, less than 1% of patients have experienced facial or trigeminal neuropathy after treatment.

Spiegelmann et al[12,13] reviewed their results of LINAC-based SRS in 44 patients with VSs who were treated between 1993 and 1997. CT scanning was selected as the stereotactic imaging modality for target definition. A single, conformally shaped isocenter was used in the treatment of 40 patients; two or three isocenters were used in four patients who harbored very irregular tumors. The radiation dose directed to the tumor margin was the only parameter that changed during the study period—in the first 24 patients who were treated, the dose was 15 to 20 Gy, whereas in the last 20 patients, the dose was reduced to 11 to 14 Gy. After a mean follow-up period of 32 months (range: 12–60 months), 98% of the tumors were controlled. The actuarial hearing preservation rate was 71% at 2 years. New transient facial neuropathy developed in 24% of the patients and persisted to a mild degree in 8%. Radiation dose correlated significantly with the incidence of cranial neuropathy, particularly in large tumors (≥ 4 cm^3).

Several reports on smaller series of patients treated with LINAC-based SRS for VSs have been published in recent years.

Martens et al reported on 14 patients with at least 1 year of follow-up after SRS on the LINAC unit in the University Hospital in Ghent, Belgium.[14] A mean marginal dose of 19.4 Gy (range: 16–20) was delivered to the 70% isodose line with a single isocenter. Mean follow-up duration was 19 months (range: 12–24 months). During this relatively short follow-up interval, 100% radiographic tumor control has been achieved (29% regressed, 71% stable, 0% enlarged). Rates of delayed facial and trigeminal neuropathy were 21 and 14%, respectively, and two of three facial nerve deficits resolved. Preoperative hearing was preserved in 50% of cases.

Valentino and Raimondi reported on 23 patients treated with LINAC-based SRS or multisession hypofractionated radiotherapy in Rome, Italy.[15] Five of these had neurofibromatosis type 2 and 7 (30%) had undergone previous surgery. Total radiation dose to the tumor margin ranged from 12 to 45 Gy (median: 30 Gy) and was delivered in one to five sessions. One or two isocenters were used and mean duration of follow-up was 40 months (range: 24–46 months). Results using this less conventional method of multisession hypofractionated radiotherapy were comparable to SRS techniques. Tumor control was achieved in 96% of patients (38% regressed, 58% stable, 4% enlarged), facial and trigeminal neuropathies each occurred at a rate of 4%, and "hearing was preserved at almost the same level as that of SRS in all patients."

The use of LINAC-based SRS for VS is briefly discussed in reports by Delaney et al[16] and Barcia Salorio et al.[17] In addition, conventionally fractionated (see Chapter 18) and hypofractionated stereotactic radiation therapy has been used as an alternative management for VS. This method is proposed as a way of exploiting the precision of stereotactic radiation delivery to minimize dose to normal brain, while employing lower fractionated doses with each session in an effort to minimize complications. Thus far, most radiosurgeons feel that optimal results can be achieved with highly conformal single-session SRS, while sparing the patient the inconvenience of a prolonged treatment course.

17.4 Conventionally Fractionated and Hypofractionated Radiotherapy for Vestibular Schwannoma

A number of groups have used multisession radiotherapy treatments in an attempt to reduce complications, especially hearing loss. Varlotto and colleagues[18] treated 12 patients with VS between June 1992 and October 1994. Follow-up ranged from 16 to 44 months. Patient age ranged from 27 to 70, with a median age of 45 years. Eight patients were treated with primary conventionally fractionated radiotherapy and four patients were treated after primary surgical intervention for recurrent ($N = 3$) or persistent ($N = 1$) disease. Tumor volumes were 1.2 to 18.4 cm^3 (median: 10.1 cm^3). Tumors received 1.8 Gy per treatment session normalized to the 95% isodose line. Patients received a minimum prescribed dose of 54 Gy in 27 to 30 fractions or sessions over a 6-week period. After a median follow-up of 26.5 months, tumor control was obtained in all tumors. Tumor regression was noted in three patients, and tumor stabilization was found in the remaining nine patients. No patient developed a new cranial nerve deficit. One patient developed worsening of preexisting trigeminal neuropathy and another experienced a decrease in hearing. However, all nine patients with useful hearing prior to radiotherapy maintained useful hearing at last follow-up.

Fuss and colleagues[19] treated 51 patients with VS with conventional fractionation using a mean total dose of 57.6 ± 2.5 Gy. Forty-two patients have been followed up for at least 12 months and were the subject of an outcome analysis. Mean follow-up was 42 months. Actuarial 2- and 5-year tumor control rates were 100 and 97.7%, respectively. Actuarial useful hearing preservation rate was 85% at 2 and 5 years. New hearing loss was diagnosed in four patients with neurofibromatosis type 2. Pretreatment normal facial nerve function was preserved in all cases. Two cases of new or impaired trigeminal nerve dysesthesia required medication and no other cranial nerve deficit was observed.

Williams[20] treated 80 consecutive patients with increased hypofractionation based on tumor size. Seventy patients having tumors less than 3.0 cm in diameter had 5 daily fractions or sessions of 5 Gy each (25 Gy total) and 10 patients having tumors ≥ 3 cm had 10 daily fractions or sessions of 3 Gy each (30 Gy total). All treatments were prescribed to the 80% isodose line and given via a dedicated 10 MeV LINAC. For both the larger and smaller tumors, the percentage decrease in volume was similar. No tumor increased in size, no patient developed facial weakness, and hearing was preserved.

Andrews and colleagues[21] compared the results of patients treated with SRS with the Gamma Knife or fractionated radiotherapy from October 1994 through August 2000. The Gamma Knife technique involved a fixed-frame, multiple isocenter, high conformality single treatment, whereas the LINAC technique involved daily conventionally fractionated treatments involving a relocatable frame, fewer isocenters, and high conformality established by noncoplanar arc beam shaping and differential beam weighting. Sixty-nine patients were treated on the Gamma Knife, and 56 patients were treated with radiotherapy. Three patients were lost to follow-up, and in the remaining 122 patients, the mean follow-up was 119 ± 67 weeks for SRS patients and 115 ± 96 weeks for radiotherapy patients. Tumor control rates were high (≥ 97%) for sporadic tumors in both groups. Cranial nerve morbidities were comparably low in both groups, with the exception of functional hearing preservation, which was 2.5-fold higher in patients who received conventionally fractionated radiotherapy.

Chang and colleagues[22] reported on 61 patients treated with the CyberKnife, a LINAC-based system, and followed up for at least 36 months. They received either 18 or 21 Gy, in three fractions or sessions (hypofractionated stereotactic radiotherapy). Only one treated tumor progressed, 74% of patients with serviceable hearing maintained hearing, and no new trigeminal or facial nerve complications developed.

Ellenbogen et al[23] reported on 50 consecutive patients treated over a 6-year period of time using a LINAC equipped with micromultileaf collimation using a tumor margin dose of 12.5 Gy in a single session. Over a median follow-up of 5.8 years, two tumors enlarged, one of which required surgery. Two patients each had facial or trigeminal nerve complications. ▸ Table 17.1 reviews additional outcomes of non-CyberKnife

Table 17.1 Select recent (2007–2017) publications reviewing LINAC-based radiosurgery and stereotactic radiotherapy for vestibular schwannoma (excludes CyberKnife)

Author	Year published	Institution	Years of study	Modality	No. of pts	SRS vs. FSRT	Dose strategy (Gy)	Tumor size	Tumor control	Follow-up	New facial neuropathy	New trigeminal dysfunction	Serviceable hearing preservation	Other
Rutten et al[24]	2007	University Hospital Maastricht, Maastricht, The Netherlands	1995–2001	LINAC X-Knife	26	1 (SRS)	Median 12 Gy (range 10–14 Gy) prescribed at the 80% isodose line	Median 18 mm (range 9–30)	88% decrease, 8% stabilized, 4% increase	Median: 49 mo (range: 16–85)	0%	8% (transient in all)	96% maintained same GR class	1 with NF1 2 with NF2 2 with prior surgery
Hsu et al[25]	2010	Chang Gung University, Taoyuan, Taiwan	1994–2006	Siemens KDS-2 (1994–1999) Varian 21Ex (2000–2006)	75	1 (SRS)	Median: 14 Gy (range: 12–20 Gy) prescribed at the 80% isodose line	Median: 1.5 cm^3 (range: 0.1–23.7)	40% decrease, 52% stabile, 8% increase	Mean: 98 mo (range: 60–163)	8%	0%	87.5% "intact hearing"	0 with NF2 46 with prior surgery
Combs et al[26]	2010	University of Heidelberg, Heidelberg, Germany	1998–2007	Stryker-Leibinger system	30	1 (SRS)	Median: 13 Gy (range, 10–20) prescribed at the 80% isodose line	NR	98% at 3 y, 96% at 5 and 10 y (SRS vs. FSRT, NSS)	Median: 75 mo (range: 2 mo–19 y)	17%	7%	85% at 1 y, 83% at 2 y, and 78% at 5 y maintained GR class I or II	14 with NF2 37 with prior surgery
					172	FSRT	Total: 57.6 Gy prescribed at the 90% isodose line (5 × 1.8 Gy per week)	2.8 mL (range, 0.2–33 mL)			2%	3%		
Roos et al[27]	2011	Royal Adelaide Hospital and University of Adelaide, Australia	1994–2010	Stryker-Leibinger system (1994–2008) BrainLAB system (2009–2010)	102	1 (SRS)	12–14 Gy prescribed at the 70–90% isodose line	22 mm (range: 11–40)	98% control; 62% decrease, 36% stable, 2% increase (defined as sustained change ≥ 2 mm in diameter)	65 mo (range: 10–184)	6% (all mild and transient)	10% (all either resolved or improved over time)	38% overall 50% at 5 y, 23% at 10 y (defined as an inter-aural difference of ≤ 50 dB PTA)	5 with NF2 6 with prior surgery 4 required VP shunt after treatment
Kopp et al[28]	2011	The Technical University of Munich, Munich, Germany	1997–2007	Adapted Siemens LINAC with micromultileaf collimator	68	1 (SRS)	12 Gy prescribed at the 100% isodose line	Mean: 1.24 cm^3 (range: 0.1–5.36)	99%	Median: 30.1 mo (range: 1.2–105.6)	6% (1.5% transient)	13%	85% at mean 30.1 mo (GR class I or II)	5 with NF2 13 with prior surgery
					47	FSRT	54 Gy, 5 × 1.8 Gy per week in 41 cases (6 with	Mean: 5.79 cm^3 (range: 0.1–19.27)	98%	Median: 32.1 mo (range: 2.4–97.2)	4% (2% transient)	8% (4% transient)	79% at mean 32.1 mo (GR class I or II)	

Table 17.1 (*Continued*)

Author	Year published	Institution	Years of study	Modality	No. of pts	SRS vs. FSRT	Dose strategy (Gy)	Tumor size	Tumor control	Follow-up	New facial neuropathy	New trigeminal dysfunction	Serviceable hearing preservation	Other
							alternate variable schedules							
Collen et al[29]	2011	Vrije Universiteit Brussel, Brussels, Belgium	2000–2008	BrainLAB	78	1 (SRS)	Median: 12.5 Gy (range: 11–14) prescribed at the 80% isodose line	Mean: 1.7 mL (range: 0.1–9.5)	95% at 5 y	Median: 56 mo (7–129)	16%	6%	82% at 48 mo	2 with NF2 14 prior surgical resection 1 prior Gamma Knife
					41	FSRT	10 × 3–4 Gy (*N* = 32), and 25 × 2 Gy (*N* = 10) prescribed at the 100% isodose line	Mean: 6.3 mL (range: 0.2–18.6)		Median: 73 mo (6–136)	3%	3%	59% at 48 mo	6 with NF2 13 prior surgical resection 1 prior Gamma Knife
Langenberg et al[30]	2011	Maastricht University Medical Center, The Netherlands	2003–2008	BrainLAB	17	SRS	12–12.5 Gy prescribed at the 80% isodose line	Mean: 2.09 cm^3 (range: 0.07–16.3)	65% decrease, 22% stabile, 13% increase (defined as volume change > 20%)	Median: 40 mo (16–80)	NR	NR	NR	0 with NF2 5 with prior surgery
					20	FSRT	54 Gy total, 30 × 1.8 Gy							
McWilliams et al[31]	2011	Allegheny General Hospital, Pittsburgh, PA	2003–2009	"6 MV LINAC with cone based or multileaf collimation"	13	1 (SRS)	12.5 Gy prescribed at the 80–90% isodose line	Median: 1.1 cm (range: 0.5–1.7)	31% decrease, 62% stable, 8% increase (growth defined as sustained change ≥ 2 mm in diameter)	Median: 13 mo (range: 3–36 mo)	0%	0%	0% maintained AAO–HNS class A or B hearing	NR
					10	FSRT	Total 25 Gy, 5 × 5 Gy prescribed at the 80–95% isodose line	Median: 1.4 cm (range: 0.5–2.2)	20% decrease, 60% stable, 20% increase (growth defined as				25% maintained AAO–HNS class A or B hearing	

Table 17.1 (*Continued*)

Author	Year published	Institution	Years of study	Modality	No. of pts	SRS vs. FSRT	Dose strategy (Gy)	Tumor size	Tumor control	Follow-up	New facial neuropathy	New trigeminal dysfunction	Serviceable hearing preservation	Other
									sustained change ≥ 2 mm in diameter)					
Matsuo et al[32]	2015	Nagasaki University School of Medicine, Nagasaki, Japan	1994–2002	Varian Clinac 2100C	44	1 (SRS)	Median: 14 Gy (range: 10–16), prescription isodose line NR	Median: 2.38 mL (range: 0.4–8.99)	82% decrease, 7% stable, 11% increase (defined as volume change > 20%)	Mean: 13.8 y (range: 5.5–19.5)	NR	NR	NR	0 with NF2
Ellenbogen et all[23]	2015	Beaumont Hospital, Dublin, Ireland	2003–2009	Elekta Precise Treatment System with micromultileaf collimator	50	1 (SRS)	12.5 Gy prescribed at the 80% isodose line	Median: 2.4 cm^3 (range: 0.24–10.59)	92% decrease, 4% stable, 4% increase	Median: 5.8 y (range: 1.4–9.2)	4%	4%	50% (defined as PTA < 50 dB)	1 with NF2 7 with previous surgery
Ikonomidis et al[33]	2015	Centre Hospitalier Universitaire Vaudois, Lausanne, Switzerland	2002–2010	BrainLab	84	1 (SRS)	Median: 12 Gy (10.8–12.8) prescribed at the 80% isodose line	Median: 2.15 mL (0.03–5.88)	84% decrease, 7% stable, 9% increase	Median: 39 mo (6–84)	1% transient	1% transient	36% retained GR grade I or II hearing	0 with NF2
Rezk et al[34]	2017	University Hospital of Cologne, Germany	NR	SL25 linear accelerator with micromultileaf collimator	50	1 (SRS)	Median: 12 Gy (range: 11–14) prescribed at the median 77% isodose (range: 65–85%)	Median: 1.4 mL (range: 0.18–7.2)	21% decrease, 75% stable, 4% increase	Median: 51 mo (range, 24–130)	4%	6%	94% did not have "deterioration of hearing"	0 with NF2 11 with prior surgery

Abbreviations: AAO–HNS, American Academy of Otolaryngology – Head and Neck Surgery; FSRT, fractionated stereotactic radiotherapy; NF2, neurofibromatosis type 2; SRS, stereotactic radiosurgery.

LINAC-based SRS and fractionated radiotherapy, published within the last 10 years.

17.5 The University of Florida Experience

As of December 2015, the University of Florida experience with VSs comprised 707 patients. The indications for SRS were age greater than 60 years ($N = 298$), failed surgery ($N = 102$), patient preference ($N = 265$), and medical infirmity ($N = 8$). With an overall median follow-up of 48 months, 202 tumors were unchanged, 279 were smaller, and 23 tumors (3%) were larger. Only eight patients have required surgery because of tumor growth after SRS (1%). Since 1994, when we reduced our treatment dose to 12.5 Gy, less than 1% of patients have experienced facial or trigeminal neuropathy after treatment.

References

[1] Leksell L. The stereotaxic method and radiosurgery of the brain. Acta Chir Scand. 1951; 102(4):316–319
[2] Betti OO, Derechinsky VE. Hyperselective encephalic irradiation with a linear accelerator. Acta Neurochir Suppl (Wien). 1984; 33:385–390
[3] Colombo F, Benedetti A, Pozza F, et al. External stereotactic irradiation by linear accelerator. Neurosurgery. 1985; 16(2):154–160
[4] Hartmann GH, Schlegel W, Sturm V, Kober B, Pastyr O, Lorenz WJ. Cerebral radiation surgery using moving field irradiation at a linear accelerator facility. Int J Radiat Oncol Biol Phys. 1985; 11(6):1185–1192
[5] McGinley PH, Butker EK, Crocker IR, Landry JC. A patient rotator for stereotactic radiosurgery. Phys Med Biol. 1990; 35(5):649–657
[6] Podgorsak EB, Olivier A, Pla M, Lefebvre PY, Hazel J. Dynamic stereotactic radiosurgery. Int J Radiat Oncol Biol Phys. 1988; 14(1):115–126
[7] Winston KR, Lutz W. Linear accelerator as a neurosurgical tool for stereotactic radiosurgery. Neurosurgery. 1988; 22(3):454–464
[8] Friedman WA, Bova FJ. The University of Florida radiosurgery system. Surg Neurol. 1989; 32(5):334–342
[9] Friedman WA, Buatti JM, Bova FJ, Mendenhall WM. LINAC Radiosurgery - A Practical Guide. Berlin: Springer-Verlag; 1998
[10] Leksell L. A note on the treatment of acoustic tumours. Acta Chir Scand. 1971; 137(8):763–765
[11] Foote KD, Friedman WA, Buatti JM, Meeks SL, Bova FJ, Kubilis PS. Analysis of risk factors associated with radiosurgery for vestibular schwannoma. J Neurosurg. 2001; 95(3):440–449
[12] Spiegelmann R, Gofman J, Alezra D, Pfeffer R. Radiosurgery for acoustic neurinomas (vestibular schwannomas). Isr Med Assoc J. 1999; 1(1):8–13
[13] Spiegelmann R, Lidar Z, Gofman J, Alezra D, Hadani M, Pfeffer R. Linear accelerator radiosurgery for vestibular schwannoma. J Neurosurg. 2001; 94 (1):7–13
[14] Martens F, Verbeke L, Piessens M, Van Vyve M. Stereotactic radiosurgery of vestibular schwannomas with a linear accelerator. Acta Neurochir Suppl (Wien). 1994; 62 Suppl:88–92
[15] Valentino V, Raimondi AJ. Tumour response and morphological changes of acoustic neurinomas after radiosurgery. Acta Neurochir (Wien). 1995; 133 (3-4):157–163
[16] Delaney G, Matheson J, Smee R. Stereotactic radiosurgery: an alternative approach to the management of acoustic neuromas. Med J Aust. 1992; 156 (6):440
[17] Barcia Salorio JL, Hernandez G, Ciudad J, Bordes V, Broseta J. Stereotactic radiosurgery in acoustic neurinoma. Acta Neurochir Suppl (Wien). 1984; 33: 373–376
[18] Varlotto JM, Shrieve DC, Alexander E, III, Kooy HM, Black PM, Loeffler JS. Fractionated stereotactic radiotherapy for the treatment of acoustic neuromas: preliminary results. Int J Radiat Oncol Biol Phys. 1996; 36(1):141–145
[19] Fuss M, Debus J, Lohr F, et al. Conventionally fractionated stereotactic radiotherapy (FSRT) for acoustic neuromas. Int J Radiat Oncol Biol Phys. 2000; 48(5):1381–1387
[20] Williams JA. Fractionated stereotactic radiotherapy for acoustic neuromas: preservation of function versus size. J Clin Neurosci. 2003; 10(1):48–52
[21] Andrews DW, Suarez O, Goldman HW, et al. Stereotactic radiosurgery and fractionated stereotactic radiotherapy for the treatment of acoustic schwannomas: comparative observations of 125 patients treated at one institution. Int J Radiat Oncol Biol Phys. 2001; 50(5):1265–1278
[22] Chang SD, Gibbs IC, Sakamoto GT, Lee E, Oyelese A, Adler JR, Jr. Staged stereotactic irradiation for acoustic neuroma. Neurosurgery. 2005; 56(6): 1254–1261, discussion 1261–1263
[23] Ellenbogen JR, Waqar M, Kinshuck AJ, et al. Linear accelerator radiosurgery for vestibular schwannomas: Results of medium-term follow-up. Br J Neurosurg. 2015; 29(5):678–684
[24] Rutten I, Baumert BG, Seidel L, et al. Long-term follow-up reveals low toxicity of radiosurgery for vestibular schwannoma. Radiother Oncol 2007; 82:83-89
[25] Hsu PW, Chang CN, Lee ST, et al. Outcomes of 75 patients over 12 years treated for acoustic neuromas with linear accelerator-based radiosurgery. J Clin Neurosci 2010; 17:556-560
[26] Combs SE, Welzel T, Schulz-Ertner D, Huber PE, Debus J. Differences in clinical results after LINAC-based single-dose radiosurgery versus fractionated stereotactic radiotherapy for patients with vestibular schwannomas. Int J Radiat Oncol Biol Phys 2010; 76:193-200
[27] Roos DE, Potter AE, Zacest AC. Hearing preservation after low dose linac radiosurgery for acoustic neuroma depends on initial hearing and time. Radiother Oncol 2011; 101:420-424
[28] Kopp C, Fauser C, Muller A, et al. Stereotactic fractionated radiotherapy and LINAC radiosurgery in the treatment of vestibular schwannoma-report about both stereotactic methods from a single institution. Int J Radiat Oncol Biol Phys 2011; 80:1485-1491
[29] Collen C, Ampe B, Gevaert T, et al. Single fraction versus fractionated linac-based stereotactic radiotherapy for vestibular schwannoma: a single-institution experience. Int J Radiat Oncol Biol Phys 2011; 81:e503-509
[30] van de Langenberg R, Dohmen AJ, de Bondt BJ, Nelemans PJ, Baumert BG, Stokroos RJ. Volume changes after stereotactic LINAC radiotherapy in vestibular schwannoma: control rate and growth patterns. Int J Radiat Oncol Biol Phys 2012; 84:343-349
[31] McWilliams W, Trombetta M, Werts ED, Fuhrer R, Hillman T. Audiometric outcomes for acoustic neuroma patients after single versus multiple fraction stereotactic irradiation. Otol Neurotol 2011; 32:297-300
[32] Matsuo T, Okunaga T, Kamada K, Izumo T, Hayashi N, Nagata I. Long-term follow-up results of linear accelerator-based radiosurgery for vestibular schwannoma using serial three-dimensional spoiled gradient-echo MRI. J Clin Neurosci 2015; 22:320-325
[33] Ikonomidis C, Pica A, Bloch J, Maire R. Vestibular Schwannoma: The Evolution of Hearing and Tumor Size in Natural Course and after Treatment by LINAC Stereotactic Radiosurgery. Audiol Neurootol 2015; 20:406-415
[34] Rezk EM, El Majdoub F, Kocher M, Treuer H, Sturm V, Maarouf M. Micro-Multileaf Collimator LINAC Radiosurgery for Vestibular Schwannomas. World Neurosurg 2017

18 Conventional Fractionation LINAC-Based Stereotactic Radiotherapy for Treatment of Sporadic Vestibular Schwannoma

Wenyin Shi, Haisong Liu, Christopher J. Farrell, and David W. Andrews

18.1 Introduction

Conventional fractionated radiotherapy refers to the fractionation schedule that uses a daily dose of 1.8 to 2.0 Gy with five daily fractions per week. The entire treatment course usually is 5 to 6 weeks with total treatment doses in the range of 45 to 54 Gy for benign intracranial tumors. This method of treatment is widely used for benign and malignant primary brain tumors, with proven efficacy and a favorable toxicity profile.

18.2 Fractionated Stereotactic Radiotherapy

Conventional fractionated radiation treatment originally utilized 3D conformal technology. Over the past several decades, the development of stereotactic radiation techniques has allowed treatment to be performed with greater conformity, fewer complications, and potentially improved tumor control. Fractionated stereotactic radiotherapy (FSRT) has the radiobiological advantages of conventional fractionated radiotherapy[1] while maintaining the same superior dose conformity, precision, and steep dose falloff outside the target volume of stereotactic radiosurgery (SRS). In essence, FSRT has the same radiation dosimetric characteristics as SRS with the only difference being the number of fractions and dose per fraction.

Currently, several different stereotactic systems are available for patient treatment, including infrared camera guidance,[2] relocatable frame,[3,4,5] implanted fiducial markers,[6] and thermoplastic mask fixation system.[7,8,9] The thermoplastic head mask is most widely used due to its convenience and patient comfort. High precision can be reproducibly achieved with the current FSRT systems. One study using the Gill-Thomas-Cosman (GTC) relocatable frame demonstrated a total 3D displacement of 1.8 mm ± 0.8 mm (mean ± SD) with a range of 0.3 to 3.9 mm[5] which is similar to mask-based systems where the 3D displacement is usually less than 2 to 2.5 mm.[7,8] Accuracy of patient positioning reproducibility with a stereotactic mask fixation system can be further improved with daily imaging guidance (image-guided radiation therapy). There are three types of in-room kilovoltage (kV) X-ray imaging guidance systems commonly used in current treatment centers. CT-on-rails is a rail-track–mounted kV tomographic imaging system that consists of a conventional CT scanner installed in the treatment room such that it can be moved into a position for acquiring helical CT scans of the patient on the treatment couch. The stereoscopic X-ray imaging system utilizes kV X-ray tubes that are mounted permanently either to the ceiling or floor such that the tube and detector locations are fixed relative to the treatment room coordinates. Examples of this type of system are ExacTRAC (BrainLab, Westchester, IL) and CyberKnife (Accuray, Sunnyvale, CA). Gantry-mounted systems, such as Varian On-Board Imager (OBI) and Elekta X-ray Volume Imaging (XVI), rely on X-ray tube and detectors that are mounted on the treatment gantry orthogonal to the central axis of the treatment beam. The kV imaging system rotates along with the gantry and shares the same isocenter as the MV treatment beam. It can generate radiographs, fluoroscopic images, as well as tomographic images such as CBCT, which uses a cone-beam X-ray source that encompasses a large volume with a single rotation about the patient. Images are then reconstructed into 3D images. The ceiling/floor-mounted stereoscopic X-ray imaging system and gantry-mounted system can also be integrated into a single treatment room, such as the Novalis Tx (BrainLab, Westchester, IL) or Truebeam STx (Varian, Palo Alto, CA) configurations.

In order to quantify the end-to-end positioning uncertainty of an image-guided fractionated stereotactic radiotherapy (IG-FSRT) procedure, several independent groups have reported their results of hidden target tests, which involved simulating a complete typical treatment of a hidden metal target in a rigid phantom with measurement of the localization accuracy. The average reported mean localization error is 0.8 mm.[10,11,12,13,14,15,16,17] As a result of the modern technology, a planned target volume (PTV) margin of 1 to 2 mm is sufficient. Such small PTV margin for vestibular schwannoma treatment allows better sparing of critical brain structures adjacent to the tumor, such as the brainstem and cochlea. Moreover, advanced radiation treatment planning, such as intensity-modulated radiation therapy (IMRT) and volumetric arc therapy (VAMT), can further carve the radiation distribution to achieve additional normal structure sparing which is unable to be performed with the 3D conformal technique[18] (▶ Fig. 18.1).

18.3 Radiobiology

Understanding the basic radiobiological rationale of FSRT will help interpret the clinical data, particularly the differences in efficacy and toxicity profile between FSRT and SRS for the treatment of vestibular schwannomas. The relationship between time, dose, fractions of FSRT, and its biological effect is based on basic principles of radiology, defined as the "4Rs" (repair, repopulation, redistribution, and reoxygenation) of radiation.[19] The most important biological principle that influences FSRT for vestibular schwannoma is "repair." Fractionation allows time between treatments for repair of sublethal damage. Due to faulty repair mechanisms, vestibular schwannomas are less efficient at repair compared to normal tissue and these differences between tumor and normal tissue are magnified with increased number of fractions.[1,20] This leads to the separation of normal tissue with highly fractionated radiation treatment. Fractionation also allows reoxygenation of tumor tissue and redistribution of cells in cell cycle. The ultimate result is an increased therapeutic index of radiation. The radiobiology of high-dose single-fraction treatment exerts major effects through lethal

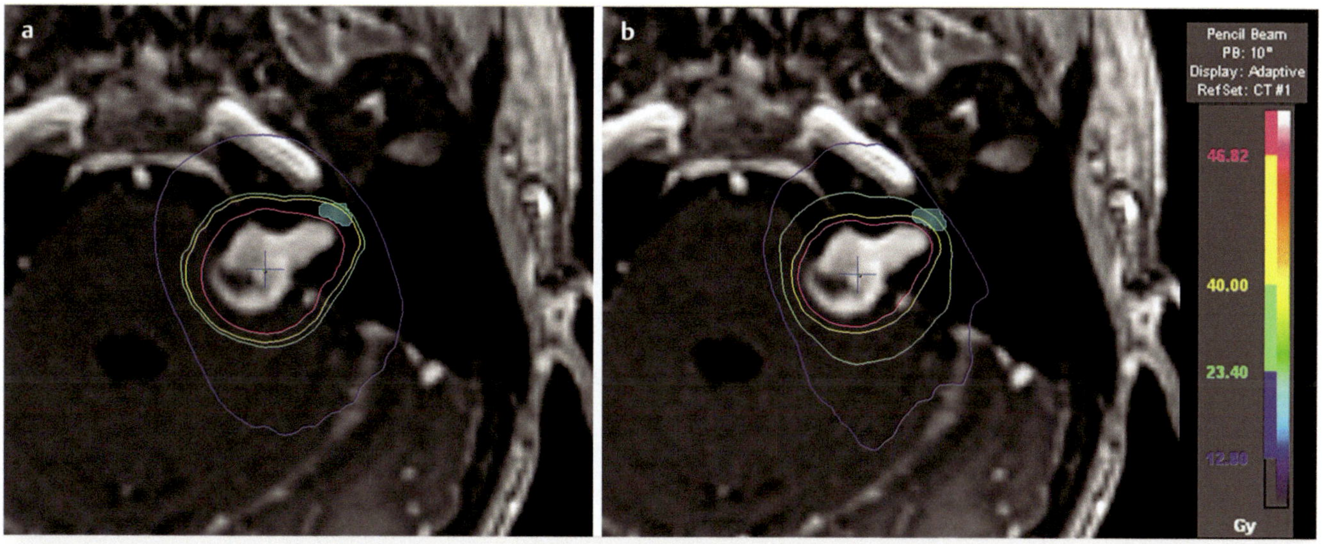

Fig. 18.1 Plan comparison of 3D conformal SRS vs. IMRT SRS, showing improved cochlea sparing with IMRT for vestibular schwannoma with a significant intracanalicular component. (**a**) 3D conformal planning with five dynamic arcs. The mean cochlea dose is 43 Gy. (**b**) Hybrid arc planning with four dynamic arcs and four IMRT beams. The mean cochlea dose is 30 Gy.

DNA damage and endothelial damage.[19] Though SRS may be favorable for tumor cell kill for vestibular schwannomas due to its low α/β ratio, it also has more adverse effects on the normal structure, such as injury to the cochlea and cochlear nerve.[1,21] Protection of normal tissue is achieved through steep dose fall off and high conformity of SRS technology. Unfortunately, due to the adjacent proximity of vestibular schwannomas to the cochlea and overlapping proximity with the cochlear nerve, these structures frequently cannot be adequately spared. Damage to the cochlear sensory cells, particularly the hair cells of organ of Corti, and cells of the stria vascularis is one major mechanism of radiation-induced hearing loss.[22]

The biological effects of SRS and FSRT on hearing can be further estimated based on the RET formula[20] which implies that the SRS dose should not exceed a threshold of around 11.2 Gy to obtain high rates of hearing preservation. Similarly, a cumulative FSRT dose above 45 Gy could result in higher rates of hearing loss. Based on our previous analysis, even a median value of 13 Gy has resulted in serviceable hearing losses ranging from 17 to 67%, while a median FSRT dose of 47.5 Gy has resulted in serviceable hearing losses ranging from 29 to 43%.[20] These findings are further supported by clinical evidence of loss of serviceable hearing as being statistically related to a threshold dose to the cochlea above 40 Gy.[23,24,25] Further discussion regarding the principles of radiobiology relevant to SRS and FSRT for vestibular schwannoma can be found in Chapter 15.

18.4 Tumor Control

FSRT was initially used as adjuvant therapy following incomplete surgical resection of vestibular schwannomas. In 1987, Wallner et al reported their initial experience, demonstrating that postoperative irradiation (> 45 Gy) decreased the recurrence rate after subtotal resection from 46 to 6%.[26] Subsequently, stereotactic radiation therapy has been demonstrated to achieve excellent tumor control equivalent to surgical resection, and may be effectively used as a definitive treatment option. The efficacy of primary radiation treatment for vestibular schwannomas was first established with Gamma Knife SRS.[27] Over the past two decades, multiple studies have reported tumor control rates utilizing FSRT comparable to those achieved with SRS, potentially with lower risk of cranial nerve morbidity (Table 18-1). A meta-analysis of 3,677 patients treated with SRS reported a 91% tumor control rate.[28] Several large retrospective series of FSRT with long-term follow-up showed local control rate exceeding 94%.[23,29,30,31,32] Other FSRT studies have reported a wider range of tumor control rates between 85 and 100% (Table 18-1). The variance in results is largely related to the length of follow-up and definitions of tumor control. It is well recognized now that after FSRT, there may be transient tumor expansion (▶ Fig. 18.2).[32,33,34] In the initial period after treatment, tumors may increase in size because of the effects of radiation, followed by a period of stabilization and often subsequent shrinkage. This transient expansion has been observed in 14 to 74% of patients at 9 to 16 months.[32,33,34] In order to properly account for this phenomenon, definition of treatment failure should involve sustained tumor growth on two consecutive follow-up MRI scans separated by an adequate time period.[23,35] Another important factor for accurate assessment of tumor control is adequate follow-up. Series with long-term follow-up demonstrated decreased local control with over time, though failure is rare after 5 years.[23,30,36]

Despite the overall high success rate of achieving long-term tumor control, the optimal dose and fractionation scheme for FSRT remains uncertain. There is a widespread variation in treatment practices at different institutions. The most commonly used radiation doses range from 45 to 57.6 Gy, administered in 1.8 to 2 Gy fractions (Table 18-1). Fuss et al reported their experience of 51 patients treated with FSRT to the dose of 57.6 Gy.[36] They demonstrated actuarial 2- and 5-year tumor control rates of 100 and 97.7%, respectively. The actuarial

Table 18.1 Outcomes of selected modern FSRT series for vestibular schwannoma

Author	Year	*n*	Dose/Fx size (Gy/Gy)	Local control	Hearing preservation	CN V neuropathy	CN VII neuropathy	Median follow-up (y)
Shirato et al[37]	1999	37	36–44/2	86.2%	53% at 5 y	0%	2.6%	2
Fuss et al[36]	2000	51	57.6/1.8	97.7%	85.2 % at 5 y	3.9%	0%	3.5
Andrews et al[38]	2001	56	50/2	97%	81% at 5 y	7%	2%	9.6
Sawamura et al[39]	2003	101	40–50/2	91.4%	71.5% at 5 y	4%	0.9%	3.8
Selch et al[40]	2004	48	54/1.8	100%	91.4% at 5 y	2.2%	2.1%	3
Chung et al[41]	2004	27	45/1.8	100%	57% at 2 y	7%	4%	2.1
Chan et al[42]	2005	70	54/1.8	98%	74%	0%	0%	4
Combs et al[43]	2005	106	57.6/1.8	95.3%	98% at 5 y	3.4%	2.3%	4
Combs et al[29]	2010	172	57.6/1.8	96%	69% at 10 y	4.6%	4%	6.3
Maire et al[44]	2006	45	51/1.8	86%	77.7%	0%	0%	6.7
Horan et al[45]	2007	42	50/1.67	96.9%	73% at 2 y	0%	3.2%	1.6
Koh et al[46]	2007	60	50/2	96%	77.3%	0%	0%	2.6
Thomas et al[47]	2007	34	45/1.8	96%	63%	0%	7%	3
McClelland et al[48]	2008	20	54/1.8	100%	100%	10%	0%	1.8
Andrews et al[49]	2009	43 46	50.4/1.8 46.8/1.8	100% 100%	68% at 3 y 79% at 3 y	0% 0%	0% 0%	1.2
Champ et al[23]	2013	154	46.8/1.8	96%	66% at 5 y	2%	1.8%	3
Kopp et al[50]	2011	47	54/1.8	97.9%	79%	0%	0%	2.7
Aoyama et al[32]	2012	201	36–50/2	96.6%	54.5% at 5 y	–	2.4%	6
Rasmussen et al[51]	2012	42	54/1.8	85%	38% at 2 y	0%	4.7%	5
Choy et al[52]	2013	103	52.2/1.8	89%	86%	–	2%	3.5
Litre et al[31]	2013	155	50.4/1.8	95.2%	54%	3.2%	2.5%	5
Woolf et al[53]	2013	93	52.2/2.1	92%	87%	1%	1%	5.7
Anderson et al[54]	2014	56	45–50.4/1.8	97%	44.4%	0%	0%	4.4
Combs et al[30]	2015	291	57.6/1.8	94%	86%	1%	1%	5.6

Abbreviations: CN, cranial nerve; f/u, follow-up; FSRT, fractionated stereotactic radiotherapy.

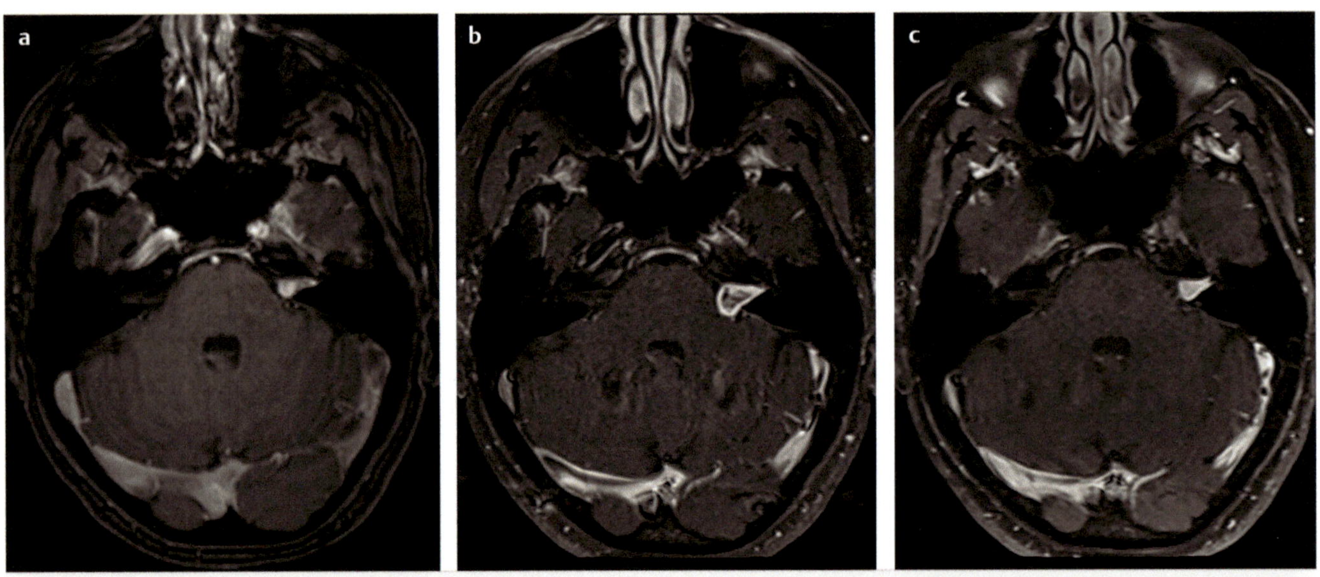

Fig. 18.2 An example of transient tumor expansion after FSRT. **(a)** Pretreatment tumor volume; **(b)** tumor expansion with central necrosis of tumor volume 3 months after FSRT; **(c)** shrinkage and restitution of enhancement, now most likely fibrosis at 2 years after FSRT. Tumor remains stable 4 years after treatment at last follow-up.

serviceable hearing preservation rate at 2 and 5 years was 85%. Lower doses were explored to reduce toxicity and improve hearing preservation, while maintaining tumor control. Andrews et al performed a nonrandomized prospective cohort analysis comparing outcomes after FSRT dose reduction from 50.4 Gy to 46.8 Gy.[49] This study successfully improved hearing outcomes without reduction of tumor control. Long-term follow-up of the low-dose 46.8 Gy cohort showed tumor control rates at 3 and 5 years of 99 and 93%, respectively. The overall serviceable hearing preservation was 67% with 3 and 5 year rates of 66 and 54%, respectively.[23] Importantly, hearing impairment after FSRT appears to have a delayed time to onset relative to SRS.[25] Several series using doses as low as 45 Gy also showed similar high tumor control probability.[41,47,54] However, doses lower than 45 Gy, particular lower than 40 Gy, appear to be associated with inferior tumor control.[26,37] Based on the current data, it seems that no dose–response relationship exists beyond 45 to 46.8 Gy, and this dose range may represent the threshold for high tumor control probability. Given the potential for reduced side effects and improved hearing preservation, low-dose FSRT (45–46.8 Gy) should be considered. Further dose de-escalation below 45 Gy should be carefully performed in the prospective setting with long-term follow-up.

18.5 Hearing Preservation

FSRT has been developed to reduce the toxicity of SRS, with improved hearing preservation as one of the main objectives. While the overall tumor control rates reported after FSRT are within a consistent narrow range, hearing preservation rates have a much wider variable, ranging from 38 to 100% for patients who received standard doses (45–57.6 Gy) (Table 18-1). For reference, the reported rates of hearing preservation from larges series of patients treated with current low-dose (12–13 Gy) SRS are 16 to 82%.[55,56] It should be noted that direct comparison of hearing preservation rates between series is difficult and unreliable. The results are confounded by multiple factors including differences in hearing assessment with many institutions failing to measure the hearing according to the American Academy of Otolaryngology–Head and Neck Surgery or Gardner–Robertson (G-R) classification. Moreover, the definition of hearing preservation also varies. Hearing is most often considered preserved when the hearing level has been maintained at G-R grade I or II after FSRT.[23] However, some series have utilized more stringent criterion, defined as the absence of any hearing decline.[52] Other studies have relied on subjective assessment of hearing rather than formal audiometry.[57] It is also important to follow these patients long term, because hearing can continue to decline for years after FSRT or other radiation therapy.[23,38,43,49] Making things more complicated, some patient factors such as age, comorbidity, and tumor size may also affect the hearing preservation rate.[30,55]

An additional factor complicating outcomes assessment of FSRT for vestibular schwannomas is the wide variety of dose fractionation schedules administered at different centers. Several studies have shown that higher doses of radiation are associated with poorer rates of hearing preservation. Our institution demonstrated this effect in a prospective cohort study of radiation dose de-escalation from 50.4 to 46.8 Gy with formal audiogram evaluations.[49] When patients with serviceable hearing were analyzed at a comparable 3-year follow-up, the raw hearing preservation rate was better in the low-dose group (79 vs. 68%), and the actuarial hearing preservation rate was significantly longer for the low-dose group than for the high-dose group (165 vs. 79 weeks).[49] In a recently reported update of our experience of 154 patients treated with the reduced FSRT dose (46.8 Gy), at a median follow-up time of 3 years, the overall hearing preservation rate was 67%. Hearing preservation rates at 3 and 5 years were 66, and 54 %, respectively.[23] We also identified more favorable hearing preservation in the patients with G-R class I hearing prior to FSRT. Among this subgroup, the overall hearing preservation rate was 82%.[23] However, the dose relationship is still unclear when compared to other groups utilizing higher radiation doses. Combs et al reported on a large cohort of patients treated with FSRT to a dose of 57.6 Gy. Their 3- and 5-year hearing preservation rates were 79 and 76%, respectively.[43] However, no formal audiometric testing was performed in their series with useful hearing defined as any serviceable hearing that allowed sufficient communication without visual aids. Comparison of series that required audiometric assessment does show similar hearing preservation rates. In a series of patients treated with a low dose of 45 Gy, the 3-year hearing preservation rate was 63%.[47] Another large series of approximately 200 patients treated with 54 Gy showed a 5-year hearing preservation rate of 54.5%.[32] A very similar overall hearing preservation rate of 54% was also reported by Litre et al in their series of 155 patients who received 50.4 Gy.[31]

Due to the aforementioned confounding factors and lack of a clear dose response relationship across compared series, no firm conclusion can be made about the optimal fractionation schedule. However, given the consistent excellent local control rates reported across the dose range examined (45–57.6 Gy), it is quite reasonable to recommend low-dose (45–46.8 Gy) FSRT for the potential benefit of better hearing preservation.

Similar challenges also exist when comparing hearing preservation outcomes between SRS and FSRT. Several authors have reported their own experiences using both SRS and FSRT for vestibular schwannomas. Andrews et al compared their experience with FSRT and SRS and reported that tumor control, facial nerve preservation, and trigeminal neuropathy rates were equivalent among the two cohorts. However, hearing preservation rates were 2.5-fold higher in the FSRT group with a crude hearing preservation rate of 81% compared to 33% in the SRS cohort.[38] Combs et al also reported their single-institution experience of FSRT and SRS for patients with vestibular schwannoma.[29] They found no statistical difference in tumor control between the groups and that the probability of maintaining the pretreatment hearing level after SRS with doses of ≤ 13 Gy was comparable to that of FSRT. A very favorable hearing preservation rate was reported in their series. The probability of preserving the same G-R hearing grade was 83, 79, 76, and 69% at 1, 3, 5, and 10 years after radiotherapy, respectively. There was no difference between SRS and FSRT patients.[29] Though the author defined serviceable (useful) hearing as G-R class I to II, the hearing assessments were retrospectively based on information available within the patient chart including hearing evaluations performed before and after radiotherapy by the patients' otolaryngologist, data collected from the follow-up visits or from the primary care physicians, as well as from the patient questionnaires rather than based entirely on formal audiometry testing.[29] The much more favorable hearing outcome, particularly at long-term follow-up at 5 and 10 years reflects the suboptimal data collection, and should be taken into consideration when interpreting the results. Combs et al also performed a pooled analysis with three German groups comparing the hearing preservation after FSRT and SRS.[30] Again, a high overall hearing preservation of 84% was reported with long-term follow-up with no difference between SRS and FSRT groups. However, the same limitation in hearing assessment with inconsistent obtainment of objective audiometric data prevents any definitive conclusions based on these data. Though no randomized trial has yet been done to address this question, prospective cohort studies with formal audiometric follow-up are needed to provide a higher level of evidence. Further discussion regarding hearing preservation with SRS and FSRT can be found in Chapter 52.

18.6 Cranial Nerve Toxicity

Facial nerve function preservation is another critical goal in the management of vestibular schwannomas. The overall risk of facial nerve neuropathy in modern series of FSRT is low, generally less than 3 to 4% (Table 18-1). For example, the combined series of three German institutions of 291 patients treated with FSRT to a dose of 57.6 Gy showed an overall facial nerve neuropathy rate of 1%.[30] Though long-term facial neuropathy risk is low, transient worsening of facial nerve function or transient new facial nerve paresis can be observed in up to 9% of patients due to transient tumor expansion[32] with the risk increased in patients harboring larger tumors.[32] Additional cranial nerve deficits following FSRT are also rare, including trigeminal neuropathy or neuralgia, with a risk of less than 3 to 4% in large modern series (Table 18-1).

18.7 Future Development

Although vestibular schwannomas are benign tumors with a frequently slow rate of growth, these tumors and their subsequent treatment are capable of resulting in significant neurologic impairment including hearing loss, tinnitus, other cranial neuropathy, and disequilibrium. Although radiotherapy offers high tumor control rates with very few side effects, there still lacks consensus for treatment selection between FSRT and SRS, particularly in patients with small tumors and excellent hearing. Though such questions are best answered through properly designed randomized trials, randomization between SRS and FSRT is difficult in practice due to institutional biases and variations in the commercially available stereotactic radiation delivery systems. However, prospective studies with long-term MRI and formal audiometric assessment can provide reliable data and may allow for improved comparison of these techniques. Furthermore, the optimal dose of FSRT that would maintain the currently reported excellent rates of tumor control while achieving the highest rates of hearing and cranial nerve preservation remains unclear. Additional factors beyond radiation dose to the cochlea that determine long-term hearing preservation including the impact of radiation on the cochlear nerve and its vascular supply and cochlear nucleus remain to be elucidated. The impact of various radiation delivery modalities on tinnitus and disequilibrium has also not been well investigated. Based on the currently available evidence, it appears that radiation doses less than 45 Gy may be below the tolerance of the cochlea and cochlear nerve; however, dose reduction beyond this level should only be considered in the clinical trial setting with careful long-term follow-up to assess for potential compromise in tumor control.

References

[1] Anker CJ, Shrieve DC. Basic principles of radiobiology applied to radiosurgery and radiotherapy of benign skull base tumors. Otolaryngol Clin North Am. 2009; 42(4):601–621

[2] Buatti JM, Bova FJ, Friedman WA, et al. Preliminary experience with frameless stereotactic radiotherapy. Int J Radiat Oncol Biol Phys. 1998; 42(3):591–599

[3] Gill SS, Thomas DG, Warrington AP, Brada M. Relocatable frame for stereotactic external beam radiotherapy. Int J Radiat Oncol Biol Phys. 1991; 20(3):599–603

[4] Graham JD, Warrington AP, Gill SS, Brada M. A non-invasive, relocatable stereotactic frame for fractionated radiotherapy and multiple imaging. Radiother Oncol. 1991; 21(1):60–62

[5] Kumar S, Burke K, Nalder C, et al. Treatment accuracy of fractionated stereotactic radiotherapy. Radiother Oncol. 2005; 74(1):53–59

[6] Kim KH, Cho MJ, Kim JS, et al. Isocenter accuracy in frameless stereotactic radiotherapy using implanted fiducials. Int J Radiat Oncol Biol Phys. 2003; 56 (1):266–273

[7] Willner J, Flentje M, Bratengeier K. CT simulation in stereotactic brain radiotherapy–analysis of isocenter reproducibility with mask fixation. Radiother Oncol. 1997; 45(1):83–88

[8] Alheit H, Dornfeld S, Dawel M, et al. Patient position reproducibility in fractionated stereotactically guided conformal radiotherapy using the BrainLab mask system. Strahlenther Onkol. 2001; 177(5):264–268

[9] Hodapp N, Nanko N, Röhner F, Frommhold H. Quality assurance for non-invasive patient fixation during stereotactic convergent beam irradiation. Acta Neurochir Suppl (Wien). 1994; 62:101–104

[10] Wurm RE, Erbel S, Schwenkert I, et al. Novalis frameless image-guided non-invasive radiosurgery: initial experience. Neurosurgery. 2008; 62(5) Suppl: A11–A17, discussion A17–A18

[11] Gevaert T, Verellen D, Engels B, et al. Clinical evaluation of a robotic 6-degree of freedom treatment couch for frameless radiosurgery. Int J Radiat Oncol Biol Phys. 2012; 83(1):467–474

[12] Ramakrishna N, Rosca F, Friesen S, Tezcanli E, Zygmanszki P, Hacker F. A clinical comparison of patient setup and intra-fraction motion using frame-based radiosurgery versus a frameless image-guided radiosurgery system for intracranial lesions. Radiother Oncol. 2010; 95(1):109–115

[13] Lamba M, Breneman JC, Warnick RE. Evaluation of image-guided positioning for frameless intracranial radiosurgery. Int J Radiat Oncol Biol Phys. 2009; 74 (3):913–919

[14] van Santvoort J, Wiggenraad R, Bos P. Positioning accuracy in stereotactic radiotherapy using a mask system with added vacuum mouth piece and stereoscopic X-ray positioning. Int J Radiat Oncol Biol Phys. 2008; 72(1):261–267

[15] Jin JY, Ryu S, Faber K, et al. 2D/3D image fusion for accurate target localization and evaluation of a mask based stereotactic system in fractionated stereotactic radiotherapy of cranial lesions. Med Phys. 2006; 33(12):4557–4566

[16] Feygelman V, Walker L, Chinnaiyan P, Forster K. Simulation of intrafraction motion and overall geometrical accuracy of a frameless intracranial radiosurgery process. J Appl Clin Med Phys. 2008; 9(4):2828

[17] Ackerly T, Lancaster CM, Geso M, Roxby KJ. Clinical accuracy of ExacTrac intracranial frameless stereotactic system. Med Phys. 2011; 38(9):5040–5048

[18] Witek M, Vahknenko Y, Siglin J, et al. Dose reduction to the scalp with hippocampal sparing is achievable with intensity modulated radiotherapy. Int J Med Phys Clin Eng Radiat Oncol. 2014; 3(3):176–182

[19] Santacroce A, Kamp MA, Budach W, Hänggi D. Radiobiology of radiosurgery for the central nervous system. BioMed Res Int. 2013; 2013:362761

[20] Andrews DW, Bednarz G, Werner-Wasik M, Downes-Phillips B. Fractionated stereotactic radiotherapy: rationale, indications, and treatment technique. In: Chin L, Regine W, eds. Principles and Practice of Stereotactic Radiosurgery. New York, NY: Springer; 2008:289–298

[21] Yeung AH, Sughrue ME, Kane AJ, Tihan T, Cheung SW, Parsa AT. Radiobiology of vestibular schwannomas: mechanisms of radioresistance and potential targets for therapeutic sensitization. Neurosurg Focus. 2009; 27(6):E2

[22] Linskey ME, Johnstone PA. Radiation tolerance of normal temporal bone structures: implications for gamma knife stereotactic radiosurgery. Int J Radiat Oncol Biol Phys. 2003; 57(1):196–200

[23] Champ CE, Shen X, Shi W, et al. Reduced-dose fractionated stereotactic radiotherapy for acoustic neuromas: maintenance of tumor control with improved hearing preservation. Neurosurgery. 2013; 73(3):489–496

[24] Pan CC, Eisbruch A, Lee JS, Snorrason RM, Ten Haken RK, Kileny PR. Prospective study of inner ear radiation dose and hearing loss in head-and-neck cancer patients. Int J Radiat Oncol Biol Phys. 2005; 61(5):1393–1402

[25] Bhandare N, Jackson A, Eisbruch A, et al. Radiation therapy and hearing loss. Int J Radiat Oncol Biol Phys. 2010; 76(3) Suppl:S50–S57

[26] Wallner KE, Sheline GE, Pitts LH, Wara WM, Davis RL, Boldrey EB. Efficacy of irradiation for incompletely excised acoustic neurilemomas. J Neurosurg. 1987; 67(6):858–863

[27] Flickinger JC, Lunsford LD, Coffey RJ, et al. Radiosurgery of acoustic neurinomas. Cancer. 1991; 67(2):345–353

[28] Pannullo SC, Fraser JF, Moliterno J, Cobb W, Stieg PE. Stereotactic radiosurgery: a meta-analysis of current therapeutic applications in neuro-oncologic disease. J Neurooncol. 2011; 103(1):1–17

[29] Combs SE, Welzel T, Schulz-Ertner D, Huber PE, Debus J. Differences in clinical results after LINAC-based single-dose radiosurgery versus fractionated stereotactic radiotherapy for patients with vestibular schwannomas. Int J Radiat Oncol Biol Phys. 2010; 76(1):193–200

[30] Combs SE, Engelhard C, Kopp C, et al. Long-term outcome after highly advanced single-dose or fractionated radiotherapy in patients with vestibular schwannomas - pooled results from 3 large German centers. Radiother Oncol. 2015; 114(3):378–383

[31] Litre F, Rousseaux P, Jovenin N, et al. Fractionated stereotactic radiotherapy for acoustic neuromas: a prospective monocenter study of about 158 cases. Radiother Oncol. 2013; 106(2):169–174

[32] Aoyama H, Onodera S, Takeichi N, et al. Symptomatic outcomes in relation to tumor expansion after fractionated stereotactic radiation therapy for vestibular schwannomas: single-institutional long-term experience. Int J Radiat Oncol Biol Phys. 2013; 85(2):329–334

[33] Kapoor S, Batra S, Carson K, et al. Long-term outcomes of vestibular schwannomas treated with fractionated stereotactic radiotherapy: an institutional experience. Int J Radiat Oncol Biol Phys. 2011; 81(3):647–653

[34] Mandl ES, Meijer OW, Slotman BJ, Vandertop WP, Peerdeman SM. Stereotactic radiation therapy for large vestibular schwannomas. Radiother Oncol. 2010; 95(1):94–98

[35] Pollock BE, Link MJ, Foote RL. Failure rate of contemporary low-dose radiosurgical technique for vestibular schwannoma. J Neurosurg. 2009; 111(4): 840–844

[36] Fuss M, Debus J, Lohr F, et al. Conventionally fractionated stereotactic radiotherapy (FSRT) for acoustic neuromas. Int J Radiat Oncol Biol Phys. 2000; 48 (5):1381–1387

[37] Shirato H, Sakamoto T, Sawamura Y, et al. Comparison between observation policy and fractionated stereotactic radiotherapy (SRT) as an initial management for vestibular schwannoma. Int J Radiat Oncol Biol Phys. 1999; 44(3): 545–550

[38] Andrews DW, Suarez O, Goldman HW, et al. Stereotactic radiosurgery and fractionated stereotactic radiotherapy for the treatment of acoustic schwannomas: comparative observations of 125 patients treated at one institution. Int J Radiat Oncol Biol Phys. 2001; 50(5):1265–1278

[39] Sawamura Y, Shirato H, Sakamoto T, et al. Management of vestibular schwannoma by fractionated stereotactic radiotherapy and associated cerebrospinal fluid malabsorption. J Neurosurg. 2003; 99(4):685–692

[40] Selch MT, Pedroso A, Lee SP, et al. Stereotactic radiotherapy for the treatment of acoustic neuromas. J Neurosurg. 2004; 101 Suppl 3:362–372

[41] Chung HT, Ma R, Toyota B, Clark B, Robar J, McKenzie M. Audiologic and treatment outcomes after linear accelerator-based stereotactic irradiation for acoustic neuroma. Int J Radiat Oncol Biol Phys. 2004; 59(4):1116–1121

[42] Chan AW, Black P, Ojemann RG, et al. Stereotactic radiotherapy for vestibular schwannomas: favorable outcome with minimal toxicity. Neurosurgery. 2005; 57(1):60–70, discussion 60–70

[43] Combs SE, Volk S, Schulz-Ertner D, Huber PE, Thilmann C, Debus J. Management of acoustic neuromas with fractionated stereotactic radiotherapy (FSRT): long-term results in 106 patients treated in a single institution. Int J Radiat Oncol Biol Phys. 2005; 63(1):75–81

[44] Maire JP, Huchet A, Milbeo Y, et al. Twenty years' experience in the treatment of acoustic neuromas with fractionated radiotherapy: a review of 45 cases. Int J Radiat Oncol Biol Phys. 2006; 66(1):170–178

[45] Horan G, Whitfield GA, Burton KE, Burnet NG, Jefferies SJ. Fractionated conformal radiotherapy in vestibular schwannoma: early results from a single centre. Clin Oncol (R Coll Radiol). 2007; 19(7):517–522

[46] Koh ES, Millar BA, Ménard C, et al. Fractionated stereotactic radiotherapy for acoustic neuroma: single-institution experience at The Princess Margaret Hospital. Cancer. 2007; 109(6):1203–1210

[47] Thomas C, Di Maio S, Ma R, et al. Hearing preservation following fractionated stereotactic radiotherapy for vestibular schwannomas: prognostic implications of cochlear dose. J Neurosurg. 2007; 107(5):917–926

[48] McClelland S, III, Gerbi BJ, Higgins PD, Orner JB, Hall WA. Safety and efficacy of fractionated stereotactic radiotherapy for acoustic neuromas. J Neurooncol. 2008; 86(2):191–194

[49] Andrews DW, Werner-Wasik M, Den RB, et al. Toward dose optimization for fractionated stereotactic radiotherapy for acoustic neuromas: comparison of two dose cohorts. Int J Radiat Oncol Biol Phys. 2009; 74(2):419–426

[50] Kopp C, Fauser C, Müller A, et al. Stereotactic fractionated radiotherapy and LINAC radiosurgery in the treatment of vestibular schwannoma-report about both stereotactic methods from a single institution. Int J Radiat Oncol Biol Phys. 2011; 80(5):1485–1491

[51] Rasmussen R, Claesson M, Stangerup SE, et al. Fractionated stereotactic radiotherapy of vestibular schwannomas accelerates hearing loss. Int J Radiat Oncol Biol Phys. 2012; 83(5):e607–e611

[52] Choy W, Spasic M, Pezeshkian P, et al. Outcomes of stereotactic radiosurgery and stereotactic radiotherapy for the treatment of vestibular schwannoma. Neurosurgery. 2013; 60 Suppl 1:120–125

[53] Woolf DK, Williams M, Goh CL, et al. Fractionated stereotactic radiotherapy for acoustic neuromas: long-term outcomes. Clin Oncol (R Coll Radiol). 2013; 25(12):734–738

[54] Anderson BM, Khuntia D, Bentzen SM, et al. Single institution experience treating 104 vestibular schwannomas with fractionated stereotactic radiation therapy or stereotactic radiosurgery. J Neurooncol. 2014; 116(1):187–193

[55] Yang I, Sughrue ME, Han SJ, et al. A comprehensive analysis of hearing preservation after radiosurgery for vestibular schwannoma. J Neurosurg. 2010; 112 (4):851–859

[56] Lunsford LD, Niranjan A, Flickinger JC, Maitz A, Kondziolka D. Radiosurgery of vestibular schwannomas: summary of experience in 829 cases. J Neurosurg. 2005; 102 Suppl:195–199

[57] Combs SE, Thilmann C, Edler L, Debus J, Schulz-Ertner D. Efficacy of fractionated stereotactic reirradiation in recurrent gliomas: long-term results in 172 patients treated in a single institution. J Clin Oncol. 2005; 23(34): 8863–8869

19 CyberKnife Radiotherapy for Treatment of Sporadic Vestibular Schwannoma

Navjot Chaudhary and Steven D. Chang

19.1 Introduction

Single-session stereotactic radiosurgery (SRS) and fractionated radiotherapy have emerged as viable alternatives to microsurgical resection for vestibular schwannoma (VS). Radiation delivery methods include SRS using the Gamma Knife (GK SRS), linear accelerator-based (LINAC) systems including CyberKnife (CK) using either single session SRS or hypofractionated and conventionally fractioned regimens, and proton beam therapy. Numerous prior publications have documented the safety and efficacy of SRS, hypofractionated radiotherapy (two to five sessions), or conventionally fractionated radiotherapy for VS (▸ Table 19.1 and ▸ Table 19.2). Single-session SRS has shown excellent rates of tumor control; however, a single higher therapeutic dose theoretically may carry a greater risk of injuring adjacent structures than multiple lower dose sessions. One large series investigated single-session GK or CK SRS to treat 386 patients with VS.[1] Tumor volume was the only predictor of trigeminal neuropathy, and no predictor of facial nerve injury was found. On the House-Brackmann scale, one patient had a permanent one-level drop and seven patients experienced a transient drop of 1 to 3 levels. Serviceable hearing was preserved in 75% of cases. In this study, there were no statistically significant differences found when comparing tumor control and toxicity between GK and CK SRS on multivariate regression.

Given excellent tumor control rates reported with SRS, there has been an increasing emphasis on minimizing cranial nerve morbidity. The marginal dose for single-fraction SRS has been reduced from 16 to 20 Gy to the currently accepted dose of 12 to 13 Gy in order to reduce the risk of cranial neuropathy and hearing loss.[2,3,4] The likelihood of hearing preservation in earlier studies was 51 to 60%.[5,6,7] However, more recent studies utilizing a lower marginal dose demonstrate improved hearing preservation rates of 71 and 73%.[8] Fractionation, administering smaller doses over multiple sessions, may help minimize cranial nerve morbidity.[8] The rationale behind multisession radiotherapy is that it allows adjacent brain tissue to recover in between doses. Also, organs at risk including the cochlea receive significantly lower doses with each treatment using multisession radiotherapy. Given these theoretical advantages, fractionated radiotherapy has become the mainstay at many institutions. The results for the frameless CK system are discussed below.

Table 19.1 Vestibular schwannomas treated with single-session stereotactic radiosurgery ($n > 100$ cases)

Authors	Year published	No. of pts	Modality	Median tumor volume, cm³	Median radiation dose at IDL, Gy	Local control, %	Median follow-up, mo	Median follow-up, no. pts	Serviceable hearing preservation, %	New trigeminal neuropathy, %	New facial neuropathy, %
Murphy et al[23]	2011	103	GK	1.95 ± 2.42	13	95.2 (3-y actuarial)	37.5	NR	NR	1	5
Fukuoka et al[24]	2009	152	GK	2	12	94 (5-y actuarial)	> 60	59	71 crude	2.6	0
Chopra et al[25]	2007	216	GK	1.3	13	98.3 ± 1 (10-y actuarial)	68	106	57–74 crude	4.2 ± 1.6	0
Friedman et al[26]	2006	295	LINAC	2.2	12.5	90 (5-y actuarial)	34	NR	NR	3.6 overall, 0.7 for dose < 12.5 Gy	4.4 overall, 0.7 for dose < 12.5 Gy
Hempel et al[27]	2006	116	GK	1.6	13	96.7 crude	Mean: 98	NR	NR	5.8	0
Hasegawa et al[28]	2005	301	GK	Mean: 5.6	13	93 (5-y actuarial)	94	19	37 crude, 68 crude for dose < 13 Gy	2	1
Wowra et al[29]	2005	111	GK	1.6	13	95 (6-y actuarial)	84	NR	NR	11.7	3
Chung et al[30]	2005	187	GK	Mean: 4.1	13	96.8 crude	31	26	60 crude	1.1	1.4
Litvack et al[31]	2003	134	GK	NR	12	98 crude	36	47	62 crude	5.8	2.3
Rowe et al[32]	2003	212	GK	3.7	15	97 crude	34	49	75 crude	3.5	4.5
Unger et al[33]	2002	100	GK	3.4	13	96 crude	76	29	55 crude	5	6
Prasad et al[34]	2000	153	GK	Mean: 2.7	13.2	92 crude	38	36	58 crude	5	2.3

Abbreviations: IDL, prescriptions isodose line; GK, Gamma Knife; NR, not reported; pts, patients.

Table 19.2 Vestibular schwannomas treated with conventionally fractionated radiotherapy

Authors	Year	No. of pts	No. of fractions	Median tumor volume, cm^3	Median radiation dose, Gy	Local control, %	Median follow-up, mo	Median follow-up, no. pts	Serviceable hearing, %	New trigeminal neuropathy, %	New facial neuropathy, %
Kopp et al[35]	2010	47	30	3.95	54	97.9 crude	32	33	79 crude	8.5	4.3
Combs et al[36]	2010	165	30	2.8	57.6	96 (5-y actuarial)	75	94	78 (5-y actuarial)	3	4
Horan et al[37]	2007	42	30	2 cm diameter	50	96.9 (2.5-y actuarial)	18.6	20	100 crude subjective hearing	0	3.2
Koh et al[38]	2007	60	25	4.9	50	96 (5-y actuarial)	31.9	22	77 crude	0	0
Maire et al[39]	2006	45	30	3.1 cm diameter	51	86 (15-y actuarial)	80	9	78 crude subjective hearing	0	0
Chan et al[40]	2005	68	30	2.4	54	92 (5-y actuarial)	45	NR	NR	4	1
Selch et al[41]	2004	48	30	2.5	54	100 crude	36	42	91 (5-y actuarial)	2.2	2.1
Sawamura et al[42]	2003	101	23	1.9 cm diameter	48	91 (5-y actuarial)	45	36	71 (5-y actuarial)	4	0
Andrews et al[43]	2001	56	25	2.8	50	97 crude	26	27	81 crude	7	2

Abbreviation: pts, patients.

19.2 CyberKnife Radiotherapy

The introduction of the frameless CK system makes it possible to deliver multiple sessions of highly conformal radiation to targeted lesions with great accuracy. CyberKnife radiotherapy (Accuray, Inc., Sunnyvale, CA) was first introduced by Dr. John Adler at Stanford University Medical Center in 1994 (▶ Fig. 19.1).[9] It is a dedicated robotic LINAC-based system, with the features of real-time image guidance, no rigid immobilization, and nonisocentric planning. This versatile system gives the ability of submillimeter accuracy when correcting in real time for changes in target position, to treat both nonisocentrically and isocentrically, to easily fractionate treatments, to treat both intracranial and extracranial targets, and to treat moving targets while preserving tight dosimetry surrounding the lesion.[9,10,11] The CK radiotherapy planning system takes advantage of the robot's six-degree-of-freedom maneuverability and allows an array of overlapping beams to be superimposed without an isocenter. An inverse planning procedure optimizes the set of beam directions and dose, and this nonisocentric planning can achieve excellent dose homogeneity even with irregularly shaped targets. Similar dose homogeneity may be difficult to achieve with multiple isocenter models. A significant benefit of a frameless system is the ability to conveniently treat patients in multiple sessions, which is especially advantageous for treating lesions in eloquent brain regions.[9] ▶ Fig. 19.2 and ▶ Fig. 19.3 provide examples of treatment plans for small and large VSs.

One of the earliest series to report CK radiotherapy outcomes for VS was performed by Ishihara et al and evaluated 38 tumors treated from 1998 to 2002.[12] Fourteen patients had Gardner-Robertson (GR) class I or II hearing (serviceable), and 24 patients had class III to V hearing. The total and marginal radiation doses were 15.0 to 20.5 Gy and 11.9 to 20.1 Gy, respectively. They found a 94% tumor control rate after a mean follow-up of 31.9 months. Only one patient in the group with nonserviceable hearing underwent additional surgical resection for an increase in tumor size. The overall hearing preservation rate was 93%. Delayed transient facial nerve paresis developed in one patient in the nonserviceable hearing group, as did one case of trigeminal neuropathy. Another early study was performed by Ju et al and evaluated 21 VS patients (14 sporadic and 7 neurofibromatosis type-2 [NF2]) treated with CK radiotherapy. Two patients experienced hearing deterioration (16.7%) in the non-NF2 group, and three patients (50%) in the NF2 group.[13] No facial or trigeminal dysfunction, brainstem toxicity, or cerebellar edema occurred. Tumor regression occurred in 43% and was stable in 57% of patients, achieving an overall tumor control rate of 100%.

One of the largest and most comprehensive experiences with CK radiotherapy for VS was reported by Hansasuta et al at the Stanford University Medical Center, in which 383 patients were treated from 1999 to 2007.[14] Ninety percent were treated with 18 Gy in three sessions, targeting a median tumor volume of 1.1 cm^3. During a median follow-up of 3.6 years, 10 tumors required additional treatment, resulting in 3- and 5-year Kaplan–Meier tumor control rates of 99 and 96%, respectively. The 5-year tumor control rate was 98% for tumors less than 3.4 cm^2. NF2 patients were associated with worse tumor control ($p = 0.02$). Of the 200 evaluable patients with preradiotherapy serviceable hearing (GR grades I and II), the rate of serviceable hearing preservation was 76%. Smaller tumor volume was associated with hearing preservation ($p = 0.001$). Two percent of patients developed trigeminal dysfunction, half of which was transient, and there were no cases of facial weakness. Another

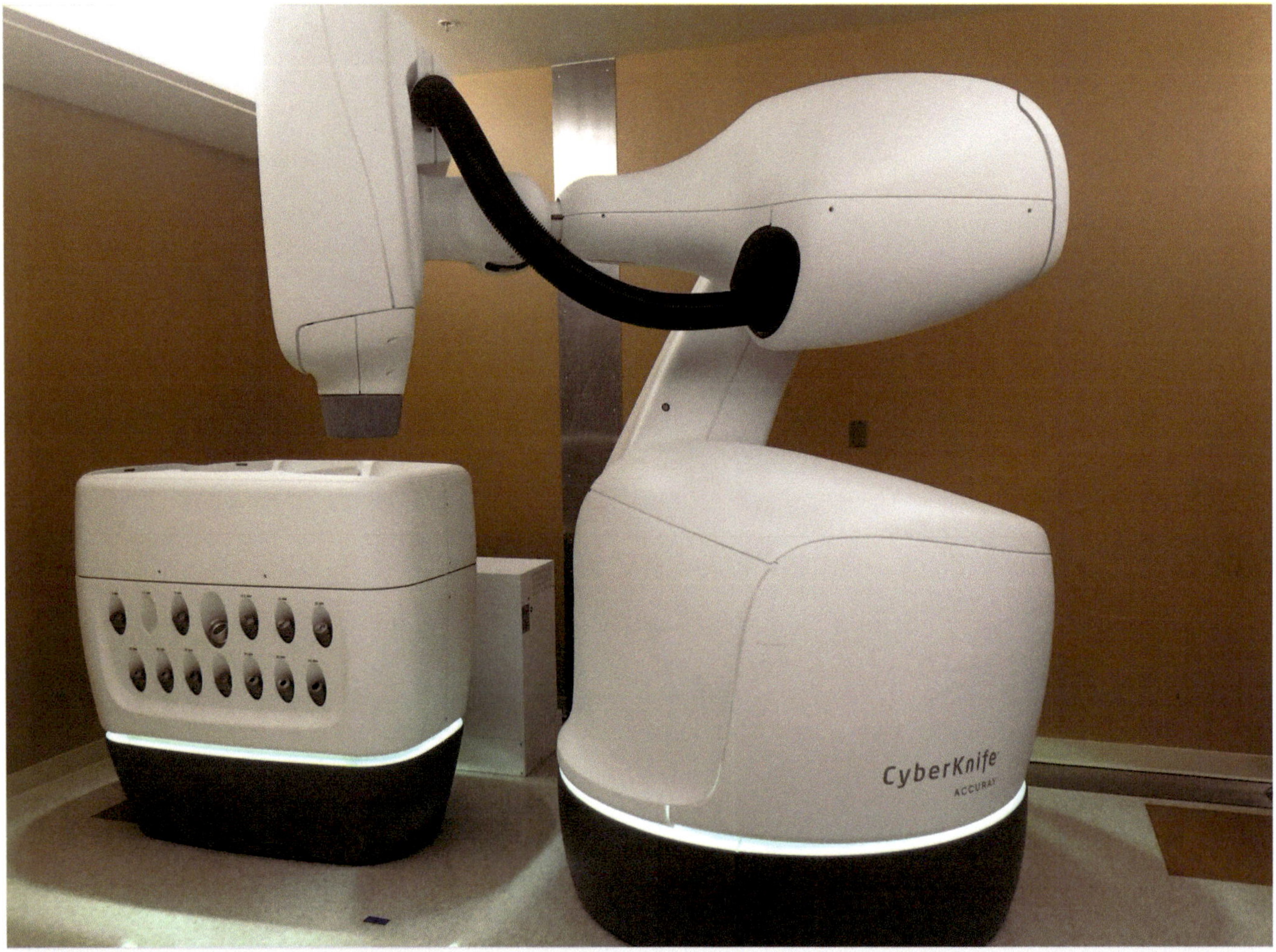

Fig. 19.1 CyberKnife treatment system. The Xchange Table for the collimators (*left*), the linear accelerator (*middle*), and manipulator (*right*).

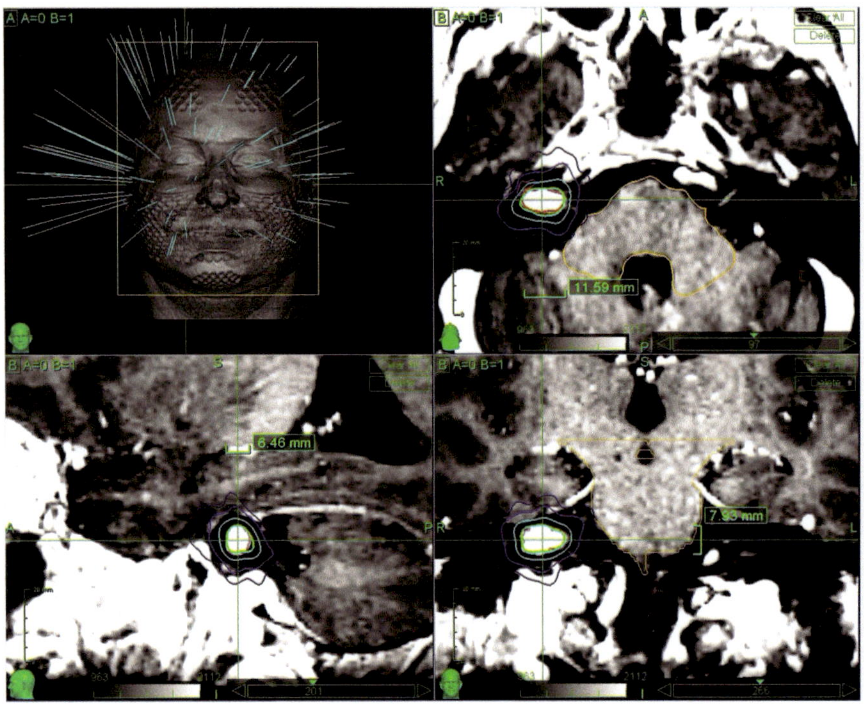

Fig. 19.2 Axial, sagittal, and coronal MRI slices demonstrating a small vestibular schwannoma that is primarily confined to the internal auditory canal.

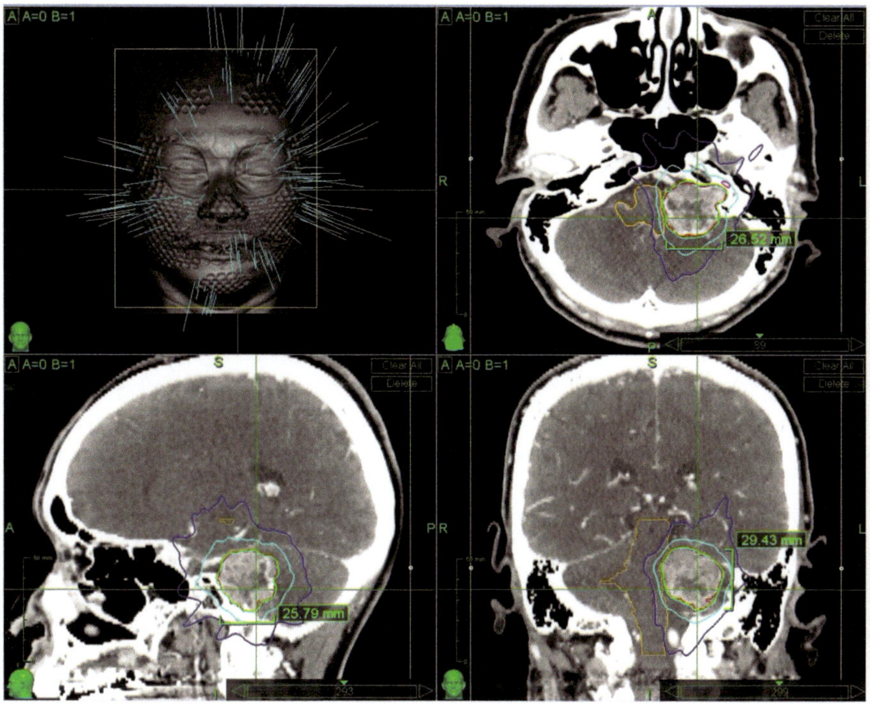

Fig. 19.3 Axial, sagittal, and coronal CT slices demonstrating a large vestibular schwannoma that extends from the IAC into the cerebellopontine angle, and compresses the brainstem.

large series published by Tsai et al at Tapei Medical University Wan-Fang Hospital evaluated 117 patients with VS who underwent CK radiotherapy between 2006 and 2012.[15] Tumors were similarly treated with a marginal dose of 18 Gy in three sessions. Tumor control rates of 99.1% were reported at a mean imaging follow-up of 61.1 months. Of the 65 patients with serviceable pretreatment hearing (GR I or II), 81.5% maintained GR grade I or II hearing after CK radiotherapy. Twelve patients experienced hearing degradation (91.6% were GR grade II pretreatment). Compared to the patients with preserved hearing, these patients appeared to have significantly larger tumor sizes and significantly smaller cochlear volumes.

Several more recent studies have demonstrated results in keeping with the two larger series discussed earlier. Vivas et al treated 73 patients with CK radiotherapy—63 patients were treated with primary CK radiotherapy and 10 were treated following microsurgery.[16] Of those treated with CK radiotherapy as the primary modality, 83% had 0 to 2 mm growth (tumor control or stable) and 17% grew more than 2 mm. Of the tumors that were stable, 29% shrank 2 mm or greater. Volumetric analysis found that 74% of tumors had less than 20% tumor volume growth, whereas 26% exhibited 20% or greater tumor volume growth. Of those deemed stable, 65% shrank 20% or greater in tumor volume, 95% did not need additional surgical intervention, 3 required salvage surgery, and 1 underwent additional radiotherapy. The majority of patients started with class D hearing (AAO-HNS hearing classification), but of those with class A or B hearing (serviceable hearing) before treatment, 53.5% maintained serviceable hearing at 3 years of follow-up. Hearing preservation was much higher (77%) in patients with pretreatment class A hearing. Similarly, Karam et al evaluated 37 patients treated with fractionated CK from 2002 to 2011.[17] The dose ranged from 12 to 30 Gy in one to three fractions. No patients required additional treatment at a median follow-up of 4.25 years. The radiographical tumor control rate was 91% in 32 patients at a median follow-up of 3 years. Of the 14 patients with serviceable hearing and audiometric data available, the hearing preservation rate was 78% at a median follow-up of 18 months. There were two patients who developed both new trigeminal paresthesia and facial spasms, but there were no cases of facial paresis.

Several smaller series also corroborate the results of the earlier and larger studies. Lin et al examined 20 patients undergoing CK radiotherapy for VS.[18] The radiological tumor control rate was 95%, and facial nerve preservation was 95% at 2-year follow-up. The percentage of cases with abnormal vestibular evoked myogenic potential tests did not significantly differ before and after CK radiotherapy, which was interpreted as preservation of vestibular nerve function. Morimoto et al examined 25 patients with 26 VSs treated with CK radiotherapy. The 7-year progression-free rate was 95%.[19] Delayed adverse events (> 3 months) were observed in six patients: grade III hydrocephalus in one patient, grade II facial nerve injury in one patient, and grades I to II tinnitus in three patients. Twelve out of 25 patients maintained pure-tone averages ≤ 50 dB before CK radiotherapy, and 50% maintained a pure-tone average at this level at the final audiometric follow-up after treatment. Mahadevan et al evaluated 10 VSs treated with CK radiotherapy. At a median follow-up of 22 months, the radiological tumor control rate was 100%.[20] On assessment of pure-tone average and speech discrimination scores before and after treatment, no patient showed a decrease in their hearing after a median follow-up of 19 months. Two patients reported improved hearing, and had a decrease in tumor volume. Wagner et al assessed 22 patients with VS treated with microsurgery, and 16 treated with CK radiotherapy.[21] Tumor size was significantly larger in the microsurgery cohort (mean: 23.64 mm) compared to the CK radiotherapy cohort (mean: 10.13 mm). The rate of hearing

Table 19.3 Large vestibular schwannomas treated with stereotactic radiotherapy

Authors	Patients	Tumor size	Modality	Follow-up (mo)	Tumor control
Casentini et al (2015)[22]	33	> 8 cm^3	CyberKnife (multisession)	Median: 48	31/33
Van de Langenberg et al (2011)[44]	33	> 6 cm^3	Gamma Knife (single session)	Median: 30	29/33
Yang et al (2011)[45]	65	> 3 cm	Gamma Knife (single session)	Median: 36	59/65
Mandl et al (2010)	25	> 3 cm	LINAC (multisession)	Mean: 36	21/25
Hasegawa et al (2005)[6]	24	> 15 cm^3	Gamma Knife (single session)	Median: 93	13/24
Inoue et al (2005)[46]	18?	> 3 cm	Gamma Knife (single session)	72–156	14/15
Litvack et al (2003)[9]	9	> 3 cm	Gamma Knife (single session)	Mean: 31.7	9/9
Rowe et al (2003)[10]	35	> 3 cm	Gamma Knife (single session)	Mean: 35	30/35
Prasad et al (2000)[12]	19	> 6.5 cm^3	Gamma Knife (single session)	Mean: 50	18/19
Lederman et al (1997)[47]	16	> 3 cm	LINAC (multisession)	Median: 20.7	16/16

preservation was significantly greater with CK radiotherapy compared to microsurgery.[21]

One recent study evaluated outcomes in 33 VSs larger than 8 cm^3 (range: 8–24 cm^3, mean: 11 cm^3, median: 9.4 cm^3) treated with CK radiotherapy, delivered in two to five sessions (hypofractionated, 14–19.5 Gy).[22] After a median follow-up of 48 months, radiological tumor control was achieved in 94% of cases—58% displayed no size variation or reduction in tumor diameter, and 36% displayed arrested growth or shrinkage after transient enlargement. Two patients required surgical debulking and two needed ventriculoperitoneal shunts. Actual progression-free survival rates at 1 and 5 years were 97 and 83%, respectively. Hearing was retained in seven of the eight patients with baseline serviceable hearing. Adverse events were limited to one case each of vertigo, tongue paresthesia, and trigeminal neuralgia. The authors concluded that CK radiotherapy may be an option for large VSs. See ▸ Table 19.3 for a summary of GK SRS and LINAC-based treatment of large VSs.

19.3 Conclusion

Given that a variety of treatment options for VS have achieved similar tumor control outcomes, cranial nerve injury and hearing loss have emerged as important factors when selecting a particular treatment modality. Hypofractionated CK radiotherapy has demonstrated excellent rates of tumor control and minimal risks to hearing, trigeminal, and facial nerve function. Multi-institutional, prospective studies are needed to better evaluate CK radiotherapy treatment outcomes compared to other radiation platforms, and to determine optimal dosing.

References

[1] Wowra B, Muacevic A, Fürweger C, Schichor C, Tonn JC. Therapeutic profile of single-fraction radiosurgery of vestibular schwannoma: unrelated malignancy predicts tumor control. Neuro-oncol. 2012; 14(7):902–909

[2] Lunsford LD, Niranjan A, Flickinger JC, Maitz A, Kondziolka D. Radiosurgery of vestibular schwannomas: summary of experience in 829 cases. J Neurosurg. 2005; 102 Suppl:195–199

[3] Flickinger JC, Kondziolka D, Niranjan A, Maitz A, Voynov G, Lunsford LD. Acoustic neuroma radiosurgery with marginal tumor doses of 12 to 13 Gy. Int J Radiat Oncol Biol Phys. 2004; 60(1):225–230

[4] Flickinger JC, Kondziolka D, Pollock BE, Lunsford LD. Evolution in technique for vestibular schwannoma radiosurgery and effect on outcome. Int J Radiat Oncol Biol Phys. 1996; 36(2):275–280

[5] Hirato M, Inoue H, Zama A, Ohye C, Shibazaki T, Andou Y. Gamma Knife radiosurgery for acoustic schwannoma: effects of low radiation dose and functional prognosis. Stereotact Funct Neurosurg. 1996; 66 Suppl 1:134–141

[6] Hirato M, Inoue H, Nakamura M, et al. Gamma knife radiosurgery for acoustic schwannoma: early effects and preservation of hearing. Neurol Med Chir (Tokyo). 1995; 35(10):737–741

[7] Lunsford LD, Kondziolka D, Flickinger JC. Radiosurgery as an alternative to microsurgery of acoustic tumors. Clin Neurosurg. 1992; 38:619–634

[8] Niranjan A, Lunsford LD, Flickinger JC, Maitz A, Kondziolka D. Dose reduction improves hearing preservation rates after intracanalicular acoustic tumor radiosurgery. Neurosurgery. 1999; 45(4):753–762, discussion 762–765

[9] Adler JR, Jr, Chang SD, Murphy MJ, Doty J, Geis P, Hancock SL. The Cyberknife: a frameless robotic system for radiosurgery. Stereotact Funct Neurosurg. 1997; 69(1–4, Pt 2):124–128

[10] Chang SD, Gibbs IC, Sakamoto GT, Lee E, Oyelese A, Adler JR, Jr. Staged stereotactic irradiation for acoustic neuroma. Neurosurgery. 2005; 56(6): 1254–1261, discussion 1261–1263

[11] Sakamoto GT, Blevins N, Gibbs IC. CyberKnife radiotherapy for vestibular schwannoma. Otolaryngol Clin North Am. 2009; 42(4):665–675

[12] Ishihara H, Saito K, Nishizaki T, et al. CyberKnife radiosurgery for vestibular schwannoma. Minim Invasive Neurosurg. 2004; 47(5):290–293

[13] Ju DT, Lin JW, Lin MS, et al. Hypofractionated CyberKnife stereotactic radiosurgery for acoustic neuromas with and without association to neurofibromatosis Type 2. Acta Neurochir Suppl (Wien). 2008; 101:169–173

[14] Hansasuta A, Choi CY, Gibbs IC, et al. Multisession stereotactic radiosurgery for vestibular schwannomas: single-institution experience with 383 cases. Neurosurgery. 2011; 69(6):1200–1209

[15] Tsai JT, Lin JW, Lin CM, et al. Clinical evaluation of CyberKnife in the treatment of vestibular schwannomas. BioMed Res Int. 2013; 2013:297093

[16] Vivas EX, Wegner R, Conley G, et al. Treatment outcomes in patients treated with CyberKnife radiosurgery for vestibular schwannoma. Otol Neurotol. 2014; 35:162–170

[17] Karam SD, Tai A, Strohl A, et al. Frameless fractionated stereotactic radiosurgery for vestibular schwannomas: a single-institution experience. Front Oncol. 2013; 3:121

[18] Lin MC, Chen CM, Tseng HM, Xiao F, Young YH. A proposed method to comprehensively define outcomes in acoustic tumor patients undergoing CyberKnife management. Stereotact Funct Neurosurg. 2013; 91(3):177–185

[19] Morimoto M, Yoshioka Y, Kotsuma T, et al. Hypofractionated stereotactic radiation therapy in three to five fractions for vestibular schwannoma. Jpn J Clin Oncol. 2013; 43(8):805–812

[20] Mahadevan A, Floyd S, Wong E, Chen C, Kasper E. Clinical outcome after hypofractionated stereotactic radiotherapy (HSRT) for benign skull base tumors. Comput Aided Surg. 2011; 16(3):112–120

[21] Wagner JN, Glaser M, Wowra B, et al. Vestibular function and quality of life in vestibular schwannoma: does size matter? Front Neurol. 2011; 2:55

[22] Casentini L, Fornezza U, Perini Z, Perissinotto E, Colombo F. Multisession stereotactic radiosurgery for large vestibular schwannomas. J Neurosurg. 2015; 122(4):818–824

[23] Murphy ES, Suh JH. Radiotherapy for vestibular schwannomas: a critical review. Int J Radiat Oncol Biol Phys 2011; 79:985-997

[24] Fukuoka S, Takanashi M, Hojyo A, Konishi M, Tanaka C, Nakamura H. Gamma knife radiosurgery for vestibular schwannomas. Prog Neurol Surg 2009; 22:45-62

[25] Chopra R, Kondziolka D, Niranjan A, Lunsford LD, Flickinger JC. Long-term follow-up of acoustic schwannoma radiosurgery with marginal tumor doses of 12 to 13 Gy. Int J Radiat Oncol Biol Phys 2007; 68:845-851

[26] Friedman WA, Bradshaw P, Myers A, Bova FJ. Linear accelerator radiosurgery for vestibular schwannomas. J Neurosurg 2006; 105:657-661

[27] Hempel JM, Hempel E, Wowra B, Schichor C, Muacevic A, Riederer A. Functional outcome after gamma knife treatment in vestibular schwannoma. Eur Arch Otorhinolaryngol 2006; 263:714-718

[28] Hasegawa T, Fujitani S, Katsumata S, Kida Y, Yoshimoto M, Koike J. Stereotactic radiosurgery for vestibular schwannomas: analysis of 317 patients followed more than 5 years. Neurosurgery 2005; 57:257-265; discussion 257-265

[29] Wowra B, Muacevic A, Jess-Hempen A, Hempel JM, Muller-Schunk S, Tonn JC. Outpatient gamma knife surgery for vestibular schwannoma: definition of the therapeutic profile based on a 10-year experience. J Neurosurg 2005; 102 Suppl:114-118

[30] Chung WY, Liu KD, Shiau CY, et al. Gamma knife surgery for vestibular schwannoma: 10-year experience of 195 cases. J Neurosurg 2005; 102 Suppl:87-96

[31] Litvack ZN, Noren G, Chougule PB, Zheng Z. Preservation of functional hearing after gamma knife surgery for vestibular schwannoma. Neurosurg Focus 2003; 14:e3

[32] Rowe JG, Radatz MW, Walton L, Hampshire A, Seaman S, Kemeny AA. Gamma knife stereotactic radiosurgery for unilateral acoustic neuromas. J Neurol Neurosurg Psychiatry 2003; 74:1536-1542

[33] Unger F, Walch C, Schrottner O, Eustacchio S, Sutter B, Pendl G. Cranial nerve preservation after radiosurgery of vestibular schwannomas. Acta Neurochir Suppl 2002; 84:77-83

[34] Prasad D, Steiner M, Steiner L. Gamma surgery for vestibular schwannoma. J Neurosurg 2000; 92:745-759

[35] Kopp C, Fauser C, Muller A, et al. Stereotactic fractionated radiotherapy and LINAC radiosurgery in the treatment of vestibular schwannoma-report about both stereotactic methods from a single institution. Int J Radiat Oncol Biol Phys 2011; 80:1485-1491

[36] Combs SE, Welzel T, Schulz-Ertner D, Huber PE, Debus J. Differences in clinical results after LINAC-based single-dose radiosurgery versus fractionated stereotactic radiotherapy for patients with vestibular schwannomas. Int J Radiat Oncol Biol Phys 2010; 76:193-200

[37] Horan G, Whitfield GA, Burton KE, Burnet NG, Jefferies SJ. Fractionated conformal radiotherapy in vestibular schwannoma: early results from a single centre. Clin Oncol (R Coll Radiol) 2007; 19:517-522

[38] Koh ES, Millar BA, Menard C, et al. Fractionated stereotactic radiotherapy for acoustic neuroma: single-institution experience at The Princess Margaret Hospital. Cancer 2007; 109:1203-1210

[39] Maire JP, Huchet A, Milbeo Y, et al. Twenty years' experience in the treatment of acoustic neuromas with fractionated radiotherapy: a review of 45 cases. Int J Radiat Oncol Biol Phys 2006; 66:170-178

[40] Chan AW, Black P, Ojemann RG, et al. Stereotactic radiotherapy for vestibular schwannomas: favorable outcome with minimal toxicity. Neurosurgery 2005; 57:60-70; discussion 60-70

[41] Selch MT, Pedroso A, Lee SP, et al. Stereotactic radiotherapy for the treatment of acoustic neuromas. J Neurosurg 2004; 101 Suppl 3:362-372

[42] Sawamura Y, Shirato H, Sakamoto T, et al. Management of vestibular schwannoma by fractionated stereotactic radiotherapy and associated cerebrospinal fluid malabsorption. J Neurosurg 2003; 99:685-692

[43] Andrews DW, Suarez O, Goldman HW, et al. Stereotactic radiosurgery and fractionated stereotactic radiotherapy for the treatment of acoustic schwannomas: comparative observations of 125 patients treated at one institution. Int J Radiat Oncol Biol Phys 2001; 50:1265-1278

[44] van de Langenberg R, Hanssens PE, Verheul JB, et al. Management of large vestibular schwannoma. Part II. Primary Gamma Knife surgery: radiological and clinical aspects. J Neurosurg 2011; 115:885-893

[45] Yang HC, Kano H, Awan NR, et al. Gamma Knife radiosurgery for larger-volume vestibular schwannomas. Clinical article. J Neurosurg 2011; 114:801-807

[46] Inoue HK. Low-dose radiosurgery for large vestibular schwannomas: long-term results of functional preservation. J Neurosurg 2005; 102 Suppl:111-113

[47] Lederman G, Lowry J, Wertheim S, et al. Acoustic neuroma: potential benefits of fractionated stereotactic radiosurgery. Stereotact Funct Neurosurg 1997; 69:175-182

20 Proton Beam Radiotherapy for Treatment of Sporadic Vestibular Schwannoma

Nina Niu Sanford, Marc R. Bussiere, Jay S. Loeffler, and Helen A. Shih

20.1 Introduction

The management of vestibular schwannomas (VSs) centers on maximizing tumor control while minimizing toxicity to adjacent normal structures including cranial nerves V, VII, and VIII. Because VSs are benign tumors and the majority grow slowly if at all,[1] many patients initially choose surveillance with serial imaging. Factors that influence the decision to undergo active treatment versus observation include patient age, tumor size, presence and severity of symptoms, genetic conditions including neurofibromatosis 2, rate of tumor growth, and status of ipsilateral and contralateral hearing. The two main treatment options include radiotherapy (RT) or surgical resection. RT is often the modality of choice in patients with significant medical comorbidities or in those who decline surgery.

For patients undergoing RT, treatment schedules range from conventionally fractionated RT, which involves the delivery of small doses (1.8–2 Gy) daily over 5 to 6 weeks, to stereotactic radiosurgery (SRS) in which a high dose of RT is given in a single treatment. Hypofractionated stereotactic radiotherapy (HSRT) represents a hybrid between these two treatment extremes in which a moderately high dose per fraction of RT, generally 5 to 7 Gy, is given over three to five fractions. Each of these treatment schedules can be delivered via photon or proton beams. Studies of SRS using photons demonstrate excellent tumor control with 0 to 5% tumor progression rates,[2,3] however, with high rates of V and VII nerve injury of upward of 30% in initial reports.[4,5] Strategies including reduction of the prescription dose[6,7] and the introduction of stereotactic hypofractionated or conventionally fractionated radiotherapy (SRT)[8,9,10] have decreased the rates of cranial neuropathy. Another approach to potentially reduce toxicities while maintaining high tumor control rates is through the use of proton RT.

20.2 Dosimetric Benefit of Protons

Charged particles such as protons have intrinsic physical properties that result in superior dosimetric distribution compared to photons. Specifically, proton beams are able to deposit nearly all their radiation dose in the target with maximal sparing of adjacent normal tissue. This is due to the Bragg peak effect of the proton beam in which there is a low entrance dose followed by a uniform maximum dose in a modulated narrow zone (Bragg peak) and then a sharp decrease to zero dose immediately distal to the peak (▶ Fig. 20.1). With this low entrance dose and nonexistent exit dose, nontargeted tissues both upstream and downstream to the tumor are preferentially spared.

Several dosimetric studies have demonstrated an advantage of protons over photons for intracranial tumors.[11,12,13,14] For example, one study compared five treatment planning techniques (3D conformal RT with photons, stereotactic arc therapy with photons, intensity modulated RT with photons, spot scanning with protons, and passive scattering with protons) for 12 intracranial tumors of various histologies.[13] The analysis showed that while all techniques resulted in acceptable target coverage, proton techniques were always superior to photon approaches in terms of normal tissue sparing. There was an increasing comparative advantage for larger tumor volumes. For VS, this benefit would be expected to translate clinically into a decreased risk of cranial neuropathy. Another theoretical benefit from reduced normal tissue exposure is a decreased risk of secondary tumors with proton RT, which has also been shown in dosimetric modeling studies.[14] Lastly, because tumor coverage in proton plans is accomplished via superimposition of the Bragg peaks from multiple proton beams, the dose distribution in the tumor is more homogeneous with protons than with photons. A comparison of proton versus photon planning for a typical VS case demonstrates the difference in dosimetric distribution (▶ Fig. 20.2).

20.3 Proton Stereotactic Radiosurgery

The primary nonoperative treatment for VS is SRS, which involves the delivery of a high single dose of RT to the tumor. Results with use of proton RT were first reported in 2002 in a prospective series of 68 patients from Massachusetts General Hospital[15] and then updated in 2003 with a total of 88 patients.[16] This endeavor was motivated by photon SRS studies that resulted in cranial nerve V and VII injury rates of greater than 30% despite highly conformal treatment planning and delivery techniques.[4,5,17] The marginal doses used in those early series were 16 to 20 Gy in a single session. To determine a proton RT dosing strategy that minimized the risk of cranial neuropathy and brainstem injury, the single fraction equivalent of the standard brainstem tolerance limit of 54 Gy at 1.8 Gy daily

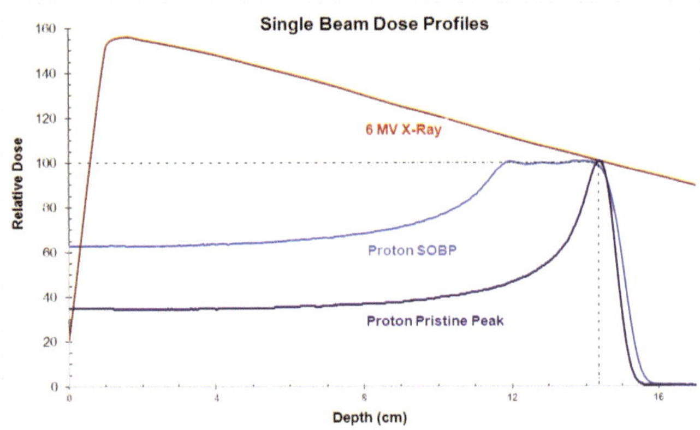

Fig. 20.1 Depth dose profiles of proton and photon beams. Graph showing depth dose profile of a 6-MV photon beam (*red*), a single proton pristine Bragg peak (*dark blue*), and a proton spread out Bragg peak (light blue) which is the sum of multiple Bragg peaks of modulated depths.

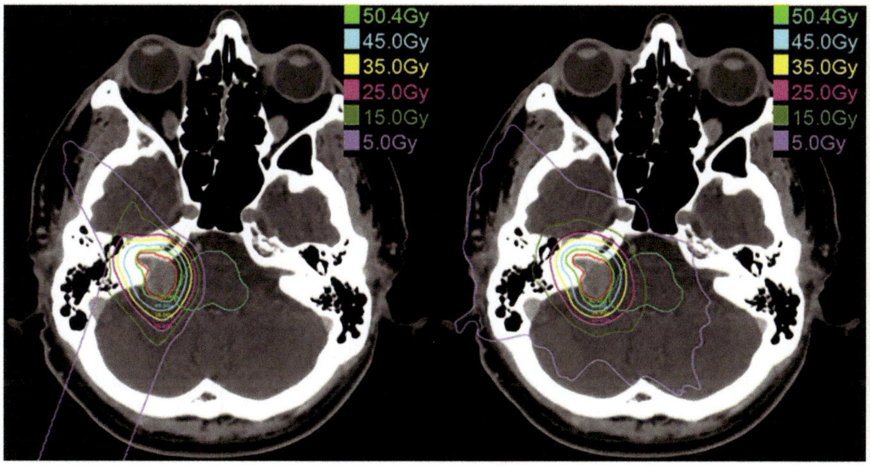

Fig. 20.2 Comparison of a proton versus a photon plan. **(a)** A proton radiotherapy plan for a patient with a vestibular schwannoma treated to 50.4 Gy (RBE: 1.1) with passively scattered protons. The tumor is outlined in *red*, the brainstem in *green*, and representative isodose lines are shown. **(b)** The same case is replanned with four photon dynamic conformal arcs. Target coverage is similar in both plans; however, the integral dose to the surrounding normal tissues is less with the proton plan.

fractions was determined using an alpha/beta ratio of 2 for the brainstem. This calculation resulted in a single fraction dose of 12 Gy (relative biological effectiveness [RBE]: 1.1), which was chosen as the dose to the tumor margin. A total of 88 patients were treated between 1992 and 2000 and were followed with neurologic evaluation and serial brain imaging (magnetic resonance imaging [MRI], or contrast-enhanced computed tomographic [CT] scans when MRI was contraindicated) at 6 months and 1 year after SRS, then annually over the next 2 years, and then once every 2 years thereafter. The median follow-up was 38.7 months. Tumor control was excellent with actuarial 2- and 5-year tumor control rates of 95.3 and 93.6%, respectively. Five-year cranial nerve V and VII function preservation rates were high at 89.4 and 91.1%, respectively. The authors did find an association between increasing prescribed dose, maximal dose, and inhomogeneity coefficient with long-term cranial nerve VII neuropathy on univariate analysis. In this cohort, 21 patients (24%) had functional hearing at baseline (Gardner–Robertson grades I and II) and only 7 (33.3%) retained serviceable hearing at last follow-up. The authors therefore proposed administering conventionally fractionated RT in patients with baseline serviceable hearing.

20.4 Fractionated Proton Radiotherapy

By providing time for normal tissue repair between treatments, conventionally fractionated RT can allow for relative organ-at-risk tissue sparing as compared to a single large dose of RT (SRS). Conventionally, fractionated proton RT was therefore explored as a strategy to reduce cranial nerve deficits, namely hearing loss, while maintaining similar excellent tumor control rates as seen with surgical resection and SRS.

The first report of conventionally fractionated proton RT was published in 2002 and assessed outcomes in 29 patients, 13 of who had useful hearing at baseline, defined as Gardner–Robertson grade I or II hearing.[18] Total dose was prescribed based on hearing status: patients with useful hearing were treated to 54 Gy (RBE: 1.1) in 30 fractions, while those without useful hearing received 60 Gy (RBE: 1.1) in 30 to 33 fractions. At a mean follow-up of 34 months, tumor control was 100% and there were no incidences of cranial nerve V or VII toxicity; however, only 4 of 13 of patients maintained useful hearing. The authors compared these outcomes to those of conventionally fractionated photon RT series, which showed higher rates of hearing preservation with lower cumulative photon doses. They concluded that these data supported a dose–response relationship for hearing preservation.

Hypofractionated RT was explored as a strategy to take advantage of both the convenience of single-session treatment and the radiobiological benefit of multisession treatment. In 2009, the group in South Africa reported their experiences with three-fraction or session proton RT for 51 patients over a 13-year period.[19] The mean dose to the tumors, prescribed to the isocenter, was 26 Gy (RBE: 1.1) in three fractions normalized to a mean of the 85% isodose line. The tumor control rate was excellent at 98% at 5 years; however, it dropped to 87% at 10 years. Forty-three percent of patients had useful hearing (Gardner–Robertson grade I or II) at baseline and of this subgroup, 2-year hearing preservation was 74%. Over time, this decreased to 42% at 5 years and remained at 42% at 10 years. The authors, however, warned the readers to view these percentages with caution since due to logistical problems, only a few patients completed the full pre- and posttreatment audiogram protocol, such that posttreatment hearing status was not graded on the Gardner–Robertson scale. The results of the three prospective proton RT series are summarized in ▶ Table 20.1.

20.5 Decision between Multisession Fractionated versus Single-Session SRS

There are no randomized controlled trials comparing proton SRS versus proton fractionated RT for VS; however, based on the available single-arm prospective data, our general recommendations are as follows:

- Conventionally fractionated proton RT (50.4–54 Gy [RBE: 1.1] in 28–30 fractions)—for patients with useful hearing, tumors greater than 2 cm, or tumors significantly abutting the brainstem.
- Proton single-session SRS (12–13 Gy [RBE: 1.1])—for patients with small tumor (≤ 2 cm diameter) and less than 50% invagination into the brainstem.

Table 20.1 Results of studies assessing proton radiotherapy for vestibular schwannoma

Author (year)	Dose (Gy, RBE 1.1)	Fractions	No. of patients	Tumor volume (cc)	Median follow-up (mo)	Tumor control (%) (y)	Cranial nerve preservation rates		
							VIII—hearing (%)[c] (y)	VII—facial (%) (y)	V—trigeminal (%) (y)
Weber et al[16] (2003)	12	1	88	1.4 (median)	38.7	95.3 (2 y) 93.6 (5 y)	79.1 (2 y) 21.9 (5 y)	91.1 (5 y)	89.4 (5 y)
Bush et al[18] (2002)	54[a] 60[b]	30[a] 30–33[b]	13[a] 17[b]	4.3 (mean)	34	100	30.8 (not reported)	100 (not reported)	100 (not reported)
Vernimmen et al[19] (2009)	26	3	51	5.9 (mean)	71	98.0 (2 y) 98.0 (5 y) 87.0 (10 y)	74.0 (2 y) 42.0 (5 y) 42.0 (10 y)	93.5 (2 y) 90.5 (5 y) 90.5 (10 y)	96.0 (2 y) 93.0 (5 y) 93.0 (10 y)

Abbreviation: RBE, relative biological effectiveness.
[a]Baseline useful hearing.
[b]Baseline nonuseful hearing.
[c]In patients with baseline useful hearing.

- Consider hypofractionated proton RT for all, with reported low morbidity and high tumor control rates with dosing regimens of three fractions of 7 Gy (RBE: 1.1) each and four or five fractions of 5 Gy (RBE: 1.1) each.

20.5.1 Treatment Method for Proton Radiotherapy

Patients first undergo a radiation planning session during which an immobilization device such as a stereotactic head frame with custom dental block is created. A planning CT scan of the brain with or without intravenous contrast is then performed. Noncontrast CT simulation scans will require subsequent fusion with a recent contrast-enhanced brain MRI. The VS and organs at risk are delineated on the planning scan. A treatment plan is created for the VS target expanded by beam path-specific planning margins, which differ in depth and lateral dimensions to account for various uncertainties. The overall effect is to approximately cover the target plus 0.5 to 1.0 mm with the prescription dose. Proton treatment plans will commonly consist of three to four proton beams from different directions. Beam angles and beam weighting are selected to maximize dose to the tumor and minimize exposure of the surrounding normal tissues. For single-session SRS, the brainstem should be constrained to a maximum dose of 12 Gy (RBE: 1.1). For any form of RT, dose to the brainstem and cochlea should be minimized. Custom apertures are used to create the desired beam shape. Daily image guidance should be employed such as by orthogonal kilovolt X-rays or cone beam CT.

20.5.2 Remaining Challenges and Future Directions

Despite the perceived benefits of proton RT, several challenges remain in ensuring accurate dose delivery and evaluating clinical outcome. First, the exact RBE of protons remains unknown. The RBE of any type of radiation is defined as the biological effect of that beam compared to a reference beam of photon radiation. The precise RBE of protons is uncertain and may vary with dose per fraction and with depth in the Bragg peak zone.[20] The reported values have mostly been in the range of 0.9 to 1.9.[21] Currently, the most widely accepted RBE correction factor is 1.1, based on experimental data from cell culture and animal systems[22,23,24]; however, further evaluation of the RBE of protons is needed.

Similarly, the optimal RT dose for VS remains to be defined. Over the past two decades, the dose for single-session SRS has been lowered from 22 to 12 Gy and for conventionally fractionated multisession RT from 60 to 46.8 Gy without a compromise in tumor control.[25] It remains to be seen if these lower doses achieve durable long-term tumor control and if further dose de-escalation is feasible and may result in decreased long-term toxicity.

Finally, although dosimetric data suggest a theoretical advantage to protons, there is no direct comparative data on proton versus photon RT to confirm a clinical benefit. Due to patient and physician biases, such a randomized controlled trial has not been successfully executed to date. We are therefore left to compare outcomes of single-arm prospective series, which is difficult due to variable treatment protocols at different facilities, and inconsistent patient follow-up, reassessment tools, and reporting. Yet because protons remain a scarce and costly resource, in the absence of randomized controlled trials, such prospective studies are needed to justify the cost and inconvenience of proton RT. Currently, there is an open trial at Massachusetts General Hospital titled "Hearing outcomes using fractionated proton RT for vestibular schwannomas" (ClinicalTrials.gov Identifier: NCT01199978). The impetus for this study is that the rate of useful hearing retention is significantly lower than the proportion of patients who retain facial or trigeminal nerve function, likely due to the proximity of the cochlea and cranial nerve VIII to the VS treatment volume. For this study, only patients with subjective useful hearing at baseline are eligible and are treated to a dose of 50.4 Gy (RBE: 1.1) in 28 fractions. The primary objective is to assess hearing preservation rates and a secondary objective is to delineate dosimetric parameters associated with hearing outcomes. Another secondary outcome is to model the secondary tumor risks after conventionally fractionated proton RT, although given the small probability of this late effect, there will likely be insufficient events to draw quantitative conclusions.

20.6 Conclusion

Proton RT for VS achieves excellent long-term tumor control and is a reasonable treatment option for patients with large or inoperable tumors. Approximately one-third of patients retain useful hearing and there is a suggestion that rates of cranial nerve injuries are reduced with conventionally fractionated multisession RT as compared to single-session SRS.

References

[1] Bakkouri WE, Kania RE, Guichard JP, Lot G, Herman P, Huy PT. Conservative management of 386 cases of unilateral vestibular schwannoma: tumor growth and consequences for treatment. J Neurosurg. 2009; 110(4):662–669

[2] Kondziolka D, Lunsford LD, McLaughlin MR, Flickinger JC. Long-term outcomes after radiosurgery for acoustic neuromas. N Engl J Med. 1998; 339 (20):1426–1433

[3] Combs SE, Welzel T, Schulz-Ertner D, Huber PE, Debus J. Differences in clinical results after LINAC-based single-dose radiosurgery versus fractionated stereotactic radiotherapy for patients with vestibular schwannomas. Int J Radiat Oncol Biol Phys. 2010; 76(1):193–200

[4] Flickinger JC, Lunsford LD, Coffey RJ, et al. Radiosurgery of acoustic neurinomas. Cancer. 1991; 67(2):345–353

[5] Mendenhall WM, Friedman WA, Buatti JM, Bova FJ. Preliminary results of linear accelerator radiosurgery for acoustic schwannomas. J Neurosurg. 1996; 85(6):1013–1019

[6] Miller RC, Foote RL, Coffey RJ, et al. Decrease in cranial nerve complications after radiosurgery for acoustic neuromas: a prospective study of dose and volume. Int J Radiat Oncol Biol Phys. 1999; 43(2):305–311

[7] Petit JH, Hudes RS, Chen TT, Eisenberg HM, Simard JM, Chin LS. Reduced-dose radiosurgery for vestibular schwannomas. Neurosurgery. 2001; 49(6):1299–1306, discussion 1306–1307

[8] Andrews DW, Suarez O, Goldman HW, et al. Stereotactic radiosurgery and fractionated stereotactic radiotherapy for the treatment of acoustic schwannomas: comparative observations of 125 patients treated at one institution. Int J Radiat Oncol Biol Phys. 2001; 50(5):1265–1278

[9] Fuss M, Debus J, Lohr F, et al. Conventionally fractionated stereotactic radiotherapy (FSRT) for acoustic neuromas. Int J Radiat Oncol Biol Phys. 2000; 48(5):1381–1387

[10] Varlotto JM, Shrieve DC, Alexander E, III, Kooy HM, Black PM, Loeffler JS. Fractionated stereotactic radiotherapy for the treatment of acoustic neuromas: preliminary results. Int J Radiat Oncol Biol Phys. 1996; 36(1):141–145

[11] Verhey LJ, Smith V, Serago CF. Comparison of radiosurgery treatment modalities based on physical dose distributions. Int J Radiat Oncol Biol Phys. 1998; 40(2):497–505

[12] Phillips MH, Frankel KA, Lyman JT, Fabrikant JI, Levy RP. Comparison of different radiation types and irradiation geometries in stereotactic radiosurgery. Int J Radiat Oncol Biol Phys. 1990; 18(1):211–220

[13] Bolsi A, Fogliata A, Cozzi L. Radiotherapy of small intracranial tumours with different advanced techniques using photon and proton beams: a treatment planning study. Radiother Oncol. 2003; 68(1):1–14

[14] Arvold ND, Niemierko A, Broussard GP, et al. Projected second tumor risk and dose to neurocognitive structures after proton versus photon radiotherapy for benign meningioma. Int J Radiat Oncol Biol Phys. 2012; 83(4):e495–e500

[15] Harsh GR, Thornton AF, Chapman PH, Bussiere MR, Rabinov JD, Loeffler JS. Proton beam stereotactic radiosurgery of vestibular schwannomas. Int J Radiat Oncol Biol Phys. 2002; 54(1):35–44

[16] Weber DC, Chan AW, Bussiere MR, et al. Proton beam radiosurgery for vestibular schwannoma: tumor control and cranial nerve toxicity. Neurosurgery. 2003; 53(3):577–586, discussion 586–588

[17] Linskey ME, Lunsford LD, Flickinger JC. Radiosurgery for acoustic neurinomas: early experience. Neurosurgery. 1990; 26(5):736–744, discussion 744–745

[18] Bush DA, McAllister CJ, Loredo LN, Johnson WD, Slater JM, Slater JD. Fractionated proton beam radiotherapy for acoustic neuroma. Neurosurgery. 2002; 50(2):270–273, discussion 273–275

[19] Vernimmen FJ, Mohamed Z, Slabbert JP, Wilson J. Long-term results of stereotactic proton beam radiotherapy for acoustic neuromas. Radiother Oncol. 2009; 90(2):208–212

[20] Tang JT, Inoue T, Inoue T, et al. Comparison of radiobiological effective depths in 65-MeV modulated proton beams. Br J Cancer. 1997; 76(2):220–225

[21] Raju MR. Proton radiobiology, radiosurgery and radiotherapy. Int J Radiat Biol. 1995; 67(3):237–259

[22] Paganetti H, Niemierko A, Ancukiewicz M, et al. Relative biological effectiveness (RBE) values for proton beam therapy. Int J Radiat Oncol Biol Phys. 2002; 53(2):407–421

[23] Paganetti H. Relative biological effectiveness (RBE) values for proton beam therapy. Variations as a function of biological endpoint, dose, and linear energy transfer. Phys Med Biol. 2014; 59(22):R419–R472

[24] Wouters BG, Skarsgard LD, Gerweck LE, et al. Radiobiological intercomparison of the 160 MeV and 230 MeV proton therapy beams at the Harvard Cyclotron Laboratory and at Massachusetts General Hospital. Radiat Res. 2015; 183(2): 174–187

[25] Andrews DW, Werner-Wasik M, Den RB, et al. Toward dose optimization for fractionated stereotactic radiotherapy for acoustic neuromas: comparison of two dose cohorts. Int J Radiat Oncol Biol Phys. 2009; 74(2):419–426

21 Secondary Radiation Treatment of Vestibular Schwannoma After Prior Microsurgery or Radiosurgery

Lucas P. Carlstrom, Avital Perry, Christopher S. Graffeo, Øystein V. Tveiten, Bruce E. Pollock, and Michael J. Link

21.1 Introduction

Primary treatment strategies for vestibular schwannoma (VS) have evolved remarkably since the advent of stereotactic radiosurgery (SRS), which has become a staple of the skull base armamentarium, alongside microsurgery (MS) and close observation. Although it is frequently a first-line treatment for growing small-to-medium-sized VS, one of the most important and well-studied indications for radiotherapy (RT) in general and SRS in particular in the VS paradigm is tumor recurrence or progression. Primary treatment strategies are reviewed in detail in preceding chapters; however, a brief overview of treatment failure, extent of resection, and recurrence/progression provides an important conceptual foundation for our discussion of the indications for secondary SRS in the VS treatment paradigm.

With respect to primary SRS, the goal of therapy is arrest of tumor growth. Therefore, we define treatment failure as serial growth on two or more follow-up magnetic resonance imaging (MRI) studies, which allows for the expected early tumor expansion and pseudoprogression that is frequently witnessed during the first 6 to 18 months after treatment, a phenomenon discussed further in Chapter 25.[1,2,3,4,5,6,7] Our institutional experience parallels most major preceding series: for single-session SRS at a margin dose of 12 to 14 Gy, long-term tumor control is 92 to 95%, with an all-comers risk of facial weakness approaching 1%, and preservation of useful hearing (i.e., AAO-HNS [American Academy of Otolaryngology—Head and Neck Surgery] class A or B) ranging from 60 to 80% at 3 years, with a decline to less than 50% at 5 years and ultimately below 25% at 10 years.[7,8,9,10]

Although the debate regarding SRS versus MS as primary treatment for slow-growing, small-to-medium-sized tumors has been hotly contested, best available evidence (level 2–3) has demonstrated nearly equivalent tumor control and improved cranial nerve outcomes after SRS at 5 years.[2,11,12,13] Correspondingly, in our practice, patients harboring tumors < 3 cm without brainstem compression and with growth rates < 2.5 mm/year are typically presented with the above data regarding the risks, benefits, and outcomes of both SRS and MS, to facilitate shared decision making and an individualized primary treatment plan. Those patients who elect primary SRS and subsequently experience a treatment failure are typically offered salvage MS, although repeat SRS or secondary RT may be considered under special circumstances, discussed in detail below.[14,15,16]

By contrast, for patients undergoing primary MS, achievement of gross total resection (GTR) is the single most important parameter for predicting the likelihood of secondary treatment, which can be defined using either surgeon's impression or absence of nodular enhancement on postoperative MRI.[17,18,19,20,21,22,23] Some attention has been directed toward separating near-total resection (NTR; defined using variable parameters to signify a minimal residual tumor volume, typically adherent to the facial nerve) from subtotal resection (STR; with definitions ranging from any postoperative residuum, to any remnant > 5% initial tumor volume, among others); however, these terms have been used inconsistently, and rarely demonstrated a statistically significant or clinically meaningful difference in long-term outcomes, particularly compared independently to GTR.[20] Consequently, the most conceptually useful parameters guiding indications for secondary treatment after primary MS are *recurrence*, defined as new nodular enhancement after clinically and/or radiographically confirmed GTR, and *progression*, defined as a ≥ 2-mm increase in size of any documented postoperative tumor residuum. Using these parameters, large preceding analyses, including our own series, have demonstrated that recurrence is rare after GTR, occurring in 0.05 to 9.2%, whereas progression after STR has been reported in up to 44%.[14,16,19,24,25,26,27,28,29]

In spite of the clear tumor control advantage associated with GTR, aggressive resection also increases the probability of unfavorable cranial nerve outcomes. Correspondingly, a variety of strategies have been advocated in an attempt to find equipoise between these competing goals, including NTR followed by observation, STR followed by either close observation or upfront SRS, and planned debulking followed by upfront SRS.[4,14,30,31,32] Although several studies have compared these treatment approaches, results have been equivocal overall, and in our own experience, among patients selected for primary MS, excellent tumor control and facial nerve outcomes have been consistently achieved by pursuing GTR, as the paramount goal of surgery, and accepting aggressive STR in markedly adherent tumors.[14,16,32]

In summary, secondary SRS is most frequently employed in the treatment of tumor progression after primary MS resulting in STR, or less frequently tumor recurrence after GTR, as well as uncommon circumstances where repeating a course of radiation is preferable to secondary MS. Although pertinent data are scattered, retrospective, and based on small patient numbers, each of these cohorts has been studied, and our chief aim herein is to describe and synthesize the key findings and their clinically significant implications.

21.2 Secondary SRS after MS

Disease recurrence/progression after primary MS is by far the most common indication for secondary SRS, as well as the best studied (▶ Table 21.1). Although increasingly large proportions of the VS population are either observed or treated with primary SRS, MS remains the most common primary treatment modality overall, particularly in younger patients, individuals desiring to avoid radiation, large tumors, or tumors producing symptomatic mass effect, via either brainstem compression/edema or hydrocephalus.[2,11,33,34,35,36] Consequently, the more widespread acceptance of SRS as a secondary modality has both historical roots (e.g., during the technology's developmental phase, patients requiring salvage therapy were considered a lower-risk/higher-reward cohort) and clinical motivations (e.g., patients requiring urgent surgery for indications described

Table 21.1 Selected studies examining outcomes of secondary radiosurgery after primary microsurgery

Authors	Year	Patients (*n*)	More than one prior operation (%)	Median time from surgery (MON)	Range time from surgery	Median tumor volume (cm^3; range)	Median tumor margin (Gy)	Median follow-up (mo)	Tumor control rate (%)	Weaker facial nerve function (%)	Serviceable hearing post-SRS (%)	Trigeminal deficits (%)
Pollock et al	1998	76 (78 tumors)	37	57 (GTR), 37 (STR)	13–312 MON	2.8 (0.2–15.7)	15 (12–20)	43 (12–101)	94	21 (23)[a]	96	12 (14)[a]
Prasad et al	2000	57				2.6 mean (0.12–12.5)	13.6 mean (10–20)	51 (12–120)	90			
Unger et al	2002	50	30	39	6–324 MON	3.4 (0.2–23.09)	13	75 (42–114)	96	0 (8)[a]	100	0 (10)[a]
Iwai et al	2003	14		3 mean	1–6 MON	18.9 mean (9.8–36.1)	12 (10–14)	32 (17–72)	93	0		0
Roche et al	2004	60	22	71.5	2–128 MON	1.6 mean (0.5–5)	13 (10–20)	56.6 (14–121)	93	0	29	0
Park et al	2006	8			0–6 MON	4.6 mean	12	69	100	0		
Pollock et al	2008	55	9	60	2–463 MON	3.0 (0.1–18.1)	14 (12–20)	47 (5–148)	94	10	23	4
Fuentes et al	2008	8		9 mean	6–12 MON	1.16 (0.31–2.2)	12 (11–13)	46 (12–73)	100	0		
Yang et al	2008	61		6	0–96 MON	3.65 mean (0.52–15.5)	13 (9–14)	54 (24.1–102.2)	98.4	5	30	
Haque et al	2011	20		47	6–92 MON	3.6 (2.5–6)	12	24 (12–53)	100	5 (15)[a]		
Pai et al	2011	7	29	66	10–84 MON			92 (41–125)	85.7			1
van de Langenberg et al	2011	50	0	8.5	2–24 MON	3.34 (0.22–11.8)	11 (9.4–11.9)	34 (12–84)	92	2 (6)[a]	98	2
Pan et al	2012	35	0	3.6 (STR), 7 (NTR)		9.35 (STR), 1.1 (NTR)	12	58 (STR), 53 (NTR)	100	0	100	0
Anaizi et al	2014	10						33	100			
Jeltema et al	2015	7	0				13			0		0
Iwai et al	2015	40	2	3	1–12 MON	3.3 (0.4–10.4)	12 (10–12)	65 (18–156)	90	0 (5)[a]	55	0 (5)[a]
Huang et al	2017	168 (173 tumors)	26	42	2–329 MON	2.7 (0.2–21.6)	13 (11–20)	74 (6–285)	95	5.5	67	5.8
Monfared et al	2016	11		35	4–74 MON		12.5		75	1		
Bailo et al	2017	90	17	31	4–174 MON	2.5 (0.03–13)	13 (11.6–14)	69 (36–156)	90	3 (8)[a]	40	3 (6)[a]
Fu et al	2018	10[b]		35	13–58 MON	3.9 (0.4–9.7)	11 (10–12.4)	94 (54–129)	100	0 (10)[a]	0	10 (20)[a]

Abbreviations: GTR, gross total resection; NTR, near-total resection; SRS, stereotactic radiosurgery; STR, subtotal resection.
[a]Temporary worsening.
[b]Received MS + SRS, then SRS after regrowth. MON = months

above have previously tipped the primary treatment balance toward MS, as have surgeon preferences to avoid MS after SRS; discussed below).[2,12,13,37] Interestingly, this balance has reversed somewhat as the fraction of incidentally diagnosed or minimally symptomatic tumors has increased alongside improved access to MRI.[38,39,40]

As a secondary modality for treatment of recurrence/progression after primary MS, SRS has demonstrated compelling tumor control results, with an overall median growth arrest rate of 94% (range, 75–100%) at a median follow-up of 69 months after secondary treatment (range, 36–156; ▶ Table 21.1). Follow-up imaging after secondary SRS demonstrated frank reduction in tumor size in 36 to 80% of cases, typically observed within 12 months of treatment.[1,6,41,42] Time-to-secondary-treatment was a median 37 months after primary MS (range, 0–329 months), with an increase of treatment interval from 37 to 57 months for patients who recurred after NTR/STR, as compared to those who recurred after GTR, respectively.[14] Durable tumor control after secondary SRS was not significantly different between patients being treated for progression and those being treated for recurrence.[30,32,43,44,45]

Median tumor margin dose was 12 Gy at secondary SRS (range, 9–20 Gy), while median tumor volume was 3.3 cm^3 (range, 0.03–36.1 cm^3), attributable to the considerable fraction of tumors that were initially too large for primary SRS (e.g., > 2.5 or 3 cm maximum diameter) that underwent STR at primary MS and subsequently progressed. Overall, these results are favorable when compared to repeat MS, the details of which are reviewed in Chapter 43, rendering SRS as the preferred secondary modality after primary MS for most cases of recurrent/progressive VS.

21.3 Secondary SRS after Primary SRS

Although SRS is currently considered an appropriate primary treatment for many small-to-medium sized, slow-growing VS in most major centers, its embrace as such is a relatively recent phenomenon. Correspondingly, data on treatment failures after primary SRS are more limited, and only a small number of studies have specifically taken up the question of long-term outcomes after repeat SRS following initial SRS failure (▶ Table 21.2).[5,46,47,48,49,50,51,52,53]

The topic of MS after SRS has been contentiously debated, and is reviewed in detail in Chapter 44. Briefly, the vast majority of surgeons describe a more challenging operation attributable to radiation-induced scarring and dense, fibrotic adhesions at the facial nerve–tumor interface. Consequently, most preceding analyses have concluded that, although GTR or aggressive STR can still be achieved via MS after SRS, the risk of cranial nerve injury is most likely to be elevated—although a small number of studies have suggested that long-term facial nerve outcomes after MS with or without preceding SRS are not significantly different.[16,24,28,54] Correspondingly, for patients who underwent primary SRS and express a strong desire to prioritize preservation of facial nerve function at secondary treatment, even at the cost of tumor control, repeat SRS presents a reasonable alternative to secondary MS. In parallel, some patients who fail primary SRS are suboptimal surgical candidates, typically due to age, comorbidities, or patient preferences, and as such may also warrant consideration for secondary treatment via repeat SRS.

Table 21.2 Selected studies examining outcomes of secondary radiosurgery after primary radiosurgery failure

Authors	Year	Patients (*n*)	Median time from initial SRS (mo)	Time from surgery (range; mo)	Tumor volume median, cm^3 (range)	Median tumor margin (Gy)	Median follow-up (mo)	Tumor control rate (%)	Weaker facial nerve function (%)	Serviceable hearing post-SRS (%)	Trigeminal deficits (%)
Norén	1998	8						88			
Hasegawa et al	2005	4	30			13	94	75	0		0
Dewan and Norén	2008	11	51	24–136	1.8 (1.2–3.1)	12		91	0	9	18
Yomo et al	2009	8	46	35–99	1.9 (0.06–21.7)	13	64 (23–121)	100	0	33	0
Liscak et al	2009	24	43	12–125	2.9 (0.7–6.5)	13	91 (22–162)	92	4	13	9
Kano et al	2010	6	63	25–169	2.1 (0.9–6.4)	11.0	29	100	0	0	0
Lonneville et al	2015	25	45	24–110	2.3 (0.2–8.3)	12	46	85	0	20	0
Fu et al	2018	28	52	19–86	2.9 (0.27–9.4)	12	66 (13–129)	100	25 (39)[a]	0	7 (14)[a]
Fu et al	2018	10[b]	35	13–58	3.9 (0.4–9.7)	11.3 (10–12.4)	94 (54–129)	100	0 (10)[a]	0	10 (20)[a]

Abbreviation: SRS, stereotactic radiosurgery.
[a]Temporary worsening
[b]Received MS + SRS, then SRS after regrowth.

Clinical outcomes after secondary SRS for treatment failure are relatively reassuring, with tumor control observed in a median 95% of cases (range, 75–100%) at a median follow-up of 66 months (range, 13–162 months; ▶ Table 21.2).[5,47,48,49,50,51,52,53] Median time-to-secondary-SRS was 46 months (range, 12–169 months), and the median secondary treatment volume was 2.3 cm^3 (range, 0.2–9.7 cm^3).

Although tumor control can be consistently achieved via repeat SRS, the potential for adverse radiation effects increases-particularly as the total radiation to surrounding tissue increases, the details of which are reviewed below. Nevertheless, the potential benefits of repeat SRS for appropriately selected patients are compelling, and may warrant consideration for a wider selection of patients in the future, particularly as strategies for dose reduction and technologies for higher fidelity conformal planning continue to improve.

21.4 Adverse Radiation Events after Secondary SRS following Primary MS or SRS

As compared to primary SRS, the risk of adverse radiation effects associated with secondary SRS is marginally worse, assuming comparable dosimetry and treatment planning parameters. With respect to hearing loss, this difference is less clinically apparent. Sustained AAO-HNS class A or B hearing at time of progression/recurrence is rare; however, where present, a routine 12- to 13-Gy dose to the tumor margin would most likely accelerate hearing loss at the upper end of the expected post-SRS 3 to 5 dB/year, with at least 50% of patients losing useful hearing by 5 years, and more than 75% by 10 years (▶ Table 21.1).[7,8,9,10] Similarly, transient trigeminal neuropathy and ataxia were each noted in up to 25% of patients after secondary SRS, with persistent symptoms remaining in approximately 5 to 10%.

Data on the risk of facial weakness after secondary SRS are more variable, but several studies have shown a significant increase relative to the expected 1% permanent decline and 6% transient decline/hemifacial spasm (HFS) at a tumor margin dose of 14 Gy.[4,14,30,31,32,43,53,55,56,57,58,59,60,61,62] In the first major series of secondary SRS after MS, Pollock et al reported new or worsened facial nerve function in 14% of patients with House–Brackmann grade I–III function post-MS pre-SRS treated with 12 to 14 Gy ($n = 3/21$). Most likely, this elevated risk reflects a multifactorial sensitization of the facial nerve attributable to intraoperative manipulation, postoperative healing and inflammation, and increased activity in the tumor immune microenvironment.[63]

Predictably, dose escalation at secondary SRS independently carries a marked increase in risk across all parameters, most prominently facial weakness, which was noted in as high as 22% of patients receiving 15 to 17 Gy and 57% of patients receiving 18 Gy or more.[32] Notwithstanding, updated analyses conducted using more conformal systems including the Gamma Knife Perfexion, as well as studies that have grouped patients by individual House–Brackmann grade, have suggested a more optimistic picture, citing overall rates of facial nerve weakness in the range of 0 to 10%.[32,55,64,65] Huang et al observed 4% ($n = 2/50$) and 11% ($n = 3/27$) declines in patients' grades I and II function pre-SRS, respectively, as well as an all-comers rate of 4% in 173 patients, 45 of whom had undergone greater than one prior resection.[45] Taken together, these findings suggest that, although a degree of facial nerve sensitization likely occurs, dose reduction strategies are likely effective at minimizing risk, while higher House–Brackmann grades post-MS pre-SRS sequentially predict higher probabilities of post-SRS facial nerve dysfunction.

As compared to secondary SRS after MS, repeat SRS is thought to carry an increased risk of postradiation deficits. Although this inference is based on limited data, it is clinically intuitive, given that higher margin doses are more frequently employed and that certain critical structures such as the cochlea or facial nerve itself typically receive additive radiation doses.[66,67] The index series by Norén et al reported eight patients undergoing secondary SRS after treatment failure: seven tumors stabilized, one progressed but was noted in post hoc analysis to have received an inadequate secondary dose, and none experienced permanent postsecondary SRS facial weakness.[32,46] By contrast, another preliminary case reported by Watanabe et al documented treating a failing patient with a combined marginal dose of 24 Gy, which resulted in complete facial paralysis while still failing to arrest tumor growth.[68]

More recent series have varied considerably regarding the cumulative risk of facial nerve dysfunction after repeat SRS, with temporary deficit or HFS reported in 0 to 39% of patients, and new permanent facial nerve weakness documented in 0 to 25% of patients (▶ Table 21.2).[5,46,47,48,49,50,51,52,53] Of note, of the nine preceding series, favorable outcomes were noted in seven, all of which documented < 4% permanent facial nerve weakness after a secondary tumor margin dose of 10 to 13 Gy at a median follow-up of 66 months (range, 13–162). Although further study is required to more definitively characterize the true risk of facial nerve weakness after repeat SRS, as well as the optimal timing and dosimetry parameters, these findings are reassuring that, in appropriately selected individuals, secondary SRS after primary SRS failure can be employed as a relatively safe alternative to salvage MS.

Whereas SRS after MS in patients with serviceable postoperative hearing carries a risk of long-term hearing loss that is comparable to primary SRS, repeat SRS all but guarantees hearing loss, with less than 9% of all patients who underwent repeat SRS reporting serviceable hearing at a median follow-up of 66 months (range, 13–162). Only one study specifically addressed the question of cochlear dose in predicting hearing outcomes after repeat SRS, with Kano et al concluding that hearing was most likely to be preserved when serial doses to the central cochlea were planned to < 4 Gy.[69]

Other miscellaneous adverse effects are less well studied in the setting of secondary SRS, including trigeminal neuropathy, ataxia, vestibulopathy /disequilibrium, lower cranial nerve dysfunction, and symptomatic hydrocephalus. Unsurprisingly, the risk for each is low overall, with less than 5% of patients reporting persistent, disabling symptoms at long-term follow-up; however, the incidence of adverse treatment effects clearly increases as radiation dose accumulates, and patients should be counseled accordingly regarding the potential for both temporary and permanent manifestations of these uncommon but potentially troublesome symptoms.[5,49,53]

Induction of a secondary neoplasm or malignant transformation of the tumor being treated is a widely discussed concern regarding SRS, yet all preceding data have convincingly demonstrated that the true risk is extremely low, as reviewed further in Chapter 24. In the setting of repeat SRS, this theoretical risk would presumably be magnified by the additional radiation delivered to the tumor, yet no such case has been reported. In our own experience with 382 VS treated with SRS from 1990 to 2009, only 1 instance of malignant transformation was observed, in a patient treated with primary SRS for presumed VS that was subsequently diagnosed as having transformed into a pleomorphic sarcoma after the treatment failure was treated with secondary MS.[70] A related analysis by Carlson et al of 9,460 eligible sporadic VS patients in the Surveillance, Epidemiology, and End Results (SEER) database with at least 5 years of follow-up after any treatment identified 66 cases of a second intracranial tumor (0.7%), of which 60 were benign and 6 were malignant, and no significant difference was appreciated between the incidences of the second tumor in patients who received primary radiation (0.5%) and primary surgery without any history of cranial radiation (0.4%).[71] This suggests that the short- and intermediate-term risk of VS patients developing a second tumor is not causally related to radiation exposure, but is in fact an incidental finding. This accords with a separate all-comers analysis of 80,000 SRS patients treated for benign disease with at least 15 years of follow-up that identified an overall combined risk of radiation-induced tumor formation or malignant transformation of 0.04%—an exponentially low incidence, particularly as compared to the accepted 1 to 2% risk associated with external beam RT (EBRT).[70,72,73]

In patients with tumors approaching or exceeding the conventional upper size limit for SRS treatment, the risk of precipitous edema at the brainstem, peduncle, or cerebellum is increased, as is the corresponding risk of hydrocephalus from fourth ventricular effacement—particularly if the tumor is growing rapidly.[2,74,75] Notwithstanding, symptomatic hydrocephalus requiring acute cerebrospinal fluid diversion is exceedingly rare after primary or secondary SRS, which is attributable to the fact that few, if any, surgeons would offer repeat SRS without debulking a patient with significant mass effect or at high risk for developing hydrocephalus.[43]

Several intuitive strategies have been advocated to allay the potential for adverse radiation effects, including both clinically oriented strategies, such as delaying treatment until both tumor growth and progressive symptoms manifest, and dose reduction techniques, such as fractionation. One more recent technical modification developed to mitigate radiation toxicity for repeat SRS reported by Fu et al is focal treatment of growing regions in isolation, which they reported in a small series of six patients, all of whom had durable tumor control with volume reduction and without new cranial nerve deficits after 42 months of follow-up—a significant improvement on comparable patients treated with whole-tumor repeat SRS at their institution previously.[53]

21.5 Consideration for Alternative RT Modalities in Secondary VS Treatment

A variety of fractionation techniques based on linear accelerator systems such as EBRT and intensity-modulated RT (IMRT) have demonstrated varying efficacy in primary VS treatment, with tumor control rates reported to be 47 to 100%, and adverse radiation effects comparable to SRS, including normal long-term facial nerve preservation rates of 81.5 to 98%.[76,77,78,79,80] Typical fractioned schemes include multiple treatments of 1.8 to 2 Gy to a total of 45 to 57.6 Gy.[2] Advocates of the technique argue that a lower cochlear dose results in superior hearing preservation; however, this has not been convincingly reproduced in studies with adequate long-term follow-up, which have suggested instead that EBRT may be associated with increased latency in hearing loss, but a similar overall incidence, as compared to SRS.[79,81,82]

Only one study by Monfared et al has compared secondary SRS after MS against secondary EBRT after MS, which documented significantly higher failure rates after EBRT as compared to SRS (67 vs. 25%).[31] Proton beam RT (PBRT) is a more novel technology, and long-term data on larger cohorts of multiply treated tumors are still being accumulated; however, in the primary treatment setting, short- and intermediate-term tumor control rates have been comparable to SRS at 93.6 to 100% after 7 to 98 months of follow-up, with similarly low rates of new postradiation cranial nerve deficits (Chapter 20).[83,84,85] Isolated reports suggest that substituting PRBT or another alternative modality for repeat SRS may be beneficial for appropriately selected patients; however, more reliable data with substantial follow-up will be required to integrate more meaningful recommendations.[31,85]

21.6 Conclusion

SRS is an essential tool in the treatment paradigm for VS, with a clear and compelling role in management of recurrence/progression after MS, as well as a range of potential indications as a secondary modality following primary SRS failure. SRS is highly effective in establishing secondary tumor control, and is associated with an acceptable adverse effect profile, which includes a minimal risk of facial nerve weakness, and a significant probability of hearing loss. Alternative radiation modalities including EBRT, IMRT, and PBRT have been less well studied.

For treatment of recurrence/progression after MS, side effect profiles favor SRS in patients who do not have a clear indication to preferentially offer repeat surgery (e.g., very large tumor causing brainstem/cerebellar compression or hydrocephalus; very rapid tumor growth; patient refusal of radiation). Repeat SRS for treatment failure after primary SRS is more fraught due to the cranial nerve risks associated with dose accumulation; however, the number of patients for whom this is the most reasonable option may be expanding, particularly as strategies for dose reduction and treatment conformity continue to improve. Recommendations regarding optimal timing of secondary treatment, dosimetry, and the role of secondary SRS in special populations such as patients with neurofibromatosis type II are not clearly established at present, and will require significant further investigation.

Taken together, the present data strongly support secondary SRS as a critically important modality for the treatment of many patients with recurrence/progression after MS or treatment failure after primary SRS, among whom the risk of adverse effects and the achievement of good outcomes will be best realized through careful patient selection and treatment planning.

References

[1] Mindermann T, Schlegel I. How to distinguish tumor growth from transient expansion of vestibular schwannomas following Gamma Knife radiosurgery. Acta Neurochir (Wien). 2014;156(6):1121-1123

[2] Link MJ, Driscoll CLW, Foote RL, Pollock BE. Radiation therapy and radiosurgery for vestibular schwannomas: indications, techniques, and results. Otolaryngol Clin North Am. 2012;45(2):353-66

[3] Pollock BE, Lunsford LD, Kondziolka D, et al. Vestibular schwannoma management. Part II. Failed radiosurgery and the role of delayed microsurgery. J Neurosurg. 1998;89(6):949-955

[4] Iwai Y, Yamanaka K, Shiotani M, Uyama T. Radiosurgery for acoustic neuromas: results of low-dose treatment. Neurosurgery. 2003;53(2):282-88

[5] Liscak R, Vladyka V, Urgosik D, Simonova G, Vymazal J. Repeated treatment of vestibular schwannomas after gamma knife radiosurgery. Acta Neurochir (Wien). 2009;151(4):317-24 discussion 324

[6] Pollock BE. Management of vestibular schwannomas that enlarge after stereotactic radiosurgery: treatment recommendations based on a 15 year experience. Neurosurgery. 2006;58(2):241-48

[7] Régis J, Delsanti C, Roche P-H. Editorial: Vestibular schwannoma radiosurgery: progression or pseudoprogression? J Neurosurg. 2017;127(2):374-379

[8] Carlson ML, Jacob JT, Pollock BE, et al. Long-term hearing outcomes following stereotactic radiosurgery for vestibular schwannoma: patterns of hearing loss and variables influencing audiometric decline. J Neurosurg. 2013;118 (3):579-587

[9] Hasegawa T, Kida Y, Kato T, Iizuka H, Yamamoto T. Factors associated with hearing preservation after Gamma Knife surgery for vestibular schwannomas in patients who retain serviceable hearing. J Neurosurg. 2011;115(6):1078-1086

[10] Roos DE, Potter AE, Zacest AC. Hearing preservation after low dose linac radiosurgery for acoustic neuroma depends on initial hearing and time. Radiother Oncol. 2011;101(3):420-424

[11] Di Maio S, Akagami R. Prospective comparison of quality of life before and after observation, radiation, or surgery for vestibular schwannomas. J Neurosurg. 2009;111(4):855-862

[12] Myrseth E, Møller P, Pedersen P-H, Lund-Johansen M. Vestibular schwannoma: surgery or gamma knife radiosurgery? A prospective, nonrandomized study. Neurosurgery. 2009;64(4):654-63

[13] Pollock BE, Driscoll CLW, Foote RL, et al. Patient outcomes after vestibular schwannoma management: a prospective comparison of microsurgical resection and stereotactic radiosurgery. Neurosurgery. 2006;59(1):77-85

[14] Pollock BE, Lunsford LD, Flickinger JC, Clyde BL, Kondziolka D. Vestibular schwannoma management. Part I. Failed microsurgery and the role of delayed stereotactic radiosurgery. J Neurosurg. 1998;89(6):944-948

[15] Slattery WH. Microsurgery after radiosurgery or radiotherapy for vestibular schwannomas. Otolaryngol Clin North Am. 2009;42(4):707-715

[16] Perry A, Graffeo CS, Copeland WR, et al. Microsurgery for Recurrent Vestibular Schwannoma After Previous Gross Total Resection. Otol Neurotol. 2017;38 (6):882-888

[17] Darrouzet V, Martel J, Enée V, Bébéar J-P, Guérin J. Vestibular schwannoma surgery outcomes: our multidisciplinary experience in 400 cases over 17 years. Laryngoscope. 2004;114(4):681-688

[18] Samii M, Matthies C. Management of 1000 vestibular schwannomas (acoustic neuromas): hearing function in 1000 tumor resections. Neurosurgery. 1997;40(2):248-62

[19] El-Kashlan HK, Zeitoun H, Arts HA, Hoff JT, Telian SA. Recurrence of acoustic neuroma after incomplete resection. Am J Otol. 2000;21(3):389-392

[20]

[21] Bloch DC, Oghalai JS, Jackler RK, Osofsky M, Pitts LH. The fate of the tumor remnant after less-than-complete acoustic neuroma resection. Otolaryngol Head Neck Surg. 2004;130(1):104-112

[22] Nakatomi H, Jacob JT, Carlson ML, et al. Long-term risk of recurrence and regrowth after gross-total and subtotal resection of sporadic vestibular schwannoma. J Neurosurg. 2017(19):1-7

[23] Seol HJ, Kim C-H, Park C-K, et al. Optimal extent of resection in vestibular schwannoma surgery: relationship to recurrence and facial nerve preservation. Neurol Med Chir (Tokyo). 2006;46(4):176-81.

[24] Freeman SRM, Ramsden RT, Saeed SR, et al. Revision surgery for residual or recurrent vestibular schwannoma. Otol Neurotol. 2007;28(8):1076-1082

[25] Hong B, Krauss JK, Bremer M, Karstens JH, Heissler HE, Nakamura M. Vestibular schwannoma microsurgery for recurrent tumors after radiation therapy or previous surgical resection. Otol Neurotol. 2014;35(1):171-181

[26] Roberson JB, Brackmann DE, Hitselberger WE. Acoustic neuroma recurrence after suboccipital resection: management with translabyrinthine resection. Am J Otol. 1996;17(2):307-311

[27] Samii M, Gerganov VM, Samii A. Functional outcome after complete surgical removal of giant vestibular schwannomas. J Neurosurg. 2010;112 (4):860-867

[28] Samii M, Metwali H, Gerganov V. Microsurgical management of vestibular schwannoma after failed previous surgery. J Neurosurg. 2016;125(5):1198-1203

[29] Ahmad RARL, Sivalingam S, Topsakal V, Russo A, Taibah A, Sanna M. Rate of recurrent vestibular schwannoma after total removal via different surgical approaches. Ann Otol Rhinol Laryngol. 2012;121(3):156-161

[30] Roche P-H, Robitail S, Delsanti C, Marouf R, Pellet W, Régis J. [Radiosurgery of vestibular schwannomas after microsurgery and combined radio-microsurgery]. Neurochirurgie. 2004;50(2-3 Pt 2):394-400

[31] Monfared A, Corrales CE, Theodosopoulos PV, et al. Facial Nerve Outcome and Tumor Control Rate as a Function of Degree of Resection in Treatment of Large Acoustic Neuromas: Preliminary Report of the Acoustic Neuroma Subtotal Resection Study (ANSRS). Neurosurgery. 2016;79(2):194-203

[32] Pollock BE, Link MJ. Vestibular schwannoma radiosurgery after previous surgical resection or stereotactic radiosurgery. Prog Neurol Surg. 2008;21:163-168

[33] Pai I, Bowman J, Thomas N, et al. Management of large and giant vestibular schwannomas. Skull Base. 2011;21(6):379-384

[34] Park C-K, Jung H-W, Kim JE, Son Y-J, Paek SH, Kim DG. Therapeutic strategy for large vestibular schwannomas. J Neurooncol. 2006;77(2):167-171

[35] Régis J, Pellet W, Delsanti C, et al. Functional outcome after gamma knife surgery or microsurgery for vestibular schwannomas. J Neurosurg. 2002;97 (5):1091-1100

[36] Sekhar LN, Gormley WB, Wright DC. The best treatment for vestibular schwannoma (acoustic neuroma): microsurgery or radiosurgery? Am J Otol. 1996;17(4):676-89

[37] Prasad D, Steiner M, Steiner L. Gamma surgery for vestibular schwannoma. J Neurosurg. 2000;92(5):745-759

[38] Carlson ML, Lees KA, Patel NS, et al. The Clinical Behavior of Asymptomatic Incidental Vestibular Schwannomas Is Similar to That of Symptomatic Tumors. Otol Neurotol. 2016;37(9):1435-1441

[39] Schmidt RF, Boghani Z, Choudhry OJ, Eloy JA, Jyung RW, Liu JK. Incidental vestibular schwannomas: a review of prevalence, growth rate, and management challenges. Neurosurg Focus. 2012;33(3):E4

[40] Hoa M, Drazin D, Hanna G, Schwartz MS, Lekovic GP. The approach to the patient with incidentally diagnosed vestibular schwannoma. Neurosurg Focus. 2012;33(3):E2

[41] Nagano O, Higuchi Y, Serizawa T, et al. Transient expansion of vestibular schwannoma following stereotactic radiosurgery. J Neurosurg. 2008;109 (5):811-816

[42] Nagano O, Serizawa T, Higuchi Y, et al. Tumor shrinkage of vestibular schwannomas after Gamma Knife surgery: results after more than 5 years of follow-up. J Neurosurg. 2010;113 Suppl:122-127

[43] Bailo M, Boari N, Gagliardi F, et al. Gamma Knife Radiosurgery for Residual and Recurrent Vestibular Schwannomas After Previous Surgery: Clinical Results in a Series of 90 Patients and Review of the Literature. World Neurosurg. 2017;98:60-72

[44] Pan H-C, Sheehan J, Sheu M-L, Chiu W-T, Yang D-Y. Intracapsular decompression or radical resection followed by Gamma Knife surgery for patients harboring a large vestibular schwannoma. J Neurosurg. 2012;117 Suppl:69-77

[45] Huang MJ, Kano H, Mousavi SH, et al. Stereotactic radiosurgery for recurrent vestibular schwannoma after previous resection. J Neurosurg. 2017;126 (5):1506-1513

[46] Norén G. Long-term complications following gamma knife radiosurgery of vestibular schwannomas. Stereotact Funct Neurosurg. 1998;70 Suppl 1:65-73

[47] Hasegawa T, Kida Y, Kobayashi T, Yoshimoto M, Mori Y, Yoshida J. Long-term outcomes in patients with vestibular schwannomas treated using gamma knife surgery: 10-year follow up. J Neurosurg. 2005;102(1):10-16

[48] Hasegawa T, Fujitani S, Katsumata S, Kida Y, Yoshimoto M, Koike J. Stereotactic radiosurgery for vestibular schwannomas: analysis of 317 patients followed more than 5 years. Neurosurgery. 2005;57(2):257-65

[49] Dewan S, Norén G. Retreatment of vestibular schwannomas with Gamma Knife surgery. J Neurosurg. 2008;109 Suppl:144-148

[50] Yomo S, Arkha Y, Delsanti C, Roche P-H, Thomassin JM, Régis J. Repeat gamma knife surgery for regrowth of vestibular schwannomas. Neurosurgery. 2009;64(1):48-54 discussion 54-5

[51] Kano H, Kondziolka D, Niranjan A, Flannery TJ, Flickinger JC, Lunsford LD. Repeat stereotactic radiosurgery for acoustic neuromas. Int J Radiat Oncol Biol Phys. 2010;76(2):520-527

[52] Lonneville S, Delbrouck C, Renier C, Devriendt D, Massager N. Repeat Gamma Knife surgery for vestibular schwannomas. Surg Neurol Int. 2015;6(1):153

[53] Fu VX, Verheul JB, Beute GN, et al. Retreatment of vestibular schwannoma with Gamma Knife radiosurgery: clinical outcome, tumor control, and review of literature. J Neurosurg. October 2017:1-9

[54] Roche P-H, Khalil M, Thomassin JM. Microsurgical removal of vestibular schwannomas after failed previous microsurgery. Prog Neurol Surg. 2008;21:158-162

[55] Unger F, Walch C, Papaefthymiou G, Feichtinger K, Trummer M, Pendl G. Radiosurgery of residual and recurrent vestibular schwannomas. Acta Neurochir (Wien). 2002;144(7):671-6 discussion 676-7

[56] Iwai Y, Ishibashi K, Watanabe Y, Uemura G, Yamanaka K. Functional Preservation After Planned Partial Resection Followed by Gamma Knife Radiosurgery for Large Vestibular Schwannomas. World Neurosurg. 2015;84(2):292-300

[57] Fuentes S, Arkha Y, Pech-Gourg G, Grisoli F, Dufour H, Régis J. Management of large vestibular schwannomas by combined surgical resection and gamma knife radiosurgery. Prog Neurol Surg. 2008;21:79-82

[58] Yang S-Y, Kim DG, Chung H-T, Park S-H, Paek SH, Jung H-W. Evaluation of tumour response after gamma knife radiosurgery for residual vestibular schwannomas based on MRI morphological features. J Neurol Neurosurg Psychiatr. 2008;79(4):431-436

[59] Haque R, Wojtasiewicz TJ, Gigante PR, et al. Efficacy of facial nerve-sparing approach in patients with vestibular schwannomas. J Neurosurg. 2011;115 (5):917-923

[60] van de Langenberg R, Hanssens PEJ, van Overbeeke JJ, et al. Management of large vestibular schwannoma. Part I. Planned subtotal resection followed by Gamma Knife surgery: radiological and clinical aspects. J Neurosurg. 2011;115(5):875-884

[61] Anaizi AN, Gantwerker EA, Pensak ML, Theodosopoulos PV. Facial nerve preservation surgery for koos grade 3 and 4 vestibular schwannomas. Neurosurgery. 2014;75(6):671-77

[62] Jeltema HR, Bakker NA, Bijl HP, Wagemakers M, Metzemaekers JDM, van Dijk JMC. Near total extirpation of vestibular schwannoma with salvage radiosurgery. Laryngoscope. 2015;125(7):1703-1707

[63] Graffeo CS, Perry A, Raghunathan A, et al. Macrophage Density Predicts Facial Nerve Outcome and Tumor Growth after Subtotal Resection of Vestibular Schwannoma. J Neurol Surg B. 2017;78:S1-S156.

[64] Yomo S, Tamura M, Carron R, Porcheron D, Régis J. A quantitative comparison of radiosurgical treatment parameters in vestibular schwannomas: the Leksell Gamma Knife Perfexion versus Model 4C. Acta Neurochir (Wien). 2010;152(1):47-55

[65] Lindquist C, Paddick I. The Leksell Gamma Knife Perfexion and comparisons with its predecessors. Neurosurgery. 2007;61(3 Suppl):130-41

[66] Ma L, Braunstein SE, Theodosopoulos PV, McDermott MW, Sneed PK. Inherent functional dependence among cochlear dose surrogates for stereotactic radiosurgery of vestibular schwannomas. Pract Radiat Oncol. 2017;7(1):e1-e7

[67] Jacob JT, Carlson ML, Schiefer TK, Pollock BE, Driscoll CL, Link MJ. Significance of cochlear dose in the radiosurgical treatment of vestibular schwannoma: controversies and unanswered questions. Neurosurgery. 2014;74(5):466-74

[68] Watanabe T, Saito N, Hirato J, Shimaguchi H, Fujimaki H, Sasaki T. Facial neuropathy due to axonal degeneration and microvasculitis following gamma knife surgery for vestibular schwannoma: a histological analysis. Case report. J Neurosurg. 2003;99(5):916-920

[69] Kano H, Kondziolka D, Khan A, Flickinger JC, Lunsford LD. Predictors of hearing preservation after stereotactic radiosurgery for acoustic neuroma. J Neurosurg. 2009;111(4):863-873

[70] Pollock BE, Link MJ, Stafford SL, Parney IF, Garces YI, Foote RL. The Risk of Radiation-Induced Tumors or Malignant Transformation After Single-Fraction Intracranial Radiosurgery: Results Based on a 25-Year Experience. Int J Radiat Oncol Biol Phys. 2017;97(5):919-923

[71] Carlson ML, Glasgow AE, Jacob JT, Habermann EB, Link MJ. The Short-Term and Intermediate-Term Risk of Second Neoplasms After Diagnosis and Treatment of Unilateral Vestibular Schwannoma: Analysis of 9460 Cases. Int J Radiat Oncol Biol Phys. 2016;95(4):1149-1157

[72] Breen P, Flickinger JC, Kondziolka D, Martinez AJ. Radiotherapy for nonfunctional pituitary adenoma: analysis of long-term tumor control. J Neurosurg. 1998;89(6):933-938

[73] Comey CH, McLaughlin MR, Jho HD, Martinez AJ, Lunsford LD. Death from a malignant cerebellopontine angle triton tumor despite stereotactic radiosurgery. Case report. J Neurosurg. 1998;89(4):653-658

[74] Roche P-H, Khalil M, Soumare O, Régis J. Hydrocephalus and vestibular schwannomas: considerations about the impact of gamma knife radiosurgery. Prog Neurol Surg. 2008;21:200-206

[75] Briggs RJ, Shelton C, Kwartler JA, Hitselberger W. Management of hydrocephalus resulting from acoustic neuromas. Otolaryngol Head Neck Surg. 1993;109(6):1020-1024

[76] Chan AW, Black P, Ojemann RG, et al. Stereotactic radiotherapy for vestibular schwannomas: favorable outcome with minimal toxicity. Neurosurgery. 2005;57(1):60-70

[77] Friedman WA, Bradshaw P, Myers A, Bova FJ. Linear accelerator radiosurgery for vestibular schwannomas. J Neurosurg. 2006;105(5):657-661

[78] Tsai J-T, Lin J-W, Lin C-M, et al. Clinical evaluation of CyberKnife in the treatment of vestibular schwannomas. Biomed Res Int. 2013;2013(2):297093-297096

[79] Mahboubi H, Sahyouni R, Moshtaghi O, et al. CyberKnife for Treatment of Vestibular Schwannoma: A Meta-analysis. Otolaryngol Head Neck Surg. 2017;157(1):7-15

[80] Vivas EX, Wegner R, Conley G, et al. Treatment outcomes in patients treated with CyberKnife radiosurgery for vestibular schwannoma. Otol Neurotol. 2014;35(1):162-170

[81] Thomas C, Di Maio S, Ma R, et al. Hearing preservation following fractionated stereotactic radiotherapy for vestibular schwannomas: prognostic implications of cochlear dose. J Neurosurg. 2007;107(5):917-926

[82] Apicella G, Paolini M, Deantonio L, Masini L, Krengli M. Radiotherapy for vestibular schwannoma: Review of recent literature results. Rep Pract Oncol Radiother. 2016;21(4):399-406

[83] Bush DA, McAllister CJ, Loredo LN, Johnson WD, Slater JM, Slater JD. Fractionated proton beam radiotherapy for acoustic neuroma. Neurosurgery. 2002;50(2):270-75

[84] Vernimmen FJAI, Mohamed Z, Slabbert JP, Wilson J. Long-term results of stereotactic proton beam radiotherapy for acoustic neuromas. Radiother Oncol. 2009;90(2):208-212

[85] Weber DC, Chan AW, Bussiere MR, et al. Proton beam radiosurgery for vestibular schwannoma: tumor control and cranial nerve toxicity. Neurosurgery. 2003;53(3):577 -88

22 Radiation Therapy and Stereotactic Radiosurgery for Large Vestibular Schwannoma

Gautam U. Mehta and Jason P. Sheehan

22.1 Introduction

Over the last three decades, radiation therapy and stereotactic radiosurgery (SRS) have become an important option in the management of vestibular schwannomas. In fact, SRS with devices such as the CyberKnife (Accuray), Edge (Varian), Gamma Knife (Elekta), and Novalis TX (Brainlab) is now first-line therapy for many growing, small-to-medium-sized tumors.[1] Comparative studies on SRS and microsurgery for vestibular schwannomas have shown that radiosurgery can be equally effective and less morbid than microsurgery for smaller tumors (≤3 cm).[2,3] During the initial years of experience, it was observed that the risks associated with SRS, specifically cranial neuropathy, were proportional to both treatment dose and extracanalicular tumor diameter (▶ Fig. 22.1).[4] These findings mirrored similar results in microsurgical series from high-volume centers, that surgical morbidity increases with tumor size.[5,6] Despite this increased morbidity for large tumors with both modalities, a threshold for choosing microsurgery over SRS similar to that applied to arteriovenous malformations was recommended (>3 cm).[1,7] Some centers with high-volume microsurgical practices have chosen slightly lower thresholds for microsurgery (>2.7 cm), while others select patients based on Koos grade (IV).[8,9] For these large lesions, the precise role of SRS in management is poorly defined. However, in selected patients radiosurgery may still have utility as first-line therapy. Recent studies using modern techniques have begun to elucidate the outcomes of SRS applied to such patients with large tumors, allowing us to better define the cohort for which it should be used.

Simultaneous clinical study has been ongoing in the use of fractionated radiotherapy for vestibular schwannomas. With advances in technique and conformal stereotactic targeting, the results of fractionated stereotactic radiotherapy (FSRT) have approached or equaled the outcomes achieved with SRS for small tumors.[10] In patients with larger tumors, FSRT and similarly multisession SRS may have potential utility in limiting cranial neuropathy and other adverse radiation effects such as hydrocephalus or parenchymal edema when treating larger volume tumors, and may help expand the range of patients who may be safely treated with radiation therapy.

22.2 Stereotactic Radiosurgery for Large Vestibular Schwannomas

22.2.1 Tumor Control

Due to current management paradigms, the majority of data available on SRS for vestibular schwannomas using contemporary dosing schedules exist for tumors less than 3 cm in diameter. Since some patients with larger tumors may be medically unfit for surgery and have been treated with SRS, several groups have recently been able to report the results of SRS on tumors greater than 3 cm.[9,11,12,13,14,15,16] Tumor control rates in this cohort at 5 years using Kaplan–Meier analyses have ranged from 82 to 92% (▶ Table 22.1).[11,14,15] These rates are lower than those typically reported for SRS-treated patients with tumors ≤3 cm in diameter, which are frequently above 95% at 5 years in large series.[17]

Complicating comparative analyses between the outcomes of SRS for small and large vestibular schwannomas is the heterogeneity of the data available. For example, nearly every study on large tumors uses a different threshold to define such lesions (▶ Table 22.1). Outcome data are similarly limited as several studies on large tumors do not perform survival analyses to define tumor control.[9,12,13] Furthermore, the length of follow-up for these studies is typically shorter than reported in studies on smaller tumors. As post-SRS tumor growth can occur up to 6 years after treatment, long-term follow-up is critical.[18]

Some larger studies that have included single institution data on the treatment outcomes of both small and large tumors allow for a more controlled comparison. One such study by Hasegawa and colleagues reported the growth outcomes of Gamma Knife radiosurgery (GKRS) in 427 patients with vestibular schwannomas, including 64 patients with tumors ≥ 10 cm^3 (e.g., equivalent to a 2.7-cm-diameter sphere).[19] Progression-free survival (PFS) in the smaller tumor group at 5 and 10 years

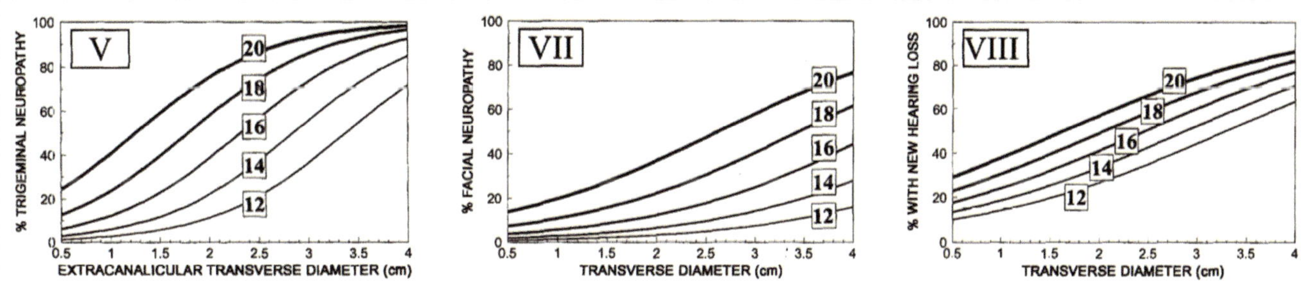

Fig. 22.1 Relationships between radiosurgery dose, extracanalicular tumor diameter, and postradiation cranial neuropathy. New trigeminal and facial neuropathy and hearing loss increase with both increasing dose and increased tumor diameter. (Reproduced with permission from Flickinger et al.[4])

Table 22.1 Tumor control after stereotactic radiosurgery for large vestibular schwannomas

Authors	Year	*N*	Definition	Volume treated (cm^3)	Dose (Gy)	Tumor control	Median follow-up (mo)
Roche et al	2004	50	Koos IV	Mean 4.3 (1.34–11.4)	Mean 10.2 (8–14)	69% at last follow-up	45.5 (14–84)
Inoue	2005	20	> 3 cm	Mean 15.2 (5.3–28.5)	Mean 11.5 (10–12)	95% at last follow-up	N/A
Chung et al	2010	53	> 3 cm	Mean 17.3 (12.7–25.2)	Mean 11.9 (11–14)	92% at 5 y	53 (12–155)
van de Langenberg et al	2011	33	> 6 cm^3	Mean 8.8 (6.1–17.7)	Mean 12.6 (12.5–13.0)	88% at last follow-up	30 (12–72)
Yang et al	2011	65	3–4 cm	Median 9 (5–22)	Median 12 (11–15)	87% at last follow-up	36 (1–146)
Milligan et al	2012	22	> 2.5 cm	Median 9.4 (5.3–19.1)	Median 12 (12–14)	82% at 5 y	66 (26–121)
Williams et al							
Large	2013	24	> 3 cm	Median 9.5 (3.1–24.7)	Median 11 (8–20)	82% at 5 y	48.5 (7–211)
Small to medium	2013	49	≤ 3 cm	Median 0.7 (0.1–6.5)	Median 12 (11–15)	90% at 5 y	100.9 (24–197)

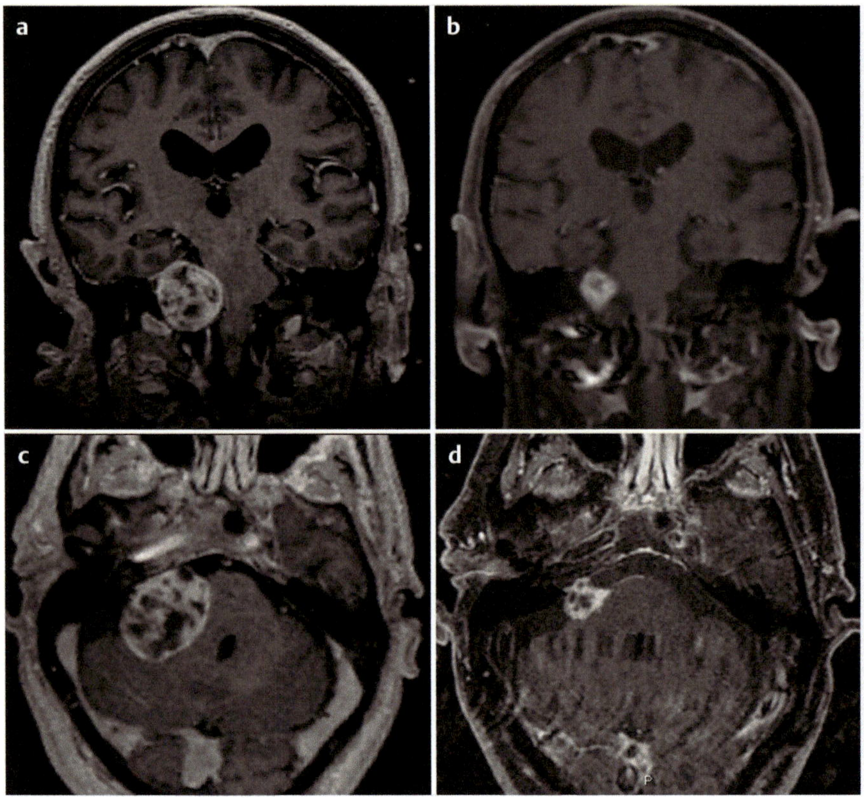

Fig. 22.2 Postcontrast T1-weighted MRI of a large, growing vestibular schwannoma in a 70-year-old man who was treated with Gamma Knife radiosurgery (Elekta) at the University of Virginia demonstrating significant tumor volume reduction between the time of treatment (**A**, coronal; **C**, axial) and 4-year postoperative follow-up (**B**, coronal; **D**, axial).

was 95 and 94%, respectively, while PFS in the larger tumor group was 79 and 77%, respectively. This was statistically significant by univariate ($p < 0.0001$), but not multivariate ($p = 0.17$) analysis. However, tumor size by Koos grade was significant on multivariate analysis ($p < 0.0001$), confirming the relationship between size and outcome. A recent study at the University of Virginia has directly compared the outcomes of GKRS for small to medium tumors (diameter ≤ 3 cm) with those of large tumors (diameter > 3 cm) using a 2:1 matched cohort design.[15] This study revealed an actuarial PFS in the smaller tumor group at 3 and 5 years of 97 and 90%, respectively, while PFS in the larger tumor group was 95 and 82%, respectively (▶ Fig. 22.2).

22.3 Complications

In addition to worsened tumor control, SRS for large vestibular schwannomas also carries a higher attendant morbidity than similar treatment for small tumors. The careful dose–diameter–cranial

Table 22.2 Complications after stereotactic radiosurgery for large vestibular schwannomas

Authors	Trigeminal neuropathy	Facial neuropathy	Hearing loss[a]	Retreatment for progression	CSF diversion
Roche et al	1/50 (0%)	0/50 (0%)	8/20 (40%)	3/50 (6%)	4/50 (8%)
Inoue	0/20 (0%)	0/20 (0%)	1/5 (20%)	1/20 (5%)	0/20 (0%)
Chung et al	0/53 (0%)	0/53 (0%)	–[b]	3/53 (6%)	2/53 (4%)
van de Langenberg et al	0/33 (0%)	0/33 (0%)	5/12 (42%)	7/33 (21%)	2/31 (6%)
Yang et al	4/65 (6%)	1/65 (1.5%)	4/22 (18%)	7/65 (11%)	4/65 (6%)
Milligan et al	3/22 (14%)	3/22 (14%)	7/10 (70%)	2/22 (9%)	3/22 (14%)
Williams et al					
Large	3/11[c] (28%)	8/24 (33%)	–[b]	6/24 (25%)	2/24 (8%)
Small to medium	–[b]	2/49 (4%)	–[b]	0/49 (0%)	0/49 (0%)

[a]Patients with useful/serviceable hearing.
[b]Not evaluated.
[c]Of patients with existing deficit.

neuropathy relationships demonstrated in the early experience by the Pittsburgh group are representative of this (▸ Fig. 22.1).[4] Similar results with cranial neuropathy led Norén to propose a lower prescription dose for larger tumors (10 Gy) than smaller tumors (12 Gy) in the early 1990s.[20] With these lower dose treatment regimens and more conformal targeting in the magnetic resonance imaging (MRI) era, the rate of trigeminal and facial neuropathy with SRS for large tumors has been very low in modern series (▸ Table 22.2).[7] The rate of hearing impairment after SRS, however, has remained high, with useful or serviceable hearing preservation rates ranging from 18 to 70% at a median of 2.5 to 5.5 years following treatment (▸ Table 22.2).

In addition to the risk of cranial neuropathy, other, potentially more serious complications may arise requiring further surgical intervention. A subset of patients with tumor progression eventually required surgical resection or debulking (5–25%; ▸ Table 22.2). Furthermore, several patients with larger tumors required cerebrospinal fluid (CSF) diversion for hydrocephalus that developed after SRS treatment (0–14%; ▸ Table 22.2). Comparatively, neither of these interventions was required in the matched cohort of 49 patients with small tumors treated with GKRS at our institution.

22.3.1 Comparison with Microsurgery

To determine the relative indications for SRS for vestibular schwannomas, it is important to understand the outcomes of the alternative therapies including microsurgery. Comparative, single-institution studies between SRS and microsurgery in small tumors (< 3 cm in diameter) have shown that SRS has a favorable risk–benefit profile when compared with microsurgery.[2,3,21] A similar comparative study for large vestibular schwannomas has not been reported to date. Numerous studies have analyzed the outcomes of microsurgery for large vestibular schwannomas alone, which allows us to understand the relative utility of this therapy. A recent systematic review of microsurgery for vestibular schwannomas has enumerated the risks of microsurgery based on size and approach.[22] With surgery for lesions greater than 3 cm, a retrosigmoid approach resulted in hearing loss in 72% of patients (91 of 127) with serviceable hearing. Facial nerve dysfunction was experienced in 36% of patients (278 of 783). While the rate of other cranial neuropathy was quite low, other complications such as CSF leak and infection may also occur.

Another option for treatment of large vestibular schwannomas is planned subtotal resection followed by SRS. A retrospective analysis of 50 patients treated with this paradigm was recently published by van de Langenberg and colleagues.[23] They found that tumor control was maintained in 90% of patients at last follow-up (median, 33.8 months). Of two patients with preoperative serviceable hearing who underwent a retrosigmoid approach, one maintained useful hearing. Facial nerve function was impaired in nine patients (18%) after treatment, with three patients (6%) having House–Brackmann grade III function or worse. No patient experienced trigeminal neuropathy. Complications included hematoma (two patients, 4%), hydrocephalus (two patients, 4%), lower cranial nerve dysfunction requiring gastronomy tube placement (one patient, 2%), and hemiparesis (one patient, 2%). Overall, this group experienced similar outcomes compared with the group that underwent SRS alone at the same institution (▸ Table 22.1, ▸ Table 22.2), despite a significantly larger mean tumor volume (14.9 vs. 8.8 cm^3).[12] This result, and specifically the requirement for postoperative SRS, must be balanced against the natural history of residual tumor after microsurgery for vestibular schwannomas. Recently, the Gruppo Otologico retrospectively analyzed the behavior of residual tumor after near-total (< 2% of tumor remaining) and subtotal (2–5% of tumor remaining) resections.[24] Among 111 patients (mean follow-up, 45.4 months), they reported a 5-year PFS of 92%. Specifically, among the 38 patients with subtotal resection, 7 (18%) experienced regrowth. Based on this result, they proposed that patients with subtotal resections should be followed for a period of 7 to 10 years postoperatively until regrowth is noted. For partial resections (> 5% of tumor remaining), they advocated second-stage surgery when possible.

22.4 Fractionated Radiotherapy for Large Vestibular Schwannomas

As vestibular schwannomas are slowly growing, benign tumors, the radiobiologic benefit of fractionation, in terms of tumor control, may be limited. However, as cranial neuropathy is a major limitation of dosing schemes for SRS, there can be an advantage to fractionation in minimizing the toxicity for the treatment of larger tumors. Similar advantage may be realized in tumors that are adjacent to or that compress the brainstem.[25]

Several studies have directly compared the results of SRS and FSRT for small to medium vestibular schwannomas within the same institution.[10,25,26,27,28] These studies have consistently demonstrated very similar tumor controls rates (≥ 95%) for both modalities. The rate of hearing preservation after treatment was reported to be worse with SRS in some studies[10,26] and worse with FSRT in others.[28] The rate of new trigeminal neuropathy was consistently higher after SRS (6–16%) than after FSRT (3–5%).[10,26,27,28] Similarly, the rate of new facial neuropathy was also consistently higher after SRS (2–17%) than after FSRT (2–3%).[10,26,27,28]

Although studies on fractionated radiotherapy for vestibular schwannomas have been reported since the 1980s, little data exist on the treatment outcomes with larger tumors.[29] Two studies on FSRT published in the 1990s have suggested a role for this treatment in large tumors. Lederman and colleagues attempted a hypofractionated scheme (20 Gy, five fractions) in 16 patients with vestibular schwannomas greater than 3 cm in diameter.[30] Over a median follow-up of 28 months, all tumors were noted to be stable or diminished in size. One patient (7%) developed a temporary facial nerve palsy; however, no patient developed permanent trigeminal or facial nerve dysfunction. Kalapurakal and colleagues analyzed hypofractionated radiotherapy (30–36 Gy, six fractions) in 19 patients with tumors that had a pons–petrous distance greater than 1 cm and a midporous transverse diameter greater than 2 cm.[31] In this study, over a median follow-up of 54 months, all patients had stable or diminishing tumors and no patient with evaluable function had trigeminal ($n = 15$) or facial ($n = 16$) neuropathy, or hearing loss ($n = 9$). A more recent study by Mandl and colleagues mixed the outcomes of fractionated radiotherapy and SRS for patients with large tumors, not allowing for evaluation of either modality individually.[32] Finally, Casentini and colleagues analyzed the outcomes of 33 patients with vestibular schwannomas greater than 8 cm^3 in volume treated with multisession SRS using CyberKnife (14–19.5 Gy, two to five fractions) over a median follow-up of 48 months.[33] PFS at 5 years was 83% and hearing was preserved in seven of eight patients with serviceable hearing. Trigeminal and facial outcomes were not clearly enumerated; however, two patients required CSF diversion and two patients required resection for tumor progression.

22.5 Patient Selection and Management

Despite an increase in the overall number of patients choosing observation, few patients (10–11%) with tumors > 3 cm do not undergo treatment.[34] Giving consideration to the outcomes described previously, the optimal patient with a large vestibular schwannoma to undergo SRS or radiation therapy is one who carries a greater risk with surgery (▶ Table 22.3). Patients who are elderly or harbor significant medical comorbidities may benefit from upfront SRS or radiation therapy over microsurgery. However, certain patient-specific risk factors may shift the balance back in favor of microsurgery, including significant brainstem compression (Koos grade IV tumors), particularly in those patients presenting with disabling symptoms. Patient preference and surgeon experience (with either microsurgery or radiation therapy) can also be important considerations in treatment choice. Emerging paradigms such as planned subtotal resection followed by SRS or radiation therapy should also be considered. Many elderly patients can tolerate a subtotal resection in which the surgeon stays within the capsule of the schwannoma and thereby preserves neurological function and later treats the residual tumor with SRS or radiotherapy.

Table 22.3 Factors in choosing therapy for large vestibular schwannomas

Favors microsurgery	Favors radiation therapy	Other considerations
Young age/healthy	Advanced age/poor medical status	Patient preference
Significant brainstem compression/giant tumors	Lack of brainstem compression	Surgeon experience
Disabling symptoms at presentation (ataxia, intractable headache, trigeminal neuralgia)	No disabling symptoms at presentation	
Useful hearing in contralateral ear	No useful hearing in contralateral ear	

For patients who do undergo SRS or radiation therapy, optimal posttreatment management of such patients may differ slightly from patients with smaller tumors. As these patients are more likely to develop hydrocephalus after radiation or to progress and cause mass effect, close posttreatment follow-up may be warranted. A greater proportion of these patients may require CSF diversion or resection due to progression and mass effect, and this potential necessity for salvage surgery should be understood by patients prior to undergoing radiation therapy.

22.6 Conclusion

Radiosurgery or radiation therapy remains a second-line option for most patients with a large (> 3 cm) vestibular schwannoma due to worsened tumor control and the greater risks associated with increased treatment volume. Regardless, recent studies have shown that SRS or radiation therapy may have utility in the appropriately selected patient. While single-session SRS is the mainstay for patients with small tumors, fractionated or hypofractionated treatment schemes may allow for similar tumor control while limiting the risk of cranial neuropathy in patients with larger tumors. This should be balanced with the comfort and convenience of single-session SRS. Overall, for patients with large vestibular schwannomas, radiation therapy affords a reasonable probability of tumor control with a low to moderate risk of cranial neuropathy and should be evaluated on a patient-by-patient basis.

References

[1] Kondziolka D, Lunsford LD, McLaughlin MR, Flickinger JC. Long-term outcomes after radiosurgery for acoustic neuromas. N Engl J Med. 1998; 339 (20):1426–1433

[2] Pollock BE, Lunsford LD, Kondziolka D, et al. Outcome analysis of acoustic neuroma management: a comparison of microsurgery and stereotactic radiosurgery. Neurosurgery. 1995; 36(1):215–224, discussion 224–229

[3] Régis J, Pellet W, Delsanti C, et al. Functional outcome after gamma knife surgery or microsurgery for vestibular schwannomas. J Neurosurg. 2002; 97 (5):1091–1100

[4] Flickinger JC, Kondziolka D, Lunsford LD. Dose and diameter relationships for facial, trigeminal, and acoustic neuropathies following acoustic neuroma radiosurgery. Radiother Oncol. 1996; 41(3):215–219

[5] Koos WT. Criteria for preservation of vestibulocochlear nerve function during microsurgical removal of acoustic neurinomas. Acta Neurochir (Wien). 1988; 92(1–4):55–66

[6] Matthies C, Samii M. Management of 1000 vestibular schwannomas (acoustic neuromas): clinical presentation. Neurosurgery. 1997; 40(1):1–9, discussion 9–10

[7] Flickinger JC, Kondziolka D, Pollock BE, Lunsford LD. Evolution in technique for vestibular schwannoma radiosurgery and effect on outcome. Int J Radiat Oncol Biol Phys. 1996; 36(2):275–280

[8] Link MJ, Driscoll CLW, Foote RL, Pollock BE. Radiation therapy and radiosurgery for vestibular schwannomas: indications, techniques, and results. Otolaryngol Clin North Am. 2012; 45(2):353–366, viii–ix

[9] Roche P-H, Robitail S, Pellet W, Devèze A, Thomassin J-M, Régis J. Results and indications of gamma knife radiosurgery for large vestibular schwannomas [in French]. Neurochirurgie. 2004; 50(2–3, Pt 2):377–382

[10] Andrews DW, Suarez O, Goldman HW, et al. Stereotactic radiosurgery and fractionated stereotactic radiotherapy for the treatment of acoustic schwannomas: comparative observations of 125 patients treated at one institution. Int J Radiat Oncol Biol Phys. 2001; 50(5):1265–1278

[11] Chung W-Y, Pan DH-C, Lee C-C, et al. Large vestibular schwannomas treated by Gamma Knife surgery: long-term outcomes. J Neurosurg. 2010; 113 (December) Suppl:112–121

[12] van de Langenberg R, Hanssens PEJ, Verheul JB, et al. Management of large vestibular schwannoma. Part II. Primary Gamma Knife surgery: radiological and clinical aspects. J Neurosurg. 2011; 115(5):885–893

[13] Yang H-C, Kano H, Awan NR, et al. Gamma Knife radiosurgery for larger-volume vestibular schwannomas. Clinical article. J Neurosurg. 2011; 114(3):801–807

[14] Milligan BD,, Pollock BE,, Foote RL,, Link MJ.. Long-term tumor control and cranial nerve outcomes following γ knife surgery for larger-volume vestibular schwannomas. J Neurosurg. 2012; 116(3):598–604

[15] Williams BJ, Xu Z, Salvetti DJ, McNeill IT, Larner J, Sheehan JP. Gamma Knife surgery for large vestibular schwannomas: a single-center retrospective case-matched comparison assessing the effect of lesion size. J Neurosurg. 2013; 119(2):463 471

[16] Inoue HK. Low-dose radiosurgery for large vestibular schwannomas: long-term results of functional preservation. J Neurosurg. 2005; 102 Suppl:111–113

[17] Chopra R, Kondziolka D, Niranjan A, Lunsford LD, Flickinger JC. Long-term follow-up of acoustic schwannoma radiosurgery with marginal tumor doses of 12 to 13 Gy. Int J Radiat Oncol Biol Phys. 2007; 68(3):845–851

[18] Prasad D, Steiner M, Steiner L. Gamma surgery for vestibular schwannoma. J Neurosurg. 2000; 92(5):745–759

[19] Hasegawa T, Kida Y, Kato T, Iizuka H, Kuramitsu S, Yamamoto T. Long-term safety and efficacy of stereotactic radiosurgery for vestibular schwannomas: evaluation of 440 patients more than 10 years after treatment with Gamma Knife surgery. J Neurosurg. 2013; 118(3):557–565

[20] Norén G. Gamma knife radiosurgery of acoustic neurinomas. A historic perspective. Neurochirurgie. 2004; 50(2–3, Pt 2):253–256

[21] Pollock BE, Driscoll CLW, Foote RL, et al. Patient outcomes after vestibular schwannoma management: a prospective comparison of microsurgical resection and stereotactic radiosurgery. Neurosurgery. 2006; 59(1):77–85, discussion 77–85

[22] Ansari SF, Terry C, Cohen-Gadol AA. Surgery for vestibular schwannomas: a systematic review of complications by approach. Neurosurg Focus. 2012; 33 (3):E14

[23] van de Langenberg R, Hanssens PEJ, van Overbeeke JJ, et al. Management of large vestibular schwannoma. Part I. Planned subtotal resection followed by Gamma Knife surgery: radiological and clinical aspects. J Neurosurg. 2011; 115(5):875–884

[24] Chen Z, Prasad SC, Di Lella F, et al. The behavior of residual tumors and facial nerve outcomes after incomplete excision of vestibular schwannomas. J Neurosurg. 2014; 120(6):1278–1287

[25] Murphy ES, Suh JH. Radiotherapy for vestibular schwannomas: a critical review. Int J Radiat Oncol Biol Phys. 2011; 79(4):985–997

[26] Collen C, Ampe B, Gevaert T, et al. Single fraction versus fractionated linac-based stereotactic radiotherapy for vestibular schwannoma: a single-institution experience. Int J Radiat Oncol Biol Phys. 2011; 81(4):e503–e509

[27] Combs SE, Welzel T, Schulz-Ertner D, Huber PE, Debus J. Differences in clinical results after LINAC-based single-dose radiosurgery versus fractionated stereotactic radiotherapy for patients with vestibular schwannomas. Int J Radiat Oncol Biol Phys. 2010; 76(1):193–200

[28] Kopp C, Fauser C, Müller A, et al. Stereotactic fractionated radiotherapy and LINAC radiosurgery in the treatment of vestibular schwannoma-report about both stereotactic methods from a single institution. Int J Radiat Oncol Biol Phys. 2011; 80(5):1485–1491

[29] Wallner KE, Sheline GE, Pitts LH, Wara WM, Davis RL, Boldrey EB. Efficacy of irradiation for incompletely excised acoustic neurilemomas. J Neurosurg. 1987; 67(6):858–863

[30] Lederman G, Lowry J, Wertheim S, et al. Acoustic neuroma: potential benefits of fractionated stereotactic radiosurgery. Stereotact Funct Neurosurg. 1997; 69(1–4, Pt 2):175–182

[31] Kalapurakal JA, Silverman CL, Akhtar N, Andrews DW, Downes B, Thomas PRM. Improved trigeminal and facial nerve tolerance following fractionated stereotactic radiotherapy for large acoustic neuromas. Br J Radiol. 1999; 72 (864):1202–1207

[32] Mandl ES, Meijer OWM, Slotman BJ, Vandertop WP, Peerdeman SM. Stereotactic radiation therapy for large vestibular schwannomas. Radiother Oncol. 2010; 95(1):94–98

[33] Casentini L, Fornezza U, Perini Z, Perissinotto E, Colombo F. Multisession stereotactic radiosurgery for large vestibular schwannomas. J Neurosurg. 2015; 122(4):818–824

[34] Carlson ML, Habermann EB, Wagie AE, et al. The changing landscape of vestibular schwannoma management in the United States–a shift toward conservatism. Otolaryngol Head Neck Surg. 2015; 153(3):440–446

23 Complications of Radiosurgery and Fractionated Radiotherapy for Vestibular Schwannoma

Clayton A. Smith and Albert Attia

23.1 Introduction

Radiotherapy for vestibular schwannoma (VS) is rarely associated with acute adverse effects. Uncommonly, patients may develop acute transient or delayed progressive ipsilateral trigeminal neuropathy or neuralgia and facial paresis or hemispasm. If the fourth ventricle becomes compressed due to peritumoral edema or cyst formation, then hydrocephalus may also occur (▶ Fig. 23.1 and ▶ Fig. 23.2). The latter complication rarely occurs with small-to-medium-sized tumors, and develops more frequently with tumors greater than 2.5 cm in maximum posterior fossa dimension. In contrast, progressive deterioration of hearing and vestibular function is common after radiotherapy; however, separating the direct effects of radiation and the natural course of disease is somewhat challenging. It is important for the treating physician and patient to be aware of these potential side effects to inform treatment decision making and manage posttreatment care.

23.2 Facial Nerve (CN VII) Paralysis

Modern series reporting outcomes for single-session stereotactic radiosurgery (SRS) performed with Gamma Knife (GK) have reported long-term facial nerve deficits ranging from 0 to 21% (▶ Table 23.1); however, reports of patients treated with a marginal dose of ≤ 13 Gy indicate facial nerve paralysis or hemifacial spasm in 0 to 5% of cases, with the majority of series observing < 2% risk of long-term facial paresis. In one of the largest patient series reported, Lunsford and colleagues[1] examined outcomes in 829 patients treated at the University of Pittsburg between 1987 and 2002. In the first 5 years of the series, patients were treated at a higher margin dose (mean, 16 Gy) resulting in 21% of patients experiencing facial nerve dysfunction at 5 years. In contrast, after reducing the margin dose to ≤ 13 Gy, facial nerve dysfunction occurred in less than 1% of cases. Similarly, Hasegawa and colleagues[2] reported their experience of 440 patients with a median follow-up of 12.5 years. For patients receiving doses > 13 Gy, long-term facial nerve dysfunction was experienced by 3.5% of patients, while 0% of patients treated to < 13 Gy experienced deficits.

A systematic analysis of the literature found that factors affecting facial nerve function preservation following GK radiosurgery included radiation dose, tumor size, and patient age.[3] Analysis of 1,908 patients from 23 published series determined facial nerve function preservation rates of 98.5% for doses ≤ 13 Gy and 94.7% for doses > 13 Gy. Similarly, patients with tumor volumes ≤ 1.5 cm^3 had preservation rates of 99.5% and those with tumor volumes > 1.5 cm^3 had a 95.5% preservation rate. Finally, patients younger than 60 years had preservation rates of 96.8%, while those older than 60 years experienced a preservation rate of 89.4%. One limitation of this study is that it did not allow for multivariable analysis to determine the impact of the various individual factors. The reader is encouraged to review Chapter 16 for a more in-depth discussion of outcomes after GK radiosurgery for VS.

While much of the early experience with radiosurgical treatment of VSs was delivered with GK, there is a growing literature for treatment outcomes for both single-session and

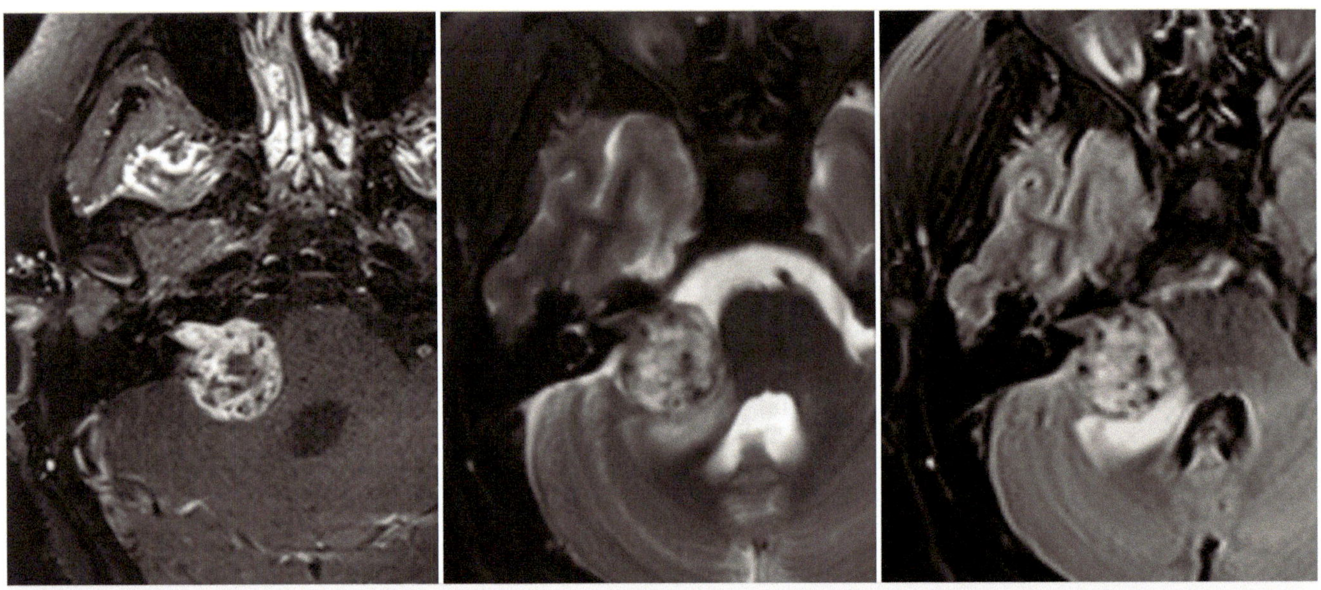

Fig. 23.1 Right-sided 2.7-cm vestibular schwannoma that was treated with five fractions of LINAC-based radiation therapy. Following treatment, the patient developed progressive vertigo, hemifacial hypoesthesia, and ataxia. The patient was initially managed with oral steroid therapy but ultimately underwent salvage microsurgery. Note the moderate amount of peritumoral edema in the adjacent brainstem and cerebellum.

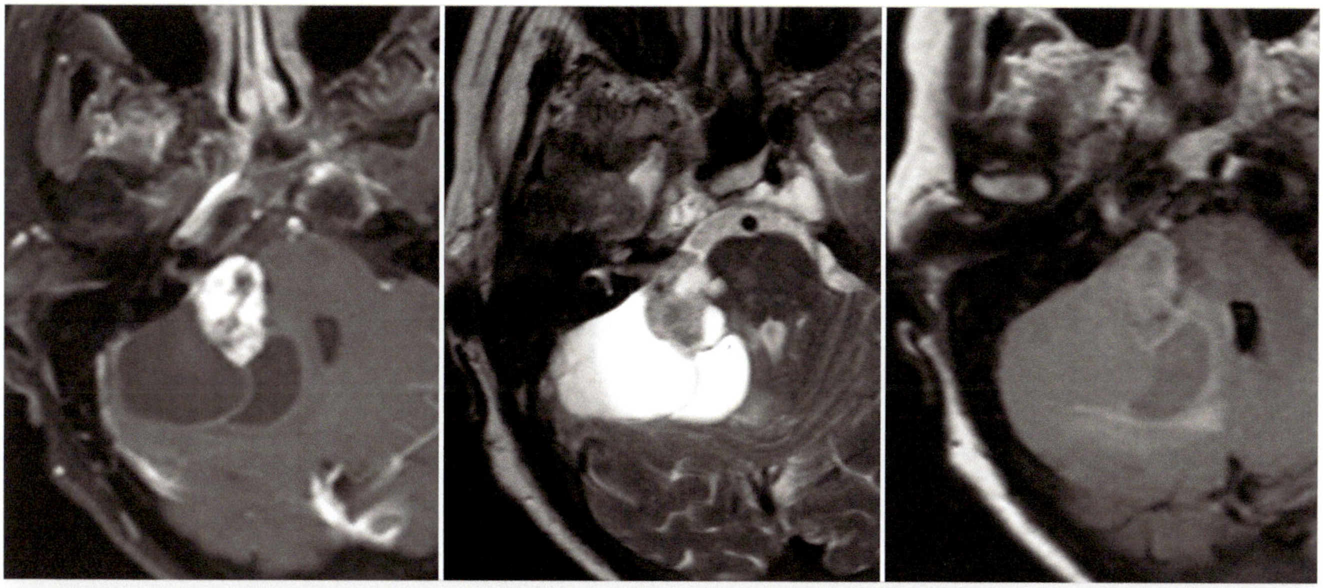

Fig. 23.2 Right-sided vestibular schwannoma that developed marked enlargement of the cystic component following Gamma Knife radiosurgery. Note the moderate amount of peritumoral edema and compression of the fourth ventricle. The patient experienced significant gait dysfunction with intractable nausea and vomiting and ultimately underwent salvage microsurgery.

multisession linear accelerator (LINAC)-based radiosurgery. Overall rates of facial nerve paresis for VS treated with single-session LINAC SRS range from 3.2 to 20% (▶ Table 23.1), though series that reported on patients treated with doses < 13 Gy generally report deficits in less than 1% of patients.[4,5] Reports of patients treated with multisession hypofractionated or conventionally fractionated radiotherapy demonstrate facial nerve paralysis rates in the range of 0 to 4% (▶ Table 23.1). Differences in dose-fractionation regimens make direct comparison difficult across series, but there appears to be a range of well-tolerated schedules. Combs and colleagues[4] reported on the outcomes of 449 patients treated at three German centers from 1990 to 2012, 291 of whom were treated with multisession conventionally fractionated radiotherapy to a median dose of 57.6 Gy. With a median follow-up of 5.6 years, only 1% of patients developed new facial nerve symptoms. Alternative dose schedules that also appear to be well tolerated include 46.8 Gy in 26 fractions,[6] 50 Gy in 25 fractions,[7,8] and 54 Gy in 30 fractions.[9,10,11] Toxicity outcomes of hypofractionated radiotherapy regimens have also been reported. In one of the largest series, Hansasuta and colleagues[12] reported on 383 patients treated with CyberKnife at Stanford between 1999 and 2007. The majority of patients (90%) were treated to a dose of 18 Gy in three fractions. No patients experienced facial weakness, though 2% of patients reported facial spasm that was transient in all but one case. Alternative hypofractionated radiotherapy regimens with < 3% toxicity include 25 Gy in 5 fractions[13,14,15] and 30 Gy in 10 fractions.[15,16] Chapters 17, 18, and 19 provide further detailed discussion regarding LINCAC-based radiosurgery and conventionally fractionated radiation for treatment of VS.

Facial nerve outcomes following proton radiotherapy treatment of VS have been mixed. In the largest series reported of 88 patients treated with single-session radiosurgery using doses of 10 to 18 Gy (median, 12 Gy) (relative biological effectiveness [RBE] 1.1), Weber and colleagues[17] observed new, permanent facial nerve deficits in 8.9% of patients. Similarly, Vernimmen and colleagues[18] reported 9.5% of patients experiencing long-term facial nerve dysfunction after hypofractionated proton treatment to 26 Gy (RBE 1.1) in three fractions. In contrast, Bush and colleagues[19] reported on the outcomes of 29 patients treated at Loma Linda University Medical Center with conventionally fractionated schedules of 54 to 60 Gy (RBE 1.1) in 30 to 33 fractions and observed no patients with long-term facial nerve dysfunction.

Transient facial nerve paresis is more common than a permanent deficit after treatment, occurring in an additional 1 to 5% of patients. Time of symptom onset varies significantly from as early as 2 months up to 2 + years, though most series report onset 3 to 6 months after radiotherapy. When reported, the decrement in facial nerve function is primarily to House–Brackmann grade II, though grade III + dysfunction has been observed. In patients who develop new or worsening facial nerve paresis following single-session radiosurgery or multisession radiotherapy for VS, the standard management approach is a trial of high-dose steroids with varying tapering schedules depending on treatment response. The above data gathered from multiple, large series of patients treated with various radiosurgical and radiotherapy techniques support the low risk of facial nerve dysfunction following treatment of VS using modern dosing strategies.

23.3 Trigeminal Nerve (CN V) Deficit

Trigeminal nerve deficits following single-session radiosurgery or fractionated radiotherapy of VS typically present as facial numbness or, less commonly, trigeminal neuralgia (▶ Fig. 23.3). Long-term trigeminal nerve dysfunction has been reported to

Table 23.1 Summary of major case series and systematic analyses reporting outcomes for long-term facial (CN VII) and trigeminal (CN V) nerve deficits after radiosurgery and radiotherapy treatment of vestibular schwannomas

Authors	Year	No. pts	Dose (Gy)	Modality	CN V deficit (%)	CN VII deficit (%)	Follow-up (years)
Andrews et al[23]	2001	69	12	GK	5	2	Mean 2.3
Chung et al[29]	2005	195	13 med	GK	1.1	0	Median 2.6
Fukuoka et al[30]	2009	152	12 med	GK	2.6	0	Minimum 5
Hasegawa et al[2]	2013	440	> 13 vs. < 13	GK	2.1: > 13 Gy; 0.3: < 13 Gy	3.5: > 13 Gy; 0: < 13 Gy	Median 12.5
Lunsford et al[1]	2005	829	10–20	GK	27: > 13 Gy; 3.1: < 13 Gy	21: > 13 Gy; < 1: < 13 Gy	n.r.
Prasad et al[31]	2000	153	13.2	GK	1.7	1.5	Median 4.2
Sughrue et al[20]	2009	5,631	Various	GK	3.15: > 13 Gy; 1.63: < 13 Gy	n.r.	Median 3
Yang et al[3]	2009	1,908	Various	GK	n.r.	3.8	Mean 4.5
Andrews et al[23]	2001	56	50/25	LINAC	7	2	Mean 2.2
Aoyama et al[7]	2013	201	46–50/23–25 (90%)	LINAC	2	2.5	Median 6
Champ et al[6]	2013	154	46.8/26	LINAC	2	2	Median 2.9
Chan et al[11]	2005	70	54/30	LINAC	4	1	Median 3.8
Choy et al[9]	2013	138	12.4 mean; 53 mean	LINAC	n.r.	20 SRS; 2 CFRT	Mean 3.5
Collen et al[16]	2011	119	11–14; 50/25; 40/10; 30/10	LINAC	4 SRS; 4 HFRT and CFRT	17 SRS; 3 HFRT and CFRT	Median 5.2
Combs et al[4]	2015	449	13 med; 57.6 med	LINAC	1.8 SRS (0.6 < 13 Gy) 1.4 CFRT	3.2 SRS (0.6 < 13 Gy) 1 CFRT	Median 5.6
Friedman et al[5]	2006	390	12.5 med	LINAC	3.6 (0.7 for < 12.5 Gy)	4.4 (0.7 for < 12.5 Gy)	Median 3.3
Hansasuta et al[12]	2011	383	18/3 (90%)	LINAC	1	0.2	Median 3.6
Koh et al[8]	2007	60	50/25	LINAC	0	0	Median 2.7
Kopp et al[10]	2011	115	12; 54/30	LINAC	18 SRS; 13 CFRT	7 SRS; 4 CFRT	Median 2.5
Lederman et al[14]	1997	38	16/4; 25/5	LINAC	0	2.6	Median 2
Meijer et al[13]	2003	80	20/5; 25/5	LINAC	2	3	Mean 2.9
Meijer et al[13]	2003	49	10–12.5	LINAC	8	7	Mean 2.5
Poen et al[24]	1999	31	21/3	LINAC	16	3	Median 2
Sawamura et al[32]	2003	101	40/20; 50/25	LINAC	4	0.9	Median 3.8
Selch et al[22]	2004	48	54/30	LINAC	2.2	2.1	Median 3
Williams[15]	2003	80	25/5; 30/10	LINAC	0	0	Median 1.6

Abbreviations: CFRT, conventionally fractionated radiotherapy; HFRT, hypofractionated multisession radiotherapy; n.r., not reported; pts, patients; SRS, single-session stereotactic radiosurgery.

occur in 0.3 to 27% of patients treated with single-session SRS by GK (▶ Table 23.1). As noted with both hearing preservation and facial nerve dysfunction, margin dose is a major determinant of long-term cranial nerve dysfunction. Lunsford and colleagues[1] observed that of the 829 patients treated between 1987 and 2002, 27% of patients treated to > 13 Gy experienced trigeminal nerve deficits. In contrast, patients treated to ≤ 13 Gy reported deficits in only 3.1% of cases. Hasegawa and colleagues[2] observed a similar difference in trigeminal nerve dysfunction after GK treatment, though to a lesser degree. In their 440 patient series, 2.1 and 0.3% of patients treated to > 13 Gy and ≤ 13 Gy, respectively, noted long-term facial numbness. In a systematic review of the literature examining non-CN VIII or CN VII morbidity of single-fraction SRS treatment of VS, CN V effects were the most common cranial nerve deficit reported.[20] Analysis of 5,631 patients revealed long-term trigeminal nerve deficits in 3.15% of patients receiving doses > 13 Gy and in 2.3% of patients treated to ≤ 13 Gy. Taken together, the available data indicate very low rates of long-term trigeminal nerve morbidity following single-session SRS.

Outcomes with multisession fractionated LINAC radiotherapy including CyberKnife have been equally encouraging, ranging from 0 to 16% in modern series (▶ Table 23.1). Several conventional dose fractionation schedules have been reported including: 46.8 to 57.6 Gy at 1.80 Gy/fraction (26 or 32 fractions) with resulting long-term trigeminal nerve dysfunction reported in

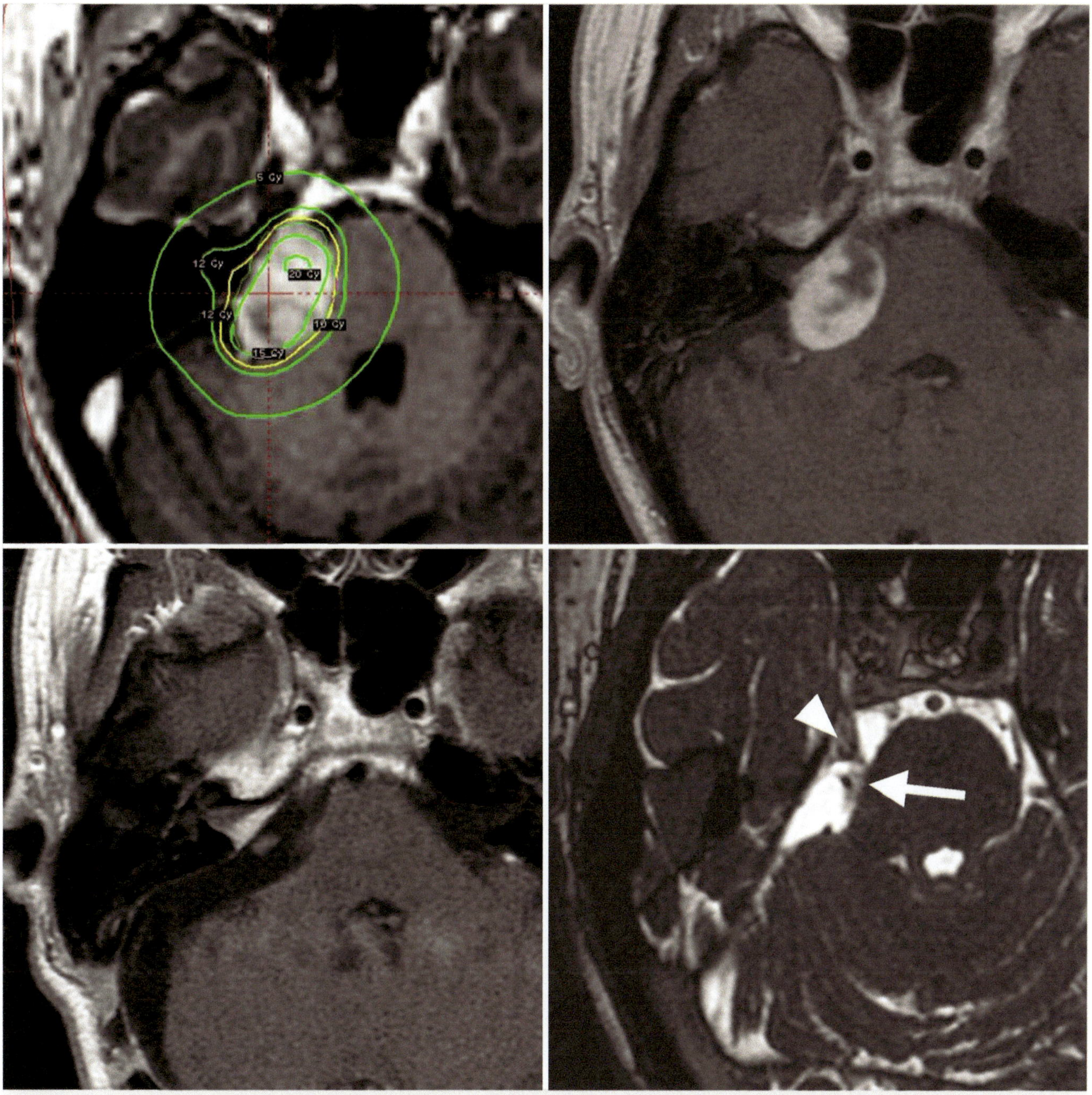

Fig. 23.3 Right-sided 2.4-cm vestibular schwannoma that underwent Gamma Knife radiosurgery using a marginal dose of 12 Gy and maximum dose of 24 Gy (top left). Following treatment, the tumor remained stable in size (top right); however, the patient experienced progressive medically refractory trigeminal neuralgia. The patient ultimately underwent subtotal resection via retrosigmoid craniotomy with microvascular decompression 5 years after radiosurgery (bottom left). A Teflon sponge (*arrow*) can be seen adjacent the offending superior cerebellar artery and trigeminal nerve (*arrowhead*).

1.4 to 4% of patients[4,6,11,21,22] and 46 to 50 Gy in 2 Gy/fraction (23 to 25 fractions) with CN V deficits in 0 to 7%.[7,8,23] Hypofractionated regimens have also been employed with limited long-term toxicity. In the early experience from Stanford treating VS to 21 Gy in three fractions with CyberKnife, Poen and colleagues[24] reported that 16% of the 31 patients developed new or worsening trigeminal neuropathy. Subsequently, a dose reduction was made to 18 Gy in three fractions, and the updated outcomes of 383 patients treated at Stanford (90% receiving the dose reduction) observed only a 1% risk of long-term trigeminal nerve dysfunction.[12] Other reported hypofractionation schedules with favorable trigeminal nerve morbidity rates of ≤ 4% toxicity include 25 Gy in 5 fractions[13,14,15] and 30 Gy in 10 fractions.[15,16]

As with the data on facial nerve outcomes, there are limited, mixed reports on outcomes for VS treated with proton radiotherapy. Reports using single-session SRS to 10 to 18 Gy (RBE 1.1)[17] or hypofractionated proton radiotherapy to 26 Gy (RBE

1.1) in three fractions[18] observed trigeminal nerve deficits in 10 and 7% of patients, respectively. In contrast, conventional fractionation to 54 to 60 Gy (RBE 1.1) in 30 to 33 fractions seemed to be well tolerated, with 0% of patients experiencing late trigeminal neuropathy in one small series.[19]

Similar to observations of facial nerve dysfunction, transient trigeminal neuropathy is reported to occur in an additional 1 to 5% of patients treated with radiotherapy in modern series. Published onset of symptoms ranges widely from 1 month to 4 years after treatment, but most symptoms develop within 6 to 15 months. Patients who develop new or worsening facial numbness are generally managed with a trial of high-dose steroids with a tapering schedule depending on response. Trigeminal neuralgia is managed first with steroids to assess for the effect of edema contributing to nerve dysfunction, and then with antiepileptics such as carbamazepine or gabapentin. The management of trigeminal neuralgia after radiation treatment of VS is discussed in greater detail in Chapter 70.

23.4 Hydrocephalus

Along with cranial nerve deficits, hydrocephalus is a reported adverse late effect following radiotherapy (▶ Fig. 23.4). When symptomatic, this may present as gait imbalance, headache, confusion, somnolence, or urinary incontinence. In a systematic review of the literature that included 5,631 patients treated with GK SRS for VS, overall 0.85% of cases experienced post-treatment hydrocephalus.[20] There was a modest association with dose; patients treated to > 13 Gy experienced hydrocephalus in 1% of cases, while patients receiving ≤ 13 Gy experienced hydrocephalus in only 0.74% of cases. A large review of 444 patients treated with GK SRS to a mean margin dose of 12.4 Gy specifically looked at factors associated with symptomatic hydrocephalus.[25] Symptomatic communicating hydrocephalus was observed in 5.6% of patients, with a median time to development of 7 months. Factors associated with development on multivariate analysis included tumor size, female gender, and brain atrophy as defined by increased cross-sectional area of the lateral ventricles.

There are fewer published series that comment on development of hydrocephalus following LINAC single-session radiosurgery or multisession radiotherapy for the treatment of VS, with rates ranging from 1 to 11.6%.[6,7,12,23] Favorable rates of 1.9 and 3.6% were observed for conventional multisession dose schedules of 46.8 Gy in 26 fractions[6] and 50 Gy in 25 fractions,[23] respectively. However, the Japanese experience with 201 patients treated to conventional multisession doses of 46 to 50 Gy in 2-Gy fractions (23–25 fractions) observed rates of new or worsening hydrocephalus in 11.6% of patients. On multivariate analysis, only the occurrence of tumor expansion (defined as increase in size > 3 mm) was significantly associated with hydrocephalus requiring shunt placement, though pretreatment tumor size (≥ 30 mm) approached significance. Hypofractionated multisession radiotherapy appears to be well tolerated, with one of the largest series of 383 patients, 90% of whom were treated to 18 Gy in three fractions, reporting only 1% requiring shunt placement to relieve hydrocephalus.[12]

23.5 Brain Necrosis

Despite delivery of relatively high radiation doses adjacent to the brainstem, reports of radiation necrosis of either the brainstem or nearby brain parenchyma following radiotherapy for VS are rare. In the series of Woolf and colleagues,[26] 1 patient out of 90 (1%) developed brainstem radionecrosis presenting with facial nerve paresis, gait imbalance, and radiologic appearance of brainstem necrosis 9 months after multisession radiotherapy. In a separate series, 3 out of 125 patients (2.4%) were noted to have MRI changes in the brainstem and cerebellum upon post-treatment imaging.[23] Only one of these patients was reported to be symptomatic with mild gait disturbance that resolved spontaneously. Another case report describes a patient treated

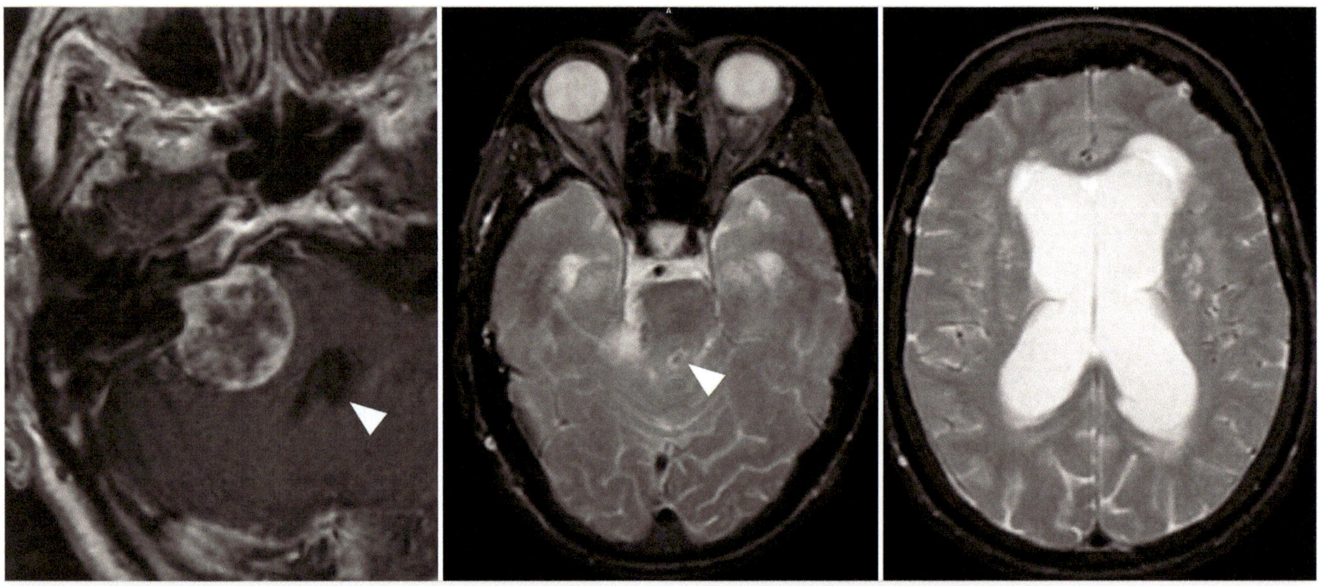

Fig. 23.4 Right-sided 2.9-cm vestibular schwannoma with development of hydrocephalus following radiosurgery. Note the loss of central enhancement indicative of treatment effect (left), and the significant effacement of the fourth vertical (*white arrowheads*).

with GK radiosurgery for VS secondary to neurofibromatosis type II who began experiencing progressive cranial neuropathies approximately 18 months later.[27] Subsequent MRI demonstrated tumor recurrence, increased edema in the pons and medial temporal lobe, and T1 postcontrast enhancement in the medial temporal lobe. The patient underwent surgical resection for recurrent VS, and pontine and medial temporal lobe edema gradually decreased over time. In a series of 11 patients treated with repeat GK for recurrent VS, 2 patients were noted to have radiologic signs of edema within the adjacent pons and cerebellar peduncle approximately 6 months after treatment.[28] Only one of these patients was symptomatic from this.

The available reports demonstrate the limited occurrence of both radiographic and symptomatic radionecrosis following either single-fraction radiosurgery or multisession radiotherapy. Management is similar to cranial nerve deficits described above with trial of high-dose steroids and taper to tolerance. Patients with radiation necrosis associated with tumor recurrence or cyst formation should have consideration of surgical management. In refractory cases that are not surgical candidates, the anti-vascular endothelial growth factor antibody bevacizumab shows some promise in ameliorating symptoms; however, we eagerly await the results of an ongoing cooperative group trial comparing the effectiveness of dexamethasone versus bevacizumab in improving radionecrosis.

23.6 Hearing Loss after Radiotherapy

One of the primary long-term side effects of VS-directed therapy is hearing loss. Defining the degree of loss due to radiotherapy can be difficult due to preexisting deficits and the expected natural progression from the disease itself. In patients with serviceable hearing prior to radiotherapy, rates of hearing preservation vary by series and by how hearing preservation is defined. As has been determined with other cranial nerve deficits described above, factors such as dose, fractionation, and tumor size all influence the rate of hearing loss after radiotherapy. For an in depth review of this topic, see Chapter 52.

23.7 Risk of Malignancy after Radiotherapy

Ionizing radiation induces double-strand breaks in DNA that can lead to cell death. One of the consequences of this damage is the potential to produce mutations that may result in tumorigenesis and malignancy, either within the treated VS or in the adjacent tissue. Though this potential is very low following radiotherapy for VS, it has been reported in case reports and series. For further review of this topic, see Chapter 24.

23.8 Conclusion

There are numerous series with large numbers of patients treated with single-session radiosurgery or multisession radiotherapy that confirm the safety and efficacy of radiosurgery and radiotherapy in the management of VS. Review of the available data indicates that rates of adverse effects including facial nerve paresis, trigeminal nerve dysfunction, and hydrocephalus are very low across radiation modalities when the appropriate patient selection and treatment planning are performed.

References

[1] Lunsford LD, Niranjan A, Flickinger JC, Maitz A, Kondziolka D. Radiosurgery of vestibular schwannomas: summary of experience in 829 cases. J Neurosurg. 2005; 102 Suppl:195–199

[2] Hasegawa T, Kida Y, Kato T, Iizuka H, Kuramitsu S, Yamamoto T. Long-term safety and efficacy of stereotactic radiosurgery for vestibular schwannomas: evaluation of 440 patients more than 10 years after treatment with Gamma Knife surgery. J Neurosurg. 2013; 118(3):557–565

[3] Yang I, Sughrue ME, Han SJ, et al. Facial nerve preservation after vestibular schwannoma Gamma Knife radiosurgery. J Neurooncol. 2009; 93(1):41–48

[4] Combs SE, Engelhard C, Kopp C, et al. Long-term outcome after highly advanced single-dose or fractionated radiotherapy in patients with vestibular schwannomas - pooled results from 3 large German centers. Radiother Oncol. 2015; 114(3):378–383

[5] Friedman WA, Bradshaw P, Myers A, Bova FJ. Linear accelerator radiosurgery for vestibular schwannomas. J Neurosurg. 2006; 105(5):657–661

[6] Champ CE, Shen X, Shi W, et al. Reduced-dose fractionated stereotactic radiotherapy for acoustic neuromas: maintenance of tumor control with improved hearing preservation. Neurosurgery. 2013; 73(3):489–496

[7] Aoyama H, Onodera S, Takeichi N, et al. Symptomatic outcomes in relation to tumor expansion after fractionated stereotactic radiation therapy for vestibular schwannomas: single-institutional long-term experience. Int J Radiat Oncol Biol Phys. 2013; 85(2):329–334

[8] Koh ES, Millar BA, Ménard C, et al. Fractionated stereotactic radiotherapy for acoustic neuroma: single-institution experience at The Princess Margaret Hospital. Cancer. 2007; 109(6):1203–1210

[9] Choy W, Spasic M, Pezeshkian P, et al. Outcomes of stereotactic radiosurgery and stereotactic radiotherapy for the treatment of vestibular schwannoma. Neurosurgery. 2013; 60 Suppl 1:120–125

[10] Kopp C, Fauser C, Müller A, et al. Stereotactic fractionated radiotherapy and LINAC radiosurgery in the treatment of vestibular schwannoma-report about both stereotactic methods from a single institution. Int J Radiat Oncol Biol Phys. 2011; 80(5):1485–1491

[11] Chan AW, Black P, Ojemann RG, et al. Stereotactic radiotherapy for vestibular schwannomas: favorable outcome with minimal toxicity. Neurosurgery. 2005; 57(1):60–70, discussion 60–70

[12] Hansasuta A, Choi CYH, Gibbs IC, et al. Multisession stereotactic radiosurgery for vestibular schwannomas: single-institution experience with 383 cases. Neurosurgery. 2011; 69(6):1200–1209

[13] Meijer OWM, Vandertop WP, Baayen JC, Slotman BJ. Single-fraction vs. fractionated linac-based stereotactic radiosurgery for vestibular schwannoma: a single-institution study. Int J Radiat Oncol Biol Phys. 2003; 56(5):1390–1396

[14] Lederman G, Lowry J, Wertheim S, et al. Acoustic neuroma: potential benefits of fractionated stereotactic radiosurgery. Stereotact Funct Neurosurg. 1997; 69(1–4, Pt 2):175–182

[15] Williams JA. Fractionated stereotactic radiotherapy for acoustic neuromas: preservation of function versus size. J Clin Neurosci. 2003; 10(1):48–52

[16] Collen C, Ampe B, Gevaert T, et al. Single fraction versus fractionated linac-based stereotactic radiotherapy for vestibular schwannoma: a single-institution experience. Int J Radiat Oncol Biol Phys. 2011; 81(4):e503–e509

[17] Weber DC, Chan AW, Bussiere MR, et al. Proton beam radiosurgery for vestibular schwannoma: tumor control and cranial nerve toxicity. Neurosurgery. 2003; 53(3):577–586, discussion 586–588

[18] Vernimmen FJAI, Mohamed Z, Slabbert JP, Wilson J. Long-term results of stereotactic proton beam radiotherapy for acoustic neuromas. Radiother Oncol. 2009; 90(2):208–212

[19] Bush DA, McAllister CJ, Loredo LN, Johnson WD, Slater JM, Slater JD. Fractionated proton beam radiotherapy for acoustic neuroma. Neurosurgery. 2002; 50(2):270–273, discussion 273–275

[20] Sughrue ME, Yang I, Han SJ, et al. Non-audiofacial morbidity after Gamma Knife surgery for vestibular schwannoma. Neurosurg Focus. 2009; 27(6):E4

[21] Andrews DW, Werner-Wasik M, Den RB, et al. Toward dose optimization for fractionated stereotactic radiotherapy for acoustic neuromas: comparison of two dose cohorts. Int J Radiat Oncol Biol Phys. 2009; 74(2):419–426

[22] Selch MT, Pedroso A, Lee SP, et al. Stereotactic radiotherapy for the treatment of acoustic neuromas. J Neurosurg. 2004; 101 Suppl 3:362–372
[23] Andrews DW, Suarez O, Goldman HW, et al. Stereotactic radiosurgery and fractionated stereotactic radiotherapy for the treatment of acoustic schwannomas: comparative observations of 125 patients treated at one institution. Int J Radiat Oncol Biol Phys. 2001; 50(5):1265–1278
[24] Poen JC, Golby AJ, Forster KM, et al. Fractionated stereotactic radiosurgery and preservation of hearing in patients with vestibular schwannoma: a preliminary report. Neurosurgery. 1999; 45(6):1299–1305
[25] Han JH, Kim DG, Chung HT, et al. The risk factors of symptomatic communicating hydrocephalus after stereotactic radiosurgery for unilateral vestibular schwannoma: the implication of brain atrophy. Int J Radiat Oncol Biol Phys. 2012; 84(4):937–942
[26] Woolf DK, Williams M, Goh CL, et al. Fractionated stereotactic radiotherapy for acoustic neuromas: long-term outcomes. Clin Oncol (R Coll Radiol). 2013; 25(12):734–738
[27] Djalilian HR, Benson AG, Ziai K, Safai Y, Thakkar KH, Mafee MF. Radiation necrosis of the brain after radiosurgery for vestibular schwannoma. Am J Otolaryngol. 2007; 28(5):338–341
[28] Dewan S, Norén G. Retreatment of vestibular schwannomas with Gamma Knife surgery. J Neurosurg. 2008; 109 Suppl:144–148
[29] Chung W-Y, Liu K-D, Shiau C-Y, et al. Gamma knife surgery for vestibular schwannoma: 10-year experience of 195 cases. J Neurosurg. 2005; 102 Suppl:87–96
[30] Fukuoka S, Takanashi M, Hojyo A, Konishi M, Tanaka C, Nakamura H. Gamma knife radiosurgery for vestibular schwannomas. Prog Neurol Surg. 2009; 22: 45–62
[31] Prasad D, Steiner M, Steiner L. Gamma surgery for vestibular schwannoma. J Neurosurg. 2000; 92(5):745–759
[32] Sawamura Y, Shirato H, Sakamoto T, et al. Management of vestibular schwannoma by fractionated stereotactic radiotherapy and associated cerebrospinal fluid malabsorption. J Neurosurg. 2003; 99(4):685–692

24 Risk of Radiation-Associated Tumorigenesis in the Treatment of Vestibular Schwannoma

Michael J. Torrens

24.1 Introduction

There has been increasing use of both fractionated radiotherapy (FRT)[1,2] and more conformal, stereotactically directed radiosurgery[3,4] for benign intracranial lesions over the last 20 years. In the case of vestibular schwannoma (VS), it has produced high control rates with few side effects compared to open surgery. Only around 60 cases were treated in North America by radiosurgery in 1990 but a prediction that over 1,000 cases per annum would be treated by 2010 has been fulfilled.[4] One of the possible disadvantages of radiosurgery has been the unknown frequency of radiation-induced secondary tumors.

The association of secondary neoplasia with therapeutic radiation is well known. A recent study[5] estimated that about 0.45% of the 298,000 new cancers registered in the United Kingdom in 2007 were associated with radiotherapy for a previous cancer. It is not so certain, however, that the conformal higher dose radiation used in radiosurgery has a similar effect. An important, prospective, controlled study from Sheffield, England,[6] followed 5,000 radiosurgery patients over 30,000 patient-years of follow-up and detected no increased risk of malignancy. However, sporadic case reports that suggest induction of malignancy by radiosurgery have been published, and in particular several cases of malignant transformation in VS (MTVS) have occurred. The purpose of this chapter is to evaluate the significance of these reports.

24.2 Radiation-Induced Tumors

The criteria for radiation-induced neoplasia as originally defined by Cahan et al[7] include: (1) the tumor must not be present at the time of irradiation; (2) there must be a prolonged latency period between radiation delivery and tumor development; (3) the tumor must arise in the irradiated region; (4) the tumor must be histologically distinct from the original tumor; and (5) the patient must not have a genetic predisposition to the development of cancer.

In the case of specific treatment of VS, the risk may be firstly of MTVS and secondly the induction of a separate secondary neoplasia in other tissue within the field of radiation.

24.3 Radiation Treatment of Vestibular Schwannoma

In this context, radiation has been delivered in three principal ways. FRT involves repeated small doses, usually less than 2 Gy and not with high conformality, being delivered over a period of weeks. Fractionated stereotactic radiotherapy (FSRT) requires more precise direction and conformality and may involve a hypofractionated regime of fewer and larger doses. Stereotactic radiosurgery (SRS) is highly selective and conformal with, classically, only one dose of around 12 Gy to the tumor margin (though the definition allows for up to five doses).

FRT has been used for the treatment of VS from at least 1945, at first usually in incompletely resected tumors, and such postoperative irradiation has been shown to decrease the chance for recurrence following subtotal resection from 46 to 6%.[8]

SRS for VS was first suggested by Leksell[9] in 1971 but did not become widespread until after 1990 when the improved delineation provided by MRI allowed conformal targeting. A recent study[10] of 440 patients followed for more than 10 years after SRS showed progression-free survival of 93% at 5 years and of 92% at 10 years, with 100% facial nerve preservation if the prescription dose was less than 13 Gy.

FSRT became an alternative after the success of SRS had been demonstrated, perhaps with the aim of improving hearing preservation. A recent large review[11] of 449 cases from Germany showed local control was 97% at 36 months, 95% at 60 months, and 94% at 120 months, with no statistical difference between FSRT and SRS. "Useful hearing" was preserved in 85% of the patients. Loss of useful hearing was observed in 14% in the FSRT group and in 16% in the SRS group.

In another recent review, Conley and Hirsch[12] also concluded that SRS and FRT are equally effective treatment modalities and that current evidence supports use of radiation for small-to-medium-sized primary and recurrent VSs with optimal dosing below 13 Gy. It is also recommended in poor surgical candidates and for those who do not desire observation or surgery.

24.4 Malignant Transformation in Vestibular Schwannoma

There have been, to date, 29 reports of MTVS after radiation (▶ Table 24.1).[13] However, the quantitated significance of this presumed radiation induction has not been clarified except in neurofibromatosis type 2 (NF2) where the incidence of malignancy is high in relation to the numbers treated.[14]

A total of 59 cases of malignant peripheral nerve sheath tumor (MPNST) of the vestibular nerve have been found reported in the literature, 29 cases occurring after radiation treatment, 25 cases arising spontaneously, and 5 cases occurring after surgery for benign disease (▶ Table 24.1, ▶ Table 24.2, ▶ Table 24.3).[13] In those irradiated cases with prior benign histology and therefore totally conforming to Cahan's criteria,[7] the mean delay to malignant expression was 68 months. A greater proportion of patients with NF2 in the irradiated group is compatible with the increased susceptibility of NF2 cases to radiation, having multiple tumors. Of the 29 cases after radiation, 11 of 26 (42%) with available information were suffering from neurofibromatosis, and of the 30 cases occurring without prior radiation, the equivalent proportion was 5 of 29 (17%).

An independent study[14] in patients with neurofibromatosis has revealed that in a population of 1,348 NF2 patients, 106 would have received radiosurgery. Malignant transformation occurred in five of these cases. This corresponds to a risk of $4{,}717 \times 10^{-5}$, a very substantially greater risk than in non-NF2 patients.

Table 24.1 Malignant transformation following radiation treatment

Authors and year	Age (y), sex	NF	Type of RT	Histological type	Cahan's criteria	Latency (mo)
Akamatsu et al 2010[32]	67, F	No	SRS	MPNST	Yes	90
Bari et al 2002[33]	28, F	Yes	SRS	MPNST		48
Baser et al 2000[34]	NS, NS	Yes	SRS	MPNST		NS
	NS, NS	Yes	SRS	MPNST		NS
	NS, NS	Yes	SRS	MPNST		NS
Carlson et al 2010[35]	25, F	Yes	SRS	Triton		120
Comey et al 1998[36]	50, M	No	SRS	Rhabdomyosarcoma		60
Demetriades et al 2010[37]	37, M	No	SRS	MPNST	Yes	120
Hanabusa et al 2001[38]	51, F	No	SRS	Sarcoma	Yes	6
Hasegawa et al 2013[10]	NS, NS	NS	SRS	MPNST		NS
Ho and Kveton 2002[39]	14, F	Yes	SRS	NS		7
Kubo et al 2005[40]	55, M	No	SRS	MPNST		NS
Maire et al 2006/Markou et al 2012[41]	45, F	No	CRT	MPNST		231
McEvoy and Kitchen 2003[42]	22, M	Yes	SRS	NS		24
Muracciole et al 2004[43]	61, F	No	SRS	Triton		72
Newell and Pollack 2012[44]	50, M	No	Yes	MPNST		NS
Norén 1998[45]	18, F	Yes	SRS	MPNST		60
Pollock et al 1998[46]	NS, NS	NS	SRS	Triton		NS
Puataweepong et al 2012[47]	34, F	No	SRS	MPNST		72
Scheithauer et al 2009[48]	32, M	Yes	CRT	MPNST		324
Schmitt et al 2011[49]	51, M	No	SRS	Sarcoma		87
Shin et al 2002; Kurita 1997[50]	26, F	No	SRS	MPNST	Yes	72
Tanbouzi Husseini et al 2011[51]	20, M	Yes	SRS	MPNST		60
Thomsen et al 2000[52]	19, F	Yes	SRS	Sarcoma	Yes	72
Van Rompaey et al 2009[53]	53, F	No	SRS	MPNST		96
Wilkinson et al 2004[54]	53, M	No	SRS	MPNST	Yes	48
Yanamadala et al 2013[55]	51, F	No	SRS	MPNST	Yes	60
Yang et al 2010[56]	74, M	No	SRS	Sarcoma	Yes	72
Seferis et al 2014[13]	34, F	No	SRS	MPNST	Yes	72

Abbreviations: CRT, conformal radiotherapy; MPNST, malignant peripheral nerve sheath tumor; NF, evidence of neurofibromatosis; NS, not stated; RT, prior exposure to radiation; SRS, stereotactic radiosurgery.
Source: Used with permission from Seferis C, Torrens M, Paraskevopoulou C, Psichidis G. Malignant transformation in vestibular schwannoma: report of a single case, literature search, and debate. J Neurosurg. 2014; 121 Suppl:160–166.[13]

However, it is less easy to quantify the risk in non-NF2 cases because the condition is very rare and the true incidence depends on the accuracy of reporting of individual cases. In particular, there may be a tendency to report MTVS after radiation more readily than cases arising spontaneously.

There are several reasons to assume that MTVS after radiation is a genuine entity. The first is the delay or latency from diagnosis to malignant expression. In the irradiated group, this is 68 months (in those with confirmative initial benign histology) or 85 months (all cases) compared with 7.2 months in those nonirradiated cases where there was a prior histological diagnosis. This would suggest that the irradiated cases are showing the delay required by the Cahan criteria for malignant induction, whereas the nonirradiated cases are already in the process of malignant expression. Secondly, the irradiated group has a larger proportion of cases in which the histology shows a sarcomatous element (8/27, or 29.6%) compared with the nonirradiated group (4/30, or 13.3%).[13] Sarcomatous differentiation is known to be associated with irradiation and the overall incidence of postradiation sarcoma in patients who survive longer than 5 years following radiation therapy is about 0.1%.[15] Thirdly, there has been a threefold increase in the number of case reports of MTVS since the year 2000 (▶ Table 24.4).[13] If a delay period of 5 to 8 years, according to Cahan's criteria, is added to the decade of 1990 when significant numbers of radiosurgical treatments began to be performed, then an increase in reported cases of MTVS would be expected from 2000 onward if radiation is a significant predisposing factor.

The most important question is to evaluate the quantitative significance of radiation in the induction of MTVS. In relation to the number of VS presenting worldwide per annum of between 72,000 and 114,000,[16] it has been calculated[13] that there is a risk of developing a spontaneous malignancy between 1.32×10^{-5} and 2.08×10^{-5}. If only the 25 cases not associated with NF2 are considered, then the chance becomes between 1.09×10^{-5} and 1.74×10^{-5}.

Table 24.2 Spontaneous occurrence of malignant vestibular nerve tumors

Authors and year	Age (y), sex	NF	RT	Histological type
Best 1987[57]	24, F	Yes	None	Triton
Caporlingua et al 2014[58]	50, F	No	None	Triton (?)
Chen et al 2008[59]	62, F	No	None	MPNST
Earls et al 1994[60]	NS, NS	NS	NS	Melanotic
Gong et al 2012[61]	55, F	No	None	Triton
Gonzalez et al 2007[62]	43, F	No	NS	MPNST
Gruber et al 1994[63]	61, F	No	None	MPNST
Han et al 1992[64]	47, F	No	None	Triton
Harada et al 2000[65]	10, M	No	None	MPNST
Hernanz-Schulman et al 1986[66]	NS, child	No	None	MPNST
Higami et al 1998[67]	45, F	Yes	None	MPNST
Hong et al 2014[68]	25, M	No	None	MPNST
Karami et al 2011[69]	23, F	No	None	MPNST
Kudo et al 1983[70]	54, M	No	None	MPNST
Kuzmik et al 2013[71]	73, F	No	None	MPNST
Maeda et al 1993[72]	38, M	No	None	MPNST
Matsumoto et al 1990[73]	54, M	No	None	MPNST
Miller et al 1986[74]	74, M	Yes (?)	None	Melanotic
Mrak et al 1994[75]	40, M	No	None	MPNST
Saito et al 2000[76]	69, M	No	None	Melanotic
Scheithauer et al 2009[77]	32, M	Yes	None	MPNST
	26, F	No	None	MPNST
	5, M	No	None	MPNST
Suresh et al 2003[78]	NS, NS	Yes	None	MPNST
Wei et al 2012[79]	41, F	No	NS	MPNST

Abbreviations: MPNST, malignant peripheral nerve sheath tumor; NF, evidence of neurofibromatosis; NS, not stated; RT, prior exposure to radiation.
Source: Used with permission from Seferis C, Torrens M, Paraskevopoulou C, Psichidis G. Malignant transformation in vestibular schwannoma: report of a single case, literature search, and debate. J Neurosurg. 2014; 121 Suppl:160 -166.[13]

Extrapolation from the records of the Leksell Gamma Knife Society[17] and a survey by the Acoustic Neuroma Association[18] suggests that a very provisional total number of VS cases treated by radiation worldwide could be 115,333. In relation to the 29 patients with postirradiation MTVS recorded over 20 years, the risk is 29 in 115,333 or 25.1×10^{-5}. If patients with neurofibromatosis are excluded from this analysis, there remain 18 patients with MPNST associated with radiation and so the risk for malignant transformation in the absence of neurofibromatosis is reduced to 15.6×10^{-5}. This represents a 9 to 14 times increased probability of malignancy in relation to the spontaneous incidence of between 1.09×10^{-5} and 1.74×10^{-5}. Compared with MTVS, the frequency of reporting other induced malignancies is smaller.

24.5 Glioblastoma

In total, 191 cases of radiation-induced glioma have been reported[19] and no doubt the true number is significantly higher but, up to now, this complication appears rarely in association with radiation treatment of VS. Balasubramaniam et al[20] collected two cases of glioblastoma following irradiation of VS, one by SRS and one by FSRT, and in both cases the dose to the area of the temporal lobe where the glioblastoma developed was 4 to 5 Gy. Neither suffered from NF2. Baser et al[14] describe a neurofibromatosis patient who developed a malignant ependymoma (glial series tumor) following radiation treatment of VS.

Table 24.4 Cases of malignant VSs presenting over time

Dates of publication of MPNST cases	No. of cases recorded
1983–1989	4
1990–1994	6
1995–1999	5
2000–2004	14
2005–2009	11
2010–2014	18

Abbreviation: MPNST, malignant peripheral nerve sheath tumor.
Source: Used with permission from Seferis C, Torrens M, Paraskevopoulou C, Psichidis G. Malignant transformation in vestibular schwannoma: report of a single case, literature search, and debate. J Neurosurg. 2014; 121 Suppl:160 -166.[13]

Table 24.3 Malignant transformation of a benign entity

Authors and year	Age (y), sex	NF	RT	Histological type	Prior benign histological type	Latency (mo)
Gousias et al 2010[80]	64, M	No	None	MPNST	No[a]	120
McLean et al 1990[81]	75, M	No	None	MPNST	Yes	11
Scheithauer et al 2009[82]	67, M	No	None	MPNST	Yes	9
	56, M	No	None	MPNST	Yes	7
Son et al 2001[83]	33, F	No	None	MPNST	Yes	2

Abbreviations: MPNST, malignant peripheral nerve sheath tumor; NF, evidence of neurofibromatosis; RT, prior exposure to radiation.
Source: Used with permission from Seferis C, Torrens M, Paraskevopoulou C, Psichidis G. Malignant transformation in vestibular schwannoma: report of a single case, literature search, and debate. J Neurosurg. 2014; 121 Suppl:160 -166.[13]
[a]No histology report available, but MRI over 120 months clearly shows a benign process that progressed to malignant disease.

24.6 Meningioma

Induction of meningiomas after radiation is well known. A first case was described in 1953.[21] The Israeli study[22] in 1988 showed that patients exposed to as little as 2 Gy at a young age for treatment of tinea capitis were at a 9.5 times higher risk of developing intracranial meningiomas. They also had an 18.8 times risk for developing nerve sheath tumors. Twenty-two percent of children with leukemia undergoing cranial irradiation were observed to develop meningiomas with a median latency of 25 years.[23]

However, a literature search performed for this communication revealed only one meningioma, of a malignant nature, following radiation treatment of VS.[14] Otherwise, though meningiomas represent 70% of radiation-induced tumors, the number induced by highly conformal radiosurgery of targets appears to be very low in comparison to conventional radiotherapy, at least at the present time. Only three reports[24,25] were found in the literature though the author is aware of one other probable case following Gamma Knife treatment of a Cushing's pituitary adenoma with a latency of 10 years.

This relatively low incidence must be regarded with caution. The latency of meningioma development after the Nagasaki atomic bomb was 35 to 40 years.[26] Many more cases, including those after radiation treatment of VS, should be expected after 2025.

24.6.1 Other Tumors

Five cases of radiation-induced tumors of the temporal bone have been described (two osteosarcomas, two fibrosarcomas, and one squamous cell carcinoma).[27] All five temporal bone tumors occurred in individuals who had previously received more than 50-Gy FRT. The initial histologic diagnoses included two astrocytomas, a jugular paraganglioma, a malignant meningioma, and a VS.

24.7 Conclusion

Despite recent more frequent reports of MTVS after radiation, it is difficult to quantitate the overall risk of malignant induction because of the unreliability of reporting and the long latency to development in some cases. The risk over 30,000 years of follow-up was said to be insignificant,[6] but the possible incidence of MTVS in non-NF2 cases noted above[13] is one to two cases in 200,000 years of follow-up. It is clear that the risk in NF2 is high in relation to the number of cases treated at $4{,}717 \times 10^{-5}$, or 4.7%.[14]

The most recent analysis of reported cases[13] reveals that after radiation treatment the overall risk of MTVS over 20 years is 25.1×10^{-5}, or 0.025%, and this reduces to 15.6×10^{-5}, or 0.016%, if cases of NF2 are excluded. In relation to spontaneous malignancy in non-NF2 cases, where the risk is between 1.09×10^{-5} and 1.74×10^{-5}, or about 0.0014%, radiation treatment increases the risk of MTVS by approximately 10 times.

Thus, radiation treatment including SRS is significant in the induction of MTVS but the risk appears small in the region of 0.01 to 0.02%. In addition, there is a relatively smaller risk of other induced neoplasia such as glioblastoma or meningioma. Reported cases suggest that this figure is only five cases, or 4.3×10^{-5}, which increases the overall risk to about 0.02%. This compares with a realistic mortality rate after craniotomy for VS of at least 1%,[28,29] although there are a few small surgical series of selected cases without mortality.[30] In comparison, the risk of developing an SRS-induced neoplasm after radiosurgery in any part of the brain has been calculated as approximately 0.04% at 15 years.[31]

These conclusions must be provisional because they depend on an unknown frequency of reporting of induced neoplasia. In addition, the long latency before the appearance of secondary neoplasms, especially of meningioma, means that the situation could be different in 10 to 20 years' time. However, it is unlikely that the mortality of surgery will fall enough, or the incidence of secondary neoplasia will rise, for the risks to become comparable in the foreseeable future. Radiation treatment of VS will remain a treatment of first choice in selected cases but it is as important that the patient be informed of the risk of tumorigenesis as it is for them to be informed of the risk of mortality after open surgery.

References

[1] Varlotto JM, Shrieve DC, Alexander E, III, Kooy HM, Black PM, Loeffler JS. Fractionated stereotactic radiotherapy for the treatment of acoustic neuromas: preliminary results. Int J Radiat Oncol Biol Phys. 1996; 36(1):141–145

[2] Litre F, Rousseaux P, Jovenin N, et al. Fractionated stereotactic radiotherapy for acoustic neuromas: a prospective monocenter study of about 158 cases. Radiother Oncol. 2013; 106(2):169–174

[3] Leksell L. Stereotactic radiosurgery. J Neurol Neurosurg Psychiatry. 1983; 46 (9):797–803

[4] Pollock BE, Lunsford LD, Norén G. Vestibular schwannoma management in the next century: a radiosurgical perspective. Neurosurgery. 1998; 43(3): 475–481, discussion 481–483

[5] Maddams J, Parkin DM, Darby SC. The cancer burden in the United Kingdom in 2007 due to radiotherapy. Int J Cancer. 2011; 129(12):2885–2893

[6] Rowe J, Grainger A, Walton L, Silcocks P, Radatz M, Kemeny A. Risk of malignancy after gamma knife stereotactic radiosurgery. Neurosurgery. 2007; 60 (1):60–65, discussion 65–66

[7] Cahan WG, Woodard HQ, Higinbotham NL, Stewart FW, Coley BL. Sarcoma arising in irradiated bone: report of eleven cases. 1948. Cancer. 1998; 82(1): 8–34

[8] Wallner KE, Sheline GE, Pitts LH, Wara WM, Davis RL, Boldrey EB. Efficacy of irradiation for incompletely excised acoustic neurilemomas. J Neurosurg. 1987; 67(6):858–863

[9] Leksell L. A note on the treatment of acoustic tumours. Acta Chir Scand. 1971; 137(8):763–765

[10] Hasegawa T, Kida Y, Kato T, Iizuka H, Kuramitsu S, Yamamoto T. Long-term safety and efficacy of stereotactic radiosurgery for vestibular schwannomas: evaluation of 440 patients more than 10 years after treatment with Gamma Knife surgery. J Neurosurg. 2013; 118(3):557–565

[11] Combs SE, Engelhard C, Kopp C, et al. Long-term outcome after highly advanced single-dose or fractionated radiotherapy in patients with vestibular schwannomas - pooled results from 3 large German centers. Radiother Oncol. 2015; 114(3):378–383

[12] Conley GS, Hirsch BE. Stereotactic radiation treatment of vestibular schwannoma: indications, limitations, and outcomes. Curr Opin Otolaryngol Head Neck Surg. 2010; 18(5):351–356

[13] Seferis C, Torrens M, Paraskevopoulou C, Psichidis G. Malignant transformation in vestibular schwannoma: report of a single case, literature search, and debate. J Neurosurg. 2014; 121 Suppl:160–166

[14] Baser ME, Evans DG, Jackler RK, Sujansky E, Rubenstein A. Neurofibromatosis 2, radiosurgery and malignant nervous system tumours. Br J Cancer. 2000; 82 (4):998

[15] Inoue YZ, Frassica FJ, Sim FH, Unni KK, Petersen IA, McLeod RA. Clinicopathologic features and treatment of postirradiation sarcoma of bone and soft tissue. J Surg Oncol. 2000; 75(1):42–50

[16] Babu R, Sharma R, Bagley JH, Hatef J, Friedman AH, Adamson C. Vestibular schwannomas in the modern era: epidemiology, treatment trends, and disparities in management. J Neurosurg. 2013; 119(1):121–130

[17] Leksell Gamma Knife Society. Indications treated from 1991 to 2014. Available at: https://www.lgksociety.com/fileadmin/groups/1/Documents/Treatment_Statistics/2014/1968–2014_Indications_Treated.pdf. Accessed January 11, 2016

[18] Acoustic Neuroma Association. ANA Survey/Registry. Available at: https://www.anausa.org/resources/patient-surveys. Accessed January 11, 2016

[19] Yamanaka R, Hayano A. Radiation-induced gliomas. In: Lichtor T, ed. Molecular Considerations and Evolving Surgical Management Issues in the Treatment of Patients with a Brain Tumor. Available at: http://cdn.intechopen.com/pdfs-wm/47617.pdf. Accessed December 22, 2015

[20] Balasubramaniam A, Shannon P, Hodaie M, Laperriere N, Michaels H, Guha A. Glioblastoma multiforme after stereotactic radiotherapy for acoustic neuroma: case report and review of the literature. Neuro Oncol. 2007; 9(4): 447–453

[21] Mann I, Yates PC, Ainslie JP. Unusual case of double primary orbital tumour. Br J Ophthalmol. 1953; 37(12):758–762

[22] Ron E, Modan B, Boice JD, Jr, et al. Tumors of the brain and nervous system after radiotherapy in childhood. N Engl J Med. 1988; 319(16): 1033–1039

[23] Banerjee J, Pääkkö E, Harila M, et al. Radiation-induced meningiomas: a shadow in the success story of childhood leukemia. Neuro Oncol. 2009; 11 (5):543–549

[24] Copeland WR, Link MJ. A radiation-induced meningioma "cures" a complex dural arteriovenous fistula. J Neurol Surg A Cent Eur Neurosurg. 2013; 74 Suppl 1:e215–e220

[25] Sheehan J, Yen CP, Steiner L. Gamma knife surgery-induced meningioma. Report of two cases and review of the literature. J Neurosurg. 2006; 105(2): 325–329

[26] Sadamori N, Shibata S, Mine M, et al. Incidence of intracranial meningiomas in Nagasaki atomic-bomb survivors. Int J Cancer. 1996; 67(3):318–322

[27] Lustig LR, Jackler RK, Lanser MJ. Radiation-induced tumors of the temporal bone. Am J Otol. 1997; 18(2):230–235

[28] Samii M, Matthies C. Management of 1000 vestibular schwannomas (acoustic neuromas): surgical management and results with an emphasis on complications and how to avoid them. Neurosurgery. 1997; 40(1):11–21, discussion 21–23

[29] Cardoso AC, Fernandes YB, Ramina R, Borges G. Acoustic neuroma: surgical results on 240 patients. Arq Neuropsiquiatr. 2007; 65 3A:605–609

[30] Shahinian HK, Ra Y. 527 fully endoscopic resections of vestibular schwannomas. Minim Invasive Neurosurg. 2011; 54(2):61–67

[31] Patel TR, Chiang VL. Secondary neoplasms after stereotactic radiosurgery. World Neurosurg. 2014; 81(3–4):594–599

[32] Akamatsu Y, Murakami K, Watanabe M, Jokura H, Tominaga T. Malignant peripheral nerve sheath tumor arising from benign vestibular schwannoma treated by gamma knife radiosurgery after two previous surgeries: a case report with surgical and pathological observations. World Neurosurg 73: 751?754, 2010

[33] Bari ME, Forster DM, Kemeny AA, Walton L, Hardy D, Anderson JR. Malignancy in a vestibular schwannoma. Report of a case with central neurofibromatosis, treated by both stereotactic radiosurgery and surgical excision, with a review of the literature. Br J Neurosurg 16:284?289, 2002

[34] Baser ME, Evans DG, Jackler RK, Sujansky E, Rubenstein A. Neurofibromatosis 2, radiosurgery and malignant nervous system tumours. Br J Cancer 82:998, 2000

[35] Carlson ML, Babovic-Vuksanovic D, Messiaen L, Scheithauer BW, Neff BA, Link MJ. Radiation-induced rhabdomyosarcoma of the brainstem in a patient with neurofibromatosis type 2. Case report. J Neurosurg 112:81?87, 2010 (Erratum in J Neurosurg 112:209, 2010)

[36] Comey CH, McLaughlin MR, Jho HD, Martinez AJ, Lunsford LD. Death from a malignant cerebellopontine angle triton tumor despite stereotactic radiosurgery. Case report. J Neurosurg 89:653?658, 1998

[37] Demetriades AK, Saunders N, Rose P, Fisher C, Rowe J, Tranter R, et al. Malignant transformation of acoustic neuroma/ vestibular schwannoma 10 years after gamma knife stereotactic radiosurgery. Skull Base 20:381?387, 2010

[38] Hanabusa K, Morikawa A, Murata T, Taki W. Acoustic neuroma with malignant transformation. Case report. J Neurosurg 95:518?521, 2001

[39] Ho SY, Kveton JF. Rapid growth of acoustic neuromas after stereotactic radiotherapy in type 2 neurofibromatosis. Ear Nose Throat J 81:831?833, 2002

[40] Kubo O, Chernov M, Izawa M, Hayashi M, Muragaki Y, Maruyama T, et al. Malignant progression of benign brain tumors after gamma knife radiosurgery: is it really caused by irradiation? Minim Invasive Neurosurg 48:334?339, 2005

[41] Maire JP, Huchet A, Milbeo Y, Darrouzet V, Causse N, Célérier D, et al. Twenty years? experience in the treatment of acoustic neuromas with fractionated radiotherapy: a review of 45 cases. Int J Radiat Oncol Biol Phys 66:170?178, 2006

[42] McEvoy AW, Kitchen ND. Rapid enlargement of a vestibular schwannoma following gamma knife treatment. Minim Invasive Neurosurg 46:254?256, 2003

[43] Muracciole X, Cowen D, Régis J. [Radiosurgery and brain radio-induced carcinogenesis: update.] Neurochirurgie 50: 414?420, 2004 (Fr)

[44] Newell K, Pollack A. Bilateral cranial nerve VII-VIII malignant peripheral nerve sheath tumors mimicking neurofibromatosis type 2. J Neuropathol Exp Neurol 71:593, 2012

[45] Norén G. Long-term complications following gamma knife radiosurgery of vestibular schwannomas. Stereot Funct Neurosurg 70 Suppl:165?173, 1998

[46] Pollock BE, Lunsford LD, Kondziolka D, Sekula R, Subach BR, Foote RL, et al. Vestibular schwannoma management. Part II. Failed radiosurgery and the role of delayed microsurgery. J Neurosurg 89:949?955, 1998

[47] Puataweepong P, Janwityanujit T, Larbcharoensub N, Dhanachai M. Radiation-induced peripheral malignant nerve sheath tumor arising from vestibular schwannoma after linac-based stereotactic radiation therapy: a case report and review of literatures. Case Rep Med 2012:648191, 2012

[48] Scheithauer BW, Erdogan S, Rodriguez FJ, et al. Malignant peripheral nerve sheath tumors of cranial nerves and intracranial contents: a clinicopathologic study of 17 cases. Am J Surg Pathol 33:325?338, 2009

[49] Schmitt WR, Carlson ML, Giannini C, et al.Radiation-induced sarcoma in a large vestibular schwannoma following stereotactic radiosurgery: case report. Neurosurgery 68:E840?E846, 2011

[50] Shin M, Ueki K, Kurita H, Kirino T. Malignant transformation of a vestibular schwannoma after gamma knife radiosurgery. Lancet 360:309?310, 2002

[51] Tanbouzi Husseini S, Piccirillo E, et al. Malignancy in vestibular schwannoma after stereotactic radiotherapy: a case report and review of the literature. Laryngoscope 121:923?928, 2011

[52] Thomsen J, Mirz F, Wetke R, Astrup J, Bojsen-Møller M, Nielsen E. Intracranial sarcoma in a patient with neurofibromatosis type 2 treated with gamma knife radiosurgery for vestibular schwannoma. Am J Otol 21:364?370, 2000

[53] Van Rompaey K, Michotte A, Ampe B, Moens M, Ates R, Chaskis C, et al. Malignant transformation of a vestibular schwannoma after radiosurgery. Surg Neurol 71:145, 2009

[54] Wilkinson JS, Reid H, Armstrong GR. Malignant transformation of a recurrent vestibular schwannoma. J Clin Pathol 57:109?110, 2004

[55] Yanamadala V, Williamson RW, Fusco DJ, Eschbacher J, Weisskopf P, Porter RW. Malignant transformation of a vestibular schwannoma after gamma knife radiosurgery. World Neurosurg 79:593.e1?593.e8, 2013

[56] Yang T, Rockhill J, Born DE, Sekhar LN. A case of highgrade undifferentiated sarcoma after surgical resection and stereotactic radiosurgery of a vestibular schwannoma. Skull Base 20:179?183, 2010

[57] Best PV. Malignant triton tumour in the cerebellopontine angle. Report of a case. Acta Neuropathol 74:92?96, 1987

[58] Caporlingua F, Lapadula G, Antonelli M, Missori P. Pleomorphic rhabdomyosarcoma of the cerebellopontine angle in an adult: a review of literature. BMJ Case Rep 2014: bcr2013203257, 2014

[59] Chen L, Mao Y, Chen H, Zhou LF. Diagnosis and management of intracranial malignant peripheral nerve sheath tumors. Neurosurgery 62:825?832, 2008

[60] Earls JP, Robles HA, McAdams HP, Rao KC. General case of the day. Malignant melanotic schwannoma of the eighth cranial nerve. Radiographics 14:1425?1427, 1994

[61] Gong L, Liu XY, Zhang WD, Han XJ, Yao L, Zhu SJ, et al. A rare case of malignant triton tumor in the cerebellopontine angle. Diagn Pathol 7:43, 2012

[62] Gonzalez LF, Lekovic GP, Eschbacher J, Coons S, Spetzler RF. A true malignant schwannoma of the eighth cranial nerve: case report. Neurosurgery 61: E421?E422, 2007

[63] Gruber B, Petchenik L, Williams M, Thomas C, Luken MG. Malignant vestibular schwannoma. Skull Base Surg 4:227? 231, 1994

[64] Han DH, Kim DG, Chi JG, Park SH, Jung HW, Kim YG. Malignant triton tumor of the acoustic nerve. Case report. J Neurosurg 76:874?877, 1992

[65] Harada K, Nishizaki T, Adachi N, Suzuki M, Ito H. Pediatric acoustic schwannoma showing rapid regrowth with high proliferative activity. Childs Nerv Syst 16:134?137, 2000

[66] Hernanz-Schulman M, Welch K, Strand R, Ordia JI. Acoustic neuromas in children. AJNR Am J Neuroradiol 7:519?521, 1986

[67] Higami Y, Shimokawa I, Kishikawa M, Okimoto T, Ohtani H, Tomita M, et al. Malignant peripheral nerve sheath tumors developing multifocally in the

central nervous system in a patient with neurofibromatosis type 2. Clin Neuropathol 17:115?120, 1998

[68] Hong W, Cheng H, Wang X, Hu X, Feng C. Study of malignant peripheral nerve sheath tumor in cerebellopontine angle. J Craniofac Surg 25:699?701, 2014

[69] Karami KJ, Kelkar PS, Verdon MP, Grills IS, Bojrab DI, Pieper DR. Malignant peripheral nerve sheath tumor of the vestibulocochlear nerve and brainstem: multimodality treatment with survival of 27 months. A case report and review of the literature. Neurosurgery 69:E1152?E1165, 2011

[70] Kudo M, Matsumoto M, Terao H. Malignant nerve sheath tumor of acoustic nerve. Arch Pathol Lab Med 107:293?297, 1983

[71] Kuzmik GA, Michaelides EM, Chiang VL, Nonaka Y, Fukushima T, Vortmeyer AO, et al. Rapidly progressive epithelioid malignant peripheral nerve sheath tumor of the vestibular nerve. Otol Neurotol 34:1739?1742, 2013

[72] Maeda M, Jozaki T, Baba S, Muro H, Shirasawa H, Ichihashi T. Malignant nerve sheath tumor with rhabdomyoblastic differentiation arising from the acoustic nerve. Acta Pathol Jpn 43:198?203, 1993

[73] Matsumoto M, Sakata Y, Sanpei K, Onagi A, Terao H, Kudo M. [Malignant schwannoma of acoustic nerve: a case report.] No Shinkei Geka 18:59?62, 1990 (Jpn)

[74] Miller RT, Sarikaya H, Sos A. Melanotic schwannoma of the acoustic nerve. Arch Pathol Lab Med 110:153?154, 1986

[75] Mrak RE, Flanigan S, Collins CL. Malignant acoustic schwannoma. Arch Pathol Lab Med 118:557?561, 1994

[76] Saito T, Oki S, Mikami T, Kawamoto Y, Yamaguchi S, Kuwamoto K, et al. [Malignant peripheral nerve sheath tumor with divergent cartilage differentiation from the acoustic nerve: case report.] No To Shinkei 52:734?739, 2000 (Jpn)

[77] Scheithauer BW, Erdogan S, Rodriguez FJ, Burger PC, Woodruff JM, Kros JM, et al. Malignant peripheral nerve sheath tumors of cranial nerves and intracranial contents: a clinicopathologic study of 17 cases. Am J Surg Pathol 33:325?338, 2009

[78] Suresh TN, Mahadevan A, Chandrashekhar Sagar B, Santosh V, Yasha TC, Shankar SK. Unusual case of multiple cellular and malignant schwannomas of the cranial and spinal nerves. Clin Neuropathol 22:23?29, 2003

[79] Wei C, Heman-Ackah SE, Newman K, Zagzag D, Golfinos JG, Roland JT Jr. Temporal bone histopathology case of the month: malignant peripheral nerve sheath tumor arising within vestibular schwannoma. Otol Neurotol 33:e83?e84, 2012

[80] Gousias K, Boström J, Kovacs A, Niehusmann P, Wagner I, Kristof R. Factors of influence upon overall survival in the treatment of intracranial MPNSTs. Review of the literature and report of a case. Radiat Oncol 5:114, 2010

[81] McLean CA, Laidlaw JD, Brownbill DS, Gonzales MF. Recurrence of acoustic neurilemoma as a malignant spindle-cell neoplasm. Case report. J Neurosurg 73:946?950, 1990

[82] Scheithauer BW, Erdogan S, Rodriguez FJ, Burger PC, Woodruff JM, Kros JM, et al. Malignant peripheral nerve sheath tumors of cranial nerves and intracranial contents: a clinicopathologic study of 17 cases. Am J Surg Pathol 33:325?338, 2009

[83] Son EI, Kim IM, Kim SP. Vestibular schwannoma with malignant transformation: a case report. J Korean Med Sci 16: 817?821, 2001

25 Imaging Follow-up After Radiosurgery of Vestibular Schwannoma

Bruce E. Pollock and Michael J. Link

25.1 Introduction

Over the past 30 years, stereotactic radiosurgery (SRS) has emerged as an accepted treatment option for patients with small-to-moderated-sized vestibular schwannomas (VSs). Over this time period, changes to VS SRS have included the use of magnetic resonance imaging (MRI) for dose planning, improved dose planning software, lower radiation doses, and an appreciation that cochlear radiation dose may affect hearing outcomes.[1,2,3,4] The most important modification in SRS technique was marginal dose reduction from 18–20 to 12–13 Gy, but the other alterations have also contributed to improved patient outcomes. Cranial nerve morbidity after contemporary VS SRS is markedly lower when compared to early studies, and facial nerve outcomes and early hearing preservation rates have been shown to be significantly better after SRS compared to surgical resection.[5,6,7,8] Based on the efficacy and safety of SRS for properly selected VSs, more than 100,000 patients have undergone VS SRS. However, misinterpretation of the follow-up imaging after VS SRS is not uncommon and physicians may prematurely conclude that SRS has failed, leading to patients having unnecessary and inappropriate surgery. In this chapter, management recommendations are presented based on the imaging characteristics of VS after SRS.

25.2 Methods of Tumor Size Assessment

After VS SRS, patients are requested to have follow-up clinical evaluation to assess cranial nerve function, audiometric testing for patients with pre-SRS serviceable hearing, and MRI to determine tumor size, evaluate for edema in the adjacent brain, and monitor for ventricular enlargement. Although each center will follow its own protocol after VS SRS, we typically request follow-up at 6, 12, 24, and 48 months, and then biyearly after the procedure. However, many patients live a long distance from the center that performed SRS, so review of clinical information and MRI from local care providers is not uncommon.

Two methods are commonly used to assess tumor response after VS SRS. Both techniques rely on comparison of the tumor size at the time of SRS to follow-up examinations. Although computed tomography (CT) is necessary in some patients who cannot undergo MRI, the vast majority of patients are followed with serial MRI. The first method is based on the comparison of linear measurements of the cerebellopontine angle (CPA) component in the right–left (x-plane), anterior–posterior (y-plane), and superior–inferior (z-plane).[9] In most cases, the intracanalicular tumor follows the CPA tumor response and is not formally compared. Tumor size is generally classified as unchanged, decreased, or increased. For most series, a change of 2 mm or greater in average tumor diameter is needed for tumors to be considered decreased or increased in size. As noted by Linskey et al,[9] the change in tumor volume necessary for tumors to be significantly changed compared to the time of SRS must account for potential measurement errors and the initial tumor size. For example, tumors with an average diameter < 1 cm must increase approximately 100% in volume before tumor enlargement can be reliably identified, whereas tumors > 2 cm in average diameter need only a 25% increase to safely state that the tumor has enlarged. Linear measurement comparisons are simple and are the most common technique utilized in both clinical practice and published VS studies.

The second method is based on comparison of tumor volumes at the time of SRS to follow-up MRI.[10,11] This technique is more sensitive to small changes in tumor size than comparison of linear measurements, but it is more time consuming, requiring segmenting (outlining) the tumor on post-SRS to determine the tumor volume. Accurate volumetric determination is closely correlated to MRI slice thickness, especially for smaller tumors. In most series, tumor volume is defined as unchanged or stable if it falls within a range of 10 to 15% of the pre-SRS volume, so that tumors that change more than 10 to 15% are defined as enlarged or regressed. To date, quantitative volumetric analysis is used primarily as a research tool that more accurately defines tumor response after SRS, but its day-to-day value in the clinical management of patients remains unclear.

25.3 Expected Imaging Changes after Vestibular Schwannoma Radiosurgery

The imaging changes seen after SRS of VS were first recognized by Georg Norén during his time at the Karolinska Institute, Stockholm, Sweden.[12,13] He noted that the majority of VS will exhibit "swelling" with a loss of central enhancement and an increase in tumor size. This pseudoprogression (also described as tumor expansion) is generally noted 3 to 12 months after SRS, and is followed by the tumor regaining its central enhancement on later imaging with a subsequent stabilization or reduction in tumor size (▶ Fig. 25.1).[10,11,14,15,16,17,18,19,20] The average increase in tumor volume during this period has been reported from 23 to 27%,[15,18] with the majority of tumors regressing to less than the pre-SRS volume on serial imaging (▶ Fig. 25.2). Previously, we described three patterns of tumor volume changes in VS patients whose tumors enlarged after SRS.[20] Type 1 patients showed eventual tumor regression to either the same or reduced volume. Type 2 patients had tumors that increased and remained larger but did not show progressive enlargement (▶ Fig. 25.3). Type 3 patients showed progressive tumor enlargement on serial studies denoting treatment failure. ▶ Table 25.1 shows the results for a number of studies on VS SRS. The range of treatment failure after VS SRS is between 2 and 12%, depending on the criteria used at each center.

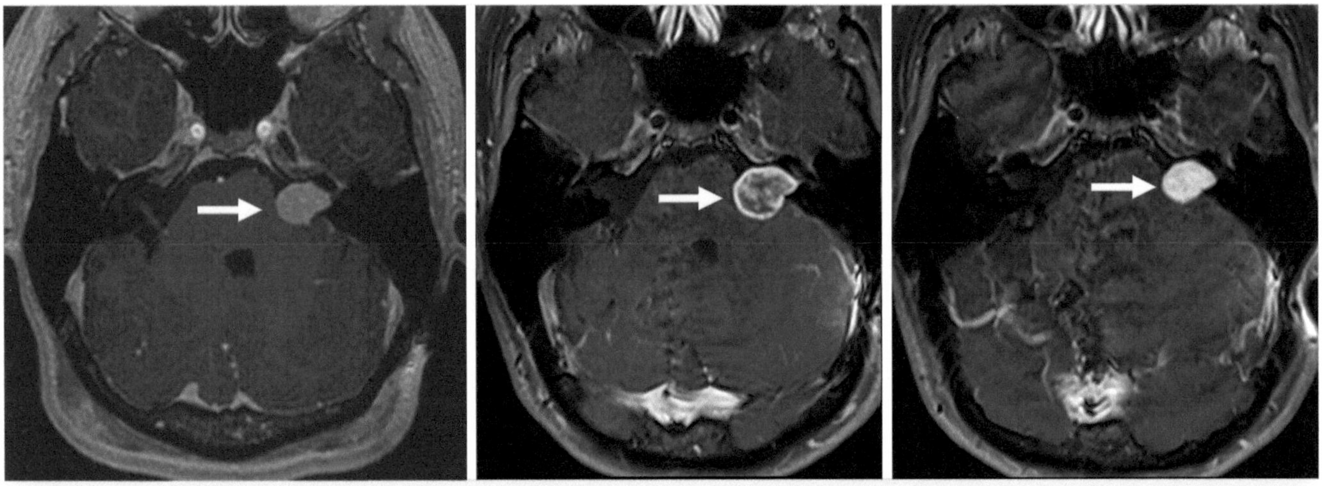

Fig. 25.1 Axial postgadolinium MRI of a 25-year-old woman with left-sided radiation-induced vestibular schwannoma. (Left) MRI at the time of radiosurgery (tumor volume, 1.5 cm^3; tumor margin dose, 13 Gy). (Middle) MRI 3 months after radiosurgery shows a loss of central enhancement and tumor expansion. (Right) MRI 1 year after radiosurgery shows the tumor has regained enhancement and returned to its original volume.

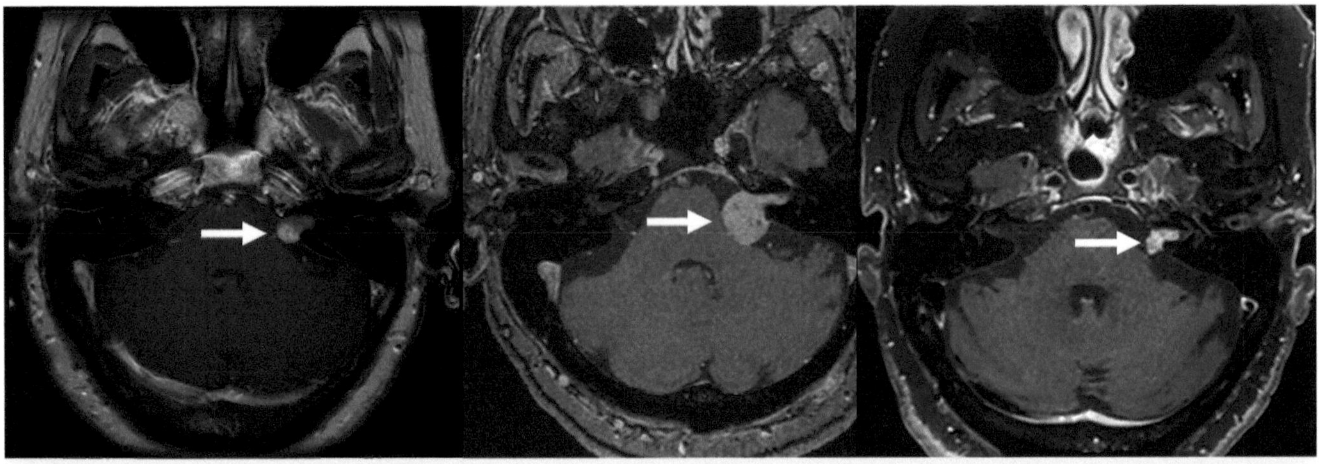

Fig. 25.2 Axial postgadolinium MRI of a 67-year-old woman with left-sided vestibular schwannoma. (Left) MRI at the time of diagnosis. Observation with serial imaging was recommended. (Middle) MRI 4 years later shows the tumor had enlarged and radiosurgery was performed (tumor volume, 3.0 cm^3; tumor margin dose, 13 Gy). (Right) MRI 8 years after radiosurgery shows the tumor significantly smaller.

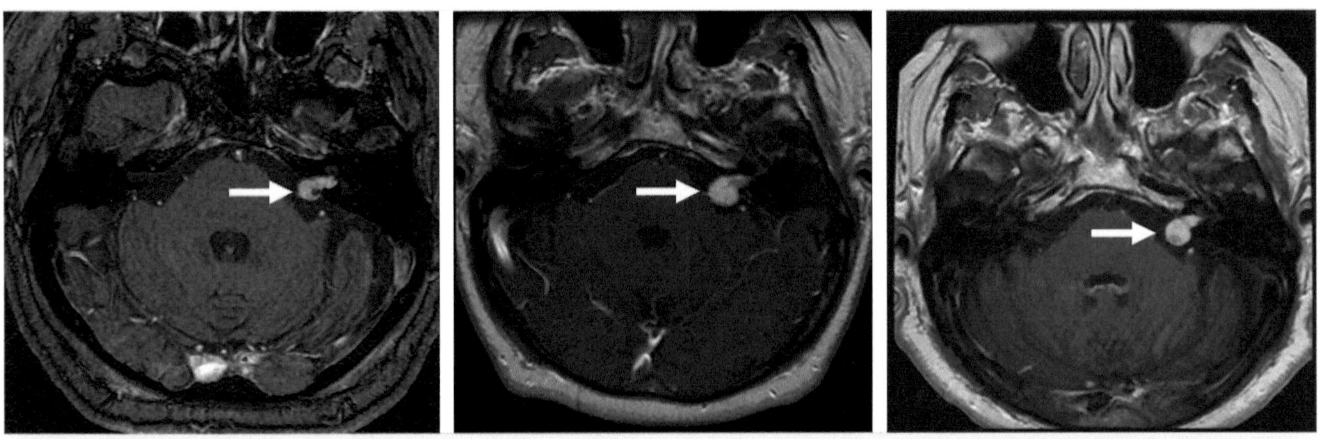

Fig. 25.3 Axial postgadolinium MRI of a 72-year-old man with left-sided vestibular schwannoma. (Left) MRI at the time of radiosurgery (tumor volume, 0.7 cm^3; tumor margin dose, 12 Gy). (Middle) MRI 2 years after radiosurgery shows the tumor is larger and the patient had developed mild hemifacial spasm. (Right) MRI 10 years after radiosurgery shows the tumor has remained enlarged but stable in size. The patient's hemifacial spasm resolved.

Table 25.1 Selected reports on vestibular schwannoma imaging after radiosurgery

Paper	No. patients	SRS	Measurement method	Pseudoprogression (%)	Failure rate (%)
Prasad et al 2000	153	GK	Volumetric	31	8[a]
Yu et al 2000	126	GK	Volumetric	62	8[b]
Okunaga et al 2005	42	LINAC	Volumetric	45	7[b]
Lunsford et al 2005	829	GK	Linear	6	2[c]
Pollock 2006	208	GK	Linear	14	2[b]
Delsanti et al 2008	332	GK	Linear	54	5[d]
Nagano et al 2008	100	GK	Volumetric	74	NS
Meijer et al 2008	45	LINAC	Volumetric	31	9[b]
Hayhurst and Zadeh 2012	75	GK	Volumetric	23	12[b]

Abbreviations: GK, Gamma Knife; LINAC, linear accelerator; NS, not stated.
[a]Defined as a tumor volume larger than at the time of radiosurgery.
[b]Defined as progressive and continuous enlargement beyond 2 years.
[c]Defined as the need for additional surgical or radiosurgical intervention.
[d]Defined as progressive and continuous growth beyond 3 years.

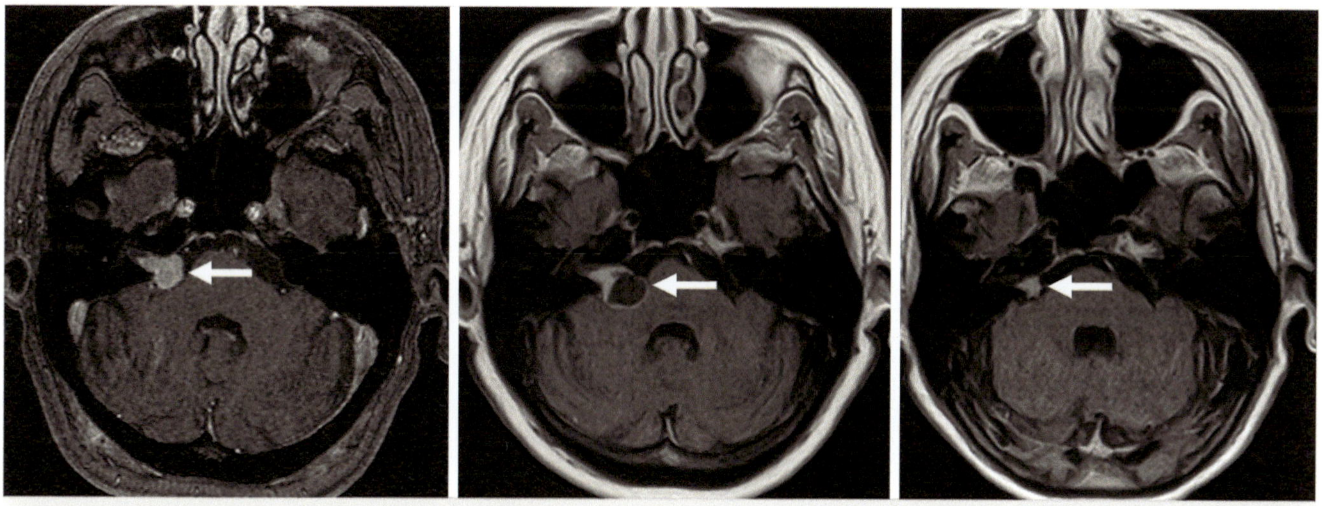

Fig. 25.4 Axial postgadolinium MRI of a 51-year-old woman with right-sided vestibular schwannoma. (Left) MRI at the time of radiosurgery (tumor volume, 1.0 cm^3; tumor margin dose, 12 Gy). (Middle) MRI 9 years after radiosurgery shows a cyst has developed and is compressing the brainstem. The patient remained asymptomatic. (Right) MRI 15 years after radiosurgery shows the cyst has resolved and the tumor is markedly smaller.

25.4 Recommendations for Enlarged Vestibular Schwannomas after Radiosurgery

The knowledge gained over the past 20 years on the expected imaging changes after VS SRS has prevented many patients from having unnecessary tumor resection after SRS. First, it is now understood that a large percentage of VS will display pseudoprogression at the same time that facial weakness or hearing loss may occur (3–12 months after SRS), but this does not equate to treatment failure. Second, a small number of patients (~2%) will develop hemifacial spasm (HFS) after VS SRS. In our experience, the onset of HFS is between 1 and 2 years and is often noted in patients whose tumor initially enlarges and remains larger than at the time of SRS. In most cases, the HFS is temporary and will resolve over several months. If bothersome, carbamazepine is generally effective in controlling the HFS and can usually be discontinued after several months. Consequently, tumor resection based on HFS after VS SRS should be avoided. Third, cyst development or enlargement can occur after VS SRS. If the patient has symptomatic mass effect secondary to the cyst formation, then surgical resection is indicated. However, we have noted cyst stabilization or regression in several patients (▶ Fig. 25.4), so in asymptomatic patients we recommend observation with serial imaging. In conclusion, additional tumor treatment should be reserved only for patients who demonstrate progressive tumor enlargement on serial imaging or those with symptomatic mass effect.

References

[1] Flickinger JC, Kondziolka D, Pollock BE, Lunsford LD. Evolution in technique for vestibular schwannoma radiosurgery and effect on outcome. Int J Radiat Oncol Biol Phys. 1996; 36(2):275–280

[2] Jacob JT, Carlson ML, Schiefer TK, Pollock BE, Driscoll CL, Link MJ. Significance of cochlear dose in the radiosurgical treatment of vestibular schwannoma: controversies and unanswered questions. Neurosurgery. 2014; 74(5):466–474, discussion 474

[3] Massager N, Nissim O, Delbrouck C, et al. Irradiation of cochlear structures during vestibular schwannoma radiosurgery and associated hearing outcome. J Neurosurg. 2007; 107(4):733–739

[4] Miller RC, Foote RL, Coffey RJ, et al. Decrease in cranial nerve complications after radiosurgery for acoustic neuromas: a prospective study of dose and volume. Int J Radiat Oncol Biol Phys. 1999; 43(2):305–311

[5] Carlson ML, Tveiten ØV, Driscoll CL, et al. Long-term quality of life in patients with vestibular schwannoma: an international multicenter cross-sectional study comparing microsurgery, stereotactic radiosurgery, observation, and nontumor controls. J Neurosurg. 2015; 122(4):833–842

[6] Myrseth E, Møller P, Pedersen PH, Vassbotn FS, Wentzel-Larsen T, Lund-Johansen M. Vestibular schwannomas: clinical results and quality of life after microsurgery or gamma knife radiosurgery. Neurosurgery. 2005; 56(5):927–935, discussion 927–935

[7] Pollock BE, Driscoll CLW, Foote RL, et al. Patient outcomes after vestibular schwannoma management: a prospective comparison of microsurgical resection and stereotactic radiosurgery. Neurosurgery. 2006; 59(1):77–85, discussion 77–85

[8] Régis J, Pellet W, Delsanti C, et al. Functional outcome after gamma knife surgery or microsurgery for vestibular schwannomas. J Neurosurg. 2002; 97 (5):1091–1100

[9] Linskey ME, Lunsford LD, Flickinger JC. Neuroimaging of acoustic nerve sheath tumors after stereotaxic radiosurgery. AJNR Am J Neuroradiol. 1991; 12(6):1165–1175

[10] Prasad D, Steiner M, Steiner L. Gamma surgery for vestibular schwannoma. J Neurosurg. 2000; 92(5):745–759

[11] Yu CP, Cheung JYC, Leung S, Ho R. Sequential volume mapping for confirmation of negative growth in vestibular schwannomas treated by gamma knife radiosurgery. J Neurosurg. 2000; 93 Suppl 3:82–89

[12] Norén G. Gamma knife radiosurgery for acoustic neuromas. In: Gildenberg PL, Tasker RR, eds. Stereotactic and Functional Neurosurgery. New York, NY: McGraw-Hill; 1998: 835–844

[13] Norén G, Arndt J, Hindmarsh T. Stereotactic radiosurgery in cases of acoustic neurinoma: further experiences. Neurosurgery. 1983; 13(1):12–22

[14] Delsanti C, Roche PH, Thomassin JM, Régis J. Morphological changes of vestibular schwannomas after radiosurgical treatment: pitfalls and diagnosis of failure. Prog Neurol Surg. 2008; 21:93–97

[15] Hayhurst C, Zadeh G. Tumor pseudoprogression following radiosurgery for vestibular schwannoma. Neuro Oncol. 2012; 14(1):87–92

[16] Lunsford LD, Niranjan A, Flickinger JC, Maitz A, Kondziolka D. Radiosurgery of vestibular schwannomas: summary of experience in 829 cases. J Neurosurg. 2005; 102 Suppl:195–199

[17] Meijer OW, Weijmans EJ, Knol DL, et al. Tumor-volume changes after radiosurgery for vestibular schwannoma: implications for follow-up MR imaging protocol. AJNR Am J Neuroradiol. 2008; 29(5):906–910

[18] Nagano O, Higuchi Y, Serizawa T, et al. Transient expansion of vestibular schwannoma following stereotactic radiosurgery. J Neurosurg. 2008; 109(5): 811–816

[19] Okunaga T, Matsuo T, Hayashi N, et al. Linear accelerator radiosurgery for vestibular schwannoma: measuring tumor volume changes on serial three-dimensional spoiled gradient-echo magnetic resonance images. J Neurosurg. 2005; 103(1):53–58

[20] Pollock BE. Management of vestibular schwannomas that enlarge after stereotactic radiosurgery: treatment recommendations based on a 15 year experience. Neurosurgery. 2006; 58(2):241–248, discussion 241–248

Part VI

Management: Microsurgery

VI

26 General Anesthesia in Vestibular Schwannoma Surgery

Michael E. Johnson

26.1 General Considerations for Craniotomy in Vestibular Schwannoma Surgery

Microsurgery for vestibular schwannoma (VS) resection involves multiple anesthetic considerations. Some are common to most craniotomies, but the use of neurophysiological monitoring, particularly electromyography (EMG), and the sitting position present particular anesthetic challenges, and will be addressed in detail.

Standard considerations for neurosurgical anesthesia are relevant.[1,2] An arterial catheter and two peripheral intravenous catheters (or a central venous catheter) suitable for vasoactive infusions should be placed. An anesthetic should be administered which provides complete immobility of the patient in a head frame and rapid emergence from anesthesia to facilitate the immediate postsurgical neurologic exam. The prolonged time required for most VS resections makes this more challenging. (See further discussion under "EMG Monitoring," below)

Because VS tumors can affect hearing and vestibular function, many are discovered and resected relatively early. Larger tumors, however, can have significant mass effect with increased intracranial pressure (ICP). Standard interventions, including dexamethasone, hyperventilation, mannitol, and head-up positioning, should then be utilized. If ICP is an issue, it will best be controlled with intravenous propofol as a primary anesthetic, rather than a volatile anesthetic. Large tumor resections can affect cranial nerves (CN) IX and X, so it is essential to confirm that protective airway reflexes (gag, swallowing) are present prior to extubation.

Corneal abrasion should be aggressively prevented. VS tumor resection has the potential to injure the trigeminal nerve (CN V) sensory innervation to the eye and eyelids, and facial nerve (CN VII) for eyelid motor and secretomotor innervation to lacrimal glands. Eyes should be carefully taped immediately after induction of anesthesia. If there is a preexisting cranial nerve deficit causing dry eye, consider instilling eye lubrication ointment before taping. Particular vigilance is required during emergence and early postanesthesia care unit (PACU) stay to prevent the patient from accidentally causing a corneal abrasion.

There is a higher incidence of postoperative nausea and vomiting (PONV) in VS surgery than in most craniotomies, from emergence from anesthesia to the PACU through at least the first postoperative day.[3] This may be related to vestibular nerve injury from tumor or surgery. Roughly half of VS patients have imbalance or vertigo as part of their initial presentation, while a history of motion sickness in any patient increases the risk of PONV.[4] Ondansetron has been shown to be highly effective, with granisetron likely to be similarly effective. Regular prophylactic treatment is beneficial for the first 24 hours postoperatively.[3]

Dexamethasone is also an effective antiemetic, as well as effective for cerebral edema related to the tumor. Intraoperative administration should be coordinated with surgical pre- and postoperative orders. A scopolamine transdermal patch may be helpful in patients at high risk of PONV. It is particularly effective in the general patient population in those with history of motion sickness.[4] It should be applied to skin near the ear, on the contralateral side, if possible, in order to be outside of the surgical area. The patch should generally be kept in place for at least 24 hours, and may be kept in place for up to 72 hours. Its main side effects are dry eyes and mouth, and blurry vision, which may affect efforts to protect against corneal abrasion and perform sequential neurological exams. Scopolamine is vestibulo-suppressive, which may help mitigate early PONV, but may also impair early vestibular compensation if used for an extended period.

Another anesthetic treatment, which usually decreases PONV, is to use a total intravenous anesthetic with propofol and without any volatile anesthetic. Surprisingly, while this is effective in preventing PONV in craniotomy for supratentorial tumors, it does not appear to decrease the incidence of PONV in craniotomy for infratentorial tumors, including VS.[5]

26.2 Neurophysiological Monitoring in Vestibular Schwannoma Surgery

The focus in this chapter is not on the detailed mechanics and theory of neuromonitoring, which are covered primarily in Chapters 27 and 28. It is rather on the effect of anesthetic technique on neuromonitoring, and how to minimize anesthetic interference with it.

26.2.1 Acoustic Nerve Monitoring

The acoustic nerve (CN VIII) is commonly monitored with brainstem auditory evoked potentials when hearing preservation surgery is attempted. Anesthetics and muscle relaxants have little effect on these potentials, so they do not need to be considered when selecting anesthetic agents.[6]

26.2.2 EMG Monitoring

In the context of VS surgery, "EMG monitoring" utilizes two different types of stimulus at the nerve[7]:

- *Spontaneous muscle activity*, also referred to as *passive or free-run EMG*. Baseline muscle activity reflects spontaneous nerve fascicle discharges. The low frequency of spontaneous muscle activity will increase with irritation or injury to the nerve. When total spike frequency exceeds 30 Hz, it is considered a neurotonic discharge and a sign of possible nerve injury.[8] In addition to the graphic display of discharges, they can be translated into a frequency-dependent audio output, thus providing immediate real-time warning to the surgeon.
- *Stimulus-evoked EMG*, also referred to as *active or triggered EMG*. Application of a stimulating electrode to a motor nerve produces a compound muscle action potential in its target

Table 26.1 EMG monitoring of nerves and target muscles during VS surgery

Cranial nerve	Target muscle[a]
Standard:	
Facial (VII)	Orbicularis oculi muscle Orbicularis oris muscle
Potentially useful depending on tumor anatomy:	
Trigeminal (V)	Masseter muscle
Vagus (X)	Vocal cords (vocalis muscle)[b,c]
Accessory (XI)	Trapezius muscle
Hypoglossal (XII)	Tongue

[a]Needle electrodes are inserted into the muscle ipsilateral to the tumor. Needle electrodes are usually secured only with tape, and present a contaminated needle stick risk to anesthesia providers if inadvertently dislodged during the case.
[b]A less invasive alternative to needle electrodes placed in the vocalis muscle is an endotracheal tube with wire electrodes on either side of the tube. There are multiple commercial products available.[55] The location of the electrodes is marked on the tube with a colored band or other marking, and the tube should be positioned with the electrodes centered between the vocal cords. Use of a videolaryngoscope for intubation may allow more accurate placement of the tube electrodes, and the endotracheal tube should be secured in the exact position it was placed. No lidocaine or other local anesthetic should be sprayed on the larynx.
[c]There is a potential risk of severe bradycardia with stimulation of the vagus (X) nerve. However, in practice, this is infrequent and treatable by discontinuing the stimulus and treating with atropine as needed.[9]

muscle.[9] This can assist in identification of the nerve, particularly if its anatomy has been distorted by the tumor. Conversely, it can be used to exclude unknown structures encountered during surgical dissection as the motor nerve is being monitored. It can also be used to evaluate functional status of the nerve, using stimulus threshold and EMG amplitude.

26.2.3 EMG Monitoring Targets

The cranial nerves most frequently monitored during VS surgery, and their target muscles, are listed in ▶ Table 26.1. Because of the close anatomic course of the facial nerve alongside the acoustic nerve, the facial nerve is at particular risk of damage during VS resection. EMG monitoring of the facial nerve has been shown to improve outcome,[7] and should always be utilized. Larger VS tumors may place other cranial nerves at risk and make EMG monitoring of them prudent.[6,9] The rostral border of a large tumor may threaten the trigeminal nerve (V). The caudal border of a large tumor may threaten the lower cranial nerves (IX–XII). There is no compelling evidence that EMG monitoring of cranial nerves other than the facial improves outcome.[10] In any event, EMG can assist in identification of cranial nerves where the tumor has distorted the nearby anatomy and thereby aid the surgical approach.

26.3 Anesthetic Selection

VS surgery imposes constraints which must be considered when selecting the anesthetic agents to use: (1) timely emergence from anesthesia at the end of long surgery, and (2) immobility with minimal paralytic muscle relaxant.

26.3.1 Timely Emergence from Anesthesia at End of Long Surgery

As in most craniotomies, it is desirable when VS surgery is concluded to have the patient awaken from anesthesia quickly and be able to undergo a rudimentary neurologic exam, so as to exclude hemorrhage or ischemia at the operative site. In other neurosurgical anesthetics, this is facilitated by using the minimal adequate dose of general anesthetic to prevent awareness and blunt hemodynamic responses, together with a dense muscle paralysis. However, dense paralysis is not compatible with EMG monitoring.

Furthermore, the characteristics of VS surgery act to increase the time to emergence from anesthesia. It is prolonged by the dose of anesthetic, which must be increased for EMG monitoring without muscle relaxant to ensure immobility, and the length of time under anesthesia.[11] VS surgery requires meticulous exposure and dissection to remove the tumor without damage to the facial and other cranial nerves. Operative time will vary with tumor size and other anatomic variables, but it is one of the longer neurosurgeries. An older study reported an average operating room time of 6.7 ± 2.0 hours for tumors ≤ 1 cm, and 10.4 ± 2.8 hours for tumors ≥ 2.5 cm.[12]

26.3.2 Immobility with Minimal Paralytic Muscle Relaxant

There are two major approaches to providing immobility without a paralytic agent preventing the muscle response necessary for EMG monitoring (except for initial, short-acting dose at intubation).

The classical approach uses infusion of muscle relaxant to achieve a submaximal paralysis allowing EMG, but preventing patient movement in combination with an anesthetic level that by itself would not ensure immobility. Given the limitations of anesthetic agents that were available previously, primarily prolonged emergence after high doses, it was reasonable to conclude that "muscle relaxation is an essential component of balanced anesthesia."[13] Most studies have been done with atracurium or a derivative at < 75% neuromuscular blockade. Its half-life is determined solely by its rate of spontaneous breakdown in the blood, independent of hepatic or renal function, giving the most stable submaximal paralytic level with an infusion.

The classical approach has two advantages related to decreasing the anesthetic depth required. Older anesthetic agents such as isoflurane and fentanyl can be used at lower levels without overly delaying time to awakening at the end of surgery. Also, lower levels of anesthetic will cause less hemodynamic depression. In a patient with severe cardiovascular disease, this may be a compelling consideration. The major disadvantage of the classical approach is that even partial paralysis can inhibit EMG. Although this is not clinically significant in all patients, it is most problematic in patients with some degree of preexisting nerve injury, or surgical anatomy putting the nerve at heightened risk of injury. If an EMG response is altered under these circumstances, it may be difficult to confidently distinguish between surgical nerve injury and drug paralytic effect. Furthermore, the effect of partial neuromuscular blockade on spontaneous EMG is poorly validated.[14]

The more recent, nonrelaxant approach uses high levels of anesthetic to provide complete immobility without administering any paralytic agent except for intubation. Its major advantage is that it removes anesthetic paralysis completely as an influence on EMG. With few exceptions, this is the author's preferred approach for VS surgery. Facial nerve paresis represents a significant morbidity and all efforts should be made to remove anesthesia as a confounding variable in EMG monitoring.

Unfortunately, there is no completely reliable predictor of movement under anesthesia. Neither hemodynamics nor the bispectral index (BIS) processed EEG monitor is a reliable predictor of movement during anesthesia.[15,16] BIS was originally designed to predict movement but was not reliable for that purpose, particularly with a narcotic as a significant component of the general anesthetic, and its algorithms were modified to provide an awareness monitor instead.[16] Interestingly, there is one study reporting that spontaneous EMG of the facial nerve may have utility as a predictor of movement under anesthesia in craniotomies, with a negative predictive value of 95%.[15]

Without a monitor that reliably predicts movement under anesthesia, it is necessary to use a supramaximal dose of anesthetic. The effect of a volatile anesthetic on movement is defined by its minimum alveolar concentration (MAC), the gas concentration in the lungs at steady state at which 50% of patients will not move in response to surgical incision. The standard deviation of volatile anesthetic dose response curves for movement is approximately 10%. To achieve no movement in 95% of patients (ED95) will then require a dose 2 SDs above the mean, or 1.2 MAC.[17] However, standard MAC values are defined for and apply only to surgical incision. The intraoperative use of EMG stimulation of the larynx and the potential for laryngeal tracheal stimulation by inadvertent movement of the endotracheal tube, directly or via attached ventilator tubing, argue for using the MAC for endotracheal intubation (MAC-EI) which is approximately 1.5 times standard MAC.

While the nonrelaxant approach is possible with volatile anesthetic as the sole anesthetic agent, a greatly prolonged time to emergence from anesthesia will result, as well as more hemodynamic instability. A more balanced approach has been made possible by the introduction of potent, ultrashort-acting anesthetics, particularly remifentanil, with a context-sensitive half-life of < 5 minutes regardless of infusion duration.[18] The nonrelaxant approach combines a dose of general anesthetic, which allows reasonably timely emergence after prolonged anesthesia, with a high-dose remifentanil infusion. Much of the data available on adequate levels of anesthetic are anecdotal. One well-designed study found that 21% of patients without relaxant moved during craniotomy when given isoflurane 0.6% (0.5 MAC) and remifentanil 0.21 µg/kg/min.[19] This has been adapted in the author's practice to successfully prevent movement with isoflurane 1.0% (measured as end-tidal concentration) and remifentanil 0.25 to 1.0 µg/kg/min, although this should also be regarded as anecdotal until further study is done.

The use of desflurane or sevoflurane rather than isoflurane during EMG monitoring would allow much faster emergence from anesthesia after a long surgery, and all of the volatile anesthetics preserve neuromuscular function and should be compatible with EMG monitoring. However, there is concern that desflurane and sevoflurane may cause a higher baseline level of spontaneous neuronal discharge than isoflurane, so that subtle neurotonic discharges may be missed. This has not been formally studied or reported. The author's current practice is to use isoflurane during EMG monitoring, and then switch to desflurane when monitoring is finished.

26.3.3 Motor Evoked Potential Monitoring

Motor evoked potential (MEP) monitoring of the facial nerve has been reported in a single study, where it correlated well with the outcome of facial nerve function.[20] Inspection of the data does not suggest a major advantage of MEP over EMG, although it has not been compared directly with EMG monitoring in a study of both monitoring methods. Since MEP imposes even more limitations on the anesthetic agents that can be used than does EMG, it does not appear to offer a significant advantage over EMG monitoring in VS surgery.

26.4 The Sitting Position for Vestibular Schwannoma Resection

VS resection can be done in the lateral or prone position, or supine with the head turned. However, the sitting position can offer surgical advantages in select cases, including better access to the tumor, less retraction and swelling, better venous drainage, better drainage of blood and cerebrospinal fluid (CSF) from the surgical site, and decreased ICP.[21] Unfortunately, it can also cause adverse effects, particularly venous air embolism (VAE), because of the increased negative pressure gradient between open veins at the surgical site and the heart. The general topic of vascular air embolism in anesthesia has been authoritatively reviewed.[22] This chapter will focus on the risks of the sitting position for VS resection.

26.4.1 Risks of Sitting Position Unrelated to Venous Air Embolism

Cervical spinal cord pathology is a relative contraindication to the sitting position. The neck will be flexed with the head in pinions for optimal surgical exposure. Overflexion has the potential to cause cord injury[23] and to impede venous return. A consensus recommendation is to preserve at least two fingerbreadths distance between the chin and the sternal notch.[21] The adequacy of this spacing should be tested in the awake patient prior to anesthetic induction. Placement of a transesophageal echocardiography (TEE) probe has the potential to place additional pressure on a compromised cervical cord, and to cause tongue swelling in an extreme flexion position. In some cases, it may be prudent to use transcranial Doppler rather than TEE as a monitor for paradoxical air embolus (PAE).

Significant cardiac disease is also a relative contraindication to the sitting position. It will limit resuscitation if a large VAE occurs. Independent of VAE, the sitting position can introduce hemodynamic instability because of venous pooling in the dependent extremities. This is worsened when a deep anesthetic is used to provide immobility without paralysis during EMG monitoring. With an uncompromised cardiovascular system, this is generally straightforward to address with intravenous fluid and vasopressor therapy guided by an arterial catheter.

26.4.2 Incidence of Venous Air Embolism

The use of the sitting position has been declining for the last several decades,[21,24,25,26] probably due to the perceived risk of VAE. The incidence of VAE in sitting craniotomies varies widely among studies, from 7 to 76%.[27] This is affected by the monitoring method and criteria for VAE used, extent of surgery, and patient selection. A frequently quoted consensus incidence for sitting suboccipital craniotomies is about 40%.[28] The only large study comparing outcome between supine and sitting positions for VS resection found no difference between the two in intraoperative and postoperative morbidity, even though the incidence of VAE was greater in sitting (28%) than in supine (5%).[29]

There will likely remain some tumors for which the sitting position offers clear advantages that compensate for its risks. While this is ultimately a surgical decision, it should be informed by consultation with the anesthesiologist. The risks are not prohibitive with appropriate monitoring and treatment by an experienced anesthesia team.[21,30,31] Assessing risks and benefits should include the risk that not using the sitting position will have adverse effects on surgical time, blood loss, adequacy of tumor resection, and preservation of cranial nerve function.[32] Avoiding the sitting position, while decreasing the risk, does not eliminate the possibility of VAE. There are multiple case reports of severe VAE in supine or prone surgeries.[33,34]

26.4.3 Pathophysiology of Venous Air Embolism

The morbidity of VAE has several etiologies.[22] Entrainment of air volume sufficient to block right ventricular outflow causes severe hemodynamic compromise. In an adult, the acute lethal dose is 200 to 300 mL of air. Slow entrainment is better tolerated because the pulmonary circulation can act as a buffer and allow some intravascular air to dissipate through the alveoli. However, passage of air through the pulmonary circulation injures the microvascular endothelium, causing release of inflammatory mediators. This can also activate the clotting cascade and result in coagulopathy. Together with physical obstruction by air, this will cause ventilation/perfusion mismatch. The lung injury may be profound and require prolonged intubation and ventilatory support.[35]

Under some conditions, VAE can also cause PAE (paradoxical air embolus), with passage of air from the venous to the systemic arterial circulation. This is a particularly feared complication. Even a small volume of air in the arterial circulation can cause ischemic infarcts in vital organs.[36,37] The most common mechanism is an interatrial right-to-left shunt (RLS) via a patent foramen ovale (PFO). Roughly 25% of the population has an asymptomatic, probe-patent, PFO.[24] Even if there is no RLS at rest, arrival of air in the right atrium can acutely increase the right atrial pressure enough to cause a new RLS.

The decision whether to utilize the sitting position when there is concern for a PAE requires careful clinical judgment informed by the incomplete studies of risk that are available. Conditions that would increase the risk of damage from paradoxical arterial air embolism are relative contraindications, including coronary artery disease, left ventricular dysfunction, elevated right heart pressure, pulmonary hypertension, and a history of stroke or transient ischemic attack or cerebrovascular disease. In contrast to a PFO, which is a tiny or only potential communication between right and left heart, the presence of an atrial septal defect or other significant pathway between right and left heart is an absolute contraindication to the sitting position.[37]

There is no consensus on how to proceed if a PFO with or without RLS is present. Two early, small studies of the sitting position where PFO was not an exclusion criterion reported a 6.6 and 14% incidence of PAE.[38,39] Most centers test for a PFO as part of the preanesthetic evaluation, and consider a PFO an absolute contraindication to the sitting position, regardless of whether an RLS can be elicited.[21,24,25] However, more recent larger studies where PFO patients were not excluded found no occurrence of PAE in sitting craniotomies.[29,30,31,40] None of these studies were large enough in terms of patients with PFO to be considered definitive. Their patients did receive extensive monitoring, including precordial Doppler and/or TEE, with immediate treatment of VAE. Since PAE is most likely with a large VAE,[39] this approach may account for the low incidence of PAE.

Another potential approach is to use a catheter-based intervention to close a PFO electively prior to surgery in the sitting position. This procedure has a low morbidity and high efficacy, but does involve a separate intracardiac procedure and anesthetic, and has not been studied beyond the few case reports available.[28,41,42] It must also be considered that excluding patients with a PFO does not guarantee against a PAE. A large or continued VAE can overwhelm the buffering defense of the pulmonary circulation and result in PAE even without an intracardiac shunt.[43,44]

In any event, the presence of a PFO or other potential intracardiac RLS should be determined prior to the surgical incision in all sitting cases, either by echocardiography[44] or by transcranial Doppler.[45,46] Even if it is not used as an exclusion criterion, the presence of a PFO will inform the anesthetic, monitoring, and treatment plans. Microbubbles are injected into the venous circulation, with passage from right to left atrium observed directly by echocardiography, or indirectly by intracranial Doppler observation of microbubbles in the cerebral arteries. The Valsalva maneuver should be used to transiently raise right atrial pressure above left atrial pressure during injection, to detect a dynamic RLS that is not present at rest.

26.4.4 Intraoperative Detection of Venous Air Embolism

Sensitive, real-time monitoring for VAE is essential in all sitting craniotomies. Even a small amount of air that does not cause

Table 26.2 Comparison of methods of detection of vascular air embolism

Method of detection	Sensitivity (mL/kg)	Availability	Invasiveness	Limitations
TEE	High (0.02)	Low	High	Expertise required, expensive, invasive
Precordial Doppler	High (0.05)	Moderate	None	Obese patients
PA catheter	High (0.25)	Moderate	High	Fixed distance, small orifice
TCD	High	Moderate	None	Expertise required
ETn_2	Moderate (0.5)	Low	None	N_2O, hypotension
$ETco_2$	Moderate (0.5)	Moderate	None	Pulmonary disease
Oxygen saturation	Low	High	None	Late changes
Direct visualization	Low	High	None	No physiologic data
Esophageal stethoscope	Low (1.5)	High	Low	Late changes
Electrocardiogram	Low (1.25)	High	Low	Late changes

Abbreviations: $ETco_2$, end-tidal carbon dioxide gas; ETn_2, end-tidal nitrogen gas; N_2O, nitrous oxide; PA, pulmonary artery; TCD, transcranial Doppler; TEE, transesophageal echo.

Source: Adapted with permission from Mirski MA, Lele AV, Fitzsimmons L, Toung TJ. Diagnosis and treatment of vascular air embolism. Anesthesiology. 2007; 106(1):164-177.[22]

serious morbidity should be treated seriously, as it may signal a surgical field susceptible to a much greater volume of air entrainment. ▶ Table 26.2 lists the major monitors available in order of sensitivity. Each has its strengths and limitations, and ideally a combination of at least three moderate-to-high-sensitivity monitors will be used.

Some of the monitors available are of limited practical utility. Most low-sensitivity monitors are not useful except to indicate that a VAE is severe. Direct visualization of vascular bubbles in the surgical field is particularly helpful in cases where VAE is low risk so that other monitors are not in place, or not functioning well. An increase in end-tidal nitrogen is more specific for VAE than a decrease in end-tidal CO_2, but many modern anesthetic machine gas analyzers do not detect nitrogen, and a separate nitrogen gas analyzer using mass spectrometry is required. Pulmonary artery pressure increase is a sensitive indicator of VAE, but of limited specificity and is mimicked by other causes of right heart failure. The small-diameter lumens of pulmonary artery catheters severely limit the ability to aspirate right heart air as treatment. Given the invasiveness and potential complications of a pulmonary artery catheter, its placement cannot be justified as a monitor for VAE.

The author's preference is to utilize TEE, precordial Doppler, and end-tidal CO_2 as primary monitors of VAE. Transcranial Doppler could be substituted for TEE as a monitor for VAE that turns into a PAE, using precordial Doppler as the only highly sensitive and specific monitor of VAE. However, this limits the ability to estimate the size of the VAE, and loses the ability to confirm the precordial signal before right to left passage of air creates a PAE, by the most sensitive monitor available for VAE. The audible signal from the precordial Doppler should be monitored continuously. The Doppler probe is positioned on the chest to interrogate blood movement in the right ventricular outflow tract, generally along the right or left sternal border between the second and fourth intercostal spaces. Correct positioning is confirmed by venous injection of microbubbles (1-mL air agitated with 9-mL fluid) and hearing a change from the regular "washing machine" turbulence of normal blood flow to an erratic high-pitched swishing roar.[22]

The TEE probe is placed so that the left and right atria can be monitored simultaneously, and position confirmed by microbubble injection as for precordial Doppler. For the nonexpert echocardiographer, the gastric short axis four-chamber view is usually easiest to obtain and maintain during the anesthetic, and allows assessment of ventricular air as well. TEE is monitored intermittently at regular short intervals, and whenever the precordial Doppler indicates a possible VAE. Continuous monitoring of TEE is not practical except for short periods, because the TEE probe generates heat when in use. As a protective mechanism to prevent esophageal burn and probe damage, the ultrasound machine will turn the probe off at a set temperature and it will not be usable until it cools below that temperature.[47] Thus, continuous TEE monitoring may create a situation where the TEE is not available when it is urgently needed.

End-tidal CO_2 is an essential monitor for VAE. It is only slightly less sensitive than precordial Doppler,[48] and should always be available as a routine monitor. It is quantitative without subjective interpretation since the decrease in end-tidal CO_2 is proportional to the amount of pulmonary arterial circulation blocked by the VAE. It is much less specific than TEE and precordial Doppler, being affected by cardiac output, metabolic rate and temperature, and ventilator settings. However, a steady state can usually be achieved during anesthesia where these factors, and hence end-tidal CO_2, are all stable. In that setting, a decrease of 2 mm Hg end-tidal CO_2 is significant and an indicator of possible VAE.[22]

26.5 Intraoperative Treatment of Venous Air Embolism

26.5.1 Ventilator Adjustment

If nitrous oxide (N_2O) is being used, it should be shut off immediately and the gas supply changed to 100% oxygen. N_2O does not increase the incidence of VAE, but will increase the size of any VAE. The source of the VAE is room air, so even if the patient has been on N_2O and is equilibrated with it, the embolus will initially contain no N_2O in it and rapidly enlarge in a patient receiving N_2O. The presence of a PFO should be considered an absolute contraindication to the use of N_2O. When isoflurane was the most rapid dispersing anesthetic available, it was reasonable to use N_2O to decrease isoflurane concentration and allow faster emergence so that a neurological exam could be done prior to extubation. With the availability of propofol, remifentanil, and desflurane, it is difficult to justify the use of N_2O in any sitting craniotomy.

High levels of positive end-expiratory pressure (PEEP) in theory can decrease the pressure gradient between the heart and the craniotomy site, and decrease the likelihood of a VAE. However, if a VAE does occur with increased right atrial pressure, the presence of PEEP will increase the right to left pressure gradient and increase the chance of RLS and PAE.

26.5.2 Surgical Treatment

When VAE is detected, the surgeon should be informed immediately. Often, the site of air entrainment will be obvious and easily treated by surgically closing or covering the venous injury. If the origin of the VAE cannot be located, careful bilateral jugular venous compression should be applied to the neck, while not compressing the carotid arteries. The increase in venous pressure will often cause the open vein to back bleed and become visible. For hemodynamically significant VAE where the site cannot be immediately located, the surgical field should be flooded with saline to prevent further air entrainment while its site is located. If the patient becomes unstable or air continues to embolize, the craniotomy should be covered or rapidly provisionally closed, and the patient repositioned with the head below the heart.

26.5.3 Aspiration of Venous Air Embolism

Placement of a large-bore (≥ 16 gauge/5 French) multiple orifice central catheter with tip at the superior vena cava–right atrial junction is effective in aspirating venous air emboli and improves survival in animal models of VAE.[49,50,51] Previously, there were several commercial brands of air aspiration catheters designed for placement from an antecubital vein with ECG-guided placement at the superior vena cava–right atrial junction, but in the United States the only catheter available is the Cook Bunegin-Albin air aspiration catheter (Cook Medical, Bloomington, Indiana), and sterile ECG adapters must be procured separately. In most cases, it is simpler and more accurate to use TEE to guide placement.[52,53] The specification of the superior vena cava–right atrial junction as the optimal site for catheter tip placement is based on studies using a Silastic casting of the human right atrium as a model.[49] In contrast, in a porcine model, placing the tip of the catheter in the right ventricle allowed the aspiration of more air than the right atrium.[54] Direct comparison of the superior vena cava–right atrial junction and the right ventricle as aspiration sites using the same large-bore catheter has not been reported, and the consensus location clinically has become the superior vena cava–right atrial junction. If the air aspiration catheter is placed through an introducer sheath with sterility sleeve cover, its location can potentially be adjusted for maximum effect with TEE guidance when a VAE occurs. For either location, the catheter should be taken out in the PACU to avoid the risk of perforation and cardiac tamponade.

There are centers that do not usually place an air aspiration catheter for sitting suboccipital craniotomy, concerned about the risk of catheter placement and believing that early detection of VAE allows effective treatment without a catheter.[31] A contrary case report has been published where TEE monitoring with immediate treatment, but without a central air aspiration catheter, did not prevent severe morbidity from two episodes of VAE, requiring a prolonged ICU stay with ventilatory support.[35]

26.5.4 Cardiovascular Support

Vasopressor and fluid support will be necessary with a large VAE. However, it should not displace efforts to locate and eliminate the source of the VAE.

References

[1] Cottrell JE, Young WL. Cottrell and Young's Neuroanesthesia. Philadelphia, PA: Mosby Elsevier; 2010

[2] Miller RD, Cohen NH, Eriksson LI, Fleisher LA, Wiener-Kronish JP, Young WL. Miller's Anesthesia. 8th ed. Philadelphia, PA: W.B. Saunders Co.; 2014

[3] Hartsell T, Long D, Kirsch JR. The efficacy of postoperative ondansetron (Zofran) orally disintegrating tablets for preventing nausea and vomiting after acoustic neuroma surgery. Anesth Analg. 2005; 101(5):1492–1496

[4] Honkavaara P. Effect of transdermal hyoscine on nausea and vomiting during and after middle ear surgery under local anaesthesia. Br J Anaesth. 1996; 76 (1):49–53

[5] Tan C, Ries CR, Mayson K, Gharapetian A, Griesdale DE. Indication for surgery and the risk of postoperative nausea and vomiting after craniotomy: a case-control study. J Neurosurg Anesthesiol. 2012; 24(4):325–330

[6] Sclabassi RJ, Balzer JR, Crammond D, Habeych ME. Neurophysiological monitoring: a tool for neurosurgery. In: Sekhar LN, Fessler RG, eds. Atlas of Neurosurgical Techniques: Brain. 1st ed. New York, NY: Thieme; 2006:50–71

[7] Minahan RE, Mandir AS. Neurophysiologic intraoperative monitoring of trigeminal and facial nerves. J Clin Neurophysiol. 2011; 28(6):551–565

[8] Oh T, Nagasawa DT, Fong BM, et al. Intraoperative neuromonitoring techniques in the surgical management of acoustic neuromas. Neurosurg Focus. 2012; 33(3):E6

[9] Schlake HP, Goldbrunner RH, Milewski C, et al. Intra-operative electromyographic monitoring of the lower cranial motor nerves (LCN IX-XII) in skull base surgery. Clin Neurol Neurosurg. 2001; 103(2):72–82

[10] Thirumala PD, Mohanraj SK, Habeych M, et al. Value of free-run electromyographic monitoring of lower cranial nerves in endoscopic endonasal approach to skull base surgeries. J Neurol Surg B Skull Base. 2012; 73(4):236–244

[11] Sinclair RCF, Faleiro RJ. Delayed recovery of consciousness after anaesthesia. Contin Educ Anaesth Crit Care Pain. 2006; 6:114–118

[12] Buchman CA, Chen DA, Flannagan P, Wilberger JE, Maroon JC. The learning curve for acoustic tumor surgery. Laryngoscope. 1996; 106(11):1406–1411

[13] Holland NR. Intraoperative electromyography. J Clin Neurophysiol. 2002; 19 (5):444–453

[14] Sloan TB. Muscle relaxant use during intraoperative neurophysiologic monitoring. J Clin Monit Comput. 2013; 27(1):35–46

[15] Jellish WS, Leonetti JP, Buoy CM, Sincacore JM, Sawicki KJ, Macken MP. Facial nerve electromyographic monitoring to predict movement in patients titrated to a standard anesthetic depth. Anesth Analg. 2009; 109(2):551–558

[16] Johansen JW, Sebel PS. Development and clinical application of electroencephalographic bispectrum monitoring. Anesthesiology. 2000; 93(5):1336–1344

[17] Aranake A, Mashour GA, Avidan MS. Minimum alveolar concentration: ongoing relevance and clinical utility. Anaesthesia. 2013; 68(5):512–522

[18] Kapila A, Glass PS, Jacobs JR, et al. Measured context-sensitive half-times of remifentanil and alfentanil. Anesthesiology. 1995; 83(5):968–975

[19] Maurtua MA, Deogaonkar A, Bakri MH, et al. Dosing of remifentanil to prevent movement during craniotomy in the absence of neuromuscular blockade. J Neurosurg Anesthesiol. 2008; 20(4):221–225

[20] Fukuda M, Oishi M, Takao T, Saito A, Fujii Y. Facial nerve motor-evoked potential monitoring during skull base surgery predicts facial nerve outcome. J Neurol Neurosurg Psychiatry. 2008; 79(9):1066–1070

[21] Jadik S, Wissing H, Friedrich K, Beck J, Seifert V, Raabe A. A standardized protocol for the prevention of clinically relevant venous air embolism during neurosurgical interventions in the semisitting position. Neurosurgery. 2009; 64(3):533–538, discussion 538–539

[22] Mirski MA, Lele AV, Fitzsimmons L, Toung TJ. Diagnosis and treatment of vascular air embolism. Anesthesiology. 2007; 106(1):164–177

[23] Hitselberger WE, House WF. A warning regarding the sitting position for acoustic tumor surgery. Arch Otolaryngol. 1980; 106(2):69

[24] Leonard IE, Cunningham AJ. The sitting position in neurosurgery–not yet obsolete! Br J Anaesth. 2002; 88(1):1–3

[25] Porter JM, Pidgeon C, Cunningham AJ. The sitting position in neurosurgery: a critical appraisal. Br J Anaesth. 1999; 82(1):117–128

[26] Jürgens S, Basu S. The sitting position in anaesthesia: old and new. Eur J Anaesthesiol. 2014; 31(5):285–287

[27] Leslie K, Hui R, Kaye AH. Venous air embolism and the sitting position: a case series. J Clin Neurosci. 2006; 13(4):419–422

[28] Fathi AR, Eshtehardi P, Meier B. Patent foramen ovale and neurosurgery in sitting position: a systematic review. Br J Anaesth. 2009; 102(5):588–596

[29] Duke DA, Lynch JJ, Harner SG, Faust RJ, Ebersold MJ. Venous air embolism in sitting and supine patients undergoing vestibular schwannoma resection. Neurosurgery. 1998; 42(6):1282–1286, discussion 1286–1287

[30] Feigl GC, Decker K, Wurms M, et al. Neurosurgical procedures in the semisitting position: evaluation of the risk of paradoxical venous air embolism in patients with a patent foramen ovale. World Neurosurg. 2014; 81(1):159–164

[31] Lindroos AC, Niiya T, Randell T, Romani R, Hernesniemi J, Niemi T. Sitting position for removal of pineal region lesions: the Helsinki experience. World Neurosurg. 2010; 74(4–5):505–513

[32] Roessler K, Krawagna M, Bischoff B, et al. Improved postoperative facial nerve and hearing function in retrosigmoid vestibular schwannoma surgery significantly associated with semisitting position. World Neurosurg. 2016; 87:290–297

[33] Gómez-Perals LF, Bayo R, Lorenzana-Honrado LM, Antona-Díaz M, Cabezudo JM. Severe intraoperative air embolism during convexity meningioma surgery in the supine position. Case report. Surg Neurol. 2002; 57(4):262–266, discussion 266–267

[34] Wei ST, Chen DC. Catastrophic venous air embolism during craniotomy in the supine position: the bleeding pattern as a warning sign? J Craniofac Surg. 2013; 24(3):e228–e229

[35] Wong AY, Irwin MG. Large venous air embolism in the sitting position despite monitoring with transoesophageal echocardiography. Anaesthesia. 2005; 60 (8):811–813

[36] Clayton DG, Evans P, Williams C, Thurlow AC. Paradoxical air embolism during neurosurgery. Anaesthesia. 1985; 40(10):981–989

[37] Furtado SV, Venkatesh PK, Murthy GK, Furtado AD, Hegde AS. Paradoxical embolus across atrial septal defect and posterior circulation infarct in neurosurgical patients. Int J Neurosci. 2010; 120(7):516–520

[38] Cucchiara RF, Nugent M, Seward JB, Messick JM. Air embolism in upright neurosurgical patients: detection and localization by two-dimensional transesophageal echocardiography. Anesthesiology. 1984; 60(4):353–355

[39] Mammoto T, Hayashi Y, Ohnishi Y, Kuro M. Incidence of venous and paradoxical air embolism in neurosurgical patients in the sitting position: detection by transesophageal echocardiography. Acta Anaesthesiol Scand. 1998; 42(6): 643–647

[40] Ganslandt O, Merkel A, Schmitt H, et al. The sitting position in neurosurgery: indications, complications and results. A single institution experience of 600 cases. Acta Neurochir (Wien). 2013; 155(10):1887–1893

[41] Laban JT, Rasul FT, Brecker SJ, Marsh HT, Martin AJ. Patent foramen ovale closure prior to surgery in the sitting position. Br J Neurosurg. 2014; 28(3): 421–422

[42] Webb ST, Klein AA, Calvert PA, Lee EM, Shapiro LM. Preoperative percutaneous patent foramen ovale closure before neurosurgery in the sitting position. Br J Anaesth. 2009; 103(2):305–306, author reply 306

[43] Butler BD, Hills BA. Transpulmonary passage of venous air emboli. J Appl Physiol (1985). 1985; 59(2):543–547

[44] Cucchiara RF, Nishimura RA, Black S. Failure of preoperative echo testing to prevent paradoxical air embolism: report of two cases. Anesthesiology. 1989; 71(4):604–607

[45] Mojadidi MK, Roberts SC, Winoker JS, et al. Accuracy of transcranial Doppler for the diagnosis of intracardiac right-to-left shunt: a bivariate meta-analysis of prospective studies. JACC Cardiovasc Imaging. 2014; 7(3):236–250

[46] Van H, Poommipanit P, Shalaby M, Gevorgyan R, Tseng CH, Tobis J. Sensitivity of transcranial Doppler versus intracardiac echocardiography in the detection of right-to-left shunt. JACC Cardiovasc Imaging. 2010; 3(4):343–348

[47] Prabhu M, Raju D, Pauli H. Transesophageal echocardiography: instrumentation and system controls. Ann Card Anaesth. 2012; 15(2):144–155

[48] English JB, Westenskow D, Hodges MR, Stanley TH. Comparison of venous air embolism monitoring methods in supine dogs. Anesthesiology. 1978; 48(6): 425–429

[49] Bunegin L, Albin MS, Helsel PE, Hoffman A, Hung TK. Positioning the right atrial catheter: a model for reappraisal. Anesthesiology. 1981; 55(4):343–348

[50] Colley PS, Artru AA. Bunegin-Albin catheter improves air retrieval and resuscitation from lethal venous air embolism in upright dogs. Anesth Analg. 1989; 68(3):298–301

[51] Mongan PD, Hinman JA. Evaluation of a double-lumen multiorifice catheter for resuscitation of swine from lethal venous air embolism. Anesthesiology. 1995; 83(5):1104–1111

[52] Jeon Y, Ryu HG, Yoon SZ, Kim JH, Bahk JH. Transesophageal echocardiographic evaluation of ECG-guided central venous catheter placement. Can J Anaesth. 2006; 53(10):978–983

[53] Kerr RH, Applegate RL, II. Accurate placement of the right atrial air aspiration catheter: a descriptive study and prospective trial of intravascular electrocardiography. Anesth Analg. 2006; 103(2):435–438

[54] Schäfer ST, Lindemann J, Neumann A, Brendt P, Kaiser GM, Peters J. Cardiac air transit following venous air embolism and right ventricular air aspiration. Anaesthesia. 2009; 64(7):754–761

[55] Medniuk A, Bareisiene D, Ahmad I. Nerve integrity monitor tubes for thyroid surgery. Anaesthesia. 2014; 69(3):287–288

27 Intraoperative Facial Nerve Monitoring During Vestibular Schwannoma Microsurgery

David R. Friedmann, Sean O. McMenomey, and J. Thomas Roland Jr.

27.1 Introduction

Facial nerve monitoring has become standard in neurotologic procedures, distinct from its more adjunctive role in other subspecialties in otolaryngology. Many of the early studies evaluating the benefits of neuromonitoring were retrospective and utilized historical matched cohorts. Control groups commonly consisted of operative cases performed before adoption of facial nerve monitoring and were compared to the same surgeon's outcomes following routine nerve monitor use. From a methodologic perspective, these studies are plagued by confounding factors such as improved skill of the surgeon over time and the benefits of other advances in skull base surgery occurring over the study period. Still, the evidence from these studies ethically precludes a randomized trial. Based on the existent data, the National Institutes of Health Consensus Statement on Acoustic Neuroma explicitly recommends the routine use of intraoperative facial nerve monitoring.[1]

With improvements in imaging modalities facilitating earlier detection of vestibular schwannomas (VSs), preservation of facial nerve function has become a primary consideration in the management of patients undergoing microsurgical resection. Two different, but complementary, techniques for facial nerve monitoring are utilized for posterior fossa skull base surgery and will be described within this chapter. Continuous facial electromyography (EMG) is in widespread use among centers conducting otologic and neurotologic procedures, while transcranial motor evoked potential (TCMEP) monitoring is utilized less frequently. These techniques may be used in a variety of ways to facilitate facial nerve preservation and to aid in decision making during VS resection.

27.2 History and Overview

The earliest and most primitive form of facial nerve monitoring is direct observation of facial nerve twitching from muscle contraction after mechanical stimulation of the facial nerve. This remains a technique commonly used among head and neck surgeons in parotid gland dissection and in settings where equipment for facial nerve monitoring is unavailable. It is only of historical interest for microsurgery of the posterior fossa. Intraoperative facial nerve EMG was first introduced in 1979.[2] Facial EMG allows for early identification and confirmation of the facial nerve either distally within the internal auditory canal or proximally at the brainstem, and provides good spatial resolution to map the nerve course at low stimulation levels. Suprathreshold stimulation levels may also be used before dissecting a particular region of the tumor capsule to confirm the nerve is not in close proximity. Continuous EMG testing detects nerve stimulation in real time, providing the surgeon with valuable feedback during the course of dissection by monitoring spontaneous EMG activity from mechanical manipulation. Finally, direct electrical stimulation of the proximal nerve following tumor resection provides some prognostic value for estimating postoperative facial nerve function and the likelihood of recovery even in the presence of immediate postoperative facial paralysis.

TCMEP monitoring of the facial nerve aims to provide a "functional" assessment of cranial nerve integrity during cranial base surgery without the need for direct proximal stimulation by the surgeon. It has been found to be of greatest help in the setting of large tumors where tumor dissection (▶ Fig. 27.1) is often necessary prior to definitive identification of the facial nerve.[3]

27.3 Monitoring Setup

Although the advent of facial nerve monitoring represents a tremendous advance in skull base surgery, there are a number of considerations critical to its effective use. Anesthetic agents that cause long-term neuromuscular blockade may interfere to varying degrees with monitoring and should be avoided. Typically, anesthetic induction with endotracheal intubation is performed using short-acting agents, namely succinylcholine, so that neuromuscular blockade will clear early before critical portions of the surgery are underway. It is important that anyone providing neuroanesthesia be comfortable managing such patients without the use of long-term muscles relaxants. Additionally, injection of xylocaine and other similar pharmacologic agents, particularly in the vicinity of the stylomastoid foramen, may induce local muscular blockade of the facial nerve, interfering with the interpretation of the facial EMG. Further discussion regarding anesthetic considerations during neuromonitoring for VS microsurgery can be found in Chapter 26.

Although an indispensable tool, there are ways in which intraoperative monitoring can be counterproductive and detrimental to surgical outcomes. Facial nerve monitoring can in no way take the place of a fundamental anatomic knowledge and of sound microsurgical dissection technique. Potential problems with intraoperative monitoring may be mitigated by routine use and specialized technical training among those involved in setting up the equipment. The ability to

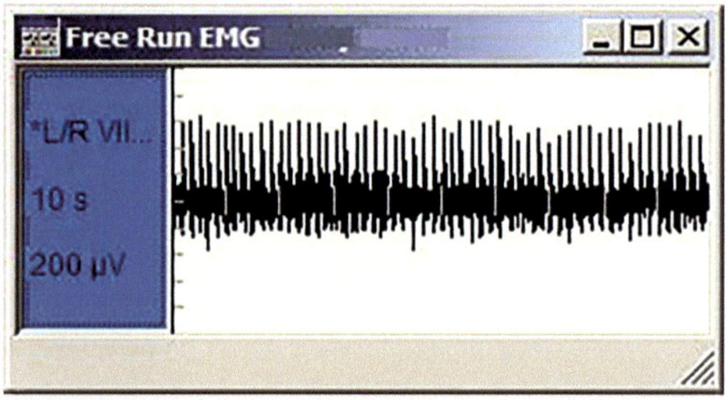

Fig. 27.1 Continuous facial electromyography (EMG) provides real-time feedback throughout tumor dissection.

troubleshoot the equipment in real time, recognize when it is not working appropriately, and proceed with the operation is an important aspect of its use.

The use of multiple EMG channels improves the sensitivity of EMG monitoring, and therefore, it is recommended to monitor at least two branches of the facial nerve. Subdermal electrodes are preferred to surface electrodes, which are more susceptible to artifact and easily displaced during surgery. Electrodes for facial EMG are most commonly placed in the orbicularis oculi and orbicularis oris muscles. Electrodes should be secured well with adhesive tape, and the orbicularis oculi subdermal needle electrode should be oriented pointing away from the globe to avoid ocular injury. Placing a small loop of redundancy in the electrode wire near the insertion site reduces the risk of accidental displacement if the proximal wires are inadvertently pulled. Additionally, a ground electrode is placed over the sternum and a return electrode for monopolar stimulation is placed on the contralateral shoulder.

Using multiple channels allows for an "internal control" for troubleshooting potential intraoperative problems. For example, increased activity in one channel and silence in other leads may indicate nonsurgical factors or faulty electrode placement. In addition, multiple leads allow for simultaneous monitoring of multiple divisions of the facial nerve, which may be particularly useful for a very splayed nerve. Mechanical trauma to the nerve may induce high tonic EMG activity, making response to direct stimulation difficult to detect. In this case, having additional electrodes will often allow for audible responses to direct stimulation on the quieter channels.

We have chosen to include the "tap test" as part of the surgical "time-out" procedure. This is performed by gently tapping on the electrodes and surrounding face to elicit EMG activity on the monitoring system. It is important to understand what information can and cannot be gleaned from this. It can confirm for the surgeon (1) the volume of the loudspeaker is at an adequate level and (2) the integrity of the equipment's connectivity. However, this response represents an artifact, and is not a compound muscle action potential (CMAP) emanating from the facial nerve. Ultimately, the surgeon or a technologist with experience in neurophysiologic intraoperative monitoring should be responsible for proper setup.

27.4 Intraoperative Use

False-positives or false-negatives resulting from an incorrect setup can be more detrimental than not using monitoring at all, as this can mislead the surgeon and may result in false assurance during dissection. At the authors' center, an electrophysiologist is responsible for monitoring equipment setup and is present throughout the case to help monitor, interpret, and troubleshoot EMG monitoring. Their presence is necessary for TCMEP and other intraoperative neuromonitoring techniques, although most EMG systems can be programmed for surgeons who may not have this luxury. Adjustable stimulating probes allow the surgeon to change the stimulation levels directly and the EMG machine settings can be programmed to provide audible feedback about stimulation parameters.

When present, the electrophysiologist should be situated in the line of sight of the surgeon and have a video monitor to visualize tumor dissection. EMG activity should be monitored via loudspeaker for acoustic feedback and an oscilloscope for visual feedback. Before stimulation, it is important for the surgeon and electrophysiologist to communicate about parameters including the stimulation level and the baseline TCMEP value. TCMEP stimulation itself results in activity detected on the facial EMG and noticeable contraction of the patient's musculature. Therefore, the electrophysiologist should confirm with the surgeon each time before employing its use to ensure it is an appropriate time in the case. A "squelch circuit" is another important feature routinely employed that allows for muting of the artifact produced with electrocautery.

27.5 Facial Electromyography

Free-running EMG, or so-called passive monitoring, involves recording CMAPs through needle electrodes in the facial muscles activated through nonelectrical stimulation of the nerve, be it mechanical or stretch activity. Continuous EMG provides the surgeon real-time immediate feedback during facial nerve dissection. Spontaneous neurotonic firing and increased irritability may suggest risk of permanent injury and can direct the surgeon to stop their current approach and work elsewhere until EMG activity returns to baseline. One should also note that if the patient is "becoming light" from inadequate anesthesia during the procedure, facial muscle fasciculation and resultant EMG activity may be one of the earlier signs—preceding gross physical movement or changes in the bispectral (BIS) monitor sometimes used to determine the depth of anesthesia.

Stimulating the nerve electrically or with gentle mechanical stimulation may result in a *burst potential* that represents a short synchronous firing of a single discharge across multiple axons. Intriguingly, sharp cutting or laceration of a facial nerve is less likely to elicit neurotonic activity, as compared to traction, compression, or gentle manipulation.[4] Traction on the nerve from mechanical stretch leading to a prolonged irregular series of EMG activity is referred to as a *train potential.* Trains represent tonic activity, often from multiple asynchronous discharges from different motor units that may last seconds to minutes. Two train patterns have been described—high-frequency trains (50–100 Hz) present acoustically similar to an airplane engine and are called "bomber potentials," while low-frequency trains (1–50 Hz) acoustically resemble popping popcorn. Trains may result from mechanical tension in the form of pressure or stretch from tumor dissection. This feedback may direct the surgeon to alter their surgical strategy to reduce the risk of permanent facial nerve injury. Unfortunately, there is often a delay in seconds to minutes between the inciting event and the development of train activity. Similar to burst potentials, train activity may also result from thermal cautery and cold irrigation.

27.6 Direct Stimulation

Direct electrical stimulation of the facial nerve is often termed "active" monitoring. Intraoperatively, direct electrical stimulation may be used for definitive nerve identification, confirmation of neural integrity, and mapping of the nerve location and course. Early use of the stimulating probe within the case allows for confirmation of correct equipment setup and reassurance that the system is responding appropriately. Before employing active stimulation, it may be checked in surrounding soft tissue rather than directly in the dissection field.

Both monopolar and bipolar electrodes can be used for direct facial nerve stimulation. Bipolar probes theoretically provide greater stimulation specificity and precision compared to monopolar probes. However, in practice, bipolar electrodes are cumbersome to use in the tight confines of the posterior fossa. In addition, stimulation efficiency is dependent on the orientation of the electrode tips in relation to the facial nerve, adding additional complexity.[5] In contrast, monopolar probes are compact and also provide submillimeter spatial resolution when using low stimulation settings. Furthermore, monopolar stimulation at higher current levels is invaluable for tumor mapping, where high sensitivity is required. Today, most available probes are insulated and monopolar in design, with the Prass probe (Medtronic Xomed, Jacksonville, FL) being most widely used. Kartush and colleagues developed a set of dissecting instruments with a noninsulated cutting surface allowing for simultaneous stimulation and dissection (Neurosign Magstim Co., Carmarthenshire, UK). This avoids the need to constantly change instruments when stimulation is desired.

Stimulation may be performed using either a constant-current or constant-voltage system. While still a topic of controversy, intraoperative skull base neuromonitoring is most commonly performed using constant-current stimulators. The primary limitation of constant-current stimulation is the potential for current shunting through surrounding fluid, including cerebrospinal fluid (CSF) and irrigant, and thus, the possibility of false-negative stimulation. However, the use of insulated flush-tip stimulating probes largely resolves this shortcoming.

The pulse parameters most commonly adjusted during VS microsurgery include the amplitude of the current (milliamp, mA) and the length of time the current is applied (pulse duration, microseconds [µs]). To characterize the magnitude of the pulse charge, both parameters must be known. For example, the charge delivered to a nerve using 0.1 mA and a 50-µs pulse duration is less than that using 0.1 mA with a 100-µs pulse duration. Usual parameters when stimulating the facial nerve directly may vary between 0.05 and 0.2 mA, and 50- and 200-µs pulse duration.

Stimulation parameters are tailored to the task at hand. Suprathreshold levels are typically employed before the nerve is definitively identified. By using higher stimulation settings, the surgeon can confirm that the nerve is not in proximity when bipolar coagulating or resecting tumor capsule. Before engaging the tumor, the entire dorsal surface of the tumor capsule should always be stimulated at higher levels to ensure the facial nerve is not splayed over the back side of the tumor and to confirm that the tumor is not in fact a facial nerve schwannoma, both of which are uncommon. The use of successively lower stimulation settings may help localize or triangulate the facial nerve at the brainstem in the case of a larger tumor with significant brainstem compression. Minimum settings are generally used to directly stimulate a previously identified nerve, to assess overall neural integrity, or to precisely locate a conduction block if proximal stimulation is lost. While preferences vary from surgeon to surgeon, there is a theoretical advantage to resecting the cerebellopontine component of the tumor before the intracanalicular portion because a nerve will always stimulate distal to an acute injury. If a significant conduction block develops within the internal auditory canal before the facial nerve is found proximally, dissection at the brainstem, cistern, and porus may be more challenging.

27.7 Transcranial Motor Evoked Potentials

TCMEP monitoring yields information about the integrity of the entire course of the facial nerve without requiring direct proximal nerve stimulation (▶ Fig. 27.2). The general technique for motor evoked potentials elsewhere in the body has been used in intraoperative monitoring of spinal cases, but its application to facial nerve surgery is more complex. Prior studies have validated the technique and suggest some utility in prognosticating facial nerve outcomes.[3] This technique is used routinely at our center in VS surgery and is felt to be most useful for larger tumors where early identification of the facial nerve at the brainstem may be difficult. Of note, TCMEP is more sensitive to inhalational anesthetic agents than EMG because of their impact on cortical excitability, and measurements must be interpreted with this in mind. Reference to the BIS monitor provides a measure of the depth of anesthesia.

The exact setup for this technique is beyond the scope of this chapter, but is described in Cosetti et al[3] and Cueva.[6] The authors stimulate from corkscrew electrodes for the cranial electrode montage and record from separate subdermal bipolar electrodes placed in the facial muscles. TCMEPs of the facial nerve are subject to artifact as the strength needed to stimulate the appropriate area of the cortex through the skull may also lead to peripheral motor responses from the face (▶ Fig. 27.3). Careful setup and interpretation of the measured response can recognize and avoid this pitfall.

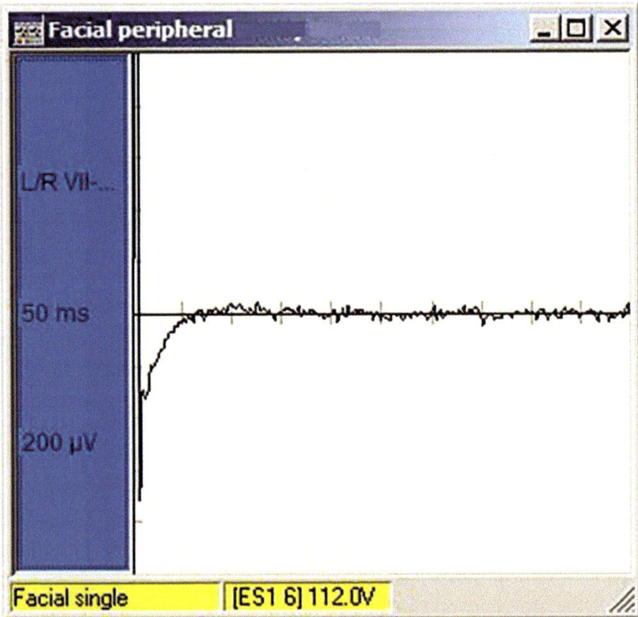

Fig. 27.2 An additional peripheral facial nerve electrode is placed to differentiate true transcranial motor evoked potential (TCMEP) from artifact.

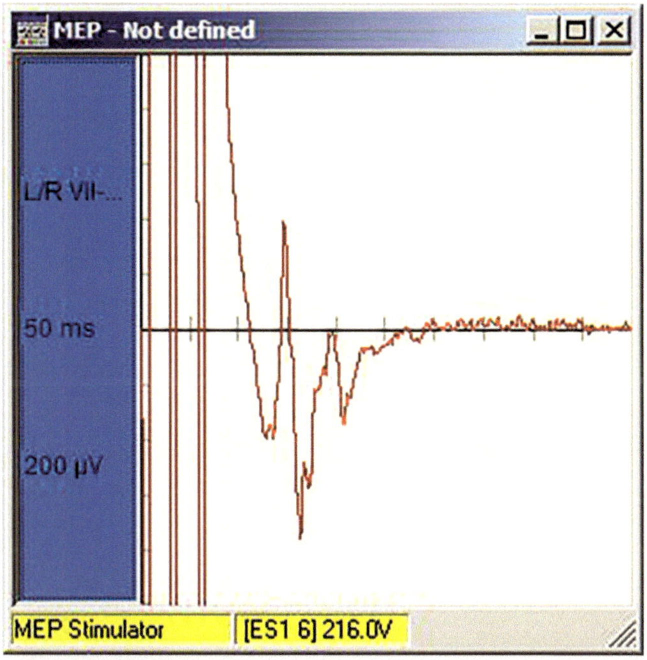

Fig. 27.3 Transcranial motor evoked response at 216 µV suggests integrity of the facial nerve.

An absent direct stimulation response but affirmed baseline TCMEP response may provide the surgeon important feedback that the thin nerve remains intact and, thus, confidence to continue the dissection. Surgeons can become "paralyzed" by absent or overly active EMG monitoring responses. It is our opinion that we are able to accomplish complete resections more often with large tumors due to the added information provided by TCMEP monitoring.

27.8 Prediction of Facial Nerve Outcome

A final utility of intraoperative facial nerve monitoring is the estimation of short- and long-term postoperative facial nerve function. Specifically, electroprognostic testing provides an objective real-time assessment of progressive neural injury that may help guide extent of resection, particularly for larger tumors (also see Chapters 32, 41, and 55), and an estimate of long-term facial nerve function for postoperative patient counseling. However, perhaps the ultimate theoretical goal of testing is to dependably identify the select group of patients who *will not* recover satisfactory facial nerve function, so that early reinnervation procedures can be considered. In many centers, it is still common practice to delay irreversible nerve transfer procedures for at least 12 or even 18 months, until final facial nerve function declares itself. However, this paradigm may lead to suboptimal outcomes since prolonged denervation results in loss of motor end plates and irreversible muscle atrophy. If intraoperative testing could reliably rule out the possibility of satisfactory recovery, then perhaps an injured segment of the facial nerve could be repaired with an interposition nerve graft or same-surgery nerve transfer using the masseteric branch of V3 or the hypoglossal nerve could be considered, for example. Unfortunately, despite great effort, no study to date has identified a testing strategy that can reliably separate those patients that will ultimately have poor function from those that will gain satisfactory recovery. Herein lies a primary limitation of facial nerve electroprognostication—at the time of acute facial nerve injury, direct facial nerve stimulation testing cannot decipher a simple conduction block that is fully reversible (neuropraxia) from a more severe nerve injury such as axonotmesis or neurotmesis. A very favorable response at the conclusion of resection provides assurance that the patient will have good long-term function; however, a very poor response does not guarantee the patient will not recover well. To demonstrate the limits of testing, in a study evaluating 11 VS cases where the facial nerve was anatomically intact at the conclusion of tumor resection, but proximal high-level stimulation (e.g., 10 mA) was lost, the median definitive postoperative House–Brackmann (HB) score was III.[7] Only three patients had HB ≥ IV and two cases even recovered HB grade II function. The authors concluded that present-day electrophysiological testing strategies are incapable of reliably predicting who will do poorly and that, if the anatomic continuity of the facial nerve is maintained, attempts at same-surgery nerve repair should not be pursued.

Several stimulation strategies, with their respective predictive values, have been published in the literature, as summarized in ▶ Table 27.1 and reviewed below. The use of the ***absolute amplitude of the evoked CMAP*** was first described by Harner et al and has since been modified by others.[8] This method of testing is based on the observation that the CMAP amplitude is directly proportional to the number of stimulated muscle fibers, which in turn reflects the number of intact axons that are able to propagate an electrical signal. With CMAP amplitude testing, the surgeon stimulates the proximal facial nerve at the brainstem following tumor resection and the absolute value, in microvolts (µV), is recorded. The chief limitation of this testing method is the wide variability in responses that can be seen from person to person, resulting from differences in facial EMG electrode placement and muscle size. Stimulation settings vary greatly between studies, but most authors favor lower stimulation levels in order to reduce the risk of unnecessary electrical injury. However, an advantage of maximal or near-maximal stimulation over low-level stimulation is that all axons are being simultaneously evaluated which provides a more complete assessment of neural integrity. Low stimulation settings are more susceptible to untoward current shunting from CSF and may only selectively stimulate a subpopulation of axons, particularly if the nerve is severely splayed.

A second method for intraoperative prediction of facial nerve function is ***minimum stimulation threshold testing***. This strategy is based on the assumption that the lowest level of stimulation required to first elicit an EMG response is related to overall facial nerve integrity. For example, after completion of tumor resection, stimulation of the facial nerve at the brainstem at 0.05 or 0.1 mA with a brisk response of 500 µV portends excellent prognosis of HB grade II or better, independent of immediate postoperative outcome[9,10] (▶ Fig. 27.4). Similar to absolute amplitude of the CMAP, variability in patient response, in addition to significant variance in parameters used by different authors, precludes consensus regarding absolute cut-off values. However, despite these limitations, minimum stimulation

Table 27.1 Select publications evaluating the utility of intraoperative electroprognostic testing of the facial nerve to predict postoperative facial nerve function

Study	Study design	Number of patients	Histology	Pulse duration (µs)	Stimulus protocol (CC/CV)	Probe	Channels, muscle	Stimulation site	IOFNM criteria	Results
Beck et al 1991[12]	Retrospective	56	VS	100	CC	Monopolar	1, oris	REZ	1. 500 µV amplitude of neurotonic discharge (trains) sustained for >30 s 2. 500 µV amplitude of orbicularis oris response using 0.05-mA stimulation at the end of tumor resection	Four groups of patients: a) <500 µV EMG and 500 µV to stimulation b) >500 µV EMG and to stimulation c) <500 µV EMG and to stimulation d) >500 µV EMG and <500 µV to stimulation Group A, at 1 wk, 97% had HB grade I
Prasad et al 1993[13]	Retrospective	34	CPA	100–200	CV	NA	2, oculi, oris	REZ	Pre- vs. posttumor resection variation <0.2 V of proximal stimulation	90%, HB I/II at 2 d 83%, HB I/II at 1–44 mo
Wolf et al 1993[14]	Prospective	25	VS	100	CC	Monopolar	3, tumor side; 1, opposite side	REZ	1. 500 µV amplitude of neurotonic discharge (trains) sustained for 30 s 2. 500 µV amplitude of muscle response using 0.1–0.4 mA stimulation at the end of tumor resection	Response < 500 µV EMG and > 500 µV to stimulation was correlated with normal facial function in 90% of the patients at 1 d
Lacombe et al 1994[15]	Retrospective	62	VS	100	CC	Monopolar	2, oculi, oris	REZ	Stimulation threshold	<0.1 mA, all HB I/II at 1 mo Between 0.1 and 0.3 mA, 71.4% HB I/II at 1 mo >0.3 mA, 20% HB I/II at 1 mo
Lalwani et al 1994[16]	Retrospective	129	VS	200	CV	Monopolar	2, oculi, oris	REZ	<0.2 V stimulation after tumor resection	Stimulation threshold was not correlated with immediate postoperative 98%, HB I/II at 1 y, if >0.2 V, 50% HB I/II
Silverstein et al 1994[17]	Retrospective	44	VS	200	CC	Monopolar	NA (EMG); oris (motion detector)	REZ	<0.1 mA stimulation after tumor resection (EMG or motion detector)	95%, HB I/II at >1 y If between 0.1 and 0.2 mA, 82% HB I/II
Hone et al 1997[18]	Prospective	27	VS	100	CC	Bipolar	2, frontalis, oris	REZ	Lowest current to elicit >250 µV for facial muscle contraction	Stimulus threshold >0.1 mA, HB >II immediately postoperative and at 6 mo
Nissen et al 1997[19]	Retrospective	81	VS	NA	CV	Monopolar	NA	IAC, REZ	Minimal voltage stimulus to elicit an EMG response (stimulus threshold)	Median threshold of 0.1 V, HB I/II at 6 mo Median threshold of 0.725 V, HB III/IV at 6 mo

Table 27.1 *(Continued)*

Study	Study design	Number of patients	Histology	Pulse duration (μs)	Stimulus protocol (CC/CV)	Probe	Channels, muscle	Stimulation site	IOFNM criteria	Results
Zeitouni et al 1997[20]	Prospective	109	VS	NA	CC	Monopolar	2, oculi, oris	REZ	1. Minimal current stimulus to elicit an EMG response (stimulus threshold) 2. CMAP amplitude	Intraoperative thresholds significantly associated with immediate and late follow-up, 87% threshold between 0.05 and 0.1 mA (HBI/II 83% at immediate and 91.6% at 1 y) CMAP amplitude failed to predict facial function
Axon and Ramsden 1999[21]	Prospective	184	VS	200	CC	Bipolar	2, oculi, oris	Proximal to the site of tumor	Minimal stimulation threshold (0.05 mA)	94% sensitivity in predicting good long-term facial function and 91% PPV
Fenton et al 1999[22]	Prospective	35	VS	100	CC	NA	NA	Medial and lateral to tumor	Minimal stimulation intensity medial and lateral to tumor after tumor resection	Medial minimal stimulation <0.1 mA, 96% HB I/II immediately postoperative >0.15 mA, 30% HB I/II is suggestive of an abnormal facial function
Fenton et al 2002[23]	Prospective	67	VS	100	CC	NA	2, oculi, oris	Medial to tumor	Minimal stimulation intensity medial and lateral to tumor after tumor resection	0.1 mA, 88% of the patients were correctly predicted to have a favorable initial outcome on the basis of tumor size and stimulation threshold
Isaacson et al 2003[24]	Retrospective	229	VS	100	CC	Monopolar	2, oculi, oris	IAC, REZ	1. Stimulus threshold 2. Proximal-to-distal CMAP amplitude ratio	<0.5 mA, 93.6% HB I/II at 6 mo Ratio >0.33, 97% HB I/II at 6 mo
Fenton et al 2004[25]	Prospective	16	CPA non-VS	100	CC	NA	NA	REZ	Stimulation threshold <0.1 mA	Good long-term FN outcome
Akagami et al 2005[26]	Prospective	71	CPA	NA	NA	NA	2, oculi, oris	NA	Proximal-to-distal CMAP amplitude ratio	Independent variable predictive of satisfactory FN outcome
Anderson et al 2005[27]	Retrospective	67	VS (3 cm)	NA	CC	Monopolar	NA	REZ	Absolute CMAP amplitude >100 μV in response to as high as 0.4 mA stimulation	93%, HB I/II at final follow-up (6 mo to 1 y)
Grayeli et al 2005[28]	Prospective	89	VS	NA	CC	Monopolar	4, oculi, oris, frontalis, platysma	Fundus, IAC, REZ	1. Lowest intensity that elicits a response of >100 μV on at least 1 channel 2. Stimulation threshold	0.01–0.04 mA, 90% HB I/II at days 1 and 8 0.05–0.2 mA, 75% HB I/II at days 1 and 8 >0.2 mA, 20% HB I/II
Neff et al 2005[29]	Prospective	74	VS	NA	CC	NA	2, oculi, oris	REZ	1. Response amplitude >240 μV or greater 2. Stimulation threshold 0.05 mA or less	One criterion, 85% HB I/II at 1 y Both criteria, 98% probability of HB I/II at 1 y Stimulus threshold or response amplitude alone had a lower probability with the same result

Table 27.1 *(Continued)*

Study	Study design	Number of patients	Histology	Pulse duration (µs)	Stimulus protocol (CC/CV)	Probe	Channels, muscle	Stimulation site	IOFNM criteria	Results
Isaacson et al 2005[30]	Retrospective	60	VS	100	CC	Monopolar	2, oculi, oris	IAC, REZ	1. Stimulus threshold 2. Proximal-to-distal CMAP amplitude ratio	Accurate in predicting increased risk of long-term FN dysfunction when a logistic regression model was used Score >0.8, all patients with final HB III or better Score <0.8, 67% do not regain eye closure
Lin et al 2006[31]	Prospective	38	VS	200	CC	Bipolar	3, oculi, oris, frontalis	REZ	Percentage ratio was calculated by dividing the CMAP response to REZ stimulation (0.05–0.3 mA) by the amplitude of distal ipsilateral transcutaneous maximal stimulus response	CMAP >50% of the maximum, 93% PPV of HB I/II immediately postoperative CMAP >20% of the maximum, 81% PPV
Bernat et al 2010[32]	Prospective	120	VS	100	CC	Monopolar	4, oculi, oris, frontalis, chin	IAC, REZ	1. Stimulation threshold 2. Response amplitude after supramaximal stimulation (2 mA) 3. Proximal-to-distal CMAP amplitude ratio	<0.04 mA, sensitivity 89% and specificity 43% CMAP amplitude >800 µV, sensitivity 38% and specificity 87% Ratio <0.6, sensitivity 78% and specificity 40% All 3 criteria, sensitivity 90% and specificity 78% to predict HB I or II at day 8

Abbreviations: CC, constant current; CMAP, compound muscle action potential; CPA, cerebellopontine angle; CV, constant voltage; EMG, electromyography; FN, facial nerve; HB, House–Brackmann; IAC, internal auditory canal; IOFNM, intraoperative facial nerve monitoring; PPV, positive predictive value; REZ, root entry zone; VS, vestibular schwannoma.
Source: Adapted with permission from Acioly MA, Liebsch M, de Aguiar PH, Tatagiba M. Facial nerve monitoring during cerebellopontine angle and skull base tumor surgery: a systematic review from description to current success on function prediction. World Neurosurg. 2013; 80(6):e271 -e300.[11]

threshold testing is likely the most common method used today for intraoperative facial nerve function prediction.

The final method of facial nerve electroprognostic testing is the *relative amplitude ratio*. Several variations of this technique have been described, but all require that consistent stimulation parameters be used to elicit the two CMAPs that are being compared. Examples include the difference in absolute amplitude when stimulating the proximal facial nerve at the brainstem both before and after tumor resection, and the difference in amplitude when stimulating the facial nerve at the brainstem compared to the fundus after tumor resection is complete (i.e., proximal-to-distal amplitude ratio). Both of these methods assess the change in the evoked EMG response attributable to neural injury from tumor dissection. The primary advantage of using a technique based on the response ratio, rather than an absolute response, is that it controls for interindividual patient differences.

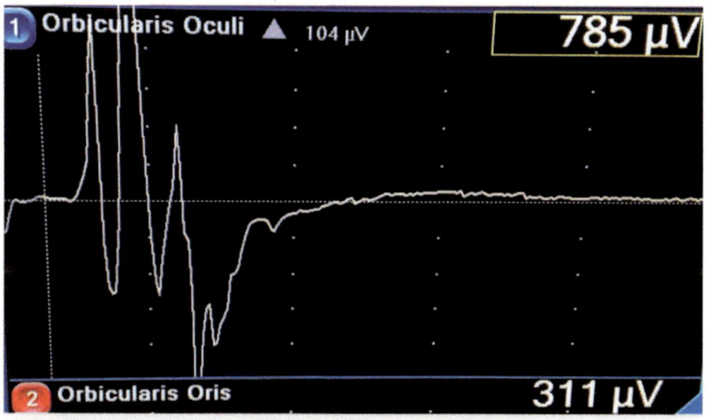

Fig. 27.4 Direct facial nerve stimulation at the conclusion of tumor dissection at 0.05 mA with brisk response to 785 µV portends an excellent facial nerve outcome.

The exact predictive parameters of TCEMP remain under investigation but may include change in threshold from baseline, the amplitude of response, the facial motor evoked potential ratio, and waveform morphology. The authors have found that an intraoperative delta TCMEP of > 57 µV may be worrisome for long-term recovery of satisfactory facial nerve function.[3] A recent publication suggests that an event-to-baseline ratio of 60% or greater is predictive of satisfactory long-term facial nerve function.[10,11] ▶ Table 27.2 summarizes select

Table 27.2 Select publications evaluating the utility of transcranial motor evoked potential monitoring to predict postoperative facial nerve function

Study	Study design	Number of patients	Histology	Pulse duration (µs)	Stimulus protocol (CC/CV)	Intensity	Channels, muscle	IOFNM criteria	Results
Zhou and Kelly 2001[33]	Prospective	50	Brain tumor	500	5, frequency 0.5–2 Hz	40–160 mA	1, oris	Persistent MEP decrease of >50%	MEP amplitude reductions were associated with postoperative motor deficits The degree of amplitude reduction was correlated with the degree of immediate postoperative worsening No mention of facial function
Dong et al 2005[10]	Prospective	76	Skull base	50/500	3–4, ISI 1 or 2 ms	100–400 V	1, oris	Final-to-baseline MEP ratio	Significant immediate postoperative facial deficits predicted 50% ratio, sensitivity 100%, specificity 88% 35% ratio, sensitivity 91%, specificity 97% 0% ratio (loss), sensitivity 64%, specificity 100% FMEP loss accounted for all patients who developed complete facial palsy postoperatively
Akagami et al 2005[26]	Prospective	71	Skull base	50	3–5, ISI 1–3 ms	200–400 V	1, oris	Final-to-baseline MEP ratio	A 50% final-to-baseline ratio predicted immediate HB I/II facial function
Fukuda et al 2008[34]	Retrospective	26	Skull base	NA	5, ISI 1 ms	180–550 V	2, oculi, oris	Final-to-baseline MEP ratio	A 50% threshold consistently predicted immediate HB I/II facial function and palsy of both muscles
Acioly et al 2010[35]	Retrospective	60	CPA	50	3 or 5, ISI 2 ms	200–600 V	2, oculi, oris	Final-to-baseline MEP ratio	Immediate postoperative facial function correlated significantly with the FMEP ratio in the orbicularis oculi muscle at 80% amplitude ratio and orbicularis oris muscle at 35% ratio; FMEP loss was always related to postoperative facial paresis

Abbreviations: CC, constant current; CPA, cerebellopontine angle; CV, constant voltage; HB, House–Brackmann; IOFNM, intraoperative facial nerve monitoring; FMEP, facial motor-evoked potential; ISI, interstimulus interval; MEP, motor-evoked potential.
Source: Adapted with permission from Acioly MA, Liebsch M, de Aguiar PH, Tatagiba M. Facial nerve monitoring during cerebellopontine angle and skull base tumor surgery: a systematic review from description to current success on function prediction. World Neurosurg. 2013; 80(6):e271 -e300.[11]

previous publications evaluating the predictive value of TCMEP. An important caveat to interpreting these data is the inherent influences that volatile anesthetics have on TCMEP monitoring, explaining a large range of values in studies to date.

References

[1] Acoustic neuroma. Consens Statement. 1991; 9(4):1–24

[2] Delgado TE, Bucheit WA, Rosenholtz HR, Chrissian S. Intraoperative monitoring of facila muscle evoked responses obtained by intracranial stimulation of the facila nerve: a more accurate technique for facila nerve dissection. Neurosurgery. 1979; 4(5):418–421

[3] Cosetti MK, Xu M, Rivera A, et al. Intraoperative transcranial motor-evoked potential monitoring of the facial nerve during cerebellopontine angle tumor resection. J Neurol Surg B Skull Base. 2012; 73(5):308–315

[4] Kartush JM. Electroneurography and intraoperative facial monitoring in contemporary neurotology. Otolaryngol Head Neck Surg. 1989; 101(4): 496–503

[5] Kartush JM, Niparko JK, Bledsoe SC, Graham MD, Kemink JL. Intraoperative facial nerve monitoring: a comparison of stimulating electrodes. Laryngoscope. 1985; 95(12):1536–1540

[6] Cueva RA. Preoperative, intraoperative, and postoperative auditory evaluation of patients with acoustic neuroma. Otolaryngol Clin North Am. 2012; 45 (2):285–290, vii

[7] Carlson ML, Van Abel KM, Schmitt WR, Driscoll CL, Neff BA, Link MJ. The anatomically intact but electrically unresponsive facial nerve in vestibular schwannoma surgery. Neurosurgery. 2012; 71(6):1125–1130, discussion 1130

[8] Harner SG, Daube JR, Beatty CW, Ebersold MJ. Intraoperative monitoring of the facial nerve. Laryngoscope. 1988; 98(2):209–212

[9] Bhimrao SK, Le TN, Dong CC, et al. Role of facial nerve motor-evoked potential ratio in predicting facial nerve function in vestibular schwannoma surgery both immediate and at 1 year. Otol Neurotol. 2016; 37(8):1162–1167

[10] Dong CC, Macdonald DB, Akagami R, et al. Intraoperative facial motor evoked potential monitoring with transcranial electrical stimulation during skull base surgery. Clin Neurophysiol. 2005; 116(3):588–596

[11] Acioly MA, Liebsch M, de Aguiar PH, Tatagiba M. Facial nerve monitoring during cerebellopontine angle and skull base tumor surgery: a systematic review from description to current success on function prediction. World Neurosurg. 2013; 80(6):e271–e300

[12] Beck DL, Atkins JS, Jr., Benecke JE, Jr., Brackmann DE. Intraoperative facial nerve monitoring: prognostic aspects during acoustic tumor removal. Otolaryngol Head Neck Surg 1991; 104:780-782.

[13] Prasad S, Hirsch BE, Kamerer DB, Durrant J, Sekhar LN. Facial nerve function following cerebellopontine angle surgery: prognostic value of intraoperative thresholds. Am J Otol 1993; 14:330-333.

[14] Wolf SR, Schneider W, Hofmann M, Haid CT, Wigand ME. [Intraoperative monitoring of the facial nerve in transtemporal surgery of acoustic neurinoma]. HNO 1993; 41:179-184.

[15] Lacombe H, Keravel Y, Peynegre R, Eshraghi A. [Value of the monitoring of the facial nerve in the evaluation of facial function in translabyrinthine surgery for acoustic neuroma]. Ann Otolaryngol Chir Cervicofac 1994; 111:89-93.

[16] Lalwani AK, Butt FY, Jackler RK, Pitts LH, Yingling CD. Facial nerve outcome after acoustic neuroma surgery: a study from the era of cranial nerve monitoring. Otolaryngol Head Neck Surg 1994; 111:561-570.

[17] Silverstein H, Willcox TO, Jr., Rosenberg SI, Seidman MD. Prediction of facial nerve function following acoustic neuroma resection using intraoperative facial nerve stimulation. Laryngoscope 1994; 104:539-544.

[18] Hone SW, Commins DJ, Rames P, et al. Prognostic factors in intraoperative facial nerve monitoring for acoustic neuroma. J Otolaryngol 1997; 26:374-378.

[19] Nissen AJ, Sikand A, Curto FS, Welsh JE, Gardi J. Value of intraoperative threshold stimulus in predicting postoperative facial nerve function after acoustic tumor resection. Am J Otol 1997; 18:249-251.

[20] Zeitouni AG, Hammerschlag PE, Cohen NL. Prognostic significance of intraoperative facial nerve stimulus thresholds. Am J Otol 1997; 18:494-497.

[21] Axon PR, Ramsden RT. Facial nerve injury caused by vestibular Schwannoma compression: severity and adaptation to maintain normal clinical facial function. Am J Otol 1999; 20:763-769.

[22] Fenton JE, Chin RY, Shirazi A, Fagan PA. Prediction of postoperative facial nerve function in acoustic neuroma surgery. Clin Otolaryngol Allied Sci 1999; 24:483-486.

[23] Fenton JE, Chin RY, Fagan PA, Sterkers O, Sterkers JM. Predictive factors of long-term facial nerve function after vestibular schwannoma surgery. Otol Neurotol 2002; 23:388-392.

[24] Isaacson B, Kileny PR, El-Kashlan H, Gadre AK. Intraoperative monitoring and facial nerve outcomes after vestibular schwannoma resection. Otol Neurotol 2003; 24:812-817.

[25] Fenton JE, Chin RY, Fagan PA, Sterkers O, Sterkers JM. Facial nerve outcome in non-vestibular schwannoma tumour surgery. Acta Otorhinolaryngol Belg 2004; 58:103-107.

[26] Akagami R, Dong CC, Westerberg BD. Localized transcranial electrical motor evoked potentials for monitoring cranial nerves in cranial base surgery. Neurosurgery 2005; 57:78-85; discussion 78-85.

[27] Anderson DE, Leonetti J, Wind JJ, Cribari D, Fahey K. Resection of large vestibular schwannomas: facial nerve preservation in the context of surgical approach and patient-assessed outcome. J Neurosurg 2005; 102:643-649.

[28] Grayeli AB, Guindi S, Kalamarides M, et al. Four-channel electromyography of the facial nerve in vestibular schwannoma surgery: sensitivity and prognostic value for short-term facial function outcome. Otol Neurotol 2005; 26:114-120.

[29] Neff BA, Ting J, Dickinson SL, Welling DB. Facial nerve monitoring parameters as a predictor of postoperative facial nerve outcomes after vestibular schwannoma resection. Otol Neurotol 2005; 26:728-732.

[30] Isaacson B, Kileny PR, El-Kashlan HK. Prediction of long-term facial nerve outcomes with intraoperative nerve monitoring. Otol Neurotol 2005; 26:270-273.

[31] Lin VY, Houlden D, Bethune A, et al. A novel method in predicting immediate postoperative facial nerve function post acoustic neuroma excision. Otol Neurotol 2006; 27:1017-1022.

[32] Bernat I, Grayeli AB, Esquia G, Zhang Z, Kalamarides M, Sterkers O. Intraoperative electromyography and surgical observations as predictive factors of facial nerve outcome in vestibular schwannoma surgery. Otol Neurotol 2010; 31:306-312.

[33] Zhou HH, Kelly PJ. Transcranial electrical motor evoked potential monitoring for brain tumor resection. Neurosurgery 2001; 48:1075-1080; discussion 1080-1071.

[34] Fukuda M, Oishi M, Saito A, Takao T, Fujii Y. [Facial nerve motor evoked potentials elicited by transcranial electrical stimulation for intraoperative monitoring]. No Shinkei Geka 2008; 36:315-321.

[35] Acioly MA, Liebsch M, Carvalho CH, Gharabaghi A, Tatagiba M. Transcranial electrocortical stimulation to monitor the facial nerve motor function during cerebellopontine angle surgery. Neurosurgery 2010; 66:354-361; discussion 362.

28 Intraoperative Eighth Nerve Monitoring During Vestibular Schwannoma Microsurgery

Joseph P. Roche and Marlan R. Hansen

28.1 Introduction

Intraoperative neurophysiologic monitoring of the cochlear division of the eighth cranial nerve (CN) provides the microsurgeon a tool to assess the impact of operative manipulations on the physiologic integrity and long-term function of the auditory system during surgical treatment of a vestibular schwannoma (VS). There are several options available to the surgeon to monitor the entire auditory system or specific portions thereof, each with advantages and disadvantages. Currently available options include auditory brainstem response/brainstem auditory evoked response (ABR/BAER), cochlear nerve action potential (CNAP), electrocochleography (ECoG), otoacoustic emissions, and cochlear blood flow estimates.[1,2,3] Several groups have utilized combinations of monitoring technique including BAER and ECoG[3,4] and BAER and CNAP.[5,6] Each monitoring technique has its proponents and published reports extolling its respective virtue. However, the two most commonly employed techniques in contemporary microsurgical treatment of VS are intraoperative BAER and CNAP. This chapter focuses on these two techniques.

28.2 Background

ABR and cochlear nerve compound potential testing measure two types of auditory evoked potentials (AEPs): electrical potentials generated by populations of neurons responding to acoustic stimuli. Various terms are used to describe each response. In this chapter, the terms brainstem auditory evoked response (BAER) and cochlear nerve action potential (CNAP) will be used. Both BAER and CNAP monitoring provide measures of the physiological functioning of the auditory system, which can also be used to infer some aspects regarding the health of the underlying neuroanatomy. In the setting of microsurgery, these responses can help guide the surgeon in making manipulations that are likely to allow for the preservation of residual auditory functioning.[1,4,7,8,9] However, neither response is a measurement of hearing per se. Hearing is the perception and processing of the acoustic environment. Complete and permanent loss of AEP responses can still be associated with preserved hearing.[9,10,11,12,13,14] Additionally, preservation of responses does not guarantee postoperative hearing.[3,9,12,15] The utility of AEPs, including BAER and CNAP, comes from the objective nature of the responses and the relative insensitivity to general anesthesia and commonly utilized muscle relaxants.[2,16] Additionally, when properly performed, these responses can give an estimate of potentially reversible damage to the auditory structures at risk or prevent further injury during surgical treatment of VS.[1]

Candidacy for hearing preservation microsurgery and outcomes are discussed in other sections, including Chapters 36, 37, and 53, and are not discussed in this chapter. However, the capacity to monitor hearing physiology can be a consideration in approach selection, though typically a small contributing factor overall. In properly selected and counseled patients, a hearing-preserving approach can be undertaken without intraoperative monitoring and successful hearing preservation can be a reasonable aspiration.[17] Indeed, the first report of hearing preservation after removal of a VS occurred in 1954, well before the description of the BAER in the early 1970s.[18,19,20,21]

Both BAER and CNAP require sufficient residual physiological functioning of the peripheral and central auditory system as these structures serve as the electrical generators of the potentials being monitored. The outer, middle, and inner ear structures, except in rare circumstances, are typically unaffected by a VS whose size and residual hearing allow for the consideration of a hearing preservation treatment option. If the patient has conductive, sensory, or mixed hearing losses, these losses may preclude the generation of waveforms to monitor regardless of the impact of the VS on the auditory physiology.

28.3 General AEP Recording Principles

The recording techniques used in AEP monitoring and recording, including BAER and CNAP, are well established and share common characteristics. These AEP signals are generated by synchronized firing of large populations of acoustically sensitive neurological structures, mainly outer and inner hair cells (transducer potentials) and the neurons of the central auditory system (action potentials).[1,19,20,21,22] Typically, an acoustic stimulus is presented to the outer ear and the voltage changes that result from the acoustically responsive elements are measured over a specific time epoch from the stimulus onset. Each stage of acoustic processing generates its own response that can be characterized by morphology (shape, polarity, and amplitude of the response) and timing in relationship to the stimulus (latency).[22] These potentials are very small, typically in the microvolt or nanovolt range.[1,7] To reliably identify these potentials, multiple technical and processing strategies are employed. There are various electrode configurations in the published literature[1,3,4,15,22,23,24,25,26]; the most common montages consist of the recording (AKA active or positive) electrode at the vertex (Cz in standard "10–20 system" electroencephalogram nomenclature) and the reference (AKA inactive or negative) electrode at or below the level of the CN (earlobe or ipsilateral mastoid, designated A1 or A2).[1,27] The ground electrode can be placed in various locations such as the midline forehead (Fz) or one of the deltoid regions. ▶ Fig. 28.1 demonstrates the typical electrode montage used at the University of Iowa during intraoperative eighth nerve monitoring. Electrodes can be skin surface contacts or subcutaneous needles. Intraoperative AEP monitoring can utilize either, but subcutaneous needle electrodes typically have lower and more stable impedances in our experience. Proper recording requires low impedances at each electrode and very small difference between all three electrodes (active,

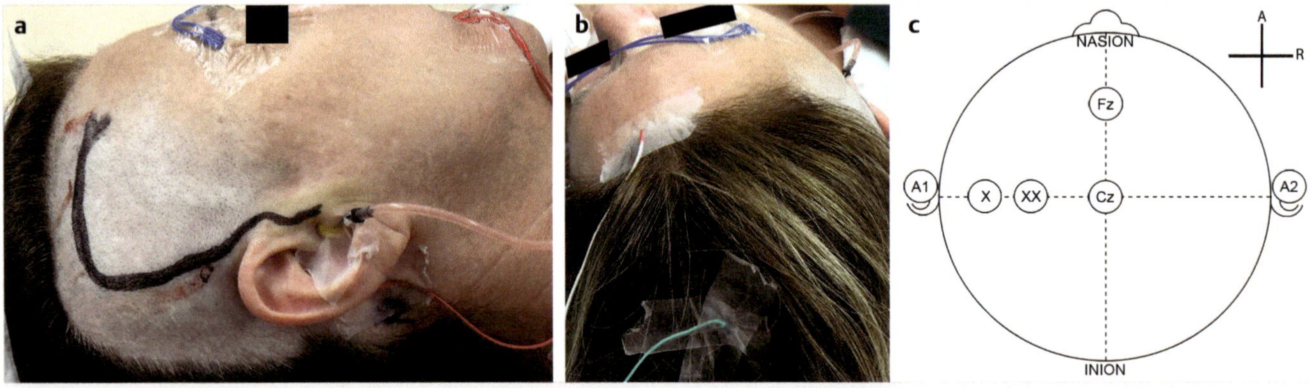

Fig. 28.1 Electrode montage used at the University of Iowa for intraoperative monitoring of the eighth cranial nerve. **(a)** Lateral view of a right ear. An insert earphone is placed in the external ear canal and sealed with a piece of occlusive tape. The inactive (Ai) electrode (*single red cable*) is placed subcutaneously at the mastoid tip and secure with tape. The facial nerve monitoring electrodes, also viable in the orbicularis oculi and orbicularis oris, can be seen as well. **(b)** Top-down view demonstrating the placement of active (*green cable*) at the vertex (Cz) and the reference (*white cable*) placed at the midline forehead (Fz). **(c)** Schematic of the setup for a left ear in the standard "10–20" EEG nomenclature. X = inactive electrode in the IAC. XX= inactive electrode placed at the brainstem. A1, left mastoid/ear placement of the inactive electrode; A2, right mastoid/ear placement of the contralateral (nontest ear) electrode.

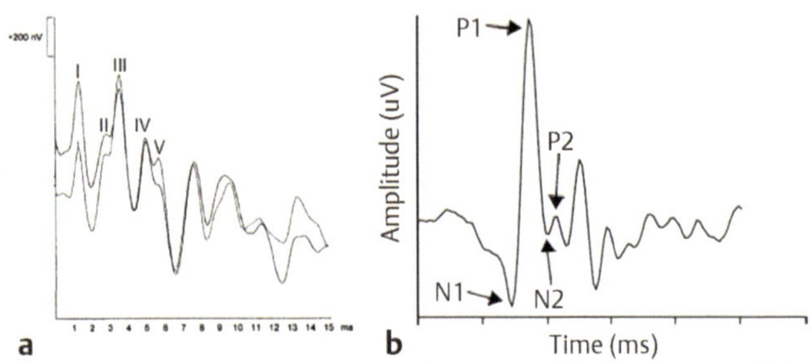

Fig. 28.2 Normal waves for both brainstem auditory evoked responses and direct cochlear nerve responses. **(a)** This figure demonstrates two averaged BAER responses with clear waves labeled with roman numerals. This response is from a patient with a very small (1 mm, normal audiometric testing) vestibular schwannoma, classed as normal. **(b)** This demonstrates the wave forms from direct eighth nerve recordings obtained from a patient with a 5-mm vestibular schwannoma. Each major wave component is labeled as vertex negative (N1 and N2) or positive (P1 and P2).

inactive, and reference). High impedances and significant differences can reduce or alter the size and morphology of the AEPs.

AEPs have many responses (often called waves) that can be recorded starting with responses from the cochlea and extending to the neocortex.[2,19,20,21,28] Intraoperative BAER and CNAP focus on five main waveforms: vertex positive waves I–V.[1,19] Each wave represents synchronized spiking of a population of neurons at progressively more central locations in the auditory system.[1,19,20,21] Each waveform has a characteristic morphology and latency, and normative data are used to class responses as normal or abnormal. Additionally, the timing between successive waves (interwave latency) can be measured and compared with normative data. When using the electrode configurations demonstrated in ▶ Fig. 28.1, there are five vertex (Cz) positive waveforms that constitute the BAER, labeled with Roman numerals as per Jewett.[19] The timescale is measured in milliseconds from the stimulus onset. ▶ Fig. 28.2 demonstrates a preoperative BAER recording from a patient with a 1-mm VS, which was classified as normal when compared to normative data. As reviewed in Martin and Stecker, the generators of each wave in human subjects have been postulated and are generally accepted.[1] Wave I represents the synchronous activation of type I afferents laterally in the modiolus with the onset of an acoustic stimulus. This has been termed the compound action potential and can be demonstrated with CNAP, BAER, and ECoG.[22] Wave II is thought to represent the proximal CN and possibly some responding cochlear nucleus neurons. Wave III is thought to represent neuronal responses in the cochlear nucleus and superior olivary complex (brainstem structures). Wave IV is thought to be produced by generators in the lateral lemniscus. Wave V is the result of spiking in the inferior colliculus (midbrain structures). There is overlap in time and space of these potentials and thus each waveform likely has some contribution from multiple generator sources. The waveforms that are utilized most frequently during intraoperative eighth nerve monitoring are waves I and V.[1] In general, wave I gives a good estimate of the cochlear function (including the modiolar nerve) and wave V an estimate of the brainstem auditory function.[3] A thorough review of the science behind the generators is beyond the scope of this chapter.

Given the small size of the recorded potentials, AEPs are exquisitely sensitive to inference from other intrinsic and extrinsic electrical sources such as skeletal muscle activity or electric instrumentation, respectively. Several strategies are used to reduce the impact of other electrical signals: averaging, artifact rejection, and filtering.[1,7,22,29] Averaging consists of performing multiple individual recordings (i.e., trials), using the same stimulus type and intensity, and then calculating the mean voltage at each time point in the trial. Signals that are synchronized to the start of the recording epoch (i.e., the AEP of interest) will remain; other nonsynchronized signals will be minimized or eliminated. For large and uniform AEPs, a low number of trials are needed to obtain a reliable response pattern. The higher the number of trials needed, the longer it will take to obtain the response pattern. Artifact rejection is a process where trials with large swings in electrical potential are automatically excluded from the averaging process due to the likelihood that these records contain significant interfering signals.[3] Artifact rejection parameters can be adjusted to be more or less selective in which records are excluded. The lower the rejection thresholds, the higher the number of trial attempts required to obtain enough data for averaging. Filtering is the process where undesired signals are removed or reduced from each trial record. This can be done during the actual recording (online) or after the record has been made (offline). Additionally, the filtering can be performed with analog circuits or with digital signal processing techniques. The most common configuration is a bandpass filter (or a combination of a low-pass and high-pass filters[1]) that allows alternating current signals with a frequency between the upper and lower cutoffs to pass unattenutated; signals that are outside the bandpass domain are attenuated or eliminated. The upper and lower bounds of the filter are generally set between 300 and 1,500 hertz (Hz)[1,2] as most of the energy from BAER is found between 400 and 1,400 Hz.[30] These settings should reduce the impact that 50- to 60-Hz signals have on the record and processed waveforms. Additional "notch" filters can be used to reduce the impact of 60-Hz electric line interference, though some authors caution against the use of these filters as there is the potential for distortion of the recorded waveforms.[1,29]

The stimuli utilized to elicit AEPs range from clicks to tone pips to pure tones. Intraoperative AEP monitoring typically utilize clicks.[1,3,4,5,6,14,15,23,25,31,32,33,34,35,36] Clicks, by virtue of their physical properties, stimulate large regions of the cochlea and give robust responses,[1] which is important as large responses make averaging more efficient. The rates of stimulation are typically between about 10 and 30 Hz; other reports have used higher rates when indicated.[2,4,5,10,33] Higher rates of stimulation allow for quicker accumulation of enough trials to generate reliable responses but may reduce the amplitude of the responses.[2,3,4] If the recorded waveforms are small, then lower stimulation rates are employed to reduce this effect.[1] Additionally, stimulus presentation rates should not be at values that are even divisors of 60 Hz to avoid confounding the responses with 60-Hz electrical line interference.[1,29] Click stimuli can be one polarity (condensation or rarefaction) or alternating polarity. Alternating polarity stimuli can be used to average out any contribution of the cochlear microphonic, if this signal is not desired.[3,4] Lastly, the stimulus intensity is typically high (> 70 db HL) as this can provide large and reproducible waveforms. Stimulation intensities as high as 95 dB HL can be required if the pure tone thresholds are significantly depressed. However, higher intensity stimulation can result in acoustic crossover and possible responses from the contralateral ear and can require a masking stimulus to the nontest ear.[3,4]

A variety of equipment and supplies are utilized in the generation and recordings of AEPs. In general, these can be broken down into three components: a stimulus source and delivery method, recording electrodes, and a signal recording and processing computer. Acoustic stimuli can be generated by a receiver placed in the external ear canal or located remotely from the external ear but delivered by insert earphones to the external ear.[2,8,29] The latter configuration has some distinct advantages: physically separated receivers allow for better electrical shielding and a time delay for the stimulus to travel to the external ear canal.[3,4,29] Shielding helps reduce the amount of electrical artifact created by the receiver as it generates the clicks (AKA stimulus artifact). The time delay due to the distance that the stimulus must travel from the receiver through the tubing to the inert earphone additionally helps reduce the impact of any stimulus artifact. This is possible because the time delay provides temporal isolation of the AEPs from any stimulus artifact.[3,4] Recording electrode can be either skin surface contacts or subcutaneous needles, as outlined above. For CNAP recording, an additional electrode needs to be placed on or near the cochlear nerve. This occurs after the craniotomy has been performed. Various electrodes have been used and designed for CNAP, and examples include a simple wire, a wire with a ball-tipped end, bipolar wire electrodes, flat contacts, and a specialized "C"-shaped electrode.[5,37,38,39] Some of these examples are fabricated each time by the surgeon or institution; others are commercially available.[1,6,7,40,41] The electrodes are connected to a recording device, typically an amplifier attached to a computer. In contemporary AEP systems, the computer drives the generation of the acoustic signals, recording and processing of any responses, and display of the waveforms for interpretation. These systems allow for the control of a variety of stimulus types and rates, filtering options, artifact rejection criteria, and recording parameters. Lastly, a skilled technician or neurophysiologist is required to assess the readout from the AEPs recording and determine if a change in the response pattern has occurred.

28.4 BAER versus CNAP

The overall goal of AEP monitoring of the eighth nerve during surgical management of VS is to identity manipulations that are resulting in physiologic changes likely to produce a decrement in residual hearing and to predict hearing function at the termination of the case.[1,3,4,7,35] The ideal monitoring system would 1) provide clear and stable electrophysiologic responses from the structures at surgical risk; 2) responses would be measured in real time and changes in these responses would be quickly, reliably, and objectively identified; 3) changes in these responses would represent reversible dysfunctions amenable to intervention; 4) changes would reflect the exact structure that is being harmed; and 5) the responses would reliably predict postoperative hearing outcomes. At this time, no system or strategy fulfills fully all or even most of these criteria. However, both BAER and CNAP can provide the meaningful estimates of residual physiologic function of the auditory system. Each has its advantages and disadvantages. ▶ Table 28.1 gives a general comparison of BAER and CNAP monitoring techniques.

BAER is a far-field recording technique, meaning that the recording electrodes are located at a distance from the neural generators of the AEP signals.[1,2,22] Advantages of BAER include the familiarity of BAER waveforms to most neurotologists and neurophysiologists, the capacity to obtain preoperative measurements, consistent placement of electrodes relative to the neural generators, and a generally stable recording environment as the electrodes are located away from the operative field. BAER is a standard technique used by many neurotologists, neurologists, audiologists, and researchers and thus the waveform morphologies, latencies, and interpretations are

Table 28.1 Comparison of BAER and CNAP characteristics

Parameter	BAER	CNAP
Inactive electrode location	Ipsilateral mastoid (Ai)/earlobe	IAC, CN, or brainstem CN
	Far-field	Near-field
Active and ground electrode locations	Active = Cz Ground = Fz/other	Active = Cz Ground = Fz/other
Stimulus type, stimulus frequency, filtering, recording	Same	Same
Waves of interest	I and/or V	N1
Approximate amplitude	<1 μV to nanovolts	1–10 μV
Latency	Variable	Variable
Trials	1,000–2,000	10–300
Typical time frame	Minutes	Seconds
Auditory system focus	Cochlea to midbrain	Distal and proximal CN

Abbreviations: BAER, brainstem auditory evoked response; CN, cochlear nerve; CNAP, cochlear nerve action potential; Cz, vertex; Fz, midline forehead; IAC, internal acoustic canal.

familiar (▶ Fig. 28.2a).[42] Preoperative recording can be compared with intraoperative findings to assess for changes or technical issues at any time in the case. The stability of the electrode placement allows for more reliable assessment of changes. When the relative position of an electrode changes, this will alter the morphology of the waves of interest and may confound the ability to determine if a change is due to a surgical manipulation. There is one main and significant disadvantage to BAER: the relatively small size of the potentials as measured by the technique (nanovolts to microvolts). This results in a need for many averaged trials to reduce the impact of other confounding signals. It is not uncommon for several thousand trials to be required to discern BAER waveforms. This can take a considerable amount of time, frequently several minutes, and reduces the temporal accuracy of BAER monitoring to alert the surgeon of a potentially injurious maneuver prior to irreversible damage.

CNAP is a near-field recording technique, meaning that one of the electrodes is located very close to the neural generators of the AEP signal.[1] This technique was introduced as a means to overcome the disadvantages of BAER, specifically the small measured amplitude, which requires significant averaging to reduce contaminating signals.[7,34,40,43] The CNAP response takes a triphasic waveform with a vertex positive initial wave and then larger negative wave, followed by a second positive wave (P1N1P2 configuration).[5] The P1 wave can be very small and there is sometimes a fourth negative wave (N2) resulting in the N1P2N2 and P1N1P2N2 configurations.[40] ▶ Fig. 28.2b demonstrates the CNAP waveform we typically identify at the University of Iowa. There is some disagreement in the published literature regarding the naming convention as some authors begin naming with the first negative wave; this is the convention used at the University of Iowa (▶ Fig. 28.2b).[7,9,41] The source generators and latencies of these responses change depending on where the inactive electrode is placed: distal CN in the internal auditory canal (IAC) or proximal CN in the medial cerebellopontine angle at or near the brainstem. In the initial description of the intraoperative CNAP, Møller and Jannetta described the latency of the CNAP matching with the wave II of the BAER, indicating a proximal CN source.[40] Several authors have described changes in the waveform morphology depending on the exact placement of the inactive electrode.[9,33,40]

When used in the middle fossa approach, the electrode is placed near the distal CN,[17,33] whereas when utilized in the retrosigmoid or suboccipital approaches the electrode is placed near the proximal CN at the brainstem, in some cases near the foramen of Luschka.[5,6,7,38,41,44] The main and significant advantage of CNAP is the relatively large evoked potentials. This allows for rapid signal identification, as the number of averaged trials can be low, resulting in near-real-time readout of auditory system physiology.[1,17,33,34,45] This near-real-time assessment may allow for the identification of an injurious surgical maneuver in time to alter the maneuver or to intervene and potentially preserve residual physiologic function. We have found that with CNAP recordings, we can identify reliable waveforms in as few as 100 trials in many patients, which is in agreement with the published literature.[5,6] Other authors have reported CNAPs requiring 100 to 300 averages to discern a waveform.[7,9,42] There are several disadvantages to CNAP: there is no method to measure CNAPs preoperatively until the tumor is exposed, the electrode placement is generally less stable than BAER, the waveforms are less familiar to most neurotologists and neurophysiologists, and there is not a currently available standard electrode. The inability to obtain preoperative CNAP measurements is not significant impediment since, if a BAER can be recorded, it is highly likely that a CNAP can be obtained[17] (unless the residual auditory physiology has been compromised by the surgical approach; see below). Many reports demonstrated CNAP responses in the setting of absent BAER either preoperatively or postoperatively.[17,33] Electrode placement and stability are significant issues. Regardless of which surgical approach is undertaken, the electrode and its wire are invariably in the surgical field, making movement or complete dislodgement possible during surgical maneuvers. With movement of the electrode, the morphology and possibly the polarity of the waves can be altered even if the physiology of the generators has not changed.[7,38] This is discussed below but it should be evident that nonphysiologic changes in the signals will make interpretation less reliable. Depending on the exact location of the electrode, different waves of the response will be accentuated or diminished. If the electrode is placed in the IAC, then wave I will be large with smaller later waves. On the other hand, electrode placement at the root entry zone will accentuate wave III. Thus, the morphology is less stable, predictable, and familiar to most neurotologists and neurophysiologists, making interpretation more difficult.

CNAP is the preferred method for intraoperative eighth nerve monitoring at the University of Iowa, despite its shortcomings, as it can provide near-real-time estimates of the physiological impact of surgical manipulations. Additionally, it is quick and easy to switch back to BAER if CNAP is not stable or reliable enough to be of practical use during the case.

28.5 Preoperative Assessment

The evaluation and diagnosis of VS, management decision making, surgical candidacy, and suitability of the patient for a hearing-preserving operation are discussed in other chapters of this book and are not reviewed in this chapter. Audiometric testing, including pure tone threshold and speech assessment, has typically been performed and occasionally BAER has been performed as well. A BAER is performed, if not already completed, to assess for the presence of the standard waves, especially waves I and V. This is normally performed with skin surface electrodes with the patient sitting still and as relaxed as possible to minimize skeletal muscle artifacts. Contralateral BAER can give valuable insight into the technical quality of the recording: normal waves from the non–tumor affected ear and poor waveforms from the index ear indicate a technically sufficient recording with physiologically disturbed BAER from the index ear. Conversely, if the contralateral ear gives a poor BAER, a technical issue may be present and resolution sought. ▶ Fig. 28.3 demonstrates normal waveforms in each ear but delayed absolute and interwave latencies in the tumor-affected ear. ▶ Fig. 28.4 provides a preoperative BAER from a patient with an attenuated BAER from the ear affected by the tumor and a normal response from the contralateral ear. This demonstrates that a technically adequate BAER recording environment was present and that the derangement seen in the response from the tumor-affected ear is likely from the tumor. Preoperative BAER is not mandatory but allows for an estimation of the stimulus parameters needed to generate a reliable AEP response as well as establish a baseline. AEPs can be obtained in the operating room after the patient is under anesthesia but significant time can be spent attempting to determine if a no-response pattern is a technical or physiological issue; a preoperative recording can help clarify this question. Additionally, a no-response AEP found with a technically satisfactory recording is not a contraindication to attempted intraoperative eighth nerve monitoring.[1,3,17] Subcutaneous needle electrodes offer lower impedances and can improve the size and reproducibility of recorded AEPs. Additionally, with the patient under general anesthesia, skeletal muscle interference is minimized.[3,35] Even in cases where no discernable waves can be found and all technical issues have been eliminated or reduced, CNAP can often be recorded in no-response BAER situations (▶ Fig. 28.5).

a

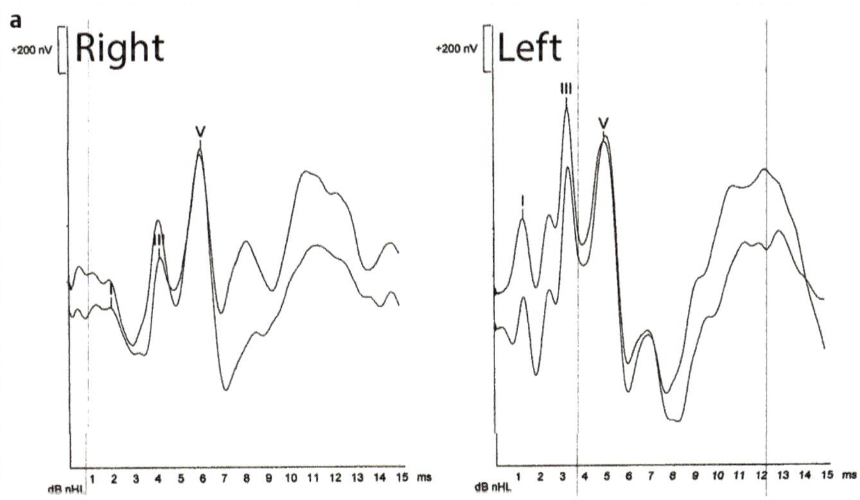

b

Ear	Absolute waveform latencies (ms)					Interwave latencies (ms)		
	I	II	III	IV	V	I- III	III -V	I-V
Right	1.93		4.13		6.03	2.20	1.90	4.10
Left	1.33		3.33		5.00	2.00	1.67	3.67

Fig. 28.3 Preoperative BAER from a patient with a right-sided vestibular schwannoma. **(a)** The right and left side demonstrate normal waveforms though the latencies are slightly prolonged on the right side. **(b)** Latency data demonstrate prolonged latencies from the right ear, both absolute and interwave latencies.

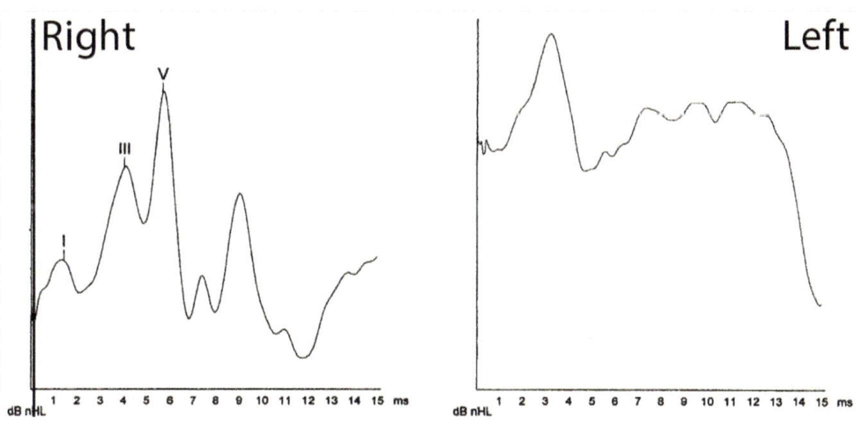

Fig. 28.4 Preoperative BAER from a patient with a left-sided vestibular schwannoma. This image demonstrates normal BAER waveforms on the right and no identifiable waveforms on the left.

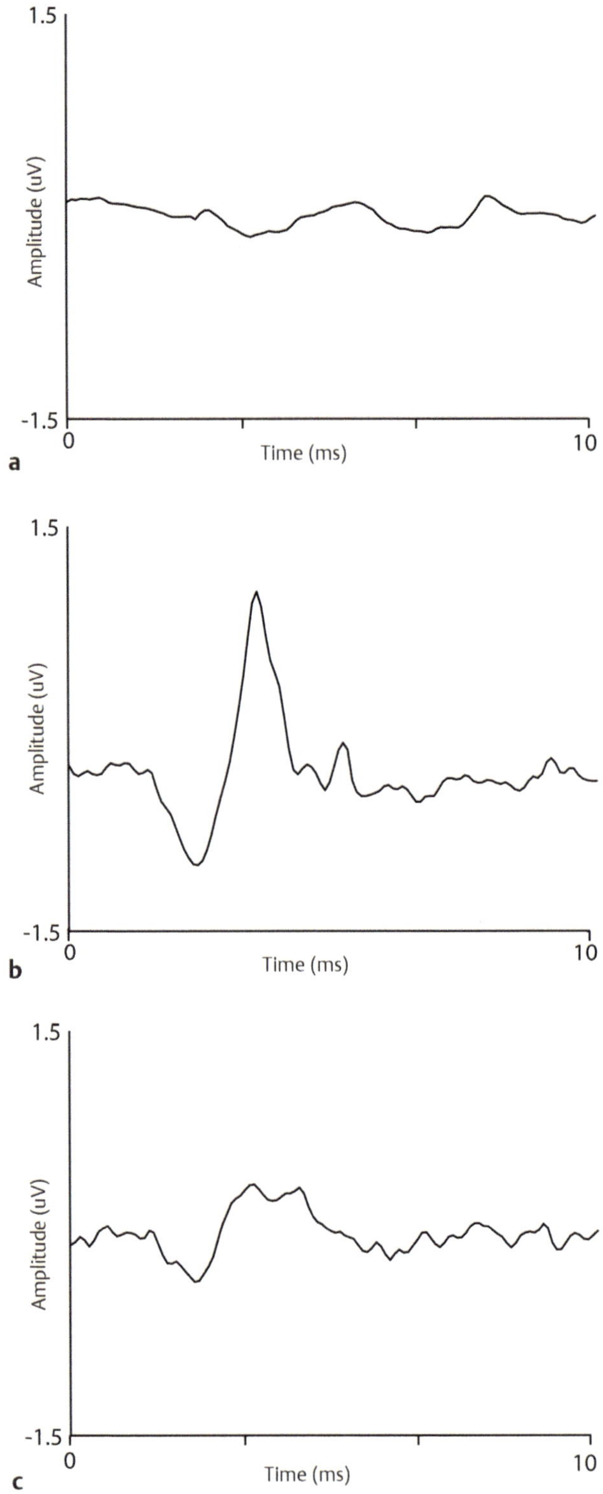

Fig. 28.5 BAER and CNAP responses from a patient with a medium-sized vestibular schwannoma. **(a)** Intraoperative BAER at the beginning of the case that fails to demonstrate identifiable waveforms. **(b)** CNAP with the inactive electrode in the distal IAC. This demonstrates a large and obvious CNAP despite the lack of demonstrable waves on BAER. **(c)** This demonstrates the presence of the CNAP response that is diminished but still present at the end of the tumor removal.

28.6 Intraoperative Setup and Performance

There are many variations to the technical aspects of the recording of intraoperative AEPs for eighth nerve monitoring. The following description is the technique used at the University of Iowa during surgical procedures where the eighth nerve is at risk and hearing preservation is desired.[39] Our preferred surgical approach for VS removal with attempted hearing preservation is the middle cranial fossa exposure of the IAC and lateral cerebellopontine angle. ▶ Table 28.2 provides the technical recording parameters used at our institution. Preoperative BAER recordings are made and examined at the initial surgical consultation. The patient is administered general anesthesia and positioned for the surgical procedure. The Natus Bio-Logic Navigator Pro (Pleasanton, CA) system is used to generate the

Table 28.2 Intraoperative eighth nerve monitoring setup utilized at the University of Iowa

Parameter	Setting/location	Features
Electrode montage	**Location**	
• Active/recording	Vertex (Cz)	
• Inactive/reference	Ipsilateral mastoid tip (Ai)	
• Ground	Midline forehead (Fz)	
• CN electrode (CNAP only)	Between IAC dura and anterior wall of the IAC	
Stimuli		
• Type/polarity	Rarefaction	
• Rate	27.7 Hz	
• Amplitude	80–90 dB nHL	
• Recording epoch	21.33 ms	
• Sampling rate	~12,500 Hz	
Filtering		
• Type	Bandpass	
• Upper bound	1,500 Hz	
• Lower bound	100 Hz	
• Notch filter	Not typically used	
Amplifier gain	100,000	
Artifact rejection		
• Threshold voltage	Not typically used	
Trials/averaging		
• Number of trails	BAER	CNAP
	1,000–2,000	Running visual assessment
Waveforms monitored		Parameter of wave(s) monitored
• BAER	Wave V	Amplitude only
• CNAP	P1[a]	Amplitude only

Abbreviations: Ai, ipsilateral mastoid cortex; BAER, brainstem auditory evoked response; CN, cochlear nerve; CNAP, cochlear nerve action potential; Cz, vertex; Fz, midline forehead; IAC, internal acoustic canal.
[a]Based on N1P1N2P2 waveform configuration.

acoustic stimuli and record any AEP responses. ▶ Fig. 28.1 demonstrates the intraoperative setup utilized at the University of Iowa for intraoperative facial and eighth nerve monitoring. Foam insert earphones are placed in each external auditory canal and the shielded speakers are taped to the shoulders such that the tubing connecting the speaker to the earphone is not kinked and is lying away from the surgical field. A small piece of occluding clear tape is placed over the conchal bowl of the operative ear to prevent prep solution or other fluids from entering the external canal. Needle electrodes are placed subcutaneously in the skin overlying each mastoid tip (inactive/reference electrodes; Ai and Ac for ipsilateral and contralateral locations, respectively), the vertex (active/recording electrode; Cz), and the midline forehead (ground electrode; Fz). These are secured with tape to minimize movement or extrusion of the needle during the case and positioned away from the operative field. The electrodes are connected to the recording system and positioned as physically far from other electrical devices as possible. A baseline BAER is performed and the waveforms assessed. This is done prior to formal prepping and draping of the surgical site so that if the electrodes or earphones need to be repositioned, this can be accomplished with ease. Another BAER is recorded after the skin incision is made to assess the impact that prepping, draping, and the initial surgical exposure have had on the BAER. Typically, there is not much alteration in the waveform morphologies and latencies between preoperative and postincisional recordings, but if changes have occurred, it is important to note these prior to tumor manipulation.

Once the IAC and tumor are exposed, a BAER is performed to serve as the pre-excisional baseline. The dura is opened and the tumor is removed, as outlined in other chapters of this book. Continuous BAER monitoring is performed and the neurophysiologist alerts the surgeon if there is a change in the waveform morphology or amplitude of wave V. There are no objective criteria used at our institution, except that the change needs to be reproducible and stable. Interpretation of the etiology of a change and possible interventions or alterations in the surgical technique is discussed below. After the tumor excision is completed, a final BAER is obtained. Representative records are saved to the patient's medical record and all data are stored. ▶ Fig. 28.6 demonstrates stable BAER waveforms throughout the procedure.

If CNAP is to be employed, the setup is the same as for BAER. Once the IAC is exposed, a needle electrode is insinuated between the anteroinferior dura of the IAC and the bony anterior IAC (▶ Fig. 28.7). This approximates the position of the distal CN and helps to hold the electrode in place. The electrode is then connected to the recording system and replaces the

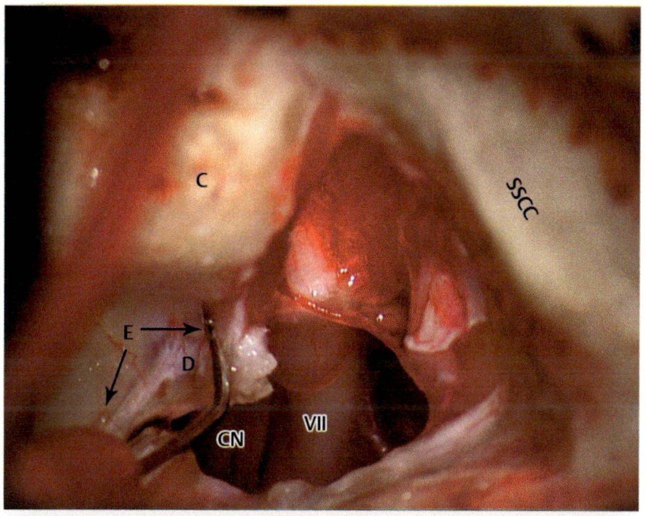

Fig. 28.7 Placement of the direct eighth nerve monitoring electrode. The electrode is tucked between the anterior bony internal auditory canal and the juxtaposed dura. We prefer to create a slight bend in the wire to facilitate the electrode angling away from the main operative field. Additionally, we also curl the tip of the electrode to prevent the needle tip from lacerating the dura or nearby cochlear nerve. C, cochlea; CN, cochlear nerve; D, anterior IAC dura; E, direct nerve monitoring electrode; SSCC, superior semicircular canal; VII, facial nerve/CN 7.

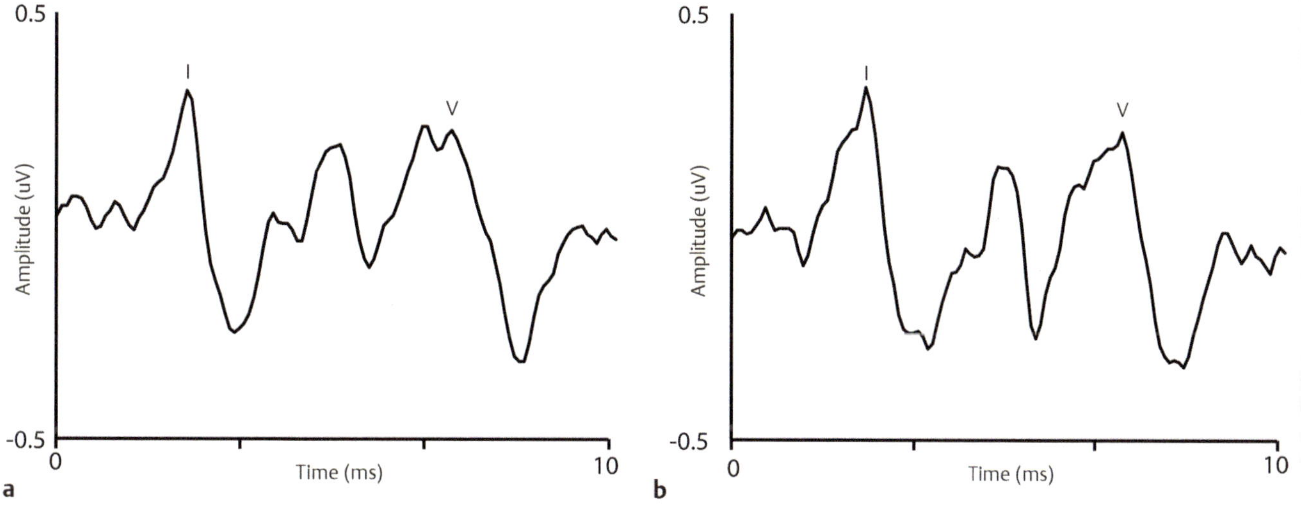

Fig. 28.6 BAER responses from a right-sided, small vestibular schwannoma. **(a)** Preincisional BAER demonstrating normal waveform morphology. Waves I and V are labeled. This patient had normal audiometric testing results at the time of surgical consultation. **(b)** BAER response after the tumor has been removed demonstrating preserved waveform morphology. This patient had stable postoperative audiometric testing results when compared to his preoperative testing.

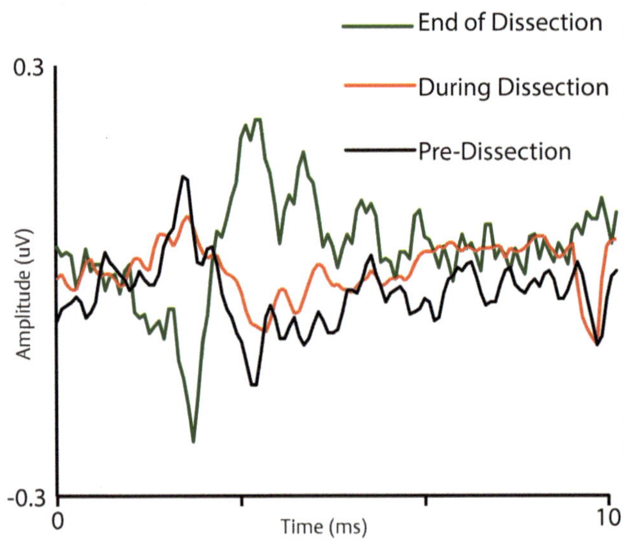

Fig. 28.8 CNAP response with diminution and then recovery. This patient had a moderate-sized vestibular schwannoma and indiscernible BAER waveforms. There is a decrease in the amplitude and increase in the latency of the response during dissection. At the end of the case, the CNAP response has recovered and is larger than that pre-excisional baseline. Audiometric testing results of this patient were reduced but still present when compared to preoperative testing.

ipsilateral mastoid electrode. The same stimulus and recording parameters are used but typically there is a significant reduction in the required number of trials needed to obtain the CNAP response. Similar interpretation strategies are used as in BAER monitoring. ▶ Fig. 28.8 demonstrates an intraoperative CNAP with a slight decline from pre-excisional baseline to postexcisional terminal recordings.

If a retrosigmoid or suboccipital approach is used to expose the tumor, the setup and recording of BAERs is the same as for the middle fossa exposure. If CNAP is used, the electrode is placed at more proximal locations including the proximal CN at the root entry zone of the eighth nerve complex.[5,6] Many times, the tumor must be debulked prior to placement of the electrode.[5,6] Additionally, most iterations of the electrode are placed directly on the nerve with little method of securing the position, thus making electrode migration a significant issue. The interpretation strategies are similar to those used with the middle fossa approach as discussed below. Further descriptions of CNAP use with the retrosigmoid approach can be found in Chapter 36.

If skin surface electrodes are to be used, the skin should be cleaned with alcohol to remove natural oils and desquamated epithelium that can increase the impedance at the contact site.[1,22] Additionally, surface electrodes should be secured, as these are more likely to be displaced or migrate during surgery, making the recordings less reliable. If metal surface electrodes are used, these should be cleaned of any residual debris or corroded material.

28.7 Interpretation of AEP Responses

The main advantage of using AEPs as an intraoperative measure of auditory system physiology is that these signals are objective and are relatively insensitive to the use of general anesthetics and commonly employed neuromuscular relaxants.[1,2] In the ideal setting, clear waveforms are identified at the start of the surgical case and are preserved without alteration throughout the case with patient confirmation upon arousal that hearing in the index ear is intact. Often, changes occur in the course of the procedure and these can be grouped into three categories[29]: (1) technical issues where the physiology of the generators has not changed but the recorded waveform is altered; (2) physiologic changes in the generators that are not due to surgical manipulation; and (3) physiologic changes due to surgical damage. Discernment of one type of physiologic change from another can be difficult as all can occur independent of each other and can result in similar waveform perturbations from baseline measures. The first two types of intraoperative changes can be thought of as false-positive changes, with the last type representing true-positive changes.

Technical recording problems include broken electrodes or wires, kinked sound conduction tubing, conductive blocks between the insert earphone and the cochlear (fluid or bone dust in the external or middle ear), stimuli that are of insufficient intensity, electrode impedances being too high or with large discrepancies between the recording and reference electrodes, filter settings that are either too broad or too narrow, artifact rejection criteria are too lax or stringent, migration or frank displacement of the electrodes, and competing electrical signals from operative equipment.[29] Broken wires will result in abnormal or absent waveforms and large and/or unstable impedances. Any type of blockage of the transmission of acoustic energy from the receiver to the inner ear (kinked sound tube, fluid in the external or middle ear) will result in small and delayed waveforms due to a lower intensity sound delivered to the sensory epithelium. Electrode impedances that are too high or disparate between the electrode montage points will distort or eliminate the AEP waveforms. Filter setting that are too wide will let competing signals into the recording, while filter setting that are too narrow will exclude some of the energy of the AEP and reduce the signal. All of these technical issues are typically stable over the course of the operation. Electrode migration is a more significant issue as changes in electrode position due to migration or displacement will alter the morphology of the waveforms, which can mimic other physiologic changes.[38] Sources of electrical interference can be from the facial nerve monitor, the operating microscope, overhead lights and lightboxes, the anesthesia machine and its various monitors, the operating room table, powered surgical instruments (e.g., ultrasonic aspirator or electric drill), the acoustic stimulation speakers/receivers, and even suctions. It can be difficult to eliminate the interference from these devices, as their use is often critical to the successful performance of the operation. Whenever possible, using shielded equipment should be employed. Additionally, the electrodes should be placed as far as possible from the interference sources. Lastly, use of powered instruments and equipment can be paused to obtain a clear recording, though this strategy may add considerable time to the procedure.

Physiologic changes due to nonsurgical manipulations include hypothermia, hypoxia, and masking.[29] As core or local temperatures decrease, there is a nonlinear decrease in amplitude and increase in latency.[1,29] Core temperature changes are less problematic as tight control can typically be achieved with contemporary anesthesia techniques/equipment as well as the relatively limited surface area exposed with skull base approaches. Local temperature decreases due to surgical irrigation that is cooler than the body can have an impact on the waveform morphology.[29] Using warmed irrigation can help reduce this impact. Hypoxia, for whatever reason, will impact the capacity to generate a synchronized response. The noise from surgical instrumentation can serve as a masking signal and reduce or eliminate a response from the index ear. Typically, this is from the otologic drill but could also occur with the noise from the suctions or ultrasonic aspiration systems. With any of these sources of physiologic change, waveforms can be altered and can confound interpretation for the surgical and monitoring team.

Surgical damage to the auditory structures can be from many surgical manipulations and represents the types of changes that are of utmost interest to the surgeon as these are most likely to result in permanent hearing loss. The damaging event can be anatomic disruption (stretching, cutting, tearing, or avulsing), thermal injury, or cauterization of the CN.[2,29] Alternatively, disruption or occlusion of the vascular supply to the CN or cochlea may result in hypoxia or infarction, or both.[2,29] Many of these events are irreversible but prompt recognition can inform the surgeon of an injurious maneuver to allow for alteration of the surgical technique to prevent further injury. Reversible changes might include stretch on the CN or vessels from retractors (which can be released) or hypoxia from vasospasm that could be treated with topical application of a vasodilator (e.g., papaverine 30 mg/mL[13,33]), raising the systemic blood pressure, and or decreasing blood viscosity.[4,12,13,33,39]

Changes in the waveforms can be either a change in waveform morphology or latencies. Physiologic changes at early stages in the auditory processing stream may impact subsequent waves even if these location have unaffected physiology.[29] For example, ischemic insults to the CN can result in delayed latencies and decreased amplitude of waves II–V or loss of these waves altogether.[29] Damage to more central locations will typically have very little impact on the earlier waveforms. For example, damage to the eighth nerve proximal to the IAC will typically not impact wave I but may attenuate wave V. However, if the injurious maneuver at the brainstem results in infarction of the cochlea (internal auditory artery damage/occlusion), then all waves could be lost. Thus, no pattern of waveform changes is precisely predictive of which neuroanatomical structure has been injured or the mechanism of injury. Additionally, an injurious maneuver may set in motion events that will, in the near future, result in an AEP waveform change or loss. Thus, an observed change may not temporally correlate with the surgical events at the time of the observation, confounding the ability to effectively alter the surgical progression.[4,9,45]

28.8 AEP Response Parameters and Criteria for Establishing an Intraoperative Change from Baseline

No universally accepted objective criteria for what constitutes a change from baseline recordings exist.[1] This is not unexpected given the wide variety of recording protocols (electrode montages, stimulus rates and intensities, etc.) and the wide variety of residual physiology due to the variable tumor presentations. A survey of the literature demonstrates that most authors monitor for changes in AEP amplitudes, the absolute presence (or loss) of an AEP waveform, and/or latency changes in an AEP waveform. When monitoring waveforms, responses can be stable (no change from baseline), temporarily altered (partially or completed lost with recovery to baseline), or permanently altered (partially or completely lost relative to baseline). Additionally, the definitions of what constitutes a change range from being undefined[4,13], to a subjective[5,34] assessment that a change has occurred in some way, to objective[23,31,37,38] criteria. Some authors define meaningful changes based on post hoc analysis of their data. Good, high-quality evidence based on prospective head-to-head comparisons of the various thresholds for establishing a change from baseline does not exist. Criteria for judging a change should be individualized to the patient's pre-op baseline and the experience of the surgical team.[29]

The most commonly followed BAER wave is wave V with waves I and III or combinations of waves being followed as well in various studies.[3,26,46,47,48] When considering wave V, the most commonly monitored parameter is the amplitude, with the absolute latency being monitored commonly but less often. Latency of wave V has been used as the sole metric,[24] but this is uncommon. A commonly used, albeit arbitrarily defined parameter, is a 50% or greater reduction in the wave amplitude.[9,10,12,23,31,49] Similar arbitrary changes in the absolute wave V latency have been used. Subjective decreases in wave V amplitude are also reported.[3,4,15,25,48] Similarly, arbitrary latency shifts between 0.1 and 1.0 ms have been considered significant by various authors.[10,15,23,31] Many authors have used both wave V amplitude decreases and latency increases together when considering if a change from baseline is significant. The American Society for Neurophysiological Monitoring (ANSM) 2007 position statement on intraoperative eighth nerve monitoring regards a > 50% reduction and/or an increase in latency of > 10% as reasonable criteria for warning the surgeon that a change has been detected but they additionally caution that the type of posterior fossa surgery and residual auditory physiology should be taken into account.[1] Indeed, reports looking at outcomes from posterior fossa surgery for non-VS reasons have found differing results when looking at the significance of waveform changes when compared to VS surgery.[10] Additionally, the ASNM 2007 position statement proposes an alternative to strict numeric criteria: any change that is reproducible (more than test–retest variability) should be reported to the surgeon.

Criteria for determining a change in CNAP waveforms are significantly more variable in the literature. As reviewed above, the position of the electrode in the IAC versus the brainstem will affect the morphology and latency of the recorded waveforms. Additionally, as the inactive electrode is in the operative field and mobile, it is prone to movement or dislodgement, all of which will degrade the detection of the changes from baseline. Published criteria for changes from baseline are variable and range from subjective changes in waveform morphology or latency to objective metrics similar to those used for BAER wave V.[5,6,9,14,37,44] Additionally, there are differing naming conventions for the components of the CNAP that make direct comparison of reports tricky. Colletti and colleagues used a > 10%

decrease in the P1:total CNAP ratio or a > 50% decrease in the total CNAP amplitude as significant changes.[37,38] Wiet and coworkers defined a > 50% decrease CNAP amplitude as significant.[9,42] The absolute latency of the N1 portion of the CNAP response has been the most commonly monitored latency metric and significant changes warranting an alert to the surgeon have been between 0.5 and 1 ms.[7,9,37,38] Given the variety of inactive electrode locations and types as well as the greater instability of the electrode position once placed, it is prudent for the neurophysiologist to have a more flexible definition of what constitutes a significant change from baseline. As for BAER monitoring, a reasonable guideline might be to report any change that is reproducible (more than test–retest variability) to the surgeon.

28.9 Prognostic Value of Intraoperative AEP Monitoring

The ultimate goal of undertaking a hearing-preserving surgical approach is to preserve hearing, not intraoperative AEP responses. As has been reviewed above, the presence of AEP responses is not perfectly predictive of postoperative hearing[3,9,12,15] and the loss of AEP responses does not preclude postoperative hearing.[9,10,11,12,13,14] The overall trend in the literature over the past 40 years has been that intraoperative AEP monitoring is useful,[5,6,7,8,9,12,14,15,17,25,33,37,38,39,42,44,50,51] though this is a source of controversy and not uniformly supported.[15,23,52,53] The definition of what this "usefulness" means varies widely from report to report. This is due to differing preoperative and postoperative definitions of hearing preservation. As discussed previously, responses can be stable (no change from baseline), temporarily altered (partially or completed lost with recovery to baseline), or permanently altered (partially or completely lost relative to baseline). Other parameters that have been assessed include the rate of change (gradual vs. abrupt) and the appearance of waves that were not present on preoperative BAER testing.

When considering BAER, the most consistent and established prognostic finding is that the presence of a stable wave V is associated with preserved hearing of some configuration.[3,4,8,14,25,31,47,50,51] However, the presence of wave V at the end of the operation may not be sufficient for hearing preservation, as Levine and colleagues demonstrated that only if wave V was stable and present (i.e., did not disappear and then reappear or had a significant amplitude decline that recovered by the end of the case) then hearing was likely to be present postoperatively.[4] Additionally, when wave V is lost, the prognosis for preserved hearing is poor.[10,13,23,25,35,48,54,55,56] However, it should be stressed again that neither situation rules in or out postoperative hearing. Other waves or metrics have been reported to be more sensitive than wave V. Matthies and Samii reported that wave III was the most sensitive wave for predicting postoperative hearing.[47] The rate of loss of waves (including wave V) has also been reported as predictive of postoperative hearing. Abrupt loss of waves (postulated to be from acute vascular occlusion) has been associated with permanent anacusis,[3,25,31,50,51] while more gradual loss of waves can be associated with a better chance of postoperative hearing.[25,48]

The prognostic value of CNAP responses has also been generally reported to be useful and predictive of postoperative hearing. The two most frequently reported metrics are the latency of the N1 portion and amplitude of response. Most authors report a favorable prognosis for postoperative hearing if CNAP is present at the end of the case.[6,9,14,37,38,39] Yamakami et al found that CNAP presence was 100% sensitive and specific as none of their 22 patients had hearing without a CNAP response and all who had a CNAP had postoperative hearing.[14] Cohen et al found similar results—no patients who had lost responses had hearing; however, they were not able to demonstrate a positive prognostic value.[53] Colletti and Fiorino felt that the latency of the N1 portion of the response was the most predictive aspect of CNAP monitoring.[7]

When comparing BAER to CNAP, the majority of the published reports find that either CNAP is better than BAER or the addition of CNAP to BAER is beneficial to the postoperative hearing outcome.[6,9,14,17,32,33,37,38,39,44] Battista et al compared patients in which BAER or CNAP was used and found that the use of CNAP improved hearing preservation rates from 18 to 40%.[9] Similarly, Colletti and colleagues have reported that the use of CNAP monitoring greatly improves the hearing outcomes, with hearing preservation rates improving from about 30 to 70% and postoperative pure tone audiometric averages improving by about 29 dB.[7,37,38,44] Further analysis revealed that CNAP monitoring had the best predictive characteristics for postoperative hearing when receiver-operator curves were constructed for BAER, ECoG, and CNAP.[38] Danner et al demonstrated that hearing preservation rates improved from 41 to 64% with the used of CNAP monitoring.[6] Lastly, Yamakami et al found that the presence of CNAP was superior to BAER in predicting hearing outcomes as outlined above (100% sensitive and specific), while ABR was not specific (12 of 14 patients with no ABR wave V had postoperative hearing).[14] While less in number, not all reports have demonstrated benefit of CNAP. In a large report of 99 patients, Piccirillo et al found no benefit with the addition of CNAP to hearing preservation rates: 21% without CNAP and 26% with CNAP.[15] Additionally, Cohen et al did not demonstrate a hearing preservation benefit with the use of CNAP monitoring.[53]

It is difficult to draw firm conclusions about the utility of intraoperative eighth nerve monitoring using either BAER or CNAP. Frankly, the predictive value of long-term hearing with either technique is not reliable enough to make firm intraoperative decisions. Additionally, it is difficult to correlate intraoperative changes of specific waves with operative manipulations as there is at least some delay from the time of the manipulation to the time that a waveform alteration is detectable. This is partially due to the requirement of many trials that need to be performed and averaged but also because certain manipulation may start in motion a cascade of events that ultimately result in a waveform change but that take time to manifest (as proposed by Levine et al[4]). However, given that both BAER and CNAP pose little risk to the patient and most authors espouse the ability of AEP monitoring to improve hearing outcomes, there seems to be little downside in utilizing this technology and we find it to be helpful during tumor dissection. Proper interpretation is key and requires a surgical and neurophysiological team that is knowledgeable in the nuances of AEP generation and recording.

28.10 Conclusion

Intraoperative eighth nerve neurophysiological monitoring offers the chance to obtain near-real-time feedback about the impact that various surgical manipulations have on the health of the residual auditory system. It is hard to formulate specific criteria that can be universally applied given the wide variety of tumor sizes, locations, residual ipsilateral hearing, operating room noise, surgical approaches used, and the experience and skill of the tumor surgeon that impact intraoperative AEP usefulness. Changes in the amplitude and/or latencies of the various waves can be used to judge perturbations from baseline recordings. Care must be taken when interpreting the intraoperative signals, as significant source of error can be present. Monitoring of CNAP responses has the advantage of larger amplitude responses and thus requires less averaging and can provide feedback more quickly than BAER but has the disadvantage that it requires a more difficult electrode placement and is more vulnerable to spurious changes in waveform morphology. BAER has the advantage of being more stable but requires significantly more averaging time to obtain meaningful waveforms, which diminishes its value as a real-time feedback system.

References

[1] Martin WH, Stecker MM. ASNM position statement: intraoperative monitoring of auditory evoked potentials. J Clin Monit Comput. 2008; 22(1):75–85
[2] Yingling CD, Ashram YA. Intraoperative monitoring of cranial nerves in skull base surgery. In: Jackler RK, Brackmann DE, eds. Neurotology. Vol 1. 2nd ed. Philadelphia, PA: Mosby; 2005:958–996
[3] Ojemann RG, Levine RA, Montgomery WM, McGaffigan P. Use of intraoperative auditory evoked potentials to preserve hearing in unilateral acoustic neuroma removal. J Neurosurg. 1984; 61(5):938–948
[4] Levine RA, Ojemann RG, Montgomery WW, McGaffigan PM. Monitoring auditory evoked potentials during acoustic neuroma surgery. Insights into the mechanism of the hearing loss. Ann Otol Rhinol Laryngol. 1984; 93(2, Pt 1):116–123
[5] Cueva RA, Morris GF, Prioleau GR. Direct cochlear nerve monitoring: first report on a new atraumatic, self-retaining electrode. Am J Otol. 1998; 19(2): 202–207
[6] Danner C, Mastrodimos B, Cueva RA. A comparison of direct eighth nerve monitoring and auditory brainstem response in hearing preservation surgery for vestibular schwannoma. Otol Neurotol. 2004; 25(5):826–832
[7] Colletti V, Fiorino FG. Vulnerability of hearing function during acoustic neuroma surgery. Acta Otolaryngol. 1994; 114(3):264–270
[8] Grundy BL, Jannetta PJ, Procopio PT, Lina A, Boston JR, Doyle E. Intraoperative monitoring of brain-stem auditory evoked potentials. J Neurosurg. 1982; 57 (5):674–681
[9] Battista RA, Wiet RJ, Paauwe L. Evaluation of three intraoperative auditory monitoring techniques in acoustic neuroma surgery. Am J Otol. 2000; 21(2): 244–248
[10] James ML, Husain AM. Brainstem auditory evoked potential monitoring: when is change in wave V significant? Neurology. 2005; 65(10):1551–1555
[11] Mustain WD, al-Mefty O, Anand VK. Inconsistencies in the correlation between loss of brain stem auditory evoked response waves and postoperative deafness. J Clin Monit. 1992; 8(3):231–235
[12] Harner SG, Harper CM, Beatty CW, Litchy WJ, Ebersold MJ. Far-field auditory brainstem response in neurotologic surgery. Am J Otol. 1996; 17(1):150–153
[13] Browning S, Mohr G, Dufour JJ, et al. Hearing preservation in acoustic neuroma surgery. J Otolaryngol. 2001; 30(5):307–315
[14] Yamakami I, Yoshinori H, Saeki N, Wada M, Oka N. Hearing preservation and intraoperative auditory brainstem response and cochlear nerve compound action potential monitoring in the removal of small acoustic neurinoma via the retrosigmoid approach. J Neurol Neurosurg Psychiatry. 2009; 80(2):218–227
[15] Piccirillo E, Hiraumi H, Hamada M, Russo A, De Stefano A, Sanna M. Intraoperative cochlear nerve monitoring in vestibular schwannoma surgery–does it really affect hearing outcome? Audiol Neurootol. 2008; 13(1):58–64
[16] Yingling CD, Gardi JN. Intraoperative monitoring of facial and cochlear nerves during acoustic neuroma surgery. 1992. Neurosurg Clin N Am. 2008; 19(2): 289–315, vii
[17] Roberson JB, Jr, Jackson LE, McAuley JR. Acoustic neuroma surgery: absent auditory brainstem response does not contraindicate attempted hearing preservation. Laryngoscope. 1999; 109(6):904–910
[18] Elliott FA, McKISSOCK W. Acoustic neuroma; early diagnosis. Lancet. 1954; 267(6850):1189–1191
[19] Jewett DL. Volume-conducted potentials in response to auditory stimuli as detected by averaging in the cat. Electroencephalogr Clin Neurophysiol. 1970; 28(6):609–618
[20] Jewett DL, Romano MN, Williston JS. Human auditory evoked potentials: possible brain stem components detected on the scalp. Science. 1970; 167 (3924):1517–1518
[21] Jewett DL, Williston JS. Auditory-evoked far fields averaged from the scalp of humans. Brain. 1971; 94(4):681–696
[22] Kileny PR, Edwards BM. Objective measure of auditory function. In: Jackler RK, Brackmann D, eds. Neurotology. Vol 1. Philadelphia, PA: Mosby; 2005:287–305
[23] Slavit DH, Harner SG, Harper CM, Jr, Beatty CW. Auditory monitoring during acoustic neuroma removal. Arch Otolaryngol Head Neck Surg. 1991; 117(10): 1153–1157
[24] Samii M, Gerganov V, Samii A. Improved preservation of hearing and facial nerve function in vestibular schwannoma surgery via the retrosigmoid approach in a series of 200 patients. J Neurosurg. 2006; 105(4):527–535
[25] Neu M, Strauss C, Romstöck J, Bischoff B, Fahlbusch R. The prognostic value of intraoperative BAEP patterns in acoustic neurinoma surgery. Clin Neurophysiol. 1999; 110(11):1935–1941
[26] Gouveris H, Mann W. Association between surgical steps and intraoperative auditory brainstem response and electrocochleography waveforms during hearing preservation vestibular schwannoma surgery. Eur Arch Otorhinolaryngol. 2009; 266(2):225–229
[27] Klem GH, Lüders HO, Jasper HH, Elger C, The International Federation of Clinical Neurophysiology. The ten-twenty electrode system of the International Federation. Electroencephalogr Clin Neurophysiol Suppl. 1999; 52:3–6
[28] Dinh CTO, Ojo R, Yilmazer R, et al. Intraoperative neurophysiologicial monitoring. In: Brackmann D, Shelton C, Arriaga M, eds. Otologic Surgery. Vol 1. 4th ed. Philadelphia, PA: Elsevier; 2016:678–689
[29] Legatt AD. Mechanisms of intraoperative brainstem auditory evoked potential changes. J Clin Neurophysiol. 2002; 19(5):396–408
[30] Fridman J, John ER, Bergelson M, Kaiser JB, Baird HW. Application of digital filtering and automatic peak detection to brain stem auditory evoked potential. Electroencephalogr Clin Neurophysiol. 1982; 53(4):405–416
[31] Harper CM, Harner SG, Slavit DH, et al. Effect of BAEP monitoring on hearing preservation during acoustic neuroma resection. Neurology. 1992; 42(8): 1551–1553
[32] Jackson LE, Roberson JB, Jr. Acoustic neuroma surgery: use of cochlear nerve action potential monitoring for hearing preservation. Am J Otol. 2000; 21(2): 249–259
[33] Roberson J, Senne A, Brackmann D, Hitselberger WE, Saunders J. Direct cochlear nerve action potentials as an aid to hearing preservation in middle fossa acoustic neuroma resection. Am J Otol. 1996; 17(4):653–657
[34] Silverstein H, McDaniel AB, Norrell H. Hearing preservation after acoustic neuroma surgery using intraoperative direct eighth cranial nerve monitoring. Am J Otol. 1985 Suppl:99–106
[35] Schramm J, Mokrusch T, Fahlbusch R, Hochstetter A. Detailed analysis of intraoperative changes monitoring brain stem acoustic evoked potentials. Neurosurgery. 1988; 22(4):694–702
[36] Levine RA, Montgomery WW, Ojemann RG. Evoked potential detection of hearing loss during acoustic neuroma surgery. Neurology. 1978; 28:339
[37] Colletti V, Fiorino FG. Advances in monitoring of seventh and eighth cranial nerve function during posterior fossa surgery. Am J Otol. 1998; 19(4):503–512
[38] Colletti V, Fiorino FG, Mocella S, Policante Z. ECochG, CNAP and ABR monitoring during vestibular schwannoma surgery. Audiology. 1998; 37(1):27–37
[39] Meyer TA, Canty PA, Wilkinson EP, Hansen MR, Rubinstein JT, Gantz BJ. Small acoustic neuromas: surgical outcomes versus observation or radiation. Otol Neurotol. 2006; 27(3):380–392
[40] Møller AR, Jannetta PJ. Compound action potentials recorded intracranially from the auditory nerve in man. Exp Neurol. 1981; 74(3):862–874

[41] Colletti V, Bricolo A, Fiorino FG, Bruni L. Changes in directly recorded cochlear nerve compound action potentials during acoustic tumor surgery. Skull Base Surg. 1994; 4(1):1–9
[42] Zappia, JJ, Wiet RJ, O'Connor CA, Martone L. Intraoperative auditory monitoring in acoustic neuroma surgery. Otolaryngol Head Neck Surg. 1996; 115(1): 98–106
[43] Silverstein H, Norrel H, Hyman SM. Simultaneous use of CO2 laser with continuous monitoring of eighth cranial nerve action potential during acoustic neuroma surgery. Otolaryngol Head Neck Surg. 1984; 92(1):80–84
[44] Colletti V, Fiorino FG, Carner M, Cumer G, Giarbini N, Sacchetto L. Intraoperative monitoring for hearing preservation and restoration in acoustic neuroma surgery. Skull Base Surg. 2000; 10(4):187–195
[45] Nedzelski JM, Chiong CM, Cashman MZ, Stanton SG, Rowed DW. Hearing preservation in acoustic neuroma surgery: value of monitoring cochlear nerve action potentials. Otolaryngol Head Neck Surg. 1994; 111(6):703–709
[46] Youssef AS, Downes AE. Intraoperative neurophysiological monitoring in vestibular schwannoma surgery: advances and clinical implications. Neurosurg Focus. 2009; 27(4):E9
[47] Matthies C, Samii M. Management of vestibular schwannomas (acoustic neuromas): the value of neurophysiology for intraoperative monitoring of auditory function in 200 cases. Neurosurgery. 1997; 40(3):459–466, discussion 466–468
[48] Tonn JC, Schlake HP, Goldbrunner R, Milewski C, Helms J, Roosen K. Acoustic neuroma surgery as an interdisciplinary approach: a neurosurgical series of 508 patients. J Neurol Neurosurg Psychiatry. 2000; 69(2):161–166
[49] Radtke RA, Erwin CW, Wilkins RH. Intraoperative brainstem auditory evoked potentials: significant decrease in postoperative morbidity. Neurology. 1989; 39(2, Pt 1):187–191
[50] Fischer G, Fischer C, Rémond J. Hearing preservation in acoustic neurinoma surgery. J Neurosurg. 1992; 76(6):910–917
[51] Watanabe E, Schramm J, Strauss C, Fahlbusch R. Neurophysiologic monitoring in posterior fossa surgery. II. BAEP-waves I and V and preservation of hearing. Acta Neurochir (Wien). 1989; 98(3–4):118–128
[52] Kveton JF. The efficacy of brainstem auditory evoked potentials in acoustic tumor surgery. Laryngoscope. 1990; 100(11):1171–1173
[53] Cohen NL, Lewis WS, Ransohoff J. Hearing preservation in cerebellopontine angle tumor surgery: the NYU experience 1974–1991. Am J Otol. 1993; 14 (5):423–433
[54] Nadol JB, Jr, Chiong CM, Ojemann RG, et al. Preservation of hearing and facial nerve function in resection of acoustic neuroma. Laryngoscope. 1992; 102 (10):1153–1158
[55] Schlake HP, Milewski C, Goldbrunner RH, et al. Combined intra-operative monitoring of hearing by means of auditory brainstem responses (ABR) and transtympanic electrocochleography (ECochG) during surgery of intra- and extrameatal acoustic neurinomas. Acta Neurochir (Wien). 2001; 143(10): 985–995, discussion 995–996
[56] Matthies C, Samii M. Management of vestibular schwannomas (acoustic neuromas): the value of neurophysiology for evaluation and prediction of auditory function in 420 cases. Neurosurgery. 1997; 40(5):919–929, discussion -929–930

29 Training in Vestibular Schwannoma Microsurgery

Alex D. Sweeney, Joseph T. Breen, and Jeffrey T. Vrabec

29.1 Introduction

Surgical training methods have evolved significantly over the last century. Early training was through an informal apprenticeship model, characterized by observation at the side of the "master." The trainee's appointment was by mutual agreement, the duration of the experience was often open ended, technical "hands-on" training was not assured, and cost was generally borne by the trainee. The development of formal residency programs allowed for more structured training, though pyramidal programs were initially common, in which a certain number of trainees showing inadequate progress would be dismissed annually.[1] In order to create consistency, governing boards were established to provide training oversight and certification of graduates. Over time, the benefit of formalized instruction has been reinforced, in part, by relationships that have been identified between training and postoperative outcomes.[2,3] This chapter will provide an overview of the past, present, and potential future of vestibular schwannoma (VS) microsurgical training, as well as insight into the advantages of a focused surgical education regimen.

29.2 History of Vestibular Schwannoma Surgical Training

Surgical resection has historically been the standard of VS management. However, initial attempts at tumor extirpation were fraught with complications. Limitations in visibility, aseptic technique, anesthetic care, and hemostasis led to significant perioperative morbidity and mortality.[4] Through the work of pioneering neurosurgeons such as Harvey Cushing, Walter Dandy, and Vilhelm Magnus, mortality rates dropped significantly. Consequently, questions began to arise regarding the factors associated with the improvement in outcomes. When visited by Magnus in 1928, Cushing was reported to have "had harsh judgment to pronounce on those surgeons who without the requisite experience undertook these operations, which in the hands of an inexperienced surgeon were desperate remedies indeed."[4] Over time, standardization emerged in terms of surgical approaches, operative techniques, and perioperative management, leading to widespread improvements in postoperative outcomes.

As in any medical discipline, new advances alter the existing management paradigm. In the early 1960s, largely through the efforts of William House, transtemporal approaches to the lateral skull base were refined. The operating microscope was introduced into tumor resection, and electrophysiology of the auditory and vestibular system was also developed, augmenting the breadth of knowledge in the nascent field of neurotology. As mortality rates associated with VS microsurgery steadily dropped, emphasis was placed on the reduction of morbidity.[4,5,6] Specifically, postoperative cranial nerve function became paramount. Increased attention was given to facial nerve outcomes, postoperative vestibular rehabilitation, and techniques to preserve hearing with tumor removal, reinforcing the importance of comprehensive, specialized training in lateral skull base surgery.

29.3 Modern Training for Vestibular Schwannoma Surgery

Demand for training in lateral skull base surgery naturally led to the expansion of training opportunities. Many early neurotologists obtained their experience under the tutelage of Dr. William House, participating in the fellowship sponsored by the House Ear Institute.[7] By the late 1980s, there were approximately 30 fellowships in otology with differing amounts of emphasis on treatment of lateral skull base tumors. Efforts to standardize neurotology training began in response to the large number of fellowship programs and a subspecialty certificate in neurotology was approved by the Accreditation Council for Graduate Medical Education (ACGME) in 1995. Accreditation of training programs required a 2-year training period with concentrated experience in lateral skull base surgery. Key elements for accreditation included association with a residency program, board-certified faculty, adequate case volume for trainees, and available time for research. The first certification examination was given in 2004 with a 10-year time-limited certificate. Established practitioners were eligible for certification early in the process, but now certificates are only issued to graduates of accredited programs. At present, there are 19 accredited programs, producing between 14 and 16 fellows annually. Nearly all fellowship positions are filled through a subspecialty match.

The ACGME has established minimum case numbers for neurotology fellows that include performance of 25 lateral skull base approaches, 20 tumor resections, 2 temporal bone resections, and 10 repairs of skull base defects with local tissue flaps or grafts. Other skull base cases, including repair of cerebrospinal fluid otorrhea and repair of superior canal dehiscence, account for another five cases. Clinical experience requires the diagnosis of 20 VSs, 3 temporal bone paragangliomas, and 2 facial nerve tumors.

Despite the established minimums, the emphasis in residency training is not on total number of cases, but rather on proficiency in achieving technical, professional, and cognitive milestones. The adoption of this form of analysis recognizes that trainees do not display equal ability to learn. Some trainees are "naturals" who rapidly internalize surgical concepts and can mimic techniques readily. Others who are less adept take longer to achieve proficiency despite a larger volume of cases. In either case, the ability of the trainee to gather, integrate, communicate, and apply data to clinical practice may best predict commitment to self-assessment and continued process improvement.

Though the American Board of Neurologic Surgery (ABNS) does not have provisions for subspecialty certification, fellowship training in skull base surgery is available following neurosurgery residency. The Society of Neurological Surgeons (SNS), often referred to as the "Senior Society," serves as an accrediting body for neurosurgical fellowships in a variety of disciplines, including neurosurgical oncology and cerebrovascular surgery. Fellowships are generally 1 year in length, and candidates are required to have completed an ACGME accredited (or Canadian equivalent) neurosurgery residency. At present, there are eight neurosurgical oncology fellowships accredited by the SNS. Neurosurgical fellowships specifically focused on skull base tumor surgery are currently not separately accredited.

29.4 How Does Experience Affect Outcomes in Vestibular Schwannoma Surgery?

Unquestionably, dedicated training in skull base microsurgery can provide a wealth of experience with the complex anatomy and pathophysiology encountered during VS resections. With gradated autonomy of the learner, a more safe transition from strict observation to independent tumor resection can be achieved. As was initially noted by Cushing and Magnus, outcomes in VS surgery may be tied to surgeon experience. After it was established that facial nerve function could be preserved during VS surgery, research began to evaluate the factors that govern successful preservation. In 1996, Moffat et al reported a single center's experience with 300 VS resections.[8] When analyzing this cohort of patients, it became apparent that better facial nerve outcomes were achieved with increasing surgeon experience. In particular, it was noted that 52% of the first 50 consecutive surgical patients in this center achieved a House–Brackmann (HB) grade I–III, while 92% of the last 50 patients evaluated had equivalent facial outcomes in the absence of a significant difference of tumor size between the two groups. Moreover, it was noted that the learning curve was more pronounced with the translabyrinthine approach relative to the retrosigmoid approach, though more recent work has identified that the existence of a learning curve is not necessarily approach-specific.[9] Nearly 20 years following the aforementioned work, Moffat et al performed a follow-up study of 652 patients undergoing VS microsurgery from the same center to evaluate the factors that influenced postoperative facial nerve function.[10] The positive correlation between experience and outcome was again observed, and specifically, it was noted that the learning curve was steepest for the first 50 cases performed through any approach. Additionally, it was reported that surgical patients were approximately four times more likely to have "satisfactory" facial nerve outcomes (HB I–III) following 10 years of surgeon experience. To quantify the learning curve further, research by Buchman[11] and Welling,[12] respectively, considered the number of cases that need to be performed to achieve consistently good postoperative facial nerve function. Welling demonstrated that HB I outcomes are more likely to be achieved after the first 20 surgical cases, whereas Buchman found that approximately 60 cases are needed before outcomes mirror those of more experienced teams. More recently, Wang et al utilized the cumulative summation test for learning curve (LC-CUSUM) to establish that approximately 56 cases are necessary before newly formed surgical teams are able to consistently achieve "satisfactory" outcomes (HB I–III).[13]

Similar to facial nerve outcomes, many factors have been shown to influence rates of hearing preservation in VS microsurgery.[14] With regard to surgeon experience, one study attempted to primarily evaluate trends in hearing preservation microsurgery over time at a single center. In 2001, Kanzaki et al reported on 127 hearing preservation surgeries over a 24-year period.[15] All cases were performed through a middle cranial fossa approach using electrocochleography or auditory brainstem response for cochlear nerve monitoring. In the last 5 years of data collection, higher rates of Gardner–Robertson grade I hearing preservation were achieved on univariate analysis compared to rates for patients with earlier surgical dates (67 vs. 33%, $p < 0.05$). Though it is likely that surgeon experience does play a role in the probability of hearing preservation during VS surgery, the relative influence of this variable compared to tumor size, tumor location, surgical approach, and the quality of preoperative hearing remains unclear.

The experience of a particular hospital or surgical team likely plays a role in postoperative outcomes, as well. In 2004, Slattery et al evaluated the California Hospital Discharge Database (CHDD) for the period 1996 to 1998 to establish a relationship between hospital volume and VS microsurgical outcomes.[16] Hospitals were categorized into four groups on the basis of the average number of VS resections performed annually. Patients undergoing surgery at the highest volume centers, performing an average of 185 cases per year, were 14.8 times more likely to have routine discharges from the hospital than those patients in centers performing 5 or fewer cases per year (95% confidence interval, 8.2–26.6). Similar findings were also reported by Mahboubi et al when evaluating the CHDD for the period 1997 to 2011.[17] In Maryland, Ward et al found that VS patients undergoing surgery at a high-volume center had a lower likelihood of postoperative readmission as well as urgent or emergent admission.[18] Also noteworthy was the finding that between 1990 and 2009, there was a decrease in the absolute number and relative percentage of cases treated at low-volume centers. It is suspected by the authors of this chapter that trends toward centralization of VS management will continue, and through these trends, multidisciplinary collaborations between neurosurgery, neurotology, audiology, speech pathology, vestibular therapy, facial plastic surgery, and radiation oncology will allow for the optimization of care for VS patients in the future.[19]

29.5 Emerging Considerations in Vestibular Schwannoma Surgical Training

The accreditation process has significantly improved training experiences, eliminating many of the inconsistencies seen in the early 1900s. As expertise accumulates, the discussion shifts to identify the appropriate number of trainees. The major factors defining subspecialization are population density, scope of practice, and disease burden. Problems that are very common allow concentration of effort in smaller areas. On the contrary, sparse population and limited incidence of a given problem dictate that techniques necessary for treatment of an uncommon problem will be infrequently performed. Over 300 individuals have passed the certification examination in neurotology. An analysis of the distribution of these specialists shows that they appropriately match to the population, with few, if any, areas that might be considered to be underserved.[20]

Changes in disease prevalence and alteration in management strategies significantly impact the ability of practitioners to maintain their surgical skills. An example of this effect is illustrated in the change in performance of stapedectomy by general otolaryngologists over time.[21] The dual impact of training program proliferation and changing practice trends in VS management has led to similar concerns with VS microsurgery.[20,22,23] The percentage of tumors being observed without treatment has increased, and these lesions are generally smaller and technically easier to remove. Radiation is also frequently used for treatment of VS less than 3 cm in size, further limiting surgical cases and potentially increasing the complexity of cases appropriate for resection.[24] Obviously, if a molecular strategy for control of tumor growth is refined, the indications for surgery may decrease further. Moving forward, the ability of all trainees to maintain appropriate lateral skull base surgical skills over time could be challenged, which lends credence to the argument that the future of VS microsurgery may involve the emergence of fewer centers performing a higher volume of cases.

The degree to which simulated surgery can contribute to surgical training remains to be seen. In temporal bone surgery, virtual simulators have been introduced to training regimens over the past few decades.[25,26,27] Initial results with this technology have identified positive correlations between experience and performance, suggesting that simulators can potentially be used as assessment tools for trainees and attending surgeons.[28,29] Furthermore, with the advent of higher resolution imaging techniques and three-dimensional printing, the ability to create accurate representations of human anatomy is also an exciting prospect.[30,31] While there is likely no substitute for clinical experience in surgical training, simulation methods may ultimately prove to be valuable addition to training and assessment paradigms for skull base surgeons

29.6 Conclusion

The training process for those who seek to perform VS surgery has become increasingly standardized. It is clear, however, that the learning process extends beyond the formal training years. Surgeon experience does appear to play a role in outcomes after VS surgery. However, the degree of experience needed to overcome the learning curve for microsurgical approaches and dissection is yet unclear, particularly as it relates to different parts of the surgical team. Furthermore, the optimal method of obtaining experience while consistently providing excellent patient care is unclear, as is the role of surgical simulation as an adjunct tool. It is suspected that multidisciplinary team-based models of patient care, in which comprehensive care can be offered to patients and mentorship can be provided to relatively inexperienced surgeons, are likely able to optimize both training and patient outcomes.

References

[1] Grover BT, Kothari SN. Fellowship training: need and contributions. Surg Clin North Am. 2016; 96(1):47–57

[2] Tu JV, Austin PC, Johnston KW. The influence of surgical specialty training on the outcomes of elective abdominal aortic aneurysm surgery. J Vasc Surg. 2001; 33(3):447–452

[3] Dueck AD, Kucey DS, Johnston KW, Alter D, Laupacis A. Survival after ruptured abdominal aortic aneurysm: effect of patient, surgeon, and hospital factors. J Vasc Surg. 2004; 39(6):1253–1260

[4] Koerbel A, Gharabaghi A, Safavi-Abbasi S, Tatagiba M, Samii M. Evolution of vestibular schwannoma surgery: the long journey to current success. Neurosurg Focus. 2005; 18(4):e10

[5] Machinis TG, Fountas KN, Dimopoulos V, Robinson JS. History of acoustic neurinoma surgery. Neurosurg Focus. 2005; 18(4):e9

[6] McRackan TR, Brackmann DE. Historical perspective on evolution in management of lateral skull base tumors. Otolaryngol Clin North Am. 2015; 48(3): 397–405

[7] Lambert PR. Neurotology: past, present, and future-the 2012 William F. House Lecture. Otol Neurotol. 2013; 34(1):1–5

[8] Moffat DA, Hardy DG, Grey PL, Baguley DM. The operative learning curve and its effect on facial nerve outcome in vestibular schwannoma surgery. Am J Otol. 1996; 17(4):643–647

[9] Elsmore AJ, Mendoza ND. The operative learning curve for vestibular schwannoma excision via the retrosigmoid approach. Br J Neurosurg. 2002; 16(5): 448–455

[10] Moffat DA, Parker RA, Hardy DG, Macfarlane R. Factors affecting final facial nerve outcome following vestibular schwannoma surgery. J Laryngol Otol. 2014; 128(5):406–415

[11] Buchman CA, Chen DA, Flannagan P, Wilberger JE, Maroon JC. The learning curve for acoustic tumor surgery. Laryngoscope. 1996; 106(11): 1406–1411

[12] Welling DB, Slater PW, Thomas RD, McGregor JM, Goodman JE. The learning curve in vestibular schwannoma surgery. Am J Otol. 1999; 20 (5):644–648

[13] Wang AY, Wang JT, Dexter M, Da Cruz M. The vestibular schwannoma surgery learning curve mapped by the cumulative summation test for learning curve. Otol Neurotol. 2013; 34(8):1469–1475

[14] Kari E, Friedman RA. Hearing preservation: microsurgery. Curr Opin Otolaryngol Head Neck Surg. 2012; 20(5):358–366

[15] Kanzaki J, Inoue Y, Ogawa K. The learning curve in post-operative hearing results in vestibular schwannoma surgery. Auris Nasus Larynx. 2001; 28(3): 209–213

[16] Slattery WH, Schwartz MS, Fisher LM, Oppenheimer M. Acoustic neuroma surgical cost and outcome by hospital volume in California. Otolaryngol Head Neck Surg. 2004; 130(6):726–735

[17] Mahboubi H, Ahmed OH, Yau AY, Ahmed YC, Djalilian HR. Complications of surgery for sporadic vestibular schwannoma. Otolaryngol Head Neck Surg. 2014; 150(2):275–281

[18] Ward BK, Gourin CG, Francis HW. Vestibular schwannoma surgical volume and short-term outcomes in Maryland. Arch Otolaryngol Head Neck Surg. 2012; 138(6):577–583

[19] Sharp MC, MacfArlane R, Hardy DG, Jones SE, Baguley DM, Moffat DA. Team working to improve outcome in vestibular schwannoma surgery. Br J Neurosurg. 2005; 19(2):122–127

[20] Vrabec JT. Workforce analysis of neurotologists in the United States. Otol Neurotol. 2013; 34(4):755–761

[21] Ruckenstein MJ, Staab JP. Who is performing stapedectomy surgery? Implications for residency and fellowship training. Laryngoscope. 2008; 118(7): 1224–1227

[22] Dobie RA. Are we training too many otologists. Am J Otol. 1997; 18(2):131–132

[23] Breen JT, Vrabec JT. Early practice: neurotology. Otolaryngol Clin North Am. 2015; 48(2):257–262

[24] Slattery WH, III. Microsurgery after radiosurgery or radiotherapy for vestibular schwannomas. Otolaryngol Clin North Am. 2009; 42(4):707–715

[25] Wiet GJ, Stredney D, Sessanna D, Bryan JA, Welling DB, Schmalbrock P. Virtual temporal bone dissection: an interactive surgical simulator. Otolaryngol Head Neck Surg. 2002; 127(1):79–83

[26] Wiet GJ, Bryan J, Dodson E, et al. Virtual temporal bone dissection simulation. Stud Health Technol Inform. 2000; 70:378–384

[27] Wiet GJ, Stredney D, Kerwin T, et al. Virtual temporal bone dissection system: OSU virtual temporal bone system: development and testing. Laryngoscope. 2012; 122 Suppl 1:S1–S12

[28] Zhao YC, Kennedy G, Hall R, O'Leary S. Differentiating levels of surgical experience on a virtual reality temporal bone simulator. Otolaryngol Head Neck Surg. 2010; 143(5) Suppl 3:S30–S35

[29] Zhao YC, Kennedy G, Yukawa K, Pyman B, O'Leary S. Can virtual reality simulator be used as a training aid to improve cadaver temporal bone dissection? Results of a randomized blinded control trial. Laryngoscope. 2011; 121(4): 831–837

[30] Mick PT, Arnoldner C, Mainprize JG, Symons SP, Chen JM. Face validity study of an artificial temporal bone for simulation surgery. Otol Neurotol. 2013; 34 (7):1305–1310

[31] Rose AS, Kimbell JS, Webster CE, Harrysson OL, Formeister EJ, Buchman CA. Multi-material 3D models for temporal bone surgical simulation. Ann Otol Rhinol Laryngol. 2015; 124(7):528–536

30 Anatomy of Vestibular Schwannoma Surgery

Albert L. Rhoton Jr.

30.1 Introduction

Vestibular schwannomas (VSs), as they expand, may involve a majority of the cranial nerves and cerebellar arteries, and the midbrain, pons, and medulla. An understanding of microsurgical anatomy of the cerebellopontine angle and internal auditory canal provides the basis for optimizing surgical results with these tumors. This chapter reviews this anatomy basic to understanding and treating VSs.

30.2 Microsurgical Anatomy

30.2.1 Neural Relationships

An understanding of microsurgical anatomy is especially important in preserving the facial and cochlear nerves, which are the neural structures at greatest risk during VS removal. A widely accepted operative precept is that, when possible, a nerve involved by a tumor should be identified both proximal and distal to the tumor, where its displacement and distortion are least, before the tumor is removed from the involved segment of nerve. This operative principle has received only a limited application in operations for VS removal. Considerable attention has been directed to the early identification of the facial and vestibulocochlear nerves distal to the tumor at the lateral part of the internal auditory canal,[1,2,3,4,5,6,7,8,9] but less attention has been directed to identification at the brainstem on the medial side of the tumor. The neural considerations are divided into sections dealing with the relationships at the lateral end of the tumor in the meatus and those on the medial end of the tumor at the brainstem.

30.2.2 Meatal Relationships

The four nerves in the lateral part of the internal auditory canal are the facial, the cochlear, and the inferior and superior vestibular nerves (▶ Fig. 30.1). The position of the nerves is most constant in the lateral portion of the meatus at the fundus, which is divided into a superior and an inferior portion by a horizontal ridge, the transverse or falciform crest. The facial and the superior vestibular nerves are superior to the crest. The facial nerve is anterior to the superior vestibular nerve and is separated from it at the lateral end of the meatus by a vertical ridge of bone, called the vertical crest (a.k.a. "Bill's bar" after William House). The cochlear and inferior vestibular nerves run below the transverse crest with the cochlear nerve located anteriorly. Thus, the lateral meatus can be divided into four portions, with the facial nerve being anterosuperior, the cochlear nerve anteroinferior, the superior vestibular posterosuperior, and the inferior vestibular nerve posteroinferior.

Because VSs most frequently arise in the posteriorly placed vestibular nerves, they usually displace the facial and cochlear nerves anteriorly (▶ Fig. 30.2). The facial nerve is most commonly stretched around the anterior half of the tumor capsule. Variability in the direction of growth of the tumor arising from the vestibular nerves may result in the facial nerve being displaced, not only directly anteriorly, but also anterosuperiorly or anteroinferiorly. Because the facial nerve always enters the facial canal at the anterosuperior quadrant of the lateral margin of the meatus, it is usually easiest to locate it here after the internal auditory canal has been exposed, rather than at a more medial location where the degree of displacement of the nerve is more variable. The cochlear nerve also lies anterior to the vestibular nerve and will usually be stretched around the anterior margin of the tumor.

30.2.3 Brainstem Relationships

The importance of early identification of the facial nerve proximal to the tumor at the brainstem has received less attention, even though there is a consistent set of relationships at the brainstem that facilitates identification of the facial nerve at this location.[10]

The neural structures most intimately related to the medial side of a VS are related to the junction of the pons, medulla, and cerebellum (▶ Fig. 30.3a, ▶ Fig. 30.4a, and ▶ Fig. 30.5a). The landmarks on these structures that are helpful in guiding the surgeon to the junction of the facial nerve with the brainstem are: the sulcus between the pons and medulla, junction of the glossopharyngeal, vagus, and accessory nerves with the medulla; the flocculus and choroid plexus protruding from the foramen of Luschka; and the inferior olive.

Pontomedullary Sulcus

The facial nerve arises from the brainstem near the lateral end of the pontomedullary sulcus. This sulcus extends along the junction of the pons and the medulla and ends just medial to the foramen of Luschka and the lateral recess of the fourth ventricle (▶ Fig. 30.3a, ▶ Fig. 30.4a, ▶ Fig. 30.5a). The facial nerve arises in the pontomedullary sulcus 1 to 2 mm anterior to the point at which the vestibulocochlear nerve joins the brainstem at the lateral end of the sulcus. The interval between the vestibulocochlear and facial nerves is greatest at the level of the pontomedullary sulcus and decreases as these nerves approach the meatus. When in the upright position, the pontomedullary sulcus is roughly horizontal. In the exposure provided by a retrosigmoid craniotomy, the junction of the facial nerve with the pontomedullary sulcus will be hidden directly anterior to the vestibulocochlear nerve, and in some cases the facial nerve can be seen only by gently elevating, depressing, or dividing the vestibulocochlear nerve.

Glossopharyngeal, Vagus, and Accessory Nerves

The facial nerve enjoys a consistent relationship to the junction of the glossopharyngeal, vagus, and accessory nerves with the lateral side of the medulla. The facial nerve arises 2 to 3 mm above the most rostral rootlet contributing to these nerves. In the suboccipital operative exposure, the rootlets of these three

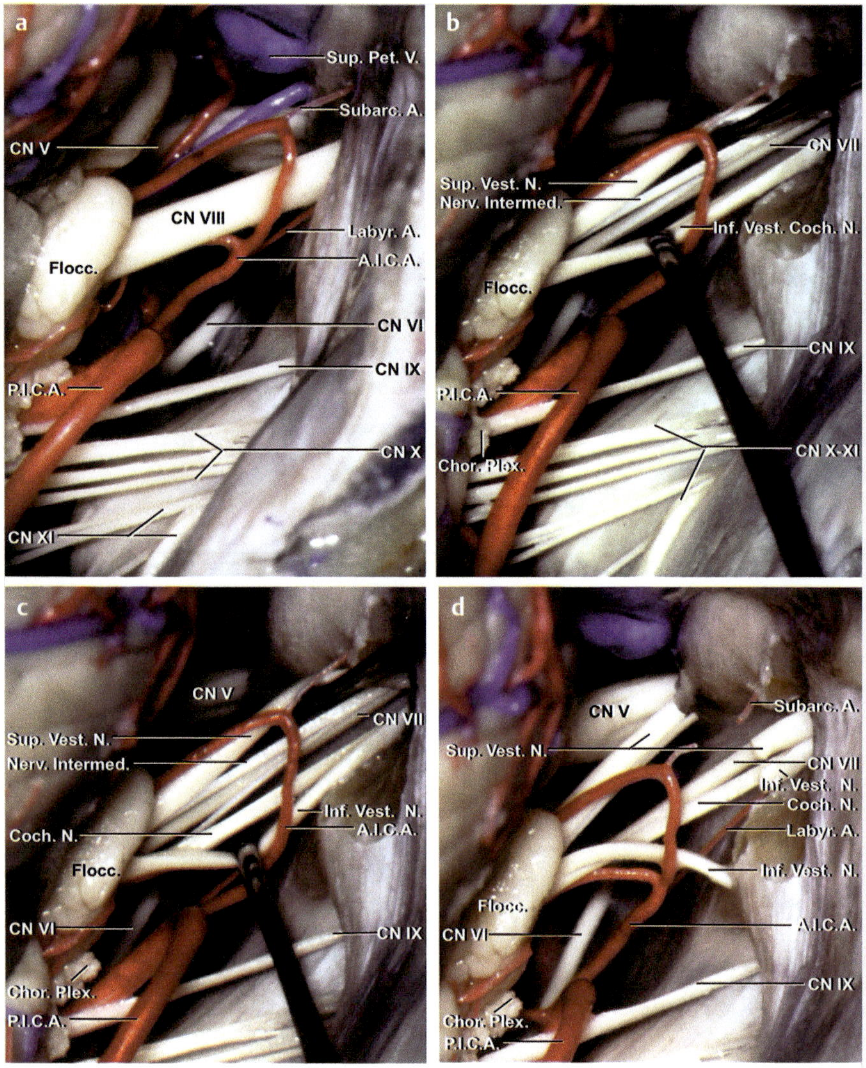

Fig. 30.1 Posterior (retrosigmoid) view of the nerves in the right cerebellopontine angle. **(a)** The vestibulocochlear nerve enters the internal auditory canal with a labyrinthine branch of the AICA. The posterior inferior cerebellar artery (PICA) courses around the glossopharyngeal, vagus, and accessory nerves. The abducens nerve ascends in front of the pons. A subarcuate artery enters the subarcuate fossa superolateral to the porus of the internal auditory canal. Choroid plexus protrudes into the cerebellopontine angle behind the glossopharyngeal and vagus nerves. **(b)** The posterior wall of the internal auditory canal has been removed. The cleavage plane between the upper bundle, formed by the superior vestibular nerve, and the lower bundle, formed by the inferior vestibular and cochlear nerves, was begun laterally where the nerves have separated near the meatal fundus and extended medially. The nervus intermedius arises on the anterior surface of the vestibulocochlear nerve, has a free segment in the cistern and/or meatus, and joins the facial nerve distally. The facial nerve is located anterior to the superior vestibular nerve and the cochlear nerve is anterior to the inferior vestibular nerve. **(c)** The cleavage plane between the cochlear and inferior vestibular nerves, which is well developed in the lateral end of the internal auditory canal, has been extended medially. Within the cerebellopontine angle, the superior vestibular nerve is posterior and superior, the facial nerve anterior and superior, the inferior vestibular nerve posterior and inferior, and the cochlear nerve anterior and inferior. **(d)** The superior and inferior vestibular nerves have been divided to expose the facial and cochlear nerves. A labyrinthine branch of the PICA enters the internal auditory canal. (Reproduced with permission from Rhoton AL Jr. The cerebellopontine angle and posterior fossa cranial nerves by the retrosigmoid approach. Neurosurgery 2000;47(3 Suppl):S93–S129.)

nerves are seen entering the brainstem below the tumor. A helpful way of visualizing the point where the facial nerve will exit from the brainstem, even when displaced by tumor, is to project an imaginary line along the medullary junction of the rootlets forming the glossopharyngeal, vagal, and accessory nerves, and upward through the pontomedullary junction. This line, at a point 2 to 3 mm above the junction of the glossopharyngeal nerve with the medulla, will pass through the pontomedullary junction at the site where the facial nerve exists from the brainstem.

Cerebellar-Brainstem Fissures

VSs are closely related to the cerebellopontine and cerebellomedullary fissures, the clefts formed by the folding of the cerebellum around the pons and medulla (▶ Fig. 30.1, ▶ Fig. 30.2, ▶ Fig. 30.3). The cerebellopontine fissure is a V-shaped fissure formed by the folding of the petrosal surface of the cerebellum around the lateral side of the pons and middle cerebellar peduncle. The petrosal surface is the cerebellar surface that faces the posterior surface of the petrous bone and is retracted to expose the nerves entering the internal auditory canal. The cerebellopontine fissure has a superior limb situated between the rostral half of the pons and the superior part of the petrosal surface, and an inferior limb located between the caudal half of the pons and the inferior part of the petrosal surface. The apex of the fissure is located laterally where the superior and inferior limbs meet. The V-shaped area between the superior and inferior limbs, which has the middle cerebellar peduncle in its floor, corresponds to the area that is referred to as the cerebellopontine angle. The trigeminal, abducens, facial, vestibulocochlear, and glossopharyngeal nerves arise between the superior and inferior limbs of the fissure. The facial and vestibulocochlear nerves arise just anterior to the inferior limb of the fissure, and just below the middle cerebellar peduncle. The trigeminal nerve arises near the superior limb of the fissure.

The cerebellomedullary fissure—the cleft between the cerebellum and medulla, which extends upward between the cerebellar tonsil and the medulla—communicates with the inferior limb of the cerebellopontine fissure near the lateral recess of

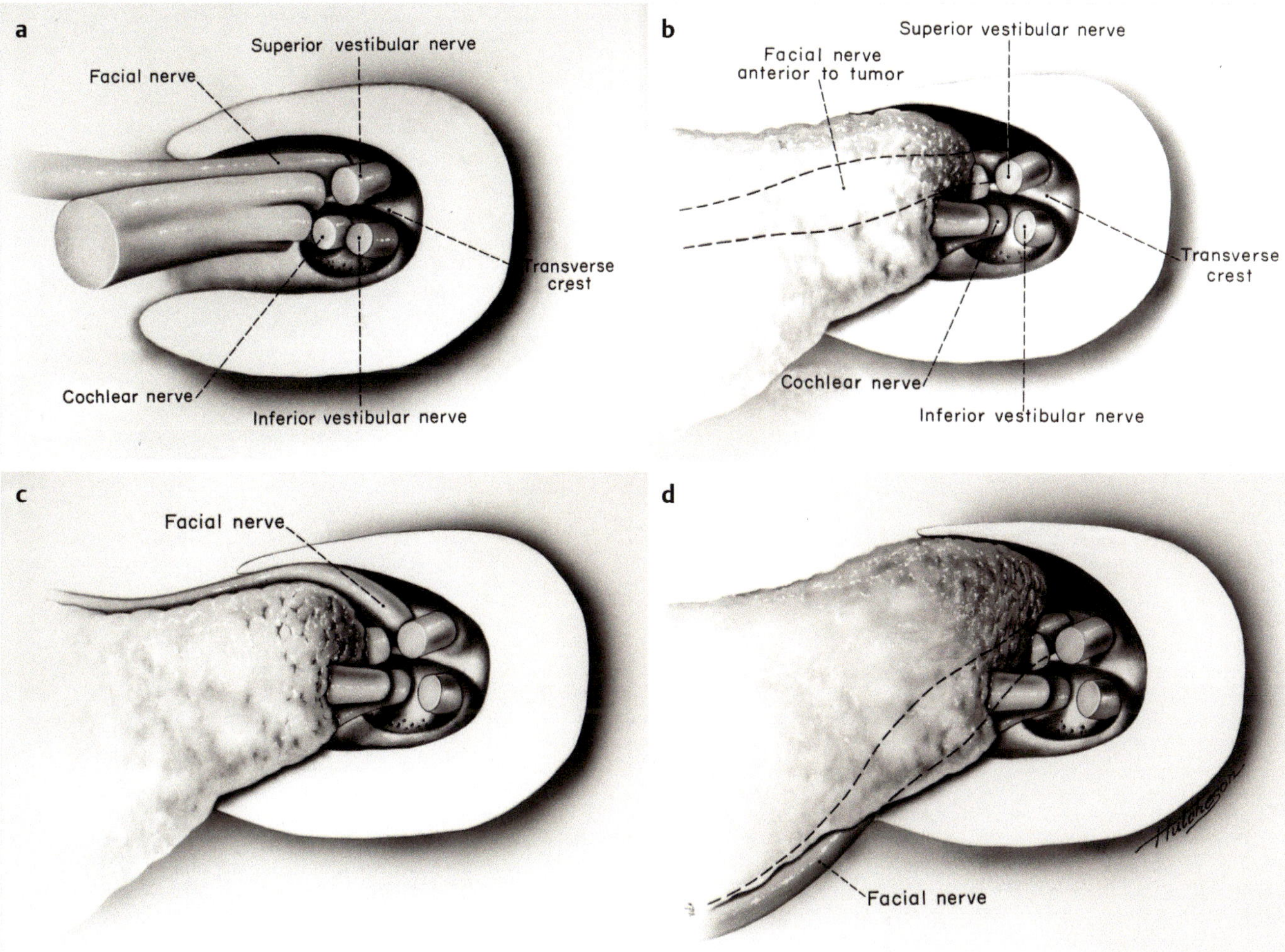

Fig. 30.2 Posterior view of right internal auditory canal with the posterior lip removed to show variable direction of facial nerve displacement by VS. **(a)** Normal neural relationships with the eighth nerve dividing into its three parts in the lateral internal auditory canal. The facial and superior vestibular nerves are above the transverse crest, and the cochlear and inferior vestibular nerves are below. The facial nerve occupies the anterosuperior quadrant of the fundus. **(b)** The facial nerve is displaced directly anteriorly. This is a frequent direction of displacement with VS. **(c)** Another frequent direction of displacement of the facial nerve is anterior and superior. **(d)** The facial nerve is displaced anteriorly and inferiorly by tumor, which erodes the superior wall of the internal auditory canal above the nerves and grows into the area above the nerves, displacing them inferiorly. (Reproduced with permission from Rhoton.[2])

the fourth ventricle. Several structures related to the lateral recess project into the cerebellopontine angle near the facial and the vestibulocochlear nerves.

Foramen of Luschka, Choroid Plexus, and Flocculus

The structures related to the lateral recess of the fourth ventricle that have a consistent relationship to the facial and vestibulocochlear nerves are the foramen of Luschka, the choroid plexus projecting from it, and the flocculus (▶ Fig. 30.6). The foramen of Luschka is situated at the lateral margin of the pontomedullary sulcus, just dorsal to the junction of the glossopharyngeal nerve with the brainstem, and immediately posteroinferior to the junction of the facial and vestibulocochlear nerves with the brainstem. The foramen of Luschka is infrequently seen from the view provided by the retrosigmoid operative exposure. However, there is consistently an identifiable tuft of choroid plexus that protrudes out of the foramen of Luschka and sits on the posterior surface of the glossopharyngeal and vagus nerves just inferior to the junction of the facial and vestibulocochlear nerves with the brainstem.

Another structure related to the lateral recess is the flocculus. It is a fan-shaped cerebellar lobule that projects from the margin of the lateral recess into the cerebellopontine angle. The flocculus, together with the nodule of the vermis, forms the primitive flocculonodular lobe of the cerebellum. The flocculus is attached to the rostral margin of the lateral recess and foramen of Luschka. The flocculus is continuous medially with the inferior medullary velum, a butterfly-shaped sheet of neural tissue that forms on the surface of the nodule and sweeps laterally above the tonsil to form part of the inferior half of the roof of the fourth ventricle. The lateral part of the inferior medullary velum narrows to a smaller bundle, the peduncle of the flocculus, which fuses to the rostral margin of the lateral recess and foramen of Luschka. The flocculus projects from the peduncle of

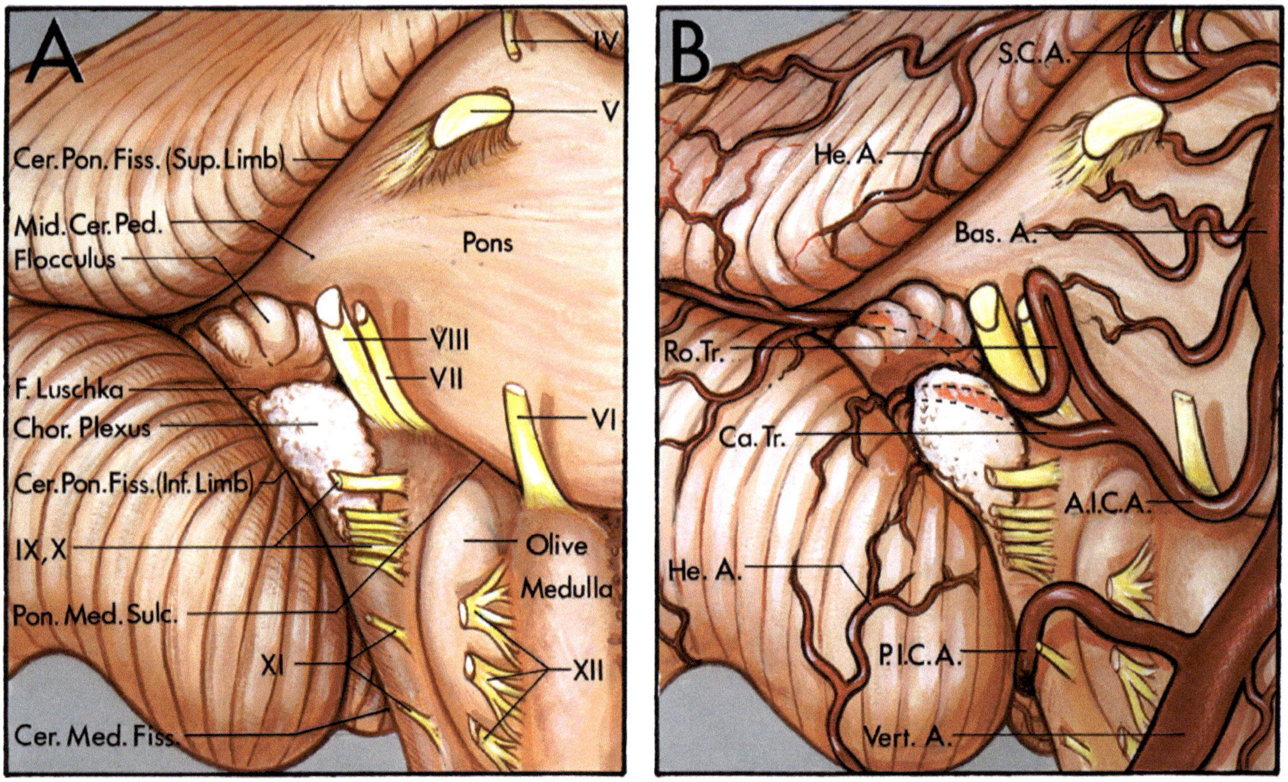

Fig. 30.3 Neurovascular relationships on the brainstem side of a VS. Anterolateral view of the right cerebellopontine angle. **(a)** Neural relationships. The facial (VII) and vestibulocochlear (VIII) nerves arise from the brainstem near the lateral end of the pontomedullary sulcus (Pon. Med. Sulc.), anterosuperior to the choroid plexus (Chor. Plex.) protruding from the foramen of Luschka (F. Luschka), anterior to the flocculus, rostral to a line drawn along the junction of the rootlets of the glossopharyngeal (IX), vagus (X), and accessory (XI) nerves with the brainstem, and slightly posterior to the rostral pole of the inferior olive. The abducens nerve (VI) arises in the medial part of the pontomedullary sulcus. The hypoglossal rootlets (XII) arise anterior to the olive. The cerebellopontine fissure (Cer. Pon. Fiss.) formed by the cerebellum wrapping around the lateral side of the pons and middle cerebellar peduncle (Mid. Cer. Ped.) has a superior limb (Sup. Limb) that passes above the trigeminal nerve (V) and an inferior limb (Inf. Limb) that extends below the foramen of Luschka. The cerebellomedullary fissure (Cer. Med. Fiss.), which extends superiorly between the medulla and cerebellum, communicates in the region of the foramen of Luschka with the cerebellopontine fissure. The trochlear nerve (IV) is above the trigeminal nerve. **(b)** Arterial relationships. The anterior inferior cerebellar artery (AICA) arises from the basilar artery (Bas. A.) and divides into rostral (Ro. Tr.) and caudal (Ca. Tr.) trunks. The rostral trunk, which is usually the larger of the two trunks, courses below the facial and vestibulocochlear nerves, and then above the flocculus to reach the surface of the middle cerebellar peduncle. The posterior inferior cerebellar artery (PICA) arises from the vertebral artery (Vert. A.) and passes first between the hypoglossal rootlets, and then between the vagus and accessory nerves on its way to the cerebellar hemisphere. The superior cerebellar artery (S.C.A.) passes above the trigeminal nerve. The cerebellar arteries give rise to hemispheric branches (He. A.). *(continued)*

the flocculus into the cerebellopontine angle just posterior to where the facial and vestibulocochlear nerves join the pontomedullary sulcus.

30.2.4 Arterial Relationships

The arteries crossing the cerebellopontine angle, especially the anterior inferior cerebellar artery (AICA), enjoy a consistent relationship to the facial and vestibulocochlear nerves, foramen of Luschka, and the flocculus (▶ Fig. 30.1, ▶ Fig. 30.3b, ▶ Fig. 30.4b, ▶ Fig. 30.5b, and ▶ Fig. 30.7).[11,12,13,14,15] The AICA originates from the basilar artery and encircles the pons near the pontomedullary sulcus. After coursing near, and sending branches to the nerves entering the internal auditory canal and the choroid plexus protruding from the foramen of Luschka, it passes around the flocculus to reach the surface of the middle cerebellar peduncle and terminates by supplying the lips of the cerebellopontine fissure and the petrosal surface of the cerebellum. The AICA may pass around the brainstem above, below, or between the facial and vestibulocochlear nerves; but after passing these nerves, the artery consistently passes back to the surface of the middle cerebellar peduncle above the flocculus. The AICA usually bifurcates near the facial and vestibulocochlear nerves to form a rostral and a caudal trunk. The rostral trunk courses along the middle cerebellar peduncle to supply the upper part of the petrosal cerebellar surface, and the caudal trunk passes near the lateral recess and supplies the lower part of the petrosal surface. If the AICA bifurcates into rostral and caudal trunks prior to reaching the region of the flocculus, it is the rostral trunk that can be followed above the flocculus to the surface of the middle cerebellar peduncle.

In most cases, the AICA passes below the facial and vestibulocochlear nerves as it encircles the brainstem, but it may also pass above or between these nerves in its course around the

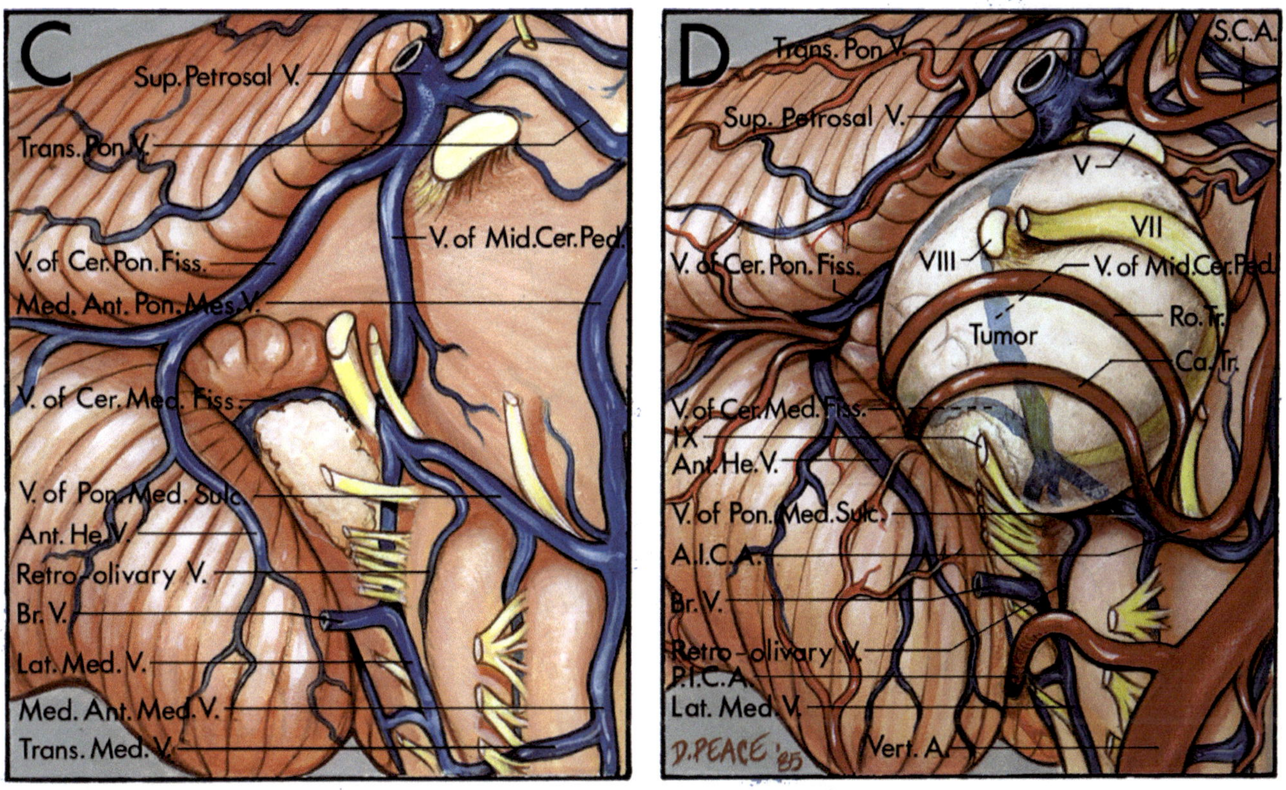

Fig. 30.3 *(continued)* **(c)** Venous relationships. The veins that converge on the junction of the facial and vestibulocochlear nerves with the brainstem are the veins of the pontomedullary sulcus (V. of Pon. Med. Sulc.), cerebellomedullary fissure (V. of Cer. Med. Fiss.), middle cerebellar peduncle (V. of Mid. Cer. Ped.), and the retro-olivary (Retro-olivary V.) and lateral medullary veins (Lat. Med. V.). The vein of the cerebellopontine fissure (V. of Cer. Pon. Fiss.), which passes above the flocculus on the middle cerebellar peduncle, is formed by the anterior hemispheric veins (Ant. He. V.) that arise on the cerebellum. Transverse pontine (Trans. Pon. V.) and transverse medullary (Trans. Med. V.) veins cross the pons and medulla. The median anterior medullary (Med. Ant. Med. V.) and median anterior pontomesencephalic veins (Med. Ant. Pon. Mes. V.) ascend on the anterior surface of the medulla and pons. The veins of the middle cerebellar peduncle and the cerebellopontine fissure and transverse pontine vein join to form a superior petrosal vein (Sup. Pet. V.), which empties into the superior petrosal sinus. A bridging vein (Br. V.) passes below the vagal rootlets toward the jugular foramen. **(d)** Neurovascular relationships of a VS. The tumor arises from the vestibulocochlear nerve and displaces the facial nerve anteriorly, the trigeminal nerve superiorly, and the vagus and glossopharyngeal nerves inferiorly. The facial nerve, even though displaced by the tumor, enters the brainstem along the lateral margin of the pontomedullary sulcus, rostral to the glossopharyngeal and vagus nerves, anterior to the flocculus, and rostral to the choroid plexus protruding from the foramen of Luschka. The rostral trunk of the anterior inferior cerebellar artery, after passing below the tumor, returns to the surface of the middle cerebellar peduncle above the flocculus. The veins displaced around the medial side of the tumor are the veins of the middle cerebellar peduncle, cerebellomedullary fissure, cerebellopontine fissure and pontomedullary sulcus, and the retro-olivary and lateral medullary veins. (Reproduced with permission from Rhoton.[10])

brainstem (▶ Fig. 30.7). In the most common case, in which the AICA passes below the nerves, the tumor would displace the artery inferiorly. If the AICA courses between the facial and vestibulocochlear nerves, a tumor arising in the latter nerve will displace the AICA forward. Tumor growth would displace the AICA superiorly if the artery passes above the nerves. In each case, once the flocculus is identified below the suprafloccular segment of the AICA, the site of entry of the facial nerve into the brainstem can be predicted because of its relationship to the AICA. The branches of the AICA that arise near the facial and vestibulocochlear nerves are: the internal auditory canal arteries, which supply the facial and vestibulocochlear nerves and adjacent structures; the recurrent perforating arteries, which may initially pass toward the meatus but subsequently turn medially and supply the brainstem; and the subarcuate artery, which enters the subarcuate fossa—a small depression on the posterior wall of the meatus.

The superior cerebellar artery, which is separated from the tumor by the trigeminal nerve, is displaced rostrally by the tumor, and the posterior inferior cerebellar artery is displaced caudally with the glossopharyngeal and vagus nerves by the tumor.

When removing the posterior meatal wall, it often is necessary to sacrifice the subarcuate artery because it passes through the dura on the posterior meatal wall to reach the subarcuate fossa (▶ Fig. 30.1 and ▶ Fig. 30.8).[15] This artery usually has a sufficiently long stem that its obliteration does not risk damage to the AICA from which it arises. In a few cases, however, the subarcuate artery and the segment of the AICA from which it arises will be incorporated into the dura covering the subarcuate fossa.[16,17] In this case, the dura and the artery will have to be separated together from the posterior meatal lip wall in preparation for opening the internal auditory canal (▶ Fig. 30.8). In rare cases, the artery will be surrounded by bone that has to be drilled to free the artery and access the meatus.

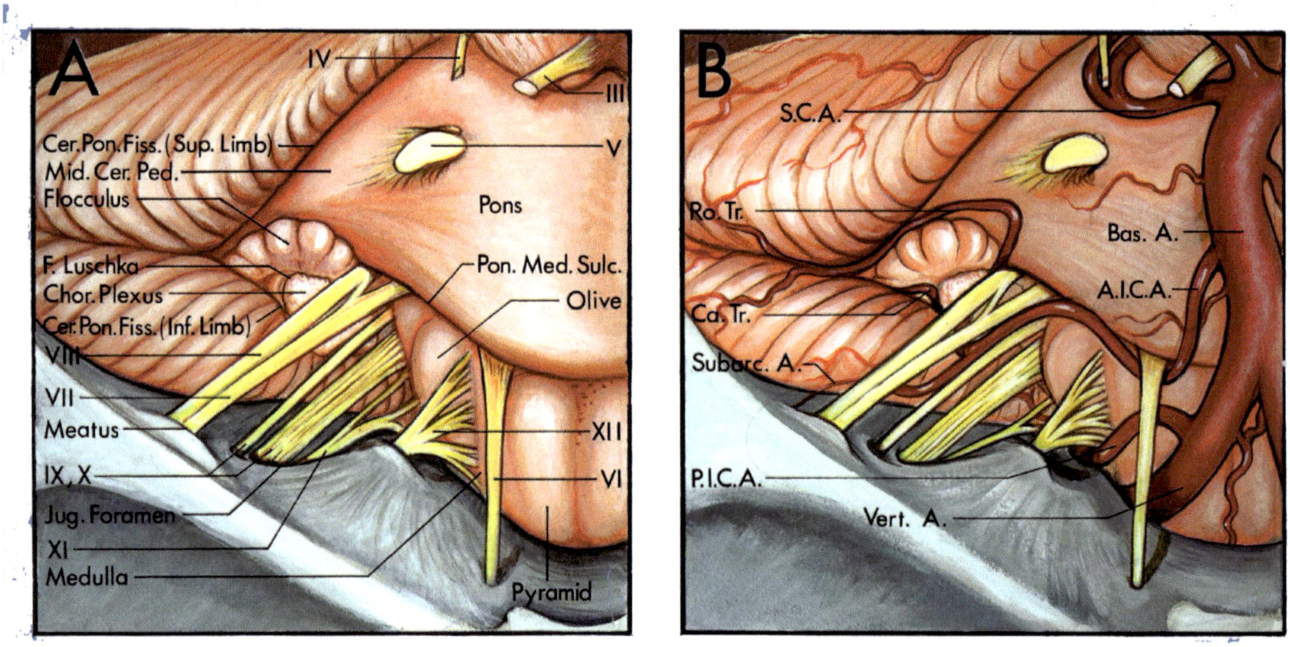

Fig. 30.4 Neurovascular relationships on the brainstem side of a VS. Anterosuperior views. **(a)** Neural relationships. The cerebrum and tentorium cerebelli have been removed, and the trigeminal (V), trochlear (IV), and oculomotor (III) nerves have been divided to allow the brainstem to be displaced posteriorly in order to expose the cerebellopontine angle from above. The facial (VII) and vestibulocochlear (VIII) nerves arise at the lateral end of the pontomedullary sulcus (Pont. Med. Sulc.) anterior to the flocculus, rostral to the glossopharyngeal (IX), vagus (X), and accessory (XI) nerves, and anterosuperior to the choroid plexus (Chor. Plex.) protruding from the foramen of Luschka (F. Luschka). The hypoglossal nerve (XII) arises anterior to the inferior olive. The abducens nerve (VI) arises from the medial part of the pontomedullary sulcus and ascends to pierce the dura mater on the clivus. The facial and vestibulocochlear nerves pass laterally to enter the internal auditory canal. The glossopharyngeal, vagus, and accessory nerves converge on the medial side of the jugular foramen (Jug. Foramen). The cerebellopontine fissure, formed where the cerebellum wraps around the lateral side of the pons and middle cerebellar peduncle (Med. Cer. Ped.), has superior (Sup. Limb) and inferior (Inf. Limb) limbs. The foramen of Luschka opens into the inferior limb near the facial and vestibulocochlear nerves. **(b)** Arterial relationships. The anterior inferior cerebellar artery (AICA) arises from the basilar artery (Bas. A.), passes below the facial and vestibulocochlear nerves, gives rise to the subarcuate artery (Subarc. A.), and divides into a rostral (Ro. Tr.) and a caudal (Ca. Tr.) trunk. The rostral trunk passes above the flocculus to course on the middle cerebellar peduncle, and the caudal trunk supplies the area below the flocculus. The posterior inferior cerebellar artery (PICA) arises from the vertebral artery (Vert. A.) and passes below the hypoglossal nerve. The superior cerebellar artery (S.C.A.) passes above the trigeminal nerve. *(continued)*

30.2.5 Venous Relationships

The veins on the side of the brainstem that have a predictable relationship to the facial and vestibulocochlear nerves are those draining the petrosal surface of the cerebellum, the pons and medulla, and the cerebellopontine and cerebellomedullary fissures (▶ Fig. 30.3c, ▶ Fig. 30.4c, and ▶ Fig. 30.5c).[18,19] The identification of any of these veins during removal of the tumor makes it easier to identify the site of the junction of the facial and vestibulocochlear nerves with the brainstem. These veins on the medial side of the tumor are: the vein of the pontomedullary sulcus, which courses transversely in the pontomedullary sulcus; the lateral medullary vein, which courses longitudinally, dorsal to the olive, along the line of origin of the rootlets of the glossopharyngeal, vagus, and accessory nerves; the vein of the cerebellomedullary fissure, which courses above the cerebellar tonsil on the inferior medullary velum and passes dorsal or ventral to the flocculus before joining the other veins in the cerebellopontine angle; the vein of the middle cerebellar peduncle, which is formed by the union of the lateral medullary vein and the vein of the pontomedullary sulcus and ascends on the middle cerebellar peduncle to join the vein of the cerebellopontine fissure; and the vein of the cerebellopontine fissure, which is formed by the union of the veins that arise on the petrosal surface of the cerebellum and converge on the apex of the cerebellopontine fissure. All these veins course near the lateral recess and the junction of the facial and vestibulocochlear nerves with the brainstem. The vein of the cerebellomedullary fissure may pass either dorsal or ventral to the flocculus before joining the other veins. If it passes ventral to the flocculus, it joins the vein of the pontomedullary sulcus and the lateral medullary vein to form the vein of the middle cerebellar peduncle; if it passes dorsal to the flocculus, it joins the vein of the cerebellopontine fissure.

The veins surrounding a VS terminate by forming bridging veins, called petrosal veins, which empty into the superior petrosal sinus. These veins crossing the cerebellopontine angle to reach the superior petrosal sinus are the ones most frequently coagulated in the course of operations in the cerebellopontine angle. Bridging veins are more frequently exposed and sacrificed in the rostral part of the cerebellopontine angle during operations near the trigeminal nerve than during operations near the nerves entering the internal auditory canal. Exposure of the trigeminal nerve through a suboccipital craniotomy

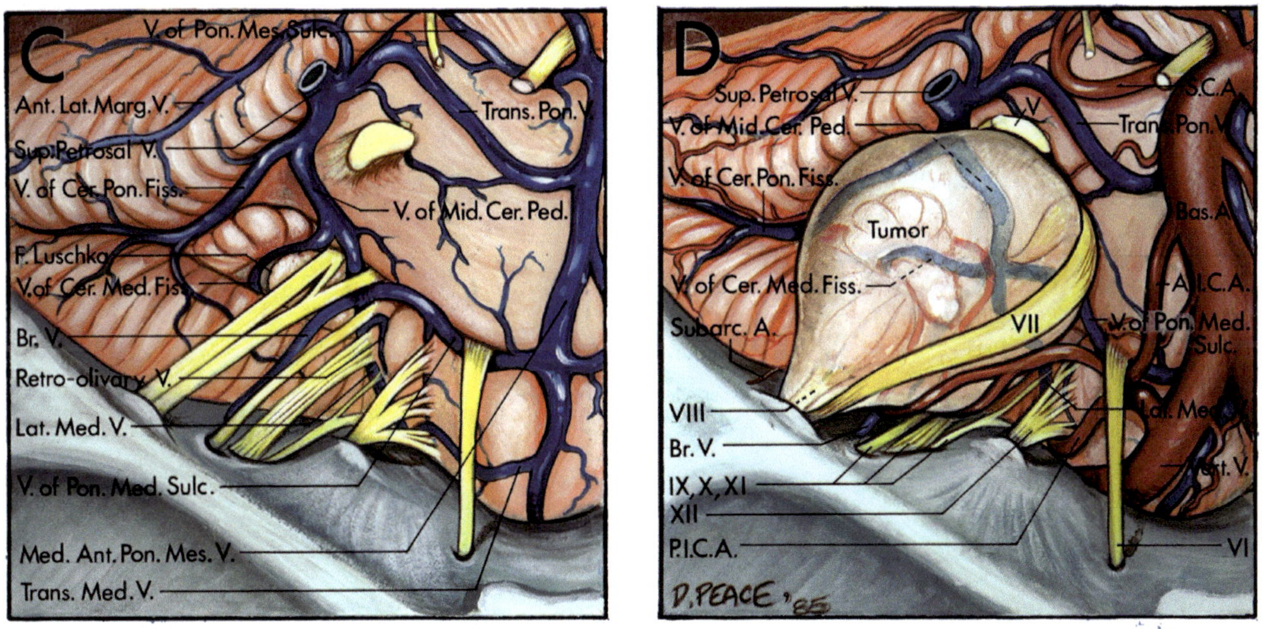

Fig. 30.4 (*continued*) **(c)** Venous relationships. The veins converging on the junction of the facial nerve with the brainstem are the lateral medullary (Lat. Med. V.) and retro-olivary (Retro-olivary V.) veins, and the veins of the pontomedullary sulcus (V. of Pon. Med. Sulc.), cerebellomedullary fissure (V. of Cer. Med. Fiss.), and middle cerebellar peduncle (V. of Mid. Cer. Ped.). The median anterior pontomesencephalic vein (Med. Ant. Pon. Mes. V.) ascends on the anterior surface of the brainstem, and the transverse pontine (Trans. Pon. V.) and transverse medullary (Trans. Med. V.) veins cross the pons and medulla. The vein of the cerebellopontine fissure (V. of Cer. Pon. Fiss.) passes above the flocculus. The transverse pontine vein and the veins of the middle cerebellar peduncle and cerebellopontine fissure join to form one of the superior petrosal veins (Sup. Pet. V.) that empty into the superior petrosal sinus. A bridging vein (Br. V.) passes from the side of the brainstem to the jugular foramen. The anterolateral marginal vein (Ant. Lat. Marg. V.) crosses the anterolateral margin of the cerebellum. The vein of the pontomesencephalic sulcus (V. Pon. Mes. Sulc.) courses in the pontomesencephalic sulcus below the oculomotor nerve. **(d)** Neurovascular relationships of a VS. The tumor arises from the vestibulocochlear nerve and displaces the facial nerve anteriorly, the trigeminal nerve superiorly, and the glossopharyngeal and vagus nerves inferiorly. The vestibulocochlear nerve disappears into the tumor. The facial nerve enters the brainstem along the lateral margin of the pontomedullary sulcus, rostral to the glossopharyngeal nerve, anterior to the flocculus, and rostral to the choroid plexus protruding from the foramen of Luschka. The anterior inferior cerebellar artery is usually displaced around the lower margin of the tumor. The veins displaced around the medial side of the tumor are the veins of the pontomedullary sulcus, middle cerebellar peduncle and cerebellomedullary fissure, and the lateral medullary and retro-olivary veins. (Reproduced with permission from Rhoton.[10])

commonly requires the sacrifice of one or more bridging veins. However, exposure of the nerves entering the internal auditory canal infrequently requires sacrifice of a bridging vein. The exposure of a VS in the central part of the cerebellopontine angle near the lateral recess, by retracting the petrosal surface of the hemisphere away from the sigmoid sinus, can usually be completed without sacrificing a bridging vein. The largest vein encountered around the superior pole of a VS is the vein of the cerebellopontine fissure, which passes from the petrosal surface of the cerebellum above the facial and vestibulocochlear nerves to join other tributaries of the superior petrosal sinus.

30.2.6 General Operative Principles

The primary surgical approaches relevant to VS microsurgery are described in ▶ Fig. 30.9, ▶ Fig. 30.10, ▶ Fig. 30.11, ▶ Fig. 30.12, ▶ Fig. 30.13, ▶ Fig. 30.14. More detailed descriptions of individual surgical approaches can be found in Chapters 33 to 39. In all operative approaches to VS, the mastoid air cells may be opened and must then be sealed to prevent cerebrospinal fluid leakage and meningitis. Craniectomy or craniotomy margins are carefully closed with bone wax. The dura is carefully closed with fat, dural graft, tissue adhesive, and sutures as needed to ensure a watertight seal.

There are landmarks that are helpful in identifying the facial and vestibulocochlear nerves at the brainstem on the medial side of the tumor. These nerves, although distorted by tumor, can usually be identified on the brainstem side of the tumor at the lateral end of the pontomedullary sulcus, just rostral to the glossopharyngeal nerve, and just anterosuperior to the foramen of Luschka, flocculus, and choroid plexus protruding from the foramen of Luschka. After the facial and vestibulocochlear nerves are identified on the medial and lateral sides of the tumor, the final remnants of the tumor are separated from the intervening segment of the nerves.

The operation for a cerebellopontine angle tumor should be planned so that the tumor surface is allowed to settle away from the neural tissue rather than the neural structures being retracted away from the tumor. The initial step is exploration of the exposed tumor surface with the facial nerve stimulator to make certain the nerve is not stretched around the exposed capsule. If the tumor is cystic, early cyst decompression may

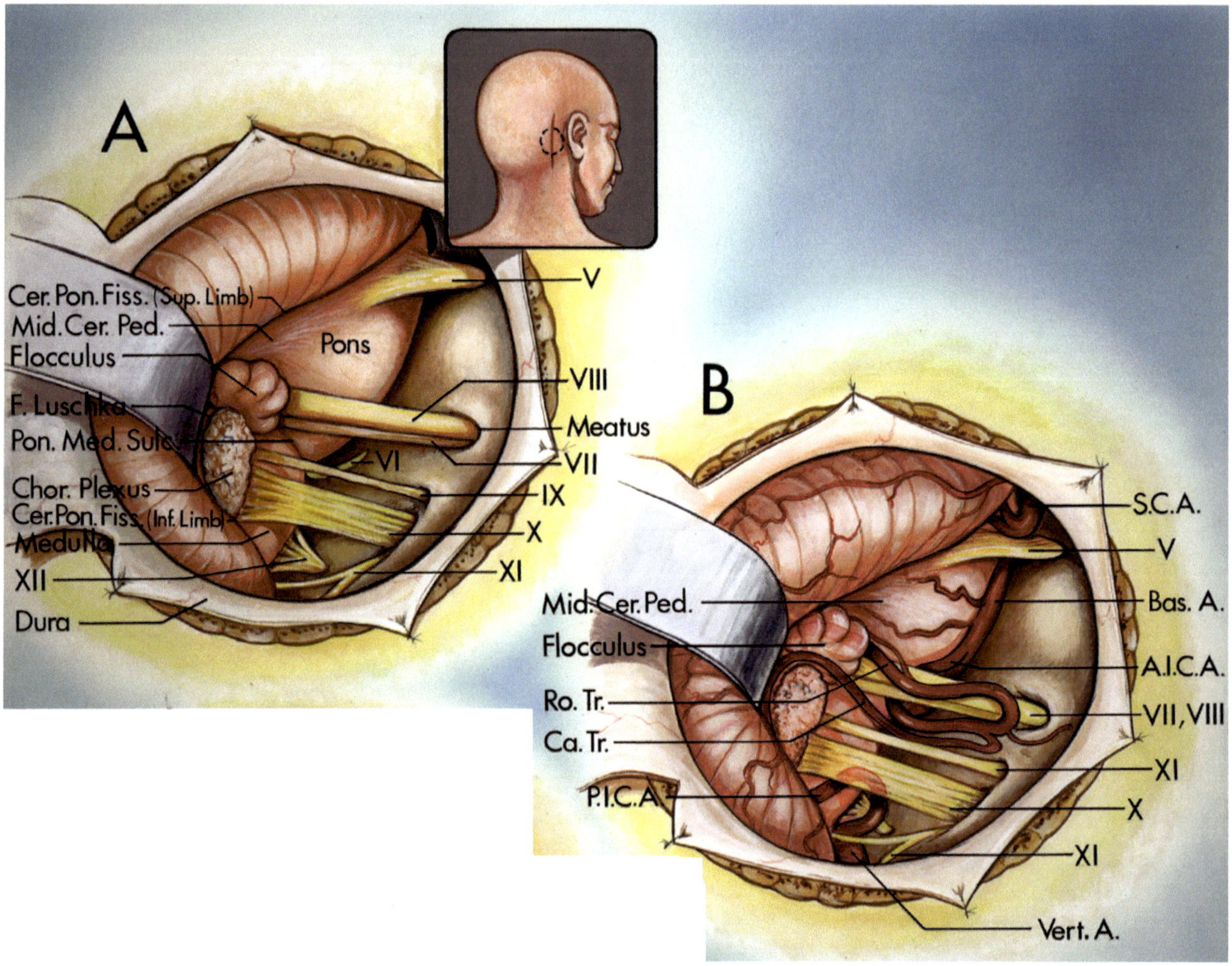

Fig. 30.5 Neurovascular relationships on the brainstem side of a VS. Posterior view through a retrosigmoid craniectomy. **(a)** Neural relationships. The orientation, skin incision (solid line), and craniectomy site (interrupted fine) are shown in the inset. The retractor is on the petrosal surface of the cerebellum. The facial (VII) and vestibulocochlear (VIII) nerves arise at the lateral end of the pontomedullary sulcus (Pon. Med. Sulc.), anterior to the flocculus, rostral to the glossopharyngeal (IX), vagus (X), and accessory (XI) nerves, and anterosuperior to the choroid plexus (Chor. Plexus) protruding from the foramen of Luschka (F. Luschka). The hypoglossal nerve (XII) arises anterior to the olive. The abducens nerve (VI) arises from the medial part of the pontomedullary sulcus. The trigeminal nerve (V) arises in the upper part of the exposure. The cerebellopontine fissure, formed where the cerebellum wraps around the lateral side of the pons and middle cerebellar peduncle (Mid. Cer. Ped.), has superior (Sup. Limb) and inferior (Inf. Limb) limbs. **(b)** Arterial relationships. The anterior inferior cerebellar artery (AICA) arises from the basilar artery (Bas. A.) and divides into a rostral trunk (Ro. Tr.), which passes above the flocculus to reach the surface of the middle cerebellar peduncle, and a caudal trunk (Ca. Tr.), which supplies the area below the flocculus. The posterior inferior cerebellar artery (PICA) arises from the vertebral artery (Vert. A.) and passes dorsally between the vagus and accessory nerves. The superior cerebellar artery (S.C.A.) courses above the trigeminal nerve. *(continued)*

greatly facilitate dissection. No attempt is made to see all of a large tumor upon initial retraction of the cerebellum. The exposed surface of the tumor is then opened and biopsied, and the intracapsular contents are removed. As the intracapsular contents are evacuated by means of a cup forceps, suction, ultrasonic aspirator, or laser, the tumor shifts laterally. This shift allows more of the tumor to be removed through the small exposure. Carefully applied fine bipolar coagulation is preferred in order to control bleeding and to shrink small deposits of tumor. In the final step, the last thin sheet of tumor capsule is removed from the neural and vascular structures by the use of fine dissecting instruments (▶ Fig. 30.12). In cases of attempted hearing preservation, the strokes of the fine dissecting instruments along the vestibulocochlear nerve should be directed from medial to lateral rather than from lateral to medial, because traction medially may tear the tiny filaments of the cochlear nerve at the site where these filaments penetrate the lateral end of the meatus to enter the modiolus (▶ Fig. 30.9b).

The most common reason for tumor appearing to be tightly adherent to the neural structures is residual tumor within the capsule wedging the tumor into position. As the intracapsular contents are removed, the tumor capsule folds inward, thus making it possible to remove more tumor through the operative corridor. If the tumor does not separate easily from neural tissue after the intracapsular contents have been removed, a brief wait often allows the

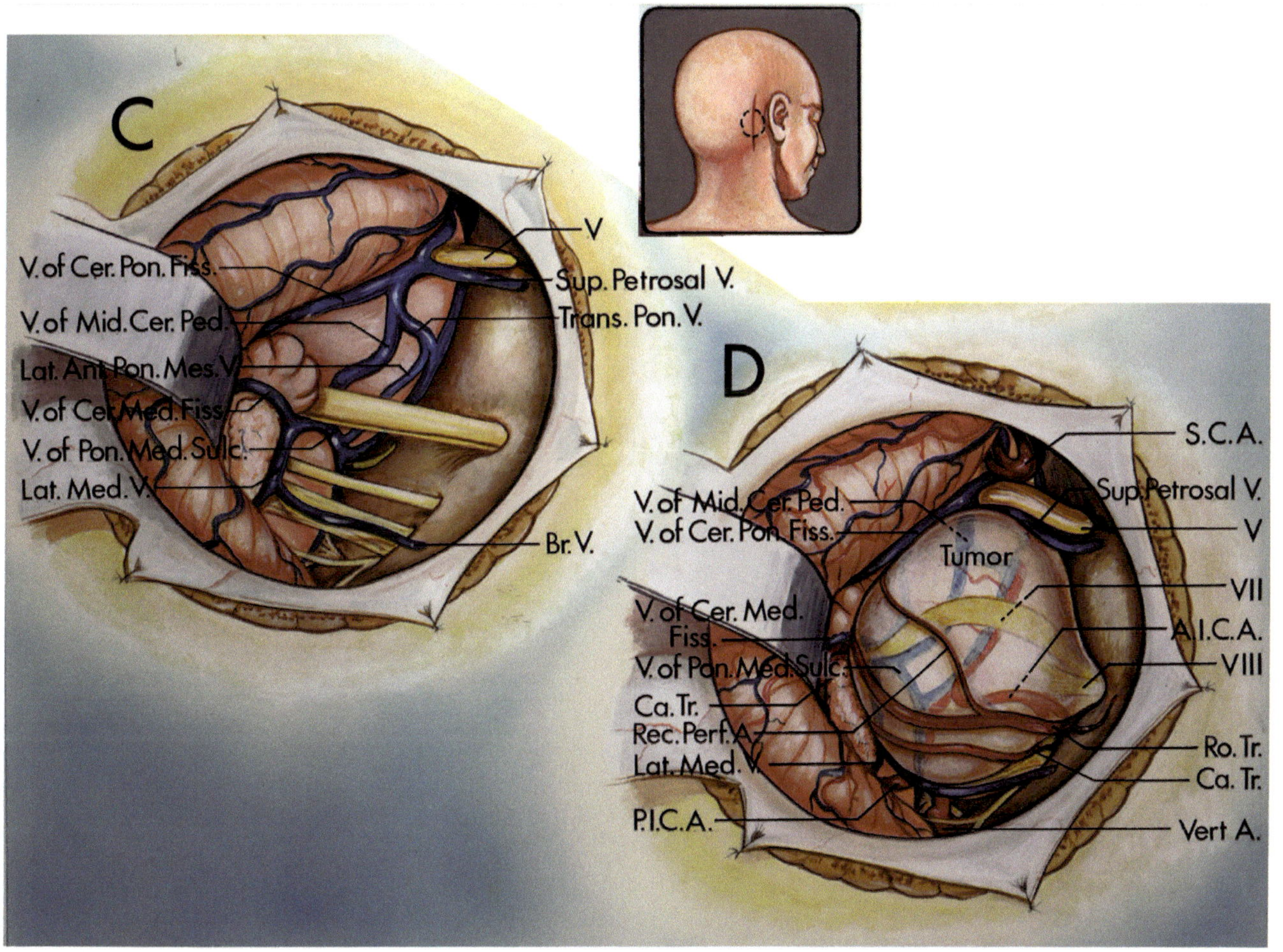

Fig. 30.5 *(continued)* **(c)** Venous relationships. The veins that join near the junction of the facial and vestibulocochlear nerves with the brainstem are the lateral medullary (Lat. Med. V.) veins and the veins of the cerebellomedullary fissure (V. of Cer. Med. Fiss.), pontomedullary sulcus (V. of Pon. Med. Sulc.), and middle cerebellar peduncle (V. of Mid. Cer. Ped.). The vein of the cerebellopontine fissure (V. of Cer. Pon. Fiss.) passes above the flocculus along the superior limb of the cerebellopontine fissure and joins the vein of the middle cerebellar peduncle and a transverse pontine vein (Trans. Pon. V.) to form a superior petrosal vein (Sup. Pet. V.), which empties into the superior petrosal sinus. A bridging vein (Br. V.) passes behind the vagus nerve. The lateral anterior pontomesencephalic vein (Lat. Ant. Pon. Mes. V.) ascends on the pons. **(d)** Neurovascular relationships of a VS. The tumor arises from the vestibulocochlear nerve and displaces the facial nerve anteriorly, the trigeminal nerve superiorly, and the glossopharyngeal and vagus nerves inferiorly. The vestibulocochlear nerve disappears into the tumor. The facial nerve enters the brainstem at the lateral margin of the pontomedullary sulcus, anterior to the flocculus and rostral to the choroid plexus protruding from the foramen of Luschka. The rostral trunk of the anterior inferior cerebellar artery courses below the tumor and above the flocculus to reach the surface of the middle cerebellar peduncle. The veins displaced around the medial side of the tumor are the lateral medullary veins and the veins of the middle cerebellar peduncle, cerebellomedullary fissure, and pontomedullary sulcus. The vein of the cerebellopontine fissure passes above the tumor. A recurrent perforating branch (Rec. Perf. A.) of the anterior inferior cerebellar artery passes across the tumor and supplies the brainstem. (Reproduced with permission from Rhoton.[10])

pulsation of the brain to dislodge the tumor into the exposure, and then more tumor frequently can be removed within the capsule. Under magnification, individual adhesions between vital structures and tumor can be divided with microinstruments. A thin remnant of tumor capsule may be left if it is so firmly adherent to vital neural or vascular structures including the facial and cochlear nerves that removing it would damage these structures.

If the pia-arachnoid is adherent to the tumor capsule or if a mass of tumor within the capsule prevents collapse of the capsule away from the pia-arachnoid, there is a tendency to apply traction to both the capsule and the pia-arachnoid and to tear vessels running on the neural structures. Prior to separating the pia-arachnoid from the capsule, it is important that the entire tumor is removed so that the capsule is so thin that it is almost transparent. If one is uncertain about the margin between the capsule and the pia-arachnoid, irrigation and fine dissection of the area often will clarify the appropriate plane for dissection. After evacuating the intracapsular contents, the remaining tumor capsule is gently separated from the side of the brainstem and the margins of the involved cranial nerve using gentle microsurgical techniques.

It is especially important that the segment of the cerebellar arteries adherent to the tumor capsule be preserved because a

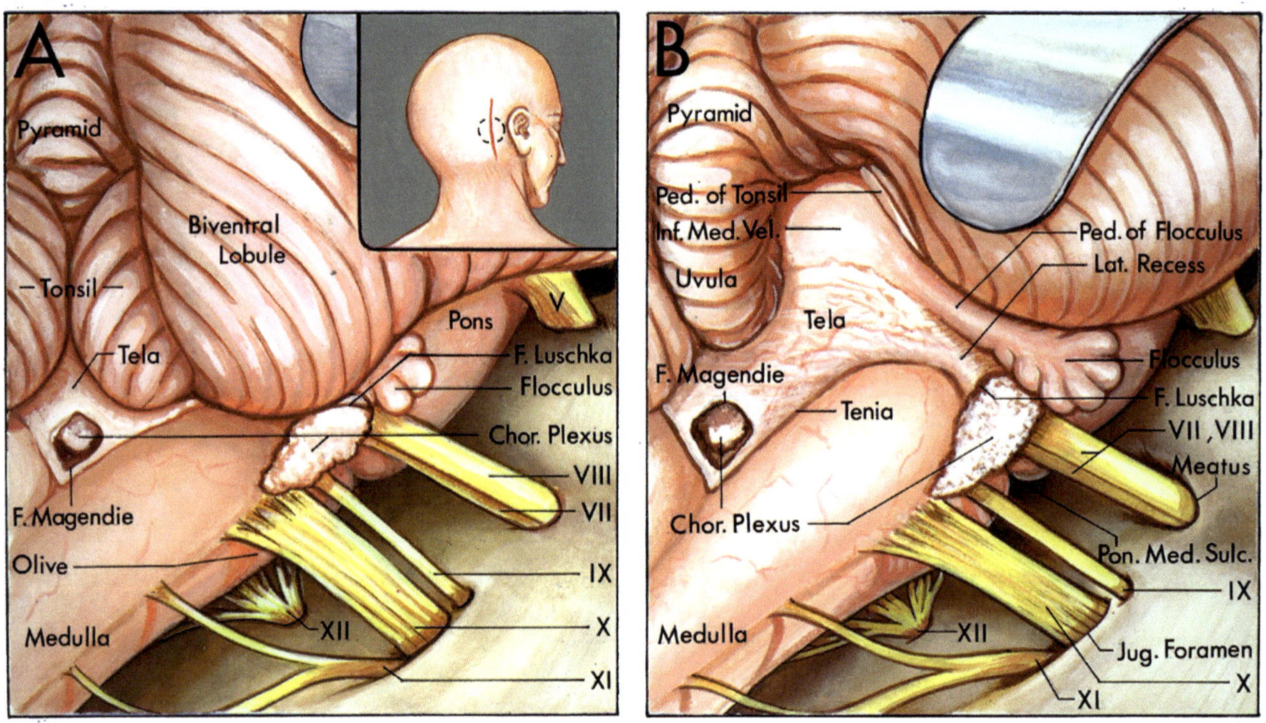

Fig. 30.6 Relationship of the foramen of Luschka and the lateral recess of the fourth ventricle to the junction of the facial and vestibulocochlear nerves with the brainstem as seen through a suboccipital craniectomy. **(a)** The orientation, skin incision (*solid line*), and craniectomy (*interrupted line*) are shown in the inset. The foramen of Magendie (F. Magendie) opens in the midline between the cerebellar tonsils and the foramen of Luschka (F. Luschka) opens into the cerebellopontine angle. The choroid plexus (Chor. Plexus) is attached to the inner surface of the tela choroidea (Tela) and protrudes from the foramen of Luschka slightly below and behind the facial (VII) and vestibulocochlear (VIII) nerves, and behind to the glossopharyngeal (IX) and vagus (X) nerves. The flocculus protrudes into the cerebellopontine angle above the foramen of Luschka. The accessory nerve (XI) arises below the vagus nerve. The hypoglossal rootlets (XII) arise ventral to the olive. The trigeminal nerve (V) crosses in the upper part of the exposure. **(b)** The right cerebellar tonsil has been removed by dividing the tonsillar peduncle (Ped. Of Tonsil) to show the relationship of the lateral recess (Lat. Recess) to the facial and vestibulocochlear nerves. The flocculus and choroid plexus protrude in the cerebellopontine angle behind the junction of the facial and vestibulocochlear nerves with the brainstem. The inferior medullary velum (Inf. Med. Vel.) stretches from the lateral side of the vermis to the flocculus and is all that remains of the connection between the flocculus and the nodulus, which form the flocculonodular lobe of the cerebellum. The inferior medullary velum stretches laterally to form the peduncle of the flocculus (Ped. of Flocculus). The tela choroidea forms the caudal part of the roof of the fourth ventricle and has the choroid plexus attached to its inner surface. Small ridges called the tenia are the site of attachment of the tela choroidea to the edge of the floor of the fourth ventricle. The glossopharyngeal, vagus, and accessory nerves pass through the jugular foramen (Jug. Foramen). The facial and vestibulocochlear nerves enter the brainstem at the lateral end of the pontomedullary sulcus (Pon. Med. Sulc.). (*continued*)

major cause of operative mortality and morbidity is loss of perforating arteries and branches of the cerebellar arteries, which may be adherent to and displaced by the tumor.[11] Any vessel that stands above or is stretched around the tumor capsule should be dealt with initially as if it were a vessel that runs over the tumor surface to supply the brain. After the tumor has been removed from within the capsule, an attempt should be made to displace the vessel off the tumor capsule using a small dissector. When dissected free of the capsule, vessels that initially appeared to be adherent to the capsule often prove to be neural vessels. The cerebellar, basilar, and vertebral arteries may be exposed in removing tumors of the cerebellopontine angle. Occlusion of a cerebellar artery is one of the most common causes of morbidity and mortality in removing cerebellopontine angle tumors.[20] The AICA is the artery most commonly involved by a VS.[11]

The number of veins sacrificed should be kept to a minimum because of the undesirable consequences of their loss. Obliteration of the petrosal veins, which pass from the surface of the cerebellum and brainstem to the superior petrosal sinus, is inescapable in reaching and removing some cerebellopontine angle tumors. Occlusion of these veins, which drain much of the cerebellum and brainstem, may infrequently cause edema of the cerebellum and the brainstem. Some of these veins may need to be sacrificed if the tumor extends into the area above the internal auditory canal. However, small VSs and other tumors in the lower part of the cerebellopontine angle may frequently be removed without sacrificing a petrosal vein.

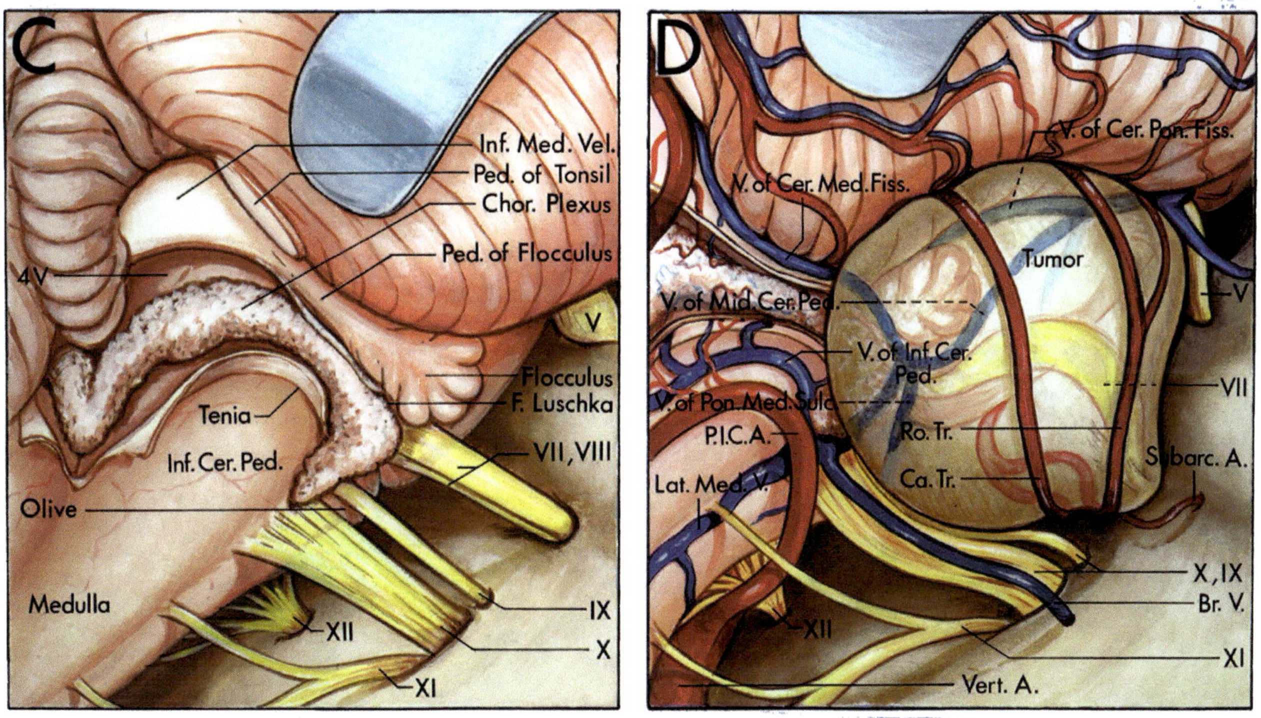

Fig. 30.6 (*continued*) **(c)** The tela choroidea has been opened, but the choroid plexus, which arises on the inner surface of the tela in the fourth ventricle (4V), has been preserved. The fringelike choroid plexus extends through the foramen of Luschka slightly below and behind the junction of the facial and vestibulocochlear nerves with the brainstem. The inferior cerebellar peduncle (Inf. Cer. Ped.) ascends on the dorsolateral margin of the medulla. **(d)** Relationships of a VS. The facial nerve is displaced anteriorly and superiorly in the cerebellopontine angle and enters the brainstem at the lateral end of the pontomedullary sulcus, anterosuperior to the choroid plexus protruding from the foramen of Luschka, and near where the flocculus is attached along the margin of the lateral recess. The tumor displaces the trigeminal nerve upward and the glossopharyngeal and vagus nerves downward. The anterior inferior cerebellar artery (AICA) gives rise to a subarcuate artery (Subarc. A.), which enters the subarcuate fossa in the posterior wall of the internal auditory canal and bifurcates into a rostral (Ro. Tr.) and a caudal trunk (Ca. Tr.). The rostral trunk courses above the flocculus to reach the surface of the middle cerebellar peduncle. The posterior inferior cerebellar artery (PICA) arises from the vertebral artery (Vert. A.) and passes around the lateral surface of the medulla. The lateral medullary vein (Lat. Med. V.) and the veins of the inferior cerebellar peduncle (V. of Inf. Cer. Ped.) and cerebellomedullary fissure (V. of Cer. Med. Fiss.) join in the area below where the facial nerve enters the brainstem to form the vein of the middle cerebellar peduncle (Mid. Cer. Ped.). A bridging vein (Br. V.) passes from the lateral surface of the medulla to the jugular foramen. The vein of the cerebellopontine fissure (V. of Cer. Pon. Fiss.) ascends along the superomedial margin of the tumor. (Reproduced with permission from Rhoton.[10])

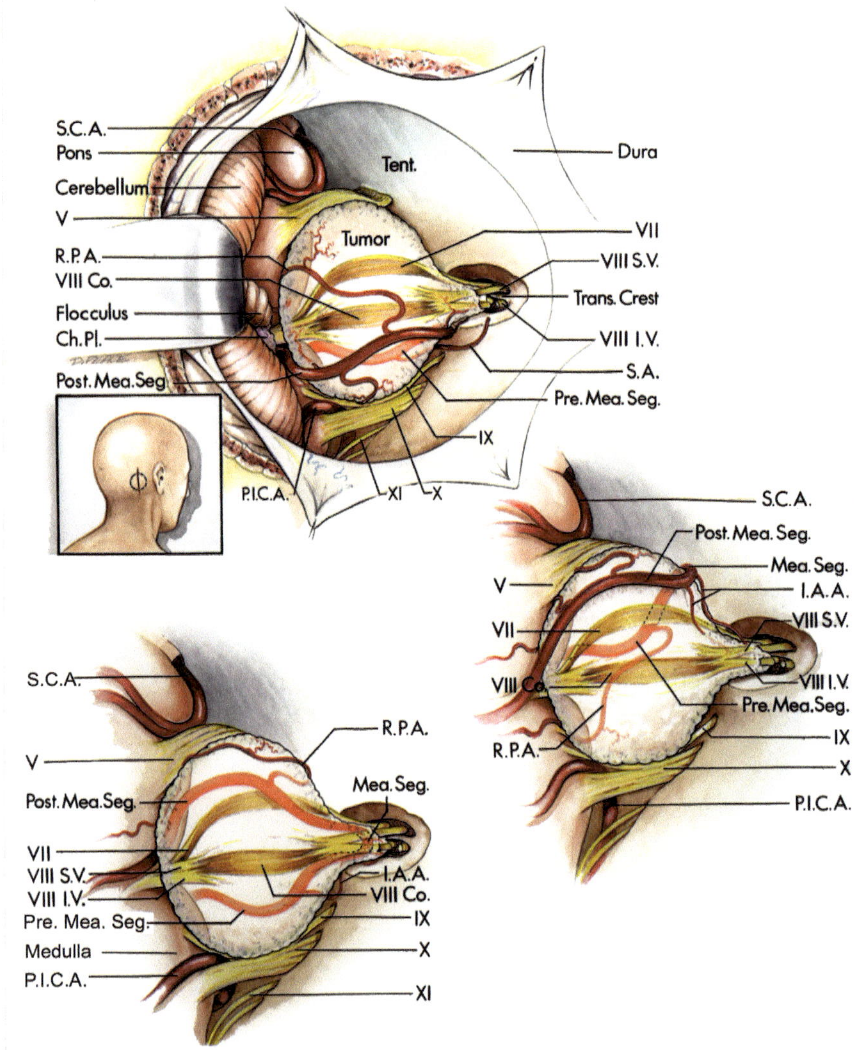

Fig. 30.7 Posterior views of the direction of displacement of the anterior inferior cerebellar artery (A.I.CA) around a VS. Top left: The inset shows the skin incision (*vertical line*) and the site of the craniectomy (*broken line*). Both the premeatal (Pre. Mea. Seg.) and the postmeatal (Post. Mea. Seg.) segments are in their most common location around the lower margin of the tumor. The premeatal segment approaches the meatus from anteroinferior, and the postmeatal segment passes posteroinferior to the tumor. The superior cerebellar artery (S.C.A.) and trigeminal nerve (V) are above the tumor, and the posterior inferior cerebellar artery (P.I.C.A.) and the glossopharyngeal (IX), vagus (X), and accessory (XI) nerves are below the tumor. The choroid plexus (Ch. Pl.) protrudes into the cerebellopontine angle medial to the tumor. The posterior wall of the internal acoustic canal has been removed to expose the transverse crest (Trans. Crest) and the superior vestibular (VIII S. V.) and inferior vestibular (VIII I.V.) nerves. The vestibular nerves disappear into the tumor; however, the cochlear (VIII Co.) and facial nerves (VII) are displaced around the anterior margin of the tumor. A subarcuate artery (S.A.) arises from the premeatal segment, and a recurrent perforating artery (R.P.A.) arises from the postmeatal segment. Center right: A less common pattern of displacement of the anterior inferior cerebellar artery in which the premeatal and postmeatal segments are above the tumor. The internal auditory arteries (I.A.A.) arise from the meatal segment (Mea. Seg.). A recurrent perforating artery arises from the premeatal segment. Bottom left: Both the premeatal and the postmeatal segments are displaced anterior to the tumor. This occurs if the anterior inferior cerebellar artery courses between the vestibulocochlear and facial nerves. The tumor arises in the vestibular nerves, and the tumor growth displaces both the premeatal and the postmeatal segments anteriorly. (Reproduced with permission from Martin et al.[15])

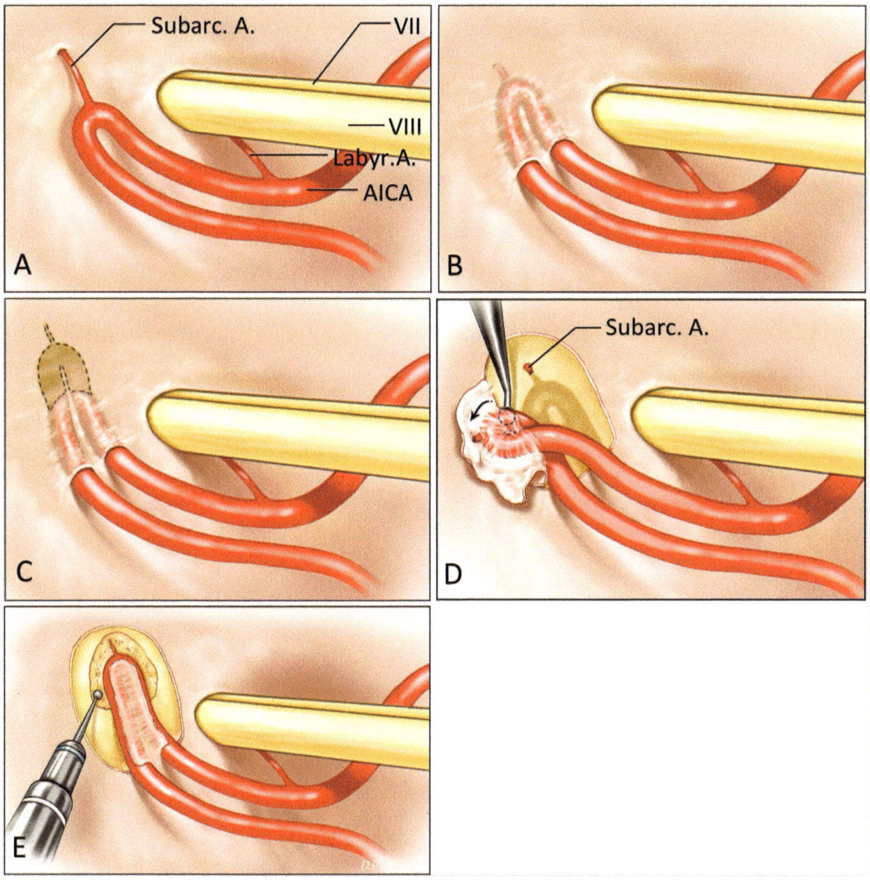

Fig. 30.8 Posterior view of the left internal auditory canal. **(a)** Subarcuate artery penetrates the dura of the subarcuate fossa lateral to the meatus. The labyrinthine artery enters the meatus with the vestibulocochlear and the facial nerves. **(b)** Laterally convex loop of the AICA is embedded in the dura covering the subarcuate fossa, where it gives off the subarcuate artery. **(c)** AICA loop is embedded in the dura and bone (*arrow*) surrounding the subarcuate fossa. **(d)** Dura over the subarcuate fossa has been incised, and the dura with the adherent loop is dissected free from the subarcuate fossa in preparation for opening the meatus. **(e)** Dura over the subarcuate fossa has been incised and remains attached to the artery. The bone surrounding the embedded AICA loop is removed with a 2-mm diamond drill to displace the artery medially for exposure of the meatus. (Reproduced with permission from Tanriover and Rhoton.[17])

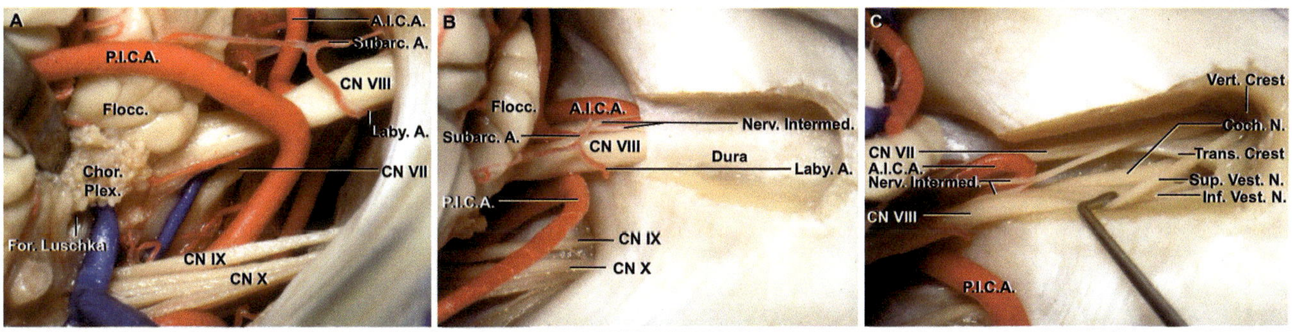

Fig. 30.9 Retrosigmoid exposure of the internal auditory canal. **(a)** The flocculus and choroid plexus, which protrude from the foramen of Luschka, have been elevated to expose the junction of the facial and vestibulocochlear nerves with the brainstem. The facial nerve is exposed below the vestibulocochlear nerve. A branch of the AICA gives rise to both the subarcuate and labyrinthine arteries. The subarcuate artery enters the dura and bone superolateral to the meatus. The junction of the facial nerve with the brainstem is easier to expose from below rather than above the flocculus and vestibulocochlear nerve. **(b)** The posterior wall of the internal auditory canal has been removed to expose the dura lining the meatus. The subarcuate artery usually has to be obliterated and divided before removing the posterior meatal wall. Two bundles from the nervus intermedius are exposed above the vestibulocochlear nerve. Care is taken to avoid entering the semicircular canals and vestibule during drilling of the posterior wall of the meatus if hearing is to be preserved. **(c)** The meatal dura has been opened, and the vestibulocochlear nerve has been depressed to expose the facial nerve coursing in the anterosuperior quadrant of the meatus. The nervus intermedius, which arises along the anterior surface of the vestibulocochlear nerve and passes laterally to join the facial nerve, is composed of several rootlets, as is common. The superior vestibular nerve passes posterior to the facial nerve, and the cochlear nerve is partially hidden anterior to the inferior vestibular nerve. The superior vestibular and facial nerves pass above the transverse crest and the inferior vestibular and cochlear nerves pass below the transverse crest. The vertical crest separates the superior vestibular and facial nerves at the fundus of the meatus. (*continued*)

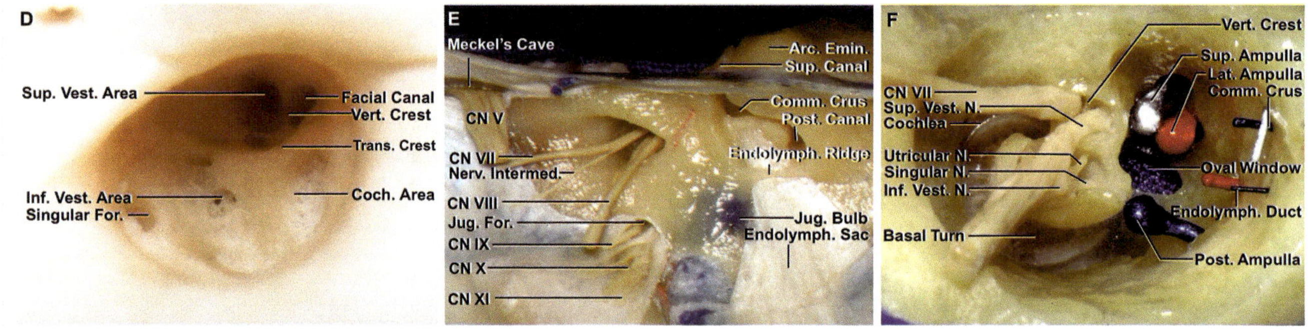

Fig. 30.9 (*continued*) **(d)** Fundus of the right internal auditory canal. The transverse crest divides the meatal fundus into superior and inferior parts. Above the transverse crest, the facial canal is anterior and the superior vestibular area is posterior. Below the transverse crest, the cochlear area is anterior and the inferior vestibular area is posterior. The singular foramen, through which the singular branch of the inferior vestibular nerve passes to innervate the posterior canal ampullae, is located posterior to the inferior vestibular area. The inferior vestibular nerve also has a saccular and, occasionally, a utricular branch. The cochlear nerve splits into tiny filaments as its fiber pass through the cochlear area. These filaments are easily torn, with a resulting loss of hearing, with medially directed retraction of the cerebellum and nerve. **(e)** The trigeminal nerve passes above the petrous apex and through the porus of Meckel's cave. The facial and vestibulocochlear nerves enter the internal auditory canal, and the glossopharyngeal, vagus, and accessory nerves enter the jugular foramen. The posterior and superior semicircular canal is positioned below the medial edge of the arcuate eminence. The upper end of the posterior canal and the posterior end of the superior canal join to form a common channel, the common crus, which opens into the vestibule. The endolymphatic duct extends downward from the vestibule and opens into the endolymphatic sac located beneath the dura inferolateral to the internal auditory canal. The endolymphatic ridge, the bridge of bone forming the lower lip of the endolymphatic duct, has been preserved. The jugular bulb can be seen through the thin bone below the internal auditory canal. Entering the posterior canal, common crus, posterior portion of the superior canal, or the vestibule during drilling of the internal auditory canal may result in loss of hearing. **(f)** Bone has been removed along the anterior margin of the fundus to open the cochlea, and along the posterior margin to expose the vestibule. The cochlear nerve penetrates the modiolus of the cochlea, where its fibers are distributed to the turns of the cochlear duct. The basal turn of the cochlea communicates below the modiolus with the vestibule. The stapes has been removed from the oval window. The promontory in the medial wall of the tympanic cavity is located lateral to the basal turn of the cochlea. A silver fiber has been introduced into the superior semicircular canal, a red fiber into the lateral canal, and a blue fiber into the posterior canal. The ampullated ends of the canals are located at the bulbous ends of the three fibers. The common crus of the superior and posterior canals is located where the tips of the blue and silver fibers cross. The superior vestibular nerve passes to the ampullae of the superior and lateral canals. The singular branch of the inferior vestibular nerve innervates the posterior ampullae. A small black fiber has been introduced into the opening of the endolymphatic duct into the vestibule.

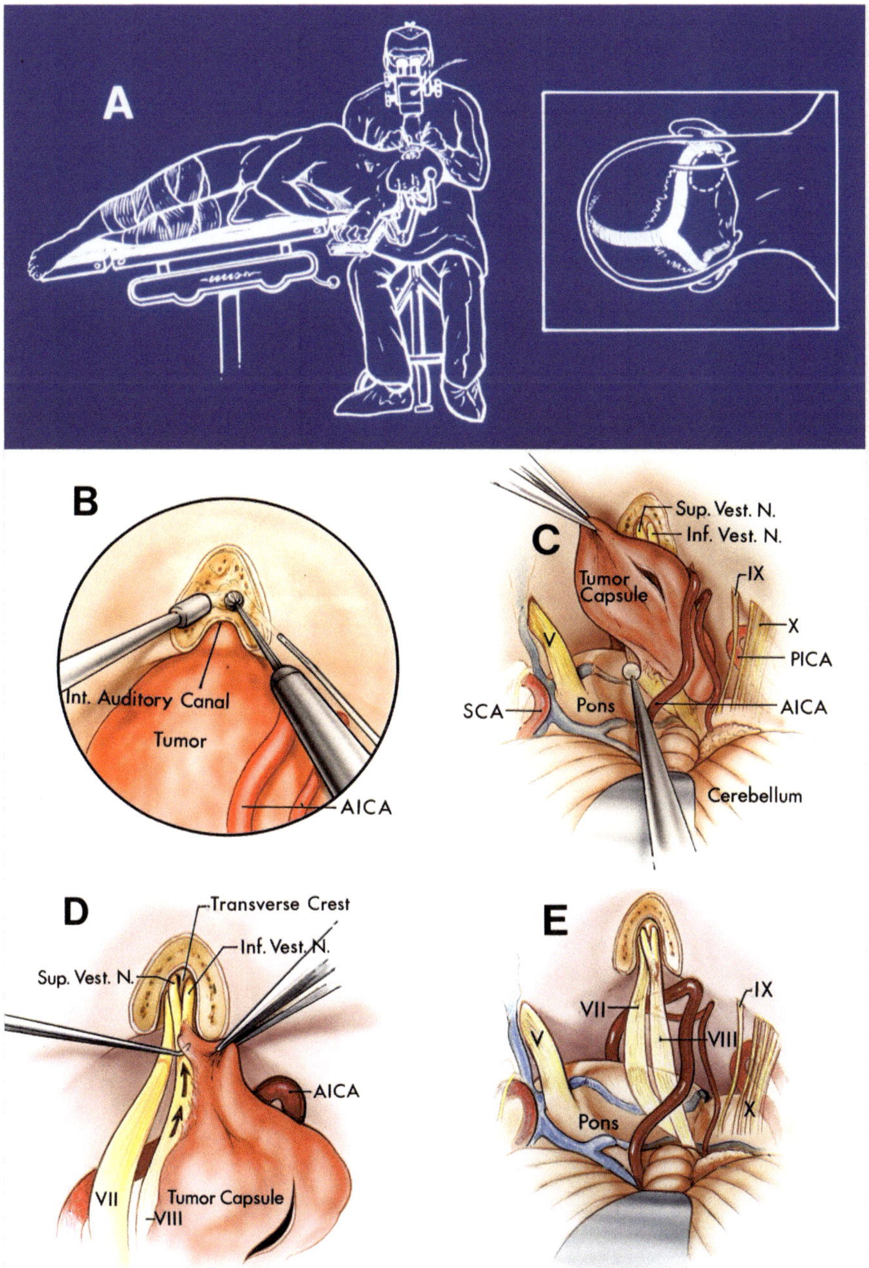

Fig. 30.10 Retrosigmoid approach. **(a)** The patient is positioned in the three-quarter prone position with the surgeon behind the head. The inset (right) shows the site of the scalp incision (continuous line) and the bony opening (interrupted line). **(b)** The posterior wall of the internal auditory canal is removed using an irrigating drill. The anterior inferior cerebellar artery (AICA) courses around the lower margin of the tumor. **(c)** The intracapsular contents of the tumor have been removed. The capsule of the tumor is being separated from the pons and the posterior surface of the part of the facial (VII) and vestibulocochlear nerves adjacent to the brainstem. The superior (Sup. Vest. N.) and inferior vestibular nerves (Inf. Vest. N.) are seen at the lateral end of the internal auditory canal. The trigeminal nerve (V) and superior cerebellar artery (SCA) are above the tumor and the glossopharyngeal (IX) and vagus (X) nerves and the posterior inferior cerebellar artery (PICA) are below the tumor. **(d)** The dissection along the eighth nerve (VIII) is done in a medial to lateral direction (*arrows*) in order to avoid tearing the tiny filaments of the cochlear nerve in the lateral end of the canal where they pass through the lamina cribrosa. The transverse crest separates the superior and inferior vestibular nerves in the lateral end of the canal. **(e)** Cerebellopontine angle and internal auditory canal after tumor removal. The facial and vestibulocochlear nerves have been preserved. (Reproduced with permission from Rhoton AL Jr. Microsurgical anatomy of acoustic neuroma. In: Sekhar LN, Janecka A, eds. Surgery of Cranial Base Tumors. Philadelphia, PA: Lippincott Williams 1993.)

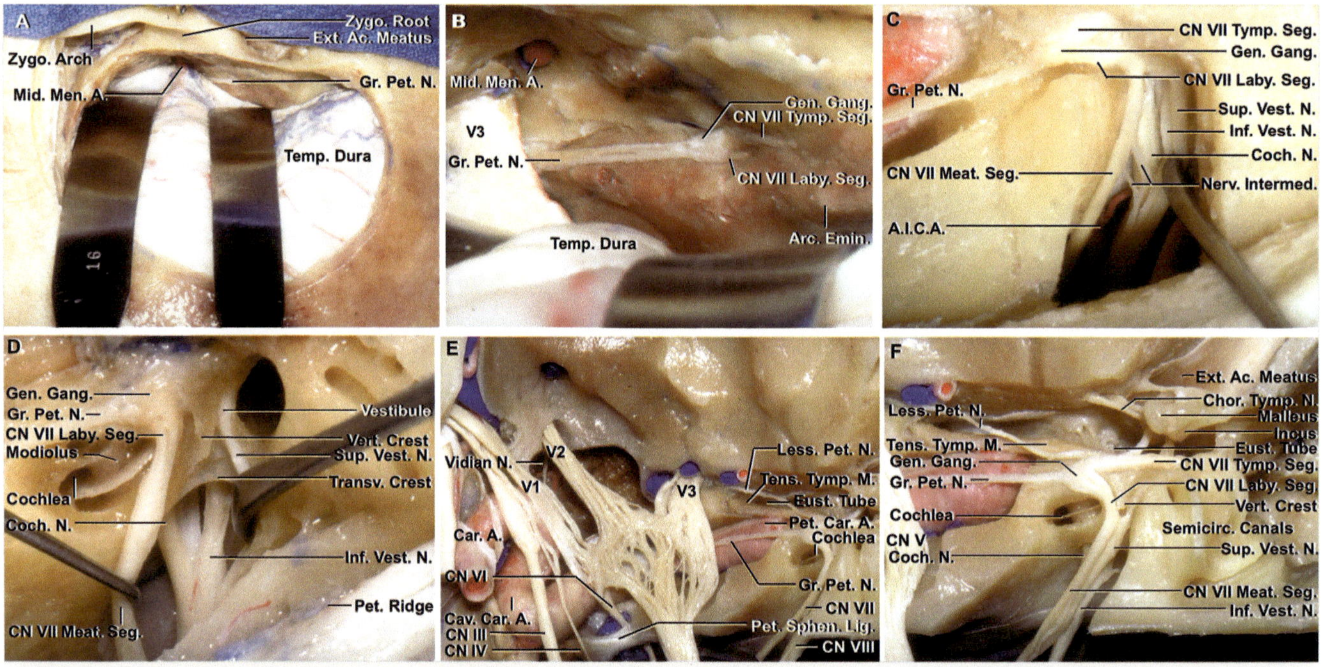

Fig. 30.11 Extradural right middle fossa exposure. **(a)** The craniotomy is positioned above the root of the zygomatic arch and extends to the middle fossa floor. The dura has been elevated from the floor of the right middle fossa to expose the greater petrosal nerve and middle meningeal artery. The middle fossa approach to the internal auditory canal is usually directed through the extradural space. **(b)** Enlarged view. The geniculate ganglion and the distal labyrinthine and proximal tympanic segments of the facial nerve are exposed directly under the dura. The ganglion is exposed without a bony covering in approximately 15% of temporal bones. Trauma to the ganglion during elevation of the dura may cause a facial palsy. The middle meningeal artery sends a small branch along the floor of the middle fossa to the geniculate ganglion and adjacent segments of the facial nerve. Occluding this small artery may cause facial paralysis. **(c)** Bone has been removed to expose the internal auditory canal and the dura has been opened. This drilling to expose the internal auditory canal usually begins at the level of the petrous ridge above the porus of the meatus and is directed laterally and forward toward the fundus of the meatus, where the exposure progressively narrows. Opening the dura lining, the internal auditory canal exposes the tumor and the nerves in the meatus and cerebellopontine angle. **(d)** The drilling has been extended to expose the cochlea along the anteromedial edge of the fundus of the meatus and the vestibule and semicircular canals along the posterolateral margin of the meatal fundus. Care must be taken in the middle fossa approach to the internal auditory canal to avoid entering the cochlea and vestibule. If either the cochlea or vestibule is entered, hearing will be lost. The transverse crest divides the fundus of the meatus into an upper and a lower compartment. The facial and superior vestibular nerves course above the transverse crest and the cochlear and inferior vestibular nerves pass below the crest. The facial nerve passes through the anterosuperior quadrant, the inferior vestibular nerve passes through the posterosuperior quadrant, the cochlear nerve passes through the anteroinferior quadrant, and the inferior vestibular nerve passes through the posteroinferior quadrant of the meatal fundus. The vertical crest (Bill's bar) separates the facial and superior vestibular nerves. **(e)** Superior view of the middle fossa. The bone above the eustachian tube, tensor tympani muscle, petrous carotid, and internal auditory canal and below the second trigeminal division has been removed. Dura has been removed from the lateral wall of the cavernous sinus to expose the trochlear, trigeminal, and oculomotor nerves in the sinus wall and the abducens nerve passing below the petrosphenoid ligament and through Dorello's canal. The greater petrosal nerve passes medially above the petrous carotid artery. The lesser petrosal nerve arises from the tympanic branch of the glossopharyngeal nerve, ascends across the promontory in the tympanic plexus, and crosses the floor of the middle fossa above the tensor tympani. The tensor tympani muscle and eustachian tube are layered along but are separated from each other from the anterior surface of the petrous carotid by a thin layer of bone. **(f)** Enlarged superior view of the junction of the eustachian tube and the internal and external meati. The mastoid air cells on the lateral side of the semicircular canals have been removed. The superior vestibular, inferior vestibular, facial, and cochlear nerves are exposed at the fundus of the meatus. The cochlear nerve enters the modiolus of the cochlea. The vertical crest (Bill's bar) separates the facial and superior vestibular nerves at the fundus of the meatus. The chorda tympani crosses the tympanic membrane and the upper part of the handle of the malleus. The greater petrosal nerve passes medially above the petrous carotid. The cochlea sits in the angle between the labyrinthine segment of the facial nerve and the greater petrosal nerve. The lesser petrosal nerve crosses above the tensor tympani and exits the cranium near the foramen ovale to reach the otic ganglion and innervate the parotid gland.

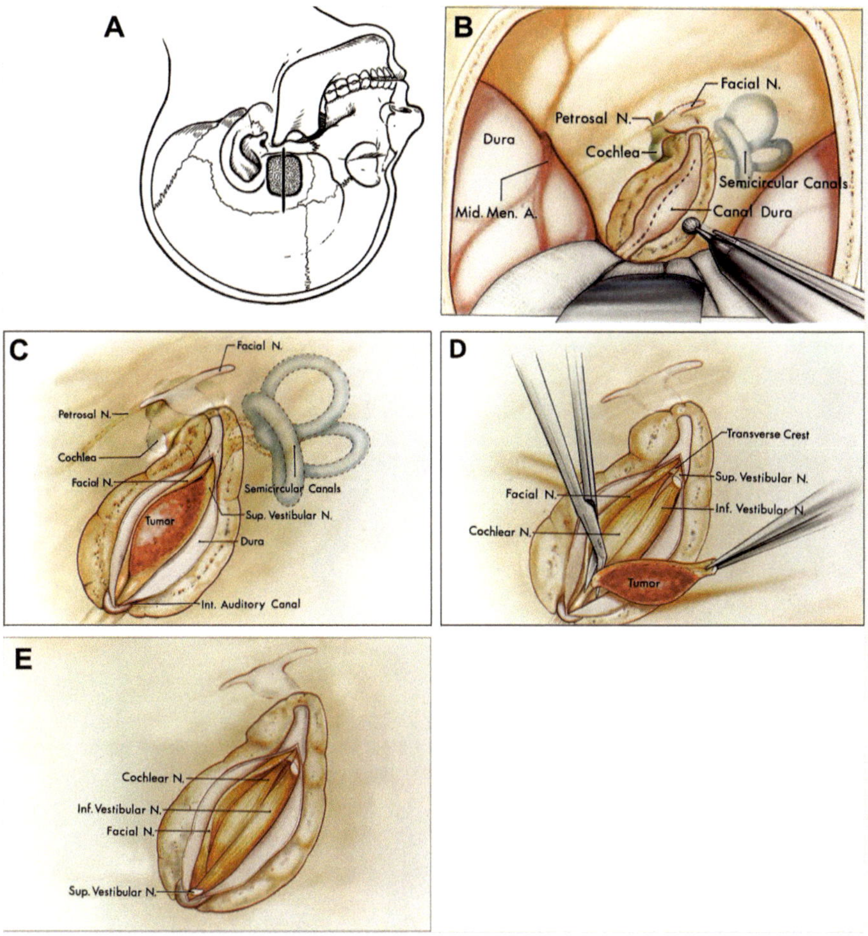

Fig. 30.12 Middle fossa approach for removing a small VS. **(a)** The vertical skin incision is located anterior to the ear and the craniotomy is situated with its base on the floor of the middle cranial fossa (stippled area). **(b)** The dura is elevated from the floor of the middle cranial fossa to identify the greater petrosal nerve (Petrosal N.). The middle meningeal artery (Mid. Men. A.) courses on the dura. Bone removal begins above the porus of the internal auditory canal and extends to the fundus lateral to the tumor. Extreme care must be taken to avoid injuring the semicircular canals located in the bone at the posterior margin of the exposure and the cochlea situated in the bone just medial and deep to the facial nerve near the fundus of the meatus. **(c)** Enlarged view of the area of bone removal. The dura has been opened to expose the tumor in the internal auditory canal (Int. Auditory Canal). The tumor arises in the superior vestibular nerve (Sup. Vestibular N.) and displaces the facial nerve anteriorly. The superior vestibular nerve has been divided above the transverse crest and elevated with the tumor. The superior vestibular nerve is being divided medial to the tumor. The facial, cochlear (Cochlear N.), and inferior vestibular (Inf. Vestibular N.) nerves are preserved. **(d)** View after removal of the tumor. (Reproduced with permission from Rhoton AL Jr. Microsurgical anatomy of VS. In: Sekhar LN, Janecka A, eds. Surgery of Cranial Base Tumors. Philadelphia, PA: Lippincott Williams 1993.)

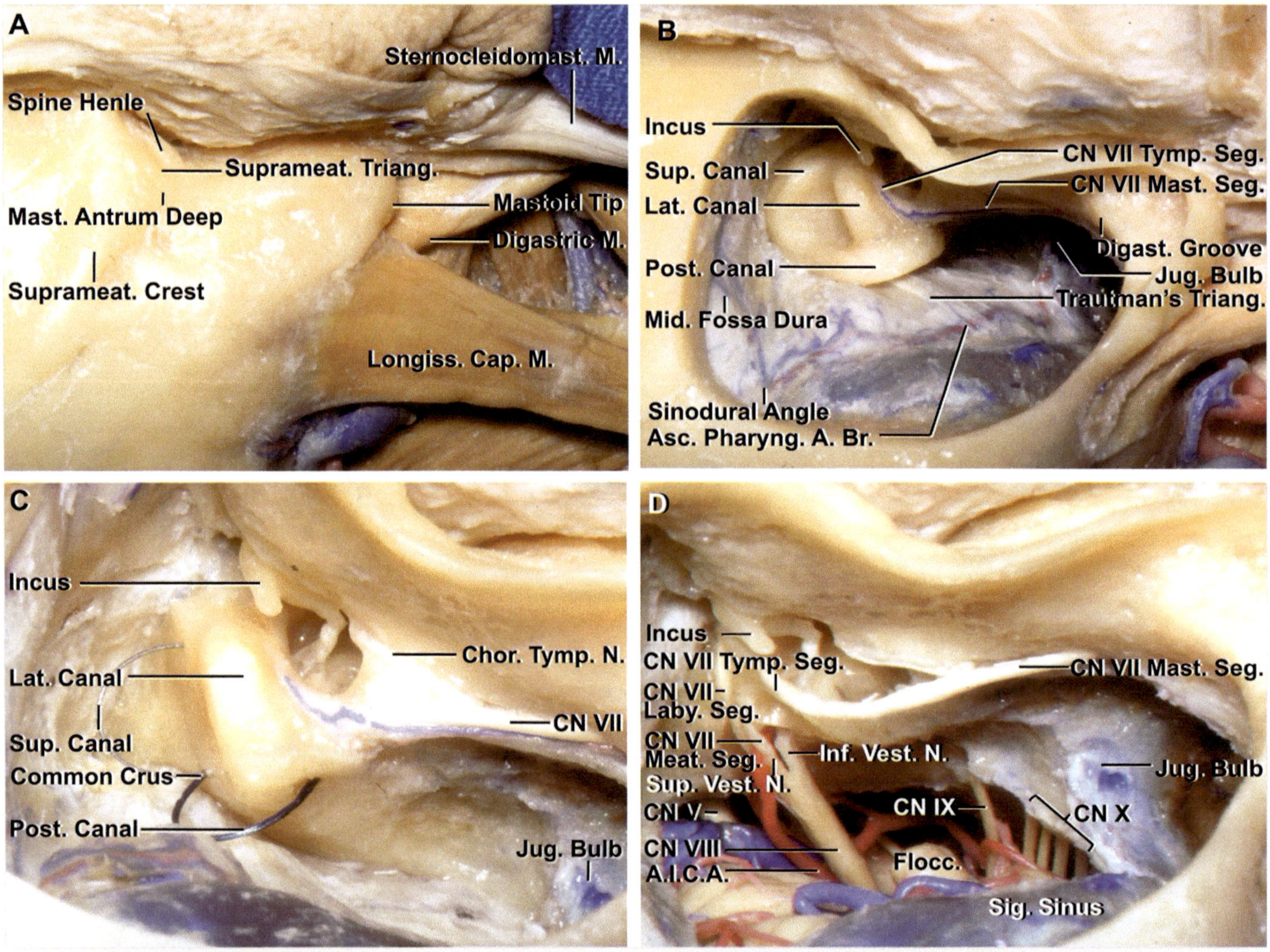

Fig. 30.13 **(a)** Mastoidectomy and retrolabyrinthine, partial labyrinthine, and translabyrinthine approaches. Right mastoid. The retroauricular flap has been reflected forward. The spine of Henle is positioned at the posterior superior margin of the external meatus and superficial to the deep site of the lateral semicircular canal and junction of the tympanic and mastoid segments of the facial nerve. The supramastoid crest, a continuation of the superior temporal line, is positioned at approximately the level of the upper margin of the transverse and sigmoid sinuses. The area below the anterior part of the supramastoid crest and behind the spine of Henle, called the suprameatal triangle, is positioned superficial to the mastoid antrum. The semicircular canals are positioned deep to the mastoid antrum. **(b)** The drilling has been extended to expose the middle fossa dura above, the sigmoid sinus posteriorly, and the jugular bulb below. The superior, lateral, and posterior semicircular canals are located deep to the mastoid antrum and suprameatal triangle. The superior canal projects upward below the arcuate eminence. The posterior canal faces the posterior fossa dura. The lateral canal is positioned above the tympanic segment of the facial nerve. The facial nerve passes below the lateral canal and turns downward to form the mastoid segment. The dura between the sigmoid sinus and the semicircular canals, named Trautmann's triangle, faces the anterior surface of the cerebellum and cerebellopontine angle. A meningeal branch of the ascending pharyngeal artery passes through the jugular foramen and ascends in the dura of Trautmann's triangle. The jugular bulb is positioned medial to the cortical bone overlying the digastric groove. The sinodural angle is positioned at the junction of the sigmoid, transverse, and superior petrosal sinuses, and where the sigmoid sinus intersects the middle fossa dura. **(c)** Enlarged view. The short process of the incus points toward the tympanic segment of the facial nerve passing between the lateral semicircular canal and the stapes sitting in the oval window. The superior and lateral canal ampullae, located at the anterior end of these canals, are innervated by the superior vestibular nerve. The posterior canal ampulla, located at the lower end of the posterior canal, is innervated by the singular branch of the inferior vestibular nerve. In the translabyrinthine approach, drilling through the anterior (ampullated) ends of the superior and lateral canals exposes the superior vestibular area and nerve at the fundus of the meatus. Drilling the lower (ampullated) end of the posterior canal exposes the inferior vestibular area and nerve at the fundus of the meatus. The posterior end of the superior canal and the upper end of the posterior canal join to form a single channel, the common crus, which opens into the vestibule. **(d)** The translabyrinthine exposure has been completed to expose the vestibulocochlear and facial nerves in the internal auditory canal. The meatal and labyrinthine segments of the facial nerve are exposed proximal to the geniculate ganglion with the tympanic and mastoid segments exposed distally. The mastoid segment of the facial nerve descends toward the stylomastoid foramen and gives rise to the chorda tympani. The dura of Trautmann's triangle has been opened to expose the trigeminal, glossopharyngeal, and vagus nerves in the cerebellopontine angle. The anterior inferior cerebellar artery loops laterally into the meatus before turning back toward the brainstem. The facial, superior, and inferior vestibular nerves are exposed at the fundus of the meatus. The cochlear nerve is hidden anterior to the inferior vestibular nerve.

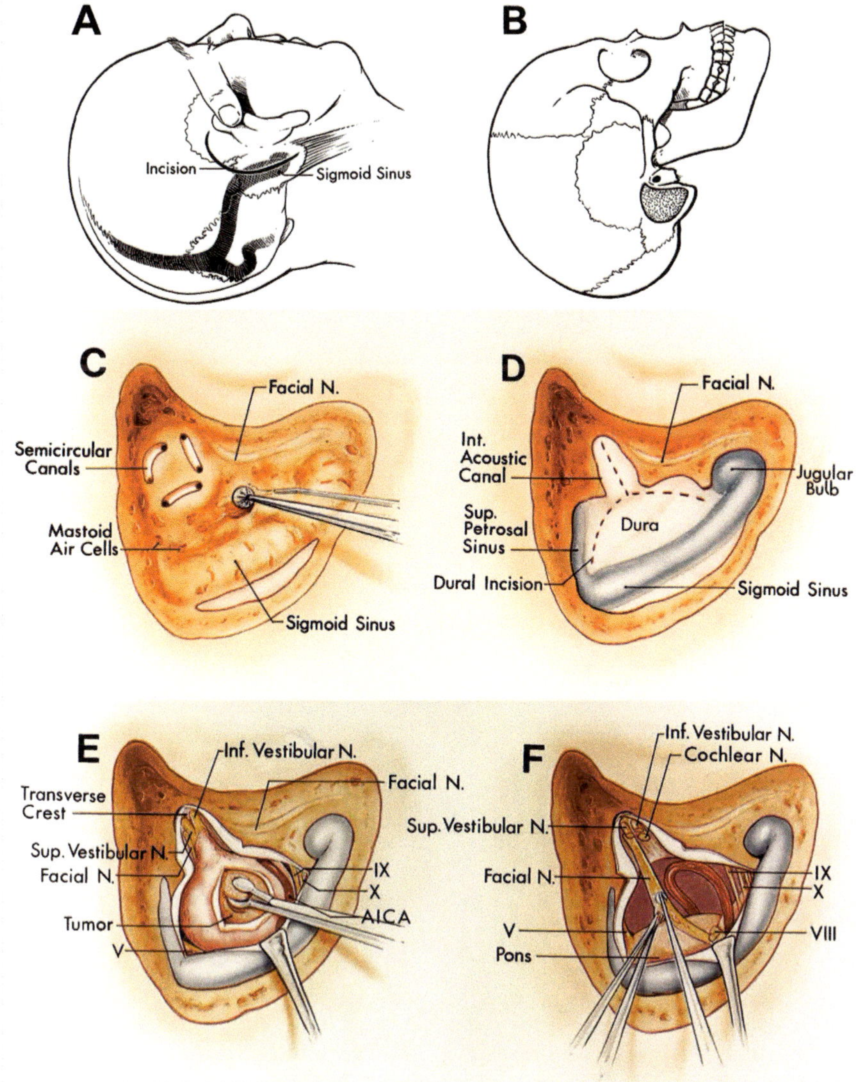

Fig. 30.14 Translabyrinthine approach. **(a)** The operation is done with the patient in the supine position with the face turned toward the side opposite the tumor. Site of the retromastoid skin incision. **(b)** The stippled area shows the site of the bony opening through the mastoid. **(c)** The mastoid air cells are being exenterated and the semicircular canals have been exposed. The drilling will be carried medially through the semicircular canals to the internal auditory canal. **(d)** The bone surrounding and including the semicircular canals has been removed to expose the dura lining the internal auditory canal. The dura between the superior petrosal (Sup. Petrosal Sinus) and sigmoid sinuses has been exposed. The interrupted lines show the site of the dural opening. **(e)** The intracapsular contents of the tumor are being removed with a cup forceps. The superior (Sup. Vestibular N.) and inferior vestibular (Inf. Vestibular N.) nerves are seen lateral to the tumor, where they are separated by the transverse crest. The anterior inferior cerebellar artery (AICA) courses around the lower margin of the tumor. The facial nerve is anterior to the tumor. The trigeminal nerve (V) is above and the glossopharyngeal (IX) and vagus nerves (X) are below the tumor. **(f)** The final fragments of tumor are being removed from the surface of the facial nerve. The superior and inferior vestibular and cochlear nerves (Cochlear N.) have been removed along with the tumor since there is no chance of saving hearing or vestibular function because the operation is directed through the semicircular canals, which leads to loss of hearing. The central stump of the eighth nerve (VIII) is exposed at the brainstem. (Reproduced with permission from Rhoton AL Jr. Microsurgical anatomy of acoustic neuroma. In: Sekhar LN, Janecka A, eds. Surgery of Cranial Base Tumors. Philadelphia, PA: Lippincott Williams 1993.)

References

[1] Pait TG, Harris FS, Paullus WS, Rhoton AL, Jr. Microsurgical anatomy and dissection of the temporal bone. Surg Neurol. 1977; 8(5):363–391

[2] Rhoton AL, Jr. Microsurgery of the internal acoustic meatus. Surg Neurol. 1974; 2(5):311–318

[3] Rhoton AL, Jr. Microsurgical removal of acoustic neuromas. Surg Neurol. 1976; 6(4):211–219

[4] Rhoton AL Jr. Microsurgery of the Temporal Bone and of Acoustic Neuromas. Tryon, NC: Paul C. Bucy & Associates; 1977

[5] Rhoton AL, Jr. Microsurgical anatomy of the posterior fossa cranial nerves. Clin Neurosurg. 1979; 26:398–462

[6] Rhoton AL, Jr. Suboccipital retrolabyrinthine removal of acoustic neuromas. J Fla Med Assoc. 1983; 70(10):895–901

[7] Rhoton AL, Jr. Microsurgical anatomy of acoustic neuromas. Neurol Res. 1984; 6(1)(-)(2):3–21

[8] Rhoton AL Jr. Microsurgical anatomy of the cerebellopontine angle by the retrosigmoid approach. In: Samii M, Gerganov V, eds. Surgery of Cerebellopontine Lesions. Berlin: Springer-Verlag; 2013

[9] Takemura Y, Inoue T, Morishita T, Rhoton AL, Jr. Comparison of microscopic and endoscopic approaches to the cerebellopontine angle. World Neurosurg. 2014; 82(3)(-)(4):427–441

[10] Rhoton AL, Jr. Microsurgical anatomy of the brainstem surface facing an acoustic neuroma. Surg Neurol. 1986; 25(4):326–339

[11] Atkinson WJ. The anterior inferior cerebellar artery; its variations, pontine distribution, and significance in the surgery of cerebello-pontine angle tumours. J Neurol Neurosurg Psychiatry. 1949; 12(2):137–151

[12] Fujii K, Lenkey C, Rhoton AL, Jr. Microsurgical anatomy of the choroidal arteries. Fourth ventricle and cerebellopontine angles. J Neurosurg. 1980; 52(4):504–524

[13] Hardy DG, Peace DA, Rhoton AL, Jr. Microsurgical anatomy of the superior cerebellar artery. Neurosurgery. 1980; 6(1):10–28

[14] Lister JR, Rhoton AL, Jr, Matsushima T, Peace DA. Microsurgical anatomy of the posterior inferior cerebellar artery. Neurosurgery. 1982; 10(2):170–199

[15] Martin RG, Grant JL, Peace D, Theiss C, Rhoton AL, Jr. Microsurgical relationships of the anterior inferior cerebellar artery and the facial-vestibulocochlear nerve complex. Neurosurgery. 1980; 6(5):483–507

[16] Tanriover N, Abe H, Rhoton AL, Jr, Kawashima M, Sanus GZ, Akar Z. Microsurgical anatomy of the superior petrosal venous complex: new classifications and implications for subtemporal transtentorial and retrosigmoid suprameatal approaches. J Neurosurg. 2007; 106(6):1041–1050

[17] Tanriover N, Rhoton AL, Jr. The anteroinferior cerebellar artery embedded in the subarcuate fossa: a rare anomaly and its clinical significance. Neurosurgery. 2005; 57(2):314–319, discussion 314–319

[18] Matsushima T, Rhoton AL, Jr, de Oliveira E, Peace D. Microsurgical anatomy of the veins of the posterior fossa. J Neurosurg. 1983; 59(1):63–105

[19] Matsushima T, Rhoton AL, Jr, Lenkey C. Microsurgery of the fourth ventricle: Part 1. Microsurgical anatomy. Neurosurgery. 1982; 11(5):631–667

[20] Rhoton AL Jr. Meningiomas and other cerebellopontine angle tumors. In: Long D, ed. Current Therapy in Neurological Surgery. Toronto: B.C. Decker Publishers; 1989:14–19

31 Surgical Approach Selection for Vestibular Schwannoma Microsurgery

Alex D. Sweeney, Matthew L. Carlson, and Colin L. W. Driscoll

31.1 Introduction

While many surgical approaches to the internal auditory canal (IAC) and cerebellopontine angle (CPA) have been described, the translabyrinthine (TL), middle cranial fossa (MF), and retrosigmoid (RS) approaches remain the most commonly employed today (▶ Fig. 31.1, ▶ Fig. 31.2, ▶ Fig. 31.3, ▶ Fig. 31.4). The decision to utilize one approach over another is influenced by tumor characteristics, anatomic factors, patient factors, and surgical team experience.[1]

The advantages and disadvantages of each surgical approach are not universally agreed upon. In fact, there are very dogmatic and opposing opinions among many highly skilled surgeons regarding the merits of each approach. This suggests there is more than one acceptable approach and that a surgeon's personal experience should play an important role in the selection. Similar to the choice between observation, surgery, and radiosurgery, it is not possible to follow a standard decision tree to arrive at a "best" surgical approach. Rather, it is important to fully understand the pros and cons of each approach in the surgeon's own hands based on personal experience. An honest assessment of one's own results with the different strategies is critical to achieving the best possible outcome for each individual patient.

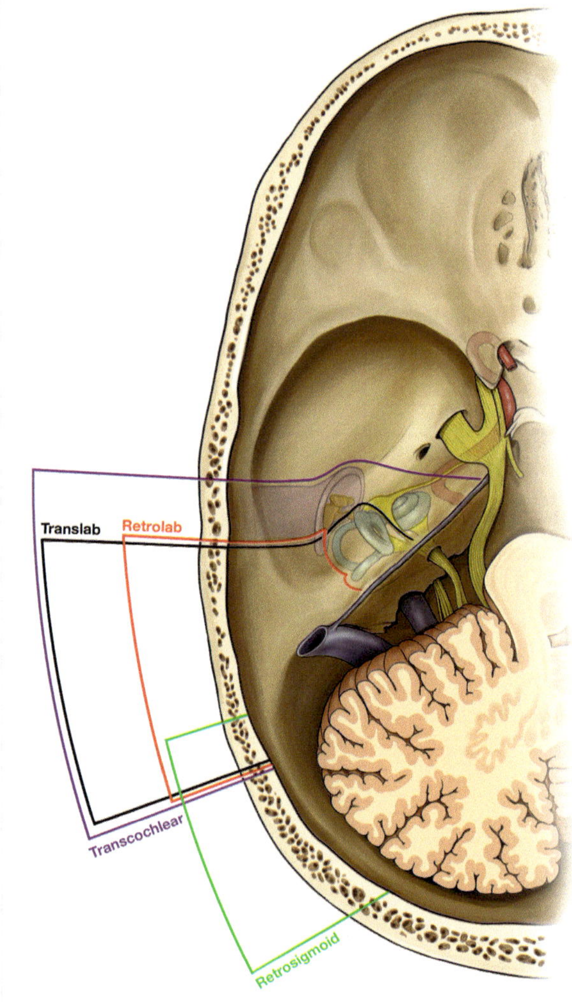

Fig. 31.1 Schematic illustrating common approaches to the lateral skull base.

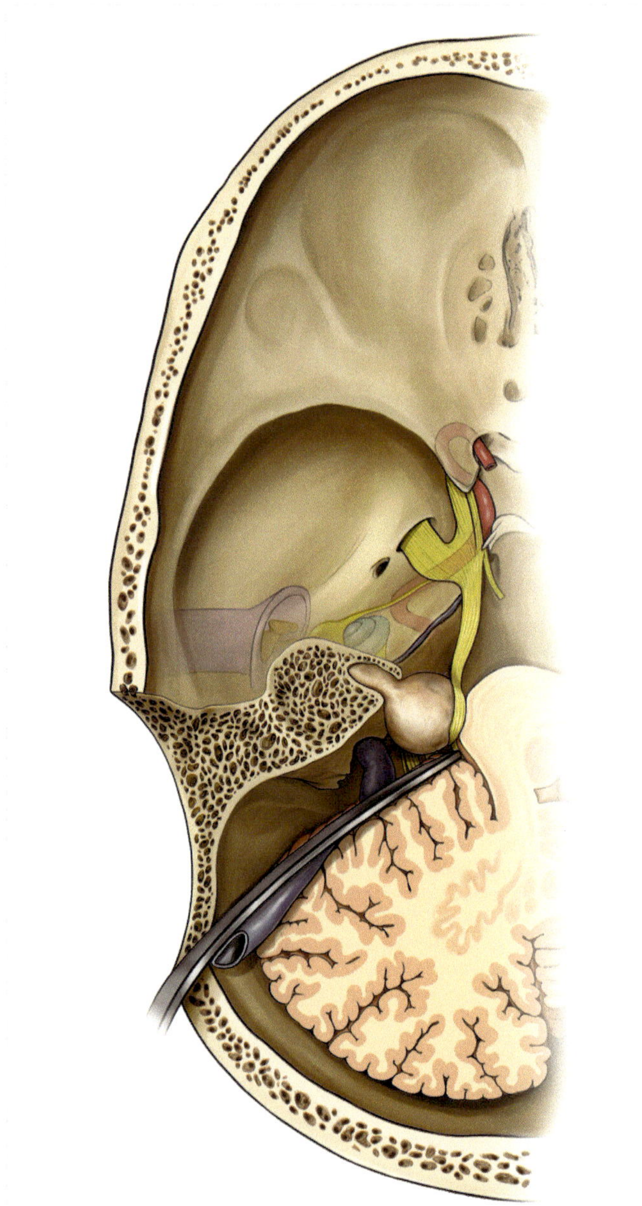

Fig. 31.2 Surgical exposure of the IAC and CPA through the translabyrinthine corridor.

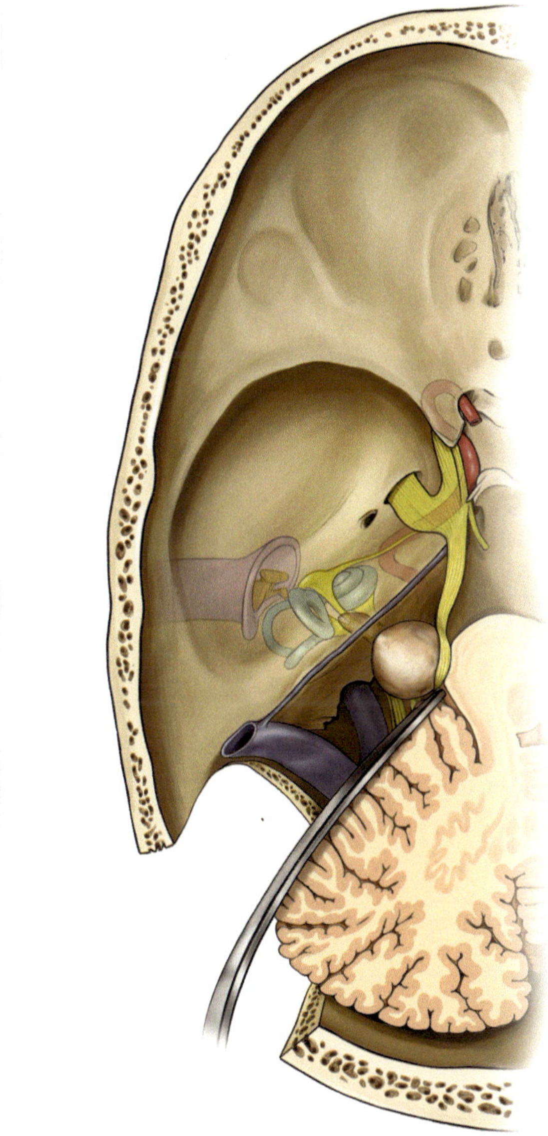

Fig. 31.3 Surgical exposure of the IAC and CPA through the retrosigmoid corridor.

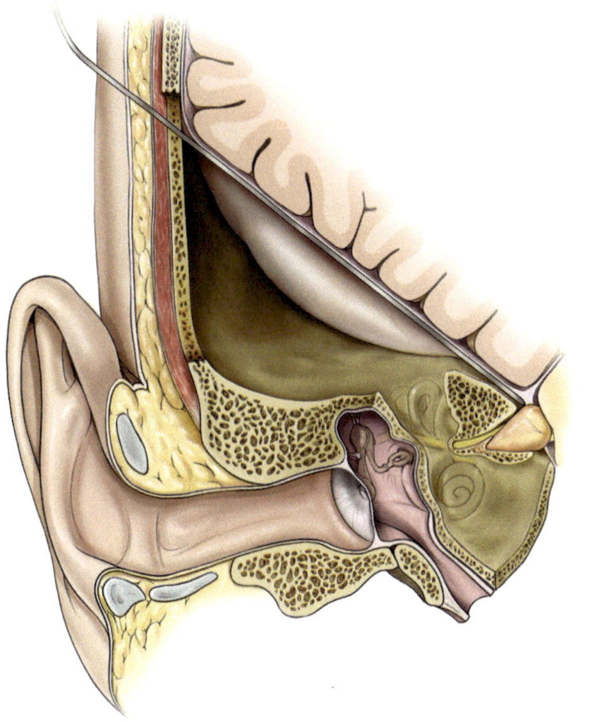

Fig. 31.4 Surgical exposure of the IAC through the middle fossa corridor.

Detailed descriptions of each surgical approach are presented in separate chapters and will not be repeated here: the TL approach is presented in Chapters 33 and 34, the RS approach in Chapters 35 and 36, the MF approach in Chapter 37, and the endoscopic transcanal transpromontorial approach in Chapter 39. Instead, this chapter will review thought processes and nuances regarding approach selection and highlight how various factors impact decision making. Our view of the suitability of the various approaches in different clinical situations has evolved over time as a result of critical analysis of our results.

Specific tumor characteristics, anatomic factors, and patient factors will exclude or favor a particular approach. Typically, there are competing factors and the weighted importance of each need to be estimated. For example, a hearing preservation approach may slightly increase the likelihood of tumor recurrence. If that is true, then we must consider how likely we are to preserve hearing in a specific case. In the following sections, we highlight the factors that ultimately drive us to a particular surgical approach. In many cases, there are equally valid options, in *our* opinion. A list of commonly referenced advantages and limitations of the three approaches is outlined in ▶ Table 31.1.

31.2 Tumor Characteristics

31.2.1 Tumor Size

Tumor size is one of the major drivers of approach selection. We do not consider tumors extending beyond the IAC to be candidates for the MF approach. The decreasing likelihood of preserving hearing and increased risk to the facial nerve make the RS approach more favorable. Assuming no other modifying anatomic or patient factors, we also prefer the RS approach for tumors greater than 3 cm due primarily to the broad exposure of the posterior fossa from tentorium superiorly, to foramen magnum inferiorly, and to the region of Meckel's cave ventrally. There are some centers that prefer the TL approach for large tumors, but this requires more extensive transapical drilling and working around the ventral corner of the porus acusticus.

31.2.2 Tumor Location

Tumor location is another important factor to consider when selecting a surgical approach. For a hearing preservation case,

Table 31.1 Advantages and limitations of the translabyrinthine, middle cranial fossa, and retrosigmoid approaches for vestibular schwannoma resection

	Advantage	Disadvantage
Translabyrinthine	• Direct exposure of the entire IAC • Early and easy identification of the distal facial nerve at the fundus • Primarily extradural and does not require brain retraction • Direct access to tumor within the labyrinth • Can combine with other procedures (e.g., facial nerve reconstruction, cochlear implantation)	• Hearing preservation is not possible • Neurosurgeon unfamiliarity • May increase surgical time • Requires abdominal adipose graft • Risk of sigmoid sinus injury
Retrosigmoid	• Wide and early exposure of the posterior fossa • Hearing preservation is possible • Early identification of the facial nerve at the brainstem in small tumors • All tumors can be removed with this one approach	• Cerebellar retraction is frequently utilized • Intradural transmeatal bone removal is necessary to access IAC • Lateral IAC access may be limited by the position of the labyrinth • Association with early postoperative headache • Potentially longer recovery
Middle cranial fossa	• The approach is primarily extradural • Hearing preservation is possible • Early exposure of the lateral IAC with relatively low risk to the inner ear	• Limited exposure of the CPA and brainstem • Limited exposure of the inferior compartment of the fundus • Unfavorable position of the facial nerve relative to the tumor • Temporal lobe retraction is required

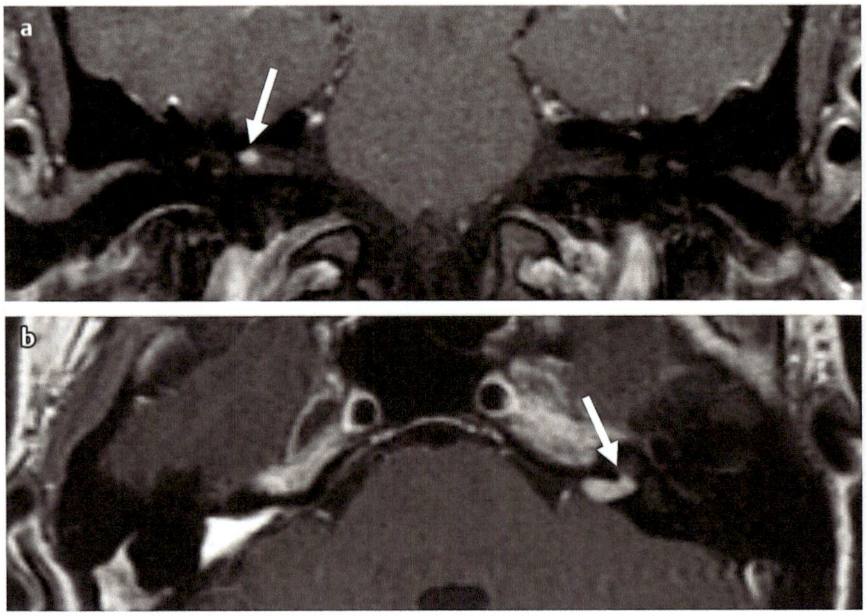

Fig. 31.5 The realistic probability of hearing preservation varies significantly according to tumor location. **(a)** Coronal contrast-enhanced T1-weighted MRI showing a small superior vestibular nerve tumor. In our experience, there is a greater than 80% chance of successfully maintaining preoperative hearing levels with the middle fossa approach. **(b)** Axial contrast-enhanced T1-weighted MRI showing a left-sided intracanalicular tumor that impacts the fundus. In our experience, this tumor is difficult to fully remove with hearing preservation regardless of surgical approach used.

an IAC tumor located at the fundus would be approached by the MF approach but that same tumor at the porus would most often be removed through the RS approach. A tumor that deeply impacts the fundus and modiolus may be very challenging to save functional hearing regardless of approach (▶ Fig. 31.5). For a large tumor that has its greatest dimension parallel to the petrous bone and anterior to the axis of the IAC, we would favor an RS approach (▶ Fig. 31.6). In contrast, the same sized tumor that is deeply indenting the brainstem is more favorably approached through the TL corridor. If there is evidence of tumor extension into the labyrinth, the TL or transotic approach provides the best access (▶ Fig. 31.7). Also, if there is the potential for needing to place an interposition graft, perform a hypoglossal-facial anastomosis, or insert a cochlear implant, the TL approach provides all the needed flexibility.

31.3 Anatomic Factors

Specific patient anatomy should influence the choice of surgical approach. The venous drainage system should always be inspected on preoperative magnetic resonance imaging (MRI) scans. There is a higher risk of injuring the sigmoid sinus and jugular bulb with the TL approach. If the patient has a highly dominant or solitary transverse sigmoid sinus system, then we are more likely to consider the RS approach (▶ Fig. 31.8, ▶ Fig. 31.9).

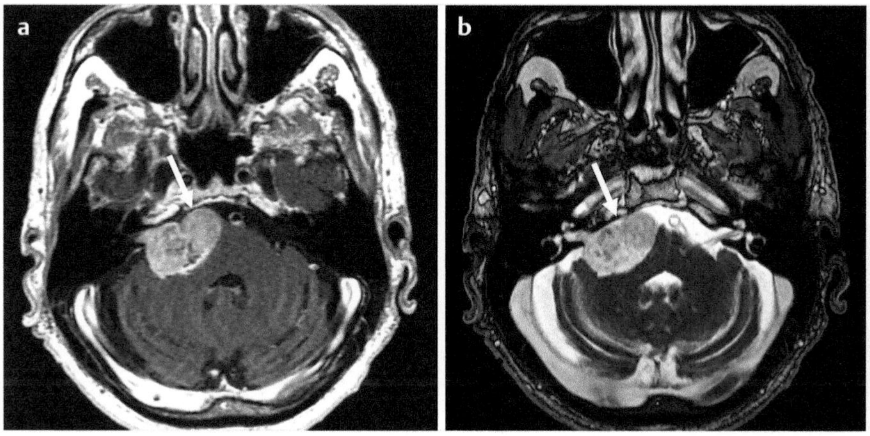

Fig. 31.6 **(a)** Axial postcontrast T1-weighted and **(b)** axial T2-weighted MRI demonstrating a large right-sided tumor. The ventral extension of this tumor anterior to the axis of the IAC (*white arrows*) makes access through the translabyrinthine approach more difficult. Unless IAC drilling is carried very far into the petrous apex, the tumor will extend around the corner and not be visible. This is particularly problematic because the facial nerve is also likely to be running over the ventral surface. The RS approach is more favorable for this tumor, although there is still a long reach as the tumor extends essentially to the clivus.

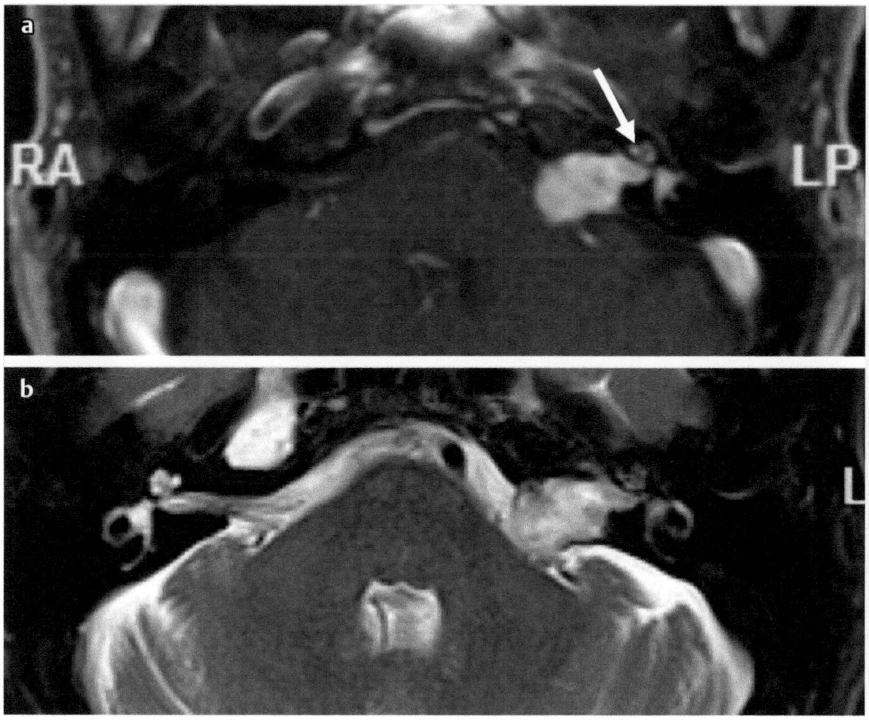

Fig. 31.7 **(a)** Axial postcontrast T1-weigthed and **(b)** axial T2-weighted MRI demonstrating a left-sided VS with involvement of the cochlea, vestibule, and semicircular canals (*white arrow*). A transotic approach allows simultaneous direct access to tumor within the inner ear, IAC, and CPA.

A "high" jugular bulb is often cited as a reason to choose the RS approach but this decision is more nuanced. We have seen the jugular bulb extend superior to the IAC, making exposure of the IAC tumor impossible without decompressing this part of the venous system and compressing the bulb inferiorly (▶ Fig. 31.10)—a very difficult task working through the RS craniotomy. In these cases of unusual venous anatomy, it is easier and safer to work through the mastoid (▶ Fig. 31.11).

A very sclerotic mastoid with an anteriorly displaced sigmoid sinus makes the TL approach more difficult and thus the RS relatively more favored (▶ Fig. 31.12, ▶ Fig. 31.13). Patients with chronic ear disease, tympanic membrane perforation, or potential to develop cholesteatoma are usually best approached by avoiding the potentially infected or diseased mastoid and middle ear. Thus, in these cases we favor the RS or MF approach. In the unusual case were the TL is still preferred, subtotal petrosectomy with ear canal closure may be used to first address any concomitant ear disease.

Prior surgical history may be a significant factor in selecting surgical approach. For recurrent tumors, we tend to favor utilizing a different approach from the original surgery.[2] This allows the initial dissection to proceed through previously untouched surgical planes, thereby avoiding scar tissue or inadvertent injury of decompressed structures. Hearing preservation is rarely a consideration when approaching a recurrent tumor; therefore, we typically use the RS or TL approach. A patient with an open mastoid cavity may be better approached through an RS craniotomy to decrease risk of infection and simplify the surgery. There are many other surgeries or procedures patients may have undergone that could impact the general advantages and disadvantages of each approach and must therefore be factored in to the final selection.

While not commonly discussed, body habitus may influence decision making regarding approach selection. A morbidly obese patient with a short neck can make the RS approach highly unpleasant. We perform most RS cases with the patient in a lateral decubitus position, which is less safe than a supine position for very large individuals. The TL approach may also be difficult but the shoulder can more easily be accommodated and in the worst cases the ear canal can be oversewn for more access. The MF approach, with the surgeon at the head of the bed, also reduces the impact of body habitus, assuming neck mobility is adequate for head rotation.

31.4 Patient Factors

Hearing status and one's desire to preserve it is the most obvious and initial patient factor to consider. If hearing preservation is considered feasible, then the TL approach is not used. As mentioned previously, the specific tumor location in the IAC will lead us to either the MF or RS approach when attempting to preserve hearing. However, there is a higher risk of temporary and permanent facial nerve weakness with the MF approach as expanded upon later in the chapter. Depending on the patient's wishes and their priority placed on facial nerve function, we may use the RS approach in the setting of a tumor at the fundus that we would typically prefer to remove through the MF approach. It may even be reasonable to sacrifice excellent hearing to maximize the chances of having normal facial nerve function in select cases. For example, some patients have felt that their careers depend on an attractive aesthetic appearance and normal facial nerve function—trial lawyers and TV personalities have been a few that we have encountered. Based on past experience, we are confident that we will achieve normal facial nerve function in over 95% of cases when the tumor is restricted to the IAC and removed through the TL approach. For us, the MF approach is less predictable (▶ Fig. 31.14).

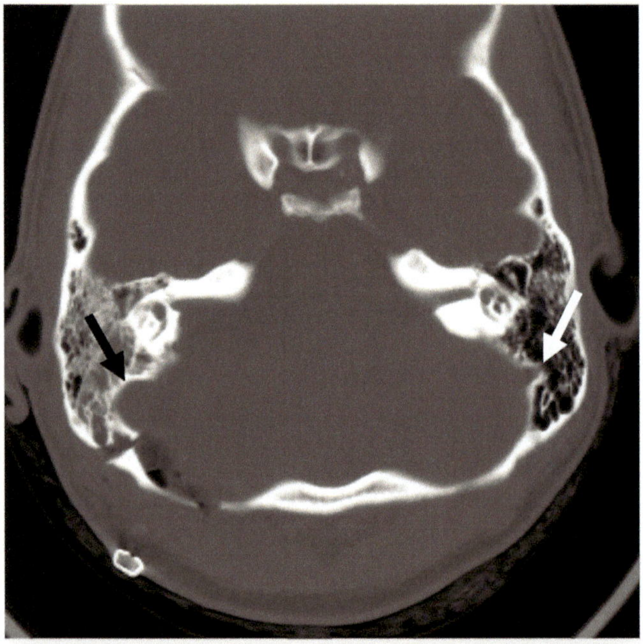

Fig. 31.8 Postoperative axial CT following a retrosigmoid approach for resection of a 3-cm right-sided VS. It was recognized preoperatively that the patient had a very underdeveloped contralateral transverse-sigmoid sinus venous system. In this case, a retrosigmoid approach was chosen to limit the risk of sigmoid sinus injury and thrombosis. Also note the variability in labyrinth position. In this case, the entire IAC could be directly accessed without violating the posterior semicircular canal or vestibule.

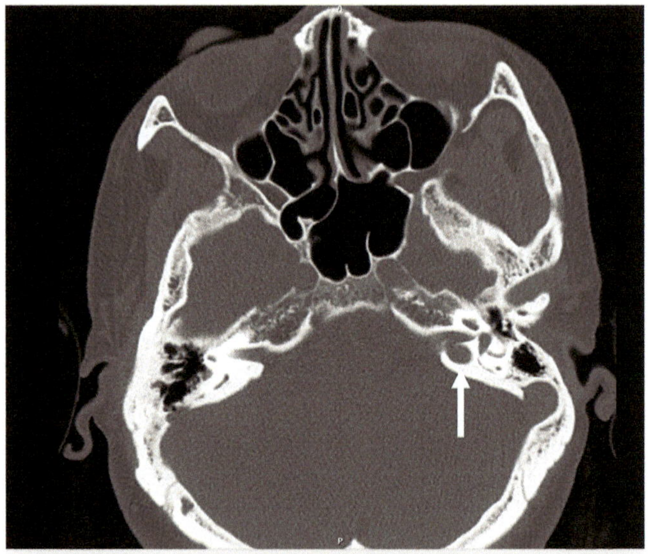

Fig. 31.10 Axial CT of the skull base demonstrating a very high-riding jugular bulb that is dehiscent with the left IAC (*white arrow*). In this case, access to the IAC is challenging regardless of approach.

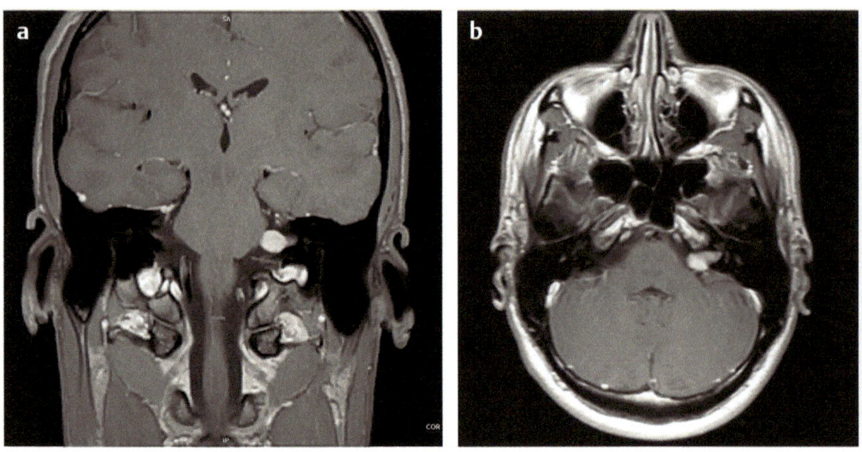

Fig. 31.9 **(a)** Coronal and **(b)** axial postcontrast T1-weighted MRI demonstrating a small left-sided VS. In this case, a well-developed mastoid with a small sigmoid sinus illustrates that a translabyrinthine approach would be the most direct and shortest route to the tumor.

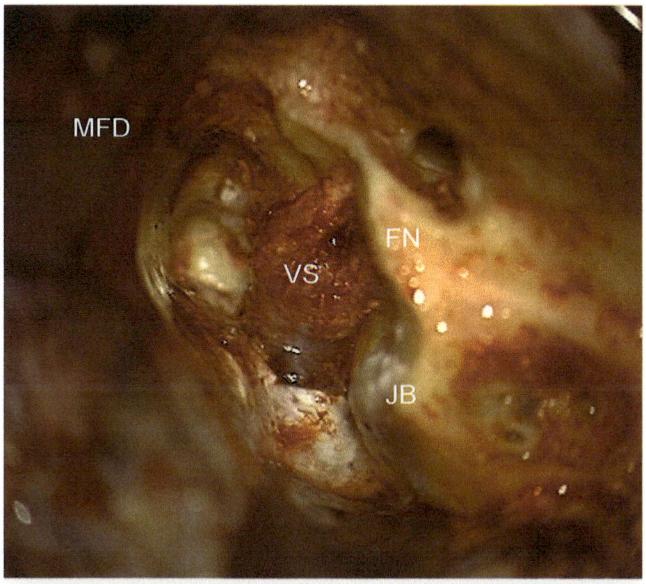

Fig. 31.11 Right translabyrinthine approach to a small tumor. Despite a large jugular bulb extending up to the inferior aspect of the IAC, there is still excellent exposure and access to the tumor without decompression and displacement of the jugular bulb inferiorly. FN, mastoid segment of the facial nerve; JB, high-riding jugular bulb; MFD, middle fossa dura; VS, vestibular schwannoma.

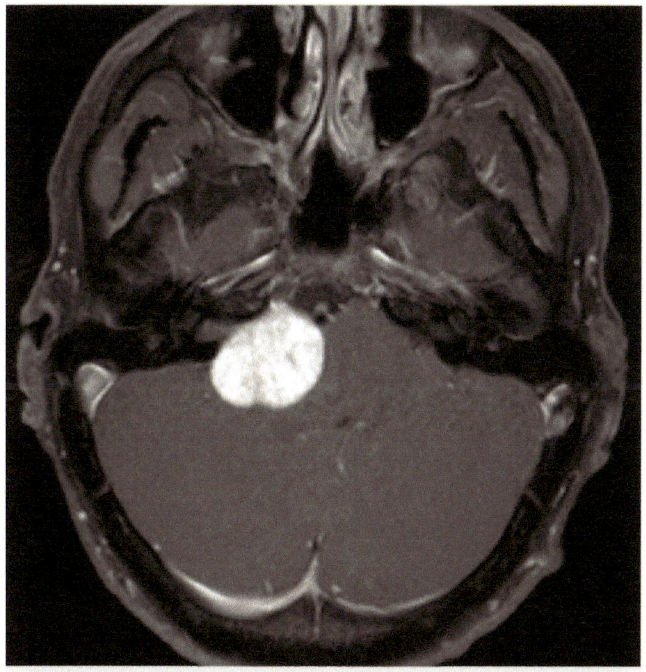

Fig. 31.12 Contrast-enhanced axial T1-weighted MRI demonstrating a right-sided medium-sized VS. Note the anteriorly displaced sigmoid sinus with a diminutive mastoid. In this case, translabyrinthine access to the tumor is more challenging and time consuming compared to the RS approach.

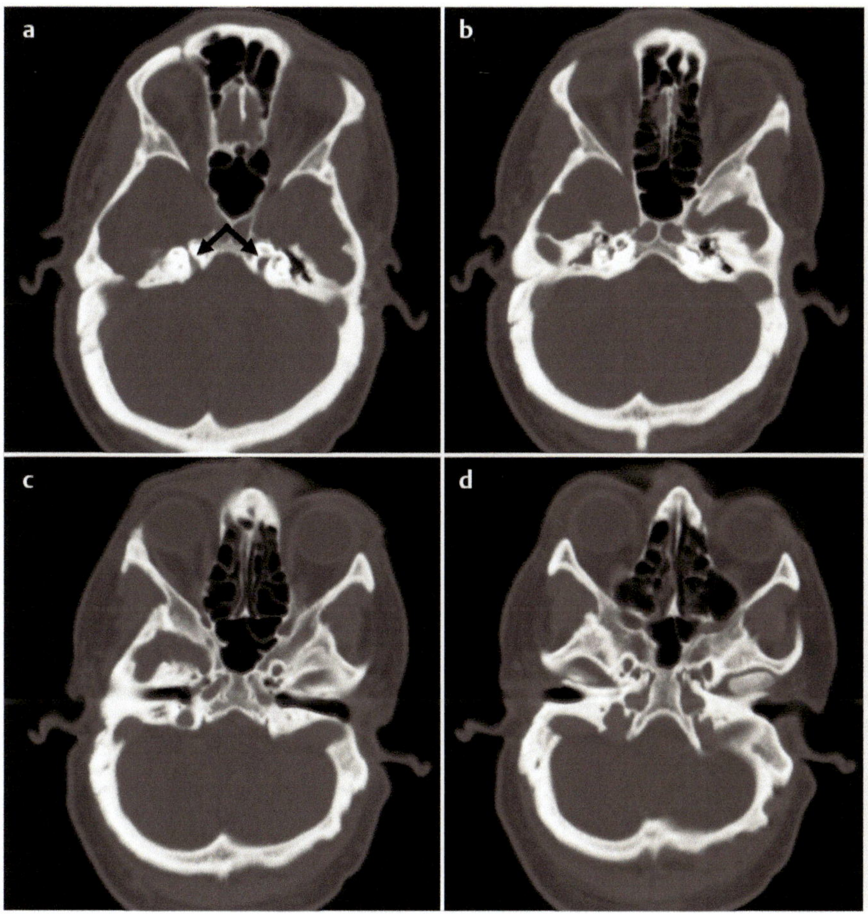

Fig. 31.13 Sequential (superior to inferior) axial CT images of the skull base demonstrating an extreme example of a sclerotic mastoid with an anteriorly located sigmoid sinus. Clearly access to the posterior fossa is best achieved through the RS approach. Note the atypical orientation of the IAC, running in an anteroposterior direction, making any approach less predictable and more complicated.

For a patient with a history of chronic headaches or migraines, we commonly prefer the TL approach when hearing preservation is not a major consideration. Although the risk of long-term headaches appears to be similar regardless of treatment approach, in our experience, patients with a headache history have more trouble in the first 3 to 6 months following RS surgery.[3]

Preoperative dizziness or the concern for postoperative dizziness is commonly cited as a reason to perform the TL approach. However, the notion that one particular approach is better than another is not strongly supported by the literature, and thus is not a factor we consider.[4,5]

The MF approach requires extradural retraction of the temporal lobe. While patients generally tolerate this quite well, we commonly avoid this approach in patients older than 65 years or in patients with a known seizure disorder. While many cite retraction of the cerebellum as a disadvantage of the RS, this does not appear to have a long-term influence on patient outcome regardless of age.[4]

There is no question that every patient wants to spend as little time as possible in the hospital and the recovery process, but this may be even more important for some. As a whole, patients undergoing TL tumor removal recover faster than the RS cohort. They tend to have less headache, neck pain, and fatigue. If there is a low likelihood of preserving hearing, it may be reasonable to forgo trying and use the TL approach with the primary goal being a quicker recovery.[6]

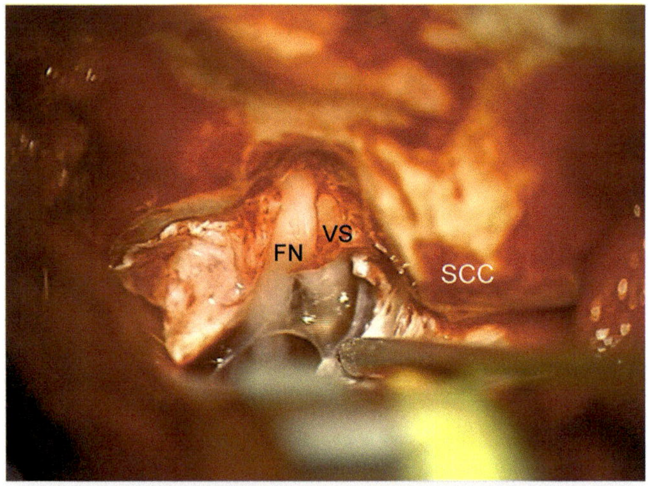

Fig. 31.14 Middle fossa approach to a small right-sided tumor illustrating the unfavorable location the facial nerve coursing over the superior aspect of the tumor. FN, facial nerve; SCC, superior semicircular canal; VS, vestibular schwannoma.

31.4.1 Facial Nerve Function: A Comparison of Approaches

While most of our decision making regarding approach selection is based on personal experience, it is often helpful to evaluate one's approach and results against the published literature and the experiences of others. It may be that altering one particular technique will change one's outcomes enough to justify shifting the balance between one approach and another. For example, a team may traditionally avoid the RS approach because of headache risk; however, modifying the incision and meticulous removal of bone particles can reduce the risk of significant headache, thereby altering the balance of pros and cons to the approach. Below we review facial nerve function outcomes based on surgical approach.

One issue that is frequently discussed in the analysis of facial preservation during vestibular schwannoma (VS) surgery is the potentially higher risk to the facial nerve with the MF approach. Considering the anatomy of the IAC, in which the facial nerve is often located superiorly, dissection from the perspective of the MF will generally necessitate working around the nerve (▶ Fig. 31.14). Conversely, dissecting the IAC from a posterior vantage, via either the TL or RS approach, generally allows the surgeon to remove the tumor without mobilizing or working around the facial nerve.[7] Though many studies suggest that long-term facial nerve outcomes are equivalent using the MF approach despite higher rates of immediate postoperative weakness (▶ Table 31.2), meta-analyses on this subject have supported the notion that the facial nerve is more vulnerable through MF exposure. Ansari et al's work from 2012 demonstrated that MF tumor excision for purely intracanalicular tumors had poorer facial function relative to the RS approach for similar sized tumors. Further, those tumors < 1.5 cm in the CPA had poorer outcomes with the MF approach relative to the TL approach. For VS > 1.5 cm in the CPA, the RS approach was superior in terms of preserving facial function.[8] Other work has found outcomes between the RS and TL approaches to be comparable.[9]

Meta-analyses of facial function preservation in VS surgery have generally reinforced the concepts that tumor size and surgeon experience are primary determinants of success. In 2004, Mangham compared the RS and MF approaches, demonstrating the former yielded significantly better facial nerve outcomes than what was seen with the MF approach. However, it was also noted that surgeon experience is at least as important as inherent differences between approaches, with certain centers achieving better facial nerve outcomes after microsurgery in general.[24]

31.4.2 Hearing Preservation: A Comparison of Approaches

Similar to facial nerve function, a variety of publications have evaluated the rates of hearing preservation between the MF and RS approaches (▶ Table 31.3). In 2012, Ansari et al reviewed data from 5,064 previously reported patients, concluding that the MF approach is superior to the RS approach for tumors extending < 1.5 cm in the CPA.[8] Beyond that size, however, results were not statistically different. Sughrue et al found the MF approach to be superior for hearing preservation even when tumor size was controlled for.[25] Noudel et al, however, found no significant difference between the approaches when only intracanalicular tumors were considered.[26] A more recent publication by Ahsan et al, reviewing publications on hearing preservation between 1980 and 2014, suggested that a hearing preservation meta-analysis cannot be feasibly performed on the basis of approach due to incompleteness of available data in previously published studies.[27]

Table 31.2 A comparison of facial nerve outcomes according to surgical approach from selected primary literature

Authors	Year	Study design	TL	RS	MF	Notes, statistical significance
Arriaga and Chen[10]	2001	*RR*	90% HB I–II	100% HB I–II	89% HB I–II	Only tumors < 1.5 cm were analyzed, no significant differences noted at last follow-up
Mamikoglu et al[11]	2001	*RR*	68% HB I–II	59% HB I–II	n/a	Only tumors between 2 and 3 cm were analyzed, no significant differences noted at last follow-up
Colletti and Fiorino[12]	2003	*PCS*	n/a	92% HB I–II	80% HB I–II	Only intracanalicular tumors < 12 mm were analyzed, no significant difference noted at last follow-up
Ho et al[13]	2003	*RR*	89% HB I–II (tumors < 1.5 cm), 81% (tumors > 1.5 cm)	89% HB I–II (tumors < 1.5 cm), 63% (tumors > 1.5 cm)	n/a	Patient age, tumor size, and date of operation were matched. No significant differences were seen for patients achieving at least HB III (calculations were not done for HB I–II).
Oghalai et al[14]	2003	*RR*	87% HB I–II	95% HB I–II	93% HB I–II	Statistical comparison not performed between approaches
Darrouzet et al[15]	2004	*RR*	34% HB I only	36% HB I only	n/a	Statistical comparison not performed between approaches
Isaacson et al[16]	2005	*RR*	93% HB I–II	n/a	92% HB I–II	Only tumors between 1 and 1.8 cm were analyzed, no significant difference noted at last follow-up
Jacob et al[17]	2007	*RR*	88% HB I–III	96% HB I–III	94% HB I–III	Statistical comparison not performed between approaches
Hillman et al[18]	2010	*RR*	n/a	90% HB I–II	88% HB I–II	HB I was more common with RS, though no significant difference in terms of achieving HB I–II at last follow-up
Sameshima et al[19]	2010	*RR*	n/a	100% HB I–II	100% HB I–II	Only tumors < 1.5 cm were analyzed, no significant differences noted at last follow-up. RS surgical time was faster
Falcioni et al[20]	2011	*RR*	86% HB I–II	96% HB I–II	68% HB I–II	MF had significantly poorer outcomes when analyzing tumors less than 1 cm
Rinaldi et al[21]	2012	*RR*	61% HB I–II	83% HB I–II	n/a	Between RS and TL, there was no significant difference at last follow-up when controlling for tumor size
Seo et al[22]	2013	*RR*	92% HB I–II	100% HB I–II	n/a	Only tumors < 2 cm were analyzed, no significant differences noted at last follow-up
Wilkinson et al[23]	2016	*RR*	n/a	100% HB I–II	97% HB I–II	HB I was more common with RS, though no significant difference in terms of achieving HB I–II at last follow-up

Abbreviations: HB, House–Brackmann; MF, middle cranial fossa; PCS, prospective cohort study; RR, retrospective review; RS, retrosigmoid; TL, translabyrinthine.

31.4.3 Cerebrospinal Fluid Leak: A Comparison of Approaches

No approach has consistently been found to be superior in terms of cerebrospinal fluid (CSF) leak risk (▶ Table 31.4). In 2004, Selesnick et al performed a meta-analysis on CSF leak rates following VS surgery.[33] CSF leaks were seen in 10.6% of RS operations (N = 2,273), 9.5% of TL surgeries (N = 3,118), and 10.6% of MF cases (N = 573). No significant difference was seen between these percentages. Ansari et al identified significantly higher rates of CSF leak after RS surgery,[8] while Sughrue et al found significantly higher rates after TL surgery.[34]

31.5 Fully Endoscopic and Endoscope-Assisted Approaches

The application of the endoscope to posterior fossa surgery may ultimately prove to be a valuable adjunct to microsurgical resection. Reports of fully endoscopic and endoscopic-assisted techniques for VS surgery are emerging, but superiority over existing microscopic techniques is not widely accepted (Chapter 40). While the microscope provides the visualization necessary for complete tumor resection in most cases, it is possible that future work could demonstrate the utility of a high-definition view from an endoscope when attempting to see structures out

Table 31.3 A comparison of hearing preservation outcomes according to surgical approach from selected primary literature

Authors	Year	Study design	RS	MF	Notes, statistical significance
Staecker et al[28]	2000	*RR*	47% maintained A–B	62% maintained A–B	Average preoperative and postoperative WRS and PTA were better in the MF patients, though no significant difference was seen in the probability of maintaining class A–B
Holsinger et al[29]	2000	*RR*	33% maintained A–B	69% maintained A–B	The mean tumor diameter was larger with RS approaches (15 vs. 9 mm); statistical comparison was not performed between approaches
Colletti and Fiorino[12]	2003	*PCS*	30% maintained A–B	33% maintained A–B	No significant difference was seen at the last reported follow-up
Oghalai et al[14]	2003	*RR*	19% maintained A–B	41% maintained A–B	Statistical comparison was not performed between approaches
Sanna et al[30]	2004	*RR*	30% maintained A–B	32% maintained A–B	Statistical comparison was not performed between approaches
Jacob et al[17]	2007	*RR*	42% maintained A–B	59% maintained A–B	Statistical comparison was not performed between approaches
Hillman et al[18]	2010	*RR*	39% maintained A–B	59% maintained A–B	No significant difference was found in maintenance of A–B, though middle fossa was more likely to preserve preoperative class A
Sameshima et al[19]	2010	*RR*	73% maintained A–B	77% maintained A–B	All tumors were less than 1.5 cm; no significant difference was seen at the last reported follow-up. RS surgical time was faster
Phillips et al[31]	2010	*RR*	49% maintained A–B	71% maintained A–B	No significant difference was seen at the last reported follow-up

Abbreviations: A–B, American Academy of Otolaryngology Class A or B hearing[32]; MF, middle cranial fossa; PCS, prospective cohort study; PTA, pure tone average; RR, retrospective review; RS, retrosigmoid; TL, translabyrinthine; WRS, word recognition score.

Table 31.4 A comparison of CSF leak outcomes according to surgical approach from selected primary literature

Authors	Study design	Year	TL	RS	MF	Notes, statistical significance
Brennan et al[35]	*RR*	2001	10%	8%	n/a	No significant difference was seen at the last reported follow-up
Leonetti et al[36]	*RR*	2001	8%	15%	0%	Data include all tumors removed by authors (not just VS); statistical comparison was not performed between approaches; MF not discussed due to small number of cases ($n=3$)
Slattery et al[37]	*RR*	2001	11%	15%	5%	Statistical comparison was not performed between approaches
Becker et al[38]	*RR*	2003	13%	10%	10%	No significant difference was seen at the last reported follow-up
Oghalai et al[14]	*RR*	2003	14%	16%	11%	Statistical comparison was not performed between approaches
Fishman et al[39]	*RR*	2004	5%	8%	8%	Statistical comparison was not performed between approaches
Sanna et al[30]	*RR*	2004	2%	18%	4%	RS had statistically higher CSF leak rate
Sameshima et al[19]	*RR*	2010	n/a	5%	5%	No significant difference was seen at the last reported follow-up; RS surgical time was faster
Mangus et al[40]	*RR*	2011	12%	12%	13%	No significant difference was seen at the last reported follow-up, though a significantly greater incidence of CSF leak was seen when multiple approaches were used
Copeland et al[41]	*RR*	2015	15%	7%	6%	TL approach had a statistically higher incidence of CSF leak

Abbreviations: CSF, cerebrospinal fluid; MF, middle cranial fossa; RR, retrospective review; RS, retrosigmoid; TL, translabyrinthine.

of a direct line-of-sight or when attempting to exploit an otherwise obscure plane of dissection between two structures.

Presently, reports of endoscopic transcanal transpromontorial approaches to the IAC and CPA are appearing in the VS literature (Chapter 39). As the number of tumors addressed in this fashion has grown, comparisons have been made between the endoscopic approach and traditional approaches.[42,43,44,45,46] Additionally, endoscopic-assisted approaches are even being proposed for tumors as large as 3 cm.[47] Over time, the indications and validity of these approaches will continue to be assessed, allowing for further comparisons between traditional approaches in terms of facial function, hearing preservation, and CSF leak risk in addition to other patient-reported outcome measures such as pain, headache, dizziness, and quality of life.

31.6 Conclusion

There are intrinsic differences in the three main surgical approaches used for VS resection. In general, the most suitable approach depends on tumor characteristics, anatomic factors, patient factors, and surgical team experience.

References

[1] Carlson ML, Link MJ, Wanna GB, Driscoll CL. Management of sporadic vestibular schwannoma. Otolaryngol Clin North Am. 2015; 48(3):407–422

[2] Perry A, Graffeo CS, Copeland WR, III, et al. Microsurgery for recurrent vestibular schwannoma after previous gross total resection. Otol Neurotol. 2017; 38(6):882–888

[3] Carlson ML, Tveiten OV, Driscoll CL, et al. Risk factors and analysis of long-term headache in sporadic vestibular schwannoma: a multicenter cross-sectional study. J Neurosurg. 2015; 123(5):1276–1286

[4] Kim HH, Johnston R, Wiet RJ, Kumar A. Long-term effects of cerebellar retraction in the microsurgical resection of vestibular schwannomas. Laryngoscope. 2004; 114(2):323–326

[5] Carlson ML, Tveiten ØV, Driscoll CL, et al. Long-term dizziness handicap in patients with vestibular schwannoma: a multicenter cross-sectional study. Otolaryngol Head Neck Surg. 2014; 151(6):1028–1037

[6] Carlson ML, Van Gompel JJ, Wiet RM, et al. A cross-sectional survey of the North American Skull Base Society: current practice patterns of vestibular schwannoma evaluation and management in North America. J Neurol Surg B Skull Base. 2018; 79(3):289–296

[7] Nejo T, Kohno M, Nagata O, Sora S, Sato H. Dorsal displacement of the facial nerve in acoustic neuroma surgery: clinical features and surgical outcomes of 21 consecutive dorsal pattern cases. Neurosurg Rev. 2016; 39(2):277–288, discussion 288

[8] Ansari SF, Terry C, Cohen-Gadol AA. Surgery for vestibular schwannomas: a systematic review of complications by approach. Neurosurg Focus. 2012; 33 (3):E14

[9] Gurgel RK, Dogru S, Amdur RL, Monfared A. Facial nerve outcomes after surgery for large vestibular schwannomas: do surgical approach and extent of resection matter? Neurosurg Focus. 2012; 33(3):E16

[10] Arriaga MA, Chen DA. Facial function in hearing preservation acoustic neuroma surgery. Arch Otolaryngol Head Neck Surg. 2001; 127(5):543–546

[11] Mamikoglu B, Esquivel C, Wiet RJ. Facial nerve functions at hospital discharge after acoustic neuroma surgery. Arch Otolaryngol Head Neck Surg. 2001; 127 (12):1518–1519

[12] Colletti V, Fiorino F. Middle fossa versus retrosigmoid-transmeatal approach in vestibular schwannoma surgery: a prospective study. Otol Neurotol. 2003; 24(6):927–934

[13] Ho SY, Hudgens S, Wiet RJ. Comparison of postoperative facial nerve outcomes between translabyrinthine and retrosigmoid approaches in matched-pair patients. Laryngoscope. 2003; 113(11):2014–2020

[14] Oghalai JS, Buxbaum JL, Pitts LH, Jackler RK. The effect of age on acoustic neuroma surgery outcomes. Otol Neurotol. 2003; 24(3):473–477

[15] Darrouzet V, Martel J, Enée V, Bébéar JP, Guérin J. Vestibular schwannoma surgery outcomes: our multidisciplinary experience in 400 cases over 17 years. Laryngoscope. 2004; 114(4):681–688

[16] Isaacson B, Telian SA, El-Kashlan HK. Facial nerve outcomes in middle cranial fossa vs translabyrinthine approaches. Otolaryngol Head Neck Surg. 2005; 133(6):906–910

[17] Jacob A, Robinson LL, Jr, Bortman JS, Yu L, Dodson EE, Welling DB. Nerve of origin, tumor size, hearing preservation, and facial nerve outcomes in 359 vestibular schwannoma resections at a tertiary care academic center. Laryngoscope. 2007; 117(12):2087–2092

[18] Hillman T, Chen DA, Arriaga MA, Quigley M. Facial nerve function and hearing preservation acoustic tumor surgery: does the approach matter? Otolaryngol Head Neck Surg. 2010; 142(1):115–119

[19] Sameshima T, Fukushima T, McElveen JT, Jr, Friedman AH. Critical assessment of operative approaches for hearing preservation in small acoustic neuroma surgery: retrosigmoid vs middle fossa approach. Neurosurgery. 2010; 67(3): 640–644, discussion 644–645

[20] Falcioni M, Fois P, Taibah A, Sanna M. Facial nerve function after vestibular schwannoma surgery. J Neurosurg. 2011; 115(4):820–826

[21] Rinaldi V, Casale M, Bressi F, et al. Facial nerve outcome after vestibular schwannoma surgery: our experience. J Neurol Surg B Skull Base. 2012; 73 (1):21–27

[22] Seo JH, Jun BC, Jeon EJ, Chang KH. Predictive factors influencing facial nerve outcomes in surgery for small-sized vestibular schwannoma. Acta Otolaryngol. 2013; 133(7):722–727

[23] Wilkinson EP, Roberts DS, Cassis A, Schwartz MS. Hearing outcomes after middle fossa or retrosigmoid craniotomy for vestibular schwannoma tumors. J Neurol Surg B Skull Base. 2016; 77(4):333–340

[24] Mangham CA, Jr. Retrosigmoid versus middle fossa surgery for small vestibular schwannomas. Laryngoscope. 2004; 114(8):1455–1461

[25] Sughrue ME, Yang I, Aranda D, Kane AJ, Parsa AT. Hearing preservation rates after microsurgical resection of vestibular schwannoma. J Clin Neurosci. 2010; 17(9):1126–1129

[26] Noudel R, Gomis P, Duntze J, Marnet D, Bazin A, Roche PH. Hearing preservation and facial nerve function after microsurgery for intracanalicular vestibular schwannomas: comparison of middle fossa and retrosigmoid approaches. Acta Neurochir (Wien). 2009; 151(8):935–944, discussion 944–945

[27] Ahsan SF, Huq F, Seidman M, Taylor A. Long-term hearing preservation after resection of vestibular schwannoma: a systematic review and meta-analysis. Otol Neurotol. 2017; 38(10):1505–1511

[28] Staecker H, Nadol JB, Jr, Ojeman R, Ronner S, McKenna MJ. Hearing preservation in acoustic neuroma surgery: middle fossa versus retrosigmoid approach. Am J Otol. 2000; 21(3):399–404

[29] Holsinger FC, Coker NJ, Jenkins HA. Hearing preservation in conservation surgery for vestibular schwannoma. Am J Otol. 2000; 21(5):695–700

[30] Sanna M, Khrais T, Russo A, Piccirillo E, Augurio A. Hearing preservation surgery in vestibular schwannoma: the hidden truth. Ann Otol Rhinol Laryngol. 2004; 113(2):156–163

[31] Phillips DJ, Kobylarz EJ, De Peralta ET, Stieg PE, Selesnick SH. Predictive factors of hearing preservation after surgical resection of small vestibular schwannomas. Otol Neurotol. 2010; 31(9):1463–1468

[32] Committee on Hearing and Equilibrium guidelines for the evaluation of hearing preservation in acoustic neuroma (vestibular schwannoma). American Academy of Otolaryngology-Head and Neck Surgery Foundation, INC. Otolaryngol Head Neck Surg. 1995; 113(3):179–180

[33] Selesnick SH, Liu JC, Jen A, Newman J. The incidence of cerebrospinal fluid leak after vestibular schwannoma surgery. Otol Neurotol. 2004; 25(3):387–393

[34] Sughrue ME, Yang I, Aranda D, et al. Beyond audiofacial morbidity after vestibular schwannoma surgery. J Neurosurg. 2011; 114(2):367–374

[35] Brennan JW, Rowed DW, Nedzelski JM, Chen JM. Cerebrospinal fluid leak after acoustic neuroma surgery: influence of tumor size and surgical approach on incidence and response to treatment. J Neurosurg. 2001; 94(2): 217–223

[36] Leonetti J, Anderson D, Marzo S, Moynihan G. Cerebrospinal fluid fistula after transtemporal skull base surgery. Otolaryngol Head Neck Surg. 2001; 124(5): 511–514

[37] Slattery WH, III, Francis S, House KC. Perioperative morbidity of acoustic neuroma surgery. Otol Neurotol. 2001; 22(6):895–902

[38] Becker SS, Jackler RK, Pitts LH. Cerebrospinal fluid leak after acoustic neuroma surgery: a comparison of the translabyrinthine, middle fossa, and retrosigmoid approaches. Otol Neurotol. 2003; 24(1):107–112

[39] Fishman AJ, Marrinan MS, Golfinos JG, Cohen NL, Roland JT, Jr. Prevention and management of cerebrospinal fluid leak following vestibular schwannoma surgery. Laryngoscope. 2004; 114(3):501–505

[40] Mangus BD, Rivas A, Yoo MJ, et al. Management of cerebrospinal fluid leaks after vestibular schwannoma surgery. Otol Neurotol. 2011; 32(9): 1525–1529

[41] Copeland WR, Mallory GW, Neff BA, Driscoll CL, Link MJ. Are there modifiable risk factors to prevent a cerebrospinal fluid leak following vestibular schwannoma surgery? J Neurosurg. 2015; 122(2):312–316

[42] Marchioni D, Soloperto D, Masotto B, et al. Transcanal transpromontorial acoustic neuroma surgery: results and facial nerve outcomes. Otol Neurotol. 2018; 39(2):242–249

[43] Marchioni D, Alicandri-Ciufelli M, Rubini A, Masotto B, Pavesi G, Presutti L. Exclusive endoscopic transcanal transpromontorial approach: a new perspective for internal auditory canal vestibular schwannoma treatment. J Neurosurg. 2017; 126(1):98–105

[44] Marchioni D, Carner M, Rubini A, et al. The fully endoscopic acoustic neuroma surgery. Otolaryngol Clin North Am. 2016; 49(5):1227–1236

[45] Wick CC, Arnaoutakis D, Barnett SL, Rivas A, Isaacson B. Endoscopic transcanal transpromontorial approach for vestibular schwannoma resection: a case series. Otol Neurotol. 2017; 38(10):e490–e494

[46] Alicandri-Ciufelli M, Federici G, Anschuetz L, et al. Transcanal surgery for vestibular schwannomas: a pictorial review of radiological findings, surgical anatomy and comparison to the traditional translabyrinthine approach. Eur Arch Otorhinolaryngol. 2017; 274(9):3295–3302

[47] Marchioni D, Carner M, Soloperto D, et al. Expanded transcanal transpromontorial approach: a novel surgical technique for cerebellopontine angle vestibular schwannoma removal. Otolaryngol Head Neck Surg. 2018; 158(4):710–715

32 Management of the Facial Nerve During Vestibular Schwannoma Microsurgery

Sampath Chandra Prasad, Alessandra Russo, Abdelkader Taibah, Enrico Pasanisi, Francesco Galletti, and Mario Sanna

32.1 Introduction

A progressive evolution in diagnostic testing and microsurgical techniques has made it possible to reduce the perioperative mortality rate of vestibular schwannoma (VS) microsurgery to less than 1%, especially at high-volume centers.[1,2,3,4] This, in part, has led to a shift in the surgeon's attention to the preservation of cranial nerve function, in particular that of the facial nerve (FN) and the cochlear nerve.[5,6,7,8] Due to the intimate association between the FN and VS capsule, surgery for this tumor is fraught with risk of FN injury. Although the anatomy of the FN is fairly consistent in the temporal bone and the cerebellopontine angle (CPA), the tumor itself may distort or displace the nerve, which may be neither evident by way of preoperative FN deficits nor discernible on preoperative imaging. In fact, the FN is very resistant to tumor stretch and compression, and more often than not, preoperative FN function is found preserved even in most giant VS. The surgeon must be prepared to deal with difficult situations wherein the nerve is thinned and stretched, is enveloped, or is found positioned between the surgeon and the tumor. Less commonly, there are intraoperative situations that may lead to interruption of FN continuity, either intentionally or otherwise. Once a nerve is interrupted, reconstruction should be performed immediately in order to obtain the best results, either by means of a primary end-to-end coaptation or by a cable nerve graft interposition.[9] In this chapter, we will discuss various pre- and intraoperative situations with regard to the FN and how to manage them.

32.2 Clinical Onset of Facial Nerve Paralysis

As discussed previously, the FN can withstand stretching imposed by tumor growth to a great deal and hence leave the patient without clinically apparent deterioration of function. The FN, as most motor nerves, is quite resistant to tumor infiltration and nerve dysfunction typically occurs very late in the course of tumor growth. Axon and Ramsden[10] found that House–Brackmann grade I FN function can be maintained with only 10% of motor neurons functioning. Neuronal degeneration and axonal demyelination is counterbalanced with the collateral sprouting and hypertrophy of the innervated muscle fibers. Furthermore, the absence of epineurium around the CPA and internal auditory canal (IAC) segments of the FN allows effacement of the nerve fibers and spreading of the nerve fascicles over large tumors.[10,11] In slow-growing pathologies such as VS and meningiomas, FN fibers are stretched slowly over many months leading to splaying of fibers over the tumor capsule (▶ Fig. 32.1).[12] Conversely, early-onset FN paralysis in cases of smaller IAC or CPA tumors should signal clinicians to a suspect FN schwannoma, cavernous hemangioma, or, much less commonly, a malignant lesion. The incidence of FN dysfunction associated with untreated VS is generally less than 10% and correlates with tumor size. FN paralysis is often preceded by facial twitch or spasm.

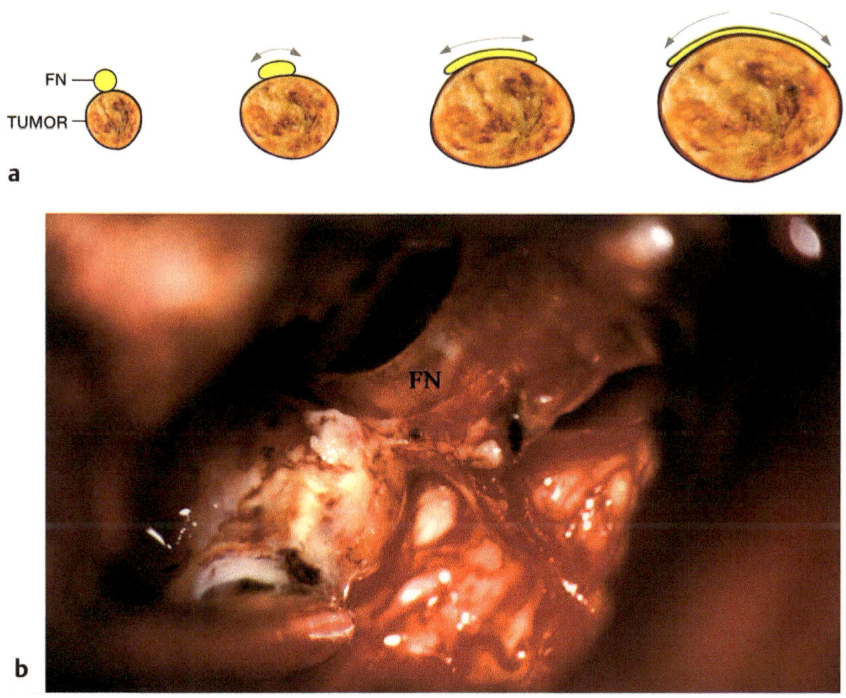

a

b

Fig. 32.1 **(a)** The FN is stretched and splayed over the tumor capsule in slow-growing tumors like VS. **(b)** Intraoperative picture of the FN after tumor removal wherein the nerve is seen to be markedly thinned and transparent.

32.3 Intraoperative Facial Nerve Monitoring

Intraoperative FN monitoring has established itself as an integral part of skull base surgery. Intraoperative electromyography (EMG) monitoring helps identify and map the FN accurately, thereby enhancing preservation. This is particularly important when tumors or anatomical variations place the nerve at a higher risk.[13] At the Gruppo Otologico, patients are routinely monitored using the Nerve Integrity Monitor (NIM-Neuro 3.0) manufactured by Medtronic Xomed (Jacksonville, FL). This is a two-channel electromyographic system used to detect FN function. The monitor displays the two channels simultaneously for detecting the activity of orbicularis oculi muscle and orbicularis oris muscle. To avoid interference and artifact, this machine is supplied with a "muting probe," which is connected around the output cable of equipment, such as bipolar cautery or other external devices that generate interfering signals. Electrical stimulation or surgical manipulation of the FN results in evoked EMG responses that provide immediate feedback to the surgeon via loudspeaker and an oscilloscope. Intraoperative FN monitoring assists with: (1) early localization of the FN, (2) definitive identification of the FN, (3) minimization of trauma during dissection, and (4) confirmation of the functional integrity of the nerve during and after tumor removal.

After tumor removal is complete, postoperative FN function can be appraised with electrical stimulation at the proximal and distal sites, usually at the root exit zone of the nerve at the brainstem and at the fundus of the IAC, respectively. The main parameters used in the evaluation of postoperative FN function are the threshold of proximal stimulation and the amplitude of the evoked response. Good function is expected when proximal stimulation between 0.05 and 0.1 mA elicits an FN response. It is important to examine the amplitude of this response and compare proximal and distal stimulation results. Amplitudes higher than 200 mV are usually indicative of good postoperative function. The presence of EMG potentials as bursts and trains during the last steps of tumor removal is another good prognostic factor. Elevation of the threshold to 0.3 mA or above is usually correlated with poor postoperative nerve function, especially if associated with low amplitude. High-amplitude bomber-type trains, especially when they arise suddenly, represent a poor prognostic factor. Finally, a "silent FN" during the last stage of tumor removal, associated with absence of response to the stimulation, is correlated with poor postoperative nerve function. Further discussion regarding intraoperative FN monitoring can be found in Chapter 27.

32.4 Preoperative Decision Making with Respect to the Facial Nerve

Though it is impossible to discuss the entire logic of preoperative decision making in this chapter, we will briefly outline our general approach and strategy. In the case of small tumors (grade I and II)[14] in patients of any age, we prefer to initially follow the tumor with a wait-and-scan approach,[15] except in a few circumstances. In the case of grade I and II tumors that have to be operated upon either due to vertigo, or evidence of fast growth on wait-and-scan, or patient preference, the choice of surgical approach will largely depend on hearing status. In cases where preoperative hearing is poor, the enlarged translabyrinthine approach (ETLA) is employed, which is the safest procedure for the FN preservation in our experience, even in larger tumors. In cases with good preoperative hearing, the retrosigmoid and middle cranial fossa approaches are preferred, with the middle fossa approach carrying a higher risk of FN paresis at least in the early postoperative period.[16,17] Surgery is the preferred choice in tumors greater than grade III. In patients older than 65 years with large tumors, if the patient is fit for surgery, we may perform sub- or near-total resection in an attempt to preserve good FN function. In older patients with debilitation or surgical contraindications, or in cases of regrowth after sub- or near-total resection, we prefer to refer for radiotherapy.[18,19]

Apart from the options discussed above, a variety of other factors including patient preference, occupation, experience of the operating team, tumor location, cerebral venous anatomy, and degree of brainstem compression are to be taken into consideration while deciding how best to treat the tumor and manage the FN.[20]

32.5 Intraoperative Decision Making with Respect to Facial Nerve

Intraoperatively, all attempts must be made to save the FN because of the physical, social, emotional, and psychological consequences of FN paralysis, especially in young patients. Whatever may be the surgical approach, care must be taken to dissect the tumor capsule from the nerve with utmost delicacy. However, even in the best hands, there will be circumstances when the FN will be injured or rarely even intentionally or unintentionally sacrificed. In the latter such cases, the nerve should be reconstructed by primary coaptation or an interposition cable graft whenever possible (Chapter 64).

32.5.1 Techniques to Improve Facial Nerve Outcomes during Surgery

A wide surgical approach improves the visual field, thereby enhancing safe and efficient tumor removal (▶ Fig. 32.2). In the ETLA, our experience indicates that the most common course of the FN in relation to the tumor capsule is in its anterior-medial-inferior surfaces, which is seen in about 70% of the cases. In about 15, 10, and 5%, the tumor displaces the nerve superiorly, inferiorly, and laterally, respectively (▶ Fig. 32.3). In VS microsurgery, the two major sites where the position of the FN is most consistent are at the fundus of the IAC (▶ Fig. 32.4) and the origin of the nerve at the level of the brainstem (▶ Fig. 32.5). The position of the FN varies at the level of the porus of the IAC, as shown in ▶ Fig. 32.3. At the porus, the nerve is generally found adherent to the surface of the tumor, and in large tumors, the FN is often splayed and thinned and hence one has to be very careful in dissecting the nerve from the tumor in this location (▶ Fig. 32.6).

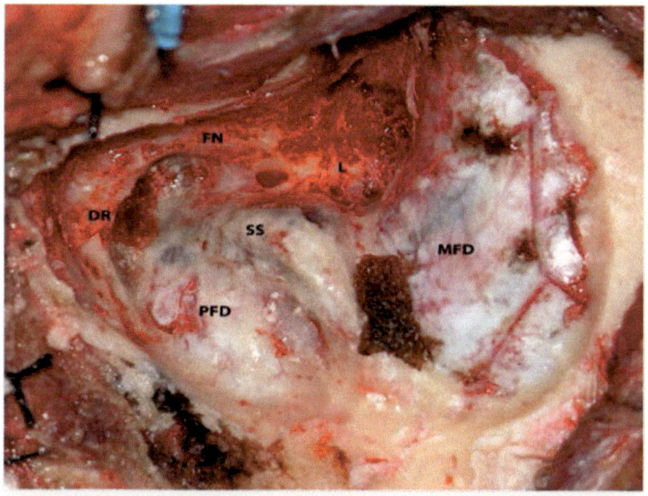

Fig. 32.2 Wide bone drilling over the middle and posterior fossa dura enlarges the visual field and allows better angles with instruments.

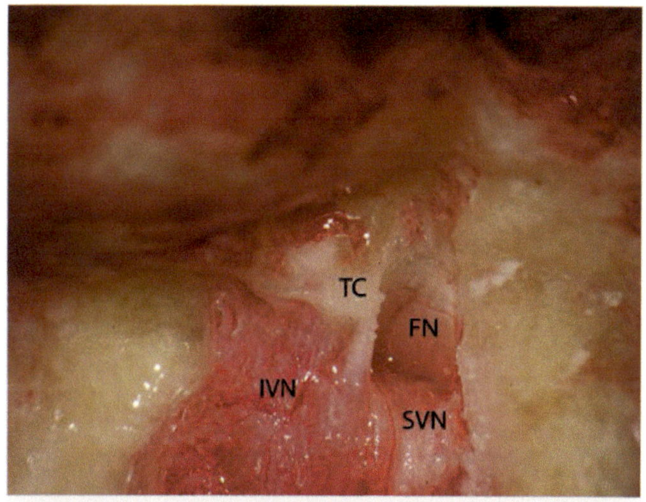

Fig. 32.4 FN in the fundus of the IAC. FN, facial nerve; IVN, inferior vestibular nerve; SVN, superior vestibular nerve; TC, transverse crest.

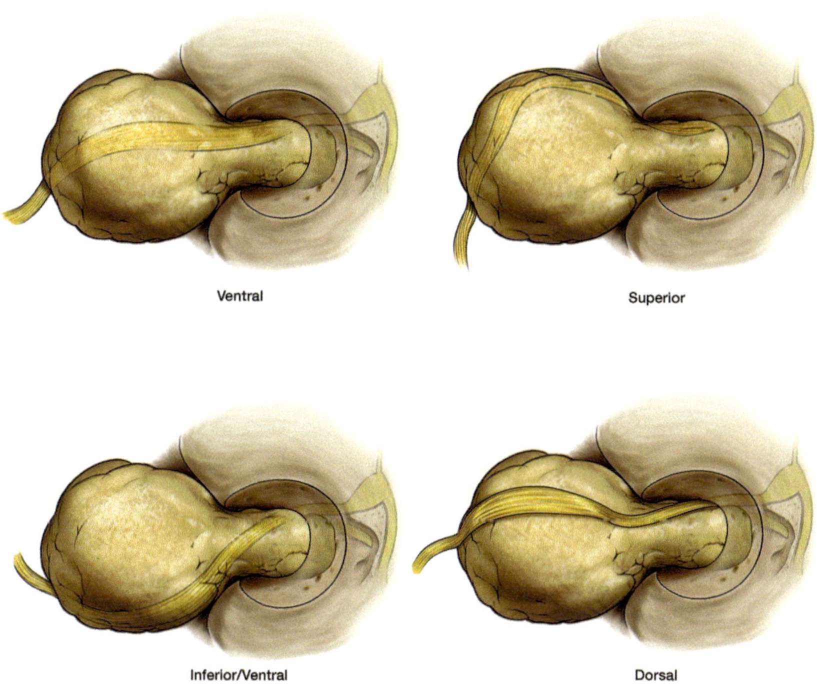

Fig. 32.3 Possible locations of the FN in relation to the tumor.

The surgeon must be able to visually identify the FN and not depend solely on intraoperative FN monitoring. In small tumors, the FN is clearly identified as a grayish glistening structure. In large tumors, however, the nerve may be difficult to identify as it is usually splayed, thinned, and translucent and cannot be differentiated from the tumor or the surrounding arachnoid. In such a situation, identification of the FN depends on tracing the nerve by strict adherence to the points of reference as described above in conjunction with use of intraoperative EMG monitoring using low intensity of stimulation (0.05 mV). Understanding the amount of expected current spread with different stimulation levels is important.

Once the nerve is identified at the level of the fundus, tumor dissection proceeds from a lateral to medial direction—or if identified at the level of the brainstem, from medial to lateral. In many cases, both techniques are used. In large tumors, dissection of the tumor from the FN should be addressed only after debulking the rest of the tumor, and traction or torsion of the tumor attached to the nerve should be avoided. A train response from EMG monitoring indicates potential trauma to the FN. When this is encountered, the inciting maneuver should be stopped or changed to avoid further damage to the nerve. One must be mindful of the fact that the train response can also be triggered by cold irrigation. Blunt dissection is performed for

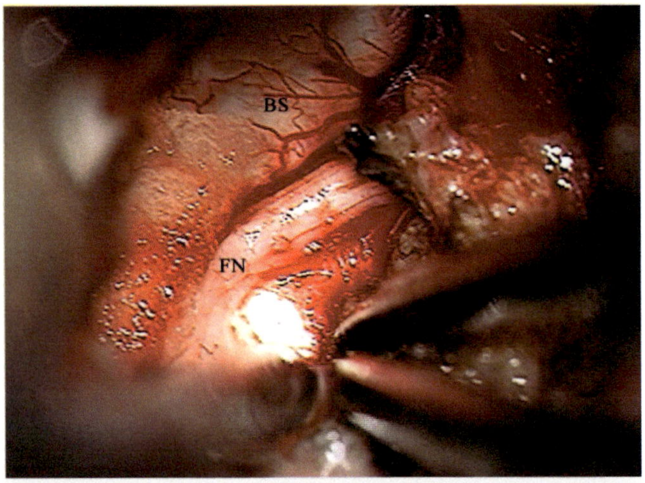

Fig. 32.5 FN at its origin from the brainstem. BS, brainstem; FN, facial nerve.

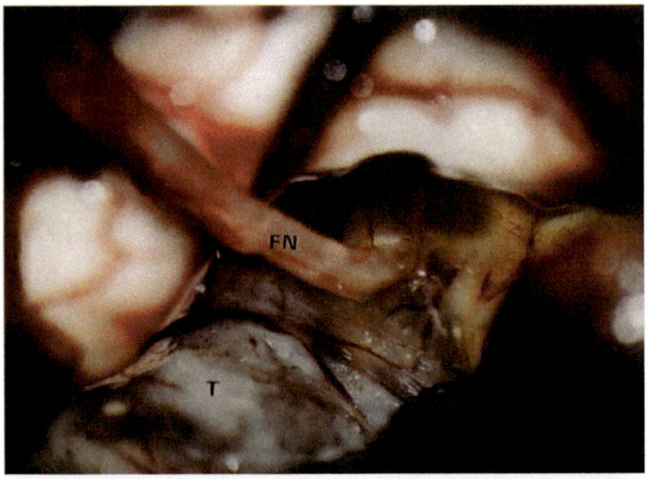

Fig. 32.6 FN at the level of the porus acusticus. FN, facial nerve; T, tumor.

most of the dissection; however, adherent attachments should be divided sharply using scissors to avoid excessive traction on the nerve. Bleeding from the FN itself is controlled by placing Gelfoam or Surgicel over the bleeding points. It cannot be overemphasized that an overall bloodless surgical field is one of the foremost factors that improves FN outcomes. Presence of blood obstructs the surgical field and also large clots may coalesce and envelope the nerves, which when suctioned could lead to inadvertent nerve injury. Precise use of fine-tip bipolar cautery on a low setting is required when near the FN, and indiscriminate cauterization should be avoided. Maintaining clean bipolar tips and use of irrigation when bipolaring can facilitate effective hemostasis while mitigating the risk of inadvertent FN injury.

In most studies, reported FN outcomes after tumor resection in cystic VS have been less favorable in comparison to results after removal of solid tumors of comparable size.[2,21,22,23,24,25,26] While our institutional series showed no statistically significant difference in FN results between solid and cystic tumors, we attribute this to our protocol of leaving behind tumor around the FN (near-total resection) if necessary in cystic tumors.[27]

32.5.2 Planned Facial Nerve Interruption

Although FN preservation is of paramount importance and every attempt should be made to maintain it, there may be instances wherein the surgeon may elect to sacrifice the FN when balancing certain priorities. These situations fall into three categories. Firstly, it may be acceptable to section the FN in difficult and emergent situations where the immediate safety of the patient takes priority, such as when there is arterial bleeding that cannot be controlled without either coagulating the nerve itself or sectioning it for access. We find these situations to be extremely rare. A second situation is the case where a patient presents with a large, multiply recurrent tumor that is associated with brainstem compression. In the rare care of a very aggressive recurrent tumor, particularly in a young patient, complete disease eradication to prevent future neurological complications may become a priority over FN preservation. In cases that have undergone prior microsurgical resection and radiation, the FN may take an unfavorable course and may be particularly adherent such that complete tumor removal with FN preservation is impossible. A third condition is the patient who presents with long-term FN paralysis, either from the tumor or from prior treatment. This must be distinguished from the case of acute FN paralysis that may often improve with steroid treatment or tumor removal.

During tumor dissection, the FN may become partially interrupted or thinned to the point that long-term viability is questioned. If the nerve can still be stimulated at a high threshold, then at least partial recovery can be expected. In some instances, although the FN appears to be anatomically intact, it will not stimulate even at high levels. In such situations, it is advisable to not sacrifice the nerve and place a graft since most patients will recover some function, with a subset regaining good function.

If the surgeon is convinced that the FN has been interrupted, immediate reconstruction should be performed to achieve the best possible result, either by means of a primary end-to-end coaptation or by a cable nerve graft interposition.[9] Cable graft interposition is a convenient and well-accepted procedure for immediate restitution of the FN. Our unpublished results, including a series of 213 patients, shows that the stitchless fibrin glue–aided anastomosis technique yields good results. This technique is discussed in detail in Chapter 64.

32.5.3 Subtotal or Near-Total Resection of Vestibular Schwannoma for Facial Nerve Preservation

The goal of surgical removal is to achieve complete tumor eradication with preservation of facial and cochlear nerve function. However, in certain instances it becomes unwise to attempt complete removal due to the tumor's intimate relationship with important structures, such as the FN, brainstem, blood vessels, and other nerves in the CPA, without compromising such structures. This is especially true in patients with large tumors, cases following failed radiation treatment, or in patients with associated severe comorbidities, where the aim of surgery may be to perform a planned sub- or near-total excision or to perform a primary debulking followed by a second-stage excision or radiosurgery. Less commonly, intraoperative vital sign changes or excessive bleeding may also force the procedure to be abandoned before total tumor excision has been achieved.

In case of involvement of the FN in particular, the dilemma that the surgeon faces is whether to preserve the nerve at the cost of leaving behind a small remnant of tumor or achieve gross total resection by sacrificing the nerve or at least putting it at high risk of long-term significant weakness. This is an important concept to discuss with the patient preoperatively. This is especially important in elderly patients and patients with comorbid conditions. The decision to leave behind tumor in an attempt to save the FN can be justified if the following two factors can be proved: (1) that the incidence and the rate of tumor regrowth is acceptably low, and (2) that there is a significant benefit in terms of postoperative preservation of FN function. Our recent article and a review of literature[28] have shown that this is indeed the case and hence there is undoubtedly merit in the concept of near-total and subtotal resection for FN preservation. When compared with subtotal resection, near-total resection has shown a lower rate of regrowth of residual tumor while having almost the same result in terms of FN function. In addition, advances in radiosurgery have provided a low-risk means of salvage if growth of the residual tumor remnant occurs. Patients with incomplete VS resection require prolonged and perhaps lifelong follow-up. Additional discussion regarding subtotal and near-total microsurgical resection can be found in Chapter 41.

32.5.4 Key Points and Summary

- The FN is resistant to stretch injury caused by slow tumor growth and, more often than not, preoperative function is normal even in patients with giant VS.
- Before surgery, the patient must be apprised of the risks of FN injury and its consequences. Full informed consent with a special emphasis on FN injury must be performed and the surgeon should clearly understand the patient's priorities.
- Intraoperative FN monitoring assists in: (1) localization of the FN, (2) definitive identification of the FN, (3) minimization of trauma during dissection, and (4) confirmation of the functional integrity of the nerve during and after tumor removal.
- The FN is frequently found adherent to the surface of the tumor at the porus acusticus, and in large tumors it is often splayed and thinned out. Therefore, one has to be particularly careful when dissecting the nerve from the tumor in this region.
- The surgeon must be able to visually identify the FN and not solely depend on intraoperative EMG monitoring.
- In cases where the nerve is transected, it should be reconstructed by a cable nerve interposition graft whenever possible.
- In certain instances, it becomes unwise to attempt complete tumor resection due to the tumor's intimate relationship with important structures, such as the FN, brainstem, blood vessels, and other nerves in the CPA. This is especially true in patients with large tumors or in those with associated severe comorbidities, where the aim of surgery may be to perform a planned sub- or near-total excision or to perform a primary debulking followed by a second-stage operation or radiation.

References

[1] Gjurić M, Wigand ME, Wolf SR. Enlarged middle fossa vestibular schwannoma surgery: experience with 735 cases. Otol Neurotol. 2001; 22(2): 223–230, discussion 230–231

[2] Samii M, Matthies C. Management of 1000 vestibular schwannomas (acoustic neuromas): surgical management and results with an emphasis on complications and how to avoid them. Neurosurgery. 1997; 40(1):11–21, discussion 21–23

[3] Sanna M, Taibah A, Russo A, Falcioni M, Agarwal M. Perioperative complications in acoustic neuroma (vestibular schwannoma) surgery. Otol Neurotol. 2004; 25(3):379–386

[4] Wiet RJ, Mamikoglu B, Odom L, Hoistad DL. Long-term results of the first 500 cases of acoustic neuroma surgery. Otolaryngol Head Neck Surg. 2001; 124 (6):645–651

[5] Brackmann DE, Cullen RD, Fisher LM. Facial nerve function after translabyrinthine vestibular schwannoma surgery. Otolaryngol Head Neck Surg. 2007; 136(5):773–777

[6] Nadol JB, Jr, Chiong CM, Ojemann RG, et al. Preservation of hearing and facial nerve function in resection of acoustic neuroma. Laryngoscope. 1992; 102 (10):1153–1158

[7] Samii M, Matthies C. Management of 1000 vestibular schwannomas (acoustic neuromas): the facial nerve–preservation and restitution of function. Neurosurgery. 1997; 40(4):684–694, discussion 694–695

[8] Sterkers JM, Morrison GA, Sterkers O, El-Dine MM. Preservation of facial, cochlear, and other nerve functions in acoustic neuroma treatment. Otolaryngol Head Neck Surg. 1994; 110(2):146–155

[9] Ozmen OA, Falcioni M, Lauda L, Sanna M. Outcomes of facial nerve grafting in 155 cases: predictive value of history and preoperative function. Otol Neurotol. 2011; 32(8):1341–1346

[10] Axon PR, Ramsden RT. Facial nerve injury caused by vestibular schwannoma compression: severity and adaptation to maintain normal clinical facial function. Am J Otol. 1999; 20(6):763–769

[11] Kartush JM, Lundy LB. Facial nerve outcome in acoustic neuroma surgery. Otolaryngol Clin North Am. 1992; 25(3):623–647

[12] Sanna M, Khrais T, Mancini F, Russo A, Taibah A. Facial nerve management in vestibular schwannoma surgery. In: The Facial Nerve in Temporal Bone and Lateral Skull Base Microsurgery. Stuttgart: Georg Thieme Verlag; 2006:149–186

[13] Sanna M, Mancini F, Russo A, Taibah A, Falcioni M, Di Trapani G. The translabyrinthine approaches. In: Atlas of Acoustic Neurinoma Microsurgery. Stuttgart: Georg Thieme Verlag; 2011:60–140

[14] Consensus meeting on systems for reporting results in acoustic neuroma. November 7–9, 2001. Tokyo, Japan. Abstracts. Keio J Med. 2001; 50 Suppl 4: 13–77

[15] Patnaik U, Prasad SC, Tutar H, Giannuzzi AL, Russo A, Sanna M. The long-term outcomes of wait-and-scan and the role of radiotherapy in the management of vestibular schwannomas. Otol Neurotol. 2015; 36(4):638–646

[16] Falcioni M, Fois P, Taibah A, Sanna M. Facial nerve function after vestibular schwannoma surgery. J Neurosurg. 2011; 115(4):820–826

[17] Rinaldi V, Casale M, Bressi F, et al. Facial nerve outcome after vestibular schwannoma surgery: our experience. J Neurol Surg B Skull Base. 2012; 73 (1):21–27

[18] Friedman WA, Bradshaw P, Myers A, Bova FJ. Linear accelerator radiosurgery for vestibular schwannomas. J Neurosurg. 2006; 105(5):657–661

[19] Sawamura Y, Shirato H, Sakamoto T, et al. Management of vestibular schwannoma by fractionated stereotactic radiotherapy and associated cerebrospinal fluid malabsorption. J Neurosurg. 2003; 99(4):685–692

[20] Goddard JC, Voelker CCJ, Brackmann DE. Facial nerve and vestibular schwannoma. In: Guntinas-Lichius O, ed. Facial Nerve Disorders and Diseases: Diagnosis and Management. Stuttgart: Georg Thieme Verlag KG; 2016:238–248

[21] Sinha S, Sharma BS. Cystic acoustic neuromas: surgical outcome in a series of 58 patients. J Clin Neurosci. 2008; 15(5):511–515

[22] Fundová P, Charabi S, Tos M, Thomsen J. Cystic vestibular schwannoma: surgical outcome. J Laryngol Otol. 2000; 114(12):935–939

[23] Benech F, Perez R, Fontanella MM, Morra B, Albera R, Ducati A. Cystic versus solid vestibular schwannomas: a series of 80 grade III-IV patients. Neurosurg Rev. 2005; 28(3):209–213

[24] Charabi S, Tos M, Børgesen SE, Thomsen J. Cystic acoustic neuromas. Results of translabyrinthine surgery. Arch Otolaryngol Head Neck Surg. 1994; 120 (12):1333–1338

[25] Moon KS, Jung S, Seo SK, et al. Cystic vestibular schwannomas: a possible role of matrix metalloproteinase-2 in cyst development and unfavorable surgical outcome. J Neurosurg. 2007; 106(5):866–871

[26] Wandong S, Meng L, Xingang L, et al. Cystic acoustic neuroma. J Clin Neurosci. 2005; 12(3):253–255

[27] Piccirillo E, Wiet MR, Flanagan S, et al. Cystic vestibular schwannoma: classification, management, and facial nerve outcomes. Otol Neurotol. 2009; 30(6):826–834

[28] Chen Z, Prasad SC, Di Lella F, et al. The behavior of residual tumors and facial nerve outcomes after incomplete excision of vestibular schwannomas. J Neurosurg. 2014; 120(6):1278–1287

33 Translabyrinthine Approach for Vestibular Schwannoma Resection

Brian S. Chen and Derald E. Brackmann

33.1 History

Descriptions of the "transtemporal approach" for vestibular schwannoma (VS) removal, which requires removal of the labyrinth for access to the cerebellopontine angle (CPA), date back to 1904 by Rudolf Panse.[1] This approach quickly fell out of favor due to the high rate of surgical mortality and the idea of spreading "dormant infections" from the unsterile mastoid air cells, "only to nibble at [the] great tumors," as described by Franciscus Quix in 1911.[2] With the introduction of the dental drill and operating microscope by William House, along with medical advances in antibiotics and anesthesia, House described his first 41 cases of VS removal through the translabyrinthine approach (TLA) in a 1964 monograph, which repopularized this approach.[3] The history of VS surgery is further expounded upon in Chapter 1.

33.2 Patient Selection

Since the reintroduction of the TLA by House, this approach has become the authors' primary approach for VS removal and is utilized in approximately 50% of our skull base cases. It is our feeling that any tumor in the internal auditory canal (IAC) and CPA, big or small, can be removed through the TLA. This approach provides the most direct route to the IAC and CPA without retraction of the cerebellum or temporal lobe by maximum bone removal—a primary tenet of skull base surgery. Furthermore, the IAC can be dissected fully in a 270-degree fashion from the porus acusticus to fundus safely without damaging the facial nerve. There are a few situations where we believe the TLA is particularly beneficial. First, we prefer any giant VS (> 3.5 cm) be removed via a TLA (▶ Fig. 33.1). Giant VSs cause brainstem and cerebellar compression, and wide exposure is required for safe dissection of these critical areas. The TLA provides direct access for tumor dissection without unnecessary retraction of the brain. Others prefer a retrosigmoid approach for very large tumors, illustrating the role for surgeon preference. We also prefer the TLA for patients who have had prior radiation or microsurgery. The exposure of the IAC in the TLA allows for wide exposure necessary for identification and dissection of the facial nerve. This is critical because the facial nerve is often encased in arachnoid scar and more adherent to the tumor in revision surgery. Finally, patients with NF2 who require tumor removal and auditory brainstem implants are also good candidates for the TLA.

33.3 Limitations of the Approach

The principal consideration for not choosing this approach is the presence of serviceable hearing. If serviceable hearing is present (pure tone average < 50 dB, speech discrimination > 50%), and the tumor is small (< 2.0 cm) and/or in a favorable position, other hearing preservation procedures are considered. Specific anatomical circumstances, most commonly related to the sigmoid sinus and jugular bulb, can make the approach less desirable. A very anterior sigmoid sinus or excessively high-riding jugular bulb can preclude good access to the tumor, unless excessive decompression is performed. If there is an absent, or very small, contralateral venous sinus system, the risk of a vascular complication rises and can be lessened by using a retrosigmoid approach.

33.4 Procedure

In most cases, surgery is performed by a six-person team: the neurotologic surgeon, neurosurgeon, anesthesiologist, circulating nurse, operating room technician, and a neural monitoring technician. After general anesthesia is administered, the patient is turned 180 degrees and prepped for surgery (▶ Fig. 33.2).

33.4.1 Monitoring

Arterial lines and a Foley catheter are placed for hemodynamic monitoring. At the start of the case, mannitol and furosemide are given to diurese the patient and lower the intracranial pressure. Facial nerve monitoring electrodes are inserted into

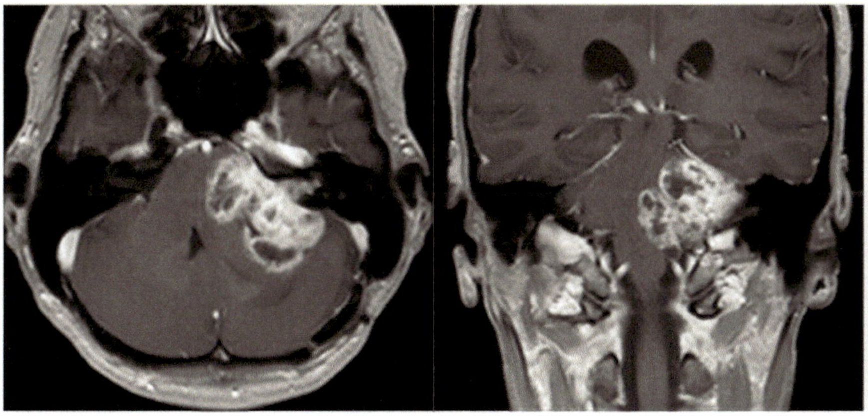

Fig. 33.1 This patient has a sporadic, 4.5-cm, large VS with brainstem and cerebellar compression. This was partially resected via a retrosigmoid craniotomy previously, but regrew. Revision surgery was conducted through a TLA approach.

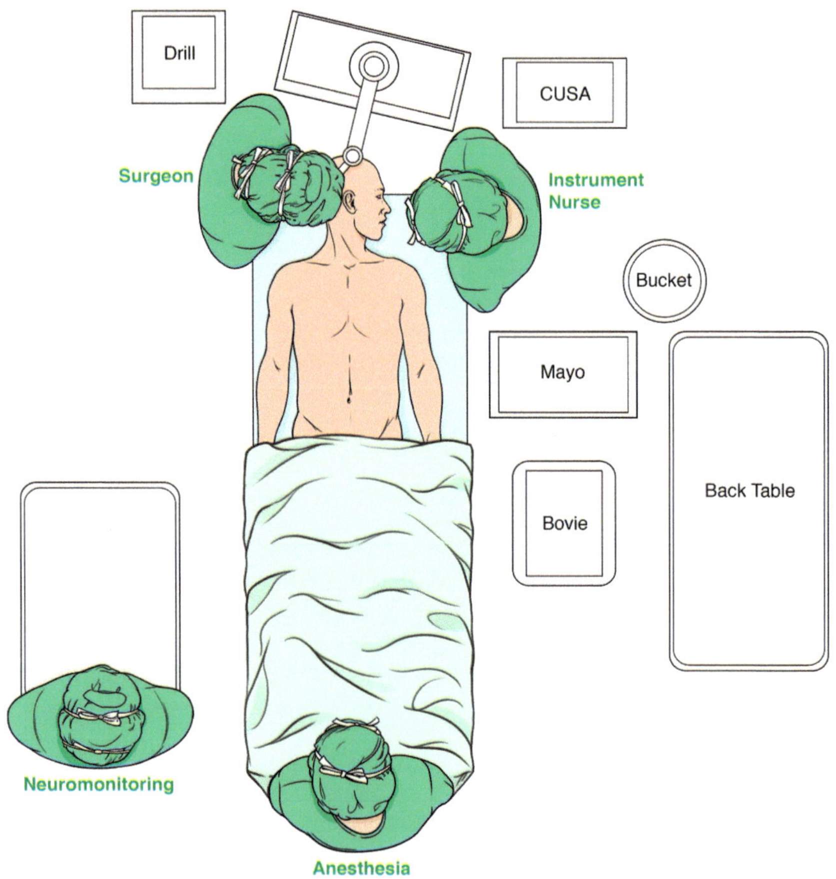

Fig. 33.2 Operating room setup for a TLA.

muscles of the facial nerve in four branches (*frontalis, orbicularis oculi, orbicularis oris,* and *mentalis*) and connected to the neuromonitoring console (NIM-Response 2.0 or 3.0, Medtronic, Jacksonville, FL). Trigeminal nerve, vagus nerve, accessory nerve, and somatosensory evoked potential monitoring can also be utilized if necessary. Finally, only short-term paralytics are used for the intubation to facilitate accurate and reliable neural monitoring.

33.4.2 Positioning

Patients remain supine for TLA surgery with their bodies positioned similar to chronic ear surgery and a gel pad is placed under the head. No pins are necessary for this procedure. The left lower quadrant of the abdomen is prepped for fat harvest.

33.4.3 Soft-Tissue Exposure

A generous shave is given behind and above the ear. Keep in mind the position of the tegmen and sigmoid sinus, which is usually inline with the zygomatic root and follows the posterior contour of the mastoid bone, respectively. The shave should be wide enough for decompression of the sigmoid sinus and post-sigmoid dura, and for decompression of the middle fossa dura superiorly. As a general rule, the skin incision should be at least two to three fingerbreadths behind the postauricular sulcus (▶ Fig. 33.3). The skin incision is made down to the level of the temporalis fascia superiorly and the mastoid periosteum inferiorly. Once the temporalis fascia is identified, the mastoid periosteum is dissected toward the ear canal. It is imperative to keep this deep layer robust, as it is used to close over the titanium plate at the end of the case. In this step, the key is to keep the periosteal incision offset from the skin incision to facilitate closure. By offsetting the incision, the risk of plate exposure and a cerebral spinal fluid (CSF) leak through the incision is also reduced.

The periosteal flaps are raised to expose the posterior edge of the ear canal anteriorly, beyond the gentle curvature of the sigmoid sinus posteriorly, above the linea temporalis superiorly, and to the digastric muscle inferiorly. Electrocautery is helpful to lift the periosteum posteriorly and superiorly. Finally, the anterior flap is retracted with silk sutures and two large self-retaining retractors are placed.

33.4.4 Bony Dissection

The bony dissection begins with identification of the tegmen mastoideum superiorly. The antrum is then identified anteriorly and the posterior canal wall is thinned and followed inferiorly to the mastoid tip. The sigmoid sinus is identified posteriorly and followed superiorly to the sinodural angle. Wide saucerization is performed along the middle fossa dura and behind the sigmoid sinus until the dura is completely uncovered and soft. If a large mastoid emissary vein is present, this

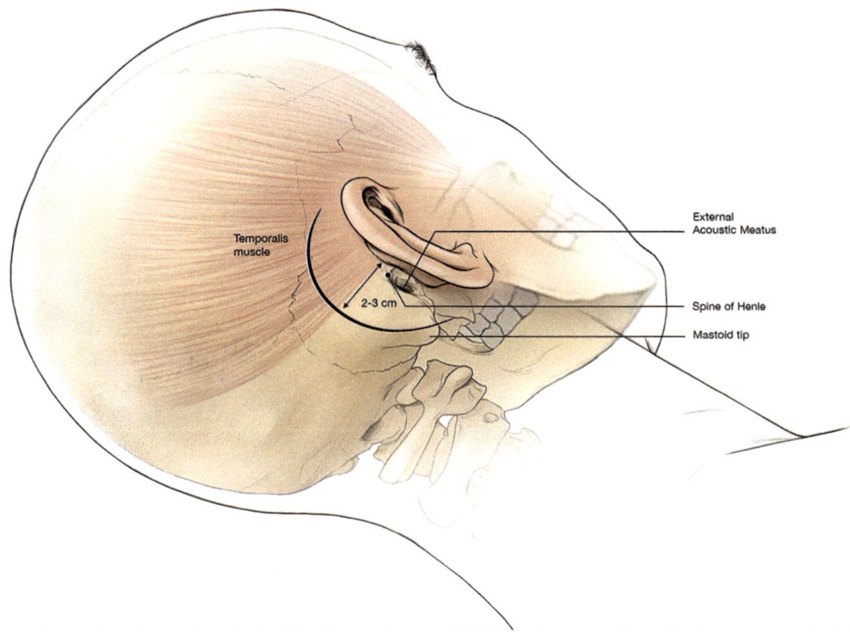

Fig. 33.3 Skin incision for a TLA. Note the position of the temporalis muscle, mastoid tip, and ear canal.

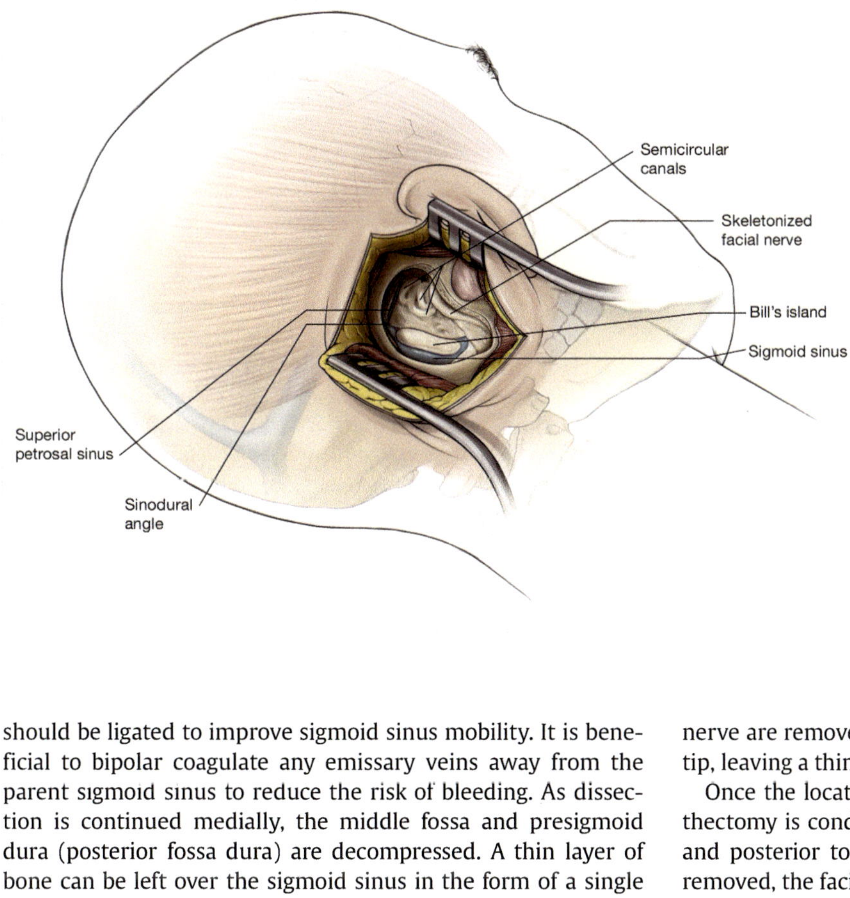

Fig. 33.4 After the mastoidectomy is complete, the facial nerve is identified. The middle fossa dura and posterior fossa dura are also decompressed and an island of bone remains over the sigmoid sinus.

should be ligated to improve sigmoid sinus mobility. It is beneficial to bipolar coagulate any emissary veins away from the parent sigmoid sinus to reduce the risk of bleeding. As dissection is continued medially, the middle fossa and presigmoid dura (posterior fossa dura) are decompressed. A thin layer of bone can be left over the sigmoid sinus in the form of a single island of bone (Bill's island) or in multiple "eggshell" pieces to protect the sinus from instrumentation or drying out as the medial temporal bone is removed (▶ Fig. 33.4).

Working anterosuperiorly, the mastoid antrum is identified where the lateral semicircular canal and incus are seen. The location of the facial nerve can then be approximated and identified in the vertical segment. The air cells overlying the facial nerve are removed and the facial nerve is traced to the mastoid tip, leaving a thin layer of bone on the facial nerve.

Once the location of the facial nerve is identified, a labyrinthectomy is conducted while decompressing the dura superior and posterior to the labyrinth. As the semicircular canals are removed, the facial nerve is at risk for injury at the second genu and vertical segment while removing the lateral canal and ampullae of the posterior canal, respectively (▶ Fig. 33.5). In particular, any undercutting of the facial nerve at the second genu, while exposing the vestibule, may result in inadvertent injury. In general, drilling superior to the lateral canal and posterior to the posterior canal can be done safely with a cutting burr. A diamond drill is then recommended to remove the

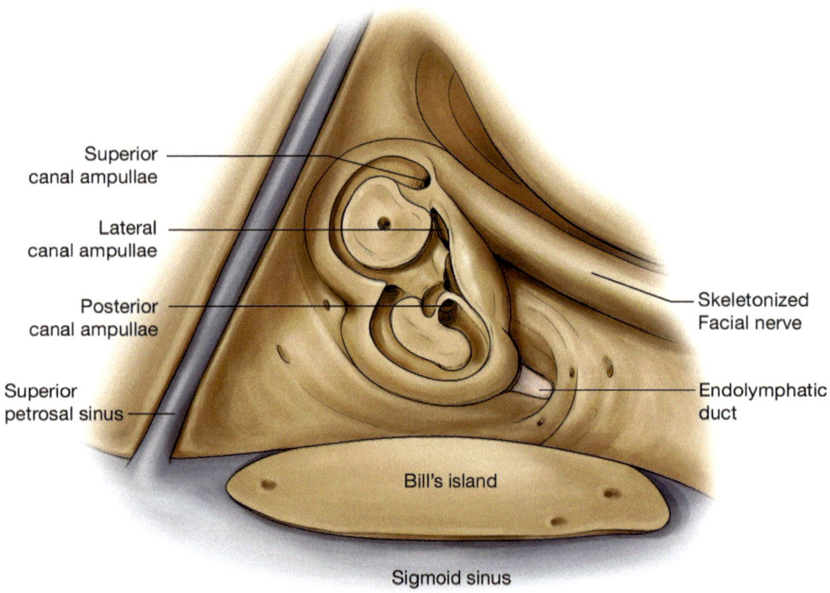

Fig. 33.5 View of the labyrinth after a partial labyrinthectomy. Note the proximity of the superior canal ampullae, lateral canal, and posterior canal ampullae to the facial nerve.

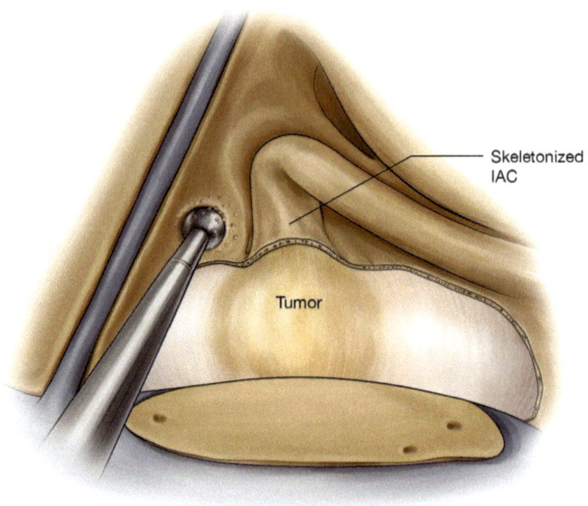

Fig. 33.6 Skeletonizing the IAC. The inferior trough should be dissected first, followed by the superior trough.

remaining labyrinth. During labyrinthectomy, the arcuate artery is invariably encountered as it passes through the subarcuate tract of the superior semicircular canal. This can be easily controlled with a diamond drill and bone wax is rarely needed. As the posterior fossa is decompressed, the endolymphatic sac is seen and should be separated from the duct, as it travels through the petrous face into the vestibule. Dividing the endolymphatic duct often allows the posterior fossa dura to fall away from the petrous bone, which facilitates exposure. As the final portions of the labyrinth are removed, keep in mind the location of the superior and posterior canal ampullae, as these are good markers for the superior and inferior borders of the IAC.

Next, the sigmoid sinus is decompressed inferiorly and the jugular bulb is identified. Once the jugular bulb is identified, the dura is decompressed superior and anterior to the bulb in order to identify the cochlear aqueduct. Once identified, a Rosen needle is used to disrupt the arachnoid in the cochlear aqueduct and CSF is released. In larger tumors, the cochlear aqueduct may be obstructed at the medial orifice in the CPA. At this juncture, drilling should not continue inferior to the cochlear aqueduct because the lower cranial nerves are in this location as they enter the neural compartment of the jugular foramen.

As the bone superior to the jugular bulb is removed, the inferior trough of the IAC is developed and the inferior edge of the IAC is identified at the porus where the bone is thickest. Once identified, the inferior border of the IAC is skeletonized laterally. As the bone is removed from the IAC laterally, the anterior face of the canal can be palpated to identify the limit of the anterior dissection. Once the inferior trough is complete, the IAC is skeletonized posteriorly and the superior trough is drilled (▸ Fig. 33.6). The superior trough is usually drilled after the inferior trough in order to protect the facial nerve, which most commonly lies in the anterior superior portion of the IAC. If the space between the tegmen and the IAC is narrow, great care must be exercised not to violate the IAC. In these situations, adequate exposure of the inferior trough will allow for tumor mobilization and facial nerve dissection. Bipolar electrocautery can also be used to contract the dura after more extensive decompression and improve surgical exposure. Some surgeons advocate reversing the drill when skeletonizing the inferior trough of a right IAC or superior trough of a left IAC to prevent the burr from "skipping" into the IAC. The final goal is to have the IAC exposed 270 degrees from the porus to the fundus. More circumferential decompression of the IAC allows for more room to dissect the tumor free from the facial nerve, but also improves visualization of the region of the porus acusticus, which is particularly important for large tumors where the risk of facial nerve splay and adherence is greater. As a general rule,

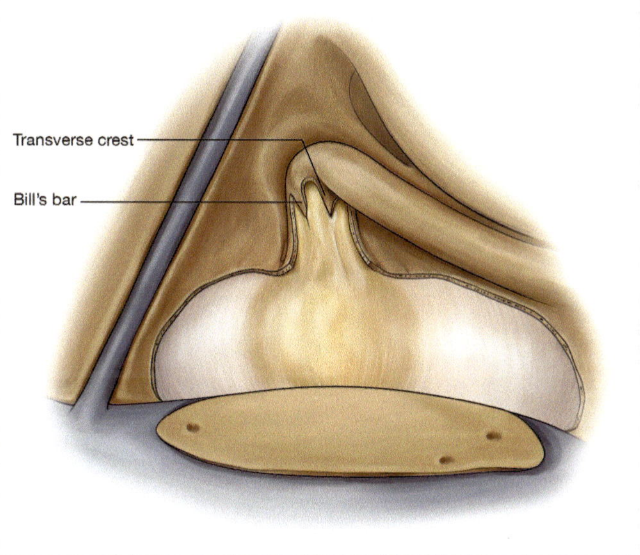

Fig. 33.7 After the IAC is fully skeletonized, Bill's bar and the transverse crest should be seen at the fundus.

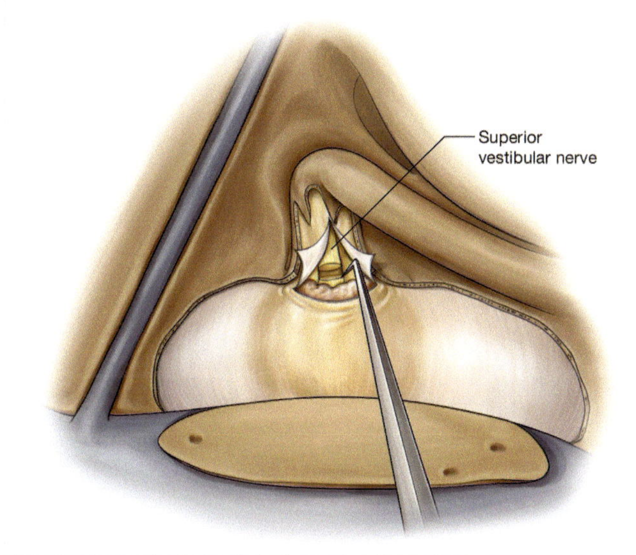

Fig. 33.8 A right-angled pick is used to take down the superior vestibular nerve once Bill's bar is exposed. The facial nerve should be seen anterior to the superior vestibular nerve as it is reflected.

all bone work should be completed before opening the dura in order to reduce the risk of facial nerve injury with the drill and to reduce intracranial bone dust dissemination.

33.4.5 Fundus Dissection

The most lateral dissection of the IAC starts inferiorly with identification of the singular nerve. The bone is carefully removed superiorly to uncover the transverse crest (or falciform crest), which separates the inferior and superior vestibular nerves. Finally, the vertical crest (or Bill's bar, named after William House) is identified superiorly, which separates the superior vestibular nerve located posteriorly from the facial nerve located anteriorly (▶ Fig. 33.7). Once identified, the most lateral portion of the IAC should be skeletonized to the labyrinthine segment. This dissection can be tedious, but is critical for facial nerve identification. Once identified, a sharp hook is used to palpate Bill's bar and take down the lateral end of the superior vestibular nerve as it enters the vestibule. While this relationship is an anatomical constant, confirmation of anatomy should still be performed with the stimulating probe prior to superior vestibular nerve avulsion. Another commonly referred to landmark for this part of dissection is Mike's dot (named after Mike Glasscock), where the terminal end of the superior vestibular nerve enters the vestibule. As the superior vestibular nerve is reflected, the facial nerve can be seen just anterior to Bill's bar (▶ Fig. 33.8).

33.4.6 Eustachian Tube Packing

Before the remaining dura is opened, the middle ear should be packed to reduce the risk of postoperative CSF leak. There are various methods of accomplishing this. Our method is to remove the incus from the antrum with a sharp hook, taking care to avoid tearing the tympanic membrane. A short facial recess is then drilled with a 2-mm diamond burr to provide direct line of sight into the eustachian tube orifice. The tensor tympani is divided and temporalis fascia is used to pack the eustachian tube opening under direct vision. This is followed by bone wax mixed with hemostatic gauze (Surgicel Nu-knit, Ethicon, Somerville, NJ). Muscle is then packed into the middle ear and bone wax is used to seal off the antrum and facial recess from the mastoid. If present, retrofacial air cells should also be sealed with bone wax.

33.4.7 Tumor Removal

The initial dural incision is made on the posterior fossa dura from the level of the midsigmoid posteriorly, to the porus acusticus, anteriorly (▶ Fig. 33.7). The arachnoid and vessels directly under the dura should be carefully swept aside and a long thin Cottonoid should be placed on the cerebellum to protect it from injury. The second dural incision is oriented along the posterior IAC. These two incisions are then connected at the porus, which can be tightly adherent and vascular. Small vessels that penetrate the dura can be cauterized and incised to release the dura as it is being lifted superiorly and inferiorly off the tumor and IAC. Sutures are then placed through the superior and inferior dural flaps to facilitate retraction.

Tumor removal is generally completed in three stages: first the CPA portion is debulked, leaving a thin layer of tumor on the facial nerve, followed by removal of the IAC portion and finally the most adherent portion in the cisternal portion of the facial nerve. To start, the avascular plane of arachnoid around the tumor in dissected, freeing the tumor from the surrounding dura and cerebellum. A nerve stimulator should be used to aid in this dissection in order to help identify the location of the facial nerve, which is most commonly in an anterior position. A small window is then removed from the posterior face of the tumor capsule in the CPA. An ultrasonic aspirator (CUSA,

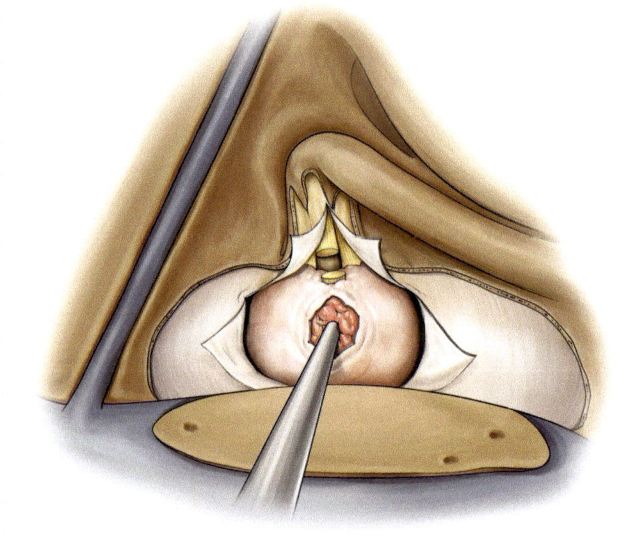

Fig. 33.9 A window is made in the posterior face of the tumor capsule in the CPA. Through this window the tumor in the CPA is debulked.

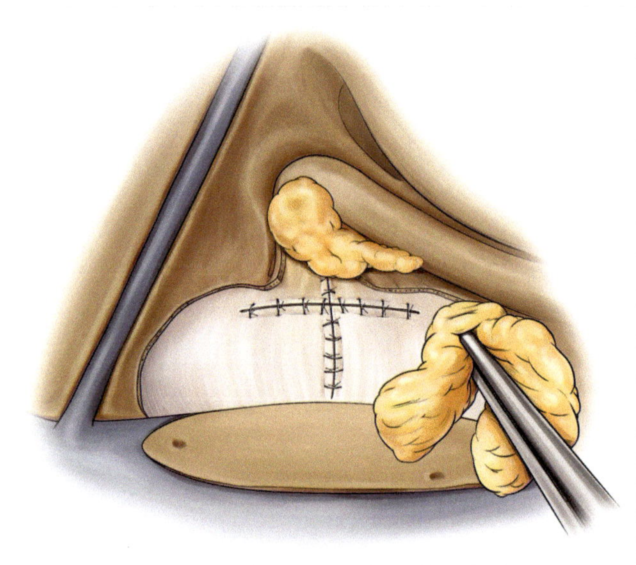

Fig. 33.10 After the dura is closed, palisading strips of abdominal fat are laid into the mastoid defect into the CPA. The mastoid should not be overpacked because this can cause sigmoid sinus occlusion or thrombosis. This figure represents an idealized view of dural closure. In most cases, primary watertight closure of the presigmoid posterior fossa dura cannot be accomplished.

Integra, Plainsboro, NJ) is then used to debulk the center of the tumor (▶ Fig. 33.9). As the intracapsular dissection continues, the planes around the periphery of the tumor should be developed medially until the facial nerve can be identified at the brainstem. Vessels that penetrate the tumor should be cauterized and incised. If they are simply on the periphery, they should be pushed aside and spared to reduce the risk of coagulating important brainstem perforators. The remaining tumor capsule should be removed piecemeal with sharp scissors and bipolar electrocautery. If the tumor capsule is firm, we prefer the CO_2 laser (BeamPath, OmniGuide Surgical, Lexington, MA) over sharp dissection to minimize traction on the tumor and facial nerve. The tumor should never be pulled anteriorly or medially, as this can inadvertently injure the facial nerve. Any movement of the tumor should be in the posterior or lateral direction.

The tumor dissection in the IAC starts when the superior vestibular nerve is separated at the fundus with a nerve hook and the posterior aspect of the facial nerve is identified. The plane between the facial nerve and superior vestibular nerve is developed from lateral to medial with blunt dissection but without medial traction on the facial nerve. The facial nerve stimulator is a helpful instrument to both dissect and differentiate nerve fibers. Dissection to the porus should be completed relatively easily. Once the IAC and CPA portion of the tumor is removed, the remaining portion of tumor is dissected off of the cisternal segment of the facial nerve in the region of the porus acusticus. This should be done gently, as the nerve can be thin, splayed, and adherent in this portion. If the tumor is too adherent to the facial nerve for safe dissection, a near-total resection (NTR) or subtotal resection (STR) should be completed to prevent facial nerve injury.

33.4.8 Closure

After tumor removal is complete, the dura is reapproximated as best as possible. Strips of subcutaneous abdominal fat from the abdomen are placed into the CPA and laid parallel to the IAC and into the mastoid defect. As a general rule, fat approximately the size of a small lime is adequate. The remainder of the mastoid defect is gently filled with strips of abdominal fat in a palisading fashion (▶ Fig. 33.10). It is important to avoid overpacking the mastoid defect, as this can compress the sigmoid sinus and facial nerve. This is especially important if the tumor is on the same side as a dominant sigmoid sinus. It is our practice to use a titanium plate to perform cranioplasty. Once the plate is secured, one should be able to observe CSF pulsations to ensure the mastoid was not overpacked but not see CSF permeate through (▶ Fig. 33.11).

The periosteal flaps are then reapproximated over the plate in a watertight fashion. If there are small gaps in this layer after it is closed, small pieces of fat can be placed to fill the defects (▶ Fig. 33.12). The skin flap is approximated and a mastoid dressing is placed. We leave the mastoid dressing on for 3 days. Ideally, one should observe a flat wound with dry, well-healing incisions once the head dressing is removed. Occasionally, a pseudomeningocele may develop. As long as the wound is not tense, this should resolve spontaneously over the following weeks.

33.5 Surgical Nuances and Pitfalls

Of the three approaches for VS microsurgery, the TLA requires the most bone removal. For this reason, having clear steps in mind and completing each step sequentially will allow for efficient and safe removal of bone. Furthermore, utilizing the largest burrs possible, minimizing the number of exchanges, and removing as much bone as safely possible with a cutting burr

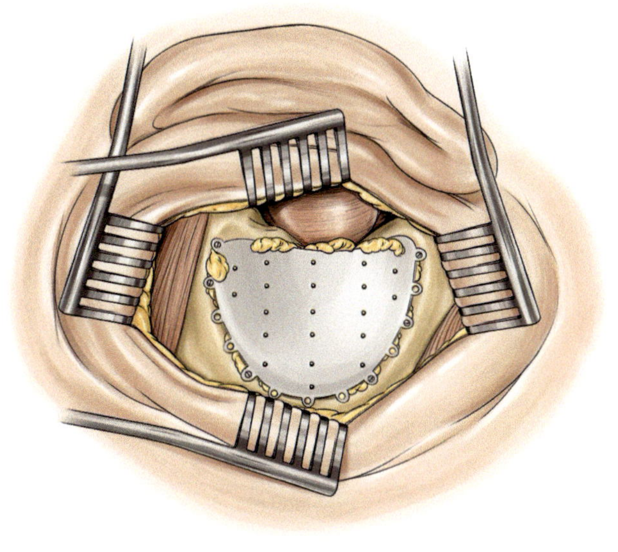

Fig. 33.11 A titanium plate is used for cranioplasty. Once the plate is secured, one should still be able to observe CSF pulsations through the fat.

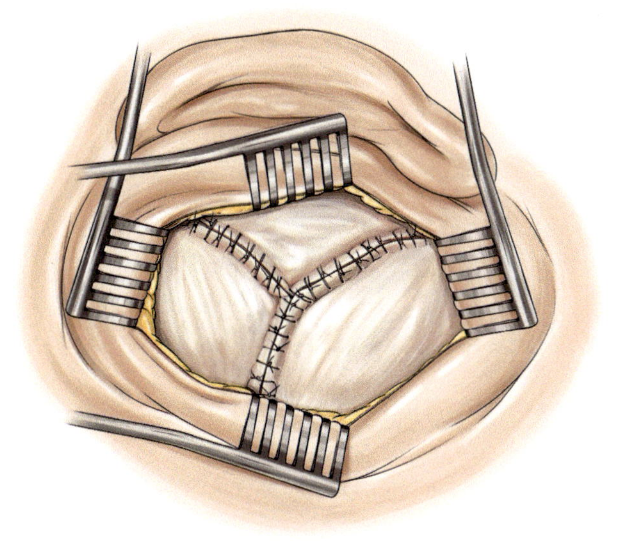

Fig. 33.12 A watertight closure of the periosteal flaps over the titanium plate is critical to prevent postoperative CSF leak. Gaps in this layer can be filled with pieces of abdominal fat.

before changing to a diamond burr will reduce surgical time. Below are few instances where one's approach may need to be modified when performing a TLA. Modifications to the traditional TLA, including the enlarged TLA and the enlarged TLA with transapical extension, are reviewed further in Chapter 34.

33.5.1 Large Vestibular Schwannoma

Large VSs can dilate the IAC and be encountered earlier than expected when drilling the inferior and superior troughs, thereby obstructing further dissection. In these situations, remove as much bone as possible, and attempt to dissect beyond the anterior wall of the IAC in the trough with more space. This will allow for mobilization of the tumor during removal. Furthermore, frequent stimulation of the dura in the IAC and CPA with the facial nerve stimulator is critical to identify the location of the nerve under the dura when the tumor is large. Although the facial nerve is typically located anterosuperiorly, large tumors can displace it to an unexpected location.

Large VSs can also extend anteriorly and inferiorly, which will make instrumentation to these areas more difficult during tumor removal. This is one primary limitation that has led some groups to prefer the retrosigmoid approach for large tumors. In these patients, wider cortical decompression along the middle and posterior fossa dura is critical—bony decompression 1 cm superior to the tegmen and 1 cm posterior to the sigmoid sinus will open a wider corridor for instrumentation anteriorly and inferiorly.

33.5.2 High-Riding Jugular Bulb

A high-riding jugular bulb can make exposure of the inferior trough and lower pole of the cisternal tumor difficult. Preoperative analysis of the magnetic resonance imaging (MRI) can be helpful to identify this. High-riding jugular bulbs may be located posterior to the IAC and will be encountered early when decompressing the posterior fossa dura. The goal is to decompress the dura in front of the jugular bulb where the inferior trough of the IAC is located. In order to achieve this, wide decompression of the cortical bone laterally over the middle fossa dura will allow for a superior to inferior trajectory for bone removal in this location. Some surgeons will also gently cauterize the jugular bulb with bipolar electrocautery in order to contract it inferiorly. This approach should be used with caution because aggressive contraction with electrocautery can cause thrombosis or, much less commonly, injury to the lower cranial nerves. Furthermore, the venous wall of the jugular bulb is more fragile than the sigmoid sinus and decompression may result in bulb injury and brisk bleeding.

33.5.3 Anterior Sigmoid Sinus

A very anterior sigmoid sinus can make dissection difficult, but can often be worked around after wide decompression of the temporal and retrosigmoid dura. Furthermore, once CSF is released and the patient is diuresed, the dura often relaxes, providing increased working room. In rare cases, where this is not enough, the external auditory canal wall can be taken down to improve surgical exposure. For these cases, a blind sac closure of the external canal and packing of the eustachian tube is performed.

33.5.4 Translabyrinthine Craniotomy after Previous Translabyrinthine Surgery

Revision TLA may be performed for growing tumors after previous STR. In these cases, identification of the facial nerve is the first priority. Once identified, the rest of the mastoid bone can be removed swiftly. After the initial skin and periosteal incisions are made, the mastoid contents should be removed carefully, as the sigmoid sinus and dura are exposed. Blunt dissection is preferred. The posterior external ear canal is identified and is a good starting landmark since it is in the same plane as the IAC. Working medially, the antrum is identified which will help identify the vertical segment of the facial nerve. Finally, just medial to this will be the fundus where the facial nerve can be found and then traced into the CPA.

33.6 Complications

33.6.1 Injury to Sigmoid Sinus

In the case of a sigmoid sinus injury, the key to hemostasis is gentle occlusion and patience. If the injury is small or on the periphery near the dura, we prefer placing a piece of Gelfoam over the sinusotomy and holding it in placed with a Cottonoid for a few minutes. The Gelfoam can be held in placed manually with the suction or cantilevered under bony spicules if present. The key is to not compress the sinus, as this will promote thrombus formation. If the hole is large and cannot be treated with Gelfoam or primary closure, a piece of Alloderm (LifeCell Corporation, Bridgewater, NJ) can also be placed over the sinus and sutured to the pre- and postsinus dura. As a last resort, the sigmoid sinus can be tied off. This requires exposure of the pre- and postsigmoid dura, opening the dura, and suture ligation. With any dural sinus bleed, it is important to alert the anesthesiologist so that they are aware of the rare but potentially serious risk of venous air embolism.

33.6.2 Injury to the Superior Petrosal Sinus

The superior petrosal sinus (SPS) may be injured directly by the drill or avulsed when the remaining sliver of petrous bone is removed between the middle and posterior fossa dura. One trick we employ is to leave this last sliver of bone over the petrous ridge and come back to it after CSF is released. After the dura relaxes, the bone is more easily dissected from the remaining bone without injuring the SPS. Nonetheless, if the SPS is violated, bleeding can be easily controlled with bipolar electrocautery and gentle packing. We prefer to pack directly into the sinus with Surgicel (Ethicon, Somerville, NJ).

33.6.3 Cerebrospinal Fluid Leak

At our institution, we have transitioned to using a titanium plate and abdominal fat for our cranioplasty with a CSF leak rate of 3.3%.[4] CSF leaks most commonly occur at the incision site, but can also present as rhinorrhea or less commonly otorrhea. It is our preference to treat incisional leaks by oversewing the incision. For rhinorrhea or otorrhea, reopening the wounds with blind sac closure of the external canal and repacking the middle ear and eustachian tube with fascia, muscle, and bone wax is used primarily. In these cases, the titanium plate and fat in the mastoid and CPA are not disturbed.

33.7 Postoperative Care

TLA patients are admitted to the intensive care unit for 24-hour observation postoperatively. Our patients are extubated in the operating room prior to arrival and they receive neurological checks every hour for the first 24 hours. A postoperative computed tomography (CT) or MRI scan is performed on postoperative day (POD) 1. The patients are then transferred to the postsurgical ward for an additional 2 to 4 days. We monitor the patient's facial grade in addition to signs and symptoms of CSF leak. Most commonly, the patients are out of bed to a chair on POD 1 and are walking with the physical therapist on POD 2. Steroids are continued and tapered for the next week. The abdominal drain is removed on POD 1 and the head wrap is removed on POD 3.

33.8 Surgical Results

Looking at the literature over the last 10 years, the rates of "good" facial nerve outcomes (House–Brackmann grade I–II) range from 59.9 to 93.7% at 1 year (▶ Table 33.1). There is also clear evidence that larger tumors have worse facial nerve outcomes. In a study at our institution that reviewed over 580 TLAs, there was a statistically significant difference between facial nerve outcomes when 3.5 cm was used as a cut-off. In tumors smaller than 3.5 cm, the rate of a good facial nerve outcome at 1 year was 84%, versus 53% in tumors larger than 3.5 cm.[5]

Overall, the other complications from TLA are very low, with CSF leak being most common, occurring in between 0.85 and 13.5% of cases, the median being 5.5% (▶ Table 33.1). The higher rate reported in this review was from the Dutch study by Springborg et al. This study, however, is unique in that it reviews patients over a 34-year span where many advances in technique, technology, and management of VS patients have occurred.[6,7,8,9,10,11,12,13]

As the microsurgical management of VS has evolved, the authors have become more willing to perform STR or NTR in lieu of long-term facial nerve injury. We aim for a gross total resection (GTR) in every case, but our final decision is based on intraoperative findings. In our most recent review of 400 patients undergoing TLA for tumors larger than 2.5 cm, 325 (81.3%) patients underwent a GTR.[7] In this cohort, the rate of good facial nerve outcome was far superior in the patients who had NTR (96.6%) and STR (96.2%) versus 76.9% in the patients who underwent GTR. Only one (2.3%) patient who underwent a NTR required a secondary intervention and only three (9.7%) patients who underwent an STR required additional treatment. Furthermore, the need for medical or surgical care of the eye was far greater in the GTR cohort. Further discussion on intraoperative decision making regarding the facial nerve and less-than-complete VS resection can be found in Chapters 32 and 41, respectively.

33.9 Conclusion

Over the last 50 years, since the reintroduction of the TLA by William House, this approach has become the workhorse for VS removal at our institution. When hearing preservation is not a

Table 33.1 TLA results reported in the literature over the last 10 years.

Article	No. of patients	Average size of tumor, cm, mean (SD)	Follow-up	Facial nerve outcome, *n* (%)	Other complications, *n* (%)	% Gross total removal, *n* (%)	Comments
Schwartz et al[7]	400	3.2 (0.7)	>1 y	HB I–II: 80.3%[a]	CSF leak: 8%; rehospitalization: 8%	325 (81.3)	
Rinaldi et al[8]	36	NA[b]	>1 y	HB I–II: 22 (61.1)	CSF leak: 4 (3)[c]	NR	Larger tumors had worse facial nerve outcomes
Springborg et al[6]	1,152	2.5 (1.3)	>1 y	HB I–II: 810 (70.3)	CSF leak: 168 (13.5); death:12 (1)	1,011 (84)	Study from single Dutch system between 1976 and 2009
Ben Ammar et al[9]	1,865	1.8 (0.97)	>1 y	HB I–II: 1,043 (59.9)	CSF leak: 16 (0.85); meningitis: 2 (0.1); post-op hemorrhage: 15 (0.8); death: 15 (0.8)	1,722 (92.33)	Single institution review over 22 years: Gruppo Otological
Charpiot et al[10]	123	NR	>1 y	HB I–III: 68.5%	CSF leak: 6.5%; meningitis: 1.6%; death: 1 (0.8)	NR	
Shamji et al[11]	128	2.3	Mean: 17 mo (range, 9–39)	HB I–III: 87%	CSF leak: 6 (5)	NR	Prognostic indicators of good FN outcome: tumor size, duration of hearing loss, and tinnitus
Jacob et al[12]	231	NR	>1 y	HB I–III: 205 (88.7)	NR	NR	No correlation between nerve of origin and FN outcome
Brackmann et al[5]	580	2.4	>1 y	HB I–II: 317 (81)	CSF leak: 28 (5.5); stroke: 5 (1); meningitis: 3 (0.6); DVT: 2 (0.4)	552 (95%)	
Isaacson et al[13]	63	1.3	>10 mo	HB I–II: 59 (93.7)[d]	NR	NR	No significant difference between FN outcome and approach (MFC vs. TLA)

Abbreviations: CSF, cerebrospinal fluid; DVT, deep vein thrombosis; FN, facial nerve; HB, House–Brackmann; MFC, middle fossa craniotomy; NA, not available; NR, not reported; TLA, translabyrinthine approach.
Note: Studies including extended TLA approaches, NF2 patients, staged surgery, giant VSs only, and meta-analysis were excluded.
[a]HB I/II at 1 year when broken down into grades of resection: gross total resection, 76.9%; near-total resection, 96.6%; subtotal resection, 96.2%.
[b]Sizes of tumors were classified into grades I–V; average size of tumor was not reported.
[c]Rate of CSF leak was reported for the entire series, including both retrosigmoid and middle fossa craniotomy approaches.
[d]Tumors < 10 mm: 100% HB I; tumors > 10 mm: 92.7% HB I/II.

concern, the TLA can be utilized to remove any sized tumor in the IAC or CPA while providing wide exposure for safe dissection of the facial nerve with minimal complications. Finally, while GTR should be goal of every case, the surgeon should weigh the risks of GTR against facial nerve injury.

References

[1] Panse R. Klinische und pathologische Mitteilungen. Eur Arch Otorhinolaryngol. 1904; 61:251–255

[2] Quix FH. Ein Acusticustumor. Arch Ohrenheilk.. 1911; 84:252–253

[3] House WF. Transtemporal bone microsurgical removal of acoustic neuromas. Evolution of transtemporal bone removal of acoustic tumors. Arch Otolaryngol. 1964; 80:731–742

[4] Fayad JN, Schwartz MS, Slattery WH, Brackmann DE. Prevention and treatment of cerebrospinal fluid leak after translabyrinthine acoustic tumor removal. Otol Neurotol. 2007; 28(3):387–390

[5] Brackmann DE, Cullen RD, Fisher LM. Facial nerve function after translabyrinthine vestibular schwannoma surgery. Otolaryngol Head Neck Surg. 2007; 136(5):773–777

[6] Springborg JB, Fugleholm K, Poulsgaard L, Cayé-Thomasen P, Thomsen J, Stangerup SE. Outcome after translabyrinthine surgery for vestibular schwannomas: report on 1244 patients. J Neurol Surg B Skull Base. 2012; 73 (3):168–174

[7] Schwartz MS, Kari E, Strickland BM, et al. Evaluation of the increased use of partial resection of large vestibular schwanommas: facial nerve outcomes and recurrence/regrowth rates. Otol Neurotol. 2013; 34(8):1456–1464

[8] Rinaldi V, Casale M, Bressi F, et al. Facial nerve outcome after vestibular schwannoma surgery: our experience. J Neurol Surg B Skull Base. 2012; 73 (1):21–27

[9] Ben Ammar M, Piccirillo E, Topsakal V, Taibah A, Sanna M. Surgical results and technical refinements in translabyrinthine excision of vestibular schwannomas: the Gruppo Otologico experience. Neurosurgery. 2012; 70(6): 1481–1491, discussion 1491

[10] Charpiot A, Tringali S, Zaouche S, Ferber-Viart C, Dubreuil C. Perioperative complications after translabyrinthine removal of large or giant vestibular schwannoma: outcomes for 123 patients. Acta Otolaryngol. 2010; 130(11):1249–1255

[11] Shamji MF, Schramm DR, Benoit BG. Clinical predictors of facial nerve outcome after translabyrinthine resection of acoustic neuromas. Clin Invest Med. 2007; 30(6):E233–E239

[12] Jacob A, Robinson LL, Jr, Bortman JS, Yu L, Dodson EE, Welling DB. Nerve of origin, tumor size, hearing preservation, and facial nerve outcomes in 359 vestibular schwannoma resections at a tertiary care academic center. Laryngoscope. 2007; 117(12):2087–2092

[13] Isaacson B, Telian SA, El-Kashlan HK. Facial nerve outcomes in middle cranial fossa vs translabyrinthine approaches. Otolaryngol Head Neck Surg. 2005; 133(6):906–910

34 Surgical Refinements to the Translabyrinthine Approach to the Cerebellopontine Angle

Sampath Chandra Prasad, Alessandra Russo, Abdelkader Taibah, Enrico Pasanisi, Francesco Galletti, and Mario Sanna

34.1 Introduction

The translabyrinthine approach (TLA) is a lateral approach used for accessing various tumors of the cerebellopontine angle (CPA), most commonly vestibular schwannoma (VS). This approach was first described by Rudolf Panse in 1904 and was first performed for VS in 1911 by Franciscus Hubertus Quix from Utrecht University, in the Netherlands. However, due to unsatisfactory results, this approach was criticized by Harvey Cushing and Walter Dandy, two of the pioneers of neurosurgery of that time, and thereafter this approach fell into disrepute.[1] After the advent of microscopes in otology, William House at the House Ear Institute in Los Angeles rediscovered the TLA, marking the beginning of the era of modern skull base microsurgery.[2,3,4,5] Subsequently, there was a developing opinion that while small tumors could be removed through the TLA, larger lesions were best approached through a suboccipital approach as the TLA failed to provide a large surgical field.[6] To overcome this limitation of the TLA, the proponents of this approach enlarged the surgical corridor by additional bone removal over the middle and posterior fossa dura and by the addition of the transapical extensions (where bone is drilled out to various degrees around the internal auditory canal [IAC]), thereby obtaining a wider surgical view and better control over the tumor and surrounding structures. This facilitated removal of even very large tumors with anterior and medial extensions.[1,7,8,9,10] Furthermore, this approach could be combined with other skull base approaches such as the transcochlear approaches described by William House[11] or transotic approaches described by Ugo Fisch[12,13] for additional exposure (Chapter 38).

Over the years, we have introduced some technical modifications to the TLA for very large tumors that have allowed us to reduce the mortality rate to < 1% with minimal morbidity.[14] Identifying the facial nerve by using the ampullary nerve as a landmark rather than the vertical crest (Bill's bar), lowering the high jugular bulb, and extending bone removal around and anterior to the IAC (transapical extension) were the major refinements added to the original technique.

The standard TLA approach is reviewed in detail in Chapter 33. This chapter will discuss the two significant modifications that have been developed at the Gruppo Otologico to the conventional TLA described by House. We refer to these modifications as the enlarged translabyrinthine approach (*ETLA*) and the *ETLA with transapical extension* (*ETLA + TAE*). Both of these approaches will be described and discussed separately. This chapter is based on the experience accumulated in the management of over 3,000 VSs using the TLA performed between 1986 and 2016 at the Gruppo Otologico.

34.2 The Enlarged Translabyrinthine Approach

34.2.1 Rationale

The limited view provided by the classic TLA prevented considering this valuable approach for the removal of large VS, more so in the presence of limiting anatomical obstacles such as a high jugular bulb, an anteriorly placed sigmoid sinus, low middle fossa dura, and a small mastoid cavity.[15]

The purpose of the ETLA approach is the same as with the conventional TLA—i.e., to obtain lateral access to the IAC and the CPA, thereby allowing removal of CPA lesions without cerebellar retraction. In the conventional TLA, a thin shelf of bone is sometimes left over the middle cranial fossa dura, the sigmoid sinus, and the jugular bulb. In the ETLA, bone is removed over these structures to completely expose the middle cranial fossa dura, the posterior fossa dura, sigmoid sinus, retrosigmoid dura, and the jugular bulb along with the contents of the IAC. This allows retraction of structures during surgery, thereby enabling exposure and hence removal of even very large VSs. The advantage in exposure obtained by the enlarged approach when compared to the conventional TLA is shown in ▶ Fig. 34.1. Another difference between the two approaches is that in the enlarged approach, the bone around the IAC is drilled by 270 degrees or more compared to 180 degrees in the conventional approach, providing the surgeon with additional anteromedial exposure (▶ Fig. 34.2).

34.2.2 Indications

- *Tumors of any size with poor preoperative hearing*: This approach is indicated for tumors wherein hearing preservation is not essential due to nonserviceable preoperative hearing. With the wide exposure that this approach provides, the surgeon can focus on disease removal.
- *Large tumors irrespective of preoperative hearing*: While opinions regarding this vary, we feel that the ETLA is indicated in VSs greater than 1.5 cm in diameter in the extracanalicular portion, regardless of the preoperative hearing, since the probability of hearing preservation with gross total resection is low. Very large tumors, even those larger than 4 cm in diameter, can be safely removed by the ETLA.
- *Neurofibromatosis type 2 (NF2) with large tumors*: NF2 commonly presents with bilateral VSs, making hearing preservation or rehabilitation very important. While hearing can be preserved in small tumors by opting for hearing

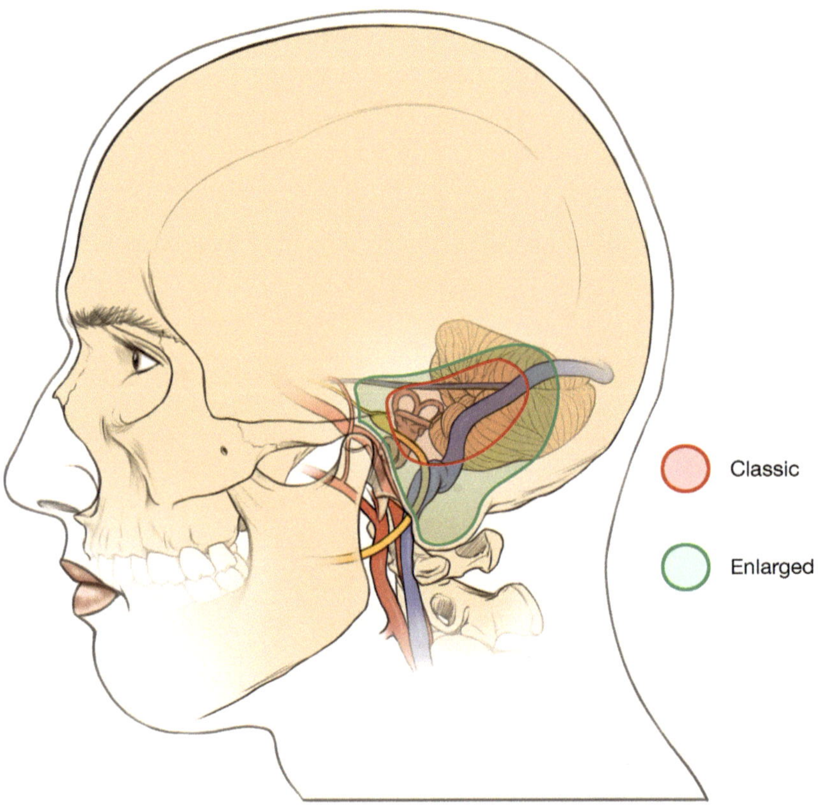

Fig. 34.1 Exposure of the CPA and the surrounding areas obtained by the ETLA is much larger than that obtained by the classic TLA.

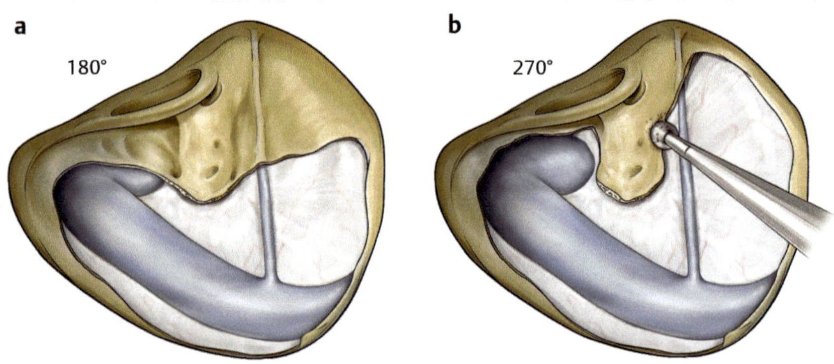

Fig. 34.2 Illustrations showing the difference between the conventional 180-degree exposure **(a)** and the 270-degree exposure **(b)** of the internal auditory canal.

preservation surgeries such as the retrosigmoid or the middle cranial fossa approaches, it is difficult to ensure this in larger tumors.[16] In such a scenario, the ETLA may be used, wherein large tumors can be removed and preservation of the cochlear nerve can be attempted for simultaneous cochlear implantation (CI). Likewise, when it is not possible to preserve the cochlear nerve, an auditory brainstem implant (ABI) can be placed in the same sitting, by this approach.[17]

34.2.3 Contraindications:

- *Only hearing ear*: This procedure is contraindicated in the only hearing ear. However, this has become a relative contraindication currently due to the option of simultaneous ipsilateral CI or ABI, as mentioned above, or a contralateral CI.[18]
- *Ipsilateral chronic otitis media*: This procedure is contraindicated in the presence of active infection. However, the approach can be used in cases of simple tympanic membrane perforation with no active infection, while the external auditory canal is closed as a cul-de-sac. If there is an active infection, a subtotal petrosectomy is performed, with eradication of the infection, obliteration of the cavity with abdominal fat, and closure of the external auditory canal as a cul-de-sac. The ETLA is then performed as a second-stage surgery.

34.2.4 Surgical Technique

Mastoidectomy (Left Ear)

A C-shaped postauricular skin incision is placed starting from 2 to 3 cm superior to the attachment of auricle, at the level of the dome of the helix, continuing 4 to 5 cm posterior to the retroauricular sulcus, and ending just below the mastoid tip (▶ Fig. 34.3). The skin flap is reflected anteriorly and maintained in position with fish hooks. The musculoperiosteal layer is incised in a T-shaped fashion using cautery (▶ Fig. 34.4) and is elevated. Monopolar cautery is applied to transect the muscles attached to the mastoid tip that helps to raise the flap. Bleeding from the mastoid emissary vein usually occurs at this step and it can be controlled by the use of bone wax. The posterior margins of the musculoperiosteal flaps are sutured to the skin, which helps in achieving hemostasis from the skin incision and at the same time keeps the flaps retracted (▶ Fig. 34.5). We do not recommend the use of the conventional retractors, which limit access and exposure.

An extended mastoidectomy is then performed. The middle cranial fossa dura and the sigmoid sinus are identified, leaving a thin shell of bone overlying them. Bone 2 to 3 cm posterior to the sigmoid sinus is also drilled using a large cutting burr (▶ Fig. 34.6). The mastoid air cells are exenterated, and the antrum is widely opened. The digastric ridge is identified, the facial nerve is skeletonized, and the retrofacial air cells are drilled out. Using a large diamond burr, the remaining bone covering the middle cranial fossa and the sigmoid sinus as well as the posterior fossa dura posterior to the sinus is further drilled and removed. The sinodural angle must be clearly exposed to know the exact location of the superior petrosal sinus exiting the sigmoid sinus. The sigmoid sinus is followed down to the jugular bulb, and the three semicircular canals are delineated.

Labyrinthectomy, access to the IAC and the CPA. The labyrinthectomy starts by opening the lateral semicircular canal using a medium-sized cutting burr. The posterior semicircular canal is next opened, followed by opening of the superior semicircular canal (▶ Fig. 34.7). The anterior end of the lateral semicircular canal is left in situ to protect the facial nerve lying anteriorly. The last part of bone over the middle cranial fossa dura adjacent

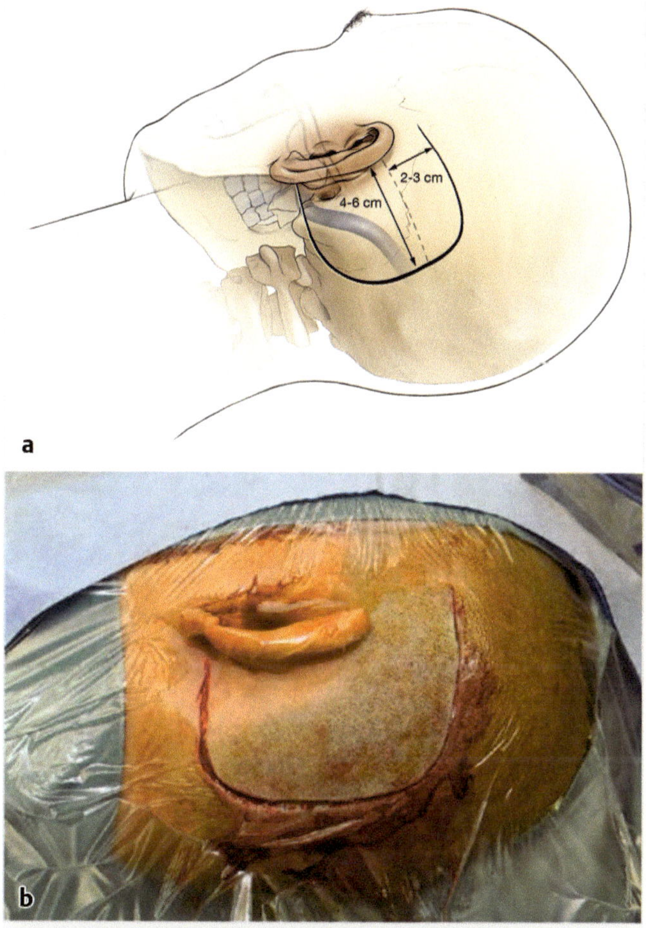

Fig. 34.3 Right postauricular skin incision for the ETLA.

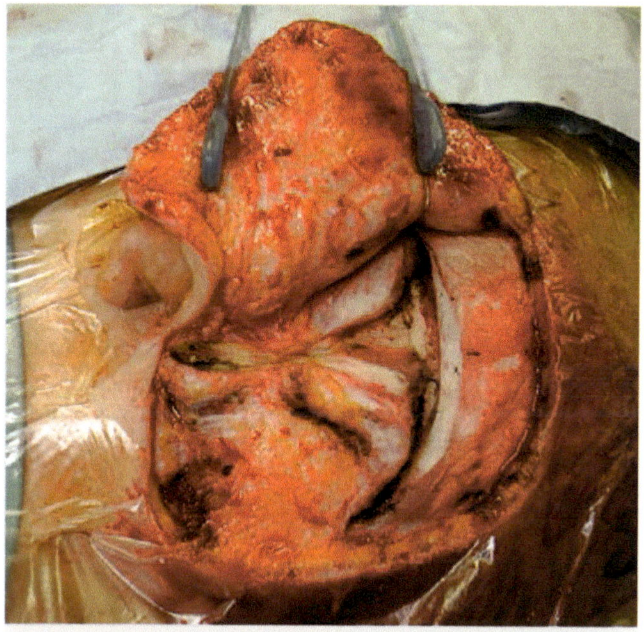

Fig. 34.4 The musculoperiosteal flap is incised using a monopolar diathermy in a "T" fashion. The vertical incision extends down to the mastoid tip.

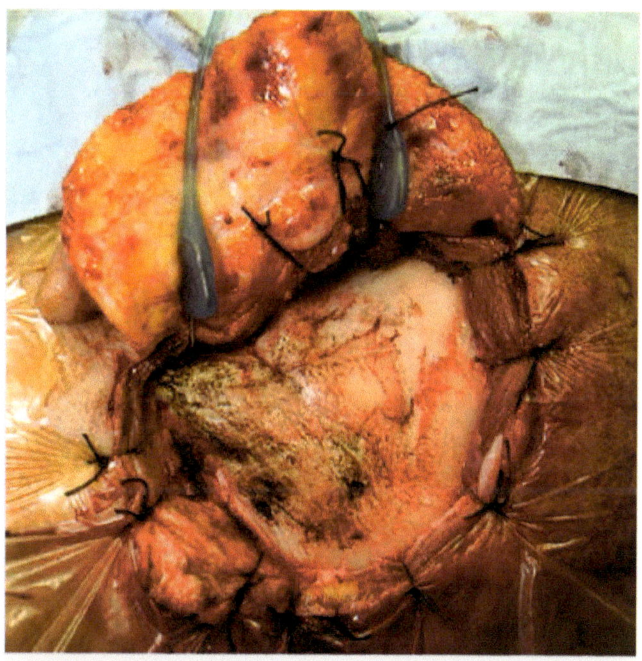

Fig. 34.5 The musculoperiosteal flaps are held by sutures.

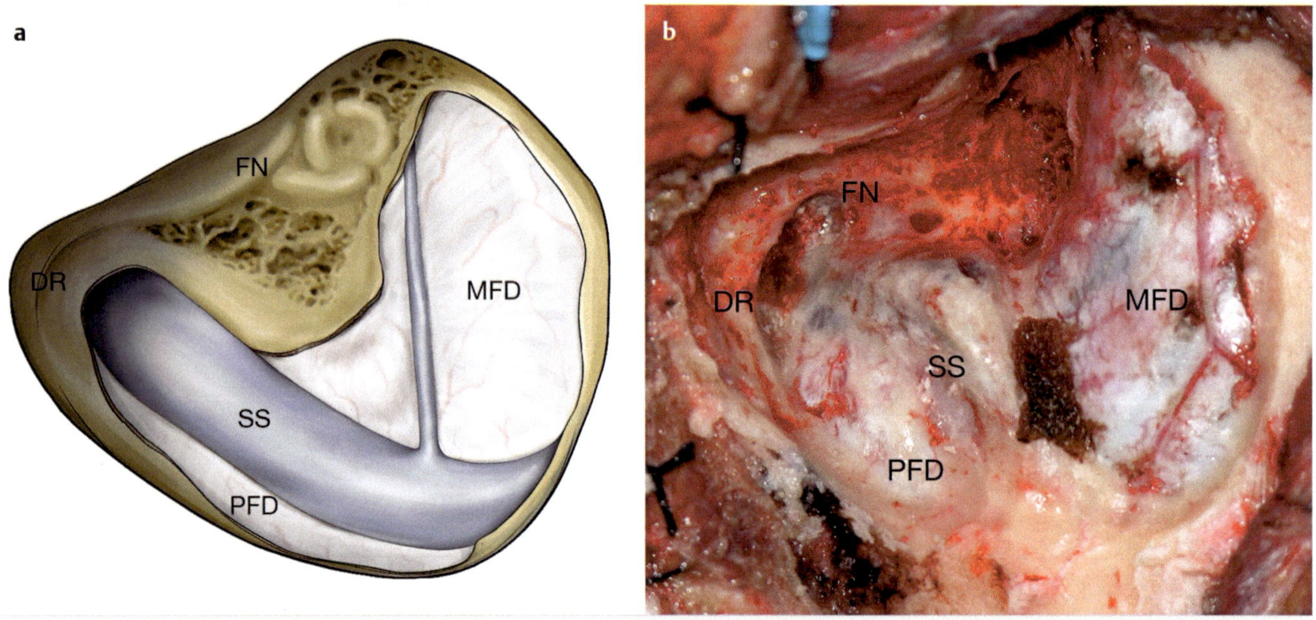

Fig. 34.6 **(a)** Extensive removal of bone over the middle cranial fossa as well as posterior to the sigmoid sinus (SS) is essential in the ETLA. **(b)** Mastoid air cells are well exenterated to demonstrate the labyrinth (L) and the mastoid segment of the facial nerve (FN). An adequate bone exposure will extend to about 3 cm posterior to the sigmoid sinus. DR, digastric ridge; MFD, middle fossa dura; PFD, posterior fossa dura.

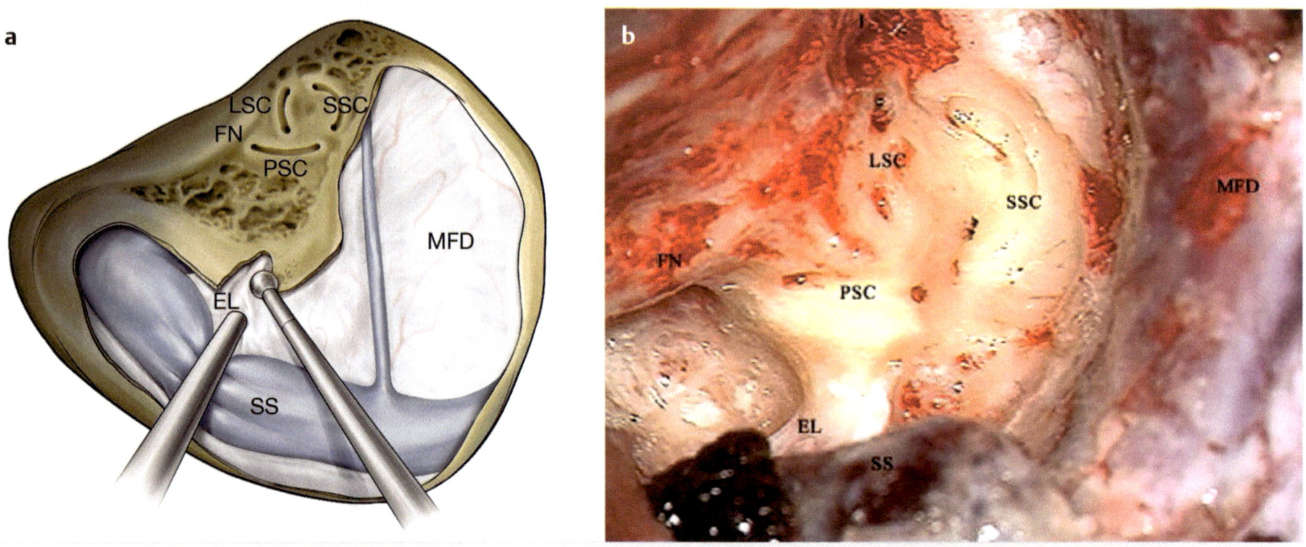

Fig. 34.7 **(a)** Note the suction-irrigator is pushing the sigmoid sinus away from the working burr. **(b)** The three semicircular canals have been opened. Note the endolymphatic duct (EL) extending from the medial surface of the posterior canal (PSC) to the posterior fossa dura (PFD). FN, facial nerve; LSC, lateral semicircular canal; MFD, middle fossa dura; SS, sigmoid sinus; SSC, superior semicircular canal.

to the labyrinth is finally removed using a rongeur after separating the bone from the dura by the use of a freer dissector. The ampullae of the lateral and superior semicircular canals are drilled. However, the anterior part of the ampullae of these two canals should be left to protect the labyrinthine segment of the facial nerve and to serve as a landmark for the superior vestibular nerve.

The vestibule is then opened widely. It is important to avoid drilling the floor of the vestibule in order to avoid inadvertent entry into the IAC. Similarly, drilling the roof of the vestibule may result in injury to the facial nerve, as the nerve runs immediately lateral to the vestibule. The endolymphatic duct is transacted by the use of Beaver knife (▶ Fig. 34.8). This step facilitates the complete drilling of bone overlying the posterior fossa dura and the subsequent dural retraction. The bone left over the posterior and middle fossa is successively drilled out. During this step, the cochlear aqueduct can be identified. This is an important landmark for the glossopharyngeal nerve, which lies immediately inferior to it. In small or medium-sized VSs, opening the cochlear aqueduct allows the cerebrospinal fluid (CSF) to drain. This does not occur in large tumors, because the duct is occluded by the tumor. After a wide exposure of the

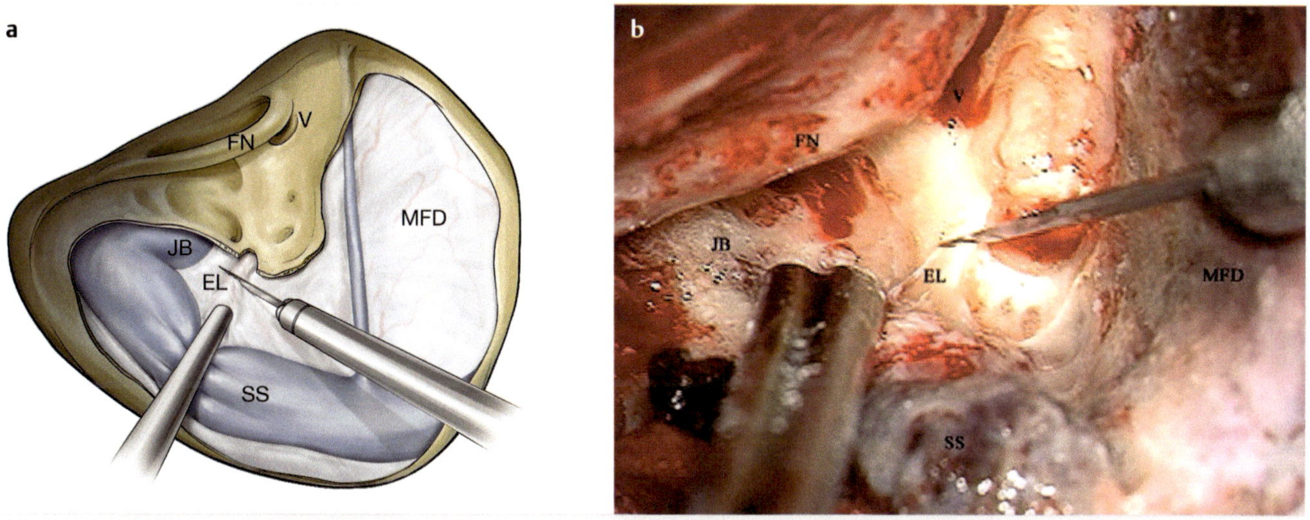

Fig. 34.8 A Beaver knife is used to cut sharply the endolymphatic duct (EL) to allow dural retraction. The semicircular canals have been drilled out and the vestibule (Ve) can be seen. FN, facial nerve; JB, jugular bulb; MFD, middle fossa dura; SS, sigmoid sinus.

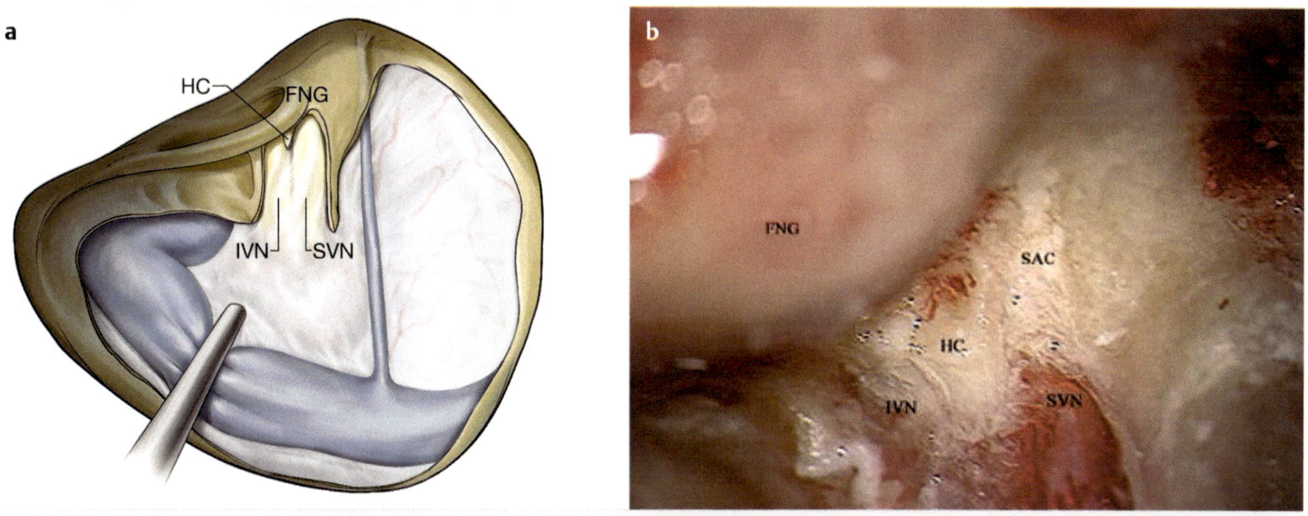

Fig. 34.9 The superior vestibular nerve (SVN) has been followed laterally into the superior ampullary nerve canal (SAC), where the superior ampullary nerve enters the lateral canal ampulla. FNG, facial nerve genu; HC, horizontal crest; I, incus; IVN, inferior vestibular nerve; LCA, ampulla of the lateral semicircular canal; SCA, ampulla of the superior semicircular canal.

dura is accomplished, following the posterior fossa dura allows the porus of the IAC to be identified. The ampulla of the superior semicircular canal serves as a landmark for the superior border of the IAC at the fundus. The inferior border of the canal is identified by drilling the retrofacial air cells up to the cochlear aqueduct. Further cautious drilling at the level of the fundus leads to the identification of the horizontal crest as well as the superior ampullary canal. Bone between the superior border of the IAC and the middle fossa dura and between the inferior border of the IAC and the jugular bulb can be further drilled, depending on the size of the tumor. We routinely drill the bone 270 degrees around the IAC (▶ Fig. 34.2).

Identification of the Facial Nerve at the Fundus

The original technique described by House for identifying the facial nerve at the fundus depends on the identification of the vertical crest (Bill's bar). However, we have modified this technique. By drilling inferiorly at the fundus, the inferior vestibular nerve is exposed, while in a more superior plane the horizontal crest is identified, which separates the inferior vestibular nerve from the superior vestibular nerve. The superior vestibular nerve is followed laterally where it leaves the fundus of the IAC. The nerve then lies in a tiny canal that enters the ampulla of the superior semicircular canal as the superior ampullary nerve (▶ Fig. 34.9). The superior ampullary nerve is dissected from its canal using a 90 degrees hook with the tip facing inferiorly (▶ Fig. 34.10a). The superior ampullary nerve is separated from the facial nerve by a vertical crest of bone, called Bill's bar, which protects the facial nerve while this step is being carried out. The hook is moved medially toward the fundus, with subsequent separation and establishment of a good plane of cleavage between the superior vestibular nerve and the anteriorly lying facial nerve. Once the superior ampullary nerve is detached and reflected medially and posteriorly, the facial

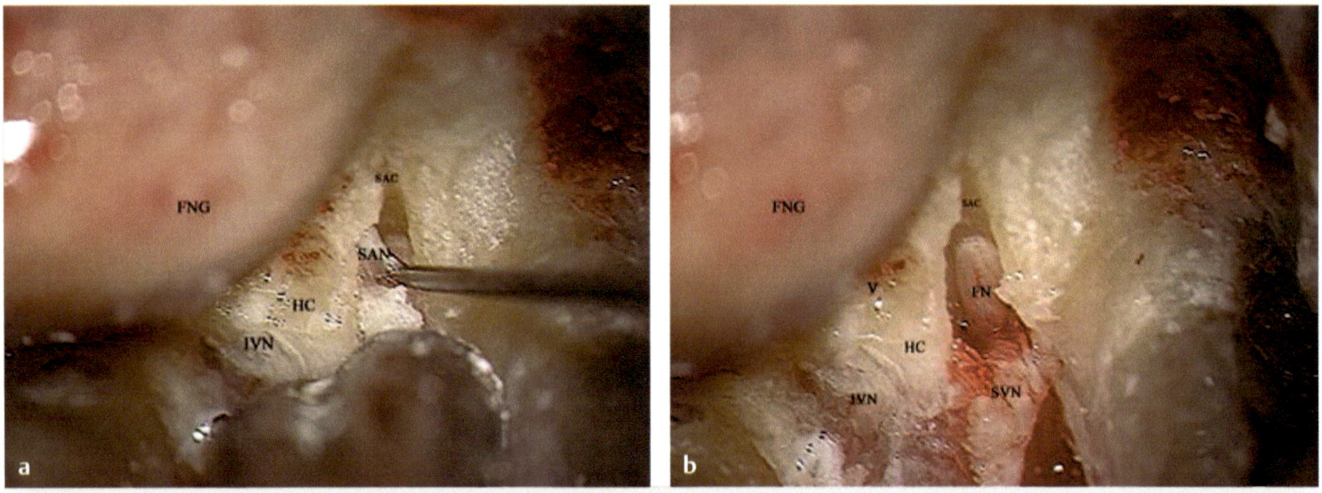

Fig. 34.10 (a) A small hook is used carefully to dislodge the superior ampullary nerve (SAN) from the superior ampullary canal (SAC). **(b)** After reflecting the superior vestibular nerve (SVN), the facial nerve (FN) can be seen anteriorly. FNG, facial nerve genu; HC, horizontal crest; I, incus; IVN, inferior vestibular nerve; LCA, ampulla of the lateral semicircular canal; SCA, ampulla of the superior semicircular canal; SVN, superior vestibular nerve; V, vestibule; VC, vertical crest (Bill's bar).

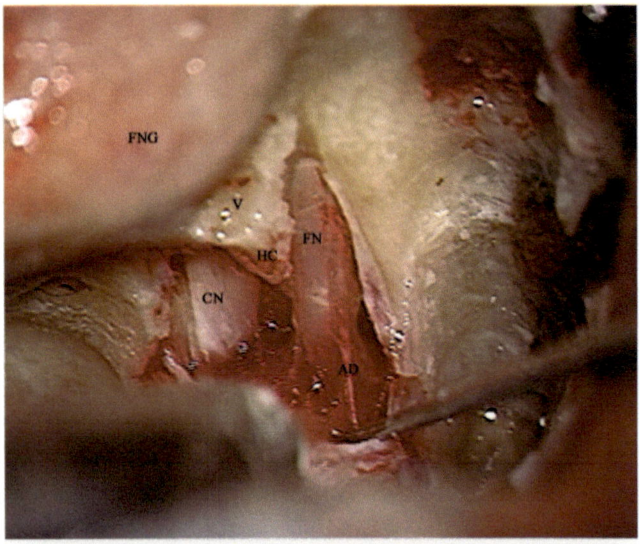

Fig. 34.11 While the dissection of the vestibular nerves is further progressed medially, adhesions (AD) between the facial nerve (FN) and the vestibular nerves start to be encountered. CN, cochlear nerve; FNG, facial nerve genu; HC, horizontal crest; I, incus; IVN, inferior vestibular nerve; LCA, ampulla of the lateral semicircular canal; SAN, superior ampullary nerve; SCA, ampulla of the superior semicircular canal; SVN, superior vestibular nerve; V, vestibule; VC, vertical crest (Bill's bar).

nerve can be clearly observed (▸ Fig. 34.10b). The relationship between the facial and cochlear nerves and the horizontal and vertical crests is well appreciated. Careful dissection of the superior vestibular nerve continues medially. Often, here, one may encounter adhesive bands between the superior vestibular nerve and the facial nerve (▸ Fig. 34.11), which may bleed on manipulation, thus obscuring the plane of dissection. To control this, a piece of dry Gelfoam is placed on the facial nerve, which also helps to protect the nerve during further dissection. Our technique of identification of the facial nerve by identification of the superior ampullary nerve and the horizontal crest rather than the vertical crest ensures proper identification and hence greater protection to the facial nerve.

Opening the Dura

Before opening the dura of the posterior fossa, the lines of incision are coagulated with a bipolar cautery. Careful coagulation over the dural surface leads to its retraction, thus providing wider access. In ▸ Fig. 34.12, the dotted red line represents the dural incision. Using the neurosurgical scissors, a small snip is made just anterior to the sigmoid sinus and immediately inferior to its junction with the superior petrosal sinus and the dura is opened. Once sufficient opening of the dura has been achieved, Merocel is inserted and slipped further in to protect the underlying structures while the dural incision is being completed. The superior dural incision runs parallel and just inferior to the superior petrosal sinus up to the limit of bony drilling. The inferior incision starts just in front of the distal part of the sigmoid sinus, and follows the sinus and jugular bulb course to the porus, where it joins the superior incision.

Bloodless Techniques for Tumor Removal

After the dura has been opened, the tumor in the CPA can be visualized, and the arachnoid of the lateral cistern is identified and opened. This allows CSF to drain out, leading to relaxation of cerebellum, which results in an increased working space. In the case of a large tumor, it is difficult to achieve this due to compression of the cistern by the tumor (▸ Fig. 34.13). In large tumors, they may be debulked at the center to reduce their size. Intracapsular debulking is performed by using microscissors and bipolar coagulation. It is extremely important to find the plane of cleavage that lies between the arachnoid adherent to the tumor capsule and the arachnoid surrounding the other structures in the CPA. Once this plane of cleavage has been obtained, Gelfoam is placed on this plane to prevent blood from entering the CPA (▸ Fig. 34.14). The outer surface of the tumor is coagulated using a bipolar. Using this maneuver in all the

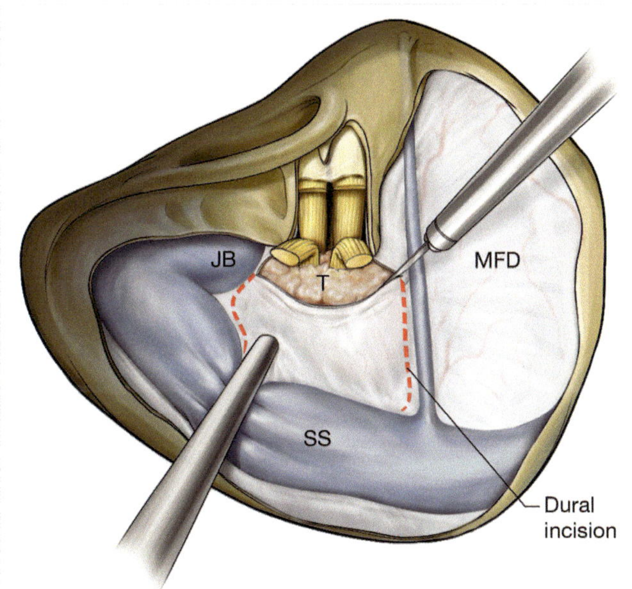

Fig. 34.12 Bipolar coagulation of the posterior fossa dura is done before incision of the dura. The dashed lines indicate the outlines of the dural incision. D, dura; JB, jugular bulb; PFD, posterior fossa dura; SS, sigmoid sinus.

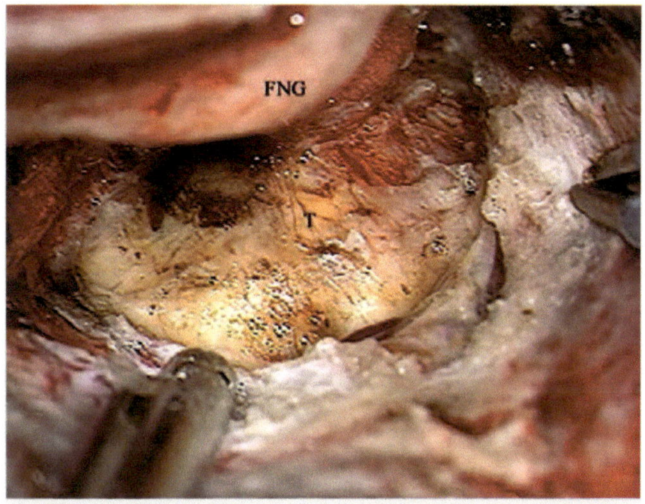

Fig. 34.13 After opening in the dura, the tumor (T) can be seen filling the cerebellopontine angle. FNG, facial nerve genu.

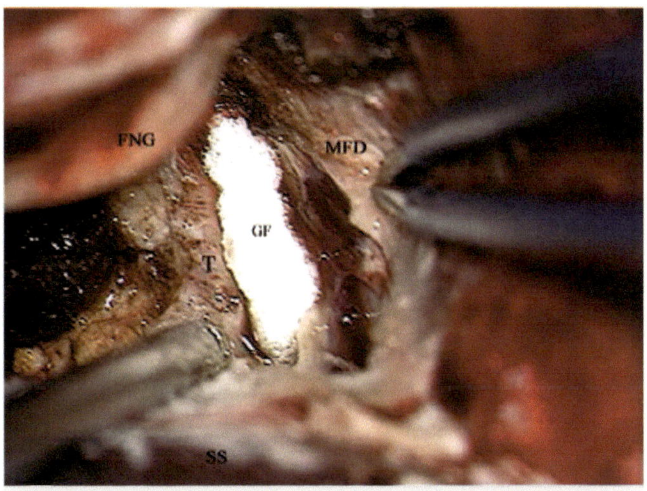

Fig. 34.14 After coagulating the arachnoid at the superior surface of the tumor (T), a plane of cleavage is looked for. A large piece of Gelfoam (GF) is used to fill the gap around the tumor (T) to prevent blood from filling the CPA. FNG, facial nerve genu; MFD, middle fossa dura; SS, sigmoid sinus.

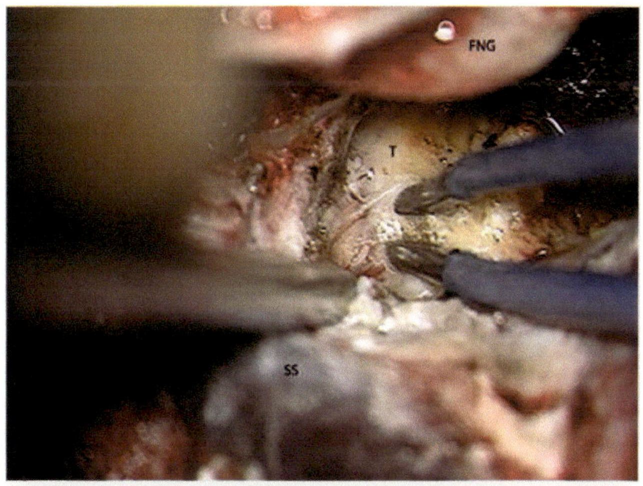

Fig. 34.15 The outer surface of the tumor is coagulated from all directions to achieve adequate tumor retraction from surrounding tissues. FNG, facial nerve genu; MFD, middle fossa dura; SS, sigmoid sinus; T, tumor; Tent, tentorium.

directions, the tumor retracts and comes separated from the surrounding structures.

The superior surface of the tumor is dissected (▶ Fig. 34.15). The trigeminal nerve is frequently found adherent to the tumor. The tumor surface is repeatedly coagulated and incised, thereby reducing the size of the tumor. The posterior aspect is further dissected and the interface between the tumor and the brainstem can be perceived. Tumor is then dissected from the facial nerve. Since the plane of cleavage between the tumor and the facial nerve has already been established at the fundus of the IAC, dissection proceeds in a lateral to medial direction. Localization of the facial nerve at the porus is achieved by following it from the fundus (▶ Fig. 34.16). Care should be taken not to force any traction on the facial nerve while carrying out the dissection. At the level of the porus, the facial nerve is usually adherent to the tumor and frequently becomes thin and splayed, thereby becoming vulnerable. Very gentle manipulation is necessary in this step (▶ Fig. 34.17). The facial nerve at the level of the brainstem is then identified and the last part of the tumor is carefully dissected from the facial nerve and the brainstem. It is important to neither coagulate nor apply traction to these important structures (▶ Fig. 34.18). The integrity of the facial nerve is determined using the facial nerve stimulator at the root exit zone. The anesthetist raises the blood pressure, and a Valsalva maneuver is performed to evaluate for bleeding points. Meticulous hemostasis is achieved.

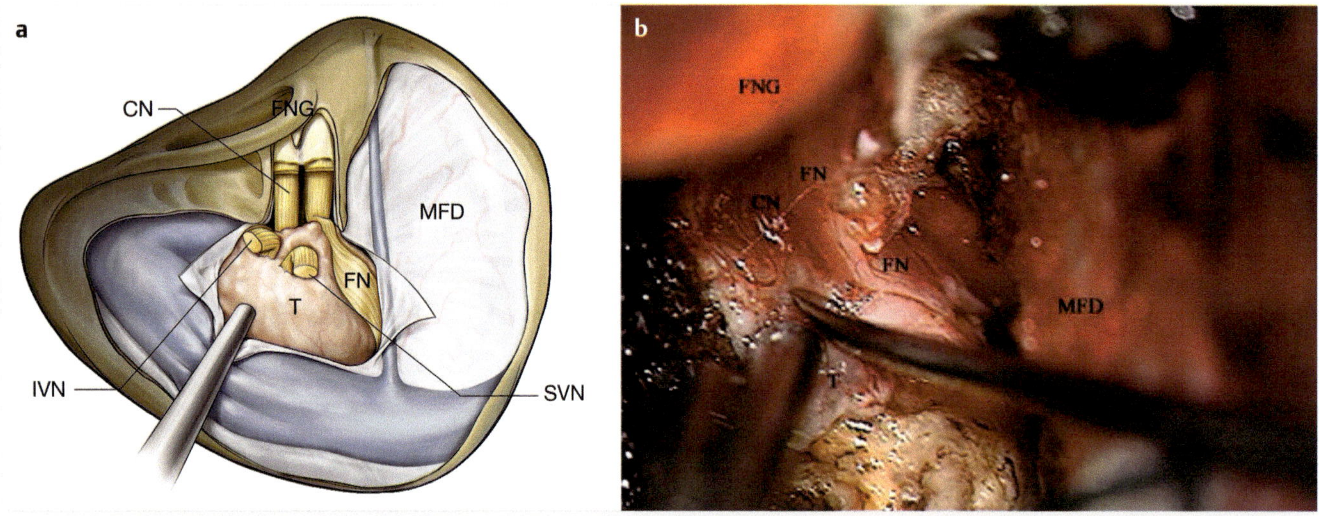

Fig. 34.16 The facial nerve (FN) can be followed from within the internal auditory canal, and it can be seen angulating anteriorly over the porus and lying adherent to the anterior surface of the tumor (T). The identification in this area where the nerve is usually adherent to the surrounding structures can be achieved with the help of transapical extension. CN, cochlear nerve; FNG, facial nerve genu; MFD, middle fossa dura; SS, sigmoid sinus; V, trigeminal nerve; VNs, superior and inferior vestibular nerves.

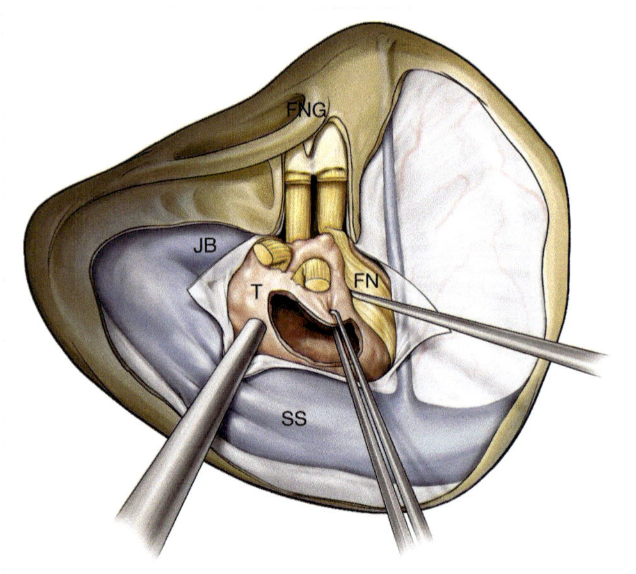

Fig. 34.17 After reducing the core and the walls of the tumor, dissection of the facial nerve is continued. Very delicate maneuvers are made in this area. FNG, facial nerve genu; MFD, middle fossa dura; SS, sigmoid sinus; T, tumor.

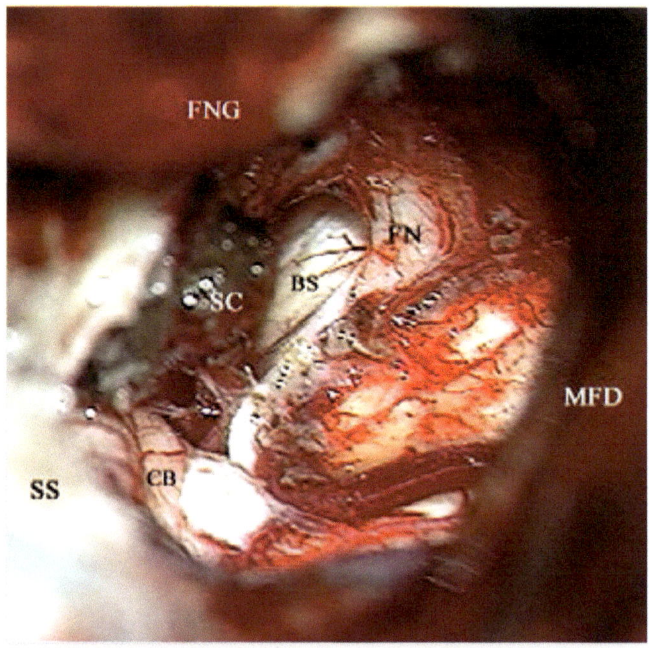

Fig. 34.18 CPA after total tumor removal. Note the integrity of the facial nerve (FN) together with its vasculature. BS, brainstem; CB, cerebellum; FNG, facial nerve genu; MFD, middle fossa dura; SC, Surgicel; SS, sigmoid sinus.

Closure

All the air cells, especially the retrofacial cells, should be observed to see if they have communication with the tympanic cavity. If so, these cells are obliterated with bone wax to avoid CSF leak postoperatively. After the incus is disarticulated and removed, the aditus is obliterated with periosteum. Abdominal fat which has been harvested is sliced into several long, thin strips, and these strips are placed inside the CPA. The musculoperiosteal layer is closed using 1–0 Vicryl (▶ Fig. 34.19). This is followed by closure of the subcutaneous tissue and skin. A pressure dressing is applied. Using this approach, our group has experienced less than a 1% rate of postoperative CSF leak.

In our experience with the ETLA, tumors of very large sizes in the CPA can be safely removed. Wide removal of bone from the middle fossa dura, as well as extensive drilling of bone between it and the IAC, provides excellent control of the upper pole of

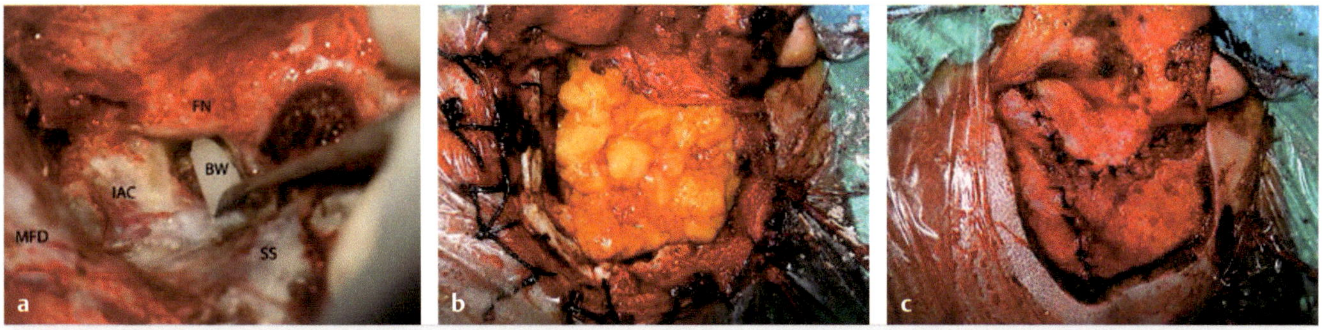

Fig. 34.19 (a) In a pneumatized temporal bone, cells superiorly and inferiorly to the internal auditory canal are obliterated with bone wax. BW, bone wax; FN, facial nerve; IAC, internal auditory canal; JB, jugular bulb; SS, sigmoid sinus. **(b)** Abdominal fat is used to close the CPA and the bony defect. **(c)** The musculoperiosteal layer is approximated using 1–0 Vicryl. After the musculoperiosteal layer is closed tightly, the skin flap is replaced and sutured.

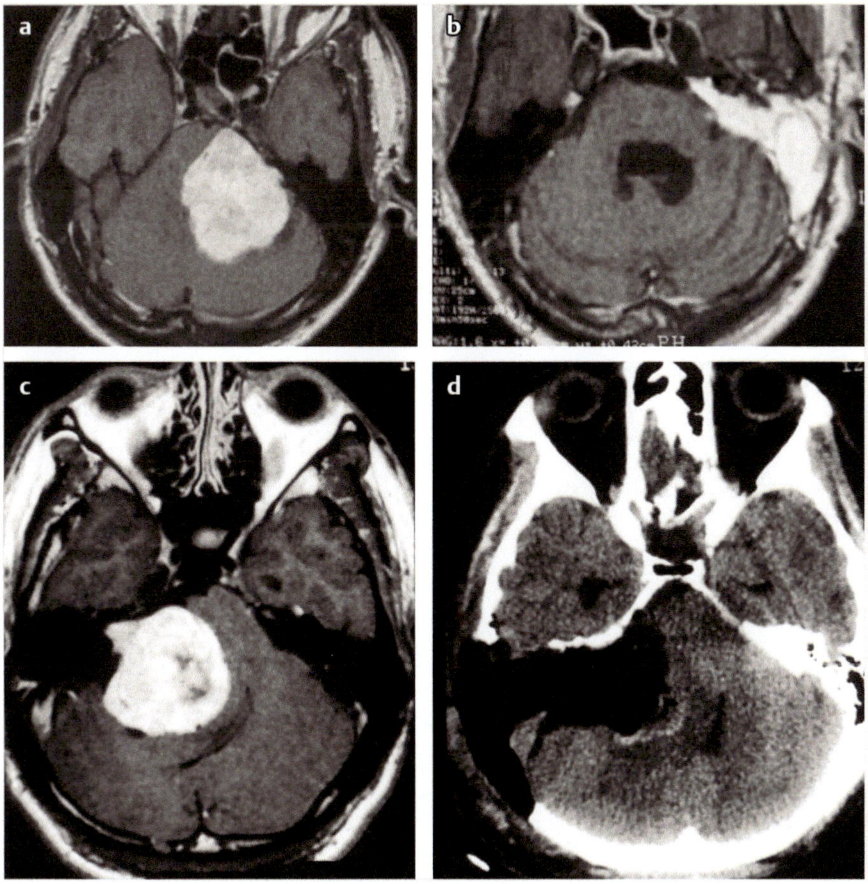

Fig. 34.20 Preoperative **(a)** and 1-week postoperative **(b)** MRI scan of a large tumor which was removed totally with the ETLA. Preoperative **(c)** and 1-year postoperative **(d)** scans of another patient with a similarly large tumor excised using a similar approach. Note that fat is inserted up to the petrous apex.

the tumor and the trigeminal nerve area. Uncovering the sigmoid sinus and bone 2 to 3 cm posterior to it, and extensive bone removal creating a deep trough inferior to the IAC, obviates the need for a suboccipital or transotic approach, and provides good control of the anterior pole of the tumor up to the lateral aspect of the prepontine cistern. In addition, extensive removal of bone between the IAC and the jugular bulb allows good visualization of the lower tumor pole. Tumors up to 6 cm in extrameatal diameter have been safely removed using this approach (▶ Fig. 34.20).

34.2.5 Pearls

- Completely uncovering the middle fossa dura, posterior fossa dura, sigmoid sinus, and the retrosigmoid area is the most important aspect of the ETLA. Uncovering the above-mentioned structures allows retraction and hence better visualization of all aspects of the tumor.
- The facial nerve lies immediately lateral to the vestibule. Utmost care should be taken not to injure the nerve during drilling to open the vestibule.

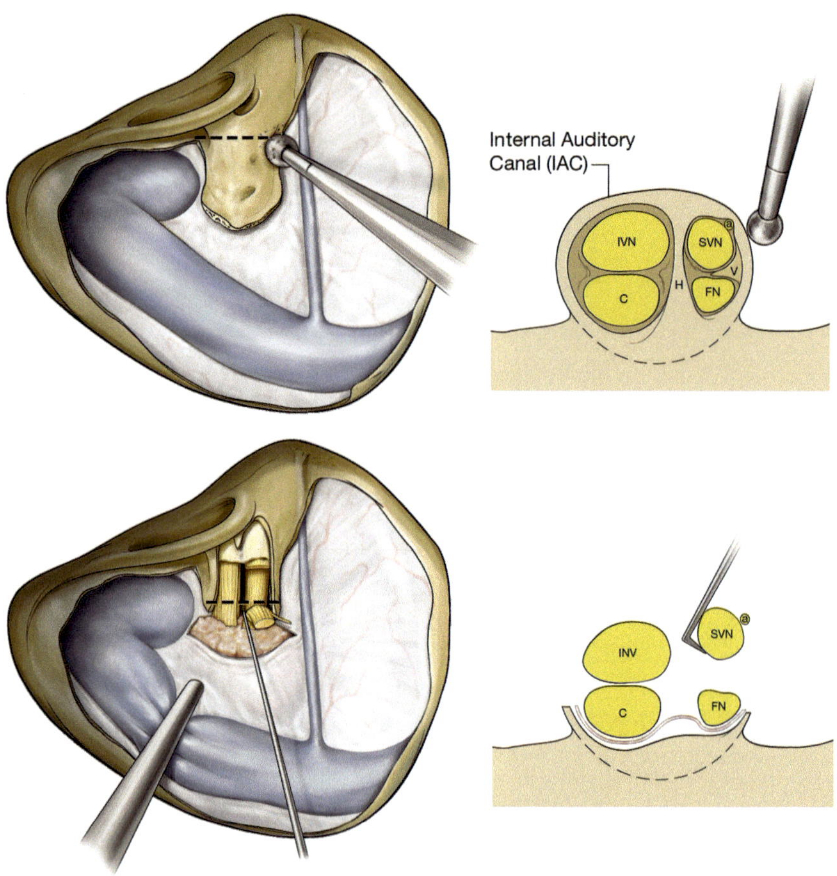

Fig. 34.21 In our technique, we first identify the superior ampullary nerve and then look for the facial nerve (FN) after dissecting out along the superior vestibular nerve. In the conventional technique described by House, the vertical crest (Bill's bar) is identified by drilling behind the superior vestibular nerve.

- The IAC should be uncovered over 270 to 310 degrees in the ETLA, creating two troughs—inferior and superior to the IAC. Sufficient removal of bone superior to the IAC is essential in order to control the area of the trigeminal nerve. Failure to do so leads to incomplete control of the superior pole of the tumor and of Dandy's vein.
- The fundus of the IAC is approached by first identifying the inferior vestibular nerve and the horizontal crest instead of the vertical crest (Bill's bar) as in the conventional TLA (▶ Fig. 34.21). Then, the superior vestibular nerve is identified and the drilling is continued laterally until the ampullary nerve is identified. Once the ampullary nerve is identified at the level of the fundus, it is dissected out and the vertical crest (Bill's bar) is identified medial to it. The facial nerve is then identified medial to Bill's bar.
- Facial nerve monitoring is helpful during tumor dissection. A train response given by the monitor indicates possible trauma to the facial nerve.
- It is important to maintain a bloodless surgical field in order to clearly visualize all vital anatomy at all times. This is ensured by dissecting the cleavage plane between the tumor surface and the arachnoid and by bipolar coagulation of the veins and small arteries on the tumor surface. Once a plane is identified, Merocel is inserted between the tumor and the arachnoid. Dissection proceeds with bipolar dissection of the tumor.
- During closure, long strips of abdominal fat are used to obliterate the CPA along with the bony defect. This is more effective in preventing CSF leakage than using the fat to obliterate the bone defect alone.
- Tumors up to 6 cm in extrameatal diameter can be safely removed using this approach.

34.2.6 Pitfalls

- The use of self-retaining retractors for the skin and subcutaneous tissue is not recommended. Retractors impede surgical access, leading to narrow working angle and deeper surgical field.
- Central debulking is important in dealing with a big tumor. Care should be taken while debulking soft or cystic tumors, so as not to penetrate the anterior or medial walls of the tumor capsule and injure the adjacent structures, particularly the facial nerve and the brainstem.
- In small tumors, the anterior inferior cerebellar artery (AICA) can be found looping around the tumor. It can also commonly traverse between the facial nerve and the vestibulocochlear nerves.
- Toward the end of surgery, care should be taken while removing the incus to avoid fracturing the footplate, since this can create a communication between the CPA and the middle ear, with subsequent postoperative CSF leakage. We prefer periosteum to fat for the closure of the attic because it is easier to manipulate and provides a better, longer lasting seal.

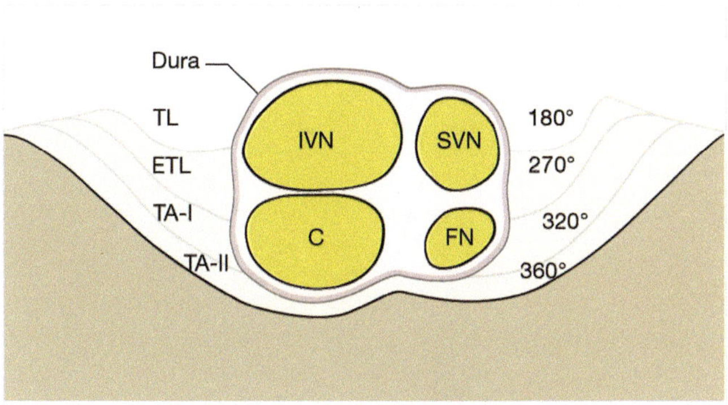

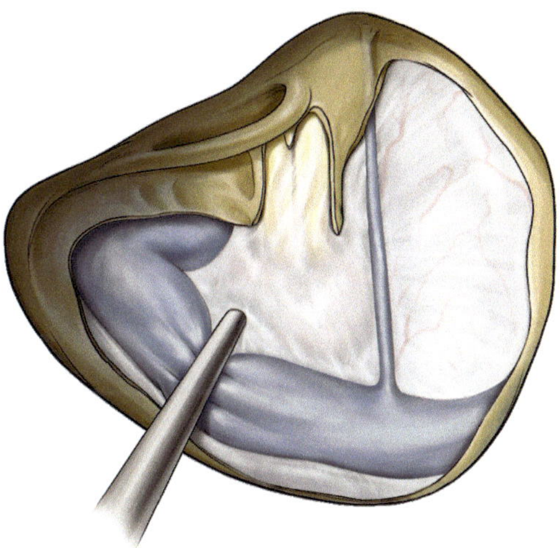

Fig. 34.22 Amount of bone removal around the internal auditory canal in the different variations of the TLA. The gray lines demonstrates the working area for extended bone removal. C, cochlear nerve; ETL, enlarged translabyrinthine; FN, facial nerve; IVN, inferior vestibular nerve; SVN, superior vestibular nerve; TA-1, enlarged translabyrinthine with transapical extension type 1; TA-2, enlarged translabyrinthine with transapical extension type 2; TL, translabyrinthine

34.3 Enlarged TLA with Transapical Extension

34.3.1 Rationale

The enlarged TLA with transapical extension (ETLA + TAE) approach is an anteromedial extension of the ETLA, in which the IAC is drilled up to 320 degrees (type I) or 360 degrees (type II) of its circumference of the IAC (▶ Fig. 34.22). This extension helps expose the anterior, superior, and medial aspects of large tumors of the CPA.

34.3.2 Indications

This approach is indicated for large CPA tumors or tumors with marked anterior extension, wherein hearing preservation is not intended. This includes large or giant VSs with anterior extension into the prepontine cistern and large meningioma of the posterior surface of the temporal bone centered on the IAC with significant anterior extension. It is also indicated in smaller tumors when marked anterior extension is present.

34.3.3 Limitations

Though this approach provides access to the prepontine cistern, it is difficult to remove tumors involving the petroclival region, such as meningiomas, wherein the modified transcochlear approach is more suitable.

34.3.4 Surgical Technique

The ETLA is performed as previously described. The IAC is identified and uncovered and bone is drilled out for 270 degrees around the canal, as previously described. Further drilling is carried superior and inferior to the IAC toward the petrous apex as required (▶ Fig. 34.23a). In the type I approach, up to 320-degree exposure around the IAC is achieved (▶ Fig. 34.23b) leaving behind a thin segment of bone anteriorly. In the type II approach, 360 degrees of the IAC circumference is exposed (▶ Fig. 34.23c). The contents of the IAC are pushed inferiorly to allow for drilling of the anterior wall of the canal (▶ Fig. 34.24). Care should be taken to avoid injury to the superior petrosal sinus. The dura is opened as previously described.

34.3.5 Pearls

- In the case of tumors extending far anteromedially, the facial nerve is markedly displaced anteriorly. The transapical extension provides enhanced visualization of the nerve.
- In the case of giant tumors causing high intracranial pressure, the dura usually bulges, hindering access. In such cases, the tumor is first debulked from inside and after this the dura is opened to allow drainage of the CSF, which leads to drop in pressure and retraction of intracranial contents.
- After introducing this approach, we have abandoned the transotic approach for removal of anteriorly located tumors limiting its use only in the case of tumors with cochlear invasion, vertical internal carotid artery involvement, or in case with very high jugular bulb and/or very advanced sigmoid sinus.

34.3.6 Pitfalls

- The facial nerve is at risk while performing the transapical drilling. Hence, a diamond burr must be used and extreme care must be taken to avoid injuring the nerve. A useful trick is to place the suction-irrigator between the drill and the nerve to afford protection.
- Care must be taken to avoid injuring the superior petrosal sinus while drilling the petrous apex superior to the IAC.

34.3.7 Difficult Situations and Special Considerations in the ETLA

Despite this being a safe surgery, one can nevertheless encounter difficult situations and complications. These problems may arise either during the approach or during removal of tumor and may be due to anatomical variants, mishaps during surgery, or tumor characteristics.

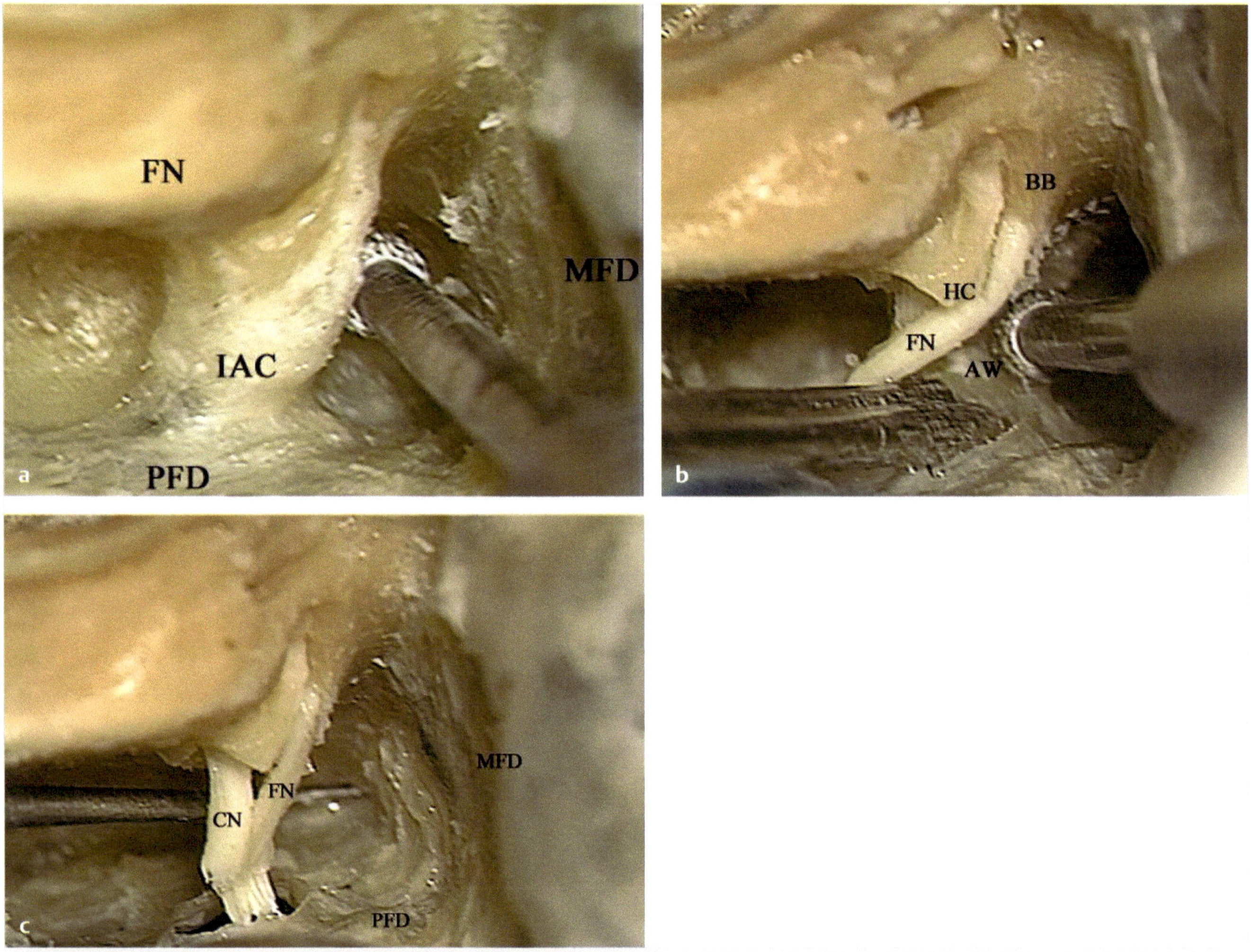

Fig. 34.23 Extended TLA **(a)** with TAE type I **(b)** and type II **(c)**. AW, anterior wall; BB, Bill's bar; CN, cochlear nerve; FN, facial nerve; HC, horizontal crest; IAC, internal auditory canal; MFD, middle fossa dura; PFD, posterior fossa dura.

High Jugular Bulb

A high jugular bulb is encountered in about 25% of cases (▶ Fig. 34.25). This may obstruct the view of the area around the lower cranial nerves. In such cases, the following steps may be followed. After the dome of the jugular bulb is completely exposed (▶ Fig. 34.26), it is gently dissected along with the periosteal layer from its wall, taking care to avoid injury to the thin bulb wall (▶ Fig. 34.27). Then the dome of the jugular bulb is pressed downward using a large piece of Surgicel and tucked in place between the bulb and the surrounding bone. Surgicel helps to control the minor bleeding that may occur during this step. A piece of bone wax is then placed over the Surgicel to keep the bulb in place and prevent entanglement of Surgicel with the burr during further drilling (▶ Fig. 34.28). By adequate inferior displacement of the jugular bulb, drilling can be safely carried out and additional surrounding bone can be removed to achieve additional exposure.

Anterior Sigmoid Sinus and Bleeding from the Sigmoid Sinus and Jugular Bulb

In the case of a forward-lying or a prominent sigmoid, it is imperative to preoperatively assess the contralateral venous drainage. If the drainage is insufficient, then working on the dominant sigmoid may be dangerous and even life threatening. One must consider avoiding surgery if possible, or if it has to be performed, it must be done so with extreme caution so as to not damage the dominant sinus. In cases with a very anterior sigmoid sinus, the retrosigmoid corridor may be particularly spacious.

Removal of bone over the sigmoid and 2 to 3 cm posterior to it over the posterior fossa dura enables the surgeon to compress any forward-lying sigmoid posteriorly. In a very prominent sigmoid, the posterior canal wall and the hypotympanic bone can be drilled out, followed by a blind sac closure, to gain additional space. It is best to place cotton patties on the sigmoid to protect

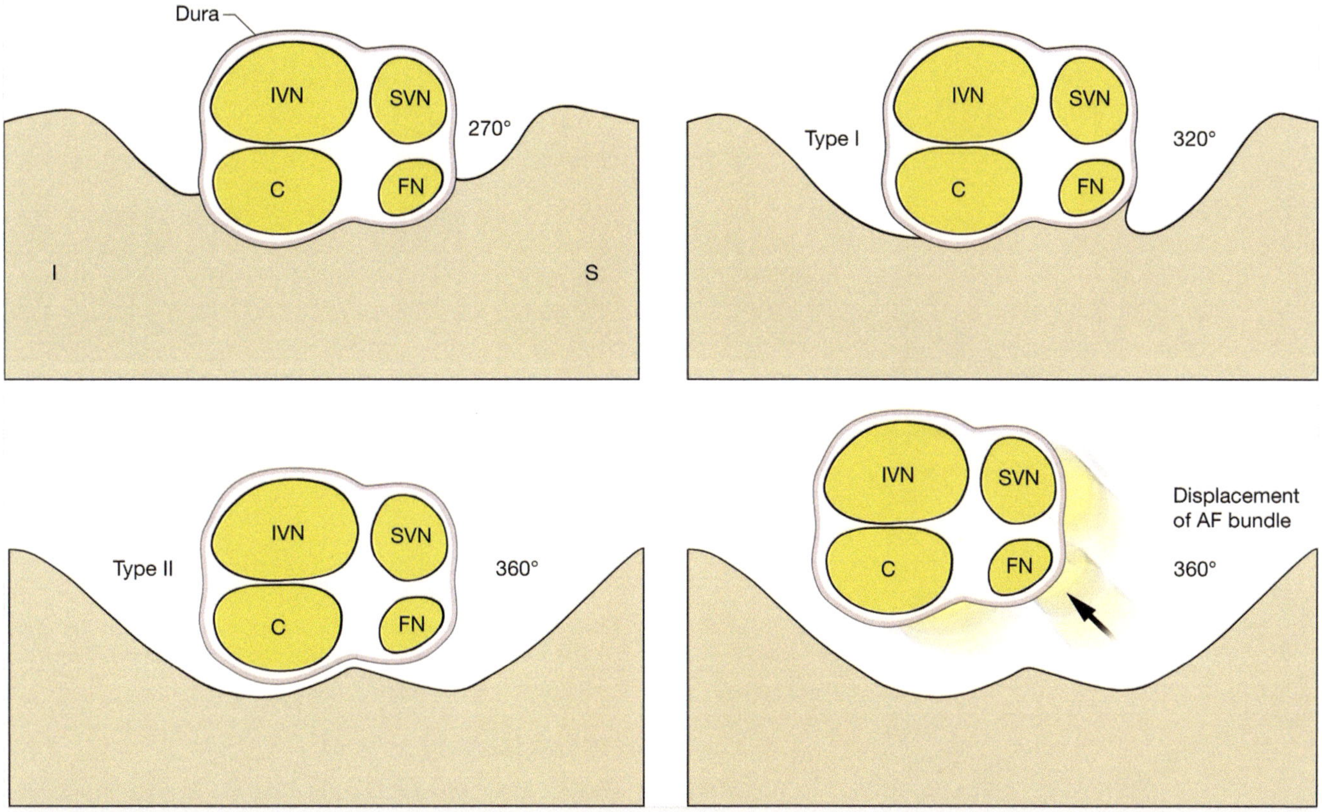

Fig. 34.24 Cross-sectional images of the internal auditory canal as seen in the ETLA exposure (270 degrees), type I (300–320 degrees), and type II TAE (360 degrees). The contents of the internal auditory canal can be moved inferiorly. C, cochlear nerve; FN, facial nerve; IVN, inferior vestibular nerve; SVN, superior vestibular nerve

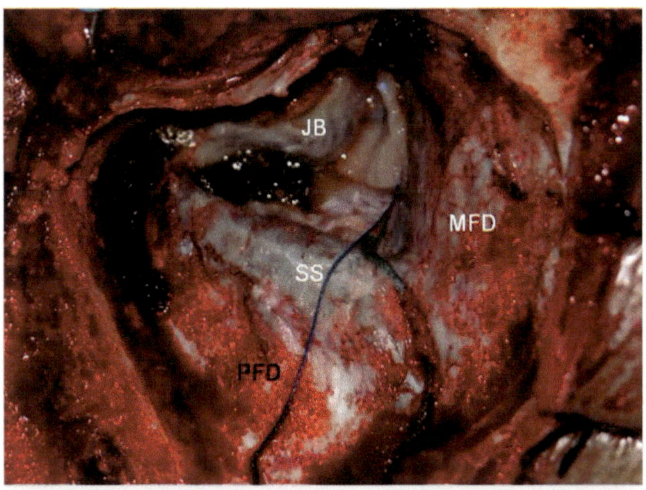

Fig. 34.25 A case of an extremely high jugular bulb that reaches the level of the labyrinth. JB, jugular bulb; MFD: middle fossa dura; PFD, posterior fossa dura; SS, sigmoid sinus.

it from the friction and heat of the instruments working over it. Small tears on the sigmoid can be controlled using bipolar coagulation. The bipolar is switched to a low setting, the edges of the tear are approximated with the bipolar tips (as if being welded), and coagulation is carried out under continuous suction irrigation. If bleeding cannot be stopped with bipolar, it can be controlled by extraluminal placement of a large piece of Gelfoam or Surgicel supported by neurosurgical Cottonoids. Large tears can be closed by suturing a free muscle graft to close the tear. Despite all these, if the bleeding is still not controlled, ligation of sigmoid sinus and internal jugular vein is the last option. This has never occurred in our practice. Bleeding from the superior petrosal sinus can be managed easily by coagulation or intraluminal packing. However, bleeding from the jugular bulb may be more challenging. Significant bleeding usually ensues after injury to the jugular bulb. Bipolar coagulation must not be attempted here, as it leads to further tearing of the very thin bulb wall and risks lower cranial nerve injury. Bleeding is best controlled by a large piece of Surgicel placed over the bulb and held in place with bone wax or Cottonoids.

Position of the Facial Nerve In Relation to the Tumor

Both the literature and our own experience indicate that by far the commonest location of the facial nerve in relation to the tumor is the anteroinferior surface of the tumor capsule. The facial nerve can be found in this position in almost 70% of cases. In 15% of cases, the facial nerve can be found adjacent to the anterosuperior surface and in another 10% it can be found adjacent to the superior surface. In the remaining 5%, the facial nerve lies on the posterior surface (▶ Fig. 34.29). There are

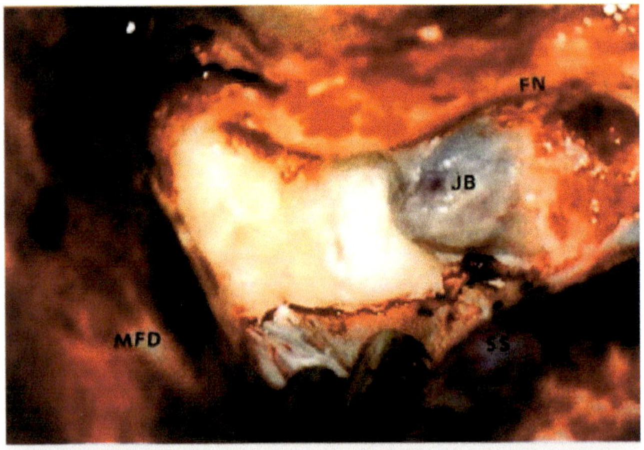

Fig. 34.26 The high bulb is uncovered. FN, facial nerve; JB, jugular bulb; MFD, middle fossa dura; SS, sigmoid sinus.

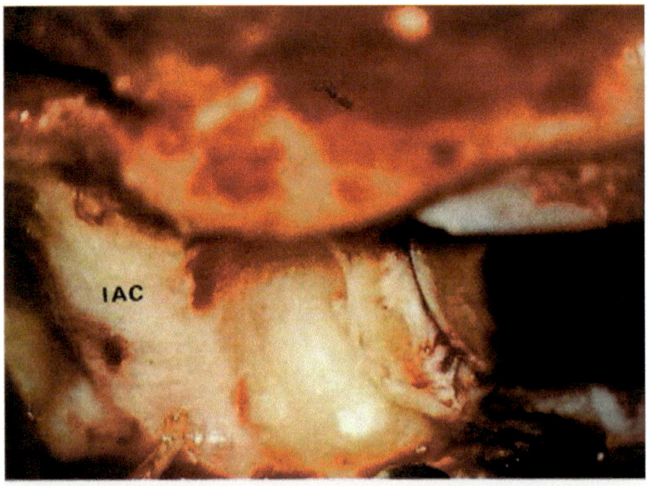

Fig. 34.27 The bulb is dissected using a large freer elevator. IAC, internal auditory canal.

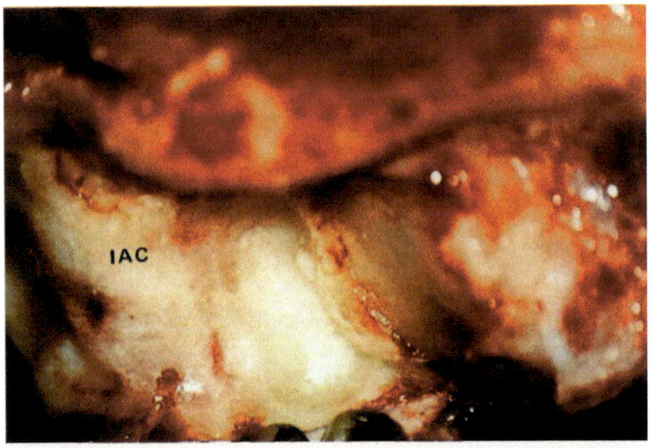

Fig. 34.28 The bulb is kept in place using Surgical and bone wax. IAC, internal auditory canal.

three sites where the facial nerve must be identified during surgery: fundus, porus, and at the level of origin of the nerve at the brainstem. The facial nerve is fairly consistent at two of these sites: the fundus of the IAC and its origin at the level of the brainstem when compared with the porus. It is prudent to identify the nerve at the fundus first, followed by the porus and the brainstem. At the porus, the tumor may cause an acute change in the thickness and direction of the nerve due to compression and adherence of the nerve to tumor (▶ Fig. 34.30). After the visual identification of the nerve, the facial nerve stimulator must be used for confirmation. Since the facial nerve in the CPA lacks the thick perineural and fibrous sheaths covering the facial nerve more distally, the lowest intensity of stimulation is used for identification.

Anterior Inferior Cerebellar Artery

Usually, large tumors tend to displace the AICA toward the inferior pole of the tumor. In some cases, the AICA may be displaced posteriorly or laterally. Rarely but more importantly, the vessel can be encountered just under the posterior fossa dura, where it is vulnerable to injury during dural incision. When the AICA is intimately in contact with the tumor, the artery is separated from the tumor by coagulating the small branches arising from the artery feeding the tumor.

Petrosal (Dandy's) Vein

Significant bleeding can arise due to injury of the petrosal vein (s). The vein can be protected during dissection of the upper pole of the tumor by keeping the arachnoid over the vein undisturbed. If bleeding does occur, it can be stopped using bipolar coagulation. Generally, no hazardous effects result from occlusion of this vein.

Tumors Associated with Arachnoid Cysts

Extratumoral arachnoid cysts result in the enclosure of arachnoid folds during tumor growth and they can often grow to a large size. Before tumor removal, the cyst is evacuated, if possible, to facilitate brain relaxation and tumor removal. An extratumoral arachnoid cyst must be differentiated from a macrocystic tumor with a thin wall. Generally, the thickness of the wall and enhancement on magnetic resonance imaging (MRI) help distinguish these two entities. The arachnoid cyst can be marsupialized, while a cystic tumor wall should be removed to prevent recurrence.

Cystic, Heterogeneous, and Irregular Tumors

Cystic tumors (▶ Fig. 34.31) are difficult to dissect due to the fact that these tumors are usually adherent to the surrounding nerves and brainstem. This also leaves the facial nerve at considerable risk. At times, it is advisable to leave behind the capsule on the facial nerve and the brainstem. VSs that are heterogeneous in appearance and/or irregular in shape are usually indicative of their fast-growing nature (▶ Fig. 34.32). Such tumors are also adherent to the surrounding structures, posing the same problems of risk of facial nerve injury.

Tumor Resection after Prior Radiation Failure

In recent times, radiotherapy has emerged as a primary treatment option for VS. Surgical removal of irradiated tumors is

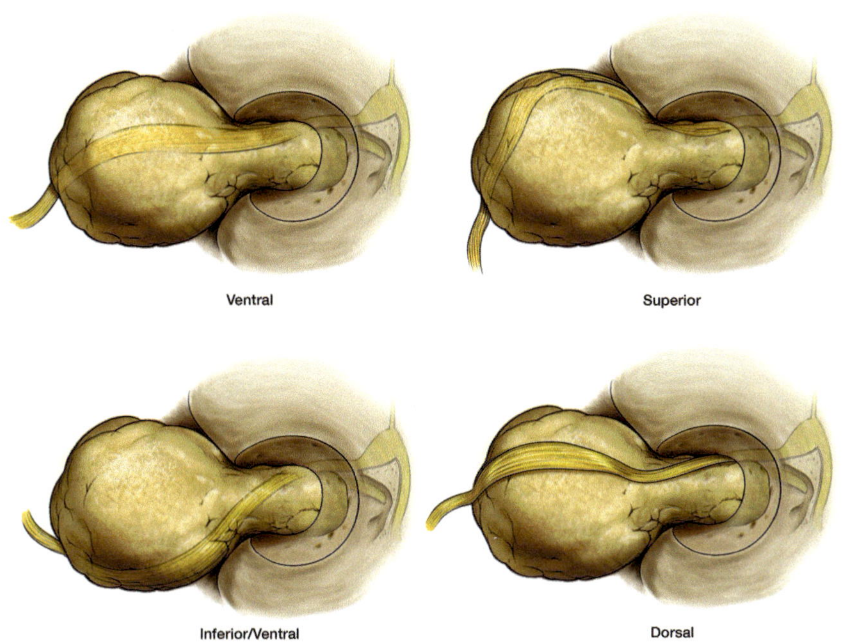

Fig. 34.29 The possible locations of the facial nerve (FN) in relation to the tumor.

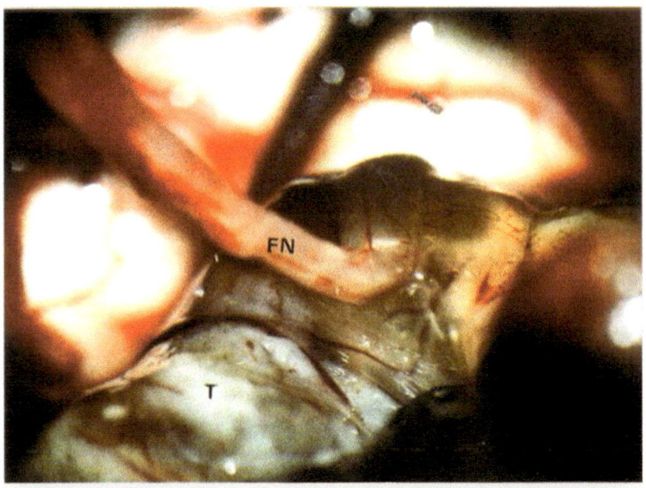

Fig. 34.30 The position of the facial nerve (FN) at the porus of the internal auditory canal is less consistent. An acute change of direction on the anterior surface of the tumor is observed.

more difficult than primary tumor resection. Usually, the arachnoid–tumor plane is nonexistent and the tumor is more adherent to the surrounding structures than nonirradiated tumors. The tumor is also usually more fibrous and firmer, making the dissection difficult. Chapter 44 reviews the topic of microsurgery after radiosurgery in greater detail.

34.4 Conclusion

The ETLA is a safe approach that provides excellent exposure for even very large tumors. The distinct advantages provided by the ETLAs are: the absence of cerebellar retraction, excellent exposure of the IAC and the CPA, extradural drilling, and reduced incidence of postoperative CSF leaks. The ETLA and the ETLA + TAE have further increased the indications of the approach and help tackled large, giant, and anteromedially located tumors more effectively. Difficult anatomical and tumor-related situations can also be managed effectively with the ETLA.

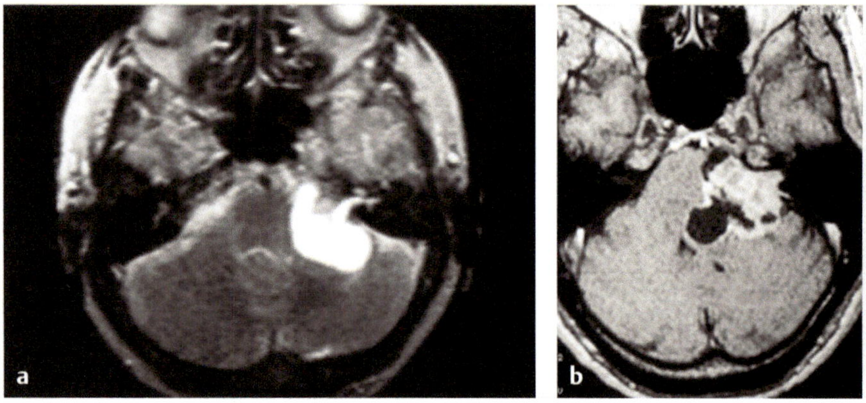

Fig. 34.31 MRI of a cystic VS. **(a)** The T2-weighted image does not show the characteristics of the tumor. **(b)** However, T1 with Gd enhancement can clearly demonstrate the tumor capsule and cystic components.

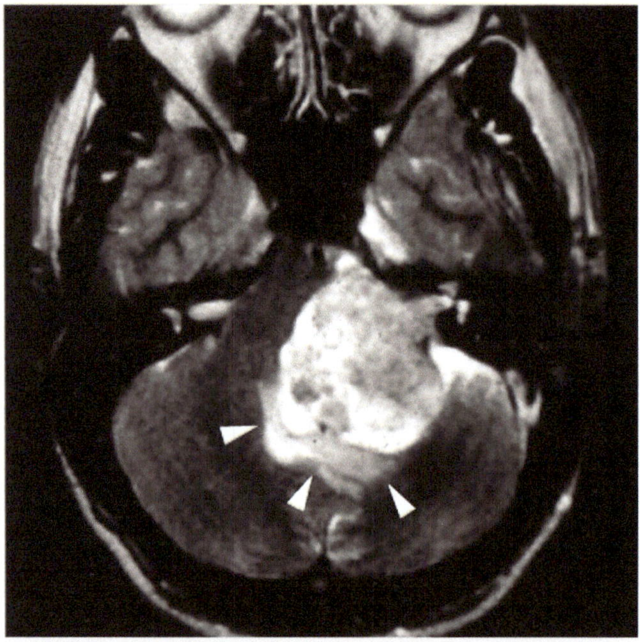

Fig. 34.32 MRI of a heterogeneous VS. This tumor is extensive and extends to the prepontine region. Planes of cleavage are not identifiable, inferring adherence to the brainstem and cerebellum (*arrowheads*).

References

[1] Ben Ammar M, Piccirillo E, Topsakal V, Taibah A, Sanna M. Surgical results and technical refinements in translabyrinthine excision of vestibular schwannomas: the Gruppo Otologico experience. Neurosurgery. 2012; 70(6): 1481–1491, discussion 1491

[2] House WF, Hitselberger WE. transtemporal bone microsurgical removal of acoustic neuromas. Morbidity and mortality of acoustic neuromas. Arch Otolaryngol. 1964; 80:752–754

[3] House WF, Belal A, Jr. Translabyrinthine surgery: anatomy and pathology. Am J Otol. 1980; 1(4):189–198

[4] House WF. Translabyrinthine approach. In: House WF, Luetje CM, eds. Acoustic Tumors. Baltimore, MD: University Parke-Davis; 1979

[5] Hitselberger WE, House WF. Transtemporal bone microsurgical removal of acoustic neuromas. Tumors of the cerebellopontine angle. Arch Otolaryngol. 1964; 80:720–731

[6] Hardy DG, Macfarlane R, Baguley D, Moffat DA. Surgery for acoustic neurinoma. An analysis of 100 translabyrinthine operations. J Neurosurg. 1989; 71(6):799–804

[7] Angeli RD, Piccirillo E, Di Trapani G, Sequino G, Taibah A, Sanna M. Enlarged translabyrinthine approach with transapical extension in the management of giant vestibular schwannomas: personal experience and review of literature. Otol Neurotol. 2011; 32(1):125–131

[8] Sanna M, Russo A, Taibah A, Falcioni M, Agarwal M. Enlarged translabyrinthine approach for the management of large and giant acoustic neuromas: a report of 175 consecutive cases. Ann Otol Rhinol Laryngol. 2004; 113(4): 319–328

[9] Falcioni M, Russo A, Mancini F, et al. Enlarged translabyrinthine approach in large acoustic neurinomas [in Italian]. Acta Otorhinolaryngol Ital. 2001; 21 (4):226–236

[10] Naguib MB, Saleh E, Cokkeser Y, et al. The enlarged translabyrinthine approach for removal of large vestibular schwannomas. J Laryngol Otol. 1994; 108(7):545–550

[11] House WF, Hitselberger WE. The transcochlear approach to the skull base. Arch Otolaryngol. 1976; 102(6):334–342

[12] Chen JM, Fisch U. The transotic approach in acoustic neuroma surgery. J Otolaryngol. 1993; 22(5):331–336

[13] Browne JD, Fisch U. Transotic approach to the cerebellopontine angle. Otolaryngol Clin North Am. 1992; 25(2):331–346

[14] Sanna MMF, Russo A, Taibah A, Falcioni M, Di Trapani G. Atlas of Acoustic Neurinoma Microsurgery. Stuttgart: Georg Thieme Verlag; 2008

[15] Gantz BJ, Fisch U. Modified transotic approach to the cerebellopontile angle. Arch Otolaryngol. 1983; 109(4):252–256

[16] Rabelo de Freitas M, Russo A, Sequino G, Piccirillo E, Sanna M. Analysis of hearing preservation and facial nerve function for patients undergoing vestibular schwannoma surgery: the middle cranial fossa approach versus the retrosigmoid approach-personal experience and literature review. Audiol Neurootol. 2012; 17(2):71–81

[17] Sanna M, Di Lella F, Guida M, Merkus P. Auditory brainstem implants in NF2 patients: results and review of the literature. Otol Neurotol. 2012; 33(2):154–164

[18] Di Lella F, Merkus P, Di Trapani G, Taibah A, Guida M, Sanna M. Vestibular schwannoma in the only hearing ear: role of cochlear implants. Ann Otol Rhinol Laryngol. 2013; 122(2):91–99

35 Retrosigmoid Approach for Medium to Large Vestibular Schwannoma

Travis C. Hill and John G. Golfinos

35.1 History and Overview of the Retrosigmoid Approach

During the early 1900s, the retrosigmoid approach was developed as a versatile technique to provide access to the posterior fossa. First described in detail by Fraenkel in 1903,[1] the retrosigmoid approach went through many iterations before reaching its current form. Early versions were associated with high morbidity and mortality resulting from poor control of intracerebral pressure, injury associated with cerebellar retraction, and blood loss. This provided impetus for development of the translabyrinthine approach in 1904, which necessarily sacrificed hearing and was thought less useful for resection of larger tumors.[2] Cushing addressed many of the problems associated with early unilateral retrosigmoid approaches by: (1) using a large bilateral suboccipital craniotomy to reduce the need for retraction and thereby limit injury to the cerebellum and medulla, (2) placing the patient in the prone position, and (3) releasing cerebrospinal fluid (CSF) from the cisterna magna or lateral ventricle to relieve intracerebral pressure. These innovations greatly reduced the mortality previously associated with the procedure.

Facial nerve injury was and is a serious complication of vestibular schwannoma (VS) resection. To avoid facial nerve dysfunction, Cushing advocated for subtotal resection and it was not until 1931 that Dandy first reported complete resection of a VS with preservation of the facial nerve. In contrast with Cushing's bilateral suboccipital approach, Dandy resurrected the small unilateral suboccipital approach, exploiting many of Cushing's morbidity-reducing innovations, but also reducing the risk to the facial nerve by carefully developing the dissection plane between the facial nerve and the tumor.

Subsequent modifications have included abandoning the prone position, use of the intraoperative microscope, and preoperative diagnostic imaging to identify patients with tumors best suited for the retrosigmoid approach as well as revealing critical anatomic details. More recent modifications of the approach include the extended retrosigmoid approach, which improves cerebellopontine angle (CPA) exposure by skeletonizing the sigmoid sinus (SS), improved intraoperative facial nerve monitoring with transcranial motor evoked potentials, and improved intraoperative monitoring of the cochlear nerve as well.

35.2 Advantages and Limitations

The retrosigmoid approach offers several advantages for appropriately selected cases (▶ Fig. 35.1). Preservation of the inner ear structures underlies the main advantage of the approach: hearing preservation remains an attainable goal of surgery even in tumors that are too large for the middle fossa approach or are predominantly extracanalicular. Whether the retrosigmoid approach is better suited for large tumors remains an area of controversy. Neurosurgeons traditionally receive more training in the retrosigmoid approach, but those trained in skull base techniques understand that the translabyrinthine approach in many ways epitomizes the tenets of skull base surgery—removing bone to obviate the need for moving or retracting the brain and removing a large tumor through a relatively small opening. Preservation of facial nerve function is possible with careful dissection techniques but may be more difficult given the more posterior approach to the anteriorly located facial nerve. The retrosigmoid approach is associated with a lower risk of CSF leak and reduced risk to vascular and nervous structures (SS, descending facial nerve). Finally, the retrosigmoid approach provides limited access to tumors that extend far into the internal auditory canal (IAC), so these lesions may be more appropriately accessed via translabyrinthine approach, especially after realistic consideration of the possibility of preserving hearing.

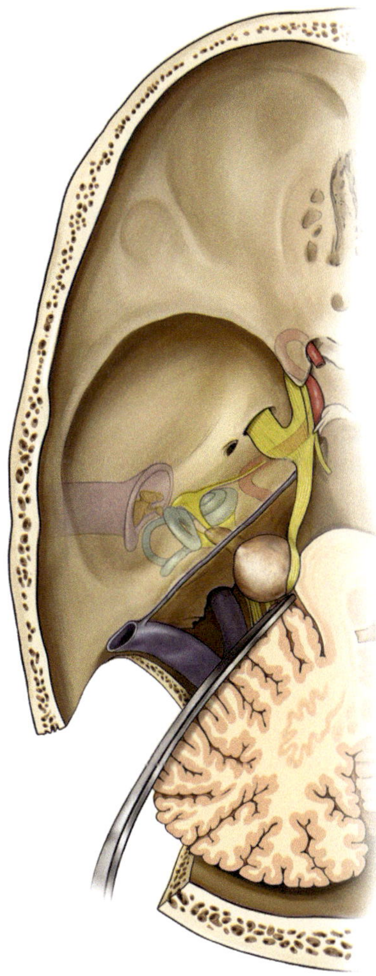

Fig. 35.1 Illustration demonstrating the retrosigmoid corridor for vestibular schwannoma resection.

Chapter 36 focuses on the retrosigmoid approach for small VS with the goal of hearing preservation. The current chapter primarily focuses on the retrosigmoid approach for medium or large-sized VS, where hearing preservation is less commonly a consideration. The interested reader is encouraged to read both chapters and review both summary tables for outcomes according to tumor size.

35.3 Patient Selection (Indications and Contraindications)

Traditionally, the retrosigmoid approach is considered best suited to tumors with a larger CPA component that do not reach to the fundus of the IAC and for whom hearing preservation is a possible goal of surgery. In our practice, however, we consider the retrosigmoid approach as primarily a hearing preservation approach and especially as a hearing preservation approach for tumors not suitable for a middle fossa approach. We prefer the middle fossa approach for hearing preservation in completely intracanalicular tumors, those within the lateral end of the canal, and tumors with less than a 10-mm extension into the CPA. For any tumor where hearing is poor or hearing preservation is very unlikely, we prefer the translabyrinthine approach, regardless of size. Finally, cases with a high-riding jugular bulb or a very anterior SS that might otherwise be suited for a translabyrinthine approach are better handled through a retrosigmoid approach. While there are no absolute contraindications to the retrosigmoid approach (save for unusual anatomic circumstances such as an obstructing developmental venous anomaly or other anatomic complication), it bears mentioning that the translabyrinthine approach can be easier in patients with an obese body habitus, since it allows access to the CSF early on without retraction of the cerebellar hemisphere.

35.4 Surgical Technique

Following intubation and Foley placement, the patient can be positioned either supine with the head turned as much as possible to the contralateral side or in full lateral decubitus position. In some locales, depending on training, neurosurgeons prefer the sitting position despite the added anesthetic complexity and risk because of the slackness of the cerebellar hemisphere. Continuous electrophysiological monitoring of the ipsilateral facial electromyogram (EMG), the ipsilateral facial motor evoked potentials, bilateral auditory brainstem responses (ABRs), and bilateral somatosensory evoked potentials should be considered. The Mayfield head holder is placed with two pins on the contralateral occiput and one pin on the ipsilateral frontal bone, with care taken to ensure adequate venous drainage with the neck rotated. This requires confirmation that the contralateral jugular vein is not compressed by the angle of the mandible. Many neurosurgeons have had the unfortunate experience of opening tight posterior fossa dura from complete occlusion of the contralateral venous drainage. We have gotten away from using the head holder altogether in routine retrosigmoid approaches for VS. In patients with a supple neck, it is easy enough to place the head on a foam donut and tape the head firmly to the bed after contralateral rotation. The tape has some natural give to it so that there is no issue with excessive neck rotation or occlusion of venous drainage. In patients lacking good neck rotation because of cervical spondylopathy or a short, thick neck, we do not hesitate to use the full lateral decubitus position with the head in pins. This position eliminates neck rotation altogether, resulting in a maximally relaxed cerebellar hemisphere even in morbidly obese patients. The supine patient should be positioned as far up and to the side of the table as possible to ensure a short reach for the surgeon. A C-shaped, anteriorly based, curvilinear incision is marked 4 cm posterior to the posterior edge of the mastoid, extending from the level of the mastoid tip to 2 cm above the pinna (▶ Fig. 35.2). Hair removal may be limited to 0.5 cm on either side of the planned incision. Perioperative antibiotics are administered and the site antiseptically prepped and draped. We prepare every patient for harvest of an autologous abdominal fat graft to be used in the closure for obstructing exposed mastoid air cells. The abdominal harvest site, either periumbilical or in the left lower quadrant, is similarly antiseptically prepped and draped.

The incision should be carried down to the periosteum covering the asterion, posterior mastoid, and the inferior surface of the occipital bone. The superficial skin flap is reflected anteriorly off the periosteum, and a periosteal flap, the so-called Palva flap, is cut with the same incision, also reflected anteriorly, and secured with fish hook retractors on rubber bands. At this point, there are many ways to expose the posterior fossa dura. For neurosurgeons, a craniectomy remains more common than a craniotomy but requires cranioplasty with foreign materials for closure. We prefer to avoid foreign materials as much as possible by performing a craniotomy. Rather than using a burr hole, we instead use the technique of exposing the SS and 2 mm of dura behind it to allow access for the craniotome footplate. Using cutting and diamond burrs, the SS is skeletonized caudally from the sigmoid–transverse junction (found deep to the asterion) to the jugular bulb, leaving only a thin layer of bone covering the posterior portion of the SS and exposing 2 to 3 mm of retrosigmoid dura. Hemostasis should be obtained by waxing air cells and with careful and definitive control of the emissary vein when it is encountered using bipolar cautery (▶ Fig. 35.3). The exposed retrosigmoid dura is now used as a starting point to free the dura from the overlying bone. Similarly, the footplate of the craniotome can now be inserted in the epidural space under direct vision without the need for additional burr holes, craniectomy, or bone loss. The craniotome is used to create a 2- to 3-cm retrosigmoid craniotomy in the occipital bone, and the bone flap is removed from the field. Some authors have touted endoscopic approaches to the CPA, claiming that the burr hole used is only 1 inch (2.54 cm) in diameter. We commonly use 2-cm craniotomies and seldom create craniotomies greater than 3 cm for the resection of VS, using the technique described.

Intracranial pressure is reduced through the usual maneuvers of low-dose mannitol (0.25–0.5 g/kg dose), temporary hyperventilation, and reverse Trendelenburg position until the dura is relaxed. The dura is then opened with a posteriorly curved incision 5 mm posterior and parallel to the sigmoid and following along the transverse sinus (▶ Fig. 35.4). The sinus is retracted anteriorly with a tack-up suture through the attached dural flap and tack-up holes drilled in the mastoid bone anteriorly. Under the operating microscope, the inferior arachnoid

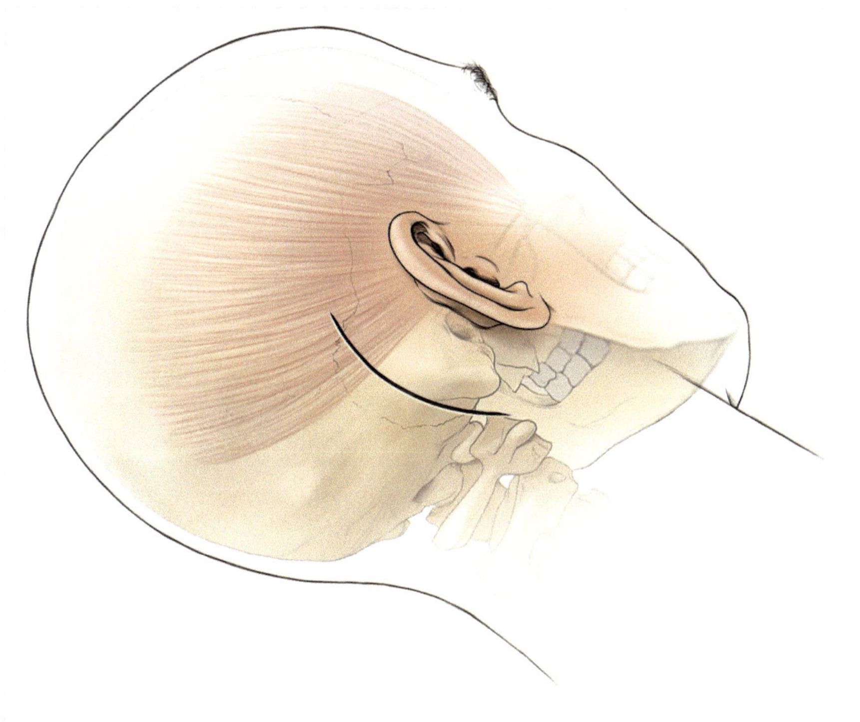

Fig. 35.2 C-shaped incision for the retrosigmoid approach.

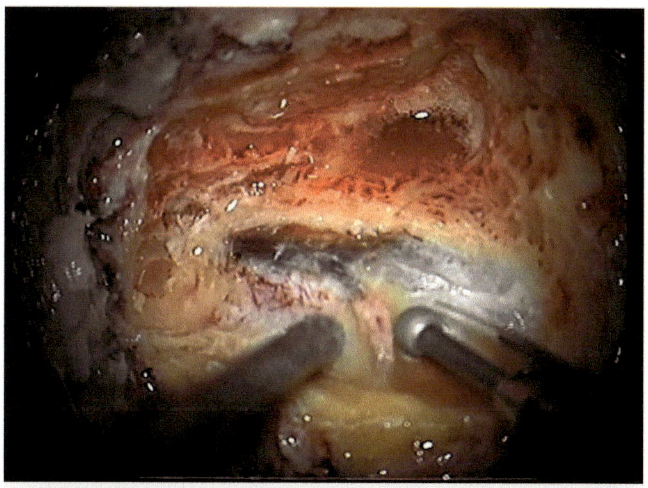

Fig. 35.3 Sigmoid sinus and exposure of the emissary vein prior to left-sided retrosigmoid craniotomy.

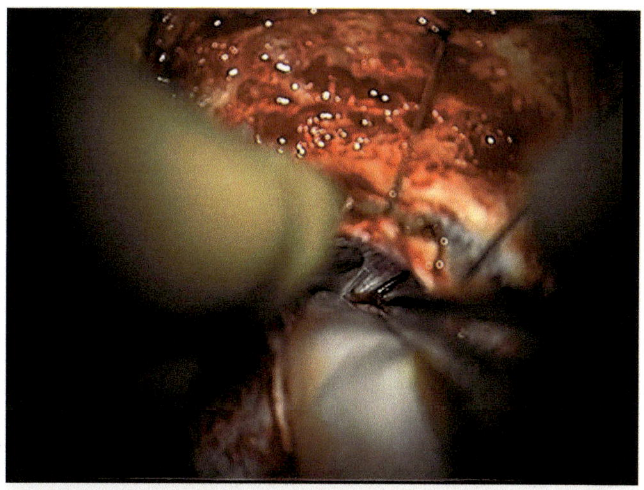

Fig. 35.4 Opening the retrosigmoid dura.

cistern either over the lower cranial nerves or over the lateral medullary cistern is opened sharply to allow CSF egress. The cerebellum will reliably relax posteriorly, eliminating the need for any retractor use after opening the cistern. The key is to rely on the microscope and to protect the inferior cerebellar hemisphere as it is lifted superiorly and posteriorly with the bipolar and microsuction. The lower cranial nerves can be identified at this point.

With the cerebellum relaxed and the sigmoid displaced slightly anteriorly, the exposure of the posterior petrous bone is exquisite and complete, and the tumor is now visible in the CPA, all without the use of a fixed retractor of any type. Even in the presence of a large tumor, opening the arachnoid cisterns and patiently draining CSF will allow the cerebellum to fall out of the way by gravity only. The cerebellar hemisphere is protected with a single Telfa strip so as to maximize the view angle and avoid any entanglement in the drills used to remove the posterior lip of the IAC. Care is taken to confirm that the facial nerve is not running over the posterior face of the tumor using direct stimulation of the nerve. Similarly, if hearing preservation is a goal of the surgery, the eighth nerve is now identified on the inferior pole of the tumor. The free-running facial nerve EMG and transcranial facial motor evoked potential are used throughout the ensuing dissection to judge the health of the facial nerve. It is always useful to note the flocculus and the relationship of the bulk of the tumor to the flocculus and the eighth cranial nerve emerging just deep to it. If, for example, the entire tumor appears to be superior to the flocculus, the

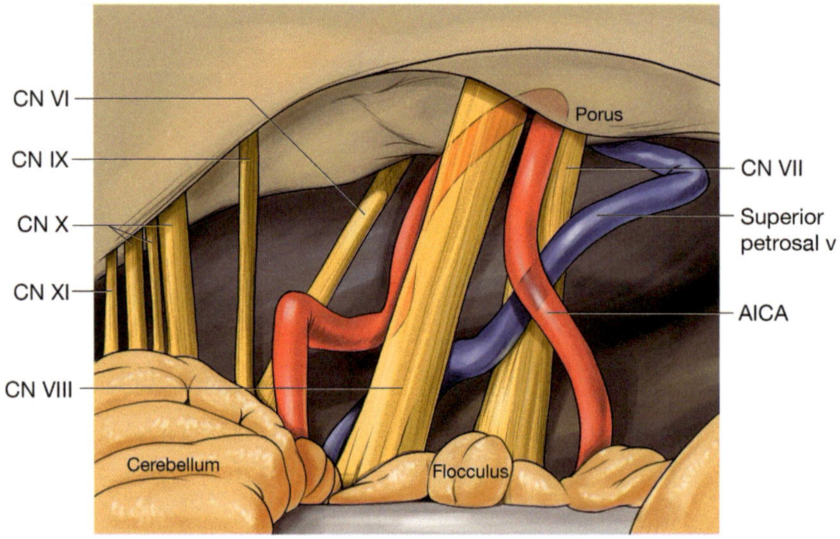

Fig. 35.5 Anatomy of the cerebellopontine angle from the perspective of a left-sided retrosigmoid approach. A branch of AICA can be seen coursing between the seventh and eighth cranial nerves. Additionally, a bridging petrosal vein is seen entering the superior petrosal sinus. The lower cranial nerves are seen on the left, as they enter the pars nervosa of the jugular foramen.

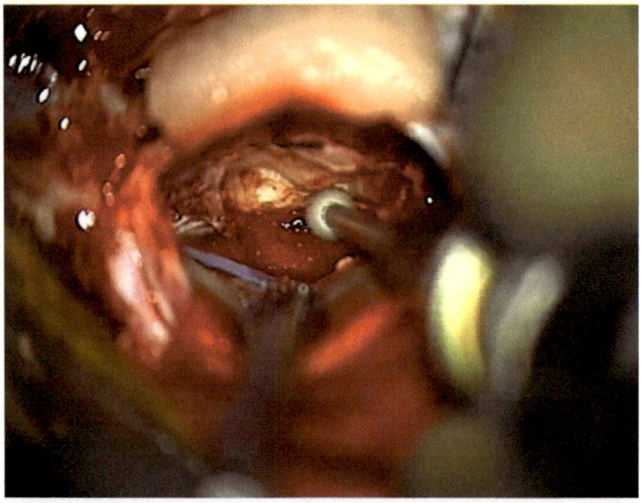

Fig. 35.6 Drilling out the IAC to expose the intracanalicular component of the tumor.

surgeon can anticipate that this is a superior vestibular nerve tumor and expect the inferior vestibular nerve to protect the cochlear nerve with no involvement of the lower cranial nerves. The tumor is now internally debulked using the ultrasonic aspirator, so that the walls of the tumor can now be collapsed inward and the tumor dissected away in turn from the cerebellar hemisphere, the flocculus, and finally the brainstem and cranial nerves. Superiorly, the tumor is dissected free of the ala of the cerebellum, the trigeminal nerve, and the petrosal vein (Dandy's vein). We make it a point to try to preserve the petrosal vein whenever possible, just to have the security of additional intact venous drainage. If, however, the petrosal vein has a short trunk and is under stretch, we coagulate and divide it sharply before it can be pulled free of the petrosal sinus with potentially voluminous bleeding. Senior residents learning the retrosigmoid removal of VS become obsessed with finding the facial nerve early and distressed at their failure to do so. No matter the size of the tumor, the eighth nerve and seventh nerve root entry zones remain in a relatively fixed relationship. Find the eighth nerve trunk and the seventh nerve will emerge from the brainstem just inferior and medial to it, separated from the eighth nerve by a small but constant recurrent branch of anterior inferior cerebellar artery (AICA; ▶ Fig. 35.5). The eighth nerve trunk will often find the inexperienced VS surgeon, rather than vice versa. More than one young surgeon has said that in removing a large VS, they elected to stop the dissection when they encountered significant venous bleeding at the brainstem. That bleeding more often than not stems from the veins of the eighth nerve trunk, which expand and dilate as the tumor is removed offering a clumsy yet effective confirmation of where the surgeon is in the dissection. On large tumors where hearing preservation is not a true goal, controlling the veins around the eighth nerve trunk allows the surgeon to coagulate and divide the thinned-out nerve, revealing the facial nerve just inferior and medial, emerging directly from the pontomedullary sulcus. Alternatively, it can be a very effective strategy to identify and maintain the flattened and splayed eighth nerve during the dissection, even if hearing preservation is not a consideration. The almost translucent eighth nerve can be kept as a veil to protect the facial nerve deep to it during the dissection. The facial nerve can now be identified by direct stimulation at the brainstem, even through the intact but splayed eighth nerve. The tumor can now be dissected off the facial nerve at the brainstem, finally freeing the tumor from all other brainstem attachments. As the tumor is now dissected off the facial nerve and eighth nerve veil along the brainstem, a point comes where the facial nerve leaves the brainstem to ascend to the superior lip of the porus acusticus. This is an area in large tumors where the nerve can be especially vulnerable. At this point, rather than lifting the tumor blindly off the nerve, it can be effective instead to find the facial nerve medially in the IAC and dissect in the other direction from lateral to medial.

The intracanalicular extension of the tumor, which is almost always present, requires that the posterior wall of the porus be drilled out; between 6 and 9 mm can usually be removed without compromising inner ear structures. An H-incision should be made in the petrous dura overlying the IAC, creating "saloon doors" which can be used for the closure. The IAC will be drilled laterally (▶ Fig. 35.6) with the limiting structures being the

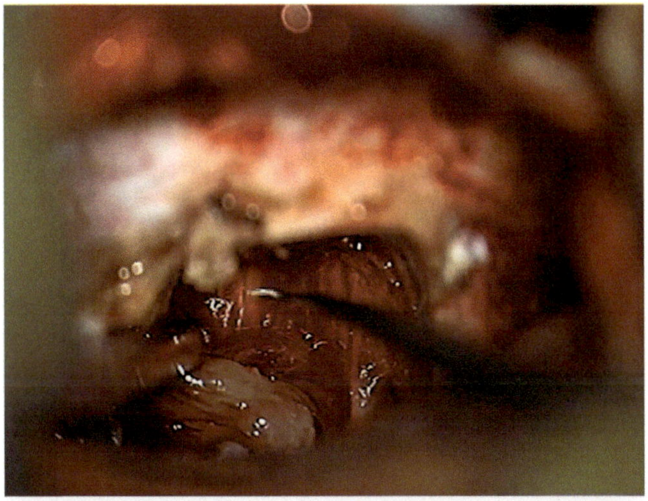

Fig. 35.7 Tumor dissection off of the cochlear nerve and transection of the vestibular nerves.

vestibule and the semicircular canals laterally and the jugular bulb inferiorly. The dura of the canal is opened longitudinally and the vestibular nerves are identified. This is a critical point of the operation in avoiding recurrences from small tumor residuals left at the fundus. The vestibular nerves are divided sharply laterally, revealing the lateral dome of the tumor. Inability to identify a smooth lateral dome suggests that the lateral tumor may have been transected with a portion left behind. A combination of tiny right-angled curettes and dissectors can be used to probe the lateral end of the canal. It is at this point in hearing preservation operations where the risk of recurrence rises because of a hesitance to dissect too roughly and blindly at the fundus of the canal in a retrosigmoid approach. Larger tumors require debulking in every phase of the operation with the ultrasonic aspirator to ease dissection off the facial and cochlear nerves, and dissection should always proceed from both ends of the facial nerve to meet at the cisternal segment (▶ Fig. 35.7). The very smallest tip of the ultrasonic aspirator is advantageous, especially when used on the IAC portion of the tumor. The superior and inferior vestibular nerves must be transected to avoid prolonged postoperative vertigo. This is another point in a hearing preservation case where the desire to protect the cochlear nerve and ABR can lead the surgeon to leave intact vestibular fibers with the possible consequence of recalcitrant dizziness. The last critical point of the dissection comes just outside or at the porus acusticus, where the facial nerve is thinnest. The experienced surgeon will preserve cochlear nerve fibers in every case at least temporarily in order to prevent the facial nerve from bearing the full weight of the remaining tumor. Once the tumor is completely removed, the field should be copiously irrigated and inspected for any residual tumor pieces. Bleeding near the facial nerve or an intact cochlear nerve with a preserved ABR should be controlled with Gelfoam and not with bipolar cautery in order to prevent inadvertent nerve injury and ruining the outcome of an otherwise exquisite dissection.

After closing the "saloon doors" of the posterior petrous dura with a single 4–0 suture, an abdominal fat graft should be harvested and placed in the IAC to seal the canal and prevent CSF leak from perimeatal air cells. Tissue glue can be used to hold the fat graft in place during healing. Hemostasis is confirmed with clear irrigation and should be meticulously maintained during closure. After closing the retrosigmoid dura and reinforcing the suture line with tissue glue, a second fat graft is placed over the SS and the bone flap is replaced with three small titanium plates. The pericranial flap is reapproximated to the surrounding periosteum. The nuchal muscles are reapproximated to the surrounding musculature and nuchal line. The skin is closed in two layers in the usual fashion. Facial nerve function should be assessed shortly after extubation whenever possible so that delayed facial paresis can be identified easily and early. Postoperative hearing assessment generally is delayed until a formal audiogram can be done and until the mastoid and middle ear are fully aerated.

In addition to standard postoperative care, patients should be monitored closely for CSF leak, which may manifest as clear fluid discharge from the incision or as rhinorrhea. Serial neurological exams should be used to monitor for cerebellar or brainstem edema, hydrocephalus, and cranial nerve dysfunction. Hearing preservation after surgery is typically durable, although studies continue in attempts to identify medications or maneuvers that can prevent postoperative hearing deterioration. We continue to use nimodipine postoperatively in patients with preserved hearing who tolerate the medication without blood pressure compromise. Depending on how much manipulation of the facial nerve was required in the dissection and how compromised the nerve was by the tumor, some facial dysfunction may be present during the immediate postoperative period. Patients should be counseled, however, to expect improvement if the nerve was intact and simulatable at a low threshold (< 0.1 mA) at the root entry zone at the end of the dissection. Additionally, a minimal change in the stimulation threshold for the facial motor evoked potential is also a predictor of intact facial nerve function postoperatively.

35.5 Outcomes and Complications (▶ Table 35.1)

35.5.1 Hearing Loss

Although patients and surgeons may intend to preserve hearing prior to surgery, hearing preservation may not prove feasible based on intraoperative observations. If the tumor is of cochlear nerve origin or the cochlear nerve is thinned or is tightly adherent to the tumor capsule, the nerve may necessarily be damaged or severed to allow complete resection. This possibility should be discussed with the patient prior to surgery so that intraoperative decision making reflects the goals of the patient. The use of intraoperative monitoring of the ABR can alert the surgeon when the nerve is in distress and thus improve outcomes.[3]

35.5.2 Headache

If one reads the internet, the most common complication of the retrosigmoid approach would seem to be postoperative headache. Usual neurosurgical headaches caused by intracranial air

Table 35.1 Select large series reporting complications and outcomes following resection of large vestibular schwannoma utilizing the retrosigmoid approach

Publication	Center	Years	Design	Number of cases	Duration of follow-up	Tumor size	Degree of resection	Recurrence	FN outcome	TN outcome	HP outcome	Management of hydrocephalus	Other complications
Jung et al 2000[12]	Chonnam National University Hospital, Dong-Ku, Kwangju, South Korea	1993–1998	Retrospective	30	At least 12 mo	All ≥ 4 cm; mean 4.9 cm (range, 4.1–7.0)	73% GTR 27% STR	3% recurrence rate	At 1 year after surgery: HB I: 32% HB II: 11% HB III: 42% HB IV: 16%	NR	NR	20% with preoperative papilledema. Postoperative hydrocephalus developed in one case (3%) and was managed by VP shunt	No mortalities 27% CSF leak 3% cerebellar hemorrhage No cases of meningitis No cases of lower cranial nerve paralysis
Yamakami et al 2004[13]	Chiba University School of Medicine, Chiba, Japan	1992–2001	Retrospective	50	Mean 58 mo (range, 12–115)	All ≥ 3 cm; mean 4.1 cm (range, 3.0–5.8)	86% GTR 14% STR	8% recurrence rate; only developed after STR	Of 46 (92%) patients with an anatomically preserved facial nerve: HB I–II: 91% HB III–IV: 7% HB V–VI: 2%	Preoperative trigeminal neuropathy improved or resolved completely in most patients after tumor removal. Hypoesthesia of the face was exacerbated in 3 patients	Useful hearing was not preserved in 49 patients; however, in 1 patient tumor removal improved the hearing from class C to class B, and useful hearing was restored	Of 15 patients with preoperative hydrocephalus, 5 (33%) required CSF diversion	No mortalities related to VS treatment 4% persistent postoperative ataxia. In 10% of cases, tumor removal caused resolution of severe preoperative ataxia
Zhao et al 2010[14]	The Second Hospital of Shandong University, Jinan, Shandong Province, China	2005–2008	Retrospective	89	At least 12 mo	All ≥ 4 cm; size not further specified	43% GTR 39% NTR 18% STR	3% recurrence rate; all developed after NTR	Early after surgery: HB I: 18% HB II: 23% HB III: 20% HB IV: 10% HB V: 16% HB VI: 14% At 1 year after surgery: HB I: 25% HB II: 29% HB III: 17% HB IV: 9% HB V: 12% HB VI: 8%	Postoperative trigeminal nerve deficit 7%	"Hearing preservation was not a consider-ation"	NR	No deaths CSF leak: 7% Cerebellar hematoma: 1% Meningitis: 3% CN IV deficit: 5% CN V deficit: 7% CN VI deficit: 6% CN IX and X deficit: 8% CN XI: deficit: 2% CN XII deficit: 1% Cerebellar ataxia: 6%
Samii et al 2010[15]	International Neuroscience Institute, Hannover, Germany	2001–2006	Retrospective	50	Mean 34 mo (range, 5–62)	All ≥ 4 cm; mean, 4.4 cm (range, 4–6.5)	All GTR	NR	Of 46 (92%) patients with an anatomically preserved facial nerve:	NR	NR using AAOHNS or Gardner–Robertson grading	43.2% with preoperative hydrocephalus. After surgery, existing hydrocephalus	No mortalities Existing lower cranial nerve dysfunction improved in all 5 patients after

Table 35.1 (Continued)

Publication	Center	Years	Design	Number of cases	Duration of follow-up	Tumor size	Degree of resection	Recurrence	FN outcome	TN outcome	HP outcome	Management of hydrocephalus	Other complications
									HB I–III: 75% HB IV: 19% HB V: 6% HB VI: 0%			did not change but was asymptomatic in 4 patients (25%), improved or resolved completely in 11 (69%), and slightly increased in 1 (6%) but needed no further therapy. New hydrocephalus developed in 1 patient and was managed by placement of a lumbar drain	surgery. New dysfunction developed in 6% but recovered in 4% Small asymptomatic hematomas managed conservatively without drainage in 8% Brainstem and cerebellar edema required temporary EVD placement in 2% Single epileptic seizure occurred in 2% CSF leak in 6%
Di Maio et al 2011[16]	Vancouver General Hospital, University of British Columbia, Vancouver, British Columbia, Canada	2003–2009	Retrospective	47	Mean 25 mo	Mean 3.6 cm (range, 3.0–5.0)	87% GTR 13% NTR	No recurrences requiring treatment	Early after surgery: HB I–II: 94%	NR	21% (6/28) retained SH after surgery. Hearing preservation rate for preoperative class A hearing was 31% (5/13). Hearing preservation was associated with CSF cleft present and when less than 35% of the tumor was located anterior to the	One patient required external ventricular drain immediately postoperatively for hydrocephalus, which was removed after a few days without requiring a VP shunt	Mortality 2%; hemorrhagic brainstem and cerebellar swelling developed after sacrifice of a large petrosal vein at the end of surgery. Despite immediate decompressive craniectomy, the patient died Temporary postoperative EVD for hydrocephalus in 2% Superficial wound infection in 2% Pseudomeningocele in 2% Mild cerebellar

Table 35.1 (*Continued*)

Publication	Center	Years	Design	Number of cases	Duration of follow-up	Tumor size	Degree of resection	Recurrence	FN outcome	TN outcome	HP outcome	Management of hydrocephalus	Other complications
											IAC axis		dysfunction affecting gait in 2%
Silva et al 2012[17]	Hospital São João, University of Porto, Porto, Portugal	2005–2010	Retrospective	29	Mean 39 mo (range, 4–73)	All ≥ 4 cm; range 4–6.1 cm, mean or median size NR	All GTR	No recurrences	Of 21 (72%) patients who did not require XIII–VII anastomosis: HB I: 19% HB II: 43% HB III: 24% HB IV: 14%	Presurgical facial dysesthesia or trigeminal neuralgia disappeared in the first 4–12 weeks after surgery	NR using AAOHNS or Gardner–Robertson grading	Although some degree of ventricular dilation was still present in postoperative MRI, hydrocephalus improved in all cases, without need for CSF diversion	No mortalities CSF leak in 14% Meningitis in 7% Lower cranial nerve dysfunction in 4% No cases of hematoma
Liu et al 2015[18]	Tongji Hospital, Tongji Medical College, Huazhong University of Science and Technology, Wuhan, China	2010–2012	Retrospective	106	All patients, 2 y	All ≥ 3 cm; mean 3.9 cm (range, 3.0–5.7)	82% GTR 14% STR 4% partial resection	18% recurrence rate; all cases of STR and partial resection regrew, but none have required treatment to date	Early after surgery: HB I: 17% HB II: 21% HB III: 30% HB IV: 15% HB V: 10% HB VI: 7 At 2 years after surgery: HB I: 56% HB II: 24% HB III: 21% HB IV: 1% HB V–VI: 0%	NR	NR	If hydrocephalus was present prior to surgery, external ventricular drainage was performed prior to craniotomy. After surgery, no patient suffered from persistent hydrocephalus	No mortalities No persistent hydrocephalus Postoperative hemorrhage requiring hematoma evacuation in 3% CSF leak 5%
Mendelsohn et al 2016[19]	University of British Columbia, Vancouver, British Columbia, Canada	2002–2013	Retrospective	85	NR	Mean 3.6 cm (range, 30–58)	NR	NR	At 6 weeks after surgery: HB I–II: 86%	NR	41% (17/42) retained SH after surgery	NR	NR
Boublata et al 2017[20]	Batna University Hospital, Batna, Algeria	2010–2015	Retrospective	151	Mean 28 mo (range, 3–54)	All ≥ 3 cm; range 3.0–6.0 cm, mean or median size NR	83% GTR 14% STR 3% partial resection	NR	Early after surgery: HB I–II: 76% HB III–IV: 18% HB V–VI: 6% At 2 years after surgery: HB I–II: 82% HB III–IV: 14% HV V–VI: 4%	NR	NR	NR	Mortality 0.7%; 1 due to postoperative hematoma and 1 due to meningitis CSF leak in 2% Meningitis in 1% Cerebellar hematoma in 3% Trochlear nerve

Table 35.1 (Continued)

Publication	Center	Years	Design	Number of cases	Duration of follow-up	Tumor size	Degree of resection	Recurrence	FN outcome	TN outcome	HP outcome	Management of hydrocephalus	Other complications
													deficit in 1% Abducens nerve deficit in 1% Lower cranial nerve dysfunction in 3% Cerebellar ataxia in 4%
Huang et al 2017[21]	Huashan Hospital, Fudan University, Shanghai	1999–2014	Retrospective	657	Mean 60 mo (range 6–191)	All ≥4 cm; size not further specified	85% GTR 15% NTR 0.3% partial resection	NR	Early after surgery: HB I–II: 33% HB III: 47% HB IV–VI: 20% Long-term facial nerve function: HB I–II: 56% HB III: 20% HB IV–VI: 24%	Postoperative facial numbness occurred in 16% of cases	7% retained SH after surgery	2% underwent CSF diversion before surgery for hydrocephalus and lateral cerebellum resection was used in 3% of cases. Delayed postoperative hydrocephalus occurred in 1% of cases	Mortality 0.6%; 2 patients died from brain hemorrhage and acute hydrocephalus. One patient died of brain edema. One patient died of severe pneumonia due to lower cranial nerve paralysis Intracranial hematoma in 1% Meningitis in 8% CSF leak in 3% Lower cranial nerve paralysis in 8%

Abbreviations: AAOHNS, American Academy of Otolaryngology–Head and Neck Surgery; CSF, cerebrospinal fluid; EVD, external ventricular drain; FN, facial nerve; GTR, gross total resection; HB, House–Brackmann; HP, hearing preservation; IAC, internal auditory canal; MRI, magnetic resonance imaging; NR, not reported; NTR, near-total resection; SH, serviceable hearing; STR, subtotal resection; VP, ventriculoperitoneal.

and blood in the spinal fluid typically resolve during the first few days postoperatively in the majority of patients. Some small proportion of patients will develop persistent headache that can be severe and may require referral to a headache specialist. We keep our incisions short and anterior curving in order to avoid severing proximal branches of the lesser and greater occipital nerves during opening (▶ Fig. 35.1). Replacing the patient's own bone flap results in a very low rate of persistent headaches as shown by our surgical series among others. The older technique of craniectomy requires a cranioplasty to keep the nuchal muscles from scarring down to the dura. Replacing the patient's own bone flap also obviates the need for any large mesh or foreign body, which can cause irritation and can also on occasion erode through the thin retroauricular skin.

35.5.3 Facial Nerve Dysfunction

Facial nerve dysfunction may result from compromise of the nerve by the tumor and subsequent intraoperative manipulation. Intraoperative facial monitoring with both the facial EMG and the transcranial motor evoked potential can minimize risk to the facial nerve by facilitating identification of the nerve and providing the surgeon with feedback when the nerve is being stretched inadvertently, leading to improved outcomes.[3] Serial facial nerve assessment during recovery is advised. We have a low threshold for placement of a gold weight in the upper eyelid to assist eyelid closure and prevent corneal abrasion, even in patients where there is a high confidence level for recovery of the facial nerve. Several options exist for repair of the facial nerve in cases where the nerve is lost or fails to recover. Our team has favored the use of a XII–VII anastomosis with excellent results.[4,5]

35.5.4 CSF Leak

Prevention of CSF leak is made more difficult in the CPA by the irregular dural topography and by the abundance of mastoid air cells. The hairs on the nape of the surgeon's neck should stand up when a preoperative temporal bone computed tomography (CT) reveals an abundantly aerated petrous bone with air cells extending into the zygoma or, worse, a CT of the head showing aerated clinoid processes and a giant frontal sinus. In addition to careful dural closure, abdominal fat grafts reduce the risk of postoperative CSF leak. When a leak occurs, the patient must have surgery to repair the defect if it does not resolve spontaneously with more conservative management (fluid, activity restriction, lumbar drain placement).

35.5.5 Cerebellar/Brainstem Edema

Using modern techniques including, above all, the banishment of retractors from the posterior fossa, brainstem or cerebellar edema is a rare complication, usually only seen with damage to branches of the superior cerebellar artery. Swelling in the posterior fossa can become an emergency, requiring urgent surgical decompression to prevent herniation and damage to brainstem structures.

35.5.6 Herniation

Now a rare complication, cerebral herniation plagued early retrosigmoid approaches. Upward cerebellar herniation seems nowadays to be more of a ghost story to scare young residents into careful neurologic surveillance of their retrosigmoid patients rather than a real complication to be feared. Still, it remains a useful rule of thumb that cerebellar swelling with brainstem compression should rarely, if ever, be treated by ventriculostomy alone instead of surgical cerebellar hemisphere decompression.

35.5.7 Infection

Despite the presence of mastoid air cells that may contain bacteria, infection is a rare complication that can be prevented with meticulous sterile technique. It is usually seen only in the presence of prolonged spinal fluid leak.

35.5.8 Vascular Injuries

Modern techniques have minimized the risk of vascular injury during retrosigmoid craniotomy. The most commonly injured structures are the sigmoid and transverse sinuses, which may thrombose secondary to prolonged compression, or may be compromised during manipulation. Intraoperatively, oozing is controlled with pressure and Gelfoam, and larger tears in the sinuses may be controlled with sutures. Injury to the AICA causes an easily identified middle cerebellar peduncle infarction with a profound ipsilateral hand dysmetria and a significant gait ataxia. Due to redundancy in cerebellar motor pathways, recovery, fortunately, is almost universal although it can take months. Injury to the posterior inferior cerebellar artery or superior cerebellar artery is rare unless dealing with massive tumors of 4 cm or greater, and even then these arteries are displaced far more often than they are intimate with the tumor.

35.5.9 Cranial Neuropathies

Cranial nerve injury may occur when normal anatomy is distorted by the tumor and nerves are improperly identified and inadvertently damaged. For nerves at high risk (VII, VIII), intraoperative electrophysiological monitoring is appropriate as discussed above. Injury to the lower cranial nerves is rare enough that monitoring is infrequently used for these nerves. The exception occurs most often in patients with neurofibromatosis type 2 where prior surgeries or multiple tumors can obscure the anatomy enough to put even the lower cranial nerves at risk.

35.5.10 Hemorrhage/Hematoma Formation

The frequency of this complication has fallen precipitously with the contemporary use of electrocautery and the availability of other hemostasis adjuvants such as thrombin-soaked Gelfoam. Meticulous hemostasis at all stages of the procedure is essential to prevent hemorrhage and postoperative hematoma formation. During closure, ensuring that irrigated fluid returns crystal clear is a reassuring sign that complete hemostasis has been achieved.

35.6 Technical Pearls and Pitfalls

35.6.1 Subtotal Resection to Preserve Facial Nerve Function

Facial nerve dysfunction should be avoided, and when the surgeon realizes the nerve is frayed or flattened, or if total resection will be difficult without risking the nerve, leaving a strip of adherent tumor along the nerve to avoid mechanical disruption may be preferable to achieving gross total resection at the cost of severe facial nerve dysfunction. Indeed, subtotal resection has been associated with better facial nerve outcomes than gross total resections,[6] but at the cost of increased risk of recurrence and the greater morbidity associated with a reoperation.[7] This possibility should be discussed with the patient preoperatively. This remains a technique that falls in the category of "easier said than done" since removing enough tumor to make a difference on larger tumors often means that the facial nerve has already been put at risk. Interpreting reported outcomes of this technique is plagued by the inescapable fact that one surgeon's subtotal resection is another surgeon's near-total resection. Further discussion regarding the merits and limitations of subtotal resection can be found in Chapter 41.

35.6.2 Fat Graft and Bone Wax to Minimize Risk of CSF Leak

The use of fat graft can significantly reduce the risk of postoperative CSF leak, as does the meticulous use of bone wax to close all violated air cells during drilling of the IAC.[8] In addition, the use of a fat graft during closure has been associated with reduced incidence of postoperative headache.

35.6.3 Intraoperative Electrophysiological Monitoring

Continuous intraoperative monitoring of evoked facial nerve EMG during VS resection[9] can help stratify risk of postoperative facial nerve dysfunction and guide surgeons in the decision to pursue early intervention for facial paralysis when warranted. When a stimulation probe is used, the ability of lower amplitude stimuli to elicit response from the facial nerve roughly correlates with preservation of good facial nerve function.[10] Similarly, cochlear nerve function may be monitored by recording the ABR or use of cochlear nerve action potential monitoring, which is more finicky but provides rapid feedback on changes to the nerve status that is better correlated with postoperative hearing status.[10,11] Chapters 27 and 28 provide further discussion on intraoperative facial nerve and intraoperative eighth nerve monitoring, respectively.

35.7 Conclusion

The retrosigmoid approach for VS resection is a versatile approach with a low complication rate. It is best suited for tumors where hearing preservation is desired yet the CPA component is too large for a safe middle fossa approach. The retrosigmoid approach is best for tumors that do not extend to the fundus of the IAC. If desired, modifications to the retrosigmoid approach, such as the extended retrosigmoid approach, may be employed to increase exposure without requiring additional retraction of the cerebellum. Where possible, collaboration between neurotologists and neurosurgeons may be employed to ensure the best outcomes for patients. Finally, the retrosigmoid approach is used for a variety of neurosurgical indications and may therefore be more familiar than other approaches to neurosurgeons who do not specialize in the treatment of VS.

References

[1] Cohen NL. Retrosigmoid approach for acoustic tumor removal. Otolaryngol Clin North Am. 1992; 25(2):295–310

[2] Cushing H. Tumors of the Nervus Acusticus and the Syndrome of the Cerebellopontile Angle. Philadelphia, PA: W. B. Saunders; 1917

[3] Samii M, Matthies C. Management of 1000 vestibular schwannomas (acoustic neuromas): the facial nerve–preservation and restitution of function. Neurosurgery. 1997; 40(4):684–694, discussion 694–695

[4] Jacobson J, Rihani J, Lin K, Miller PJ, Roland JT, Jr. Outcomes of direct facial-to-hypoglossal neurorrhaphy with parotid release. Skull Base. 2011; 21(1):7–12

[5] Roland JT, Jr, Lin K, Klausner LM, Miller PJ. Direct facial-to-hypoglossal neurorrhaphy with parotid release. Skull Base. 2006; 16(2):101–108

[6] Gurgel RK, Dogru S, Amdur RL, Monfared A. Facial nerve outcomes after surgery for large vestibular schwannomas: do surgical approach and extent of resection matter? Neurosurg Focus. 2012; 33(3):E16

[7] Cerullo L, Grutsch J, Osterdock R. Recurrence of vestibular (acoustic) schwannomas in surgical patients where preservation of facial and cochlear nerve is the priority. Br J Neurosurg. 1998; 12(6):547–552

[8] Fishman AJ, Marrinan MS, Golfinos JG, Cohen NL, Roland JT, Jr. Prevention and management of cerebrospinal fluid leak following vestibular schwannoma surgery. Laryngoscope. 2004; 114(3):501–505

[9] Amano M, Kohno M, Nagata O, Taniguchi M, Sora S, Sato H. Intraoperative continuous monitoring of evoked facial nerve electromyograms in acoustic neuroma surgery. Acta Neurochir (Wien). 2011; 153(5):1059–1067, discussion 1067

[10] Yingling CD, Gardi JN. Intraoperative monitoring of facial and cochlear nerves during acoustic neuroma surgery. Otolaryngol Clin North Am. 1992; 25(2): 413–448

[11] Oh T, Nagasawa DT, Fong BM, et al. Intraoperative neuromonitoring techniques in the surgical management of acoustic neuromas. Neurosurg Focus. 2012; 33(3):E6

[12] Jung S, Kang SS, Kim TS, et al. Current surgical results of retrosigmoid approach in extralarge vestibular schwannomas. Surg Neurol 2000; 53:370-377; discussion 377-378.

[13] Yamakami I, Uchino Y, Kobayashi E, Yamaura A, Oka N. Removal of large acoustic neurinomas (vestibular schwannomas) by the retrosigmoid approach with no mortality and minimal morbidity. J Neurol Neurosurg Psychiatry 2004; 75:453-458.

[14] Zhao X, Wang Z, Ji Y, et al. Long-term facial nerve function evaluation following surgery for large acoustic neuromas via retrosigmoid transmeatal approach. Acta Neurochir (Wien) 2010; 152:1647-1652.

[15] Samii M, Gerganov VM, Samii A. Functional outcome after complete surgical removal of giant vestibular schwannomas. J Neurosurg 2010; 112:860-867.

[16] Di Maio S, Malebranche AD, Westerberg B, Akagami R. Hearing preservation after microsurgical resection of large vestibular schwannomas. Neurosurgery 2011; 68:632-640; discussion 640.

[17] Silva J, Cerejo A, Duarte F, Silveira F, Vaz R. Surgical removal of giant acoustic neuromas. World Neurosurg 2012; 77:731-735.

[18] Liu SW, Jiang W, Zhang HQ, et al. Intraoperative neuromonitoring for removal of large vestibular schwannoma: Facial nerve outcome and predictive factors. Clin Neurol Neurosurg 2015; 133:83-89.

[19] Mendelsohn D, Westerberg BD, Dong C, Akagami R. Clinical and Radiographic Factors Predicting Hearing Preservation Rates in Large Vestibular Schwannomas. J Neurol Surg B Skull Base 2016; 77:193-198.

[20] Boublata L, Belahreche M, Ouchtati R, et al. Facial Nerve Function and Quality of Resection in Large and Giant Vestibular Schwannomas Surgery Operated By Retrosigmoid Transmeatal Approach in Semi-sitting Position with Intraoperative Facial Nerve Monitoring. World Neurosurg 2017; 103:231-240.

[21] Huang X, Xu J, Xu M, et al. Functional outcome and complications after the microsurgical removal of giant vestibular schwannomas via the retrosigmoid approach: a retrospective review of 16-year experience in a single hospital. BMC Neurol 2017; 17:18.

36 Retrosigmoid Approach for Hearing Preservation Vestibular Schwannoma Microsurgery

Roberto A. Cueva and Bill Mastrodimos

36.1 Introduction

The modern retrosigmoid (RS) approach for resection of vestibular schwannomas (VSs) is the result of an evolution from the classical suboccipital approach initially used for VS debulking/resection. The surgical pioneers of the mid to late 1800s and early 1900s who endeavored to save the lives of patients with advanced VSs were focused on avoiding operative mortality and facial paralysis.[1,2,3] While Krause advocated for a unilateral suboccipital approach, Cushing favored bilateral suboccipital exposure (▶ Fig. 36.1). Following the description of unilateral hearing loss as the most common first symptoms of VS by Cushing,[2] awareness of the characteristic symptoms and diagnostic advances allowed subsequent surgeons to address smaller tumors, shifting focus from avoidance of death to preservation of function. Smaller tumor size at the time of diagnosis increased likelihood of facial nerve survival. By the 1970s, the prospect of hearing preservation with complete tumor removal was being discussed and reported in the literature.[4,5,6] Initially, the unilateral suboccipital/transmeatal approach was favored for hearing preservation. However, William House demonstrated good results with the middle fossa (MF) approach.[7] In the subsequent decades, the MF approach was reported to be more successful for hearing preservation[8,9,10] until reports of equally successful hearing preservation were reported for the RS approach.[11,12,]

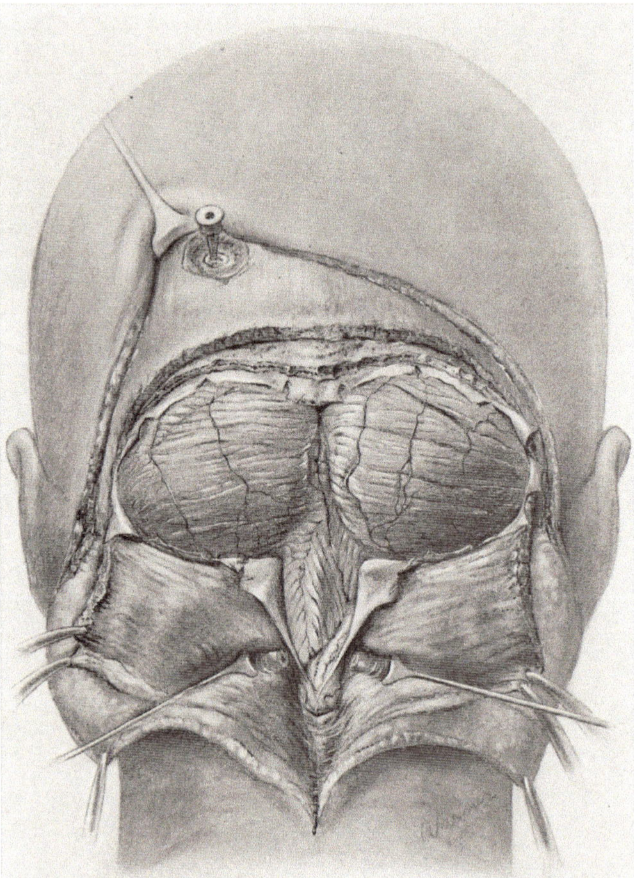

Fig. 36.1 Bilateral suboccipital craniectomy from Cushing's 1917 treatise on vestibular schwannoma. (Reproduced with permission from Cushing HW. Tumors of the Nervous Acusticus and the Syndrome of the Cerebellopontine Angle. Philadelphia, PA: W.B. Saunders; 1917:262.)

Currently, equally good hearing preservation results are achieved by surgical centers using MF and RS approaches by experienced teams adept at their chosen techniques. Each approach has its advantages and disadvantages. The MF approach allows complete exposure of the superior compartment of the internal auditory canal (IAC). However, the lateral aspect of the inferior compartment is obscured by the position of the facial nerve, the surgical angle, and the falciform crest.[13,14] The RS approach provides an early view of the more medial aspect of the tumor and the course of the internal auditory artery with minimal facial nerve manipulation during tumor removal. However, the distal 2 to 3 mm of the IAC are not directly visible.[15] Other differences in the approaches pertain to rates of temporary and permanent facial nerve paresis/paralysis, cerebrospinal fluid (CSF) leak rates, and chronic postoperative headache. The MF approach is reported to have a slightly higher rate of transient and permanent facial paresis. This is due to the facial nerve traveling over the superior aspect of the tumor and necessary mobilization to achieve tumor removal.[16,17] The RS approach is associated with a higher rate of lingering postoperative headaches that range from 5 to 16%.[18,19]

Regardless of surgical approach, intraoperative monitoring of hearing is of vital importance. A variety of studies have demonstrated the advantage of direct monitoring of the cochlear nerve action potential over auditory brainstem response (ABR) monitoring in achieving higher rates and quality of postoperative hearing preservation.[11,20,21] Further descriptions of eighth nerve monitoring techniques during VS microsurgery can be found in Chapter 28.

36.2 Patient Selection

Patients with tumors of any size up to 25 mm are candidates for RS approach for VS resection with attempted hearing preservation. The success rate for hearing preservation is inversely proportional to increased tumor size. The best rates of hearing preservation are achieved in patients with good preoperative hearing and tumors of ≤ 10 mm.[10,12,22] As tumor size increases, the rate of hearing preservation decreases fairly rapidly. Patients with tumors larger than 25 mm rarely have hearing preserved following tumor removal.[23] However, in the authors' practice, a well-informed patient with a tumor ≥ 25 mm who demands an attempt at hearing preservation is accommodated with the understanding that tumor recurrence and the facial nerve are placed at some small increased risk for the effort of hearing preservation.[23]

Some reports indicate that involvement of the fundus by tumor is an indicator of reduced success in hearing preservation.[24] Other authors find that overall tumor size is more important than fundal involvement.[12] Other factors such as quality of hearing present at the time of surgery may suggest better or worse prognosis for hearing preservation. The authors do not advocate preoperative ABR or video nystagmography to aid in the decision-making process for hearing preservation since such information is not as important as tumor size and patient desires. The absence of preoperative ABR waveforms does not preclude intraoperative monitoring with direct eighth nerve monitoring (DENM) since a cochlear nerve action potential is commonly obtained even in patients with absent ABR.[20]

All patients evaluated for VS are counseled regarding the options of: observation with serial magnetic resonance imaging (MRI); stereotactic radiosurgery/radiotherapy; and microsurgical resection. If hearing preservation is a priority in a patient with a small tumor, either observation or microsurgical resection may yield better long-term results. Radiation treatment is associated with a loss of useful hearing within 5 to 10 years of treatment in greater than 75% of cases.[25,26] For patients with small tumors and word recognition scores (WRS) of 100%, observation results in preservation of good quality hearing in 88% over the decade following diagnosis. However, only 55% of patients with even modest initial WRS decline maintained good hearing during observation.[27] For select tumors ≤ 10 mm, the likelihood of hearing preservation with microsurgical removal may be as high as 80 to 85% when performed by an experienced team.[10,12,22] The interested reader is directed to Chapter 53 for a review of hearing preservation outcomes according to surgical approach, Chapter 51 for observation, and Chapter 52 for radiosurgery.

36.3 Surgical Technique

The patient is positioned on the operating table in the supine position. After induction of general anesthesia and placement of facial and cochlear nerve monitoring leads, the patient is positioned for surgery. Some surgeons place a shoulder roll under the ipsilateral shoulder but the authors find that this is counterproductive to achieving access to the retroauricular scalp. Park-bench position is advocated by some surgeons but is awkward and time consuming to perform, and may increase the risk of pressure sores and transient neuropathy. Lumbar CSF drainage is not employed. The patient's head is placed in pin fixation and turned toward the contralateral shoulder. The head is brought above the plane of the ipsilateral shoulder, if possible, and then nodded toward the contralateral shoulder (▶ Fig. 36.2). This rotates the suboccipital skull away from the shoulder, facilitating surgical access to the postauricular scalp. Care must be taken not to overrotate the head, which can impair cerebral venous outflow. Furthermore, overrotation can cause stretch injury to the brachial plexus. Finally, space must remain between the mandible and contralateral clavicle to avoid creating pressure sores.

A small area of hair is clipped from behind the ear to allow placement of a 6- to 7-cm incision line roughly two fingerbreadths behind the auricular crease. The mastoid tip is usually the lower limit of the incision. A tangent along the upper margin of the ear canal approximates the plane of the transverse sinus and usually demarcates the upper one-third of the incision from the lower two-thirds (▶ Fig. 36.3). Local anesthetic consisting of 1 or 2% xylocaine with 1:100,000 epinephrine is injected into the skin and subcutaneous tissues primarily for hemostatic purposes. Preincision intravenous medications include dexamethasone 10 mg, mannitol 75 g, and cefazolin 2 g.

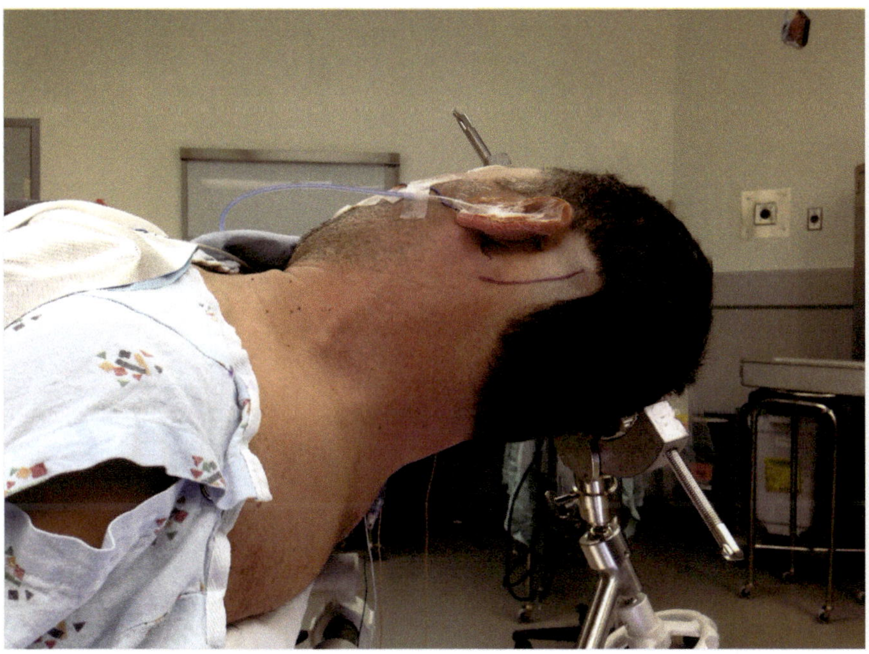

Fig. 36.2 Position of head relative to ipsilateral shoulder for left-sided procedure.

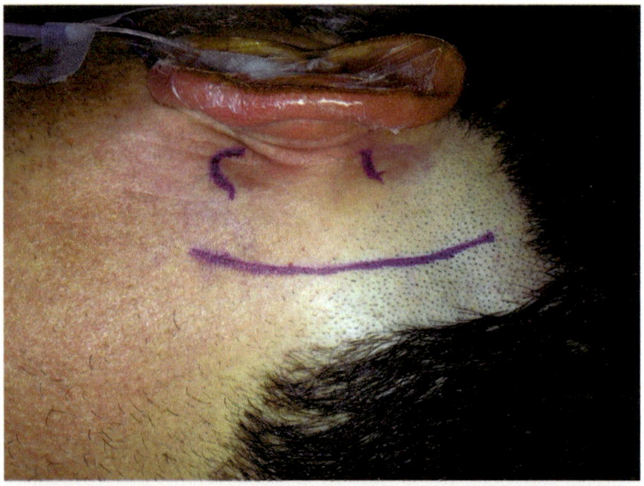

Fig. 36.3 Location of postauricular incision with mastoid tip and top of ear canal marked.

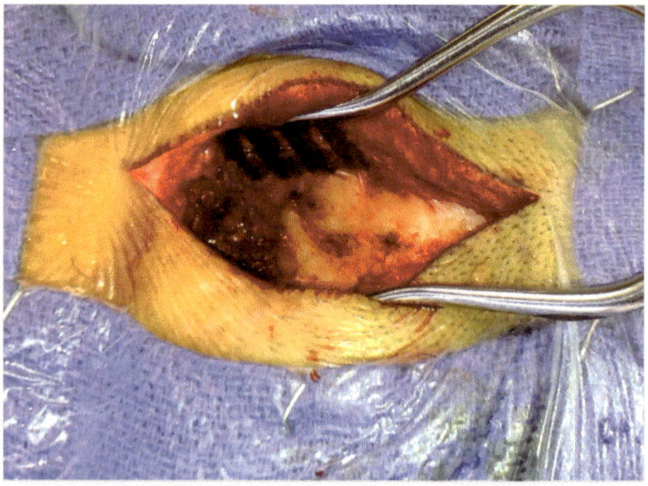

Fig. 36.4 Retromastoid skull exposed with posterior aspect of digastric groove visible.

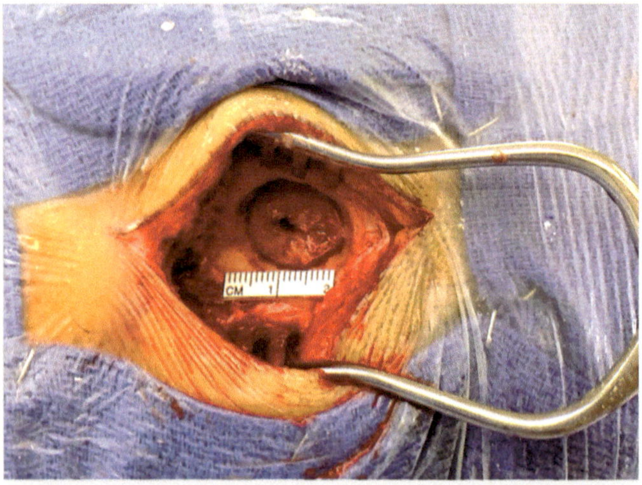

Fig. 36.5 Craniectomy completed at transverse–sigmoid junction.

Facial nerve and ABR monitoring electrodes are placed on the patient and connected to their respective devices. The electrode and ear speaker setup for ABR is used for DENM as well. The skin is prepared antiseptically. The authors prefer DuraPrep which, when dry, leaves the skin sticky, facilitating drape adhesion. The skin and underlying muscle are incised down to the calvarium, keeping the trajectory perpendicular to the skin. Periosteal elevation is directed mostly anterior to expose the posterior aspect of the mastoid process. The posterior aspect of the digastric groove is visualized and serves as a guide to the posterior edge of the sigmoid sinus (▶ Fig. 36.4). The 2-cm craniectomy is undertaken in a position near where the sigmoid–transverse junction is expected. The anterior limit of bone removal is the posterior aspect of the sigmoid sinus. Superiorly the limit of bone removal is the inferior aspect of the transverse sinus (▶ Fig. 36.5). Any mastoid air cells that are opened during the craniectomy are carefully occluded with bone wax to reduce the chance of CSF leak.

The dura is opened in a cruciate fashion and the dural flaps held aside with tacking sutures. The cerebellum is next elevated from the floor of the posterior cranial fossa to access the basal cistern and CSF is released. This results in cerebellar relaxation and facilitates posterior retraction of the cerebellum. The cerebellum is initially held in place with a retractor, but as the case proceeds, the retractor often becomes unnecessary as the cerebellum remains relaxed. The anatomy of the cerebellopontine angle (CPA) is next inspected to identify the lower cranial nerve (glossopharyngeal, vagus, spinal accessory) entering their pars nervosa. The trigeminal nerve is typically anterosuperior to the cochleovestibular nerve/facial nerve bundle and/or tumor. If no tumor is present in the CPA, the facial nerve is usually found anterior to the cochleovestibular nerve. If tumor is present in the angle, the facial nerve stimulating probe is used to stimulate the posterior surface of the tumor to ensure the facial nerve is not traveling on this side of the tumor.

Usually, ABR is used during CPA tumor debulking; however, if the tumor in the angle is small, placement of a cochlear nerve electrode for DENM during this activity is feasible. The capsule of the tumor in the CPA is then opened sharply and internal debulking of the tumor is then undertaken. As the capsule becomes more mobile and can be collapsed into the space created by debulking, identification of the cochlear and facial nerves is undertaken. Once significant debulking of the CPA portion of the tumor is performed, attention turns to the posterior surface of the petrous bone. The location of the operculum of the endolymphatic sac (ELS) is often well seen as a dimple on the surface of the posterior petrous bone. The double-layer dura of the ELS is typically whiter than the adjacent single-layer dura. An inverted U-shaped incision is made in the dura centered on the IAC with the lateral limit of the incision being the operculum. This dural flap is then elevated and excised. Direct visualization of where the ELS enters the bone at the operculum is achieved and bony dissection of the IAC is undertaken. If the DENM electrode was placed during CPA tumor debulking, it is removed during drilling to avoid potential entanglement with the drill.

The CPA cisterns above and below the cochleovestibular nerve are filled with papaverine-impregnated BICOL collagen sponges to reduce dispersion of bone dust. Using constant suction–irrigation and a 4-mm diamond burr, the bone on the posterior surface of the petrous bone is removed in a semicircle

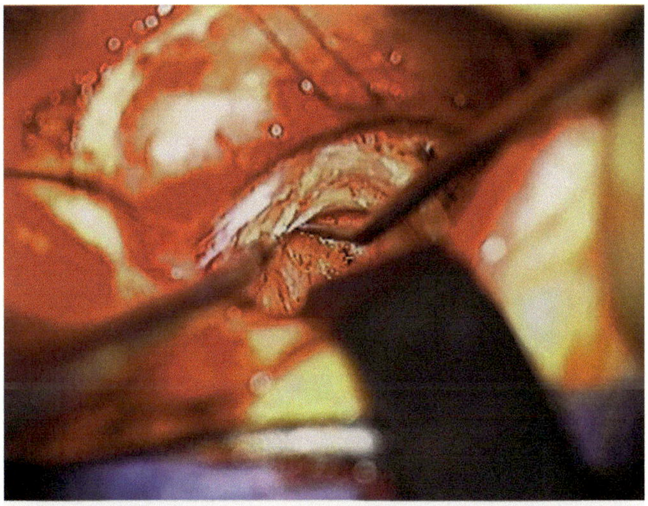

Fig. 36.6 Initial course of the endolymphatic sac/duct indicated by instrument.

pattern until the dura of the posterior aspect of the IAC can be seen through thin bone. The location of the operculum is kept in sight during this dissection to avoid labyrinthine injury. Once the dura of the posterior surface of the IAC is clearly seen, corridors of bone removal are developed superior and inferior to the IAC. As bone removal around the IAC proceeds from medial to lateral, burr size is changed to accommodate the anatomic limitations of the spaces being worked. To determine the lateral limit of bony dissection, the course of the ELS and duct are carefully exposed and followed for a short distance toward the labyrinth (▶ Fig. 36.6, ▶ Fig. 36.7). Staying medial to this important landmark will prevent labyrinthine injury.[15] The goal for the extent of bone removal is to achieve 270-degree (or greater) circumferential IAC exposure to within 2 to 3 mm of the fundus.

In addition to using the ELS and duct as guides to the lateral limit of bone removal, specially designed IAC dissectors (available from Grace Medical, Memphis, TN) are employed to separate the dura from the bony IAC and extradurally estimate the remaining amount of unexposed IAC. This direct measurement is very useful at determining the adequacy of exposure relative to the tumor's degree of fundal extension. The markings on the dissectors are millimeter markers allowing fairly precise determination of remaining unexposed IAC. The falciform crest is routinely palpated and dissection commonly taken to within 2 mm of the inferior compartment, and within 3 mm of the superior compartment of the IAC (▶ Fig. 36.8). Once the bony work has been finished, preparation is made to open the IAC dura and remove tumor from the canal.

Direct cochlear nerve monitoring is always employed during the removal of the IAC portion of the tumor. A specially designed electrode (available from AD Tech Medical Instrument Corporation, Racine, WI) provides stable positioning of the electrode that is not displaced by CSF pulsations. DENM provides the most rapid feedback regarding cochlear and cochlear nerve status of all the hearing monitoring modalities. Waveform amplitudes are one to two orders of magnitude larger than ABR, allowing capture of a cochlear nerve action potential with 10 to 20 sweeps (1–2 s). The earliest changes in DENM that may signal cochlear/cochlear nerve stress is a prolongation of action potential latency

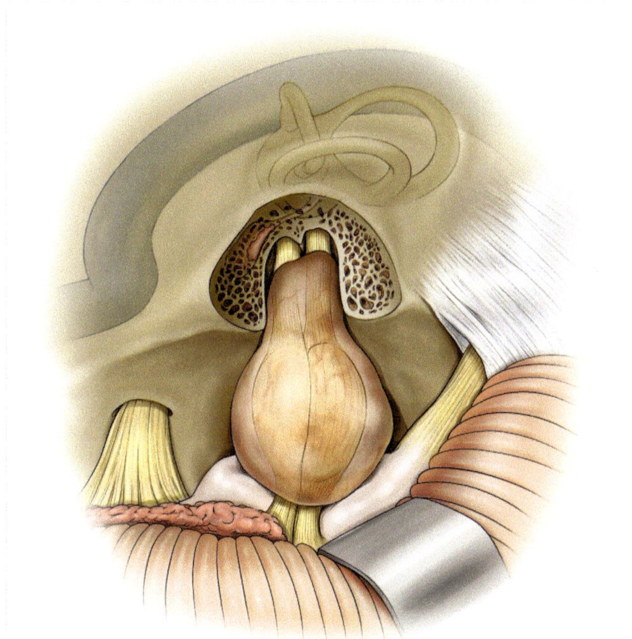

Fig. 36.7 Surgical view following retrosigmoid transmeatal drilling to expose a medium-sized left-sided VS. The endolymphatic sac + duct is a useful landmark that can be used to maximize lateral exposure of the internal auditory canal without violating the posterior semicircular canal or vestibule in cases where hearing preservation is a goal.

with decline in amplitude occurring later. Amplitude changes without latency prolongation may be due to blood in between the electrode contact surface and the cochlear nerve.

Once the cochlear nerve electrode is placed, the dura of the IAC is sharply opened to form superior and inferior rectangular flaps. The dural flaps are laid into the superior and inferior bony corridors created during bony IAC dissection. Dissection progresses from medial to lateral to diminish any sheering force on the cochlear nerve at the habenula perforata. Additionally, the course of the internal auditory artery (also known as the labyrinthine artery) is kept in mind. Should the artery travel directly on the tumor surface, dissection may result in arterial spasm which will often respond to suspension of dissection and application of papaverine. As in the CPA, the IAC tumor is centrally debulked once the facial and cochlear nerves are identified. The superior and inferior vestibular nerves are purposefully sacrificed as these are the nerves of origin in the vast majority of these tumors. Additionally, prior experience with trying to preserve these nerves during VS removal was found to result in a higher incidence of prolonged postoperative imbalance problems.

As the tumor dissection approaches the fundus of the canal, the IAC dissectors are most useful in separating tumor from the facial and cochlear nerves. Additionally the spoon shape of the dissecting tip facilitates delivery of tumor from the portion of the fundus that is not directly visible (▶ Fig. 36.9). Endoscopic inspection of the canal fundus may be employed following completion of tumor removal if the surgeon desires. In most cases, it is clear by the shape/contour of the tumor delivered from the fundus whether residual tumor may remain. A careful systematic dissection of the distal IAC is undertaken to ensure no tumor remains.

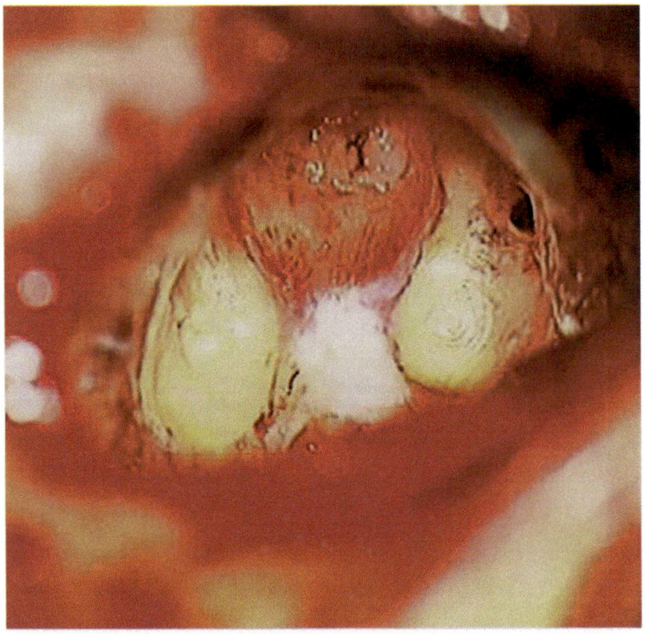

Fig. 36.8 Bony internal auditory canal dissection completed with tumor visible through intact dura.

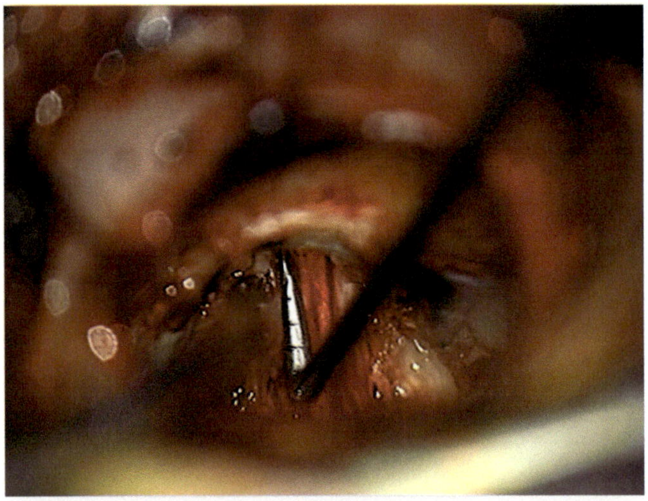

Fig. 36.9 Use of specially designed internal auditory canal dissector for tumor removal in distal IAC.

Once tumor removal has been completed, the cochlear and facial nerves are transiently covered with papaverine-impregnated Gelfoam or BICOL. All bony surfaces that were drilled during the IAC exposure are carefully coated with bone wax pressed into place with a micro-Cottonoid to reduce the risk of CSF leak. The papaverine-impregnated Gelfoam or BICOL is removed and methylprednisolone acetate (Depo-Medrol)-impregnated Gelfoam/BICOL is placed on the IAC nerves for a few moments. The latter is removed and then copious irrigation of the CPA is undertaken to remove any bone dust or blood. Careful survey to ensure hemostasis has been achieved is performed before initiating dural closure.

The dura is closed with a combination of interrupted and continuous 4–0 braided nylon (Neurolon) suture. Layered microfibrillar collagen hemostat (Avitene) which is then saturated with venous blood is used to fill the small craniectomy defect. This serves to seal the dural suture-line and will be replaced by scar in the healing process. The muscular fascia layers are approximated with interrupted 2–0 braided absorbable sutures. The same suture is used in an inverted, interrupted fashion to approximate the dermal layer of the skin. Staples are then used to approximate the epidermis. The skin is then cleansed and dried. A small quantity of antibiotic ointment is applied along the staple line and a nonstick gauze, adhesive island dressing is placed over the closed incision. The patient is then taken out of pin fixation and allowed to awaken from general anesthetic.

36.4 Complications

A summary of published outcomes for VS resection using the RS approach is presented in ▶ Table 36.1. Specific to approaches in which hearing preservation is attempted, statistically the highest risk of surgery is the loss of hearing. The risk of hearing loss increases significantly with increase in tumor size, as discussed in the section on patient selection. Risk of temporary facial paresis/paralysis likewise escalates with increased tumor size. The focus on the management of postoperative facial weakness centers on keeping the cornea of the ipsilateral eye well lubricated.

Frequent use of moisturizing eye drops during the day and ophthalmological ointment at night is usually sufficient to prevent excess corneal exposure/dryness which may lead to ulceration and potential blindness. If corneal lubrication cannot be sufficiently maintained with these measures, then urgent referral to an ophthalmologist is made. CSF leak is an additional risk and, in the author's series of patients, is in the range of 1%.[28] If CSF leak occurs via the skin incision, oversewing with suture or application of cyanoacrylate skin adhesive followed by application of a pressure dressing will often resolve the leak. Should CSF leak via the ear/eustachian tube occur within the first few weeks of surgery, then admission to the hospital for a trial of lumbar drainage will successfully resolve such leaks in roughly 50% of patients. The leaks not resolved with lumbar drainage will require surgical exploration to ensure the area of bone dissection around the IAC and any mastoid air cells opened during the craniectomy have been adequately waxed. Risk of major hemorrhage is quite small, with average blood loss of less than 100 mL. Risk of brainstem stroke or retraction injury to the cerebellum is less than 1%. The risk of death is much less than 1% but not zero. Specific to RS craniectomy for VS is the increased risk of lingering postoperative headache. Patients with an existing history of headache or cervical spine stiffness are at increased risk compared to those without such existing problems. A specific subset of postoperative headaches are related to occipital neuralgia and are amenable to targeted injection of a combination of xylocaine and steroid. These patients will often be able to identify a trigger point when palpated that will send a "zing" of pain from the area of the trigger toward the ipsilateral temporal area. Injection of a mixture of 1 mL of 1% xylocaine and 1 mL of 40 mg/mL Kenalog in the area of the trigger point and the adjacent musculature will often provide significant relief of this type of headache. Such trigger point injection may need to be repeated to achieve permanent relief. In severe cases, referral to pain management specialists may be required.

Table 36.1 Reported rates of hearing preservation following vestibular schwannoma removal via retrosigmoid approach

Publication	Center	Years	Design	Number of cases	Duration of follow-up	Tumor size	Degree of resection	Recurrence	FN outcome	HP outcome	Other complications
Goel et al 1992	Presbyterian University Hospital, Pittsburgh, Pennsylvania	NR	Retrospective	42 with SH	Median 2.5 y	Reported categorically, median or mean size NR	NR	No recurrences	NR	31% (13/42) retained SH. Hearing preservation outcomes were better in patients with smaller tumors	NR
Post et al 1995	Mount Sinai School of Medicine, New York, New York	NR	NR	46 with SH	Mean 2.5 y	Reported categorically, median or mean size NR	89% GTR	4%	96% HB I–II	39% (18/46) retained SH. Hearing preservation outcomes were better in patients with smaller tumors	No mortalities, 18% CSF leak
Rowed et al 1997	Sunnybrook Health Sciences Centre, University of Toronto, Toronto, Ontario, Canada	1985–1996	NR	23 with intracanalicular VS and SH	Minimum of 1 y	Intracanalicular	All GTR	No recurrence requiring treatment	96% HB I–II	48% (11/23) retained SH	NR
Colletti et al 2000	University of Verona, Verona, Italy	1990–1998	Retrospective	106 with SH	NR	Mean 20 mm (range, 4–50 mm)	NR	NR	NR	55% (58/106) retained SH	NR
Lee et al 2002	UMDNJ-Robert Wood Johnson University Hospital, New Brunswick, New Jersey	1995–2001	Retrospective	58 with SH	Mean 24 mo (range, 3 mo to 4.8 y)	Reported categorically, median or mean size NR	73% GTR 14% NTR 11% STR	2%	87% HB I–II 10% HB III–IV 3% HB V–VI	19% (11/58) retained SH at last follow-up. The probability of hearing preservation was greatest in smaller tumors (25%) compared to large tumors (0%)	0.6% mortality,11% CSF leak, 6% meningitis, 4% wound infection, 3% cerebellar contusion
Maw et al 2003	Frenchay Hospital, Bristol, United Kingdom	1991–2000	Prospective	33 with SH	Median or mean not reported (range, 6 mo to 9 y)	Mean or median NR; range, 0.7–4.5 cm	95% GTR 5% STR	NR	90% HB I 10% HB III	42% (14/33) retained SH	NR
Chee et al 2003	Sunnybrook & Women's College Health Science Centre, Toronto, Ontario, Canada	1978–1997	Retrospective	29 with SH	Mean 113.4 mo (range, 36–264 mo)	NR	All GTR	No recurrences	NR	79% (23/29) retained SH	NR
Lassaletta et al 2003	La Paz University Hospital, Madrid, Spain	1990–2000	Retrospective	29 with SH	Minimum of 1 y	Mean 24.1 mm (range, 8–50 mm)	NR	No recurrences	60% HB I 12% HB II 16% HB III 6% HB IV	17% (5/29) retained SH. Age, gender, side of the tumor, or tumor	10 patients developed CSF leak 2 patients

Table 36.1 (*Continued*)

Publication	Center	Years	Design	Number of cases	Duration of follow-up	Tumor size	Degree of resection	Recurrence	FN outcome	HP outcome	Other complications
									4% HB V 2% HB VI	size was not significantly associated with hearing preservation	developed cerebellar and epidural hematoma
Mohr et al 2005	Sir Mortimer B. Davis–Jewish General Hospital, McGill University, Montreal, Quebec, Canada	1981–2004	NR	128 with SH	NR	Reported categorically, median or mean size NR	NR	NR	NR	24% (31/128) retained SH. Tumor size and extent of meatal filling were associated with development of nonserviceable hearing, while pretreatment hearing level was not	NR
Betchen et al 2005	Mount Sinai School of Medicine, New York, New York	1985–2002	Retrospective	142 with SH	Mean 7 y	NR	NR	NR	97% HB I–II	27% (38/142) retained SH. The results of hearing preservation were independent of tumor size	19% CSF leak, 2% meningitis
Yamakami et al 2009	Chiba University, Chiba, Japan	1998–2007	Retrospective	18 with SH	Mean 48 mo (range, 1–110 mo)	NR	All GTR	No recurrences	100% HB I–II	78% (14/18) retained SH	NR
Phillips et al 2010	Weill Medical College of Cornell University, New York, New York	1991–2009	Retrospective	23 with SH[a]	NR	Mean 0.52 cm (range, 0–1 cm)	83% GTR 17% > 90% resected	NR	NR	48% (11/23) retained SH. Patient age, sex, preoperative hearing status, tumor size, laterality, extent of IAC filling, surgical approach, and extent of resection were not significant predictors of hearing preservation	NR
Sameshima et al 2010	Carolina Neuroscience Institute, Raleigh, North Carolina	1998–2007	Retrospective	82 with SH[a]	Median or mean NR (range, 13–42 mo)	Mean 12.4 mm	All GTR	No recurrences requiring treatment	99% HB I 1% HB II	73% (60/82) retained SH	5% CSF leak, 4% meningitis
Tringali et al 2010	Hospices Civils de Lyon, Pierre-Bénite,	1993–2007	Retrospective	213 with SH	NR	Koos grade I and II	NR	No recurrences	90% HB I	41% (87/213) retained SH.	NR

Table 36.1 *(Continued)*

Publication	Center	Years	Design	Number of cases	Duration of follow-up	Tumor size	Degree of resection	Recurrence	FN outcome	HP outcome	Other complications
	France									Regression analysis showed that degree of lateral extension in the IAC was a strong predictor of hearing preservation	
Mazzoni et al 2012	Ospedali Riuniti Bergamo, Italy	1976–2000	Retrospective	189 with SH	Mean 14 y (range, 6–21 y)	Reported categorically, median or mean size NR	NR	NR	NR	29% (54/189) retained SH. 44% (39/89) of patients with pretreatment class A hearing retained SH	NR
Nguyen et al 2012	Kaiser Permanente, San Diego, California	2001–2010	Retrospective	53 AAOHNS Class A, B, or C	NR	Mean 7.2 mm (range, 3–10 mm)	NR	NR	NR	79% (42/53) retained AAOHNS class A, B, or C	NR
Freitas et al 2012	Gruppo Otologico Piacenza, Roma, Italia	1988–2008	Retrospective	82 with SH[a]	Minimum of 1 y	Mean size 8.0 mm	All GTR	NR	97% HB I–II	24% (20/82) retained SH	No mortalities, 6 cases of CSF leak, 1 case of meningitis, 1 case of cerebellar edema with intracranial pressure elevation that required shunting
Yamakami et al 2014	Chiba University, Chiba, Japan	1998–2012	Retrospective	36 with SH	Mean 81 mo (range, 5–181 mo)	Small (intracanalicular or < 1.5 cm)	All GTR	No recurrences	100% HB I	72% (26/36) retained SH. 84% (16/19) of patients with pretreatment class A hearing retained SH	No mortalities or other postoperative complications occurred
Anaizi et al 2016	University of Cincinnati College of Medicine, Cincinnati, Ohio	2003–2012	Retrospective	35 with SH[a]	Mean 34 mo	Koos grade I and II	89% GTR 11% NTR	NR	95% HB I–II	37% (13/35) retained SH	5% CSF leak

Abbreviations: AAOHNS, American Academy of Otolaryngology–Head and Neck Surgery; CSF, cerebrospinal fluid; FN, facial nerve; GTR, gross total resection; HB, House–Brackmann; HP, hearing preservation; IAC, internal auditory canal; NR, not reported; NTR, near-total resection; SH, serviceable hearing (AAOHNS class A or B, Gardner–Robertson grade I or II; WRS > 50%, and PTA or STR < 50 dB HL).
[a]Only includes those that underwent retrosigmoid approach.

References

[1] Ballance CA. Some Points in the Surgery of the Brain and Its Membranes. London: Macmillan & Co.; 1907:276

[2] Cushing H. Tumors of the Nervus Acusticus and the Syndrome of the Cerebellopontine Angle. Philadelphia, PA: W.B Saunders Co.; 1917

[3] Krause, f. Zur Freilegung der hinteren Felsenbeinflache und des Kleinhirns. Beitr Klin Chir. 1903;37:728-764

[4] MacCarty CS. Acoustic neuroma and the suboccipital approach (1967–1972). Mayo Clin Proc. 1975; 50(1):15–16

[5] Mackay IS, King IJ. Pre- and post-operative brainstem responses in a case of acoustic neuroma, sparing the VIII nerve. Clin Otolaryngol Allied Sci. 1977; 2 (3):233–238

[6] Cohen NL. Acoustic neuroma surgery with emphasis on preservation of hearing. Laryngoscope. 1979; 89(6, Pt 1):886–896

[7] Belal A, Jr, Linthicum FH, Jr, House WF. Acoustic tumor surgery with preservation of hearing. A histopathologic report. Am J Otol. 1982; 4(1):9–16

[8] House WF, Shelton C. Middle fossa approach for acoustic tumor removal. Otolaryngol Clin North Am. 1992; 25(2):347–359

[9] Brackmann DE, House JR, III, Hitselberger WE. Technical modifications to the middle fossa craniotomy approach in removal of acoustic neuromas. Am J Otol. 1994; 15(5):614–619

[10] Arts HA, Telian SA, El-Kashlan H, Thompson BG. Hearing preservation and facial nerve outcomes in vestibular schwannoma surgery: results using the middle cranial fossa approach. Otol Neurotol. 2006; 27(2):234–241

[11] Yamakami I, Yoshinori H, Saeki N, Wada M, Oka N. Hearing preservation and intraoperative auditory brainstem response and cochlear nerve compound action potential monitoring in the removal of small acoustic neurinoma via the retrosigmoid approach. J Neurol Neurosurg Psychiatry. 2009; 80(2):218–227

[12] Nguyen QT, Wu AP, Mastrodimos BJ, Cueva RA. Impact of fundal extension on hearing after surgery for vestibular schwannomas. Otol Neurotol. 2012; 33 (3):455–458

[13] Haberkamp TJ, Meyer GA, Fox M. Surgical exposure of the fundus of the internal auditory canal: anatomic limits of the middle fossa versus the retrosigmoid transcanal approach. Laryngoscope. 1998; 108(8, Pt 1): 1190–1194

[14] Driscoll CLW, Jackler RK, Pitts LH, Banthia V. Is the entire fundus of the internal auditory canal visible during the middle fossa approach for acoustic neuroma? Am J Otol. 2000; 21(3):382–388

[15] Domb GH, Chole RA. Anatomical studies of the posterior petrous apex with regard to hearing preservation in acoustic neuroma removal. Laryngoscope. 1980; 90(11, Pt 1):1769–1776

[16] Colletti V, Fiorino F. Middle fossa versus retrosigmoid-transmeatal approach in vestibular schwannoma surgery: a prospective study. Otol Neurotol. 2003; 24(6):927–934

[17] Hillman T, Chen DA, Arriaga MA, Quigley M. Facial nerve function and hearing preservation acoustic tumor surgery: does the approach matter? Otolaryngol Head Neck Surg. 2010; 142(1):115–119

[18] Schessel DA, Nedzelski JM, Rowed D, Feghali JG. Pain after surgery for acoustic neuroma. Otolaryngol Head Neck Surg. 1992; 107(3):424–429

[19] Harner SG, Beatty CW, Ebersold MJ. Headache after acoustic neuroma excision. Am J Otol. 1993; 14(6):552–555

[20] Jackson LE, Roberson JB, Jr. Acoustic neuroma surgery: use of cochlear nerve action potential monitoring for hearing preservation. Am J Otol. 2000; 21(2): 249–259

[21] Danner CJ, Mastrodimos B, Cueva RA. A comparison of direct eighth nerve monitoring and ABR in hearing preservation surgery for vestibular schwannoma. Otol Neurotol. 2004; 25(5):826–832

[22] Woodson EA, Dempewolf RD, Gubbels SP, et al. Long-term hearing preservation after microsurgical excision of vestibular schwannoma. Otol Neurotol. 2010; 31(7):1144–1152

[23] Yates PD, Jackler RK, Satar B, Pitts LH, Oghalai JS. Is it worthwhile to attempt hearing preservation in larger acoustic neuromas? Otol Neurotol. 2003; 24 (3):460–464

[24] Goddard JC, Schwartz MS, Friedman RA. Fundal fluid as a predictor of hearing preservation in the middle cranial fossa approach for vestibular schwannoma. Otol Neurotol. 2010; 31(7):1128–1134

[25] Roos DE, Potter AE, Brophy BP. Stereotactic radiosurgery for acoustic neuromas: what happens long term? Int J Radiat Oncol Biol Phys. 2012; 82(4): 1352–1355

[26] Carlson ML, Jacob JT, Pollock BE, et al. Long-term hearing outcomes following stereotactic radiosurgery for vestibular schwannoma: patterns of hearing loss and variables influencing audiometric decline. J Neurosurg. 2013; 118 (3):579–587

[27] Stangerup SE, Caye-Thomasen P, Tos M, Thomsen J. Change in hearing during 'wait and scan' management of patients with vestibular schwannoma. J Laryngol Otol. 2008; 122(7):673–681

[28] Cueva RA, Mastrodimos B. Approach design and closure techniques to minimize cerebrospinal fluid leak after cerebellopontine angle tumor surgery. Otol Neurotol. 2005; 26(6):1176–1181

37 Middle Cranial Fossa Approach for Hearing Preservation Vestibular Schwannoma Microsurgery

Ravi N. Samy, Jennifer Kosty, and Bruce J. Gantz

37.1 Introduction

Discussing the middle cranial fossa (MCF) approach for vestibular schwannoma (VS) resection would be incomplete without acknowledging Dr. William F. House, who first introduced this technique in 1959.[1] In his initial 1961 publication with the neurosurgeon Theodore Kurze, House described the MCF approach for four patients; initial pathologies that were treated included cochlear otosclerosis through decompression of the cochlear nerve, a facial nerve tumor, tinnitus, and Ménière's disease for vestibular nerve section. The authors reported no resulting facial paralysis or major intracranial complications. House intuitively realized the utility of the MCF approach for VS resection after incidentally discovering a small VS during a vestibular nerve section. Believing the patient's symptoms were related to Ménière's disease, he discovered the small tumor and removed it, resulting in an improvement in the patient's hearing.

Based on countless hours of cadaveric dissection, House further refined his ideas about the MCF dissection. For example, he identified the internal auditory canal (IAC) by exposing the geniculate ganglion and then tracing the labyrinthine segment of the facial nerve to the canal. Other advancements still used today were the use of diamond burrs and continuous irrigation to reduce risk of injury to neurovascular structures in the IAC.

House's initial experience developed without modern skull base techniques, such as intraoperative monitoring of facial or cochlear function or preoperative magnetic resonance imaging (MRI) scans. He favored early treatment of smaller intracanalicular VS to reduce risk of neurologic injury and increase rates of hearing and facial nerve preservation. He correctly realized that bleeding, damage, or thrombosis of the labyrinthine artery could cause profound hearing loss, and he also noted that the vascularity of the facial nerve was more resilient than that of the cochlear nerve. By 1968, the time of his second MCF publication, House had resected nearly 200 VS by a variety of approaches.[2] Hearing was preserved in 4 of 5 (80%) patients with tumors limited to the IAC, and 3 of 14 (21%) patients with larger tumors extending up to 1 cm into the cerebellopontine angle (CPA).[2]

37.2 Advantages and Limitations of the MCF Approach

Since House's initial studies on the MCF approach, the treatment for VS has evolved to include observation, stereotactic radiation, and surgery. If surgery is selected, three main approaches can be used—translabyrinthine (TL), retrosigmoid (RS), and, the focus of this chapter, the MCF approach.[3]

The main advantage of the MCF approach is direct access to the contents of the IAC, allowing for preservation of both hearing and facial nerve function with excellent exposure of small, primarily intracanalicular, tumors. For this subset of VS, rates of hearing preservation tend to be higher in the MCF approach compared to the RS approach, although the rate of transient facial nerve paresis may conversely favor the RS approach.[4,5,6,7] The advantage for hearing preservation using the MCF may be size dependent. In a systematic review of 35 studies with more than 5,000 patients who underwent VS surgery, Ansari et al concluded that the MCF approach was significantly less likely than the RS approach to cause loss of serviceable hearing for tumors ≤ 15 mm (44 vs. 64%, respectively, $\underline{p} < 0.001$).[7] However, for tumors larger than 15 mm, the MCF approach tended to result in worse hearing outcomes, with 82% of cases losing serviceable hearing versus 71% for the RS approach, though this difference was not statistically significant.[7] There are likely several reasons for improved hearing results with the MCF approach for small VS confined to the IAC. First, many intracanalicular tumors extend to the fundus, which is more directly visualized with the MCF approach. With the RS approach, the posterior semicircular canal and vestibule obscure visualization of the lateral third of the IAC. Conversely, more fundus can be directly accessed with the middle fossa, although the extreme inferior compartment of the fundus may still be blocked by the transverse crest.[4] Additionally, it has been theorized that the vessels of the IAC are more easily seen and protected via the MCF approach as opposed to the RS approach. Finally, the cochlear nerve is located deep in dissection with the MCF, compared to the RS approach.

Compared to stereotactic radiosurgery, which is often offered as an alternative to surgery for comparably sized tumors, long-term hearing preservation rates may be better with the MCF approach. Several authors have reported 5-year hearing preservation rates of 65 to 89%.[8,9,10] By comparison, hearing degrades over time following radiosurgery. In a recent study of this modality with long-term follow-up, Carlson et al reported a 5-year hearing preservation rate of 48% and a 10-year preservation rate of 23%.[11] Further discussion regarding hearing preservation following radiosurgery is presented in Chapter 52.

Some authors have found early postoperative facial paresis to be more common after the MCF compared to the RS approach; however, no difference is usually seen at 1 year after surgery.[4,5] Others have found no difference in facial nerve preservation with these two approaches.[7] The facial nerve is often located over the superior pole of the tumor within the lateral IAC, between the surgeon and the tumor with the MCF, explaining this finding.

The MCF approach offers limited exposure to the CPA; therefore, significant extension (i.e., greater than 0.5–1 cm) of the tumor into this compartment is a relative contraindication to this procedure and is associated with lower rates of hearing preservation and a potentially higher risk of intracranial complications.[4,12]

37.3 Patient Selection

With the increased utilization of contrast-enhanced MRI, increasingly smaller VS are being diagnosed every year. Given the fact that the smaller tumors may have a period of quiescence, an initial period of observation is generally warranted for the asymptomatic tumor.[13] If growth is observed or the tumor becomes symptomatic, surgical resection or stereotactic radiosurgery are offered to the patient. Older patients, or those not amenable to surgery, can anticipate excellent tumor control rates and modest long-term hearing preservation with stereotactic radiosurgery.[14] For young, healthy patients with serviceable hearing, surgical resection via the MCF approach may provide the best opportunity for long-term hearing preservation and facial nerve function (▶ Table 37.1).[9,12,15,16,17,18,19,20,21,22] In those patients classified as having nonserviceable hearing (i.e., American Academy of Otolaryngology–Head and Neck Surgery class C or D), the MCF approach may still be offered in an attempt to preserve some hearing, which can later be augmented with a cochlear implant or even traditional or nontraditional hearing aids. Even marginal hearing may be valuable to the patient with contralateral hearing loss and, for others, may still be useful to facilitate sound localization. Although somewhat controversial, the MCF approach may also be used for IAC decompression in order to maximize the duration of hearing preservation in patients at risk for bilateral, profound hearing loss such as those with neurofibromatosis type 2 or VS in an only hearing ear.[23]

37.4 Surgical Technique

37.4.1 Preoperative Preparation

After review of the patient's history, physical examination, audiogram, and MRI scan with contrast, the surgeon discusses the potential risks, benefits, complications, hazards, and types of surgical procedures. Preoperative anesthesia clearance ensures the patient is a good surgical and anesthetic candidate. Coronal computed tomography (CT) scans or plain films with Stenvers views are obtained to assess the pneumatization pattern overlying the IAC and superior semicircular canal.[24]

37.4.2 Surgical Steps

The patient is intubated with appropriate anesthetic monitors as well as intravenous and arterial lines. Intraoperative monitoring electrodes are placed to monitor brain function, facial nerve function, and cochlear function, as previously discussed. After the patient's hair is trimmed for an anteriorly based skin flap, antibiotics and intravenous steroids are administered.

With the patient prepped and draped in a supine position, the skin flap is created (▶ Fig. 37.1). Hemostasis of the skin flap is achieved with electrocautery. The temporalis fascia is harvested and kept in a moist sponge for placement at end of the case along the middle fossa floor to reduce the risk of postoperative cerebrospinal fluid (CSF) leak. Next, an anteriorly based temporalis muscle flap is created and elevated off the squamosa of the temporal bone. The zygomatic root is identified.

Using a 4-mm cutting burr, a 4 × 5 cm craniotomy is made, centered over the zygomatic root (▶ Fig. 37.2 and ▶ Fig. 37.3). During the craniotomy, the patient is hyperventilated and given mannitol as an osmotic diuretic to reduce intracerebral pressure. The bone flap is held in a moist sponge. Hemostatic agents (FloSeal and Oxycel) are used for hemostasis. The dura is elevated from the inner cortex of the skull and along the middle fossa floor in a posterior-to-anterior direction in order to reduce the risk of inadvertent avulsion of the facial nerve particularly at the geniculate ganglion, or traction on the geniculate from greater superficial petrosal nerve (GSPN) pull.

The anatomic limits of dissection are the sigmoid sinus posteriorly, the superior petrosal sinus medially, and the middle meningeal artery/foramen spinosum anteriorly (▶ Fig. 37.4). Most surgeons prefer to blue line the superior semicircular canal in order to provide a reliable landmark for meatal drilling. If the canal is inadvertently entered, bone wax can be used to reduce the risk of sensorineural hearing loss. The otic capsule bone has a characteristic yellow or ivory appearance compared to the surrounding tegmen, which facilitates safe dissection. Though not completely reliable, the arcuate eminence is usually located over, or in close proximity, to the apex of the superior semicircular canal. The GSPN is also identified, and the angle between the GSPN and blue-lined superior canal is bisected to determine the location of the IAC.

Drilling commences anteromedially at the porus acusticus with a 4-mm diamond burr, where risk of inadvertent injury to the inner ear is least. Using progressively smaller diamond burrs, the surgeon continues drilling laterally until Bill's bar, the vertically oriented wedge of bone separating the facial nerve from the superior vestibular nerve, is encountered. The IAC is decompressed at least 180 degrees along the entire length. Troughs anterior and posterior to the IAC can be enlarged, particularly at the medial IAC, to improve surgical access when needed. While rarely required, division of the tentorium can facilitate access to the CPA. A 2-mm diamond burr is also used to decompress the labyrinthine segment of the facial nerve. At this point, care should be taken to avoid entering the cochlea or vestibule. An electrode to monitor the near-field response (cochlear nerve action potential [CNAP]) is wedged in a trough between meatal bone and dura anterior to the facial nerve.

The IAC dura is opened posteriorly in the region of the superior vestibular nerve. After allowing egress of CSF to facilitate additional temporal lobe relaxation, the MCF retractor blade is removed to improve access to the CPA. With reflection of the dura anteriorly, the facial nerve is identified at the labyrinthine segment and traced medially (▶ Fig. 37.5 and ▶ Fig. 37.6). Tumor is removed piecemeal with the goal of total tumor removal. Care is taken to make sure the fundus is free of any residual tumor. When performing tumor resection, use of bipolar cautery should be minimized to reduce risk of injury to the facial nerve and labyrinthine artery. If changes in the CNAP or auditory brainstem response (ABR) are encountered, pieces of papaverine-soaked Gelfoam are placed on the nerve to augment blood flow and the signals are given time to recover.

Several methods have been described for closure. We have had the most success with laying a piece of temporalis muscle over the defect and covering the floor of the middle fossa with a piece of temporalis fascia to reduce the risk of postoperative CSF leak. Opened air cells are occluded with bone wax. Temporalis fascia is placed along the middle fossa floor and the subtemporal retractor is removed. The bone flap is replaced, and titanium plates can be used for cranioplasty, if desired. The incision is closed in anatomical layers according to surgeon preference.

Table 37.1 Summary of contemporary series (2000–2016) using the middle fossa approach

Reference	No. of patients	Pre-op serviceable hearing[a]	Serviceable hearing preservation rate	Postoperative AAO-HNS classification *N* (%)[b]		Facial nerve function at last follow-up		Complications		
				A	B	HB I	HB II	CSF leak	Infection	Other
Arts et al (2006)	73	62 (85%)	45 (72%)	21 (33%)	24 (39%)	61 (85%)	8 (11%)	–	1 (1%)	4 (5%) aseptic meningitis; 1 (1%) transient expressive aphasia; 1 (1%) deep venous thrombosis; 1 (1%) transient ulnar neuropathy
Brackmann et al (2000)	333	300 (90%)	188 (62%)	108 (36%)	80 (26%)	–	–	–	–	–
Ginzkey et al (2013)	89	65 (82%)	48 (74%)	25 (39%)	23 (35%)	82 (89%)	3 (3%)	–	–	–
Gjurić et al (2001)	735	423 (58%)	188 (33% total preservation rate; 52% preservation rate for patients with IAC tumors only)	114 (23%)	74 (15%)	463 (72%; 90% for IAC tumors, 78% for tumors < 1 cm)	129 (20%; 9% for IAC tumors)	16 (2.2%)	9 (1.2%)	3 (0.4%) mortality; 2 (0.3%) CPA hematoma; 2 (0.3%) temporal lobe contusion; 1 (0.1%) seizures; 45 (5.7%) transient neurologic deficits
Goddard et al (2010)	101	92 (91%)	56 (44%)	27 (26%)	29 (29%)	–	–	–	–	–
Hillman et al (2010)	88	59 (67%)	35 (59%)	32 (54%)	3 (5%)	63 (72%)	14 (16%)	–	–	–
Hilton et al (2011)	78	78 (100%)	51 (65%)	22 (28%)	29 (37%)	–	–	–	–	–
Meyer et al (2006)	162	124 (77%)	61 (57%)	45 (36%)	16 (21%)	140 (86%)	17 (10%)	9 (5.6%)	–	2 (1.2%) aseptic meningitis; 2 (1.2%) aphasia; 2 (1.2%) seizures
Raheja et al (2016)	60	49 (81%)	38 (77%)	14 (30%)	23 (47%)	50 (76%)	9 (14%)	0	3 (3.8%)	0
Vincent et al (2012)	77	73 (95%)	46 (60%)	25 (32%)	21 (27%)	96% for HB I or II	–	–	–	–

Abbreviations: AAO-HNS, American Academy of Otolaryngology–Head and Neck Surgery; CPA, cerebellopontine angle; CSF, cerebrospinal fluid; HB, House–Brackmann; IAC; internal auditory canal.
[a]Serviceable hearing defined as word recognition score ≥ 50% and pure tone average ≤ 50 dB HL.
[b]Percentages are expressed as a percentage of patients with preoperative serviceable hearing.

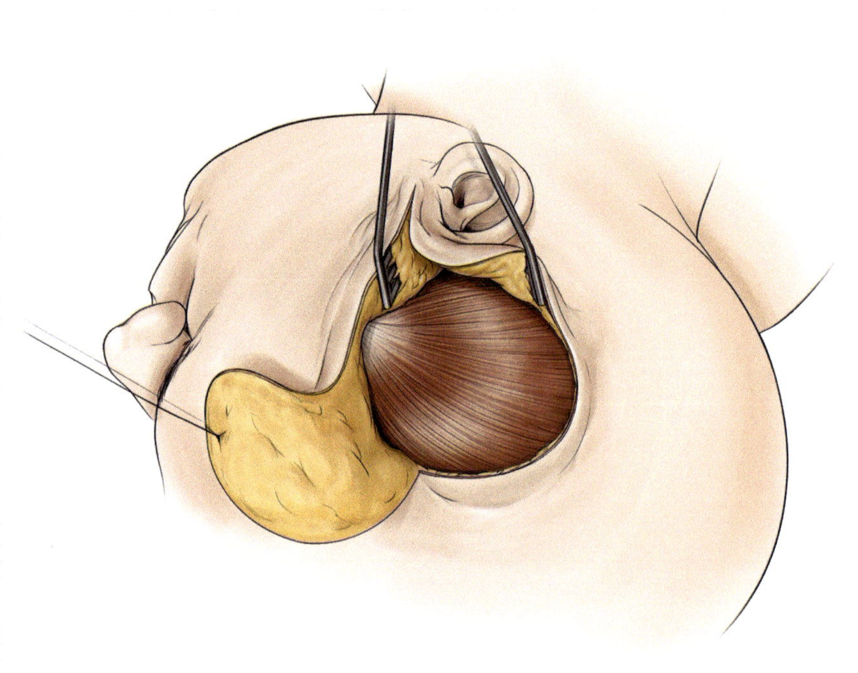

Fig. 37.1 An anteriorly based skin flap is created and the temporalis muscle is exposed. Alternatively, a posterior based skin flap can be created according to the preference of the surgeon.

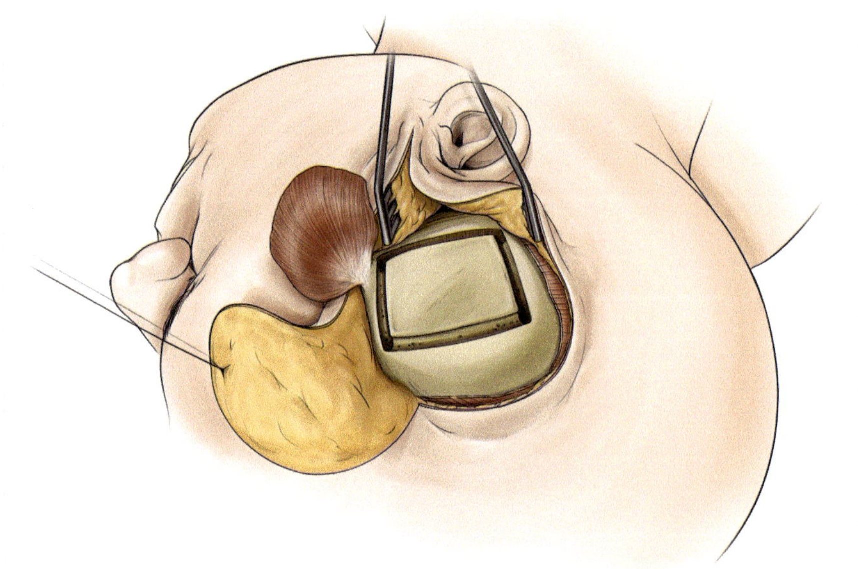

Fig. 37.2 An anteroinferiorly based temporalis muscle flap is created so that it remains attached to its vascular pedicle derived the deep temporal arteries. The temporalis muscle flap must be mobilized enough to permit access to the root of the zygoma for craniotomy, which approximates the middle fossa floor.

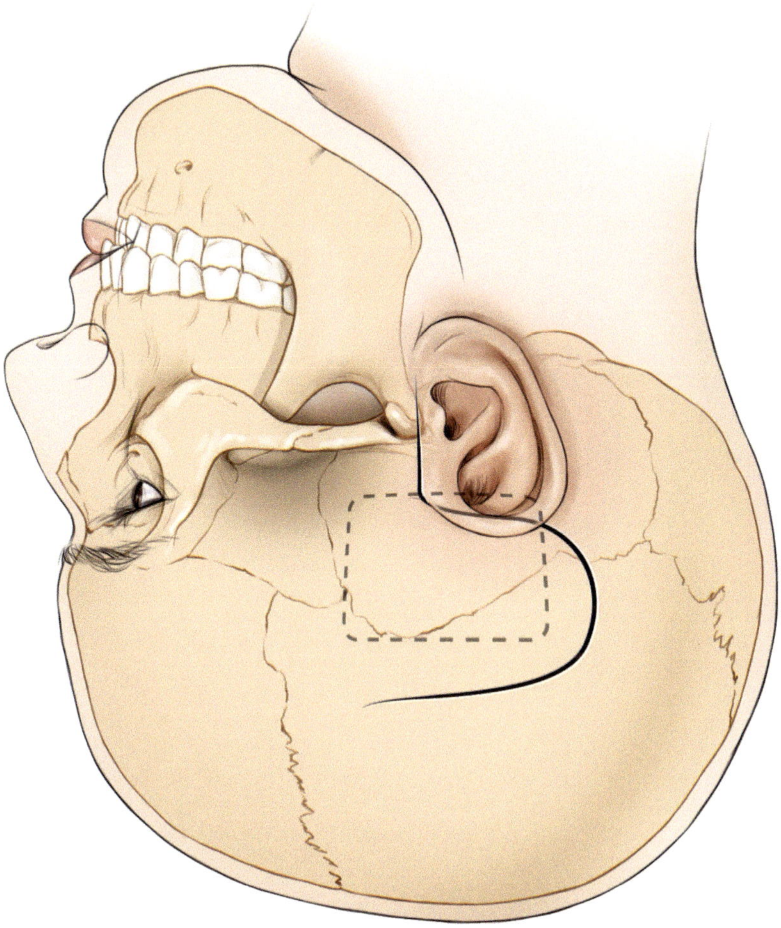

Fig. 37.3 This illustration depicts the design of the skin incision and craniotomy. Note that the craniotomy is centered over the zygomatic root. It is important to have the craniotomy centered anterior to the external auditory canal for optimal exposure of the middle fossa floor and internal auditory canal.

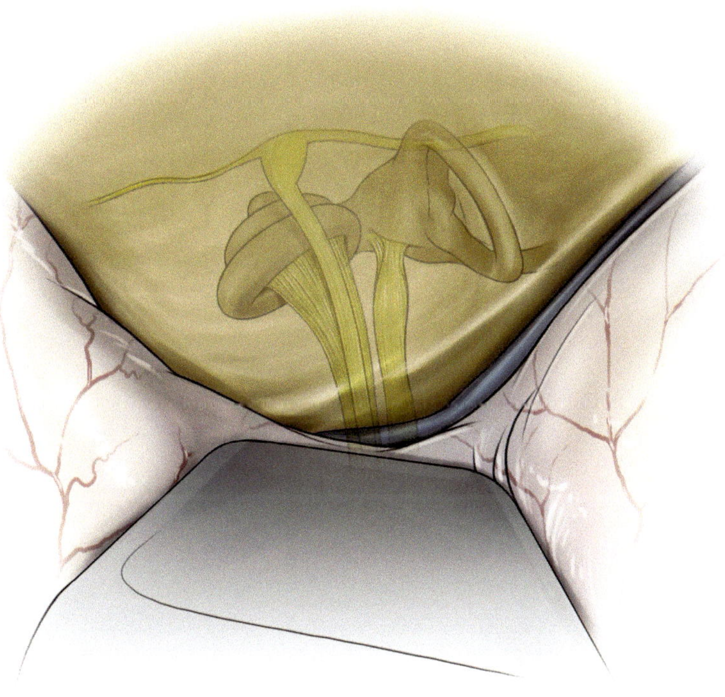

Fig. 37.4 The subtemporal dura is elevated off the middle fossa floor from a posterior-to-anterior direction to avoid traction or avulsion of the greater superficial petrosal nerve. It is important to identify the true petrous ridge medially, where the groove of the superior petrosal sinus is located. This improves surgical exposure and facilitates placement of the middle fossa retractor. Dissection should be carried anteriorly to the middle meningeal artery at the foramen spinosum.

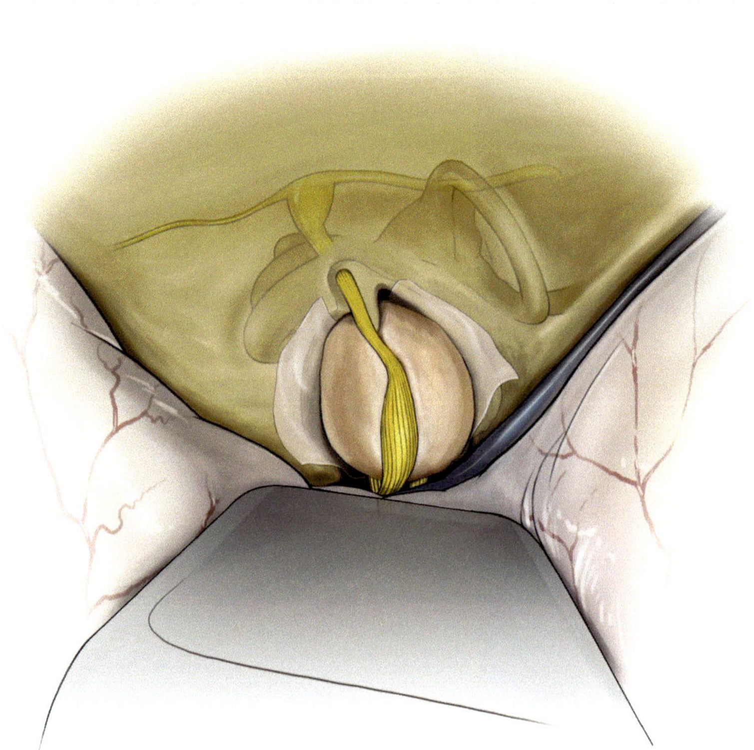

Fig. 37.5 Following bony decompression of the internal auditory canal, the dura is opened and the facial nerve is identified. The medial course of the facial nerve is somewhat variable, but often acquires a position anterior or superior to the tumor capsule. Knowledge of this relationship is important to avoid injury to the facial nerve during drilling, opening of dura, or tumor removal.

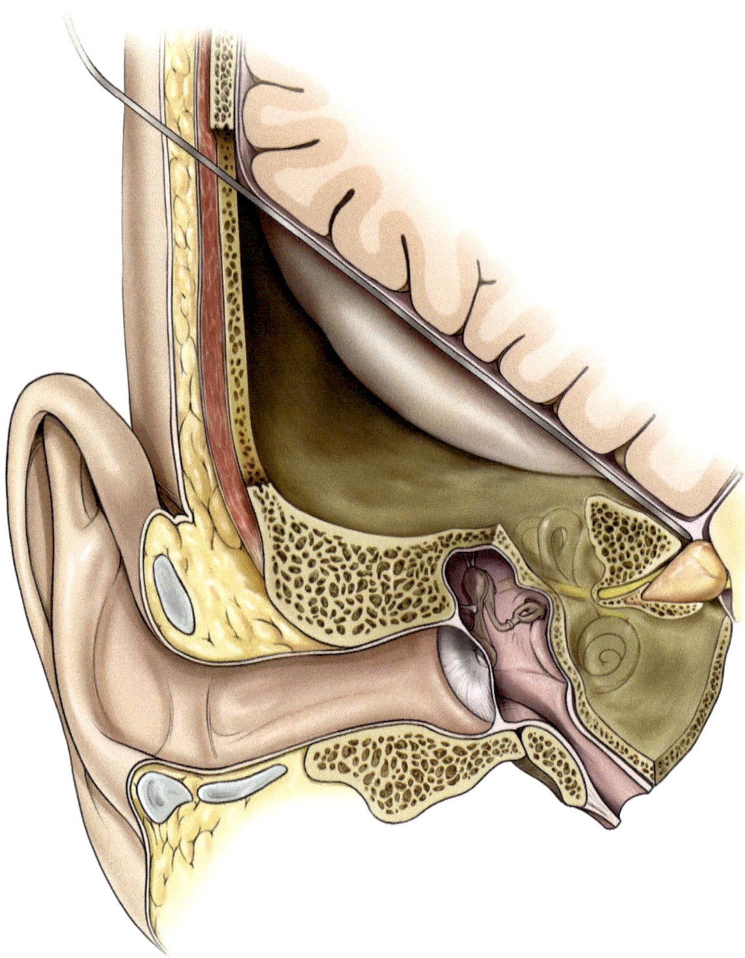

Fig. 37.6 Schematic demonstrating surgical exposure of the internal auditory canal via the middle fossa corridor.

37.4.3 Postoperative Care

At closure, a pressure dressing is applied, and the patient is admitted to the intensive care unit. On postoperative day 1, oral intake and ambulation begins. Physical therapy can lessen the patient's risk of falls and safely increase activity levels. Compression stockings and pneumatic devices can reduce the risk of deep vein thrombosis. Patients are typically discharged home on postoperative day 3. An initial postoperative audiogram is obtained at the third postoperative month. At 1-year follow-up examination, a postoperative MRI with gadolinium is performed to assess for residual tumor.

37.5 Surgical Learning Curve

Of the various surgical procedures for VS resection, the MCF approach is arguably the most challenging. When attempting gross total resection, one is aiming to preserve facial function and hearing function while avoiding intracranial complications. Accomplishing all goals at the same time is not easy. Several authors have described a learning curve in VS surgery, including the MCF approach, whereby the first 25 to 50 cases may have poorer outcomes as the surgeon and team become adept at the procedure.[24,25] Outcomes, however, improve with experience. Given the learning curve of this procedure, early difficulties should not dissuade the surgeon from using this technique. Mastery yields rewarding results. The interested reader is encouraged to review Chapter 29 regarding the learning curve of VS microsurgery.

37.6 Intraoperative Monitoring

Intraoperative monitoring is standard of care for skull base surgery utilizing the MCF approach. Both the facial and cochlear nerves are monitored throughout the case. Cochlear nerve monitoring consists of both CNAP and ABR testing. Active and passive facial nerve monitoring can map the facial nerve in relation to the tumor.[26] At the end of the operation, a constant-current stimulator probe can be used to assess for facial nerve continuity and estimate postoperative facial nerve outcomes.[27] Further discussion regarding intraoperative facial nerve and eighth nerve monitoring are reviewed in Chapters 27 and 28, respectively.

37.7 Facial Nerve and Hearing Preservation Outcomes

Preservation of facial nerve function following the MCF is generally excellent (▶ Table 37.1), with House–Brackmann grade I–II scores ranging from 90 to 96%.[9,12,15,16,17,18,19,20,21,22] As previously mentioned, long-term facial nerve function is generally comparable to the RS and TL approaches when comparing equal-size tumors.[4,5,28]

Hearing preservation varies by study, though most groups report serviceable hearing rates (AAO-HNS [American Academy of Otolaryngology–Head and Neck Surgery] class A or B) of 50 to 75% (▶ Table 37.1).[9,12,15,16,17,18,19,20,21,22] These results are durable, with 65 to 89% of patients maintaining this hearing level 5 years after surgery.[8,9,10] Risk factors for hearing loss include worse preoperative hearing, tumor originating from the inferior vestibular nerve, tumor size, and degree of extension into the CPA.[16,20] Chapter 53 reviews the topic of long-term hearing preservation following microsurgery in greater detail.

37.8 Surgical Complications

The most common complication following the MCF approach is CSF leak, with reported rates of 0 to 12%.[12,20,22,29] In one series of 1,922 patients treated with the RS, MCF, or TL approaches, the CSF leak rate did not differ significantly between approaches.[29] Critics of the MCF approach discuss the risk of temporal lobe aphasia and/or seizures, which may result from the retraction needed to access the IAC and CPA. However, this is an uncommon complication, reported in 0.3 to 1% of patients.[12,15,20]

Other rare complications of the MCF approach are comparable with other intracranial procedures for VS, and include wound infection, cranial nerve injury, death, intracranial bleeding (epidural or subdural hematoma), wound infection, meningitis, deep venous thrombosis, and pulmonary embolism.

37.9 University of Iowa Experience with the MCF Approach

Gantz et al first reported the University of Iowa experience with the MCF approach in 1986. In this series, the hearing preservation rate for 43 patients with tumors extending ≤ 15 mm outside the porus acusticus was 50%.[30] This was updated with a second series spanning 1986 to 1996, in which an improved hearing preservation rate of 69% was noted.[31] In their latest 2006 report, some level of hearing was preserved in 72% of patients. A word recognition score (WRS) greater than 70% was preserved in 77% of patients with a tumor measuring 1 cm or less.[20] Smaller tumor size and better preoperative hearing were associated with higher rates of hearing preservation. Notably, 12 additional patients experienced an improvement in WRS to > 70% following surgery.

In a 2010 review of long-term hearing preservation for 49 patients who underwent MCF resection from 1994 to 2007, Woodson et al categorized four groups based on WRS: grade I (> 70%), grade II (50–70%), grade III (< 50%), and grade IV (0 score).[10] WRS grade I hearing was present in 42 (86%) of 49 patients with a minimum 2-year follow-up, 38 (91%) of 42 patients at last follow-up, and 23 (88%) of 26 patients followed beyond 5 years.[32]

37.10 University of Cincinnati: A Decade of Experience

As the first author of this chapter transferred the skill set he acquired during fellowship to a new institution, these results of the MCF approach have continued. Of 46 patients who underwent an MCF approach for VS resection, 27 (58%) patients had hearing preservation and 45 (98%) patients had HB grade I or II facial function. During this period, one patient had a tumor recurrence requiring treatment. Complications included one

(2%) epidural hematoma, one (2%) subcutaneous wound infection requiring washout, and four (9%) CSF leaks, all managed by lumbar drain insertion (unpublished data).

37.11 Conclusion

The MCF approach for resection of small, primarily intracanalicular, VS results in excellent rates of hearing and facial nerve preservation with minimal morbidity and mortality in experienced hands. We prefer this approach for young healthy patients with good hearing, and even in select cases with poorer hearing in order to preserve some cochlear nerve function.

References

[1] House WF. Surgical exposure of the internal auditory canal and its contents through the middle, cranial fossa. Laryngoscope. 1961; 71:1363–1385

[2] House WF, Gardner G, Hughes RL. Middle cranial fossa approach to acoustic tumor surgery. Arch Otolaryngol. 1968; 88(6):631–641

[3] Chamoun R, MacDonald J, Shelton C, Couldwell WT. Surgical approaches for resection of vestibular schwannomas: translabyrinthine, retrosigmoid, and middle fossa approaches. Neurosurg Focus. 2012; 33(3):E9

[4] Irving RM, Jackler RK, Pitts LH. Hearing preservation in patients undergoing vestibular schwannoma surgery: comparison of middle fossa and retrosigmoid approaches. J Neurosurg. 1998; 88(5):840–845

[5] Colletti V, Fiorino F. Middle fossa versus retrosigmoid-transmeatal approach in vestibular schwannoma surgery: a prospective study. Otol Neurotol. 2003; 24(6):927–934

[6] Mangham CA, Jr. Retrosigmoid versus middle fossa surgery for small vestibular schwannomas. Laryngoscope. 2004; 114(8):1455–1461

[7] Ansari SF, Terry C, Cohen-Gadol AA. Surgery for vestibular schwannomas: a systematic review of complications by approach. Neurosurg Focus. 2012; 33 (3):E14

[8] Friedman RA, Kesser B, Brackmann DE, Fisher LM, Slattery WH, Hitselberger WE. Long-term hearing preservation after middle fossa removal of vestibular schwannoma. Otolaryngol Head Neck Surg. 2003; 129(6):660–665

[9] Hilton CW, Haines SJ, Agrawal A, Levine SC. Late failure rate of hearing preservation after middle fossa approach for resection of vestibular schwannoma. Otol Neurotol. 2011; 32(1):132–135

[10] Woodson EA, Dempewolf RD, Gubbels SP, et al. Long-term hearing preservation after microsurgical excision of vestibular schwannoma. Otol Neurotol. 2010; 31(7):1144–1152

[11] Carlson ML, Jacob JT, Pollock BE, et al. Long-term hearing outcomes following stereotactic radiosurgery for vestibular schwannoma: patterns of hearing loss and variables influencing audiometric decline. J Neurosurg. 2013; 118 (3):579–587

[12] Gjurić M, Wigand ME, Wolf SR. Enlarged middle fossa vestibular schwannoma surgery: experience with 735 cases. Otol Neurotol. 2001; 22(2):223–230, discussion 230–231

[13] Stangerup SE, Caye-Thomasen P, Tos M, Thomsen J. The natural history of vestibular schwannoma. Otol Neurotol. 2006; 27(4):547–552

[14] Régis J, Carron R, Park MC, et al. Wait-and-see strategy compared with proactive Gamma Knife surgery in patients with intracanalicular vestibular schwannomas: clinical article. J Neurosurg. 2013; 119 Suppl:105–111

[15] Arts HA, Telian SA, El-Kashlan H, Thompson BG. Hearing preservation and facial nerve outcomes in vestibular schwannoma surgery: results using the middle cranial fossa approach. Otol Neurotol. 2006; 27 2:234–241

[16] Brackmann DE, Owens RM, Friedman RA, et al. Prognostic factors for hearing preservation in vestibular schwannoma surgery. Am J Otol. 2000; 21(3):417–424

[17] Ginzkey C, Scheich M, Harnisch W, et al. Outcome on hearing and facial nerve function in microsurgical treatment of small vestibular schwannoma via the middle cranial fossa approach. Eur Arch Otorhinolaryngol. 2013; 270(4):1209–1216

[18] Goddard JC, Schwartz MS, Friedman RA. Fundal fluid as a predictor of hearing preservation in the middle cranial fossa approach for vestibular schwannoma. Otol Neurotol. 2010; 31(7):1128–1134

[19] Hillman T, Chen DA, Arriaga MA, Quigley M. Facial nerve function and hearing preservation acoustic tumor surgery: does the approach matter? Otolaryngol Head Neck Surg. 2010; 142(1):115–119

[20] Meyer TA, Canty PA, Wilkinson EP, Hansen MR, Rubinstein JT, Gantz BJ. Small acoustic neuromas: surgical outcomes versus observation or radiation. Otol Neurotol. 2006; 27(3):380–392

[21] Vincent C, Bonne NX, Guerin C, et al. Middle fossa approach for resection of vestibular schwannoma: impact of cochlear fossa extension and auditory monitoring on hearing preservation. Otol Neurotol. 2012; 33(5):849–852

[22] Raheja A, Bowers CA, MacDonald JD, et al. Middle fossa approach for vestibular schwannoma: good hearing and facial nerve outcomes with low morbidity. World Neurosurg. 2016; 92:37–46

[23] Slattery WH, Hoa M, Bonne N, et al. Middle fossa decompression for hearing preservation: a review of institutional results and indications. Otol Neurotol. 2011; 32(6):1017–1024

[24] Wang AY, Wang JT, Dexter M, Da Cruz M. The vestibular schwannoma surgery learning curve mapped by the cumulative summation test for learning curve. Otol Neurotol. 2013; 34(8):1469–1475

[25] Welling DB, Slater PW, Thomas RD, McGregor JM, Goodman JE. The learning curve in vestibular schwannoma surgery. Am J Otol. 1999; 20(5):644–648

[26] Rinaldi V, Casale M, Bressi F, et al. Facial nerve outcome after vestibular schwannoma surgery: our experience. J Neurol Surg B Skull Base. 2012; 73 (1):21–27

[27] Schmitt WR, Daube JR, Carlson ML, et al. Use of supramaximal stimulation to predict facial nerve outcomes following vestibular schwannoma microsurgery: results from a decade of experience. J Neurosurg. 2013; 118(1):206–212

[28] Seo JH, Jun BC, Jeon EJ, Chang KH. Predictive factors influencing facial nerve outcomes in surgery for small-sized vestibular schwannoma. Acta Otolaryngol. 2013; 133(7):722–727

[29] Mangus BD, Rivas A, Yoo MJ, et al. Management of cerebrospinal fluid leaks after vestibular schwannoma surgery. Otol Neurotol. 2011; 32(9):1525–1529

[30] Gantz BJ, Parnes LS, Harker LA, McCabe BF. Middle cranial fossa acoustic neuroma excision: results and complications. Ann Otol Rhinol Laryngol. 1986; 95 (5, Pt 1):454–459

[31] Weber PC, Gantz BJ. Results and complications from acoustic neuroma excision via middle cranial fossa approach. Am J Otol. 1996; 17(4):669–675

[32] Scheich M, Ginzkey C, Reuter E, Harnisch W, Ehrmann D, Hagen R. Quality of life after microsurgery for vestibular schwannoma via the middle cranial fossa approach. Eur Arch Otorhinolaryngol. 2014; 271(7):1909–1916

38 Transotic Approach for Vestibular Schwannoma Resection

Edwin M. Monsell, Yin Xia, and Ugo P. Fisch

38.1 Introduction

In 1979, Ugo Fisch introduced the transotic approach to improve surgical exposure and other aspects of the translabyrinthine approach of William House. The translabyrinthine approach is primarily a posterior approach to the internal auditory canal (IAC) and cerebellopontine angle, whereas the transotic approach is the widest lateral approach, bounded by the sigmoid sinus, the superior petrosal sinus, the internal carotid artery, and the jugular bulb (▶ Fig. 38.1, ▶ Fig. 38.2). The transotic approach also incorporates a subtotal petrosectomy, which may reduce the risk of cerebrospinal fluid (CSF) leakage and associated intracranial infection. Today, the translabyrinthine and retrosigmoid approaches are the most commonly used, though the transotic approach continues to have significant advantages in cases of constricted temporal bone anatomy, including cases with a high jugular bulb, prominent or anteriorly located sigmoid sinus, low tegmen, or a combination of these variations. The extra time required to develop the transotic approach compared to the translabyrinthine approach is at least partially mitigated because less time is required for tumor removal. The transotic, like the translabyrinthine approach, does not spare hearing, so it is only used when there is no intent to preserve hearing in the operated ear.

In the transotic approach, the entire circumference of the IAC is exposed except for a bar of bone that protects the meatal segment of the facial nerve superiorly. The transotic approach provides an improved direct view of the intracranial course of the facial nerve, including the interface between the tumor and the facial nerve just proximal to the porus acusticus, where most injuries to the nerve occur. In the transotic approach, the facial nerve is extensively skeletonized but left in place; however, in the transcochlear approach of House and Hitselberger, it is transposed posteriorly to help expose the clivus, a maneuver that increases the risk of facial nerve injury.

38.2 Surgical Technique

38.2.1 Preparation

The patient is positioned in the supine position with the head turned 45 degrees away, and general anesthesia is induced. A neurosurgical head holder may be used. The hair surrounding the surgical site is clipped close to the skin widely above and behind the pinna. The surgical site is prepared with povidone-iodine scrub and paint. The abdomen is prepared for harvesting abdominal fat. The contralateral leg is prepared if a sural nerve graft is anticipated. The facial nerve is monitored.

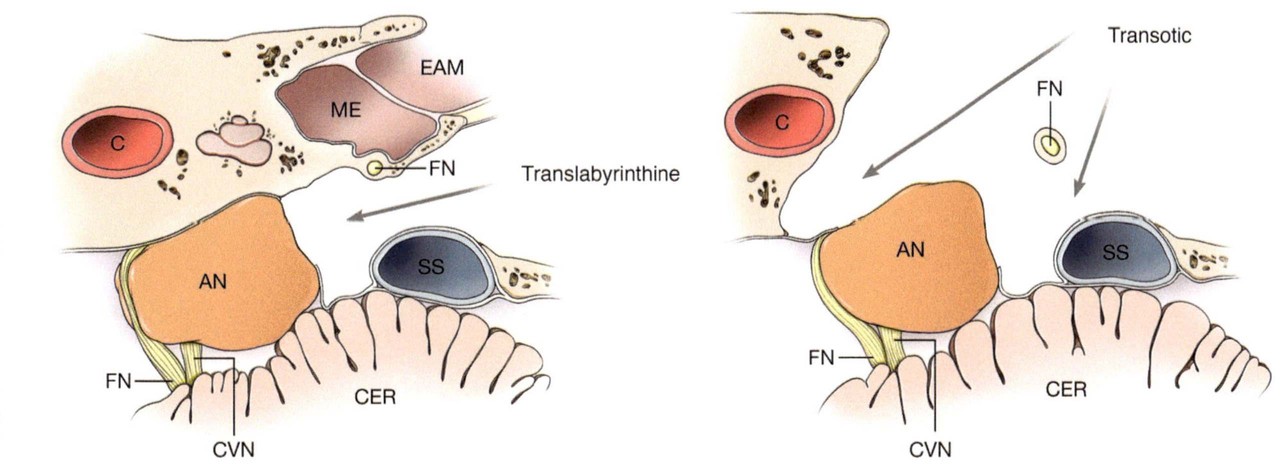

Fig. 38.1 Diagrammatic view from the superior position showing the exposure of the translabyrinthine approach (left) and the wider transotic approach (right), redrawn from Chen and Fisch.[2] AN, acoustic neuroma (vestibular schwannoma); C, carotid artery; CER, cerebellum; CVN, cochlear-vestibular nerve; EAM, external auditory meatus; FN, facial nerve; ME, middle ear; SS sigmoid sinus in an unusually anterior position that constricts the translabyrinthine exposure.

38.2.2 Skin Incision

The operative techniques for the subtotal petrosectomy and transotic approach are described in detail with indications for surgical instrumentation in *Microsurgery of the Skull Base* by Fisch and Mattox, from which most of the illustrations in this chapter are reproduced.[1] The skin incision begins superior to the pinna (▶ Fig. 38.3), continues behind the postauricular hairline, and extends over the mastoid tip. The superior portion of the incision (▶ Fig. 38.3) is made after tumor resection, and provides exposure to develop the temporalis muscle flap.

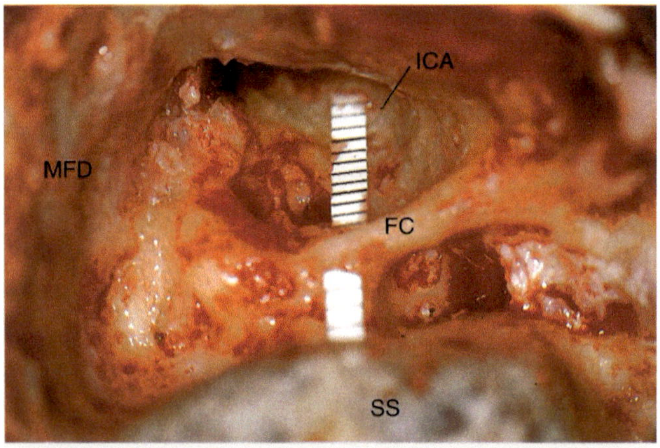

Fig. 38.2 Intraoperative photomicrograph in a case of right vestibular schwannoma with a large, anterior sigmoid sinus (large blue object in the foreground, SS). The white measuring tape passes medial to the mastoid segment of the facial nerve. In this case the approach provides 4 mm of posterior and 12 mm of anterior exposure from the facial nerve. FC, fallopian canal of the facial nerve; ICA, internal carotid artery; MFD, middle fossa dura. (Reproduced with permission from Fisch and Mattox.[1])

38.2.3 Blind Sac Closure of the External Auditory Canal

A mastoid periosteal flap is developed (▶ Fig. 38.4). The external auditory canal (EAC) is transected at the bony–cartilaginous junction. The EAC skin is separated from the cartilage, everted externally, and closed with sutures. The periosteal flap is rotated to cover the lateral end of the EAC, and is sutured to the EAC cartilage (▶ Fig. 38.4). This creates a watertight closure of the EAC. The skin of the EAC is elevated to the annulus, the middle ear space is entered, and the chorda tympani nerve is divided. The incudostapedial joint is separated and the malleus neck is cut. The tympanic membrane, manubrium, and remaining EAC skin are removed as a continuous block of tissue. The operative site is again carefully inspected to be sure that all squamous epithelium has been removed, because the cavity will be obliterated (▶ Fig. 38.5).

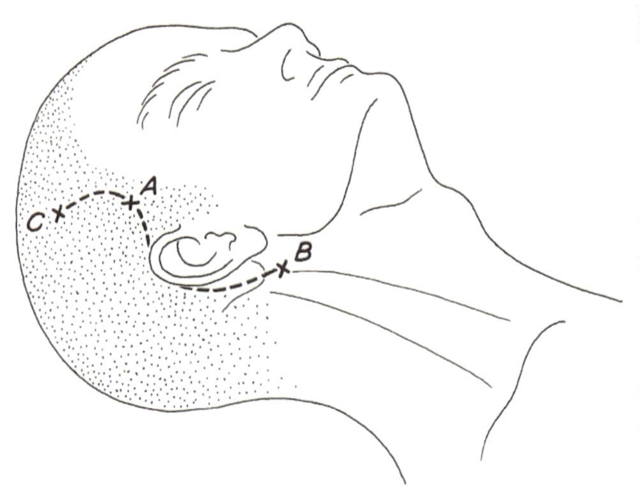

Fig. 38.3 The postauricular incision used for the transotic approach. (Reproduced with permission from Fisch and Mattox.[1])

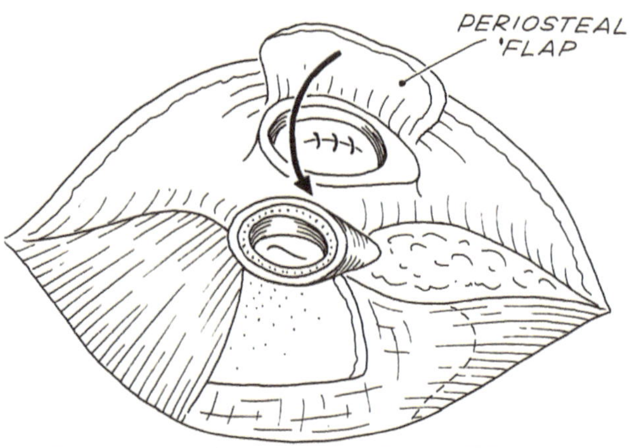

Fig. 38.4 The periosteal flap is located inferiorly from the temporal line, and is pedicled anteriorly to the soft tissues posterior to the auricle. (Reproduced with permission from Fisch and Mattox.[1])

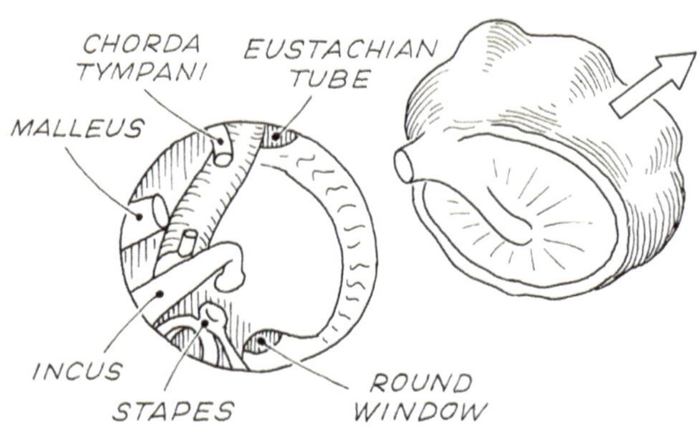

Fig. 38.5 The ossicular chain is separated and the chorda tympani nerve is sectioned. The tympanic membrane, fibrous annulus, and remaining skin of the external auditory meatus are removed en bloc. (Reproduced with permission from Fisch and Mattox.[1])

38.2.4 Subtotal Petrosectomy

The inferior temporalis muscle is elevated off the squamous temporal bone to facilitate exposure of the tegmen in the mastoid, and the attachments of the sternocleidomastoid muscle are removed to expose the entire mastoid tip. A complete mastoidectomy is carried out (▶ Fig. 38.6). The EAC wall is removed and lowered to the level of the facial nerve. All accessible air cells are systematically and completely exenterated. The tympanic end of the eustachian tube is opened to the isthmus and obliterated. The mastoid tip is removed (▶ Fig. 38.6).

38.2.5 Transotic Approach

A labyrinthectomy is performed, the cochlea is removed, and the tumor and IAC are skeletonized. The sigmoid sinus and jugular bulb are skeletonized, and the posterior fossa dura is exposed medial and anterior to the facial nerve. The facial nerve is skeletonized from the geniculate ganglion to the stylomastoid foramen, and remains in place covered with bone. The anterior bony annulus is removed. The internal carotid artery is skeletonized as the anterior limit of the dissection (▶ Fig. 38.7). The labyrinthine segment of the facial nerve is identified at the meatal foramen (▶ Fig. 38.8). Note that special care must be exercised in this maneuver to avoid damage to the tympanic segment of the facial nerve. This step is important for providing additional exposure when separating the facial nerve during tumor removal. The dura of the posterior fossa is exposed above the porus along the superior petrosal sinus, and the tympanic segment of the facial nerve is skeletonized (▶ Fig. 38.8).

38.2.6 Tumor Removal

After initial tumor debulking, the posterior fossa dura is opened between the sinodural angle and the posterior edge of the porus acusticus. This maneuver exposes the posterior pole of the tumor and the petrosal vein (▶ Fig. 38.9). The incision is extended anteriorly from the porus to the vertical segment of the internal carotid artery, providing exposure of the inferior and anterior poles of the tumor, the region of the origin of the seventh and eighth cranial nerves, and the anterior inferior cerebellar artery (AICA; ▶ Fig. 38.10). Vessels on the surface of the tumor are cauterized with bipolar forceps. The tumor is separated from the facial nerve in the IAC using a microraspatory or fine right-angle pick, and an atraumatic suction tip is applied indirectly through a neurosurgical cottonoid. The AICA is carefully displaced posteriorly after coagulation and section of its tumor branches. Remaining larger vessels are coagulated on the surface of the tumor. Until this point, the meatal dura is left attached to the tumor to help protect the facial nerve. Following sufficient intracapsular debulking of the tumor, the meatal dura is separated from the tumor, allowing the remaining tumor to be positioned inferiorly (▶ Fig. 38.11).

In some cases, there is a small amount of residual tumor attached to the nerve due to adherence or infiltration of the nerve (▶ Fig. 38.12). In the presence of dense tumor adherence or infiltration, the surgeon can then decide whether to remove the remaining tumor or to make an informed choice to leave a small amount of tumor, balancing the risk of tumor regrowth versus the risk of trauma to the nerve.

The key to management of large tumors is extensive reduction of tumor volume from intracapsular removal. In large

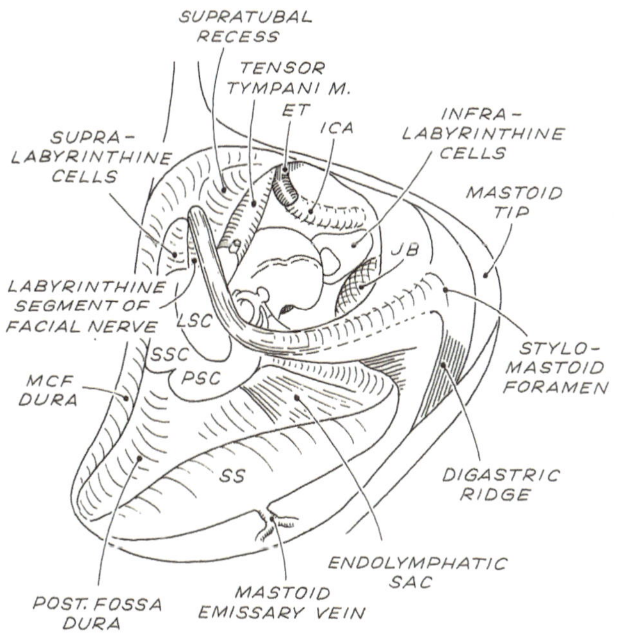

Fig. 38.6 The mastoidectomy has been completed. The canal wall has been removed and lowered to the level of the facial nerve, which has been skeletonized. The jugular bulb and internal carotid artery have been skeletonized. The eustachian tube has been obliterated. All pneumatic cell tracts have been exenterated. ICA, internal carotid artery; JB, jugular bulb; LSC, lateral semicircular canal; SS, sigmoid sinus. (Reproduced with permission from Fisch and Mattox.[1])

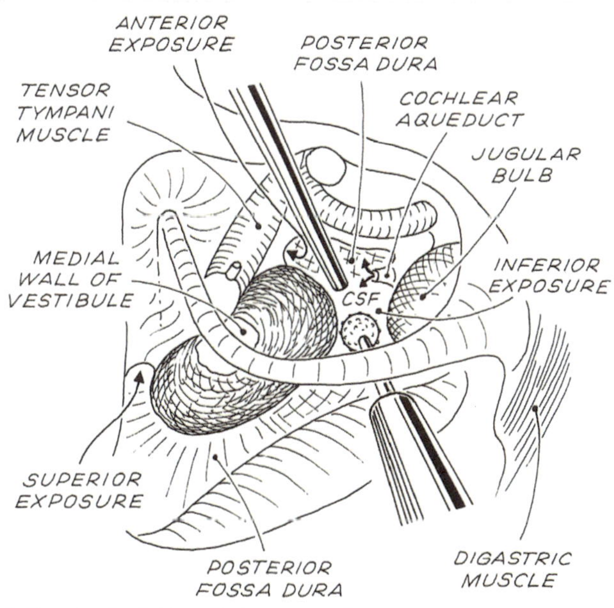

Fig. 38.7 The labyrinthectomy is complete. The cochlea has been removed (also the tensor semicanal if necessary) and the dura of the IAC and tumor has been exposed. The dura of the middle and posterior fossa has been exposed from the sigmoid sinus to the internal carotid artery and from the jugular bulb to the tensor tympani muscle. CSF is released by opening the cochlear aqueduct before the dura is opened. (Reproduced with permission from Fisch and Mattox.[1])

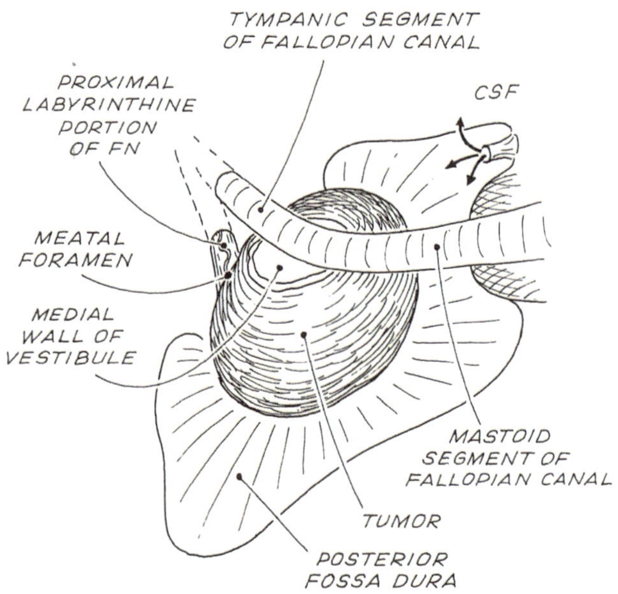

Fig. 38.8 The labyrinthine segment of the facial nerve is identified at the meatal foramen. (Reproduced with permission from Fisch and Mattox.[1])

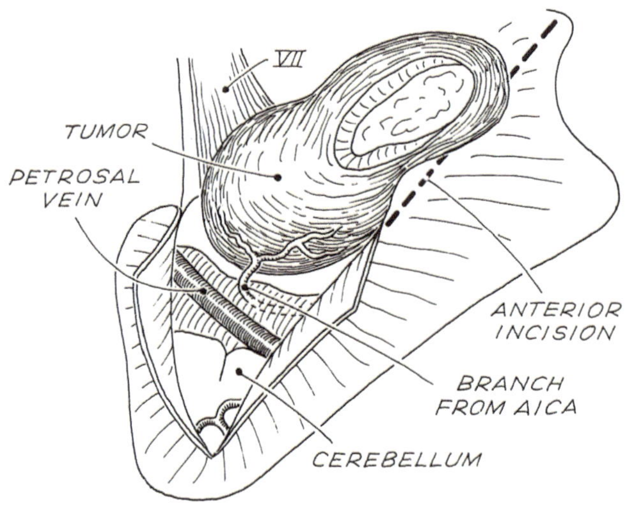

Fig. 38.9 The first part of the dural incision has been made, exposing the petrosal vein. (Reproduced with permission from Fisch and Mattox.[1])

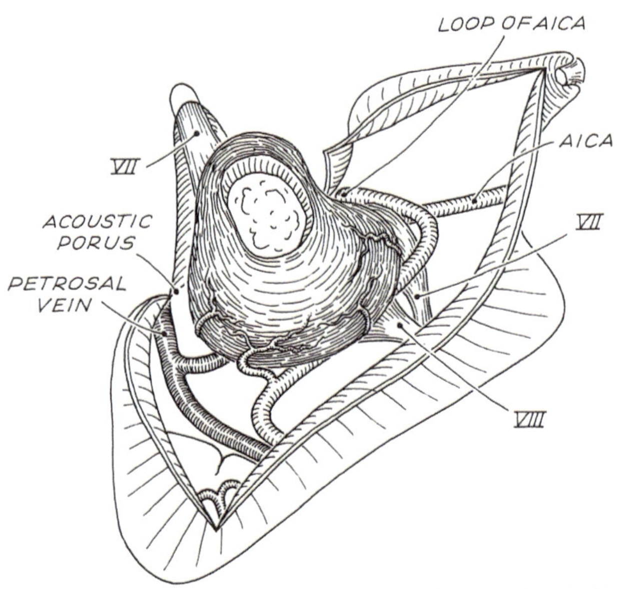

Fig. 38.10 The dural incision has been extended, potentially exposing the AICA and the inferior pole of the tumor. (Reproduced with permission from Fisch and Mattox.[1])

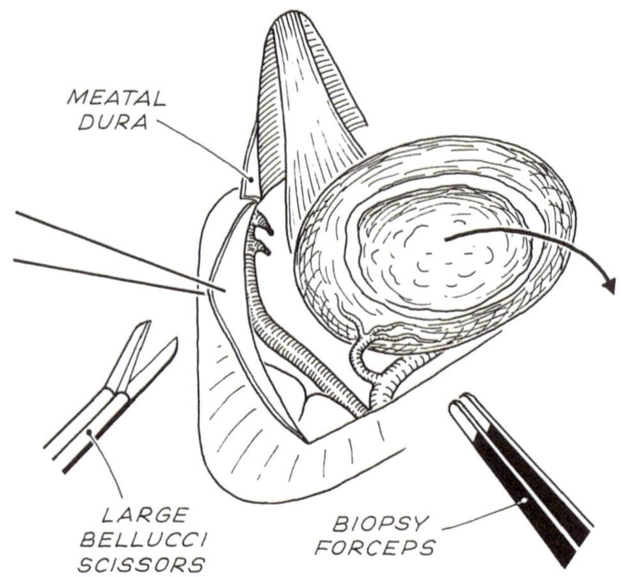

Fig. 38.11 The meatal dura is separated from the facial nerve at the porus acusticus. (Reproduced with permission from Fisch and Mattox.[1])

tumors, the region around the origin of the eighth nerve may be crowded with branches of the AICA or the petrosal vein. Extreme care is necessary when working in this region.

The more anterior exposure provided by the transotic approach has a distinct advantage over the translabyrinthine approach in cases with a high jugular bulb. Even when the jugular bulb extends to the inferior pole of the IAC, a few millimeters of posterior fossa dura can always be exposed between the porus and the dome of the jugular bulb by working medial to the fallopian canal.[1]

38.2.7 Wound Closure

A temporalis musculofascial graft is harvested and sutured medial to the dura, affording space for the large graft of abdominal fat that is placed medial to the mastoid segment of the facial nerve, filling the surgical defect in the temporal bone. A temporalis muscle flap is developed, rotated over the temporal bone, and sutured to the sternocleidomastoid muscle (► Fig. 38.13). The wound is closed in layers.

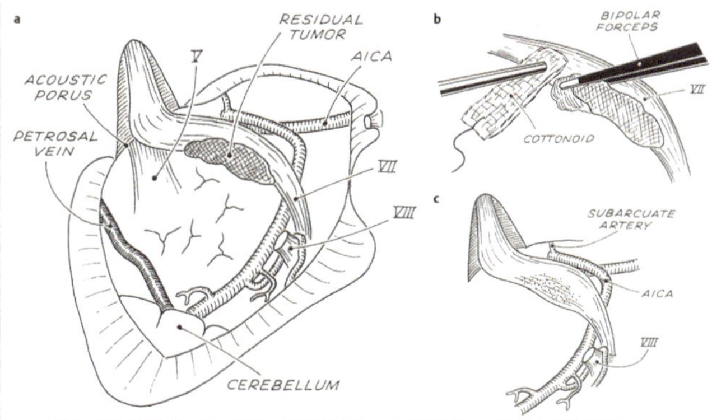

Fig. 38.12 The tumor has been removed except for a small remnant adherent to the facial nerve. (Reproduced with permission from Fisch and Mattox.[1])

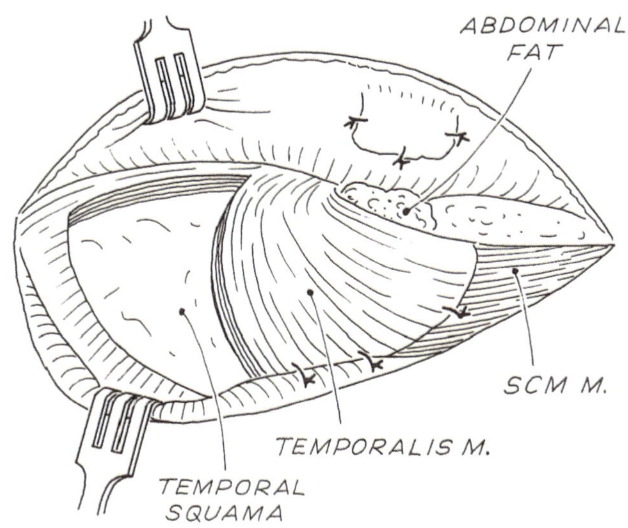

Fig. 38.13 The wound is closed by suturing a plug of fascia and muscle to the posterior fossa dura, filling the mastoid wound cavity with abdominal fat, and closing the temporalis muscle to the sternocleidomastoid muscle over the fat. (Reproduced with permission from Fisch and Mattox.[1])

38.2.8 Dressing and Postoperative Care

A large compression dressing is applied. Patients are monitored in the intensive care unit for at least 24 hours until they are awake enough to ensure that they are neurologically intact. They are usually discharged to home several days after surgery.

38.3 Technical Pearls and Pitfalls

38.3.1 Subtotal Petrosectomy

When transecting the anterior EAC skin, avoid damaging the superior branches of the facial nerve in the parotid, as these may lie close to the anterior skin of the EAC. Elevate at least 1 cm of EAC skin so there will be adequate skin to evert. Trim any excess so the closure will be uniform and heal well. Be careful to leave no remnants of skin in the EAC or middle ear. Complete exenteration of all air cells requires complete skeletonization of the labyrinthine capsule, facial nerve, jugular bulb, and internal carotid artery.

38.3.2 Transotic Approach

When developing the anterior exposure, skeletonize and expose the posterior fossa dura from the tensor tympani semicanal superiorly to the internal carotid artery anteriorly and to the jugular bulb inferiorly. This exposure is necessary to view the facial nerve anterior to the tumor. Use bone wax to control bleeding of spongiotic bone around the jugular bulb. Most of the blood supply to the tumor comes from vessels traveling with the eighth nerve, which can usually be seen well from the inferior side of the transotic exposure. Be alert that the AICA may give off the subarcuate artery entering the temporal bone. When sectioning the eighth nerve, be careful to avoid damaging the underlying AICA. Sectioning of the eighth nerve may be necessary to expose the entry zone of the facial nerve. When a high jugular bulb is present, special care must be taken with the AICA and its branches and with small veins at the inferior pole of the tumor.

Table 38.1 Two-year postoperative facial nerve results in 66 of the original 147 consecutive patients via a transotic approach, with permission.

Tumor size (cm)	*n*	Percent recovery				
		100	99–80	79–60	59–40	39–0
1–1.4	14	100	–	–	–	–
1.5–2.5[a]	52	61	19	12	4	4
Total	66	70	15	9	3	3

[a]No difference was noted in facial function following removal of tumors 1.5–1.9 cm vs. 2–2.5 cm.

Source: Used with permission from Chen JM, Fisch U. The transotic approach in acoustic neuroma surgery. J Otolaryngol. 1993;22(5):331-336.

38.3.3 Complications and Clinical Outcomes

The complications and outcomes from Fisch's original series of 147 solitary vestibular schwannomas (1.0–2.5 cm in the largest medial–lateral extent) removed by the transotic approach (1979–1990) were compared to a similar series of 114 tumors removed by the translabyrinthine approach (Table 38.1).[2,3] The tumor was completely removed in all cases. Mortality from pulmonary embolism was 1% in each series. There were no major intracranial complications. CSF leak occurred through either the nose or the wound in 3% of the transotic cases and 22% of the translabyrinthine cases ($p < 0.001$). All of the leaks in the transotic cases occurred in the immediate postoperative period; only one required operative revision. CSF leakage occurred in 22% of the translabyrinthine cases. The leakage was immediate in 15% of the operated cases, and in 7% it was delayed. Three of the translabyrinthine cases presented with meningitis more than 4 years after surgery. Facial nerve outcomes in 66 patients with data at 2 years postoperatively are shown in Table 38.1.

Table 38.2 Short-term postoperative facial nerve results in 36 consecutive patients with the transotic approach

Tumor size (cm)	Number of patients (%)	Facial nerve function (House-Brackmann)/detailed evaluation of facial nerve symmetry[4] (mean % score)					
		Preoperative			Postoperative (6 wk)		
		I/100%	II/76–99%	III/51–75%	I/100%	II/76–99%	III/51–75%
0.5–2.0	13 (36%)	13/100%	0	0	6/100%	7/83%	0
2.1–4.0	18 (50%)	15/100%	3/87%	0	1/100%	17/81%	0
4.1–5.0	5 (14%)	0	4/82%	1/66%	0	3/77%	2/59%
Total	36 (100%)	28/100%	7/84%	1/66%	7/100%	27/81%	2/59%

Source: Used with permission from Xia Y, Zhang W, Li Y, Ma X, Lui Q, Shi J. The Transotic Approach for Vestibular Schwannoma: Indications and Results. Eur Arch Otorhinolaryngol 2017; 274(8):3041-3047.[5]

Xia et al recently described outcomes in a series of 36 tumors ranging from 0.5 to more than 4.1 cm in largest lateral–medial dimension, all in temporal bones with restricted anatomy operated by the transotic approach.[5] The tumor was totally removed in 94%, and there was one case of CSF leakage. The tumor in this case was larger than 4 cm; surgical revision was required to close the leakage. There were no deaths in this series. One patient required reoperation due to intracranial bleeding. There were no intracranial infections or other severe complications. The facial nerve was preserved anatomically in all cases. Short-term facial nerve outcomes are shown in ▶ Table 38.2.

38.4 Conclusion

The transotic approach has several potential advantages over the translabyrinthine approach, including enhanced surgical exposure and a lower CSF leakage rate. Compared to other transtemporal approaches, the transotic approach is particularly advantageous in cases with an anterior sigmoid sinus, high jugular bulb, low tegmen, or tumors with significant anterior extension.

References

[1] Fisch U, Mattox D. Microsurgery of the Skull Base. New York, NY: Thieme Medical Publishers; 1988

[2] Chen JM, Fisch U. The transotic approach in acoustic neuroma surgery. J Otolaryngol. 1993; 22(5):331–336

[3] Browne JD, Fisch U. Transotic approach to the cerebellopontine angle. Otolaryngol Clin North Am. 1992; 25(2):331–346

[4] Rickenmann J, Jaquenod C, Cerenko D, Fisch U. Comparative value of facial nerve grading systems. Otolaryngol Head Neck Surg. 1997; 117(4): 322–325

[5] Xia Y, Zhang W, Li Y, Ma X, Liu Q, Shi J. The transotic approach for vestibular schwannoma: indications and results. Eur Arch Otorhinolaryngol. 2017; 274 (8):3041–3047

39 Transcanal Transpromontorial Endoscopic Approach for Vestibular Schwannoma Resection

Daniele Marchioni, Davide Soloperto, and Livio Presutti

39.1 Introduction

Totally endoscopic surgery is now a well-accepted minimally invasive technique for the treatment of many anterior skull base pathologies. While in these cases endoscopic approaches have become well established, totally endoscopic approaches to other areas of the skull base such as the cerebellopontine angle (CPA) and the internal auditory canal (IAC) have been limited. Currently, endoscopy in CPA surgery is primarily used as an adjunct to conventional microscopic surgical techniques for vestibular schwannoma (VS) treatment. The first application of the endoscope to IAC surgery was to assist in visualization with the retrosigmoid approach. After removal of the CPA component, the intracanalicular portion was removed under endoscopic visualization, trying to avoid extensive drilling of the posterior aspect of the petrous bone,[1,2] or using a keyhole retrosigmoid approach.[3] Endoscope-assisted microsurgery (EAM) of the CPA has provided an excellent initiation of the endoscope into posterior fossa surgery,[3] and the advances in the application of endoscopy in the surgical treatment of middle ear cholesteatomas and neoplasms[4,5,6,7] have further improved its acceptance in otology and lateral skull base surgery. With the gradual development and progression of middle ear endoscopic surgery, greater comfort and skill with endoscopic inner ear anatomy and surgery has come.[8] Microscopic approaches for treatment of VS have been firmly established and their outcomes widely studied, including the retrosigmoid/suboccipital, transmastoid-translabyrinthine, and subtemporal middle cranial fossa approach.[9] All these methods require external incisions with variable degrees of temporal bone drilling to adequately expose the IAC and CPA. Recently, progression from EAM to a fully endoscopic technique to the IAC for VS resection has been described and clinically applied.[10,11] In 2012, an exclusive endoscopic approach, the transcanal transpromontorial endoscopic approach (TTEA), to the IAC was described and used to resect a cochlear schwannoma (CS) involving the IAC.[10] Since this time, several publications documenting VS resection using the TTEA have emerged.

39.2 Transcanal Transpromontorial Endoscopic Approach to the IAC

In the TTEA, the external auditory canal (EAC) is used as natural surgical corridor to reach the fundus of the IAC, passing through the cochlea and the vestibule and exposing the entire IAC (▶ Fig. 39.1). From an anatomical point of view, this approach allows the surgeon to work on the medial wall of the tympanic cavity and lateral skull base, avoiding cerebellum and middle and posterior fossa manipulation and potentially reducing the morbidity related to standard approaches. Since cochlear drilling is mandatory in order to access the IAC, any residual hearing is sacrificed with this procedure (▶ Fig. 39.2).

39.3 Indications

- Growing or symptomatic VS limited to the IAC with nonserviceable hearing (type C or D, according to AAO-HNS [American Academy of Otolaryngology–Head and Neck Surgery] classification).
- CSs, with or without IAC involvement.
- Residual or recurrent VS involving the IAC, after prior microsurgical resection.

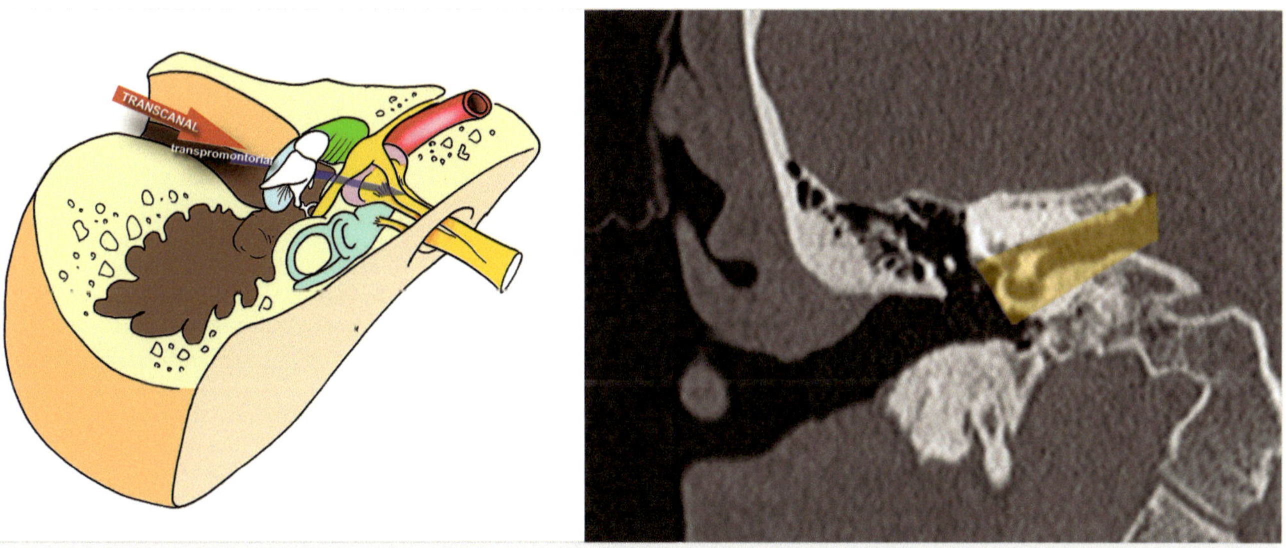

Fig. 39.1 Schematic drawing on the left representing the surgical corridors; the EAC is used as natural corridors in order to reach the IAC: on the right, a CT scan in coronal view showing in yellow the working area.

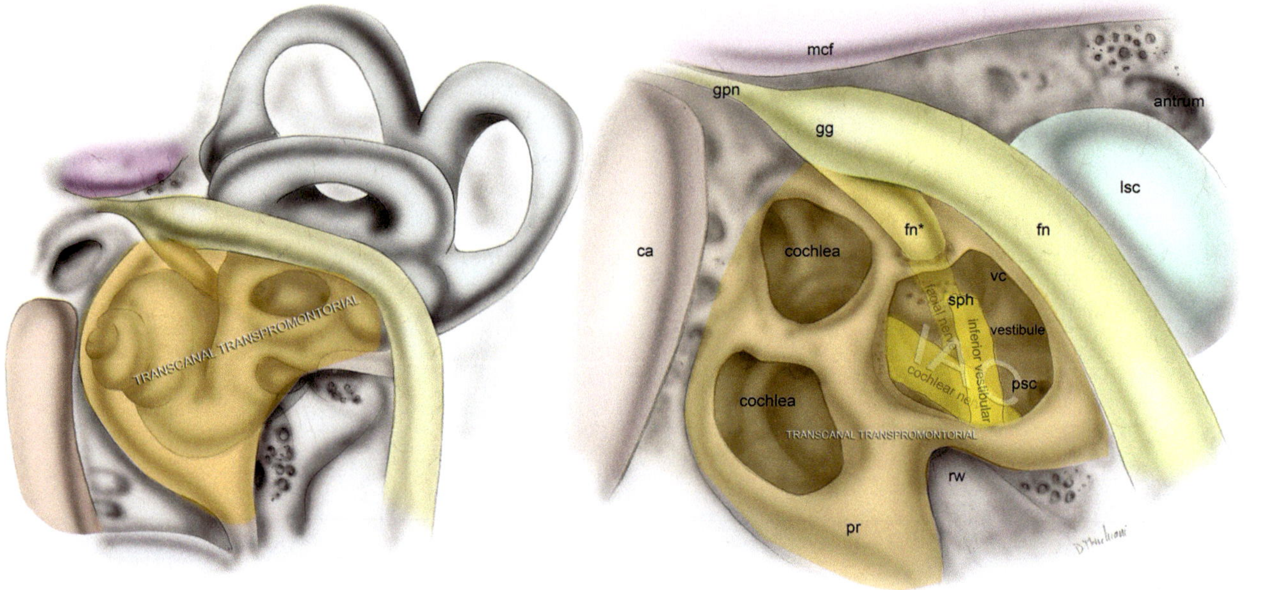

Fig. 39.2 Left ear: anatomical landmarks of the transpromontorial transcanal endoscopic approach. The reader can note the position of the facial nerve into the fundus of the IAC and the close relationships between the vestibule, the cochlea, and the IAC. ca, carotid artery; fn, facial nerve; fn*, labyrinthine portion of facial nerve; gg, geniculate ganglion; gpn, greater petrosal nerve; lsc, lateral semicircular canal; mcf, middle cranial fossa; pr, promontory; psc, posterior semicircular canal opening; rw, round window; sph, spherical recess; vc, vestibular crest.

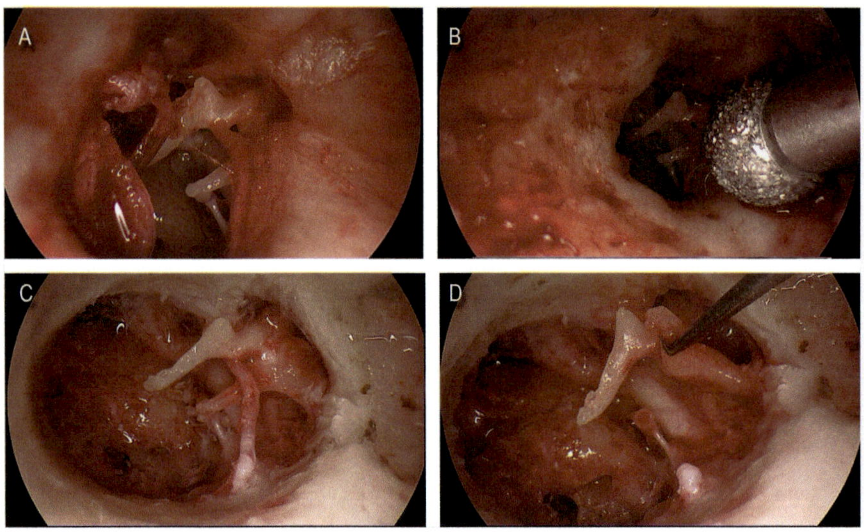

Fig. 39.3 Left ear: TTEA. **(a)** The eardrum is removed; **(b)** a diamond burr is used to enlarge the EAC; **(c)** after widening of the EAC, the tympanic cavity is under endoscopic control; **(d)** ossicular chain removal.

39.4 Surgical Technique

A 0-degree rigid endoscope (Karl Storz, Tuttlingen, Germany) is used, 15 cm in length and 3 mm or 4 mm in diameter. An AIDA three-chip high-resolution monitor and camera (Karl Storz, Tuttlingen, Germany) are employed. The patient is positioned supine, the head gently rotated to the other side, with facial nerve monitoring (NIM) applied. A circumferential skin incision of the EAC is made with a round knife under 0-degree endoscopic view, between the cartilaginous and bony portions of the EAC. The skin is elevated circumferentially with the tympanic membrane, detaching the annulus from the bony ring. The flap, pedicled on the umbus, is transposed laterally and then detached from the malleus using a microscissors ensuring that all skin is removed to avoid iatrogenic cholesteatoma. After the tympanic cavity is exposed (▶ Fig. 39.3a), the bony EAC is drilled (▶ Fig. 39.3b), with the anterior limit being the temporomandibular joint and the posterior limit being the mastoid segment of the facial nerve, providing maximum surgical access to the medial wall of the tympanic cavity. The bony annulus is then circumferentially drilled, progressively exposing the hypotympanum, protympanum, retrotympanum, and attic spaces, with the ossicular chain and promontory region well visualized (▶ Fig. 39.3c). Ossicular chain disarticulation is then performed

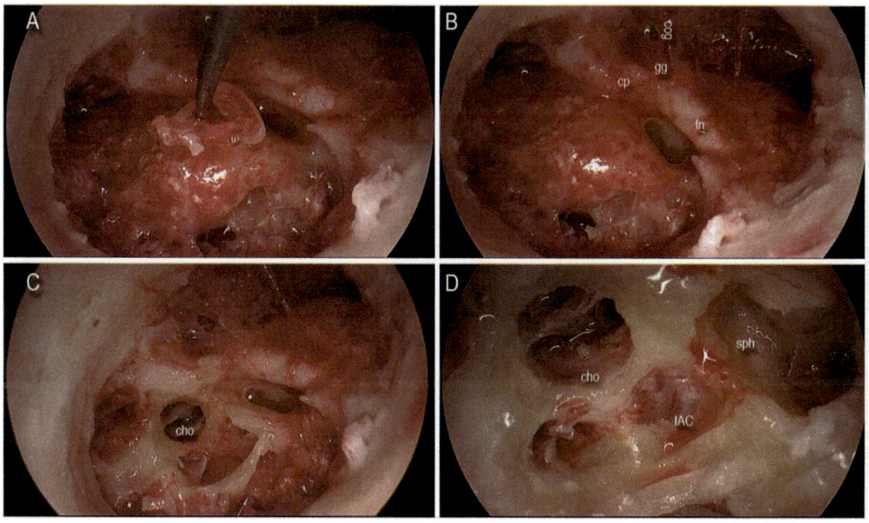

Fig. 39.4 Left ear: TTEA. **(a)** Stapes removal entering into the vestibule; **(b)** the vestibule now is opened and the tympanic portion of the facial nerve until the geniculate ganglion is under endoscopic view; **(c)** the promontory is progressively drilled, exposing cochlear turns; **(d)** the fundus of the IAC is opened between the spherical recess and the cochlea. cho, cochlea; cp, cochleariform process; gg, geniculate ganglion; IAC, internal auditory canal; sph, spherical recess.

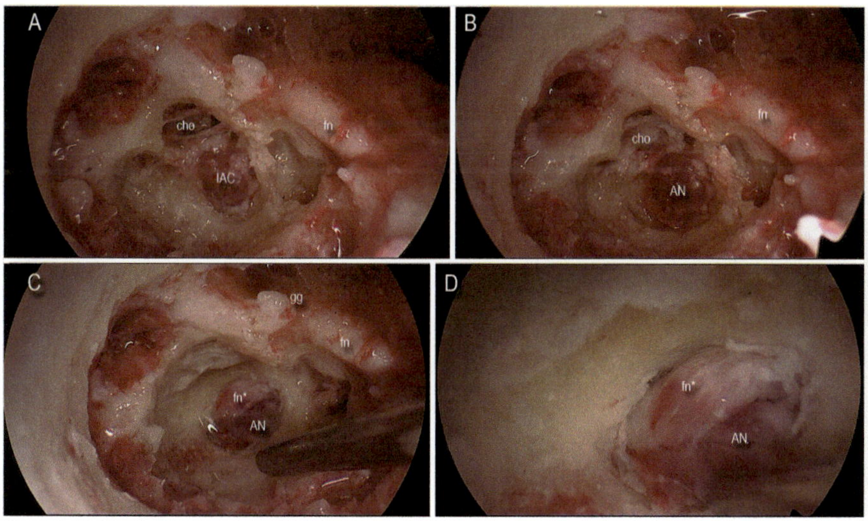

Fig. 39.5 Left ear: TTEA. **(a)** The IAC is skeletonized progressively; **(b)** the dura of the IAC is opened exposing the VS; **(c)** the facial nerve into the IAC is detected; **(d)** the VS is removed, preserving the facial nerve integrity. AN, acoustic neuroma (vestibular schwannoma); cho, cochlea; fn*, facial nerve into the IAC; gg, geniculate ganglion; IAC, internal auditory canal.

as a necessary step to access the entire medial tympanic cavity. The incus and the malleus are removed, leaving the stapes undisturbed (▶ Fig. 39.3d). The tympanic segment of the facial nerve is exposed from the second genu to the geniculate ganglion, located between the cog and the cochleariform process. After this, the stapes is removed, entering into the vestibule and identifying the saccule (▶ Fig. 39.4a,b). The spherical recess in the saccular fossa is endoscopically identified, since this structure marks the end of the inferior vestibular nerve and represents an important landmark for the localization of the fundus of the IAC. The bony overhang of the round window niche is drilled, exposing the membrane of the round window. Using a piezosurgery instrument (Mectron, Carasco/Genova, Italy), the promontory with lateral aspect of the otic capsule is removed at the cochlear level, identifying the basal, middle, and upper turns of the cochlea (▶ Fig. 39.4c). After exposing the cochlear turns, the bony wall between the cochlea and the spherical recess is carefully drilled, entering the fundus of the IAC (▶ Fig. 39.4d). Dissection of the IAC is performed, following the dura of the IAC from the fundus to the porus, progressively exposing the VS (▶ Fig. 39.5a). The bones between the IAC and the internal carotid artery anteriorly, the IAC and the mastoid portion of the facial nerve posteriorly, the IAC and the jugular bulb inferiorly, and the IAC and the tympanic segment of the facial nerve superiorly are removed circumferentially. The bone of the otic capsule is removed from lateral to medial, thereby exposing the dura of the medial surface of the temporal bone, representing the deepest limit of the dissection. After IAC exposure, the dura is opened and the VS is more fully exposed (▶ Fig. 39.5b). At this time, identification of the facial nerve in the IAC is mandatory in order to avoid facial nerve injury (▶ Fig. 39.5c); the use of a facial nerve stimulator can help the surgeon during dissection. The tumor is then carefully dissected and removed in piecemeal fashion while maintaining the integrity of the facial nerve (▶ Fig. 39.5d). When the VS has limited extension into the CPA, the bone of the porus can be enlarged using a diamond burr so that the last portion of the tumor can be safely dissected in the angle. Once tumor dissection is complete, an inspection of the IAC is performed to confirm complete tumor resection (▶ Fig. 39.6a–c). Closure is performed with abdominal fat, packing the promontorial defect and closing the communication between the inner ear and middle ear (▶ Fig. 39.6d). Fibrin glue is used to fix the fat graft into the promontorial defect; a piece of muscle is used to close the

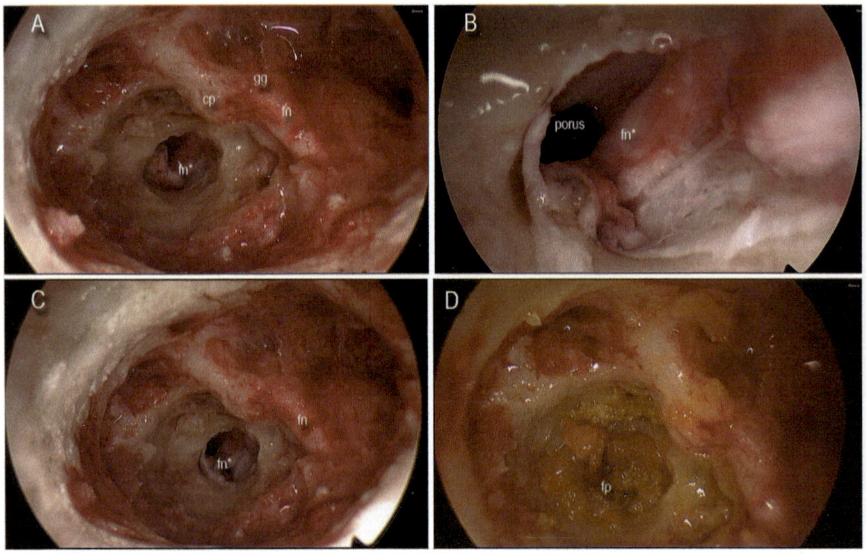

Fig. 39.6 Left ear: TTEA. **(a)** Final cavity after VS removal; **(b)** a close view on the IAC until the porus after tumor removal; **(c)** the defect on the promontory area is detected; **(d)** a fat pad is used in order to close the promontorial defect. cp, cochleariform process; fn, facial nerve; fn*, facial nerve into the IAC; fp, fat pad; gg, geniculate ganglion.

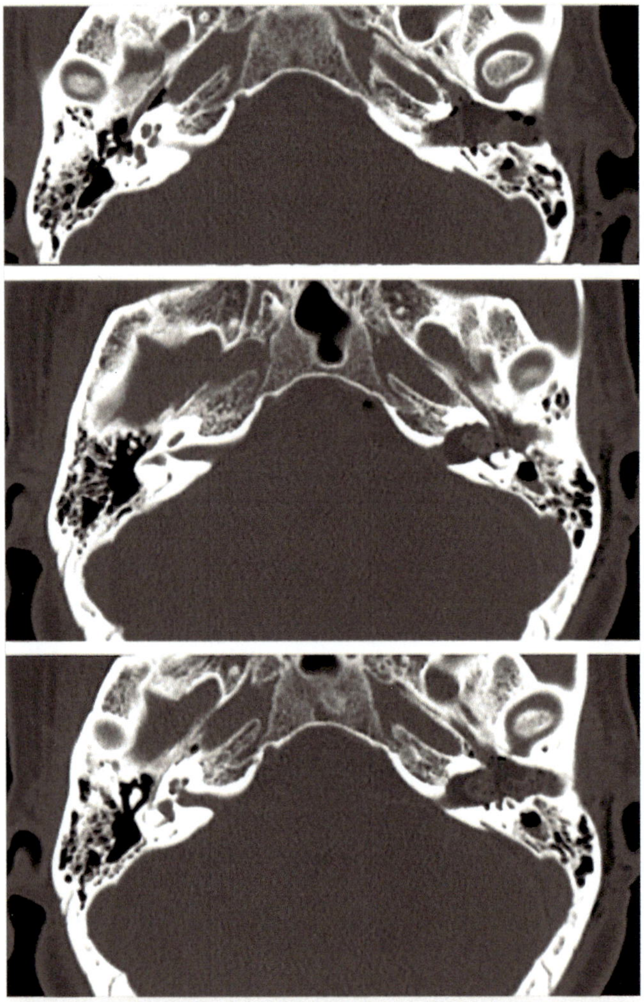

Fig. 39.7 Axial view CT scan after surgery on left ear showing the surgical route from the external to internal auditory canal.

eustachian tube orifice. The whole EAC is filled with fat, and a blind sac closure of the skin of the EAC is performed. The authors do not routinely employ intensive care unit observation, and a computed tomography (CT) scan of the brain is performed 6 hours after the surgery (▶ Fig. 39.7).

39.5 Discussion

Traditionally, retrosigmoid, middle cranial fossa, and transmastoid-translabyrinthine approaches are the most widely used for microsurgical resection of VS. The retrosigmoid approach guarantees optimal control of the CPA, although exposure of the IAC requires drilling of the posterior aspect of the petrous bone and, sometimes, complete visualization of the fundus is difficult to obtain.[9] The middle cranial fossa approach is classically utilized for small intracanalicular VS in patients with good hearing; however, this approach requires temporal lobe retraction and provides limited exposure of the CPA.[9] Translabyrinthine surgery guarantees good exposure of the IAC and CPA with limited or no brain retraction, but results in profound hearing loss and requires extensive drilling of the petrous bone.[9] Thus, all traditional microscopic approaches necessitate external incisions and soft-tissue dissection, with variable degrees of morbidity related to the craniotomy, brain retraction, and more extensive temporal bone drilling, depending on the approach.

Prior to clinical application, several cadaveric dissections were performed to verify the safety and reliability of the TTEA, in order to delineate surgical limits and landmarks.[10–11] Since the fully endoscopic approach is through a natural surgical corridor (i.e., the EAC), bone work is performed on the medial wall of the tympanic cavity and lateral skull base, from lateral to medial, avoiding cerebellum and brain retraction. The TTEA technique can be considered a minimally invasive procedure, with low morbidity in experienced hands. It is always important that these procedures be performed by qualified surgeons, with years of training in endoscopic middle ear procedures.

Regarding the surgical technique of the TTEA, several considerations should be highlighted. An important aspect of the surgery is vascular control as in some cases the anterior inferior cerebellar artery (AICA) may be encountered during IAC dissection. Achieving hemostasis from an arterial source may be very challenging with the TTEA as space is very limited compared to standard microsurgical corridors. This issue is frequently emphasized by the scientific community discussing risks of exclusive endoscopic retrosigmoid procedures by "keyhole" technique. At present, this is the main criticism to a fully endoscopic approach, but it is possible to avoid such complications by careful case selection based on preoperative imaging. Another important consideration pertains to facial nerve dissection. Since the TTEA utilizes "one-hand technique," management of the facial nerve in the IAC requires the expertise of an experienced surgeon especially when adhesions between the nerve and the tumor are encountered. Finally, there are a few potential complications unique to this approach. Cholesteatoma may develop with closure of the ear canal, the internal carotid artery is placed at some risk due to proximity, more segments of the facial nerve are vulnerable during drilling, and the temporomandibular joint may be exposed. All of these considerations must be examined over time in larger studies with greater follow-up. Based on the authors' experience, preliminary results for the TTEA are promising.[12]

39.6 Conclusion

The TTEA to the IAC provides a minimally invasive corridor to directly access intracanalicular VS through the EAC. By this innovative approach, some of the complications and morbidity observed in traditional microscopic approaches can be reduced, including external incisions and brain retraction. Indications for fully endoscopic VS surgery are currently limited to pathology involving the anterior labyrinth and/or the IAC. These procedures should be performed by very experienced surgeons, with several years of training in endoscopic middle ear procedures.

References

[1] Magnan J, Chays A, Lepetre C, Pencroffi E, Locatelli P. Surgical perspectives of endoscopy of the cerebellopontine angle. Am J Otol. 1994; 15(3):366–370

[2] Presutti L, Magnaguagno F, Pavesi G, et al. Combined endoscopic-microscopic approach for vestibular schwannoma removal: outcomes in a cohort of 81 patients. Acta Otorhinolaryngol Ital. 2014; 34(6):427–433

[3] Shahinian HK, Ra Y. 527 fully endoscopic resections of vestibular schwannomas. Minim Invasive Neurosurg. 2011; 54(2):61–67

[4] Marchioni D, Alicandri-Ciufelli M, Molteni G, Genovese E, Presutti L. Endoscopic tympanoplasty in patients with attic retraction pockets. Laryngoscope. 2010; 120(9):1847–1855

[5] Marchioni D, Alicandri-Ciufelli M, Piccinini A, et al. Surgical anatomy of transcanal endoscopic approach to the tympanic facial nerve. Laryngoscope. 2011; 121(7):1565–1573

[6] Marchioni D, Villari D, Alicandri-Ciufelli M, Piccinini A, Presutti L. Endoscopic open technique in patients with middle ear cholesteatoma. Eur Arch Otorhinolaryngol. 2011; 268(11):1557–1563

[7] Marchioni D, Alicandri-Ciufelli M, Gioacchini FM, Bonali M, Presutti L. Transcanal endoscopic treatment of benign middle ear neoplasms. Eur Arch Otorhinolaryngol. 2013; 270(12):2997–3004

[8] Marchioni D, Alicandri-Ciufelli M, Mattioli F, et al. From external to internal auditory canal: surgical anatomy by an exclusive endoscopic approach. Eur Arch Otorhinolaryngol. 2013; 270(4):1267–1275

[9] Bennett M, Haynes DS. Surgical approaches and complications in the removal of vestibular schwannomas. Otolaryngol Clin North Am. 2007; 40(3):589–609, ix–x

[10] Presutti L, Alicandri-Ciufelli M, Cigarini E, Marchioni D. Cochlear schwannoma removed through the external auditory canal by a transcanal exclusive endoscopic technique. Laryngoscope. 2013; 123(11):2862–2867

[11] Marchioni D, Alicandri-Ciufelli M, Rubini A, Presutti L. Endoscopic transcanal corridors to the lateral skull base: initial experiences. Laryngoscope. 2015; 125 Suppl 5:S1–S13

[12] Marchioni D, Alicandri-Ciufelli M, Rubini A, Masotto B, Pavesi G, Presutti L. Exclusive endoscopic transcanal transpromontorial approach: a new perspective for internal auditory canal vestibular schwannoma treatment. J Neurosurg. 2016; 11:1–8

40 Endoscopic Vestibular Schwannoma and Lateral Skull Base Surgery

Beth N. McNulty, Seilesh C. Babu, and Daniel R. Pieper

40.1 Introduction

Since the late 1800s, skull base surgeons have been pioneering the use of endoscopes in order to enhance visualization and reduce operative morbidity. The first use of the endoscope in the cerebellopontine angle (CPA) was in 1917 by Doyen in London.[1] Early neuroendoscopy was limited to the ventricular system, treating hydrocephalus and small tumors.[2] Early endoscopes had a limited depth of field, poor optic quality, and low illumination from flames or small electric bulbs.[3] A great advantage of the modern endoscope is the wide field of view—4-mm straight and angled endoscopes allow the surgeon to see beyond or around obstructing anatomical structures, thus limiting the degree of surgical exposure required. This is particularly useful in posterior fossa surgery by improving visualization around the cerebellum without the use of retractors or visualizing the lateral internal auditory canal (IAC), for example. The xenon light source is now standard within the industry, with peak wavelengths in the 800- to 1,000-nm range, improving visualization by increasing light output while minimizing heat production compared to a halogen light source.[3]

Endoscopic sinus and anterior skull base surgery began as a result of the work of Messerklinger and Stammberger in Europe in the 1970s and then Kennedy in the United States, who described "functional endoscopic sinus surgery" in 1985.[4,5] Many of the advancements seen in surgical technique and instrumentation in sinus and anterior skull base surgery were subsequently adopted by lateral skull base surgeons. Initially used as an adjunct to the operating microscope, it was not until 2001 that fully endoscopic approaches to the CPA were reported.[6,7] Although the majority of the publications in the current literature regarding the endoscopic approach to the CPA pertain to microvascular decompression, several groups have published cases of arachnoid cyst, epidermoid, vestibular schwannoma (VS), and meningioma resection.[8,9,10,11,12,13] The endoscope is particularly helpful for those tumors or cysts that cross the midline, or extend above the incisura or below the foramen magnum.[14] Marchioni et al have also recently described a fully endoscopic transcanal transpromontorial approach for resection of VSs that are limited to the IAC (refer to Chapter 39).[15]

40.2 Advantages and Limitations

The endoscopic approach to the lateral skull base offers the obvious possible advantages of a smaller incision and smaller craniotomy, in addition to less soft-tissue dissection and cerebellar retraction. These factors may contribute to a shorter hospital stay and quicker recovery.[16,17]

Illumination with the endoscope can be problematic. The light is not dispersed as it is with the microscope, creating a focused intensity with the possibility of overheating critical structures within the CPA. This issue has been addressed with the design of a water-cooled sleeve to line the outside of the endoscope. The use of a foot pedal allows this device to periodically cool the scope and clean the distal end (Endoscrub).[14] Furthermore, when a fixed endoscope holder is not used, the endoscope is frequently moved around the field, thereby limiting focal or prolonged heating of important structures.

Surgical instrumentation for neuroendoscopy has evolved to overcome early limitations, such as a limited trajectory for opposable grip instruments. Straight, "pistol-grip" retractable or guarded blades, instruments with 360-degree rotational capabilities, dual functioning suction curettes, and stimulating dissectors are now available. A great technical obstacle is the need for bimanual surgical technique and scope stabilization. A rigid endoscope holder is often used for endoscopic ventricular cases. However, visualization of the CPA requires constant changes to the field of view, making the rigid system less practical. In addition, the confined working space makes the use of an assistant scope holder challenging. A pneumatic endoscope holder with a multi-jointed, polyaxial arm (UniARM, Mitaka Kohki Co., Tokyo) has been utilized to overcome these obstacles.[14] The possibility of head movement while a rigid endoscope is fixed in position is of utmost concern for potential injury to critical structures. For this reason, rigid fixation of the patient's head in a neurosurgical head holder is recommended.

Lastly, for most lateral skull base surgeons who are mainly familiar with microscope use, endoscopic depth of field requires practice to become accustomed to. In contrast to surgical microscopes, most endoscopic systems only utilize a single optic and therefore three-dimensional images are not possible. Similar to endoscopic sinus surgery, movement of the instruments in and out of the field helps develop a sense of working depth.

40.3 Patient Selection

Patient selection is evolving as lateral skull base endoscopic techniques improve. Tumor size is one important consideration when choosing surgical approach. In our series of endoscopic VS cases, tumors ranged from 1 to 2 cm in size.[8] Initially, patients with serviceable hearing and small tumors (< 1 cm) with limited IAC involvement were considered ideal candidates. As experience has grown, criteria for patient selection have expanded to include cases with larger sized tumors (< 2 cm). In our opinion, for patients with poor preoperative hearing, the translabyrinthine approach should be considered, as it provides direct tumor access, low risk of facial nerve injury, and short convalescence. Currently, IAC tumor extension is still a challenge in cases where hearing preservation is attempted, although meatal drilling can be performed and visualization with an angled endoscope can be helpful. In our opinion, a relative contraindication to endoscopic CPA surgery would be a tumor that results in significant mass effect and associated hydrocephalus, or one that is very vascular. A microscopic approach should be considered in these cases, as it allows for early access to the cisterna magna in order to relax the brain and provides more working room.[14]

40.4 Relevant Anatomy

The endoscope provides a wide view of the CPA, with the tentorium as the superior limit, the pons and medulla medially, the temporal bone with the porus acusticus laterally, and the foramen magnum inferiorly (▶ Fig. 40.1; see Chapter 30 for further anatomical descriptions).

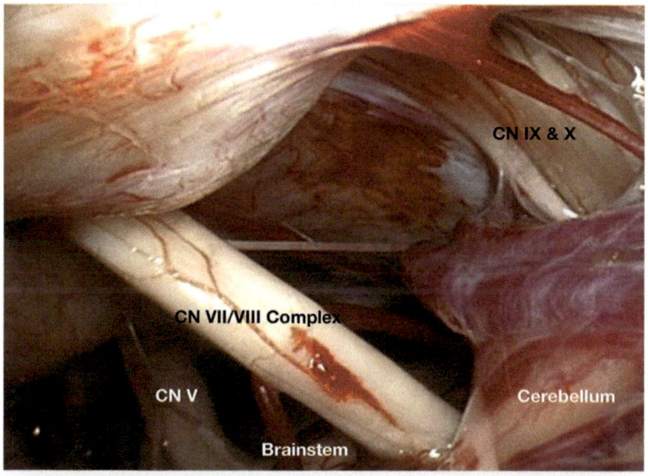

Fig. 40.1 Right-sided endoscopic view of cerebellopontine angle anatomy.

40.5 Surgical Technique

1. The patient is turned 180 degrees, placed in a supine position with the head turned to the opposite side, and secured in rigid fixation using a head holder with pins. The head of the bed is then elevated approximately 30 degrees to reduce intracranial pressure and facilitate exposure (▶ Fig. 40.2).
2. Prior to making the incision, the intracranial pressure is reduced with the administration of intravenous mannitol (0.5-1 g/kg) and 20 mg of intravenous Lasix. The arterial pCO_2 is reduced to 28 to 30 mm Hg. In the authors' opinion, these steps are critical in endoscopic approaches.
3. An oblique linear incision, about 3 cm in length, is centered over the transverse–sigmoid sinus (TS) junction. This location is based on the intersection of two reliable landmarks: (i) a line drawn from the root of the zygoma to the inion and (ii) a line drawn from the squamosal–parietomastoid suture junction to the tip of the mastoid.
4. The craniotomy is designed with the TS junction at the anterosuperior limit. A 14-mm perforator may be used; however, we prefer using standard fluted cutting and diamond burrs to minimize the risk of injury to the TS junction (▶ Fig. 40.3). A 1.5-cm craniotomy is sufficient in cases of microvascular decompression or neurectomy (▶ Fig. 40.4). For VS resection, an additional 5 to 10 mm is necessary to more easily accommodate the endoscopic drills and ultrasonic aspirators. The drilling should carefully skeletonize the TS junction.
5. The dural incision is made parallel to the transverse and sigmoid sinuses, but as close to the sigmoid sinus as possible to allow maximum anterior exposure, with care to preserve an adequate cuff to allow for dural closure.

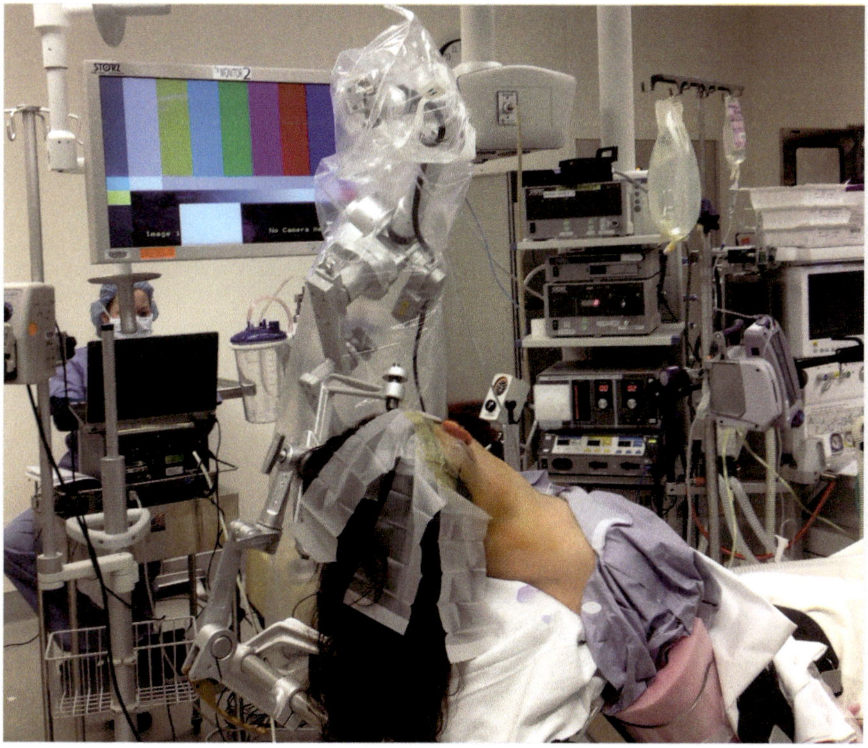

Fig. 40.2 Patient positioning: supine with the head elevated to 30 degrees and turned to the opposite side, secured in rigid fixation using a Mayfield head clamp.

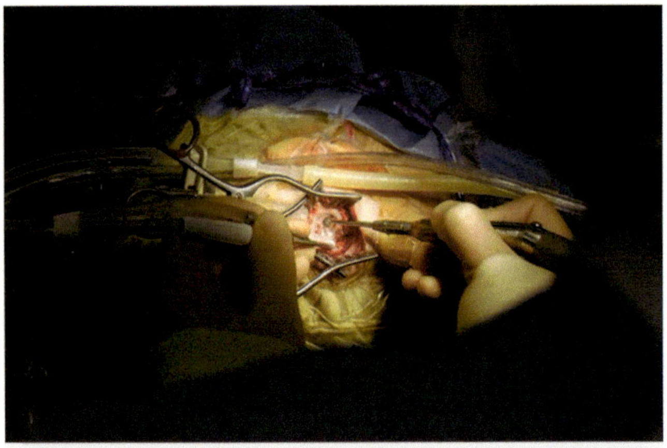

Fig. 40.3 The craniotomy is made using fluted cutting and diamond burrs to minimize the risk of injury to the transverse–sigmoid sinus junction.

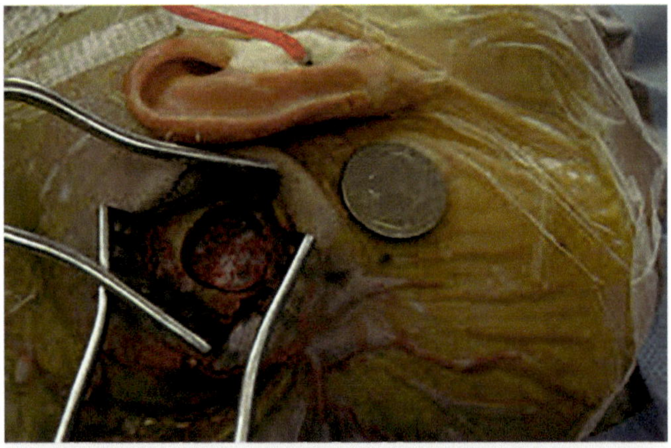

Fig. 40.4 A 1.5-cm craniotomy, approximately the size of a quarter, is used in cases of microvascular decompression or vestibular neurectomy.

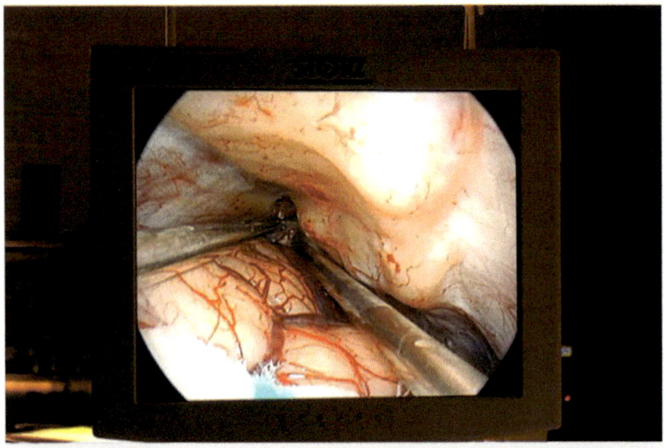

Fig. 40.5 Intraoperative view in which the endoscope is placed ventrally along the cerebellar hemisphere accessing the prepontine cistern.

6. A rigid 4-mm 0-degree endoscope is then carefully introduced (▶ Fig. 40.5). The endoscope is advanced slowly to allow for identification of the petrosal veins. These veins are varied in their location and may either be mobilized or cauterized as necessary to enable adequate visualization. Angled endoscopes may be utilized to view into the IAC and assist in tumor resection when necessary.
7. Next, the arachnoid is released using sharp microsurgical technique. Adequate time must be allotted for this important step, which allows for egress of cerebrospinal fluid (CSF) and maximal cerebellar relaxation.
8. Cranial nerves IV through XI, along with the critical vascular structures, are then identified and the endoscope is secured in position over the area of interest using the pneumatic endoscopic holder (▶ Fig. 40.6a,b).
9. Tumor resection: the cochlear nerve may be splayed along the tumor capsule and is identified along the inferior aspect of the tumor (▶ Fig. 40.7). The facial nerve and nervus

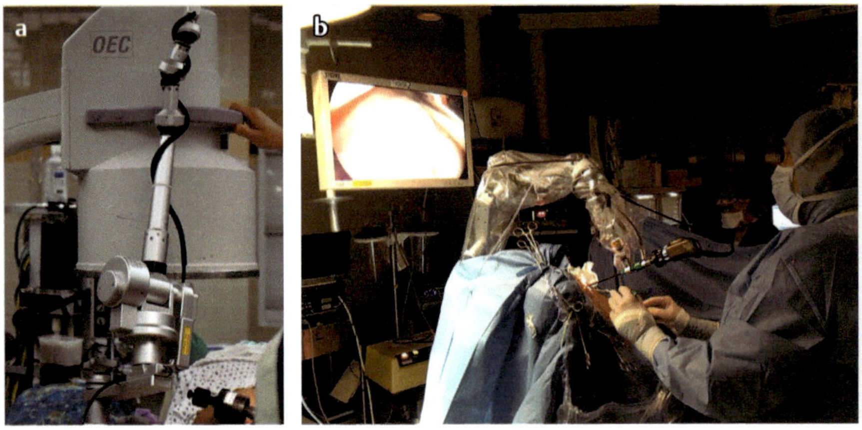

Fig. 40.6 **(a)** A pneumatic endoscope holder with a multi-jointed, polyaxial arm (UniARM, Mitaka Kohki Co., Tokyo). **(b)** Operating room setup with endoscope holder and surgeon operating off of a high definition monitor.

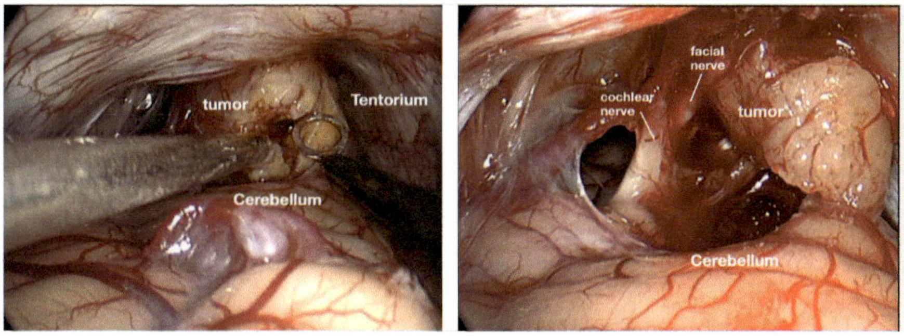

Fig. 40.7 Endoscopic view of the left cerebellopontine angle, with vestibular schwannoma easily visualized and mobilized (left side of picture). The tumor is resected and the neurovascular structures are preserved (right side of picture).

intermedius are next identified along the ventral aspect. Care should be taken to coagulate any vessels that may be supplying the tumor. The meatal bone is then removed to expose the medial IAC dura using a high-speed endoscopic drill, with care to avoid entering the labyrinth. Large pieces of Gelfoam are placed on the cerebellum and overlying the CPA to limit spread of bone particles while drilling. Drill speed is reduced to minimize skipping while maintaining adequate visualization with irrigation. The Endoscrub is also helpful in maintaining visualization while drilling. Once the tumor is isolated, the capsule is entered sharply and intratumoral debulking ensues. Stimulating dissectors or an ultrasonic aspirator may be used, depending on surgeon preference and tumor vascularity. Capsular dissection is done so that the cochlear nerve is preserved, reflecting the tumor off the cochlear and facial nerves.

10. In preparing for closure, the facial nerve is stimulated at the root exit zone and a Valsalva maneuver is performed to ensure hemostasis. The dura is closed in a watertight fashion. Synthetic dural substitutes or sealants, autologous fascia, muscle, or fat may be used in cases in which a watertight dural closure is not possible.
11. The craniotomy bone plate is fixed with titanium plates, mesh, or hydroxyapatite cement.
12. Skin closure is performed in layers and a mastoid compressive dressing is applied.[14]

40.6 Complications

Risks of bleeding, infection, and scarring inherent to any surgical intervention remain, but are rarely reported. The major complications of endoscopic CPA surgery, and more specifically VS resection, relate to the involved cranial nerves or critical structures in close proximity. Postoperative dizziness, hearing loss, and facial paresis/paralysis may result from all approaches to the CPA.[5,17,18] A CSF leak is a rare complication, noted in only one patient (2.7%) in our series of fully endoscopic tumor resection.[14] We observed tumor recurrence in one patient (2.7%), who ultimately underwent an open translabyrinthine approach for resection.[8] There are no reported cases of injury due to use of the endoscope, such as trauma from the scope itself or thermal injury to structures. In order to maintain patient safety, occasionally the endoscopic case is converted to a standard, open approach (► Table 40.1).

Table 40.1 Published outcome data for endoscope-assisted and fully endoscopic vestibular schwannoma resection

Study	No. of patients	Surgical approach	Tumor size	% Gross total resection	Facial nerve preservation	Hearing preservation	Morbidity	Mean length of stay
Göksu et al,[19] endoscope assisted	32	Combined retrosigmoid–retrolabyrinthine	Mean = 20.9 mm	96.8% (*n* = 31)	100%	15.7% (*n* = 5)	3.1% (*n* = 1, CSF leak)	NA
King and Wackym,[2] endoscope assisted	10	Suboccipital	Mean = 22.4 mm	90% (*n* = 9)	100%	0%	0%	NA
Magnan et al,[20] endoscope assisted	119	Retrosigmoid	Small/medium (< 25 mm)	NA 1 case had tumor recurrence	100%	48.7% (*n* = 58)	10.9% (*n* = 13, 10 CSF leaks, 2 persistent HA, 1 abducens palsy)	8 d
Shahinian and Ra[13] and Kabil and Shahinian,[21] fully endoscopic	527	Keyhole retrosigmoid	Mean = 28 mm	94% (*n* = 495)	100%	57% (*n* = 300)	0%	NA
Pieper,[14] fully endoscopic	23	Keyhole retrosigmoid	NA	NA	100%	92% (*n* = 29)	13% (*n* = 3, 1 CSF leak, 2 wound infections)	NA
Iacoangeli et al,[22] endoscope assisted	10	Presigmoid retrolabyrinthine	Medium-large	80% (*n* = 8)	100%	60% (*n* = 6)	20% (*n* = 2)	NA
Setty et al,[8] fully endoscopic	12	Keyhole retrosigmoid	Mean = 15 mm	100% 1 case had tumor recurrence	92% (*n* = 11)	67% (*n* = 8)	0%	3.6 d

Abbreviations: CSF, cerebrospinal fluid; HA, headache; NA, not available.

References

[1] Doyen E. Surgical Therapeutics and Operative Techniques. Vol. 1. London: Balliere, Tindall, and Cox; 1917:599–602

[2] King WA, Wackym PA. Endoscope-assisted surgery for acoustic neuromas (vestibular schwannomas): early experience using the rigid Hopkins telescope. Neurosurgery. 1999; 44(5):1095–1100, discussion 1100–1102

[3] Chandra RK, Conley DB, Kern RC. Evolution of the endoscope and endoscopic sinus surgery. Otolaryngol Clin North Am. 2009; 42(5):747–752, vii

[4] Kennedy DW. Functional endoscopic sinus surgery. Technique. Arch Otolaryngol. 1985; 111(10):643–649

[5] Artz G, Rosen M, Evans J, Pieper D. Minimally invasive and endoscopic approaches to the skull base. In: Babu S, ed. Practical Neurotology and Skull Base Surgery. San Diego, CA: Plural Publishing; 2013:47–57

[6] Eby JB, Cha ST, Shahinian HK. Fully endoscopic vascular decompression of the facial nerve for hemifacial spasm. Skull Base. 2001; 11(3):189–197

[7] Jarrahy R, Eby JB, Cha ST, Shahinian HK. Fully endoscopic vascular decompression of the trigeminal nerve. Minim Invasive Neurosurg. 2002; 45(1):32–35

[8] Setty P, D'Andrea KP, Stucken EZ, Babu S, LaRouere MJ, Pieper DR. Endoscopic Resection of Vestibular Schwannomas. J Neurol Surg B Skull Base. 2015; 76 (3):230–238

[9] Setty P, D'Andrea KP, Stucken EZ, Babu S, LaRouere MJ, Pieper DR. Fully endoscopic resection of cerebellopontine angle meningiomas. J Neurol Surg A Cent Eur Neurosurg. 2015

[10] de Divitiis O, Cavallo LM, Dal Fabbro M, Elefante A, Cappabianca P. Freehand dynamic endoscopic resection of an epidermoid tumor of the cerebellopontine angle: technical case report. Neurosurgery. 2007; 61(5) Suppl 2:E239–E240, discussion E240

[11] Krass J, Hahn Y, Karami K, Babu S, Pieper DR. Endoscopic assisted resection of prepontine epidermoid cysts. J Neurol Surg A Cent Eur Neurosurg. 2014; 75 (2):120–125

[12] Shahinian HK, Eby JB, Ocon M. Fully endoscopic excision of vestibular schwannomas. Minim Invasive Neurosurg. 2004; 47(6):329–332

[13] Shahinian HK, Ra Y. 527 fully endoscopic resections of vestibular schwannomas. Minim Invasive Neurosurg. 2011; 54(2):61–67

[14] Pieper DR. The endoscopic approach to vestibular schwannomas and posterolateral skull base pathology. Otolaryngol Clin North Am. 2012; 45(2):439–454, x

[15] Marchioni D, Alicandri-Ciufelli M, Rubini A, Presutti L. Endoscopic transcanal corridors to the lateral skull base: initial experiences. Laryngoscope. 2015; 125 Suppl 5:S1–S13

[16] O'Donoghue GM, O'Flynn P. Endoscopic anatomy of the cerebellopontine angle. Am J Otol. 1993; 14(2):122–125

[17] Kabil MS, Eby JB, Shahinian HK. Endoscopic vascular decompression versus microvascular decompression of the trigeminal nerve. Minim Invasive Neurosurg. 2005; 48(4):207–212

[18] Artz GJ, Hux FJ, Larouere MJ, Bojrab DI, Babu S, Pieper DR. Endoscopic vascular decompression. Otol Neurotol. 2008; 29(7):995–1000

[19] Göksu N, Bayazit Y, Kemaloğlu Y. Endoscopy of the posterior fossa and dissection of acoustic neuroma. J Neurosurg. 1999; 91(5):776–780

[20] Magnan J, Barbieri M, Mora R, et al. Retrosigmoid approach for small and medium-sized acoustic neuromas. Otol Neurotol. 2002; 23(2):141–145

[21] Kabil MS, Shahinian HK. A series of 112 fully endoscopic resections of vestibular schwannomas. Minim Invasive Neurosurg. 2006; 49(6):362–368

[22] Iacoangeli M, Salvinelli F, Di Rienzo A, et al. Microsurgical endoscopy-assisted presigmoid retrolabyrinthine approach as a minimally invasive surgical option for the treatment of medium to large vestibular schwannomas. Acta Neurochir (Wien). 2013; 155(4):663–670

41 Subtotal Resection of Sporadic Vestibular Schwannoma

Ashkan Monfared and Robert K. Jackler

41.1 Background

The controversy over partial resection of large vestibular schwannomas (VSs) is in no way a new topic. The question dates back to two of the earlier protagonists of VS surgery, namely, Harvey Cushing and Walter Dandy. Possibly fueled by aversion to one another's growing prominence, this issue became one of the central points of their feud.[1] Dandy, advocated a total resection of these tumors,[2] whereas Cushing was the main proponent of partial resection.[3] While every one of Dandy's patients suffered complete facial paralysis, many of Cushing's patients demised from recurrence of large remnants a few years after surgery.[4] With the advances in microsurgery over the next century, most surgeons came to endorse total resection in all but select elderly and fragile patients.[5,6] However, as the focus of surgery has now shifted from preservation of life to preservation of function, many surgeons are more willing to entertain less-than-total resection of larger tumors in favor of preservation of facial function.

41.2 Definition of Subtotal and Near-Total Resection

Currently, there is no widely acceptable definition of degree of resection when the entire tumor has not been extirpated. One encounters terms such as "partial," "subtotal," "near-total," "intracapsular," and "radical subtotal" for various degrees of less-than-total resection. The most widely accepted terms are "near-total" and "subtotal" resection (▶ Fig. 41.1). Many surgeons resort to descriptive terms and do not provide exact dimensions or percentage of the tumor resected when using subtotal (STR) or near-total (NTR) designation.[7,8,9] Few have adopted criteria established by the consensus meeting in 2003.[10] In this consensus statement, NTR was defined as tumor residual measuring less than 2% of the original tumor by volume, and partial resection deemed as up to 5% of the tumor and any larger tumor remnant was designated as STR. As the authors attested, this classification is very subjective[11] and there are major issues with its adoption. First, it is very difficult for most surgeons to make a precise measurement of the tumor remnant during surgery. Several studies have confirmed the poor relation between postoperative MRI findings and surgeon's estimation of tumor remnant volume.[12,13] Second, using percentage as a defining criterion is faulty as 5% of a tumor measuring 2 cm in diameter (volume of approximately 4.19 cm^3) is 0.21 cm^3 but 5% of a 4-cm tumor (volume of approximately 33.51 cm^3) measures 1.67 cm^3. The latter tumor remnant is eight times larger than the former. Others have proposed a definition based on actual size of the remnant. For example, Bloch et al recommended a remnant of 5 × 5 × 2 mm or smaller to be considered a NTR and anything larger to be categorized as STR (▶ Fig. 41.2). What this definition does not account for is the potential clinical outcome difference between remnants measuring 0.5 and 5 cm^3 both of which are considered STRs.

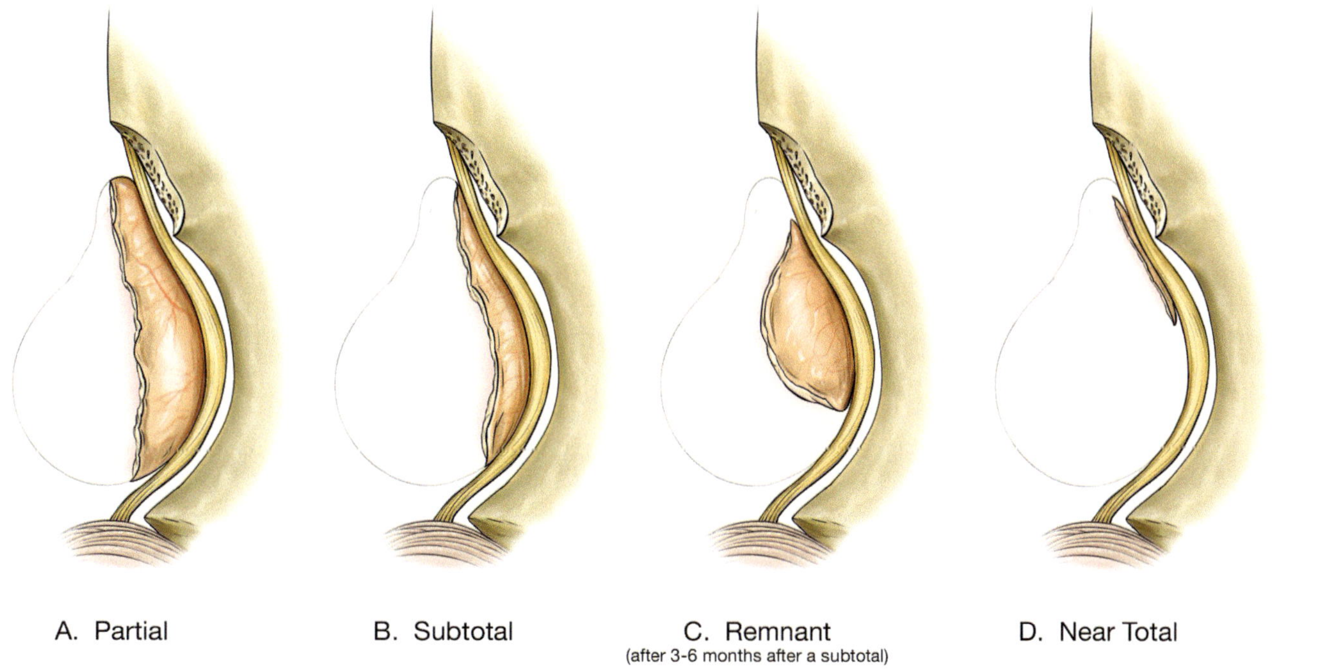

Fig. 41.1 (**a**) Partial resection of a large vestibular schwannoma. (**b**) Subtotal resection of a large vestibular schwannoma with nodular enhancement along the course of the facial nerve. (**c**) Tumor residual 6–12 months after subtotal resection. Note the tumor has coalesced, or "balled up," into a shorter and wider remnant. (**d**) Near-total resection of vestibular schwannoma, with a small thin pad of tumor in the region of the porus acusticus.

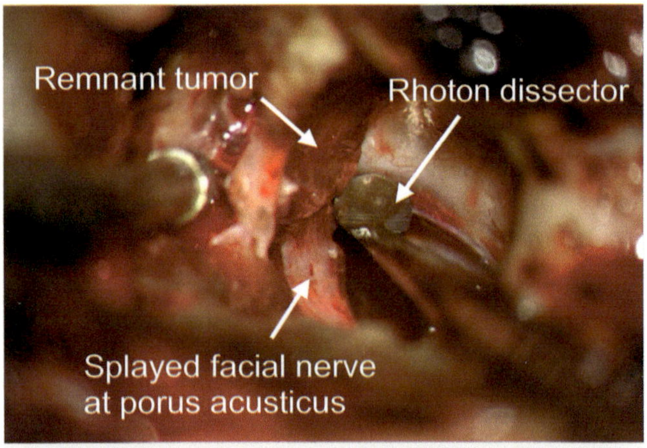

Fig. 41.2 Near-total resection of a left-sided vestibular schwannoma. A small residual tumor pad was left of the facial nerve at the porus acusticus in order to preserve neural integrity. (Used with permission, Jacob et al. Volumetric analysis of tumor control following subtotal and near-total resection of vestibular schwannoma. Laryngoscope 2016;126(8):1877–1882.)

41.3 Facial Nerve Outcomes as Related to Degree of Resection

The impetus behind a less-than-total resection is mostly preservation of facial nerve function. The majority of the literature demonstrates that excellent short-term and long-term facial nerve preservation rates are not optimal for larger tumors after gross-total resection (GTR). Surgeons with large series have reported rates between 33 and 73% of good facial nerve outcomes (i.e., House–Brackmann [HB] grades I–II) following more definitive surgery.[14,15,16,17,18,19,20,21] Conversely, when surgeons have performed planned STR as first stage of treatment to be followed by radiation or a second-stage operation, they have achieved much better results. It is not surprising that rates of 85 to 100% good facial nerve function are achieved when the plane between the tumor and thinned-out frail facial nerve or the brainstem is not engaged.[7,12] In a systematic review of studies on resection of large VSs, the extent of tumor resection was reported on 471 of the 1,688 patients eligible for the analysis. The review demonstrated a strong and significant association between degree of resection and good/excellent facial nerve outcome (HB grades I–II). The rate of good facial nerve function was 92.5% for the 80 patients receiving STR, compared to 74.6% ($n = 55$) for NTR and 47.3% ($n = 336$) for GTR.[17]

The intraoperative decision as to when any further dissection would result in deterioration of the facial nerve has been largely left to the surgeon discretion. As one can imagine, this point is highly dependent on surgeon's comfort and experience as well as what they envision appropriate based on patient's demographics and wishes. More recently, some surgeons have advocated use of electrophysiologic properties of the nerve to help guide the extent of resection. In the study of Haque et al, the authors advocated for STR if a minimum of 0.3 mA was needed to stimulate the nerve at the brainstem or an increase of 0.1 mA from baseline was observed.[22] In a similar study, continuous intraoperative evoked facial nerve electromyography (EMG) demonstrated worse outcome when the amplitude fell 50% below the initial value.[23] Schmitt et al reported reliable prognostic value using pulsed constant-current stimulation at supramaximal levels at the root exit zone compared to the peripheral segment exiting the stylomastoid foramen. They reported that for patients who had proximal-to-distal drop off of over 69%, the rate of long-term poor facial function was 44% compared to 6% for patient with values less than 69%. This method was suggested by the authors as a potential viable method to guide degree of less-than-total resection.[24] Further discussion regarding facial nerve function prognostication using intraoperative stimulation testing is reviewed in greater detail in Chapter 27.

41.4 Tumor Control Rate as a Function of Degree of Resection

The main concern with performing less-than-total resection is that the remnant tumor would require treatment within a few years. As is the case with defining the degree of resection, currently no universal definition exists for "growth of remnant" or "failure of treatment" in our literature. Studies have used radiologic definitions anywhere between 1 and 5 mm of growth in the diameter of the tumor as clinical definition of failure.[13,22,25] This is one reason why the rates of recurrence after less-than-total resection vary so widely in the literature.[8,13,22,26,27] A second source of variance in reporting is the duration of follow-up. It is clear in the literature that the reported rate of recurrence increases as the duration of follow-up is extended. Thus, the risk of recurrence is best summarized using time to event analysis, such as the Kaplan–Meier method. On average, approximately one-third of patients who have undergone STR would develop tumor regrowth, whereas the regrowth rate among GTR and NTR patients is usually in single digits. For example, Bloch et al found that the rate of regrowth for their NTR population was 3% compared to 32% for STR.[26] Similarly Seol et al reported statistically significant regrowth rates of 3.8, 9.4, and 27.6% in their GTR, NTR, and STR population, respectively.[27] ▸ Table 41.1 summarizes select large publications reporting rates of regrowth following less-than-complete VS resection.

41.5 Adjuvant Radiation Therapy

As the rate of STR among larger VSs has grown, more patients require treatment of a growing residual. Facial nerve prognosis for surgical salvage of a tumor remnant is usually associated with much worse outcome compared to the primary operation.[28] Considering the efficacy of stereotactic radiation in controlling small- and medium-sized tumors, now verified over sufficient length of time,[29,30] a combined modality treatment has become a more attractive option. Several studies have reported good facial nerve outcome (HB grades I–II in 78–94%) as well as adequate tumor control rates (79–100%) using a less-than-total approach followed by radiation therapy.[31,32,33,34] Unfortunately, all these studies are retrospective, some have very few subjects and others have relatively short follow-up. Also, use of radiation therapy was routine in every patient in some studies and prescribed only in case of tumor growth by others. In the only prospective study on the subject, the tumor

Table 41.1 Select large published series reporting rates of facial nerve function and regrowth following less-than-complete vestibular schwannoma resection

Study	Center	Design	Number	Duration of follow-up	Definition STR/ NTR	Facial function	Recurrence rate	Predictors of recurrence
Bloch et al (2004)	University of California, San Francisco, CA	Retrospective	50 NTR, 29 STR	Mean: 4.3 y (range: 1–13 y)	NTR: residual ≤ 25 mm^2 and 2 mm thick STR: residual larger than NTR	Good FN function (HB I–II) at 1 y postoperatively in 81% of patients Logistic regression analysis demonstrated no statistically significant difference in good facial nerve function between the NTR and STR groups when controlling for age, tumor size, and operative approach	NTR: 3% recurrence STR: 32% recurrence	After adjustment for follow-up time and tumor size, the odds ratio for recurrence was 12 times larger for STR than for NTR ($p = 0.033$)
Godefroy et al (2009)	Leiden University Medical Centre, Leiden, The Netherlands	Retrospective	29 NTR, 8 STR	Mean: 48 mo	NTR: < 5% of initial tumor volume remaining, but not GTR STR: > 5% of initial tumor volume remaining	NTR: 76% with good FN function (HB I–II) STR: 100% with good FN function (HB I–II)	NTR + STR: 6%; did not differentiate between NTR and STR	
Sughrue et al (2011)	University of California, San Francisco, CA	Prospective	89 NTR, 112 STR	Median 37 mo	NTR: only a thin layer of tumor attached to one or more nerves; the amount of residual tumor appears similar to GTR on imaging STR: imaging studies or intraoperative impression revealing gross evidence of residual disease	NR	NTR: 84% tumor control at 5 y, 81% tumor control at 10 y STR: 82% tumor control at 5 y, 82% tumor control at 10 y	
Fukuda et al (2011)	University of Niigata, Japan	Retrospective	25 STR, 8 PR	Mean: 104.1 mo (range: 60–241 mo)	STR: 1–10% of initial tumor volume remaining PR: > 10% of initial tumor volume remaining	STR: 60% with good FN function (HB I–II) PR: 88% with good FN function (HB I–II)	NTR: 52% recurrence STR: 63% recurrence Times to recurrence ranged from 6 to 76 mo (median 31.9 mo)	Univariate and multivariate analyses of various factors revealed that thickness of the residual tumor, based on MR imaging after surgery, and the MIB-1 index were positively related to residual tumor regrowth. The receiver operating characteristic curves, plotted for both the thickness of the

Table 41.1 *(Continued)*

Study	Center	Design	Number	Duration of follow-up	Definition STR/ NTR	Facial function	Recurrence rate	Predictors of recurrence
								residual tumor and the MIB-1 index, identified the optimal cutoff points for these values as 7.4 mm (sensitivity 83.3%, specificity 86.7%) and 1.6 (sensitivity 83.3%, specificity 66.7%), respectively
Carlson et al (2012)	Mayo Clinic, Rochester MN	Retrospective	32 NTR, 27 STR	Mean: 3.5 y (range: 0.3–9.3 y)	NTR: residual less than 5 × 5 × 2 mm STR: residual larger than NTR	NR	NTR: 3% overall recurrence; 93% estimated recurrence-free survival rate at 5 y following surgery STR: 22% overall recurrence; 71% estimated recurrence-free survival rate at 5 y following surgery	STR, nodular enhancement, nodule volume > 0.4 cm^3, and maximum nodule dimensions > 15 mm were statistically significantly associated with recurrence. Patients treated with STR were more than nine times more likely to develop recurrence compared with those treated with GTR (hazard ratio, 9.4; $p < 0.001$), and subjects with nodular enhancement on baseline postoperative MRI were at a 16-fold increased risk for later recurrence compared to those with linear patterns (hazard ratio, 16.5; $p = 0.008$)
Schwartz et al (2013)	The House Clinic, Los Angeles CA	Retrospective	44 NTR, 31 STR	Mean: 3.7 y (range: 1.0–9.8 y)	NTR: only thin layer of tumor capsule (< 1 cm) remaining on the facial nerve STR: ≥ 1 cm residual remaining	NTR: 78 and 97% with good FN function (HB I–II) at the postoperative and 1-y follow-up time points, respectively STR: 71 and 96% with good FN function (HB I–II) at the postoperative and 1-y follow-up time points, respectively	NTR: 21% recurrence STR: 22% recurrence The mean times to recurrence for those tumors that grew, based on first to last MRI, were 4.0 and 4.3 y in the NTR and STR groups, respectively	The NTR and STR groups had a significantly higher rate of regrowth than GTR resection (21 and 22% vs. 3%) at average follow-up times of 3.7, 3.7, and 5.1 y, respectively Need for further treatment occurred at a higher rate, although infrequently, in NTR and STR (2 and 10% vs. 0%)
Chen et al (2014)	Gruppo Otologico, Piacenza-Rome, Italy	Retrospective	73 NTR, 38 STR	Mean: 45.4 mo (range: 12–156 mo)	NTR: < 2% of initial tumor volume remaining, but not GTR STR: 2–5% of initial tumor volume remaining PR: > 5% of initial tumor volume remaining	NTR: 49% with good FN function (HB I–II) at 1 y postoperatively STR: 47% with good FN function (HB I–II) function at 1 y postoperatively There was no significant difference in good, intermediate, and unsatisfactory facial nerve function between groups	NTR: 0% recurrence STR: 18% recurrence The 5-y tumor regrowth–free survival was 92%, with a mean tumor regrowth–free period of 140 mo (95% CI: 127–151 mo)	

Table 41.1 *(Continued)*

Study	Center	Design	Number	Duration of follow-up	Definition STR/NTR	Facial function	Recurrence rate	Predictors of recurrence
Jacob et al (2015)	Mayo Clinic, Rochester MN	Retrospective	50 NTR, 53 STR	Mean: 56.1 mo (range: 12–150 mo)	NTR: residual < 5 × 5 × 2 mm STR: residual larger than NTR	NTR: 82% with good FN (HB I–II) function STR: 81% with good FN (HB I–II) function Postoperative FN function was not statistically significantly different between groups even after adjusting for tumor size in a multivariable setting	NTR: Estimated recurrence-free survival rates (95% CI; number still at risk) at 24, 48, 72, 96, and 120 mo were 100% (100–100; 45), 100% (100–100; 25), 100% (100–100; 15), 100% (100–100; 10), and 90% (73–100; 6), respectively STR: Estimated recurrence-free survival rates (95% CI; number still at risk) at 24, 48, 72, and 96 mo were 96% (90–100; 42), 71% (57–89; 17), 67% (51–86; 10), and 67% (51–86; 6), respectively The median time to recurrence following NTR was 124 mo (range: 98–136) compared to only 32 mo (range: 21–55) after STR ($p < 0.001$)	STR was 13 times more likely to recur compared to NTR (HR: 13.31; 95% CI: 1.71–103.91; $p = 0.014$)
Monfared et al (2015)	Multicenter	Prospective	22 NTR, 39 STR	Mean: 38 mo (range: 12–96 mo)	NTR: residual < 5 × 5 × 2 mm STR: when the tumor was resected 80–90% by volume and 60–70% by surface area	FN function at the first postoperative visit and at the ≥ 1 year postoperative visit was not associated with degree of resection as reported by the surgeon or as determined by postoperative MRI	NTR: 9.1% STR: 28.2% The average time from surgery until regrowth was 35 mo (range: 4–74 mo)	Tumor regrowth was related to longer follow-up ($p = 0.0002$), noncystic tumor (29 vs. 5%; $p = 0.02$), larger residual tumor percentage by volume ($p = 0.003$), and STR as defined by the surgeon ($p = 0.02$)
Nakatomi et al (2017)	Mayo Clinic, Rochester MN	Retrospective	18 STR	Median 7.1 y (range: 1.0–26.3 y)	STR: anything less than GTR	NR	STR: 83% recurrence at a median of 2.7 y following resection (IQR: 1.9–8.9, range: 1.2–18.7) Estimated recurrence-free survival rates at 5, 10, and 15 y following STR were 47% (95% CI: 28–78, 7 patients still at risk), 17% (5–55, 2), and 8% (1–52, 1), respectively	STR with nearly an 11-fold greater risk of recurrence than GTR (HR: 10.55, $p < 0.001$)

Abbreviations: HB, House–Brackmann; GTR, gross-total resection; NTR, near-total resection; STR, subtotal resection.

response rate of remnants to radiation therapy was much lower than what has been reported for primary radiation treatment.[35,36,37] The failure rate was especially high for patients who received intensity-modulated radiation therapy (IMRT) due to the large size of tumor remnant instead of stereotactic radiation.[13]

Several studies now have demonstrated that the majority of patients who have undergone NTR and about two-thirds of patients who have undergone STR may not experience tumor regrowth. Admittedly, most of these studies have limited follow-up and longer follow-up in a larger number of patients is required to validate these promising, but preliminary, data. Based on these results, universal application of radiosurgery after less-than-total resection may not be necessary. Instead, diligent follow-up using serial MRI scans may obviate the expense and potential morbidity associated with radiation in a portion of patients.

41.6 Postoperative Surveillance

Studies have demonstrated that the degree of concordance between the extent of resection estimated intraoperatively by the surgeon and what is found on the postoperative MRI is far from perfect.[12,13] This particularly holds true of NTR cases. It is possible that in certain cases, a very thin small remnant may be devitalized and, although present at the time of surgery, may not enhance with contrast on the postoperative MRI scan.[9] More commonly, it seems the surgeons underestimate the volume of the remnant at the end of operation.

The timing of the first postoperative MRI is an important issue. Most centers do not routinely employ MRI immediately following surgery, within the first 24 hours, as acute devascularization may limit contrast uptake and underestimate the residual tumor volume. On one hand, it should be delayed until the resolution of early inflammatory products creating enhancement in the surgical field. On the other, it cannot be postponed for too long because one may miss early regrowth of select tumors. As enhancement in the surgical bed may last for years to come,[34,38,39,40] the initial study would only serve as the baseline to be compared to future studies. Carlson et al demonstrated that in some cases, the rind of the tumor left after surgery may consolidate into a more spherical mass by 3 months.[41] For both clinical and research purposes, it is much easier to follow the tumor remnant as it has matured. One could argue that it is then best to delay obtaining the first "baseline" study for 6 months to a year, but few cases of very early growth of tumor remnants have been reported few months from surgery particularly with cystic tumors or very large remnants.[13,41] It thus seems that an MRI with gadolinium obtained at 3 months from surgery would serve as the best baseline allowing for immediate inflammatory material to resolve and the tumor rind to consolidate into a mass without great risk of missing rare instances of early tumor regrowth.

The other less studied issue is the length of time required for follow-up of tumor remnants. Studies have reported cases of late recurrence up to nearly a decade after GTR or a stable tumor remnant.[13,33,41] Considering such late recurrences, it may be wise to follow up all patients undergoing less-than-total resection, and even GTR, for at least 10 years or perhaps indefinitely. Generally, most institutions utilize more frequent imaging in the first years following surgery and increase the time interval between studies after remnant quiescence has been observed. A further discussion regarding recommended postoperative surveillance intervals and duration of follow-up is presented in Chapter 49.

A major question concerning postoperative MRI of less-than-total resection is whether the size or imaging characteristics of the remnant could be used to assess risk of regrowth. In one study, thickness of the residual tumor beyond 7.4 mm was associated with an increased rate of regrowth.[42] In this particular study, initial tumor size and cystic nature of the tumor were not independent predictors of growth. In another study of 350 patients, Carlson et al reported that nodular enhancement of the remnant on the first postoperative MRI was associated with a 16-fold increased chance of tumor regrowth compared to a linear enhancement pattern.[41] In terms of absolute measurements and volume, the same study found that residuals measuring 15 mm in maximum diameter or volume beyond 0.4 cm^3 are associated with five times higher rate of regrowth as well.

41.7 Conclusion

Previous studies have demonstrated that patients with large tumors who undergo STR or NTR generally have better facial nerve outcomes compared to those who undergo GTR. An obvious concern for patients who undergo STR is that they are simply trading better immediate facial nerve function for a higher chance of tumor regrowth in the future. Tumor recurrence treated with salvage surgery often results in poor facial nerve outcome.

Much is left to be discovered in the area of STR of VS. Some progress could be readily made by a consolidated effort on the part of surgeons to define and adopt a universal vocabulary for variables such as size of tumor, degree of resection, tumor regrowth, and failure of treatment. Ultimately, diligent prospective studies may be required to ascertain optimum degree of resection, timing and frequency of imaging studies, as well as a clinically relevant and prognostic-based definition of STR and NTR. There are limitations that make performing a double-blinded randomized study on STR virtually impossible. These larger tumors are relatively scarce and even tertiary centers may not have enough patients to achieve statistical significance. A more challenging issue is that it would be unethical to randomize patients into the GTR or STR group, as surgeons would certainly complete the resection when the planes are favorable and would not transect nerves if the tumor was strongly adherent. Because of this issue, there is an inherent bias comparing STR and GTR patients as the level of adherence may be a function of tumor physiology—meaning that tumors with faster and more aggressive growth patterns may more commonly receive STR.

From our limited data, one may consider the following statements: First, radiation treatment could be used only in case of tumor remnant growth, as a number of true NTR and STR tumor remnants do not grow for extended periods following surgery. Second, an initial baseline MRI of the tumor remnant following less-than-complete resection is likely best obtained around 3 to 6 months after surgery. Third, patients who have undergone NTR and STR (or GTR in case of very large tumors) should receive long-term follow-up of at least 10 years, or perhaps indefinitely, with MRI scans. Fourth, if GTR is not possible at the time of first operation, the surgeon should attempt to reduce the residual tumor to a very thin, small remnant as much as possible. In such cases, a true NTR may offer a better facial nerve outcome without increased risk of recurrence.

References

[1] Flamm ES. New observations on the Dandy-Cushing controversy. Neurosurgery. 1994; 35(4):737–738, discussion 738–740

[2] Dandy W. Results of removal of acoustic tumors by the unilateral approach. Arch Surg. 1941; 42:1026–1033

[3] Cushing H. Intracranial Tumors. Springfield, IL: C. C. Thomas; 1932

[4] Eisenhardt L. Long postoperative survivals in cases of intracranial tumor. Proc Assoc Res Nerv Ment Dis. 1935; 16:390

[5] House WF. Partial tumor removal and recurrence in acoustic tumor surgery. Arch Otolaryngol. 1968; 88(6):644–654

[6] Horrax G. A comparison of results after intracapsular enucleation and total extirpation of acoustic tumors. J Neurol Neurosurg Psychiatry. 1950; 13(4): 268–270

[7] Roland JT, Jr, Fishman AJ, Golfinos JG, Cohen N, Alexiades G, Jackman AH. Cranial nerve preservation in surgery for large acoustic neuromas. Skull Base. 2004; 14(2):85–90, discussion 90–91

[8] Sughrue ME, Kaur R, Rutkowski MJ, et al. Extent of resection and the long-term durability of vestibular schwannoma surgery. J Neurosurg. 2011; 114 (5):1218–1223

[9] Hahn CH, Stangerup SE, Caye-Thomasen P. Residual tumour after vestibular schwannoma surgery. J Laryngol Otol. 2013; 127(6):568–573

[10] Angeli RD, Piccirillo E, Di Trapani G, Sequino G, Taibah A, Sanna M. Enlarged translabyrinthine approach with transapical extension in the management of giant vestibular schwannomas: personal experience and review of literature. Otol Neurotol. 2011; 32(1):125–131

[11] Kanzaki J, Tos M, Sanna M, Moffat DA, Monsell EM, Berliner KI. New and modified reporting systems from the consensus meeting on systems for reporting results in vestibular schwannoma. Otol Neurotol. 2003; 24(4):642–648, discussion 648–649

[12] Godefroy WP, van der Mey AG, de Bruine FT, Hoekstra ER, Malessy MJ. Surgery for large vestibular schwannoma: residual tumor and outcome. Otol Neurotol. 2009; 30(5):629–634

[13] Monfared A, Corrales E, Theodosopoulos P, et al. Facial nerve outcome and tumor control rate as a function of degree of resection in treatment of large acoustic neuromas: preliminary report of the Acoustic Neuroma Subtotal Resection Study. Neurosurgery. 2015(Nov):28

[14] Darrouzet V, Martel J, Enée V, Bébéar JP, Guérin J. Vestibular schwannoma surgery outcomes: our multidisciplinary experience in 400 cases over 17 years. Laryngoscope. 2004; 114(4):681–688

[15] Falcioni M, Fois P, Taibah A, Sanna M. Facial nerve function after vestibular schwannoma surgery. J Neurosurg. 2011; 115(4):820–826

[16] Lanman TH, Brackmann DE, Hitselberger WE, Subin B. Report of 190 consecutive cases of large acoustic tumors (vestibular schwannoma) removed via the translabyrinthine approach. J Neurosurg. 1999; 90(4):617–623

[17] Gurgel RK, Dogru S, Amdur RL, Monfared A. Facial nerve outcomes after surgery for large vestibular schwannomas: do surgical approach and extent of resection matter? Neurosurg Focus. 2012; 33(3):E16

[18] Anderson DE, Leonetti J, Wind JJ, Cribari D, Fahey K. Resection of large vestibular schwannomas: facial nerve preservation in the context of surgical approach and patient-assessed outcome. J Neurosurg. 2005; 102(4):643–649

[19] Samii M, Gerganov VM, Samii A. Functional outcome after complete surgical removal of giant vestibular schwannomas. J Neurosurg. 2010; 112(4):860–867

[20] Sanna M, Russo A, Taibah A, Falcioni M, Agarwal M. Enlarged translabyrinthine approach for the management of large and giant acoustic neuromas: a report of 175 consecutive cases. Ann Otol Rhinol Laryngol. 2004; 113(4):319–328

[21] Jung S, Kang SS, Kim TS, et al. Current surgical results of retrosigmoid approach in extralarge vestibular schwannomas. Surg Neurol. 2000; 53(4): 370–377, discussion 377–378

[22] Haque R, Wojtasiewicz TJ, Gigante PR, et al. Efficacy of facial nerve-sparing approach in patients with vestibular schwannomas. J Neurosurg. 2011; 115 (5):917–923

[23] Amano M, Kohno M, Nagata O, Taniguchi M, Sora S, Sato H. Intraoperative continuous monitoring of evoked facial nerve electromyograms in acoustic neuroma surgery. Acta Neurochir (Wien). 2011; 153(5):1059–1067, discussion 1067

[24] Schmitt WR, Daube JR, Carlson ML, et al. Use of supramaximal stimulation to predict facial nerve outcomes following vestibular schwannoma microsurgery: results from a decade of experience. J Neurosurg. 2013; 118(1):206–212

[25] Schwartz MS, Kari E, Strickland BM, et al. Evaluation of the increased use of partial resection of large vestibular schwannomas: facial nerve outcomes and recurrence/regrowth rates. Otol Neurotol. 2013; 34(8):1456–1464

[26] Bloch DC, Oghalai JS, Jackler RK, Osofsky M, Pitts LH. The fate of the tumor remnant after less-than-complete acoustic neuroma resection. Otolaryngol Head Neck Surg. 2004; 130(1):104–112

[27] Seol HJ, Kim CH, Park CK, et al. Optimal extent of resection in vestibular schwannoma surgery: relationship to recurrence and facial nerve preservation. Neurol Med Chir (Tokyo). 2006; 46(4):176–180, discussion 180–181

[28] Freeman SR, Ramsden RT, Saeed SR, et al. Revision surgery for residual or recurrent vestibular schwannoma. Otol Neurotol. 2007; 28(8):1076–1082

[29] Hasegawa T, Kida Y, Kobayashi T, Yoshimoto M, Mori Y, Yoshida J. Long-term outcomes in patients with vestibular schwannomas treated using gamma knife surgery: 10-year follow up. J Neurosurg. 2013; 119 Suppl:10–16

[30] Lunsford LD, Niranjan A, Flickinger JC, Maitz A, Kondziolka D. Radiosurgery of vestibular schwannomas: summary of experience in 829 cases. J Neurosurg. 2013; 119 Suppl:195–199

[31] Fuentes S, Arkha Y, Pech-Gourg G, Grisoli F, Dufour H, Régis J. Management of large vestibular schwannomas by combined surgical resection and gamma knife radiosurgery. Prog Neurol Surg. 2008; 21:79–82

[32] Iwai Y, Yamanaka K, Ishiguro T. Surgery combined with radiosurgery of large acoustic neuromas. Surg Neurol. 2003; 59(4):283–289, discussion 289–291

[33] Park CK, Jung HW, Kim JE, Son YJ, Paek SH, Kim DG. Therapeutic strategy for large vestibular schwannomas. J Neurooncol. 2006; 77(2):167–171

[34] van de Langenberg R, Hanssens PE, van Overbeeke JJ, et al. Management of large vestibular schwannoma. Part I. Planned subtotal resection followed by Gamma Knife surgery: radiological and clinical aspects. J Neurosurg. 2011; 115(5):875–884

[35] Chung WY, Pan DH, Lee CC, et al. Large vestibular schwannomas treated by Gamma Knife surgery: long-term outcomes. J Neurosurg. 2010; 113 Suppl: 112–121

[36] Inoue HK. Low-dose radiosurgery for large vestibular schwannomas: long-term results of functional preservation. J Neurosurg. 2005; 102 Suppl: 111–113

[37] Mandl ES, Meijer OW, Slotman BJ, Vandertop WP, Peerdeman SM. Stereotactic radiation therapy for large vestibular schwannomas. Radiother Oncol. 2010; 95(1):94–98

[38] Weissman JL, Hirsch BE, Fukui MB, Rudy TE. The evolving MR appearance of structures in the internal auditory canal after removal of an acoustic neuroma. AJNR Am J Neuroradiol. 1997; 18(2):313–323

[39] Mueller DP, Gantz BJ, Dolan KD. Gadolinium-enhanced MR of the postoperative internal auditory canal following acoustic neuroma resection via the middle fossa approach. AJNR Am J Neuroradiol. 1992; 13(1):197–200

[40] Brors D, Schäfers M, Bodmer D, Draf W, Kahle G, Schick B. Postoperative magnetic resonance imaging findings after transtemporal and translabyrinthine vestibular schwannoma resection. Laryngoscope. 2003; 113(3): 420–426

[41] Carlson ML, Van Abel KM, Driscoll CL, et al. Magnetic resonance imaging surveillance following vestibular schwannoma resection. Laryngoscope. 2012; 122(2):378–388

[42] Fukuda M, Oishi M, Hiraishi T, Natsumeda M, Fujii Y. Clinicopathological factors related to regrowth of vestibular schwannoma after incomplete resection. J Neurosurg. 2011; 114(5):1224–1231

42 Staged Resection of Large Vestibular Schwannoma

Aaron Metrailer and Michael J. LaRouere

42.1 Introduction

Large vestibular schwannomas, defined as ≥ 3 cm in greatest posterior fossa dimension, pose a challenge to surgeons as they are associated with higher perioperative complications and worse facial nerve outcomes following surgery than for smaller tumors.[1] Due to tumor size, growth, and subsequent mass effect, conservative management is rarely a treatment option. Likewise, radiosurgery is seldom used to manage large tumors due to the potential for radiation damage to surrounding critical structures as well as risk of inducing hydrocephalus from tumor swelling or parenchymal vasogenic edema. Therefore, the majority of large vestibular schwannomas are managed with surgical extirpation.

In the current era of cranial base microsurgery, mortality is exceedingly rare and outcomes are primarily measured according to extent of resection, recurrence, complication rates, as well as hearing and facial nerve preservation. Hearing preservation continues to remain a challenge in large tumors, and its importance falls far behind tumor control and facial nerve function. One of the primary cited advantages of microsurgical resection over radiosurgery and observation is definitive cure when gross-total resection is achieved. However, complete tumor removal with preservation of good facial nerve function with large vestibular schwannomas is challenging. Historically, long-term facial nerve outcomes after resection of large vestibular schwannomas have been poor, with only approximately half of patients achieving House-Brackmann (HB) grade I or II function according to pooled data (▶ Table 42.1).[2,3,4,5,6,7,8,9] These disappointing results have led many groups to advocate for subtotal resection, with or without adjuvant radiosurgery. However, several studies have demonstrated that many tumors regrow following incomplete removal and subtotal resection alone should not be viewed as a long-term or definitive treatment. An evolving technique of staged microsurgical resection of large tumors has allowed for tumor removal while reducing the risk of poor long-term facial nerve outcome.

Table 42.1 Posttreatment facial nerve outcomes after single-stage microsurgery for large vestibular schwannomas with historical means

Study	Publication date	Tumor size (cm)	Total patients	Postoperative HB grade I or II (%)
Tos and Thomsen	1989	> 4	149	64
Briggs et al	1994	> 4	143	42
Naguib et al	1995	> 2.5	30	30
Lanman et al	1999	> 3	95	53
Wu and Sterkers	2000	> 3	40	65
Sluyter et al	2001	> 2	116	47
Mamikoglu et al	2002	> 3	70	45
Godefroy et al	2009	> 2.6	50	78
Historical summary			693	53

42.2 Staged Microsurgery

Dandy first discussed the advantages of staged surgery for vestibular schwannomas in 1925. He noted the "residual tumor was soft, necrotic, and avascular" making it more amendable to resection on a second surgery.[10] In 1979, Sheptak and Jannetta first published a series on resection of large vestibular schwannomas via two-staged suboccipital approaches. Like Dandy, they noted less tumor adherence and vascularity on the second surgery. They concluded that certain advantages for staged microsurgery exist, and the decision to perform staged surgery should be based on intraoperative findings.[11]

Multiple series of staged vestibular schwannoma resection followed the initial report by Sheptak and Jannetta. Advances in microsurgical instrumentation and neuromonitoring have allowed for the development of more objective intraoperative criteria for staged vestibular schwannoma surgery. Commonly cited reasons to perform staged surgery include facial nerve splaying, tumor adherence to the facial nerve or brainstem, and changes in facial nerve excitability. Less commonly, unfavorable changes in vital signs may also require early termination of the primary surgery. The approach to staged resection has largely evolved from strictly suboccipital approaches to include suboccipital removal followed by a translabyrinthine approach for the second stage. Translabyrinthine approaches have now been used for both stages as well. The advantages of staged surgery include a more robust facial nerve on the second stage, less facial nerve splaying, and residual tumor shrinkage. That is, the first surgery results in a large reduction in mass effect, which allows the facial nerve fibers to regroup and any surrounding edema to improve or resolve. In addition, the facial nerve has an opportunity to recover from any potential neuropraxia. Finally, during the time interval between surgeries, the residual tumor may coalesce or "ball up" from a blanket to a more nodular configuration that may facilitate dissection. These factors may hypothetically lead to higher rates of facial nerve preservation with near-total or total resection.

42.2.1 Indications and Preoperative Considerations

Staged resection is generally reserved for large vestibular schwannomas; however, if intraoperative factors dictate, it may be considered for medium-sized tumors as well. Patients and families should be educated preoperatively on the possibility of staged surgery with the goal of improved long-term facial nerve function. Although the decision for staged surgery is usually made intraoperatively, it is our opinion that it is acceptable to preoperatively plan a staged resection based on tumor size alone. Our experience has been that patients and families are accepting of more than one surgery if it offers improved long-term quality of life and facial nerve outcomes. Often, the patient's recovery after subsequent surgeries is shorter and easier due to prior vestibular function loss and compensation.

42.2.2 First-Stage Surgery

Traditionally, first-stage surgery has consisted of a retrosigmoid approach. The medial tumor is debulked and removed from the cerebellopontine angle (CPA) with preservation of neurovascular structures. Advantages of the first-stage retrosigmoid approach include keeping an undissected plane around the facial nerve in the internal auditory canal (IAC). If the tumor has favorable intraoperative factors for tumor removal and neural preservation, bone can then be removed over the IAC and dissection continued. If intraoperative factors dictate a staged resection, the bony IAC is not drilled and Silastic sheeting (0.004") is placed within the CPA to reduce adhesions between the cranial nerves, brainstem, cerebellum, and the residual tumor.

More recently, a first-stage translabyrinthine approach instead of a retrosigmoid approach has been advocated.[12] Even if the preoperative plan was to stage the tumor because of very large size, we generally still pursue near-total or gross-total resection if intraoperative factors permit. If the resection does not favor a single-stage surgery, eggshell thin bone overlying the IAC is left intact, and the tumor is removed from the CPA and Silastic sheeting placed. Preserving the bony IAC allows virgin dissection planes during the subsequent surgery.

42.2.3 Intraoperative Factors

Since the first series published by Sheptak and Jannetta, intraoperative factors have served as driving forces for staged microsurgery. As mentioned earlier, some surgeons may decide preoperatively to perform a staged resection, based on patient's health, tumor size, and degree of brainstem compression. Most often, however, intraoperative factors are used as an "ending point" for the first surgery. Early reports cited tumor adherence to the brainstem as the primary indication for staged resection; however, with technological advancements, further criteria have been found beneficial as outlined later.

The advent of facial nerve monitoring has dramatically improved facial nerve outcomes in large tumors. At the author's institution, we routinely employ the use of stimulating dissectors to maximize the benefit of facial nerve monitoring. These instruments include stimulating needles, round knifes, and other instruments which are insulated to the tips (▶ Fig. 42.1). These instruments allow for "active" monitoring in which the surgeon is alerted to the proximity of the nerve by continuous electrical stimulation. This is in contrast to intermittent stimulation with a neurostimulator probe, or "passive" monitoring that only provides feedback to the surgeon when there is stretching or mechanical injury. Higher levels of current (e.g., 1 mA) are used to map the general location of the facial nerve, whereas low levels (e.g., 0.1 mA) are used to differentiate tumor from the adjacent neurovascular structures. The use of stimulating dissectors allows for more confident dissection of the tumor and more precise localization of the facial nerve, both of which reduce intraoperative injury to the nerve and facilitate efficient dissection.

Changes in facial nerve excitability will often lead surgeons to temporarily or definitively stop resection. Prolonged or train EMG potentials indicate nerve irritation and potential damage, and should prompt the surgeon to modify dissection. An increase in the threshold of stimulation signifies facial nerve injury and serves as an indicator to stop tumor resection and consider staged surgery. The tumor and facial nerve relationship is also important in determining whether large tumors need to be staged. A thinned or splayed facial nerve and a densely adherent facial nerve are commonly cited indications for staged resection. Additionally, a meandering course of the facial nerve over the superior pole of the tumor, or much less commonly over the dorsal tumor capsule, portends a poorer facial nerve outcome and may benefit from staged surgery. Other less common indications to stage tumor resection include vital sign changes (abrupt bradycardia), prohibitive cerebellum or brainstem edema, or peritumoral bleeding.

Considering the aforementioned criteria, the guiding principle for staged surgery is the concept of "taking only what the tumor gives." A single-stage, "conventional surgery" is ideal when facial nerve function can reasonably be preserved; however, a staged surgery or multimodality treatment (e.g., adjuvant stereotactic radiosurgery) should be considered if facial nerve preservation or patient health is potentially compromised. The use of intraoperative monitoring with stimulating instruments and surgeon experience allows the surgeon to know when facial nerve injury is imminent and modify or terminate the surgery. Understanding the above factors including the principle of "taking only what the tumor gives" should guide surgeons in making the appropriate intraoperative decision to stage tumor resection or continue with a single-stage surgery. The interested reader may also review Chapter 27 on intraoperative facial nerve monitoring, Chapter 32 on intraoperative management of the facial nerve, and Chapter 41 on subtotal resection.

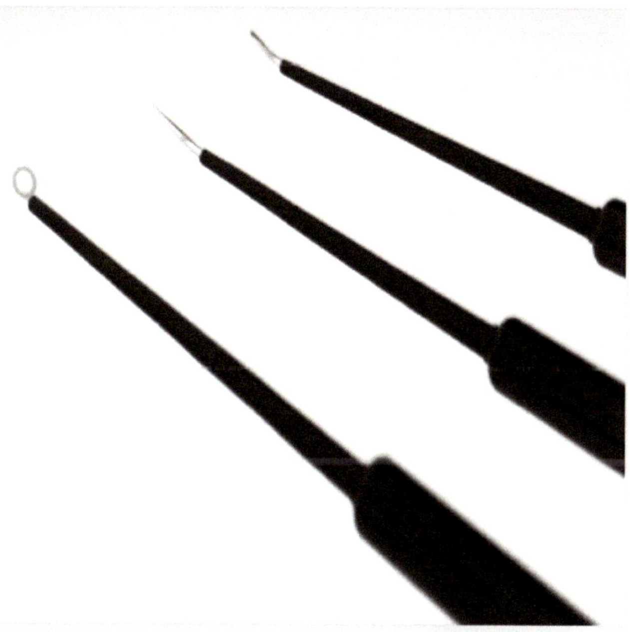

Fig. 42.1 Kartush stimulating dissectors.

42.2.4 Second-Stage Surgery

Optimal timing between surgeries has not been established; however, most published reports recommend performing the second stage within 6 months of the initial surgery. Raslan et al recommended second-stage surgery within 2 to 4 weeks of initial surgery if the immediate postoperative facial nerve function is HB grade I or II; otherwise, a typical interval of 6 months was followed to allow for facial nerve recovery.[13] We generally recommend waiting 4 to 6 months after initial surgery to allow for facial nerve recovery. If the second surgery is pursued early, the surgeon may encounter more granulation tissue and acute inflammation.

At the authors' center, second-stage surgery is performed via a translabyrinthine approach in all cases. One cited advantage of using alternate approaches with staged resection (e.g., retrosigmoid then translabyrinthine) is that a virgin or undissected surgical corridor exists for both approaches. If the patient underwent a retrosigmoid craniotomy for the first stage, a standard translabyrinthine approach is performed. For patients who had a first-stage translabyrinthine resection, the second stage is approached through the same incision. It is important to prep the abdomen for fat harvest as a new fat graft will replace the prior graft. Exposure is obtained and the prior fat graft is dissected free from surrounding structures with stimulating dissectors. Once the bony IAC is exposed, the overlying eggshell bone is removed allowing exposure of the facial nerve via undisturbed dissection planes. The facial nerve is readily identified at the meatal foramen, and we often perform meatal foramen decompression to reduce the risk of delayed facial paresis. Silastic sheeting placed during the first-stage surgery is then removed from the CPA. The remaining lateral portion of the vestibular schwannoma, including tumor near the porous acusticus is removed. The facial nerve is almost always more robust on the second stage; hence, it is easier to identify and more resistant to stretch injury. Tumor resection is completed and the wound is closed in a standard fashion (▶ Fig. 42.2).

Rarely, surgeons will not achieve near-total or gross-total resection of the residual vestibular schwannoma on the second-stage surgery, and future operations or radiosurgery may be considered. Alternatively, a very small tumor remnant may be observed with serial imaging and treated only if growth occurs. Adhering to the principle of "taking only what the tumor gives" as well as previously described intraoperative factors should guide this decision process in order to preserve facial nerve function at satisfactory levels, HB grade I or II.

42.3 Results

Historically, near-total and gross-total resection of large vestibular schwannoma has been associated with poor facial nerve outcomes. On the other hand, subtotal resection has been associated with high regrowth rates above 50% in some series.[14] Staged resection of vestibular schwannomas have allowed for near-total and gross-total removal of tumor with high facial nerve preservation rates.

42.3.1 Facial Nerve Outcomes

Excellent facial nerve outcomes, HB grade I or II, after staged vestibular schwannoma surgery range from 81 to 94% (▶ Table 42.2). In 2004, Patni and Kartush reported their series of 34 patients who underwent staged resection of large vestibular schwannomas from 1989 to 2002.[15] In this series, 32 (94%) patients had excellent long-term facial function of HB grade I. One patient had long-term HB grade III function, while another one patient had HB grade VI function. The mean follow-up for all patients was 6 years after their last surgery.

In 2012, Raslan et al reported their series of 28 patients undergoing two-stage vestibular schwannoma resection.[13] Good facial nerve outcome, HB grade I or II, at last follow-up was achieved in 23 (82%) patients. The remaining five patients

Table 42.2 Posttreatment facial nerve function for staged microsurgery compared to historical mean for resection of large vestibular schwannomas

Study	Posttreatment HB grade I or II facial nerve function
Patni and Kartush	94%
Raslan et al	82%
Porter et al	81%
Historical mean	53%

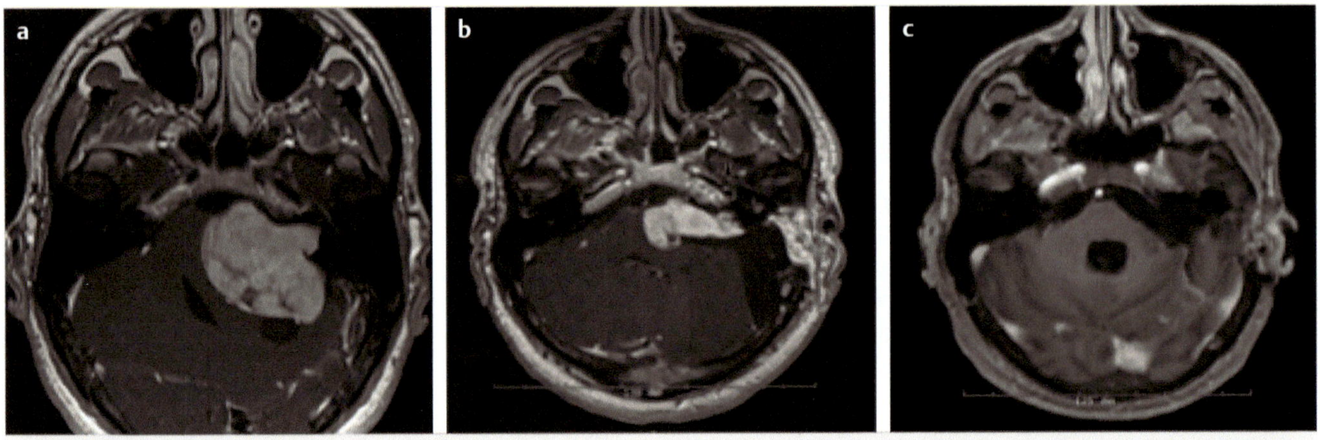

Fig. 42.2 (**a**) Preoperative MRI of a large left-sided vestibular schwannoma. (**b**) MRI obtained after first-stage surgery demonstrating tumor volume reduction. (**c**) Post second-stage MRI demonstrating no residual tumor.

had poorer long-term facial nerve outcomes, which were graded HB grade III or worse. The average follow-up time was 3 years after the last surgery. Finally, in 2013, Porter et al reported on 75 patients undergoing staged surgery for large vestibular schwannomas between 2000 and 2009.[12] Sixty-one patients (81%) undergoing staged resection had HB grade I or II function at 1 year, 7 patients (9%) had HB grade III function, while the remaining 7 patients had HB grade IV function or worse at 1 year. These retrospective series report long-term facial nerve outcomes that are better than single-stage conventional surgery for large vestibular schwannoma, which have a historical mean of 53% of patients achieving HB I or II function (▶ Table 42.1).

42.3.2 Tumor Removal

Contemporary literature for single-stage resection reports high percentages of near-total and gross-total tumor resection rates but often at the expense of long-term facial nerve function. Outcomes after staged resection reveal that over 95% of cases achieve near-total or gross-total resection with improved facial nerve outcomes. In the series reported by Patni and Kartush, the average tumor size was 4.4 cm in largest dimension on preoperative magnetic resonance imaging (MRI). All 34 patients had near-total or gross-total tumor resection after their final surgery. No recurrences were noted on follow-up MRI scans with an average follow-up of 6 years.

In the series reported by Raslan et al, the average tumor size was 3.9 cm (range: 3.2–7 cm). Total and near-total resection was achieved in 27 patients (96.4%); one patient had subtotal resection followed by postoperative radiosurgery for residual tumor. No recurrences were noted on follow-up MRI scans with an average follow-up of 3 years. All tumors in the series by Porter et al measured greater than or equal to 3 cm. In patients undergoing staged resection, complete tumor removal was achieved in 26 (35%) patients, while the remaining 49 patients (65%) had a near-total tumor removal, defined as greater than 95% resection.

42.4 Complications

Surgical resection of large vestibular schwannomas has historically been associated with higher rates of perioperative complications than resection of smaller tumors. Cerebrospinal fluid (CSF) leaks are reported to occur in 11 to 18% of operated patients with up to 5% requiring reoperation.[1,2,3,4,5,6,7,8,9,16,17] Meningitis, intracranial bleeding, stroke, cerebellar injury, other cranial nerve injuries, and death can occur in up to 3% of patients with large tumors. For staged surgery, one must consider whether repeat surgery increases complication rates.

Seventy-one operations were performed by Patni and Kartush with no reports of meningitis, vascular accidents, intracranial bleeding, hydrocephalus, or death. Five patients (7%) had a postoperative CSF leak; all were successfully managed conservatively with either lumbar drain or pressure dressing alone. Two patients had a transient abducens nerve palsy that resolved by 1 year. One wound infection was reported, while two patients had abdominal seromas managed effectively with needle aspiration. No patient had the same complication twice.

Table 42.3 Common complications of staged microsurgery compared to single-stage microsurgery historical averages

Complication	Staged microsurgery rate	Single-stage microsurgery historical rate
Cerebrospinal fluid leak	11%	11–15%
Abducens nerve palsy	2%	3%
Meningitis	1.7%	3%
Wound infection	1.2%	3%
Hydrocephalus	1.2%	3%

Raslan et al performed a total of 56 surgeries in their 28 patient series. There were no reports of death or hydrocephalus. All patients had placement of a lumbar drain postoperatively to reduce CSF leak rates. The most common complication was CSF leakage occurring in eight patients—four patients required a lumbar peritoneal shunt to treat pseudomeningocele. The next most common complication, wound infection, occurred in two patients followed by one case of both meningitis and dural sinus thrombosis.

The most common complication in the series by Porter et al was CSF leak occurring after 6 of 45 (13%) surgeries. In this series, lumbar drains were only placed postoperatively if a CSF leak occurred. Two patients developed meningitis, while two patients required a temporary ventriculostomy for hydrocephalus. No patient required a permanent shunt for CSF diversion. Two patients had transient abducens nerve palsy postoperatively. There were no strokes, deaths, or significant vascular injuries in this study population.

The most common complication for all three studies was postoperative CSF leak at an average rate of 11%. This rate is comparable to historical averages for single-stage surgery for vestibular schwannomas, ranging from 11 to 18%. The next most common complication was temporary abducens nerve palsy (2%) followed by meningitis (1.7%; ▶ Table 42.3).

42.5 Conclusion

Management of large vestibular schwannomas remains a significant challenge. Staged microsurgery allows experienced surgeons to obtain near-total or gross-total resection in most cases while maintaining excellent long-term facial nerve function. Staged surgery may be approached via either a first-stage retrosigmoid or translabyrinthine approach. Intraoperative factors including a reduction in facial nerve stimulation response, facial nerve splaying, tumor adherence to the facial nerve and brainstem, surgeon experience, and less commonly vital sign changes dictate when to terminate the first-stage surgery.

While there are no definitive guidelines on when to perform the second-stage surgery, most surgeons wait for 4 to 6 months after the initial surgery. Staging the operation after significant tumor debulking may reduce brainstem and cerebellar edema, allows a thin splayed facial nerve to recover between cases, and provides time for the residual tumor to "ball up" or coalesce—all these factors increase the probability of near-total or gross-total tumor resection with good facial nerve outcome. Multiple surgeries do not predispose patients to increased complication rates.

Future areas of investigation include subtotal tumor resection followed by planned stereotactic radiotherapy. Interestingly, in a recent pilot study, 4 of 11 patients treated with postoperative radiation for growing residual tumor required subsequent surgical salvage.[18] It is possible that large tumors behave differently from small- or medium-sized tumors in that they have a high propensity for regrowth.

References

[1] Glasscock ME, III, Kveton JF, Jackson CG, Levine SC, McKennan KX. A systematic approach to the surgical management of acoustic neuroma. Laryngoscope. 1986; 96(10):1088–1094

[2] Tos M, Thomsen J. The translabyrinthine approach for the removal of large acoustic neuromas. Arch Otorhinolaryngol. 1989; 246(5):292–296

[3] Briggs RJ, Luxford WM, Atkins JS, Jr, Hitselberger WE. Translabyrinthine removal of large acoustic neuromas. Neurosurgery. 1994; 34(5):785–790, discussion 790–791

[4] Naguib MB, Saleh E, Cokkeser Y, et al. The enlarged translabyrinthine approach for removal of large vestibular schwannomas. J Laryngol Otol. 1994; 108(7):545–550

[5] Lanman TH, Brackmann DE, Hitselberger WE, Subin B. Report of 190 consecutive cases of large acoustic tumors (vestibular schwannoma) removed via the translabyrinthine approach. J Neurosurg. 1999; 90(4):617–623

[6] Wu H, Sterkers J. Translabyrinthine removal of large acoustic neuromas in young adults. Auris Nasus Larynx. 2000; 27(3):201–205

[7] Sluyter S, Graamans K, Tulleken CA, Van Veelen CW. Analysis of the results obtained in 120 patients with large acoustic neuromas surgically treated via the translabyrinthine-transtentorial approach. J Neurosurg. 2001; 94(1): 61–66

[8] Mamikoglu B, Wiet RJ, Esquivel CR. Translabyrinthine approach for the management of large and giant vestibular schwannomas. Otol Neurotol. 2002; 23(2):224–227

[9] Godefroy WP, van der Mey AG, de Bruine FT, Hoekstra ER, Malessy MJ. Surgery for large vestibular schwannoma: residual tumor and outcome. Otol Neurotol. 2009; 30(5):629–634

[10] Dandy WE. An operation for the total removal of cerebellopontine (acoustic) tumors. Surg Gynecol Obstet. 1925; 76:129–148

[11] Sheptak PE, Jannetta PJ. The two-stage excision of huge acoustic neurinomas. J Neurosurg. 1979; 51(1):37–41

[12] Porter RG, LaRouere MJ, Kartush JM, Bojrab DI, Pieper DR. Improved facial nerve outcomes using an evolving treatment method for large acoustic neuromas. Otol Neurotol. 2013; 34(2):304–310

[13] Raslan AM, Liu JK, McMenomey SO, Delashaw JB, Jr. Staged resection of large vestibular schwannomas. J Neurosurg. 2012; 116(5):1126–1133

[14] El-Kashlan HK, Zeitoun H, Arts HA, Hoff JT, Telian SA. Recurrence of acoustic neuroma after incomplete resection. Am J Otol. 2000; 21(3):389–392

[15] Patni AH, Kartush JM. Staged resection of large acoustic neuromas. Otolaryngol Head Neck Surg. 2005; 132(1):11–19

[16] Bryce GE, Nedzelski JM, Rowed DW, Rappaport JM. Cerebrospinal fluid leaks and meningitis in acoustic neuroma surgery. Otolaryngol Head Neck Surg. 1991; 104(1):81–87

[17] Mangham CA. Complications of translabyrinthine vs. suboccipital approach for acoustic neuroma surgery. Otol Head Neck Surg. 1998; 99:396–400

[18] Monfared A, Corrales CE, Theodosopoulos PV, et al. Facial nerve outcome and tumor control rate as a function of degree of resection in treatment of large acoustic neuromas: preliminary report of the Acoustic Neuroma Subtotal Resection Study (ANSRS). Neurosurgery. 2016; 79(2):194–203

43 Microsurgery for Recurrent and Residual Vestibular Schwannoma

Avital Perry, Christopher S. Graffeo, William R. Copeland III, Brian A. Neff, Matthew L. Carlson, Colin L. W. Driscoll, and Michael J. Link

43.1 Introduction

Vestibular schwannoma (VS) recurrence after prior microsurgery (MS) is rare, with an estimated incidence of 0.05 to 9.2% following gross total resection (GTR) at the primary operation.[1,2,3,4,5,6,7] Recurrence is defined as occurring specifically after GTR, in comparison to progression of residual tumor—a considerably more common occurrence, with an incidence of 44% after subtotal resection (STR).[8,9] This distinction is emphasized in planning for repeat surgery, as it is generally held that a prior GTR or an aggressive STR will have a higher risk of scaring and adhesions along the facial nerve–tumor interface (FNTI), given that it was previously dissected along its full length. By contrast, a less aggressive primary STR that was limited to a biopsy or debulking may not have significantly engaged the FNTI, resulting in a less perilous repeat operation. Furthermore, the capacity of the facial nerve to withstand a second dissection may be significantly diminished, particularly if it was previously subject to substantial manipulation during the primary operation.

Various tactics are employed in treating recurrent or progressive residual VS after MS, including stereotactic radiosurgery (SRS), fractionated radiotherapy, repeat MS, and observation—a strategy reserved for those patients with slow-growing tumors and without brainstem compression. For the majority of patients, SRS is the treatment of choice, which has been demonstrated to provide excellent tumor control in VS recurrence after MS.[10] Notwithstanding, repeat MS after MS may warrant consideration in specific patient populations, in particular those individuals with brainstem compression requiring more urgent treatment, in patients with secondary trigeminal neuralgia who would benefit from direct decompression of the trigeminal nerve, tumors with large macrocystic changes, or individuals strongly desiring surgical treatment in lieu of radiation.

43.2 Example—Recurrent Vestibular Schwannoma

A healthy 28-year-old man experienced progressive hearing loss in his left ear over 12 months. Neurologic workup included magnetic resonance imaging (MRI) of the brain, which revealed a left 3.5-cm cerebellopontine angle (CPA) mass with extension into the internal auditory canal (IAC) and homogenous gadolinium enhancement, consistent with VS (▸ Fig. 43.1a). The fourth ventricle was effaced and signs of early hydrocephalus were apparent. The patient was taken to the operating room for a retrosigmoid (RS) craniotomy and drilling of the IAC, during

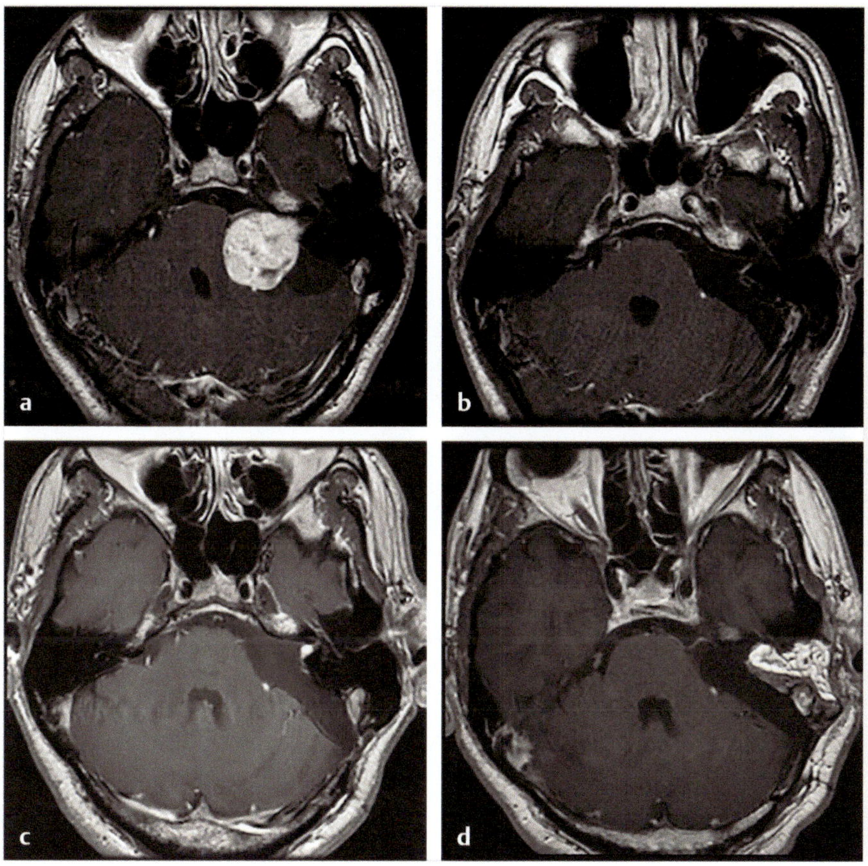

Fig. 43.1 Example 1, reoperation for recurrent VS after prior gross total resection.

which GTR was achieved, and baseline facial nerve stimulation at the brainstem was preserved. The patient awoke with House–Brackmann (HB) grade I facial nerve function, and underwent a routine postoperative recovery. Follow-up MRI at 6 months was negative for nodular enhancement or any other evidence of residual tumor (▶ Fig. 43.1b).

Further follow-up continued uneventfully until surveillance imaging at 7 years after initial resection demonstrated a new, small area of enhancement within the left IAC (▶ Fig. 43.1c). Treatment options including SRS, repeat MS, and observation were discussed, and the patient elected surgery. Repeat MS was planned via a translabyrinthine (TL) approach; the IAC dura was opened in the typical fashion, and a clear nodular recurrence was identified along the distal superior vestibular nerve. Dissection was readily carried out along the FNTI, and GTR was achieved without marked difficulty. Postoperatively, the patient maintained HB grade I facial nerve function; his immediate postoperative course was complicated by cerebrospinal fluid (CSF) rhinorrhea, which resolved after placement of a lumbar drain and 48 hours of intermittent CSF diversion. Follow-up MRI 3 months after surgery confirmed GTR, and the patient has continued to remain recurrence free over more than 5 years of subsequent follow-up (▶ Fig. 43.1d).

43.3 Review of the Literature—Recurrent Vestibular Schwannoma

Four studies have described individual outcomes after repeat MS for recurrent VS in radiation-naive, non-neurofibromatosis type 2 (NF2) patients with no history of facial reanimation surgery, documenting a total of 50 patients (▶ Table 43.1).[3,7,11,12] For the overall patient cohort, mean time-to-revision was 73 months, employment of the same approach for repeat surgery was common (90%), extent of resection was GTR in most patients (95%), and unfavorable (HB grades III–VI) facial nerve function after revision surgery was frequently reported (68%). Additional complications were rare, and predominantly limited to CSF leak (4%).

In the largest preceding series, Samii et al reported outcomes in 36 radiation-naive individuals undergoing repeat MS after primary GTR, as well as a second 17-patient cohort of patients who had previously undergone SRS during the interval between primary GTR and repeat MS.[7] To provide a control, outcomes in both groups were compared to a randomly selected group of 30 primary VS resections with no history of prior radiation. All operations were via RS craniotomy, and GTR was universally achieved. Within the MS-after-MS only group, favorable HB grades I to II preoperative facial nerve function was present in 25 (69%) at the time of repeat surgery; this was preserved in 12 (48%). No second recurrences were reported, and the mean follow-up period after repeat MS was 60 months. Of particular interest, Samii et al did not detect a significant difference in their comparison between patients undergoing repeat MS with and without a prior history of SRS, with respect to facial nerve, extent of resection, or tumor control outcomes.

A series of six recurrences without a history of radiation therapy or facial reanimation were reported by Roche et al; three each underwent enlarged TL after primary TL surgery, or repeat surgery via TL after primary RS.[11] In the enlarged TL group, GTR was achieved in two (67%), and favorable HB grades I to II facial nerve function was preserved in the only patient who had favorable preoperative function (100%). By contrast, of the three patients who underwent repeat TL surgery after primary RS,

Table 43.1 Published outcomes following repeat microsurgery for recurrent vestibular schwannoma

Author	Year	Initial EoR	*n*	Mean time-to-repeat (mo)	Mean size at repeat (cm)	Repeat extent of resection (GTR)	Pre-repeat favorable facial nerve function (HB I/HB II)	Post-repeat favorable facial nerve function (HB I/HB II)	Same approach at repeat surgery	Post-repeat CSF leak	Second recurrence	Mean post-repeat follow-up (mo)
Shelton	1995	GTR	4	128	3	4 (100%)	2 (50%)	1 (25%)	4 (100%)	–	–	–
Freeman et al	2007	GTR	4	23	3	3 (75%)	2 (50%)	1 (25%)	2 (50%)	2 (50%)	0 (0%)	47
Roche et al	2008	GTR	6	80	–	4 (67%)	4 (67%)	2 (33%)	3 (50%)	–	–	24
Ahmad et al	2012	GTR	1	108	1	1 (100%)	0 (0%)	0 (0%)	1 (100%)	–	–	–
Samii et al	2016	GTR	36	25	–	36 (100%)	25 (69%)	12 (33%)	36 (100%)	–	0 (0%)	60
Summary	–	GTR	50	73	2	48 (96%)	33 (66%)	26 (52%)	45 (90%)	4 (4%)	0 (0%)	44
Sakaki et al	1991	STR	2	32	–	1 (50%)	0 (0%)	0 (0%)	1 (50%)	–	1 (50%)	–
Ramina et al	2007	STR	12	36	4	12 (100%)	3 (25%)	1 (13%)	–	3 (25%)	–	73
Freeman et al	2007	STR	21	43	3	11 (52%)	12 (57%)	7 (33%)	6 (29%)	1 (5%)	8 (38%)	118
Roche et al	2008	STR	2	72	–	1 (50%)	2 (100%)	1 (50%)	1 (50%)	–	–	78
Chen et al	2014	STR	3	47	–	1 (33%)	–	0 (0%)	–	–	–	–
Summary	–	STR	40	46	3.5	26 (65%)	17 (43%)	9 (23%)	8 (20%)	4 (10%)	9 (23%)	90

Abbreviations: CSF, cerebrospinal fluid; EoR, extent of resection; GTR, gross total resection; HB, House–Brackmann; STR, subtotal resection.

GTR was again achieved in two (67%), but HB grades I to II function was preserved in only one of three patients with favorable preoperative facial nerve function.

Four recurrences after GTR were reported by Freeman et al, within a larger series of both recurrent and residual tumors undergoing repeat surgery.[3] Two underwent same-approach repeat surgery, both of who deteriorated from favorable pre-repeat surgery facial nerve function to unfavorable post-repeat surgery favorable nerve function. Of the two patients in whom an alternate approach was utilized, one maintained stable HB grade III facial nerve function, while the other improved from HB grades III to II. No complications or second recurrences were reported after a mean of 47 months of follow-up. Another small series of four repeat surgeries was reported by Shelton, who employed the TL approach at both primary and repeat surgery.[12] GTR was achieved in all four patients (100%), and favorable postoperative facial nerve function was preserved in one of two patients with preoperative HB grades I to II function (50%); no other complications were reported.

Hong et al reported a series of 15 patients undergoing repeat MS; unfortunately, detailed analysis is prohibited by pooled reporting of outcomes between these patients and three others who had growth of residual tumors, rather than true recurrences.[4] Although 14 of these patients underwent alternate-approach repeat surgery, detailed outcomes are not specified on an individual patient basis, and so the outcomes by approach cannot be compared. Notwithstanding, overall outcomes were encouraging, with preservation of favorable preoperative HB grades I to II facial nerve function in seven of ten patients (70%), and GTR in ten of fifteen patients (67%).

43.4 Review of the Literature—Residual Vestibular Schwannoma

As with recurrences, progressive residual tumors treated with repeat MS rather than SRS are uncommon, with five prior series reporting patient-specific outcomes on a total of 40 individuals (▶ Table 43.1). Looking at the cohort at large, mean time-to-revision was 46 months, alternate surgical approaches for the second surgery were more dominant (80%), favorable postoperative facial nerve function was uncommon (23%), and multiple instances of both CSF leak (10%) and second recurrence (23%) were reported.

Freeman et al and Roche et al's series described earlier also included subpopulation of progressive residual tumors that underwent repeat MS. Among Freeman et al's 21 primary STR patients, favorable facial nerve function was present prior to reoperation in 12 (57%), and preserved in 7 (33%), a modest but not statistically significant improvement on their results after primary GTR.[3] By contrast, extent of resection was less robust, with GTR achieved in only 11 (52%). An alternate surgical approach was selected in 15 (71%), and a second recurrence was observed in eight (38%)—a marked increase from the zero noted in Freeman et al's primary GTR population, although this most likely reflects longer follow-up and fewer repeat GTRs in the primary STR group, rather than inherent differences in the tumor biology. Roche et al reported two additional patients who had undergone primary STR, with broadly comparable results to those after primary GTR.[11] One patient underwent an alternate-approach repeat operation, during which favorable facial nerve function was preserved and GTR was achieved.

Three additional small series reported individual outcomes after repeat MS for progressive residual VS. Chen et al's series of three patients reported very limited clinical data: pre-repeat facial nerve function was not clearly documented, but all three had post-repeat HB grade VI function, and GTR was achieved in one only.[13] Similarly, in a longer series focused on VS recurrence, Sakaki et al described in detail two patients who underwent repeat MS after STR; facial nerve function was unfavorable prior to repeat surgery in both, GTR was achieved in the first patient, but in the second, STR at repeat surgery ultimately led to further progression of the residual tumor.[14] Ramina et al reported 12 patients, all of who underwent GTR after primary STR; favorable facial nerve function was preserved in one of three individuals who had HB grade I to II function prior to repeat surgery.[15]

43.5 General Operative Considerations in Repeat MS for Recurrent or Residual VS

For most patients presenting with recurrent or progressive residual VS after primary MS, SRS is the mainstay of treatment, providing a safe and reliable means to establish good tumor control without exposing the facial nerve to undue risk. However, in those patients with large, macrocystic tumors compressing the brainstem or causing intractable trigeminal mediated neuralgic pain, or individuals who strongly prefer surgery to SRS, excellent outcomes can also be achieved via repeat MS, with respect to tumor control, extent of resection, and operative morbidity. As the preceding literature demonstrates and our experience confirms, a host of factors may contribute to these outcomes, including application of an alternate surgical approach to the primary operation where appropriate, as well as deferral to STR in lieu of GTR where a particularly attenuated facial nerve may be placed in jeopardy by more aggressive surgery.

The decision regarding surgical approach selection for repeat MS is complex and nuanced, and should be individualized to the specific patient, recurrence pattern, and details from the primary surgery (where available). The literature at large demonstrates that satisfactory results can be achieved using the full range of technical strategies—although overall conclusions are somewhat skewed by the significant contributions from Samii et al, particularly as their practice exclusively uses the RS approach, and takes a more aggressive tactic toward extent of resection.[6,16,17] In our experience, we have observed that an alternate approach may reduce the extent of scar requiring dissection during the approach aspect of the operation for recurrent tumor. Large tumors with significant brainstem compression or a large CPA component benefit the most from this advantage; however, specific circumstances frequently require exception to our preference for alternate-approach repeat surgery. This is particularly evident when a recurrence is limited to the IAC fundus, for example, which would be most effectively tackled via repeat TL approach, regardless of the original trajectory.

Another important consideration in repeat MS for recurrent VS is striking an appropriate balance between the chief goals of surgery—extent of resection, and postoperative facial nerve function and avoidance of other postoperative morbidity such as stroke, bleeding, or CSF leak. A salient concept in this intraoperative calculus is facial nerve reserve—in other words, the amount of manipulation that a thinned and possibly previously dissected nerve can withstand before a significant, permanent functional deterioration is sustained. For many patients, a clear dissection plane can be established, particularly, in our experience, if an alternate approach is used in exposing the FNTI. However, in a small but significant subset of cases, a dramatically attenuated, splayed, or scarred nerve will be encountered in a patient with favorable preoperative facial nerve function. In these circumstances, if an acceptable plane cannot be developed, we recommend consideration for deliberate STR, to be followed by upfront SRS to the post-repeat surgery residual tumor. This practice is distinct from the typical approach to STR after primary resection, in which SRS is deferred until progressive growth is proven; rather, here we recommend proactive treatment, as these patients have already failed MS, suggesting an aggressive tumor phenotype potentially warranting upfront radiation.

Complications have not been proven to occur at a higher rate in repeat MS; however, anecdotal evidence suggests a higher rate of CSF leak and second recurrence, and we correspondingly underscore the importance of a thorough and scrupulous closure, as well as very close clinical and radiographic follow-up. Where required, routine management strategies for CSF leak are efficacious after repeat MS, including lumbar drain placement, wound revision, abdominal fat grafting, or overclosure of the external auditory canal with packing of the Eustachian tube.

43.6 Special Considerations Regarding Prior Approach Complications

In addition to VS that underwent either GTR or STR at primary MS, a third population of tumors may present for repeat MS—those individuals whose initial operations were aborted before the tumor was ever engaged or even biopsied, due to complications encountered during the approach. The underlying causes of such an event are diverse, ranging from an inappropriately planned craniotomy resulting in an unfavorable trajectory to malignant edema precipitating rapid cerebellar or temporal lobe swelling that prohibited safe exposure of the CPA, to excessive bleeding resulting from injury to a venous sinus or other structure. Although the details of each individual circumstance will govern more detailed planning for salvage MS in these patients, several general concepts have proven useful in our experience.

Owing to the generally unfavorable conditions under which these primary operations are typically aborted, medical and neurologic complications are commonplace after approach complications. Correspondingly, we recommend a low threshold of suspicion to work-up any concerning findings, and a thorough preoperative assessment prior to attempting a second surgery. Similarly, the postoperative recovery period after repeat MS requires heightened vigilance for complications, and patients should be appropriately counseled regarding the risk profile of a salvage operation. As compared to repeat MS after an otherwise unremarkable primary MS, in which we typically suggest that planning an alternate approach might be preferred in certain circumstances, after an approach complication we emphasize the near-universal importance of selecting an alternate approach whenever possible. This is largely attributable to our expectation that the original approach may not have been optimally executed, and further reinforced by the high risk of a repeat complication if the same approach is taken once again.

Finally, in spite of the elevated risks and unconventional planning inherent to salvage surgery in the wake of an approach complication, it has been our experience that excellent outcomes can nevertheless be achieved in these patients, particularly with respect to extent of resection, facial nerve function, and overall complication rates. We hold that high-volume experience with complex tumors in a multidisciplinary environment is at the core of these successes, and strongly recommend that similarly challenging cases be undertaken by dedicated VS teams at tertiary referral centers staffed by highly experienced neurosurgery and neurotology specialist teams. Perhaps most importantly, although limited to a small number of patients, our empiric evidence suggests that approach complications occur almost exclusively in low-volume centers—and that this specific subset of bad outcomes may be entirely avoidable if VS surgery is carried out in centers of excellence, whenever possible.

43.7 Example—Approach Complications

A 40-year-old man with a history of LEOPARD syndrome originally presented with progressive falls and was discovered to have a large, heterogeneous CPA tumor consistent with hemorrhagic VS, for which he underwent surgery at an outside hospital (▶ Fig. 43.2a). A left occipital craniectomy and inadvertent supratentorial exploration was carried out and ultimately aborted due to significant bleeding. Ten days later, he developed a CSF leak, for which he was referred to our emergency department. Clinical assessment confirmed signs concerning for wound infection, as well as nearly complete blindness resulting from the primary operation. Head CT showed extensive intracranial bilateral pneumocephalus with intraventricular extension and mass effect on the left hemisphere (▶ Fig. 43.2b–d). MRI of the brain showed an intact CPA lesion, and a large meningoencephalocele at the surgical site (▶ Fig. 43.2e, f). Vascular imaging demonstrated occlusion of the right transverse sinus. The patient was first taken for wound exploration, washout, and debridement; resection of meningoencephalocele; and dural repair with autologous fascia lata (▶ Fig. 43.2g, h). He subsequently developed hydrocephalus, requiring placement of a right frontal External ventricular drain (EVD). Ultimately, he was returned to the operating room for TL resection of VS; the facial nerve could not be preserved, but GTR was achieved (▶ Fig. 43.2i, j). Hydrocephalus did not resolve postoperatively, requiring placement of a ventriculoperitoneal shunt prior to final hospital disposition. Follow-up at 3

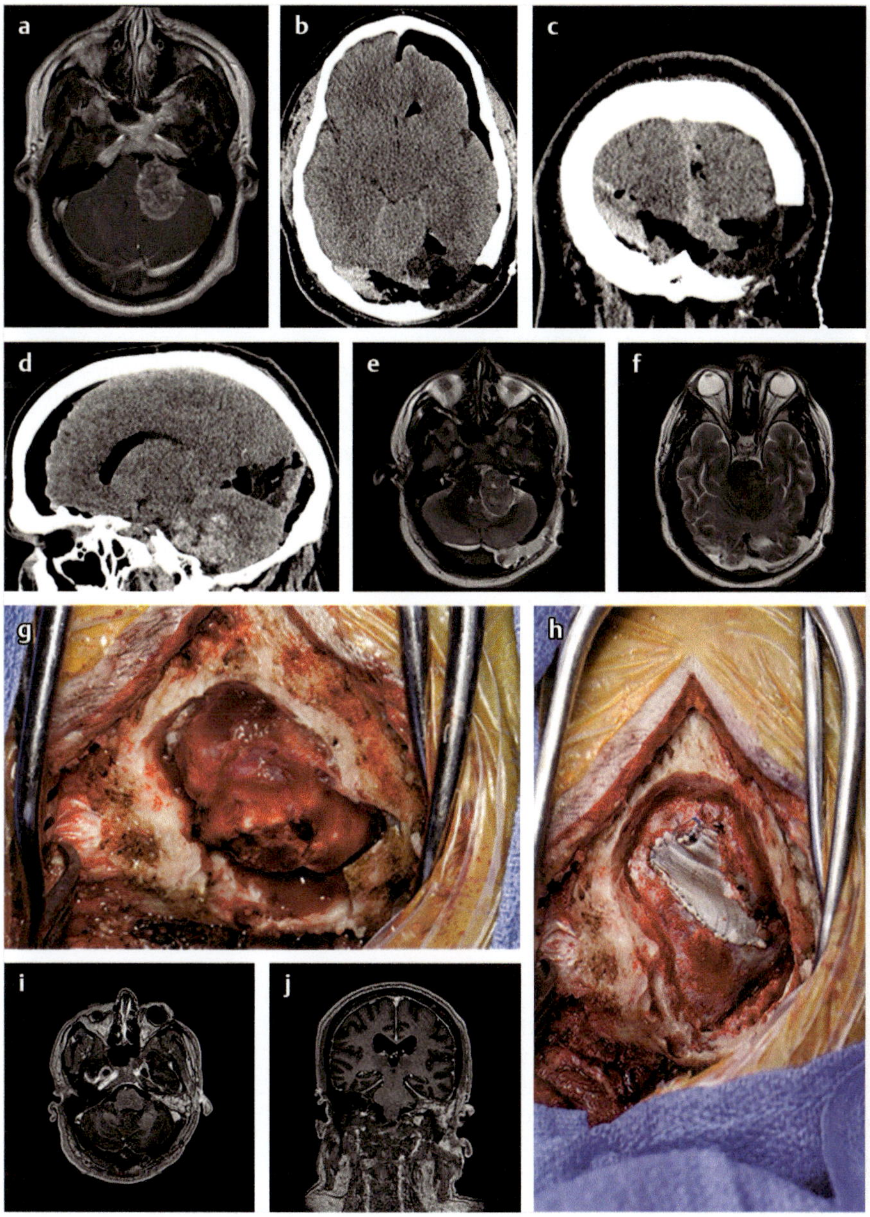

Fig. 43.2 Example 2, reoperation after complicated original surgery.

months confirmed GTR, with HB grade VI facial nerve function, and well-healed wounds; unfortunately, the patient regained no meaningful visual function, and had developed recurrent hallucinations, requiring psychotherapy and residence in a group home.

43.8 Conclusion

Repeat MS for truly recurrent or residual VS is technically demanding, due in large part to the extensive scarring frequently encountered along the full length of the FNTI, particularly if GTR was achieved at the initial operation. Although the clinical indications are infrequently encountered, repeat MS is an essential component of the VS treatment armamentarium, and may be of particular value in patients with large, macrocystic recurrences, patients with intractable trigeminal neuralgia and recurrent VS, or those who express a marked preference for surgical management. Repeat surgery after initial approach complications represents a special instance within the sphere of repeat MS, and should be tackled with trepidation, and only by highly qualified surgeons. In all circumstances, we recommend that surgical plans be tailored using an adaptive framework, with a general preference for alternate-approach surgery where appropriate—particularly following an approach complication—and consideration given to deliberate STR followed by upfront proactive SRS where GTR would clearly and permanently threaten favorable postoperative facial nerve function or risk other postoperative complications.

References

[1] Ahmad RA, Sivalingam S, Topsakal V, Russo A, Taibah A, Sanna M. Rate of recurrent vestibular schwannoma after total removal via different surgical approaches. Ann Otol Rhinol Laryngol. 2012; 121(3):156–161

[2] El-Kashlan HK, Zeitoun H, Arts HA, Hoff JT, Telian SA. Recurrence of acoustic neuroma after incomplete resection. Am J Otol. 2000; 21(3):389–392

[3] Freeman SR, Ramsden RT, Saeed SR, et al. Revision surgery for residual or recurrent vestibular schwannoma. Otol Neurotol. 2007; 28(8):1076–1082

[4] Hong B, Krauss JK, Bremer M, Karstens JH, Heissler HE, Nakamura M. Vestibular schwannoma microsurgery for recurrent tumors after radiation therapy or previous surgical resection. Otol Neurotol. 2014; 35(1):171–181

[5] Roberson JB, Jr, Brackmann DE, Hitselberger WE. Acoustic neuroma recurrence after suboccipital resection: management with translabyrinthine resection. Am J Otol. 1996; 17(2):307–311

[6] Samii M, Gerganov VM, Samii A. Functional outcome after complete surgical removal of giant vestibular schwannomas. J Neurosurg. 2010; 112(4):860–867

[7] Samii M, Metwali H, Gerganov V. Microsurgical management of vestibular schwannoma after failed previous surgery. J Neurosurg. 2016; 125(5):1198–1203

[8] Jacob JT, Carlson ML, Driscoll CL, Link MJ. Volumetric analysis of tumor control following subtotal and near-total resection of vestibular schwannoma. Laryngoscope. 2015

[9] Matthies C, Samii M. Management of 1000 vestibular schwannomas (acoustic neuromas): clinical presentation. Neurosurgery. 1997; 40(1):1–9, discussion 9–10

[10] Pollock BE, Lunsford LD, Flickinger JC, Clyde BL, Kondziolka D. Vestibular schwannoma management. Part I. Failed microsurgery and the role of delayed stereotactic radiosurgery. J Neurosurg. 1998; 89(6):944–948

[11] Roche PH, Khalil M, Thomassin JM. Microsurgical removal of vestibular schwannomas after failed previous microsurgery. Prog Neurol Surg. 2008; 21:158–162

[12] Shelton C. Unilateral acoustic tumors: how often do they recur after translabyrinthine removal? Laryngoscope. 1995; 105(9, Pt 1):958–966

[13] Chen Z, Prasad SC, Di Lella F, et al. The behavior of residual tumors and facial nerve outcomes after incomplete excision of vestibular schwannomas. J Neurosurg. 2014; 120(6):1278–1287

[14] Sakaki S, Nakagawa K, Hatakeyama T, Murakami Y, Ohue S, Matsuoka K. Recurrence after incompletely resected acusticus neurinomas. Med J Osaka Univ. 1991; 40(1–4):59–66

[15] Ramina R, Coelho Neto M, Bordignon KC, Mattei T, Clemente R, Pires Aguiar PH. Treatment of large and giant residual and recurrent vestibular schwannomas. Skull Base. 2007; 17(2):109–117

[16] Samii M, Gerganov V, Samii A. Improved preservation of hearing and facial nerve function in vestibular schwannoma surgery via the retrosigmoid approach in a series of 200 patients. J Neurosurg. 2006; 105(4): 527–535

[17] Samii M, Matthies C, Tatagiba M. Management of vestibular schwannomas (acoustic neuromas): auditory and facial nerve function after resection of 120 vestibular schwannomas in patients with neurofibromatosis 2. Neurosurgery. 1997; 40(4):696–705, discussion 705–706

44 Salvage Microsurgery After Radiation Treatment of Vestibular Schwannoma

Morten Lund-Johansen, Erling Myrseth, and Øystein V. Tveiten

44.1 Introduction

Surgeons regularly treating patients with vestibular schwannoma (VS) are familiar with cases where radiosurgery fails. Typically, persistent growth is noted on routine magnetic resonance imaging (MRI) examinations after radiosurgery, and the patient may present with increasing symptoms. Although the success rate of radiosurgery is high, it is not 100%—so with more than 80,000 cases of VS treated by Gamma Knife radiosurgery (GKRS), there are many cases in which surgery may be necessary with time.[1] The number of published cases on patients treated with microsurgery following radiation therapy is, however, low. This chapter aims at discussing what time point salvage surgery should be considered for patients who have undergone radiosurgery and what surgical challenges one may encounter, and finally it summarizes the present literature.

44.2 Volume Changes in Vestibular Schwannoma following Radiation

If a VS expands following radiation, the volume increase is usually succeeded by stagnation or regression later on. In 2008, Pollock reported on tumor volume changes in 208 VS patients who had undergone GKRS.[2] He found initial tumor enlargement in 31 (14%) of these, but only 2 cases underwent salvage surgery. In the remaining, expansion was followed by regression in 16, and cessation of growth in 8. In 2008, Nagano and coworkers reported that transient expansion was much more frequent, occurring in up to 75% of cases; a finding later confirmed by others.[3,4] It is now generally accepted that a volume increase following GKRS is a normal phenomenon for a period of up to 2 years and if well tolerated by the patient, it does not indicate the need for additional treatment. Further discussion regarding "pseudoprogression" following radiosurgery is detailed in Chapter 25.

44.3 Radiation-Induced Tissue Changes

Tissue fibrosis and damage to normal cells are consequences of radiotherapy.[5] It is generally acknowledged that whole brain irradiation affects cognition.[6] Cell death from radiation is caused by double-strand DNA damage leading to loss of mitotic activity. Most of the literature on radiation changes in nerve tissue deals with cell death, edema, and gliosis following fractionated therapy. However, typical doses delivered outside the target by stereotactic radiosurgery (SRS) are much lower and the body of literature on histopathological effects in normal tissue caused by a single SRS treatment is limited. As a rule of thumb, necrosis is seen in spot doses ≥ 18 Gy delivered by (single fraction) GKRS. The typical tumor margin dose in VS is 11 to 13 Gy at the 50% isodose line, yielding a maximum dose of 22 to 26 Gy to the tumor center. In the early days of radiosurgery, high tumor periphery doses led to cranial nerve and brainstem damage, but such adverse events are nowadays rare.[7] The histological appearance of postirradiated VS is reported by several authors: Lee et al, Iwai et al, and Hong et al did not see any histological changes attributable to radiation in their cases of postirradiated VS.[8,9,10] Pollock and coworkers on the other hand saw collagen and hemosiderin deposits and sclerotic vessels that they ascribed to radiation in most cases.[11] Understandably, histology specimens from the interphase between tumor and adjacent nervous structures may not be obtained. Still, it is possible that even low-dose single-fraction SRS may induce fibrosis, gliosis, and damage to normal cells and thus render irradiated patients more vulnerable than others if they need surgery later on. Many authors report that when operating on previously irradiated VS patients, they find unusual amounts of fibrous scarring causing adherence between the tumor and adjacent neural tissue.[12,13,14]

44.4 When Is Salvage Surgery Indicated?

In order to decide whether radiation for VS has been a success or a failure, the clinician has to review MRI findings and monitor for possible development of new clinical symptoms over a certain time frame. Some patients may experience an increase in symptomatology due to transient tumor expansion, but if tolerable this does not indicate the need for salvage treatment. In these cases, closer radiological and clinical follow-up, for instance, every 6 months instead of annually, may be necessary until stabilization. If the tumor continues to grow on several serial imaging intervals or starts growing after 2 years postradiation, this is likely to imply failed SRS (▶ Fig. 44.1).[15] If salvage treatment is decided upon, the first choice is usually surgery. Factors favoring surgery are young age, large tumor size, and symptom progression. In select cases, older patients and smaller tumors may be considered for reirradiation instead.[16,17,18,19,20]

44.5 Review of Literature

The main bulk of studies dealing with patient outcomes from postradiation VS surgery are presented in ▶ Table 44.1.[21,22,23] The results are not reported in a homogeneous way, and most publications contain few cases: neurofibromatosis type 2 and sporadic VS are frequently grouped together and in some cases, the criteria used to denote "previous radiosurgery" include patients who had microsurgery plus radiosurgery before final surgery.[11,12,19,24] Similarly, various radiation treatments, usually SRS and fractionated radiotherapy (FRT), are grouped together as "radiation" and dose plan details are often missing or

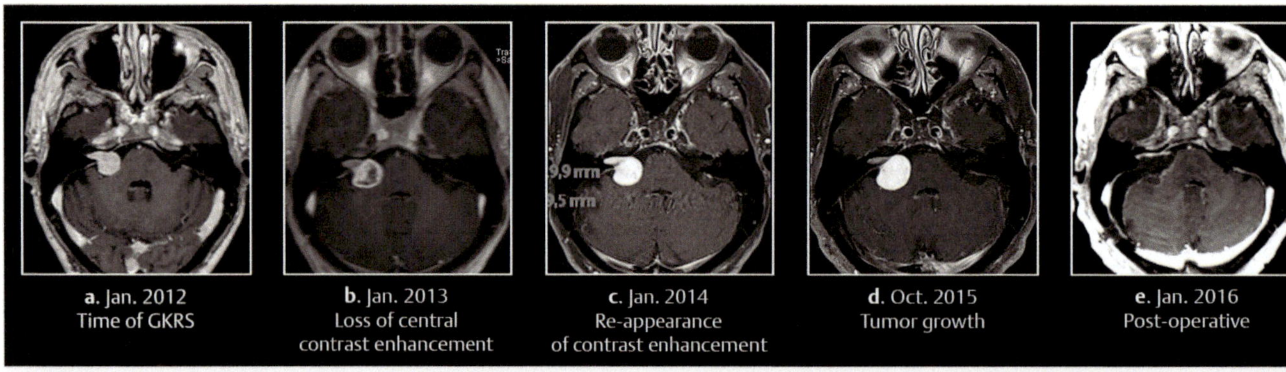

Fig. 44.1 (**a**) January 2012: A male patient, 56 years old, underwent Gamma Knife radiosurgery for growing vestibular schwannoma; 12 Gy was given to the tumor periphery. (**b**) January 2013: 1 year post-GKRS, showing loss of central contrast enhancement. (**c**) January 2014: Reappearance of central enhancement and slight volume increase. Patient is experiencing facial numbness. (**d**) October 2015: Growth of tumor is evident. Patient is scheduled for surgery. (**e**) January 2016: The patient underwent tumor resection via a suboccipital craniotomy. Images are from post-op day 2. A small remnant was left along the facial nerve due to adherence between facial nerve and tumor capsule. The facial nerve function was HB 2 at discharge and he experienced immediate improvement of facial sensation.

incomplete.[12,14,24,25] All are retrospective and there is an obvious risk of bias in the reporting on operative difficulties. Allegedly, in centers where SRS is advocated as the primary treatment of choice, the authors may be less prone to describe particular difficulties encountered when operating on tumors after radiation. Still, the majority of studies conclude that in irradiated cases, surgery is more difficult because of arachnoid scarring (▶ Table 44.1). Separating the tumor from the facial nerve (FN) is reported as being particularly difficult. Authors disagree on the importance of achieving gross total removal (GTR) in these cases, and FN outcomes vary.[14,24] Any increased risk of recurrence associated with subtotal removal (STR) versus GTR has not been established.

The five largest series on surgery for VS following single radiation treatment are as follows: two from the House Institute in Los Angeles; one from Hannover, Germany; one from the Gruppo Otologico in Italy; and a joint study between Bergen, Norway, and Rochester, MN.[12,14,24,25,26] These five studies comprising altogether 114 cases include matched control groups.[12,14,25,26,27] The studies by Limb et al and Wise et al describe dose plan details, but these data are incomplete or missing in the others. Patients treated by SRS and FRT are grouped together in all except the study from Hannover.[14] Friedman et al found severe arachnoid adherence in 89% of cases in the radiation group.[12] Although this was significantly higher than in the control group, as much as 63% of the control cases showed similar findings. FN outcomes were poorer in the irradiated series, but when the authors reviewed only those with normal preoperative House–Brackmann (HB) grade, FN function was not significantly different between groups.[14] Limb et al as well as Gerganov et al encountered extensive arachnoid scarring during surgery in all previously irradiated patients. Limb et al reported poorer "average" FN outcomes, whereas Gerganov et al found that FN function and complication rates were not significantly different between irradiated and nonirradiated cases. The proportion of control cases showing adherence is not reported in the latter. Several of the publications mentioned earlier report only patients undergoing gross total tumor removal, and conclude that surgery became more difficult than usual if the patient had undergone previous radiosurgery.[12,14,27] In their follow-up study, Friedman and colleagues were less aggressive in removing all tumors at the FN interface.[24] They showed that if aiming at a STR, the FN outcomes improved significantly (85.7% in STR group, 50% in GTR group). The patients were followed up for 1 year postsurgery and the authors reported that none had received any additional treatment at their institution. To avoid FN damage, STR was used in a significantly larger proportion of irradiated than control cases in the study by Wise and coworkers.[25] FN outcomes were similar in both groups following this strategy. In the study by Husseini et al, GTR was achieved in 13 out of 14, with good FN results, although more cases of facial paresis were found in the irradiated group. The remaining studies presented in ▶ Table 44.1 are without matched controls or contain less than 10 patients and are not reviewed further.

Surgeons operating on previously irradiated VS cases may have assumed a cause-and-effect relation between radiation and scarring, although it is only an association from a strictly scientific standpoint. It is established that conventional radiotherapy causes fibrosis.[5] A cause-and-effect relation between VS radiosurgery and adherences is thus likely, but adherences are common findings in large nonirradiated tumors as well. It must be remembered that radioresistance is uncommon in VS; only a few percentage of those undergoing radiosurgery need additional surgery. These tumors may be more difficult to operate on than others not only because they have been irradiated but also because they constitute a biologically separate group.

44.6 Conclusion

GKRS for VS fails in a small but significant proportion of cases. Due to transient expansion after radiation, one should wait for at least 2 years posttreatment before deciding on salvage therapy if this can be tolerated by the patient. When necessary, surgery has been the treatment of choice in most published series —albeit repeat GKRS may also be an option. Authors report more tumor adherence to surrounding structures and therefore

Table 44.1 Summary of literature describing salvage microsurgery after failed radiosurgical treatment of vestibular schwannoma

Author	*n*	Control group	Time to recurrence (mo)	Radiation dose, GK/CK[a] (*n*)	Radiation dose, fractionated (*n*)	GTR/STR	HB1–3/HB4–6	Authors' conclusion
Slattery and Brackmann (1995)	5	No	41 (8–120)	(3)	(2)	5/0	4/1	Difficult
Pollock et al (1998)	6	No	27 (7–72)	11–20 Gy, (6)	–	nr	nr	More difficult in some cases
Lee et al (2003)	4	No	19 (12–24)	13–14 Gy (2)	25–45 Gy (2)	nr	3/1	Difficult
Roche et al (2004)	20	No	36 (10–83)	nr (20)	–	14/6	17/3	–
Limb et al (2005)	9	Yes	nr	nr (3)	10 × 300c Gy (6)	3/6	nr	"Average" HB grade poorer in RS group
Friedman et al (2005)	38	Yes	40 (5–190)	13–20 Gy (13)	13–20 Gy, (7)[b]	30/8	13/17	Poorer FN in RT group
Pollock (2006)	5	No	9 (5–60)	12–14 Gy	12–14 Gy	2/3	3/2	Not reported
Iwai et al (2007)	6	No	28 (4–74)	11 Gy	–	0/6	4/2	Difficult
Shuto et al (2008)	8	No	29 (7–120)	12.3 Gy (8)	–	nr	4/4	Difficult
Liscak et al (2009)	2	No	29 (22–48)	12.5 Gy, 60% isodose	–	nr	0/2	Not reported
Lee, 2010	7	No	26 (3–72)	12.4 Gy, 60% isodose (7)	–	0/7	nr	Difficult
Yang, 2011	4	No	23 (4–50)	12 Gy (11–15), 50% isodose	–	nr		No more difficult
Friedman et al (2011)	73	No	41 (5–138)	12.8–20 Gy, mean 12.8 (18)[c]	16–61 Gy, mean 27.6 total dose (18)[b]	58/15	40/22	More difficult in RT group
Gerganov et al (2012)	15	Yes	30.7 (6–60)	nr (12)	nr (3)	15/0	10/4[b]	More difficult, similar HB outcomes
Husseini et al (2013)	15	Yes	34 (12–120)	nr (15)	nr	13/1	11/4	More difficult, "Average" HB grade poorer in RS group
Hong et al (2014)	5	No	10.5 (2–13)	nr (3)	nr (2)	3/2	4/nr	Difficult
Wise et al (2016)	37	Yes	36 (9–124)	12 Gy (12–14 Gy) (35)	(2)	28/9	27/10[b]	Lower proportion of GTR in RS group than in control, similar HB outcomes
	259		28 (4–190)					

Abbreviations: FN, facial nerve; GTR, gross total removal; HB, House–Brackmann; nr, not reported; RS, radiosurgery; RT, radiotherapy.
[a]Dose to periphery, unless specified.
[b]HB grade not different between groups.

more difficult surgery following previous GKRS, but FN outcomes and complication rates are in the same range as otherwise reported. The importance of obtaining total removal has not been documented yet, but STR yields better FN outcomes.

References

[1] Leksell Gamma Knife Society. Indications Treated 1968 to 2014, Accumulated Treatments by Region and Indication 2014. Available: https://www.lgksociety.com/library/annual-treatment-statistics/. Accessed February 8, 2016

[2] Pollock BE. Management of vestibular schwannomas that enlarge after stereotactic radiosurgery: treatment recommendations based on a 15 year experience. Neurosurgery. 2006; 58(2):241–248, discussion 241–248

[3] Nagano O, Higuchi Y, Serizawa T, et al. Transient expansion of vestibular schwannoma following stereotactic radiosurgery. J Neurosurg. 2008; 109(5): 811–816

[4] Varughese JK, Wentzel-Larsen T, Pedersen PH, Mahesparan R, Lund-Johansen M. Gamma Knife treatment of growing vestibular schwannoma in Norway: a prospective study. Int J Radiat Oncol Biol Phys. 2012; 84(2):e161–e166

[5] Stubblefield MD. Radiation fibrosis syndrome: neuromuscular and musculoskeletal complications in cancer survivors. PM R. 2011; 3(11): 1041–1054

[6] Balentova S, Adamkov M. Molecular, cellular and functional effects of radiation-induced brain injury: a review. Int J Mol Sci. 2015; 16(11): 27796–27815
[7] Foote KD, Friedman WA, Buatti JM, Meeks SL, Bova FJ, Kubilis PS. Analysis of risk factors associated with radiosurgery for vestibular schwannoma. J Neurosurg. 2001; 95(3):440–449
[8] Lee DJ, Westra WH, Staecker H, Long D, Niparko JK, Slattery WH, III. Clinical and histopathologic features of recurrent vestibular schwannoma (acoustic neuroma) after stereotactic radiosurgery. Otol Neurotol. 2003; 24(4):650–660, discussion 660
[9] Iwai Y, Yamanaka K, Yamagata K, Yasui T. Surgery after radiosurgery for acoustic neuromas: surgical strategy and histological findings. Neurosurgery. 2007; 60(2) Suppl 1:ONS75–ONS82, discussion ONS82
[10] Hong B, Krauss JK, Bremer M, Karstens JH, Heissler HE, Nakamura M. Vestibular schwannoma microsurgery for recurrent tumors after radiation therapy or previous surgical resection. Otol Neurotol. 2014; 35(1):171–181
[11] Pollock BE, Lunsford LD, Kondziolka D, et al. Vestibular schwannoma management. Part II. Failed radiosurgery and the role of delayed microsurgery. J Neurosurg. 1998; 89(6):949–955
[12] Friedman RA, Brackmann DE, Hitselberger WE, Schwartz MS, Iqbal Z, Berliner KI. Surgical salvage after failed irradiation for vestibular schwannoma. Laryngoscope. 2005; 115(10):1827–1832
[13] Shuto T, Inomori S, Matsunaga S, Fujino H. Microsurgery for vestibular schwannoma after Gamma Knife radiosurgery. Acta Neurochir (Wien). 2008; 150(3):229–234, discussion 234
[14] Gerganov VM, Giordano M, Samii A, Samii M. Surgical treatment of patients with vestibular schwannomas after failed previous radiosurgery. J Neurosurg. 2012; 116(4):713–720
[15] Mindermann T, Schlegel I. How to distinguish tumor growth from transient expansion of vestibular schwannomas following Gamma Knife radiosurgery. Acta Neurochir (Wien). 2014; 156(6):1121–1123
[16] Yomo S, Arkha Y, Delsanti C, Roche PH, Thomassin JM, Régis J. Repeat Gamma Knife surgery for regrowth of vestibular schwannomas. Neurosurgery. 2009; 64(1):48–54, discussion 54–55
[17] Lonneville S, Delbrouck C, Renier C, Devriendt D, Massager N. Repeat Gamma Knife surgery for vestibular schwannomas. Surg Neurol Int. 2015; 6:153
[18] Kano H, Kondziolka D, Niranjan A, Flannery TJ, Flickinger JC, Lunsford LD. Repeat stereotactic radiosurgery for acoustic neuromas. Int J Radiat Oncol Biol Phys. 2010; 76(2):520–527
[19] Liscak R, Vladyka V, Urgosik D, Simonova G, Vymazal J. Repeated treatment of vestibular schwannomas after Gamma Knife radiosurgery. Acta Neurochir (Wien). 2009; 151(4):317–324, discussion 324
[20] Dewan S, Norén G. Retreatment of vestibular schwannomas with Gamma Knife surgery. J Neurosurg. 2008; 109 Suppl:144–148
[21] Roche PH, Régis J, Devèze A, Delsanti C, Thomassin JM, Pellet W. [Surgical removal of unilateral vestibular schwannomas after failed Gamma Knife radiosurgery]. Neurochirurgie. 2004; 50(2–3, Pt 2):383–393
[22] Slattery WH, III, Brackmann DE. Results of surgery following stereotactic irradiation for acoustic neuromas. Am J Otol. 1995; 16(3):315–319, discussion 319–321
[23] Yang HC, Kano H, Awan NR, et al. Gamma Knife radiosurgery for larger-volume vestibular schwannomas. Clinical article. J Neurosurg. 2011; 114(3):801–807
[24] Friedman RA, Berliner KI, Bassim M, et al. A paradigm shift in salvage surgery for radiated vestibular schwannoma. Otol Neurotol. 2011; 32(8):1322–1328
[25] Wise SC, Carlson ML, Tveiten ØV, et al. Surgical salvage of recurrent vestibular schwannoma following prior stereotactic radiosurgery. Laryngoscope. 2016; 126(11):2580–2586
[26] Husseini ST, Piccirillo E, Taibah A, Almutair T, Sequino G, Sanna M. Salvage surgery of vestibular schwannoma after failed radiotherapy: the Gruppo Otologico experience and review of the literature. Am J Otolaryngol. 2013; 34 (2):107–114
[27] Limb CJ, Long DM, Niparko JK. Acoustic neuromas after failed radiation therapy: challenges of surgical salvage. Laryngoscope. 2005; 115(1):93–98

45 Avoidance and Management of Vascular Complications During Vestibular Schwannoma Surgery

Jacob B. Hunter, George B. Wanna, and David S. Haynes

45.1 Introduction

The risks of hearing loss and facial nerve injury associated with microsurgical resection of vestibular schwannomas (VSs) have been extensively studied; yet, neurovascular complications that can arise and lead to devastating consequences have received little attention by comparison. Intracranial vascular injury remains an uncommon, yet gravely feared complication of VS surgery. Vascular complications including arterial or venous stroke, intraoperative hemorrhage, hematoma formation, and venous thrombosis can result in significant perioperative morbidity and mortality.

Vascular complications associated with microsurgical resection of VS are uncommon and have been reported in up to 7 to 10.1% of patients.[1,2] Mahboubi et al reviewed 6,553 VS resections, reporting a 2.1% risk for requiring a blood transfusion, 0.8% risk of stroke, 0.7% risk of cerebral edema, and 0.6% risk of intracranial hemorrhage.[3] Betka et al reported hemorrhages occurred in 5% of 317 consecutive patients undergoing microsurgery—with cerebellopontine angle (CPA) hematomas reported in 8 (2.5%) patients and intracerebellar hematomas in 4 (1.3%) patients, all of which were managed with immediate reoperation.[4] In 2001, Slattery et al reported that 0.9% (15/1,687) of patients developed intracranial hemorrhage postoperatively, with 6 occurring within 24 hours of surgery.[5] Interestingly, at the time of revision surgery, the origin of bleeding was not identified in most cases. In 1994, Briggs et al reviewed 167 VSs greater than 4 cm that underwent translabyrinthine (TL) resection and reported a vascular complication rate of 4.8%; four patients demonstrated brainstem or cerebellar infarcts, three required exploration for evacuation of intracranial hematoma, and one had a cerebellar hematoma.[6]

To date, studies have not demonstrated differences in vascular complication rates when comparing surgical approaches. Sade et al compared the incidence of vascular complications in a total of 413 retrosigmoid and TL approaches for VS resection, noting that vascular complications occurred in 2.7% of patients, regardless of the approach.[1] Similarly, Ansari et al performed a systematic review, noting no significant differences in developing a major neurological complication, including stroke, seizure, and persistent cerebellar dysfunction, between the three most common microsurgical approaches to the CPA.[7]

45.2 Hemorrhage/Hematoma

Intraoperative and postoperative hemorrhage with hematoma formation is a rare, albeit potentially devastating, complication of VS microsurgery (▶ Fig. 45.1). The reported incidence of hemorrhage ranges from 0.8 to 2.4%,[5,8,9] with rates of 0.8% for both subdural and extradural hematomas.[10] Barker et al, utilizing data from the Nationwide Inpatient Sample hospital discharge database, representing about 20% of all inpatient admissions to nonfederal hospitals, noted that hematomas occurred in 1.1% of VS cases, while postoperative neurological complications, attributed to either infarction or hemorrhage, developed in 10.1% of all patients.[2] Springborg et al reviewed 1,244 patients within the Denmark centralized clinical database who underwent TL VS resection and reported a mortality rate of 0.96%.[11] Within this series, eight (0.64%) deaths were the result of postoperative hematomas, which prompted the authors to routinely obtain postoperative head CT scans to hopefully identify these complications early in the course of development.[11] In a review of approximately 1,600 VS cases from a single institution, Slattery et al described one patient who developed bleeding under the temporalis muscle following a middle fossa approach, medializing the bone flap and requiring surgical evacuation, and two other patients who developed postoperative bleeding 10 and 14 days following surgery. In the latter two cases, both were monitored and treated with steroids, with resolution in symptoms prior to discharge.[5]

To evaluate for any bleeding at the end of the procedure, Sanna et al performed at least 10 minutes of continuous suction irrigation, including a Valsalva maneuver, to identify occult bleeding and to help achieve hemostasis. In addition, they stress the importance of immediate extubation at the conclusion of the procedure when possible, since deterioration in mental status is one of the most reliable early clinical indicators

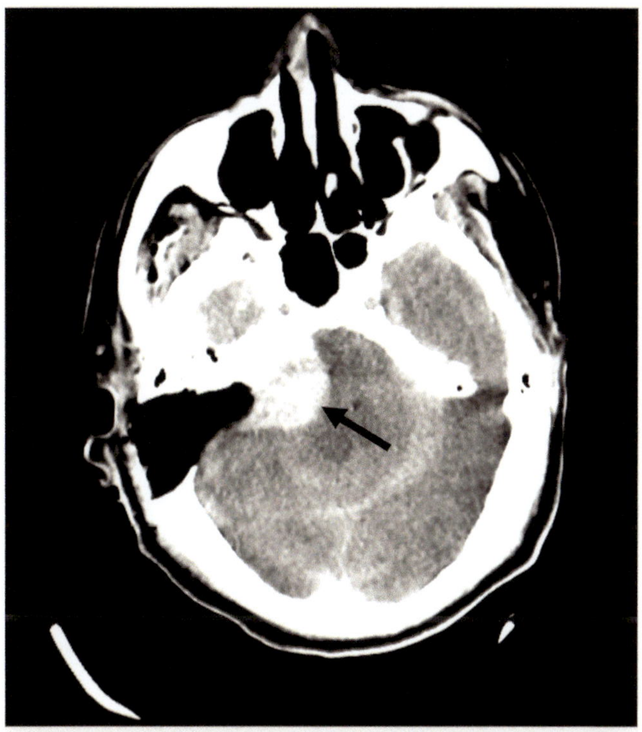

Fig. 45.1 Axial CT head with contrast obtained 8 hours following right translabyrinthine craniectomy for a VS with noted right cerebellopontine angle hematoma development.

of intracranial hematoma.[12] Several other publications have reported that postoperative intracranial hemorrhage is noted within the first 24 hours in only 33 to 40% of cases, requiring intervention in about half of all cases.[5,12,13] As for the presenting symptoms, Sade et al noted that all patients with hemorrhage presented with progressive signs of cerebellar dysfunction, cranial nerve deficits, headache, vomiting, and deterioration in their level of consciousness within 72 hours.[1]

In most cases, the likely explanation for early hematoma development is poor intraoperative hemostasis, where an arterial or more likely venous bleeding source was not adequately recognized or managed. If the source was arterial, rapid blood accumulation would most likely produce immediate clinical effects identifiable in the recovery room. Furthermore, arterial bleeding almost always requires surgical intervention, while venous bleeding will generally tamponade when the hematoma becomes large enough. Elevated blood pressure (BP) and increased intracranial pressure from coughing, emesis, or constipation is not uncommon after VS surgery and therefore meticulous hemostasis is mandatory. Less commonly, bleeding diathesis, pharmacologic anticoagulation, or antiplatelet therapy may contribute to perioperative hemorrhage.

While we are unaware of any studies evaluating the risk of venous thromboembolism (VTE) prophylaxis and hemorrhage in patients undergoing VS surgery, several studies have evaluated VTE prophylaxis in intracranial meningioma patients undergoing excision. Eisenring et al compared two regimens between 724 meningioma patients: cohort A included 5,000 international units (IUs) of low-molecular-weight heparin (LMWH) every 24 hours on the first postoperative day, while cohort B included intraoperative leg elevation to facilitate venous backflow, as well as unfractionated heparin on the day of surgery, replaced with 5,000 IU of LMWH on the first postoperative day.[14] While there were significantly more pulmonary embolisms in cohort A (8 vs. 2.5%), there were no significant differences in deep venous thrombosis, hemorrhage, or death.[14] Additional studies with meningioma patients have looked at the initiation of preoperative pharmacologic prophylaxis, as well as the addition of intraoperative hemodilution and the initiation of LMWH 12 hours postoperatively with mixed results.[15,16]

In regards to hypertension, defined as sustained BPs greater than or equal to 160/90, Basali et al reviewed 11,214 patients who underwent craniotomies at one institution, and noted that patients who had either intraoperative or postoperative hypertension within the first 12 hours were significantly more likely to develop an intracranial hemorrhage.[17] While rare, features intrinsic to the tumor itself may risk postoperative hemorrhage when subtotal resection is performed, including increased tumor vascularity, dilation and thinning of intratumoral vessels, or cystic tumors, with two known case reports of intratumoral hemorrhage following subtotal VS resections, which may have been the result of intrinsic tumor factors or inadequate hemostasis.[2,18,19,20] Lastly, one should always be aware of the risk with excessive cerebrospinal fluid (CSF) removal with lumbar drain placement in older patients with tenuous bridging subdural vessels. In such cases, a subdural bleed may occur even outside the surgical field of view and may carry grave consequences.

45.3 Petrosal Vein and Superior Petrosal Sinus Injuries

The transverse pontine vein and veins of the cerebellopontine fissure and middle cerebellar peduncle all join to form a superior petrosal vein, also known as Dandy's vein, which drains into the superior petrosal sinus, usually lateral to the trigeminal nerve.[21] There are a variety of reports on the number of petrosal veins present, ranging from 40 to 69.1% for a single vein, 27.3 to 60% for two or more veins, with some even reporting the absence of a petrosal vein.[22,23] With significant debate within the literature regarding the consequences of sacrificing the petrosal vein, Ebner et al conducted a cadaveric study after injection of the petrosal vein, finding that following petrosal vein occlusion, compensatory venous blood drainage is directed toward anastomotic supratentorial deep vein pathways.[21] Nonetheless, Sampath and colleagues routinely sacrifice the rostral bridging petrosal vein in larger size VS in order to reduce the risk of bleeding during surgery, and to allow easier retraction of the superior cerebellar hemisphere to aid in exposure of the tumor.[24]

While we are not aware of any VS articles discussing outcomes following petrosal vein sacrifice, other pathologies have several reported complications associated with petrosal vein occlusion, including hearing loss, cerebellar venous infarction, peduncular hallucinosis, cerebellar and brainstem edema, brainstem and cerebellar hemorrhage, hydrocephalus, and transient organic psychosyndrome (comparable to presenile dementia with a reduction in memory and intellect), and death.[4,21,22,23] Assessing the sectioning of the petrosal vein in petrous apex meningiomas, Koerbel et al retrospectively assessed cerebellar edema, ventriculomegaly, and/or cerebellar infarction following petrosal vein obliteration via video recordings in 57 cases, noting that in 30 cases, at least one vein was not preserved, with nine of those patients developing venous-related complications.[22] Interestingly, when compared to those patients in whom the petrosal vein complex was preserved, there were no significant differences in complications associated with venous congestion.[22] However, they found that those patients who developed complications following superior petrosal vein sectioning tended to have petrosal veins larger than 1.2 mm as compared to those patients whose veins were sectioned but did not develop complications.[22] Nonetheless, while some reports suggest complication rates as high as 30% in CPA surgery when the superior petrous vein is sacrificed, many surgeons, especially in VS resections, experience much lower complication rates.

Several groups have looked at the relationship between superior petrosal vein injury and hearing loss with conflicting results. Strauss et al noted postoperative hearing loss following injury to the superior petrosal vein during a microvascular decompression.[25,26] However, Gharabaghi et al found no differences in hearing preservation and hearing loss with petrosal vein sacrifice during petroclival meningioma resections, further reporting that the size of the vein had no significant impact.[23] They concluded that superior petrosal vein occlusion is not related to postoperative hearing loss, but its preservation should be attempted since other significant complications, such as venous congestion and hemorrhage, have been reported.[23]

It is routine in our institution to preserve the petrosal vein in CPA surgery when feasible, while avoiding any stretching that may lead to inadvertent tearing, avulsion, or thrombosis. The risk of inadvertent injury is greatest while using a cerebellar retractor, delivering the superior pole of the tumor, or drilling intracranially. Drilling should be avoided at all costs while pledgets or other loose hemostatic agents are present within the surgical field due to the significant damage that can occur if the drill was to capture the substrate while rotating at approximately 60,000 RPM. Small tears of the vein may be spot-welded on a low bipolar setting or effectively managed with Gelfoam or Floseal (Baxter, Hayward, CA), while larger tears may require vein sacrifice.

45.4 Dural Sinus Thrombosis and Vein of Labbé

Another venous complication associated with lateral skull base surgery is the development of dural or lateral sinus thrombosis, with a reported incidence rate between 0.1 and 4.7% (▶ Fig. 45.2 and ▶ Fig. 45.3).[5,10,27,28,29,30] While lateral sinus thrombosis may develop without clinical signs or subjective complaints, dural venous thrombosis may cause increased intracranial pressure, retinal hemorrhage, papilledema, headache, visual loss, dizziness, brain edema, and mental status changes, particularly when involving a dominant venous outflow system.[5,29,31]

De Bruijn et al prospectively studied prognostic factors in patients with cerebral venous sinus thrombosis, noting that patient age older than 33 years, involvement of the straight sinus, papilledema, diagnostic delay greater than 10 days, impaired consciousness, coma, and intracerebral hemorrhage were all associated with poor outcomes, while a negative or empty delta sign on CT, where contrast outlines a triangular filling defect of the superior sagittal sinus, and isolated intracranial hypertension, were associated with good outcomes.[32]

Ohata et al reviewed 174 presigmoidal-transpetrosal approaches, identifying five cases of sigmoid sinus occlusion.[30] They documented that the sinus was injured in seven cases, five of which developed occlusions postoperatively.[30] However, it must be noted that the superior petrosal sinus was transected in all cases, followed by division of the tentorium.[30] In one patient, a large hemorrhage developed in the ipsilateral temporal lobe 4 hours following the procedure, which required immediate drainage, with the patient subsequently developing a large intracerebral hematoma in the contralateral frontoparietal region 1 week later.[30] Given the risks regarding dural sinus thrombosis, many authors have attempted to classify venous configurations of the torcular herophili,[33] transverse sinus,[34] sigmoid sinus,[35] as well as documenting if one transverse sinus is dominant as compared to the other.[36] Ohata et al commented that occlusion of the ipsilateral sigmoid sinus in cases of hypoplastic or atretic transverse sinuses can lead to vein of Labbé congestion.[30] The vein of Labbé, also known as the inferior anastomotic vein, arises from the midpoint of the Sylvian fissure and travels posteroinferiorly to enter the transverse sinus at least 7 mm posterior to the superior petrosal sinus, draining the lateral temporal lobe.[37] Injury or occlusion to the vein can lead to disturbances in memory, speech, and contralateral motor deficits.[37] It is most frequently at risk with prolonged temporal lobe retraction and during combined middle and posterior fossa approaches, with the tentoriotomy placing the vein at risk. Multiple methods have been described to avoid injury to the vein of Labbé, including working above and below the tentorium with two operative fields, transecting the sigmoid sinus and ligating the transverse sinus distally to the vein of Labbé, cutting the tentorium in a posteroanterior direction, among other techniques.[37]

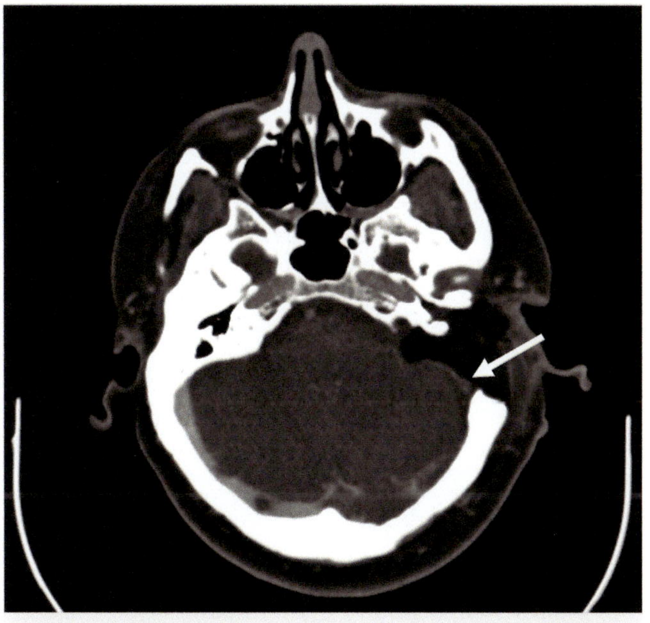

Fig. 45.2 Axial CT head with contrast demonstrates a left sigmoid and transverse sinus thrombosis (*white arrow*) following left translabyrinthine craniectomy for a VS.

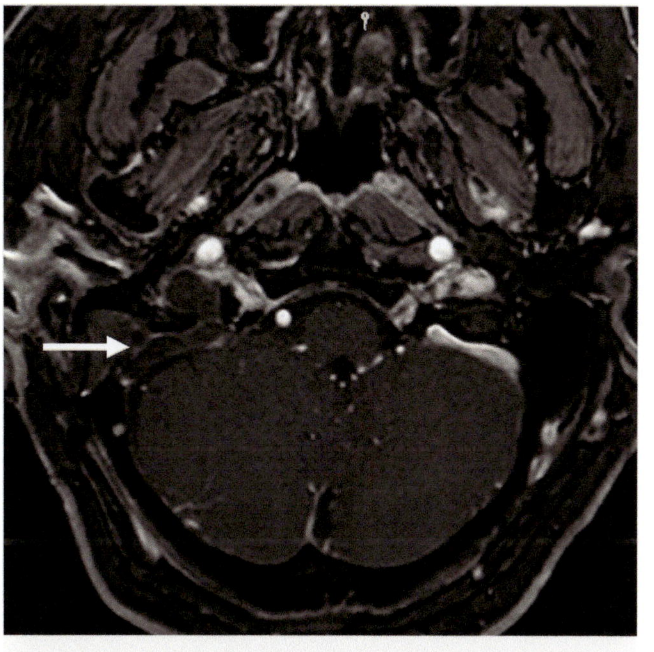

Fig. 45.3 Axial T1-weighted MRI with contrast, obtained on postoperative day 1 following a right translabyrinthine craniectomy for a VS, demonstrates right sigmoid sinus and jugular bulb thrombosis (*white arrow*).

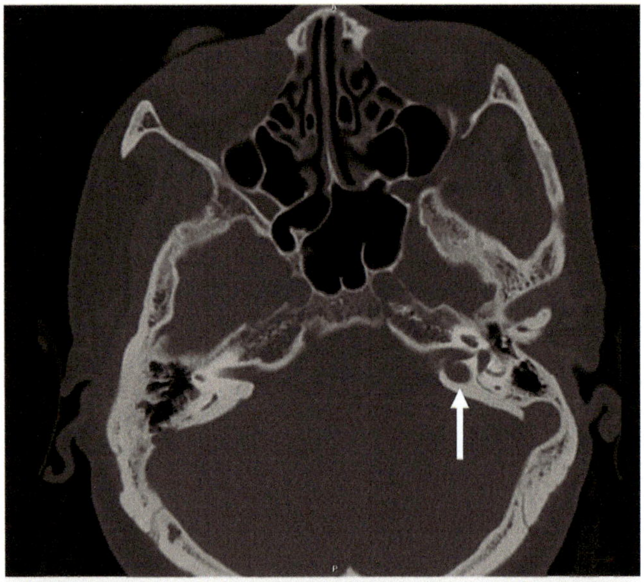

Fig. 45.4 Axial CT temporal bone without contrast demonstrates a high-riding left jugular bulb (*white arrow*) abutting the left internal auditory canal.

To avoid sinus thromboses, various authors have suggested maintaining adequate hydration during and after surgery, limiting the bony exposure to what is necessary to prevent desiccation, minimizing retraction against venous structures, and maintaining the integrity of a dominant sinus.[9,29] Preoperative sinus anatomy should be examined to determine the best approach. In some cases, for example, a very high jugular bulb or anterior sigmoid sinus may indicate that a retrosigmoid approach would be advantageous over a TL approach (▶ Fig. 45.4). If the sigmoid sinus is injured, bipolar cautery with irrigation may be used to spot-weld a small tear, or extraluminal collagen, gelatin sponge, or oxidized cellulose packing may be used to control bleeding from a small- or medium-sized venotomy without immediate occlusion.[30,38] In rare cases, a large sinus laceration may be amenable to suture repair, with or without a patch graft. Intraluminal packing or ligation should only be used as a last resort. Collagen and gelatin sponges work by providing mild mechanical compression via absorption of blood and fluids leading to swelling of the sponge, while oxidized cellulose reacts with blood to precipitate an artificial coagulum, covering the venous injury to provide hemostasis.

Though there are studies investigating a possible association between hemostatic agents and an increased risk of deep venous thromboses and pulmonary emboli in patients undergoing meningioma resections,[39] other large studies have reported no complications associated with gelatin-thrombin materials.[40] Thrombin, which is used in Floseal, and in association with collagen or gelatin sponges, assists with the clotting cascade by converting fibrinogen to fibrin, activating factor XIII which stabilizes clots, and inhibiting fibrinolysis. While rare, acquired factor V antibodies can develop, which can lead to life-threatening bleeding.[41] In our experience, sigmoid sinus injuries can almost always be controlled with a large piece of absorbable gelatin sponge covered by a cottonoid pledget with mild compression. The gelatin sponge should always be large enough to prevent inadvertent entry into the lumen of the vein and vascular system. Direct suturing is rarely needed, and extraluminal packing with ligation of the jugular vein in the neck is essentially never required.[38]

Further postoperative management options include steroids, anticoagulation, volume repletion, carbonic anhydrase inhibitors, direct endovascular thrombolysis, and surgical thrombectomy depending on patient condition and risk of clot propagation.[31] Other predisposing factors such as smoking, pregnancy, contraceptive use, or underlying coagulopathies (e.g., antiphospholipid syndrome, proteins C and S deficiency, lupus anticoagulant, or factor V Leiden mutation) should be investigated.

45.5 Venous Air Embolism

Injury to posterior fossa dural sinuses and diploic veins may lead to venous air embolism (VAE) in 1.6 to 50% of posterior fossa surgeries.[42] If large enough, VAEs are associated with the simultaneous onset of tachycardia, hypotension, and frequent premature ventricular contractions, leading to hemodynamic instability due to rapid entry or large volumes of air, putting strain on the right ventricle, increasing pulmonary arterial pressures, diminishing pulmonary venous return, decreasing left ventricular preload, and thus lowering the cardiac output.[43,44] Slbin et al evaluated the incidence of VAE by using a Doppler transducer in 180 posterior fossa procedures.[43] While a VAE was suspected on 61 occasions, it was confirmed only in 46, and only 2 of those patients developed clinical signs, both of who had the two largest volumes of aspirated air (50 mL).[43] Duke et al analyzed the incidence of VAE in sitting position as compared to supine positioned patients, noting that sitting patients experienced VAE significantly more frequently than supine patients, 28 to 5%, respectively.[45] However, Himes and colleagues reviewed 1,792 neurosurgical procedures that were performed in the sitting position and found the incidence rate of VAE was 1.06%, leading them to conclude that with modern anesthetic techniques, the sitting position provides a safe means of surgical access.[46] Comparing positions, Spektor et al reported on 130 VS patients, or 243 total neurosurgical patients, who were operated in the sitting or lateral positions, and found there were no significant differences in VAE between all patients (6.5% in the sitting position and 4.4% in the lateral position).[47] While the systemic treatment of VAE is beyond the scope of this chapter, prevention rests on the shoulders of the surgeon in collaboration with the neuroanesthesiologist. The appropriate monitoring and treatment for VAE is emphasized in Chapter 26. When a large sinus injury is identified, the site should be covered immediately with a wet gauze, bone wax, or Gelfoam. Prolonged suctioning and the reverse Trendelenburg position improve visualization, but increase the risk of VAE and should therefore be minimized if a major VAE occurs.[42]

45.6 Dural Arteriovenous Fistula

When dural venous thrombosis or stenosis occurs, venous hypertension can develop with retrograde flow leading to opening of capillaries and subsequent development of dural arteriovenous fistulas (DAVF) in very rare circumstances.[48,49]

While DAVF can occur anywhere, they exhibit a unique predilection for the transverse-sigmoid sinus junction. While many fistulas may be asymptomatic, patients can present with ipsilateral eye proptosis and conjunctival injection, tinnitus, headache, seizures, increased intracranial pressure, focal neurological deficits, dementia, strokes, and hemorrhage depending on the venous drainage from the fistula.[48,49] DAVF are diagnosed with digital subtraction angiography and may be managed with observation, surgical disconnection, endovascular embolization, or stereotactic radiosurgery.[48,49]

Several case reports exist regarding the development of DAVFs several years following TL VS resections.[48,49] Ushewokunze et al reported a case of DAVF following TL VS resection 2 years previously, in a patient who presented with eye proptosis and conjunctival injection.[49] Similarly, Li et al presented two cases of DAVF presenting 2 years following TL craniectomies.[48]

45.7 Anterior Inferior Cerebellar Artery/Posterior Inferior Cerebellar Artery Infarction

The anterior inferior cerebellar artery (AICA; ▶ Fig. 45.5) is usually the first large branch off the basilar artery, dividing into a rostral and caudal trunk. The rostral branch is typically larger and courses below the facial and vestibulocochlear nerves, eventually looping superiorly to the flocculus, supplying the lateral middle cerebellar peduncle and cerebellum. The caudal branch courses inferiorly to supply the lower cerebellum and portions of the middle peduncles. The subarcuate, labyrinthine, and recurrent perforating branches all arise from the AICA. Two other important arteries include the posterior inferior cerebellar artery (PICA), which arises from the vertebral artery, passing between the hypoglossal rootlets, as well as the vagus and accessory nerves, and the superior cerebellar artery (SCA), which passes above the trigeminal nerve. Detailed neurovascular anatomy of the posterior fossa is further described in Chapter 30.

Full AICA distribution stroke, also known as the lateral pontomedullary syndrome, may result in hearing loss, vertigo, ataxia, nausea, and contralateral beating nystagmus. Patients can also experience ipsilateral facial weakness and or numbness, ipsilateral Horner's syndrome, and contralateral body paresthesias.[50] Nonetheless, many authors suggest that distal AICA infarcts (▶ Fig. 45.6) can be relatively benign due to a limited pontocerebellar infarction.[6,50] Graffeo and colleagues identified 4 cases of AICA infarct in a large retrospective review of 591 VSs, 3 of which were clinically asymptomatic.[51] In the same study, of 61 patients who met radiographic criteria for having a cerebrovascular complication, 93% were asymptomatic: 79% had findings involving the middle cerebellar peduncle on T2 MR imaging, 54% had new posterior fossa encephalomalacia, and 16% had multiple discrete areas of T2 MRI changes.

Recent reports suggest that cerebellar peduncle infarctions (▶ Fig. 45.7) occur between 0.2 and 2.1% of VS resections, with an incidence rate of 13% in large tumors.[5,50] Hegarty et al reviewed 12 patients who developed distal AICA syndrome following VS resection and observed that the most common symptom was dysmetria, which usually resolved over months, with gait ataxia improving in about half of patients.[50] However,

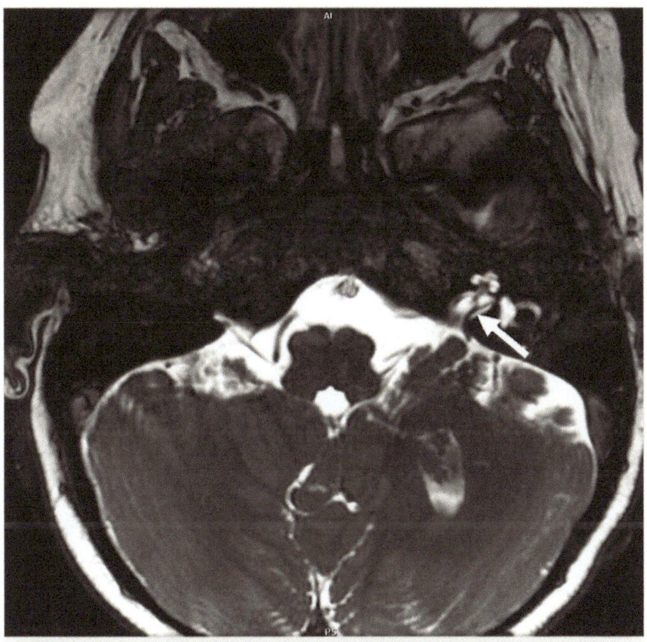

Fig. 45.5 Axial MRI FIESTA sequence, highlighting anterior inferior cerebellar artery loop (*white arrow*) entering the left internal auditory canal.

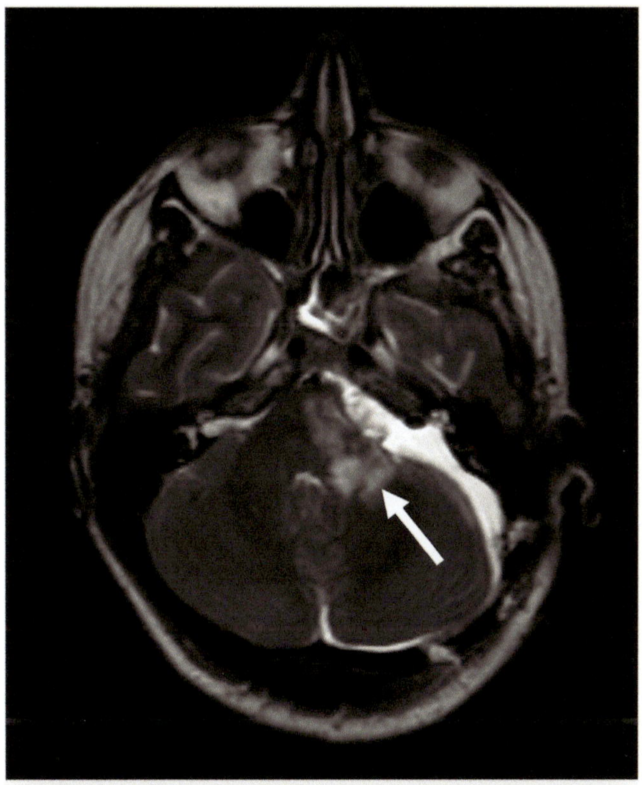

Fig. 45.6 Axial MRI brain FLAIR sequence obtained on postoperative day 1 following a retrosigmoid craniectomy for VS resection demonstrating edema within the left pons and middle cerebellar peduncle. Patient exhibited right hemiparesis, as well as left facial and vocal fold paresis.

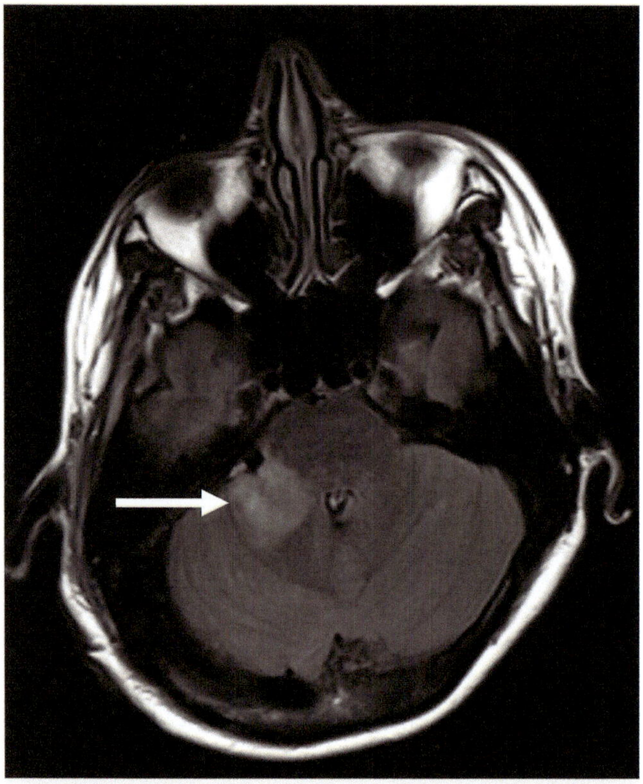

Fig. 45.7 Axial MRI brain FLAIR sequence demonstrating right middle cerebellar peduncle edema.

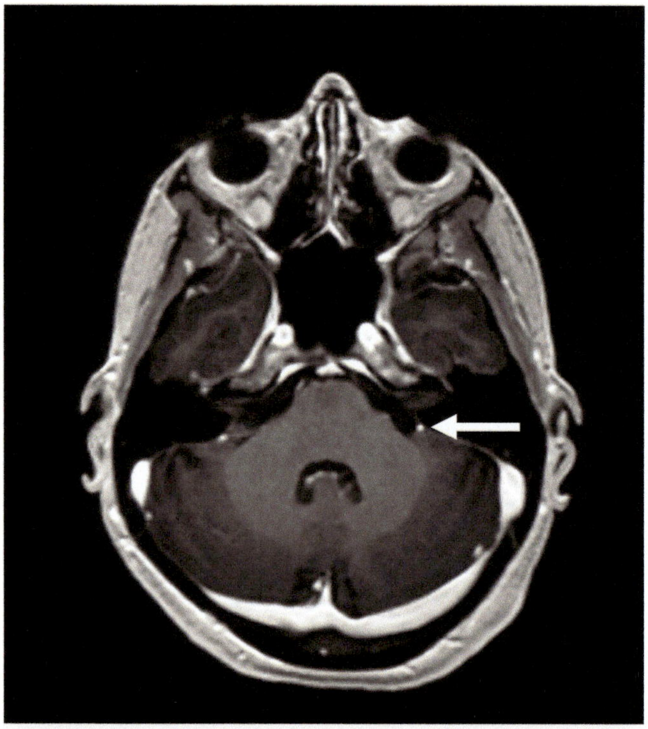

Fig. 45.8 Axial T1-weighted MRI with contrast, highlighting a branch of anterior inferior cerebellar artery (*white arrow*) adherent, or in close proximity to the posterior fossa dura.

other morbidities can coexist, including dysarthria and ataxia, which the authors attribute to flocculonodular lesions, while dysmetria, tremor, motor weakness, and dysdiadochokinesia all localize to cerebellar neocortex lesions and all of which may also be the result of distal AICA branch injuries.[50] MRI findings document an ischemic parenchymal lesion of the superior and middle cerebellar peduncles, extending from the lateral wall of the fourth ventricle to the lateral pial surface.[50] Though historically many surgeons routinely resected the lateral one-third of the cerebellum with large tumors with minimal consequences, the lack of associated comorbidity in these cases is thought to be secondary to preservation of the cerebellar peduncles.[50]

Preventive measures to avoid arterial vascular injury include meticulous hemostasis and careful microsurgical dissection of the tumor capsule, preserving all adherent arterial brainstem perforators and only coagulating those vessels directly feeding the tumor.[50,52] Internal debulking of the tumor with an ultrasonic aspirator or microdebrider must be performed with care to avoid inadvertently passing through the anterior tumor capsule. In rare cases, a branch of AICA may penetrate the subarcuate fossa or adhere to the posterior fossa dura (▶ Fig. 45.8); thus, great care must be undertaken when opening the posterior fossa dura or drilling the posterior petrous bone.[53,54]

45.8 Conclusion

Intracranial vascular injury remains an uncommon, yet feared, complication of VS surgery. Meticulous hemostasis and careful microsurgical dissection are paramount to avoid arterial and venous injury. Though injury is rare, all surgeons should retain intimate knowledge on immediate and long-term management of these injuries.

References

[1] Sade B, Mohr G, Dufour JJ. Vascular complications of vestibular schwannoma surgery: a comparison of the suboccipital retrosigmoid and translabyrinthine approaches. J Neurosurg. 2006; 105(2):200–204

[2] Barker FG, II, Carter BS, Ojemann RG, Jyung RW, Poe DS, McKenna MJ. Surgical excision of acoustic neuroma: patient outcome and provider caseload. Laryngoscope. 2003; 113(8):1332–1343

[3] Mahboubi H, Ahmed OH, Yau AY, Ahmed YC, Djalilian HR. Complications of surgery for sporadic vestibular schwannoma. Otolaryngol Head Neck Surg. 2014; 150(2):275–281

[4] Betka J, Zvěřina E, Balogová Z, et al. Complications of microsurgery of vestibular schwannoma. BioMed Res Int. 2014; 2014:315952

[5] Slattery WH, III, Francis S, House KC. Perioperative morbidity of acoustic neuroma surgery. Otol Neurotol. 2001; 22(6):895–902

[6] Briggs RJ, Luxford WM, Atkins JS, Jr, Hitselberger WE. Translabyrinthine removal of large acoustic neuromas. Neurosurgery. 1994; 34(5):785–790, discussion 790–791

[7] Ansari SF, Terry C, Cohen-Gadol AA. Surgery for vestibular schwannomas: a systematic review of complications by approach. Neurosurg Focus. 2012; 33 (3):E14

[8] Sluyter S, Graamans K, Tulleken CA, Van Veelen CW. Analysis of the results obtained in 120 patients with large acoustic neuromas surgically treated via the translabyrinthine-transtentorial approach. J Neurosurg. 2001; 94(1):61–66

[9] Roche PH, Ribeiro T, Fournier HD, Thomassin JM. Vestibular schwannomas: complications of microsurgery. Prog Neurol Surg. 2008; 21:214–221

[10] Charpiot A, Tringali S, Zaouche S, Ferber-Viart C, Dubreuil C. Perioperative complications after translabyrinthine removal of large or giant vestibular schwannoma: Outcomes for 123 patients. Acta Otolaryngol. 2010; 130(11): 1249–1255

[11] Springborg JB, Fugleholm K, Poulsgaard L, Cayé-Thomasen P, Thomsen J, Stangerup SE. Outcome after translabyrinthine surgery for vestibular schwannomas: report on 1244 patients. J Neurol Surg B Skull Base. 2012; 73 (3):168–174

[12] Sanna M, Taibah A, Russo A, Falcioni M, Agarwal M. Perioperative complications in acoustic neuroma (vestibular schwannoma) surgery. Otol Neurotol. 2004; 25(3):379–386

[13] Samii M, Matthies C. Management of 1000 vestibular schwannomas (acoustic neuromas): surgical management and results with an emphasis on complications and how to avoid them. Neurosurgery. 1997; 40(1):11–21, discussion 21–23

[14] Eisenring CV, Neidert MC, Sabanés Bové D, Held L, Sarnthein J, Krayenbühl N. Reduction of thromboembolic events in meningioma surgery: a cohort study of 724 consecutive patients. PLoS One. 2013; 8(11):e79170

[15] Sjåvik K, Bartek J, Jr, Solheim O, et al. Venous thromboembolism prophylaxis in meningioma surgery: a population-based comparative effectiveness study of routine mechanical prophylaxis with or without preoperative low-molecular-weight heparin. World Neurosurg. 2016; 88:320–326

[16] Moussa WM, Mohamed MA. Prophylactic use of anticoagulation and hemodilution for the prevention of venous thromboembolic events following meningioma surgery. Clin Neurol Neurosurg. 2016; 144:1–6

[17] Basali A, Mascha EJ, Kalfas I, Schubert A. Relation between perioperative hypertension and intracranial hemorrhage after craniotomy. Anesthesiology. 2000; 93(1):48–54

[18] Carlson ML, Tombers NM, Driscoll CL, et al. Clinically significant intratumoral hemorrhage in patients with vestibular schwannoma. Laryngoscope. 2016

[19] Misra BK, Rout D, Bhiladvala DB, Radhakrishnan V. Spontaneous haemorrhage in acoustic neurinomas. Br J Neurosurg. 1995; 9(2):219–221

[20] Chee CP, Bailey IC, Refsum SE. Spontaneous massive haemorrhage into acoustic neuroma during anticoagulation therapy. Br J Neurosurg. 1987; 1(4):489–493

[21] Ebner FH, Roser F, Shiozawa T, et al. Petrosal vein occlusion in cerebellopontine angle tumour surgery: an anatomical study of alternative draining pathways. Eur J Surg Oncol. 2009; 35(5):552–556

[22] Koerbel A, Gharabaghi A, Safavi-Abbasi S, et al. Venous complications following petrosal vein sectioning in surgery of petrous apex meningiomas. Eur J Surg Oncol. 2009; 35(7):773–779

[23] Gharabaghi A, Koerbel A, Löwenheim H, Kaminsky J, Samii M, Tatagiba M. The impact of petrosal vein preservation on postoperative auditory function in surgery of petrous apex meningiomas. Neurosurgery. 2006; 59(1) Suppl 1: ONS68–ONS74, discussion ONS68–ONS74

[24] Sampath P, Rini D, Long DM. Microanatomical variations in the cerebellopontine angle associated with vestibular schwannomas (acoustic neuromas): a retrospective study of 1006 consecutive cases. J Neurosurg. 2000; 92(1):70–78

[25] Strauss C, Naraghi R, Bischoff B, Huk WJ, Romstöck J. Contralateral hearing loss as an effect of venous congestion at the ipsilateral inferior colliculus after microvascular decompression: report of a case. J Neurol Neurosurg Psychiatry. 2000; 69(5):679–682

[26] Strauss C, Neu M, Bischoff B, Romstöck J. Clinical and neurophysiological observations after superior petrosal vein obstruction during surgery of the cerebellopontine angle: case report. Neurosurgery. 2001; 48(5):1157–1159, discussion 1159–1161

[27] Hadeishi H, Yasui N, Suzuki A. Mastoid canal and migrated bone wax in the sigmoid sinus: technical report. Neurosurgery. 1995; 36(6):1220–1223, discussion 1223–1224

[28] Crocker M, Nesbitt A, Rich P, Bell B. Symptomatic venous sinus thrombosis following bone wax application to emissary veins. Br J Neurosurg. 2008; 22 (6):798–800

[29] Keiper GL, Jr, Sherman JD, Tomsick TA, Tew JM, Jr. Dural sinus thrombosis and pseudotumor cerebri: unexpected complications of suboccipital craniotomy and translabyrinthine craniectomy. J Neurosurg. 1999; 91(2):192–197

[30] Ohata K, Haque M, Morino M, et al. Occlusion of the sigmoid sinus after surgery via the presigmoidal-transpetrosal approach. J Neurosurg. 1998; 89(4): 575–584

[31] Heman-Ackah SE, Golfinos JG, Roland JT, Jr. Management of surgical complications and failures in acoustic neuroma surgery. Otolaryngol Clin North Am. 2012; 45(2):455–470, x

[32] de Bruijn SF, de Haan RJ, Stam J, For the Cerebral Venous Sinus Thrombosis Study Group. Clinical features and prognostic factors of cerebral venous sinus thrombosis in a prospective series of 59 patients. J Neurol Neurosurg Psychiatry. 2001; 70(1):105–108

[33] Ishizaka H. [Anatomical study of the torcular Herophili]. Neurol Med Chir (Tokyo). 1985; 25(11):873–880

[34] Zouaoui A, Hidden G. Cerebral venous sinuses: anatomical variants or thrombosis? Acta Anat (Basel). 1988; 133(4):318–324

[35] Ichijo H, Hosokawa M, Shinkawa H. Differences in size and shape between the right and left sigmoid sinuses. Eur Arch Otorhinolaryngol. 1993; 250(5): 297–299

[36] Browning H. The confluence of dural venous sinuses. Am J Anat. 1953; 93(3): 307–329

[37] Lustig LR, Jackler RK. The vulnerability of the vein of Labbé during combined craniotomies of the middle and posterior fossae. Skull Base Surg. 1998; 8(1): 1–9

[38] Arriaga MA, Lin J. Translabyrinthine approach: indications, techniques, and results. Otolaryngol Clin North Am. 2012; 45(2):399–415, ix

[39] Safaee M, Sun MZ, Oh T, et al. Use of thrombin-based hemostatic matrix during meningioma resection: a potential risk factor for perioperative thromboembolic events. Clin Neurol Neurosurg. 2014; 119:116–120

[40] Fiss I, Danne M, Stendel R. Use of gelatin-thrombin matrix hemostatic sealant in cranial neurosurgery. Neurol Med Chir (Tokyo). 2007; 47(10):462–467

[41] Yao HH, Hong MK, Drummond KJ. Haemostasis in neurosurgery: what is the evidence for gelatin-thrombin matrix sealant? J Clin Neurosci. 2013; 20(3): 349–356

[42] Gracia I, Fabregas N. Craniotomy in sitting position: anesthesiology management. Curr Opin Anaesthesiol. 2014; 27(5):474–483

[43] Slbin MS, Babinski M, Maroon JC, Jannetta PJ. Anesthetic management of posterior fossa surgery in the sitting position. Acta Anaesthesiol Scand. 1976; 20(2):117–128

[44] Muth CM, Shank ES. Gas embolism. N Engl J Med. 2000; 342(7):476–482

[45] Duke DA, Lynch JJ, Harner SG, Faust RJ, Ebersold MJ. Venous air embolism in sitting and supine patients undergoing vestibular schwannoma resection. Neurosurgery. 1998; 42(6):1282–1286, discussion 1286–1287

[46] Himes BT, Mallory GW, Abcejo AS, et al. Contemporary analysis of the intraoperative and perioperative complications of neurosurgical procedures performed in the sitting position. J Neurosurg. 2017; 127:182–188

[47] Spektor S, Fraifeld S, Margolin E, Saseedharan S, Eimerl D, Umansky F. Comparison of outcomes following complex posterior fossa surgery performed in the sitting versus lateral position. J Clin Neurosci. 2015; 22(4):705–712

[48] Li PL, Mao Y, Zhu W, Zhao NQ, Zhao Y, Chen L. Surgical strategies for petroclival meningioma in 57 patients. Chin Med J (Engl). 2010; 123(20): 2865–2873

[49] Ushewokunze SO, Thomas A, Lamin S, Irving RM, Walsh AR. An unusual complication following translabyrinthine resection of an acoustic neuroma. Br J Neurosurg. 2011; 25(2):303–305

[50] Hegarty JL, Jackler RK, Rigby PL, Pitts LH, Cheung SW. Distal anterior inferior cerebellar artery syndrome after acoustic neuroma surgery. Otol Neurotol. 2002; 23(4):560–571

[51] Graffeo C, Perry A, Rayan T, et al. Cerebrovascular complications during vestibular schwannoma surgery. Skull Base. 2018; 79:A021

[52] Kunimoto Y, Lauda L, Falcioni M, Taibah A, Hasegawa K, Sanna M. Staged resection for vestibular schwannoma. Acta Otolaryngol. 2015; 135(9):895–900

[53] Tanriover N, Rhoton AL, Jr. The anteroinferior cerebellar artery embedded in the subarcuate fossa: a rare anomaly and its clinical significance. Neurosurgery. 2005; 57(2):314–319, discussion 314–319

[54] Warren DT, Warren MD, Malfair D, Akagami R. An incidence of anteroinferior cerebellar artery/posteroinferior cerebellar artery anatomic variants penetrating the subarcuate fossa dura: operative technique and identification with 3-dimensional fast imaging employing steady-state acquisition magnetic resonance imaging. Neurosurgery. 2010; 66(6) Suppl Operative:199–203, discussion 204

46 Perioperative Management of Hydrocephalus

Nickalus Khan, Jon Robertson, and L. Madison Michael III

46.1 Introduction

Hydrocephalus occasionally develops in patients with vestibular schwannomas (VS). Reports of the association between hydrocephalus and VS date back to the early 20th century. A historical piece by the Mayo Clinic in 1956 cited both Cushing's[1] and Dandy's[2] experience when treating VS.[3] They described a 44-year-old woman who had a VS resected via an intracapsular approach and underwent a prolonged treatment of over a year for communicating hydrocephalus. Bucy further added one of his cases into this seminal report of a 41 year-old-woman who developed hydrocephalus following a similar procedure.[3]

The incidence of hydrocephalus associated with VS has been reported to be between 3.7 and 13.7%.[4,5,6,7,8,9] There is a significant positive correlation of tumor size and hydrocephalus.[7] Some studies show that complete removal of the tumor can resolve hydrocephalus without requiring further modalities of cerebrospinal fluid (CSF) diversion,[4,7,8] while other studies[4,5] show that even with complete resection, hydrocephalus may still persist and warrant treatment.

To better understand this phenomenon, one must classify hydrocephalus in the setting of VS as either communicating or noncommunicating. If noncommunicating hydrocephalus exists —as in the case of large cerebellopontine angle tumors causing mass effect on the fourth ventricle—then complete removal of the tumor should cause resolution of the associated hydrocephalus. However, in the setting of small tumors with associated ventriculomegaly, the theory of mechanical compression of the CSF pathways fails to explain the etiology of the hydrocephalus.[5] There is evidence to suggest that schwannomas with an extracanalicular component may produce protein that is associated with communicating hydrocephalus.[5,10,11] This is further supported by documented reports of spinal schwannomas being associated with communicating hydrocephalus.[12,13,14,15] A study in 2003 by Tanaka et al found that the incidence of communicating hydrocephalus was higher in elderly patients.[16] The authors of this study hypothetically attributed the communicating hydrocephalus to slower tumor growth and increased CSF exposure to the tumor.[16] This hypothesis has been recently supported by a study in 2013 by Miyakoshi and colleagues that showed a significant association of elevated CSF protein and extended periods of tumor growth with concomitant hydrocephalus.[17] The focus of this chapter is on the preoperative, intraoperative, and postoperative management of hydrocephalus associated with VS.

46.2 Preoperative Management of Hydrocephalus

There are four possible clinical scenarios for patients with hydrocephalus secondary to VS: (1) asymptomatic communicating hydrocephalus, (2) symptomatic communicating hydrocephalus, (3) asymptomatic noncommunicating hydrocephalus, and (4) symptomatic noncommunicating hydrocephalus. Patients presenting with communicating hydrocephalus are typically older (> 60 years old) than those with obstructive hydrocephalus. Symptoms that can occur are those commonly found in normal pressure hydrocephalus, namely, cognitive impairment, urinary incontinence, and gait disturbance.

For patients with symptomatic communicating hydrocephalus, CSF shunting without tumor removal may be the optimal treatment (▶ Fig. 46.1). As these patients are older and often have significant comorbidities, shunting with a low-pressure or programmable valve may result in symptom resolution, obviating the need for tumor resection. Patients with communicating hydrocephalus—whether asymptomatic or symptomatic—who are deemed appropriate for surgery are not treated preoperatively with external CSF drainage. This approach is also taken with patients with asymptomatic noncommunicating hydrocephalus.

Patients who present with acute noncommunicating hydrocephalus and rapidly developing symptoms of elevated intracranial pressure (ICP) are treated with an external ventricular drain (EVD) or endoscopic third ventriculostomy (ETV) prior to surgery. These patients are taken to surgery after their

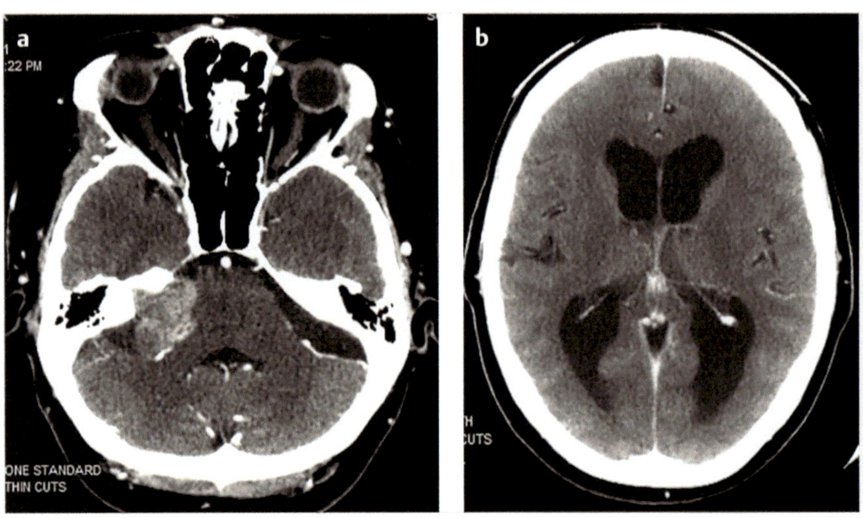

Fig. 46.1 (a) CT of the head with contrast reveals a moderate-size vestibular schwannoma without compression of the adjacent cerebrospinal fluid pathways. **(b)** Overt development of communicating hydrocephalus is demonstrated.

presenting symptoms resolve, usually within 1 to 2 days. In patients who cannot undergo surgery during the same hospital visit, and who fail an ETV, a permanent ventriculoperitoneal (VP) shunt is placed with plans for future surgical resection.

46.3 Intraoperative Management of Hydrocephalus

For patients with communicating hydrocephalus, the choice of approach is commonly dictated by the status of hearing and tumor size. With nonfunctional hearing, a translabyrinthine approach is preferred by the authors. A lumbar drain is placed prior to the incision and is opened prior to dural opening. Approximately 20 mL of CSF is removed, and the drain typically remains clamped throughout the remainder of the case. With functional hearing, a retrosigmoid approach is typically utilized. As with all approaches to the posterior fossa, it is essential to obtain relaxation of the cerebellum. This is accomplished by gaining access to the cerebellomedullary cistern. Immediately following opening of the dura, dissection should proceed toward the foramen magnum. The cerebellomedullary cistern is opened widely to allow sufficient drainage of CSF. It is maintained open to allow egress of CSF throughout the procedure. For patients with noncommunicating hydrocephalus, who typically have larger tumors (▶ Fig. 46.2), we favor the retrosigmoid approach. Historically, placement of a bur hole at Frazier's point (3–4 cm lateral to midline and 6 cm above inion) was uniformly performed prior to beginning the suboccipital exposure. In the face of cerebellar herniation, this allows emergent access to the ventricular system and promotes relaxation of the posterior fossa. We now perform this in selective cases. In a majority of cases, accessing the cerebellomedullary cistern prior to tumor exposure achieves relaxation of the cerebellum, such that removal of the tumor can be performed safely.

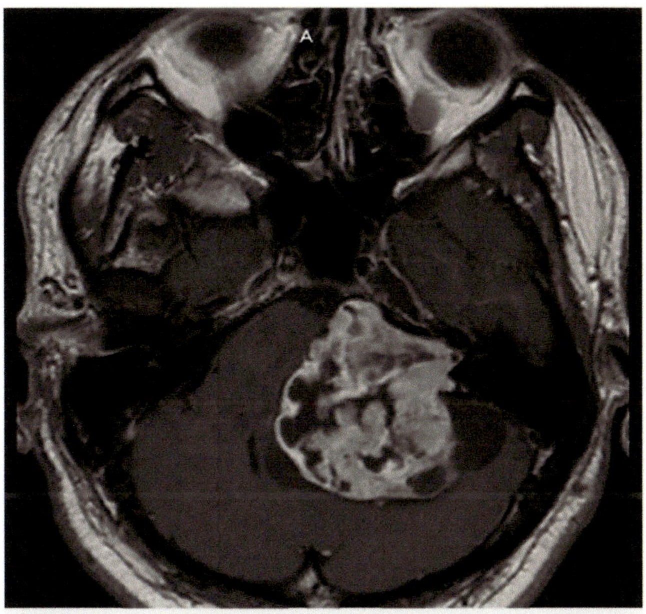

Fig. 46.2 MRI of the brain with contrast reveals a large left-sided vestibular schwannoma with marked displacement and compression of the adjacent fourth ventricle.

46.4 Postoperative Management of Hydrocephalus

The majority of patients who have communicating or noncommunicating hydrocephalus associated with VS will not need permanent CSF diversion. In those patients with persistent signs and symptoms of hydrocephalus, an EVD is placed. The EVD is set at 10 cm H_2O above the ear and weaned gradually by raising the EVD and monitoring for signs and symptoms of hydrocephalus or raised ICP. Those patients who tolerate this process have the EVD removed, and those who do not tolerate the EVD wean proceed to permanent VP shunt placed. For patients with symptomatic communicating hydrocephalus, placement of a VP shunt with a low-pressure or programmable valve is performed.

46.5 Endoscopic Third Ventriculostomy in the Management of Hydrocephalus

The role of ETV in the management of hydrocephalus associated with VS deserves mention. In 2006, Hayhurst et al published an article using ETV to treat noncommunicating hydrocephalus secondary to cerebellopontine angle tumors. A total of five VS were treated utilizing the procedure. Two patients were treated primarily with stereotactic fractionated radiotherapy and experienced postirradiation hydrocephalus. One was successfully treated with ETV, while the other experienced recurrent symptoms secondary to hydrocephalus 2 years after ETV, requiring placement of a VP shunt. Two patients presented with symptomatic noncommunicating hydrocephalus and were treated with ETV prior to tumor resection. Neither patient required external CSF drainage after the surgical operation and currently both remain shunt free. A single elderly patient was treated with an ETV alone, and her tumor was managed with observation. Her symptoms secondary to hydrocephalus resolved after the procedure. In our own personal series, we have used ETV in two patients with symptomatic noncommunicating hydrocephalus secondary to large VS. The procedure was performed prior to the surgical approach for removal of the tumor. In both situations, the need for perioperative EVD was avoided, and neither patient required a shunt procedure. For patients presenting with noncommunicating hydrocephalus secondary to VS, ETV appears to be a viable alternative to EVD and can be considered.

46.6 Discussion

In a recent retrospective cohort of 400 patients with VS, Gerganov et al found 53 patients with associated hydrocephalus (13.3%), with the majority having communicating hydrocephalus (79.3%).[18] In their series, they concluded that complete removal of the tumor is the optimum treatment for associated hydrocephalus and that large tumor size, irregular tumor surface, and severe preoperative hydrocephalus correlated with the need for hydrocephalus treatment after tumor removal.[18] They also found a significantly increased rate of CSF leak in older patients with longer durations of symptoms and those VS with a polycyclic shape. They proposed that the length of exposure to VS-related protein could have led to irreversible CSF alterations.[18] This is supported by a study from 2003, which specifically looked at hyperproteinorrhachia as an etiology for nonobstructive hydrocephalus associated with VS. This study found elevated protein levels in all patients analyzed. The authors hypothesized that the elevated protein level may impair reabsorption at the level of the pacchionian granulations. They further postulated that elderly patients may have less tolerance to CSF composition changes and could be more prone to developing this type of nonobstructive hydrocephalus.[10] The conclusions of Tanaka et al in 2003, which found an increased incidence of communicating hydrocephalus in older patients with VS, corroborates these findings.[16] In a more recent series of 43 patients in 2007, multivariate regression found that only the CSF protein concentration was predictive for development of hydrocephalus.[19] The latest study from 2013 by Miyakoshi et al analyzed 376 patients and found that extended disease duration and elevated CSF protein contribute to the occurrence of hydrocephalus, and maximal tumor resection avoids unnecessary shunting procedures.[17]

46.7 Conclusion

The optimal management of hydrocephalus related to VS is best determined by evaluating the underlying cause of the imbalance between CSF production and absorption. For noncommunicating hydrocephalus, removal of the component causing obstruction of CSF pathways will result in restoration of flow in many cases. In smaller tumors with communicating hydrocephalus, shunting without tumor resection may be considered, particularly in older patients with a small tumor and significant medical comorbidities. If surgical management of the tumor is pursued, permanent CSF diversion is performed only in those patients who remain symptomatic following the operation. We hypothesize that—based on currently available evidence—the likely etiology in most instances of communicating hydrocephalus in the setting of VS is increased CSF protein impairing CSF dynamics and the ability of pacchionian granulations to reabsorb CSF effectively.

References

[1] Cushing H. Tumors of the Nervus Acusticus and the Syndrome of the Cerebellopontile Angle. Philadelphia, PA: W.B. Saunders Co.; 1917

[2] Dandy WE. An operation for the total removal of cerebellopontile (acoustic) tumors. Surg Gynec Obstet. 1925; 41:129–148

[3] Love JG, Dodge HW, Jr, Remine WH, Wellman WE, Campagna MJ. Acoustic neuroma with meningitis and secondary communicating hydrocephalus: successful treatment; report of case. J Neurosurg. 1956; 13(4):312–316

[4] Pirouzmand F, Tator CH, Rutka J. Management of hydrocephalus associated with vestibular schwannoma and other cerebellopontine angle tumors. Neurosurgery. 2001; 48(6):1246–1253, discussion 1253–1254

[5] Kühne D, Schmidt H, Janzen RW, Lachenmayer L. [Communicating hydrocephalus due to acustic neurinoma (author's transl)]. Radiologe. 1977; 17(11):478–481

[6] Steenerson RL, Payne N. Hydrocephalus in the patient with acoustic neuroma. Head Neck Surg. 1992; 107(1):35–39

[7] Atlas MD, Perez de Tagle JR, Cook JA, Sheehy JP, Fagan PA. Evolution of the management of hydrocephalus associated with acoustic neuroma. Laryngoscope. 1996; 106(2, Pt 1):204–206

[8] Briggs RJ, Shelton C, Kwartler JA, Hitselberger W. Management of hydrocephalus resulting from acoustic neuromas. Head Neck Surg. 1993; 109(6): 1020–1024

[9] Hoffman RA. Cerebrospinal fluid leak following acoustic neuroma removal. Laryngoscope. 1994; 104(1, Pt 1):40–58

[10] Bloch J, Vernet O, Aubé M, Villemure JG. Non-obstructive hydrocephalus associated with intracranial schwannomas: hyperproteinorrhachia as an etiopathological factor? Acta Neurochir (Wien). 2003; 145(1):73–78

[11] Gardner WJ, Spitler DK, Whitten C. Increased intracranial pressure caused by increased protein content in the cerebrospinal fluid; an explanation of papilledema in certain cases of small intracranial and intraspinal tumors, and in the Guillain-Barre syndrome. N Engl J Med. 1954; 250(22):932–936

[12] Kudo H, Tamaki N, Kim S, Shirataki K, Matsumoto S. Intraspinal tumors associated with hydrocephalus. Neurosurgery. 1987; 21(5):726–731

[13] Zavala LM, Adler JR, Greene CS, Winston KR. Hydrocephalus and intraspinal tumor. Neurosurgery. 1988; 22(4):751–754

[14] Ohta K, Gotoh F, Amano T, Obara K. Normal pressure hydrocephalus associated with cauda equina neurinoma. Ann Neurol. 1990; 27(4):441–443

[15] Dario A, Dorizzi A, Marra A, Scamoni C, Crivelli G, Fachinetti P. Lumbar neurinoma associated with hydrocephalus. Case report. J Neurosurg Sci. 1993; 37(3):179–182

[16] Tanaka Y, Kobayashi S, Hongo K, Tada T, Sato A, Takasuna H. Clinical and neuroimaging characteristics of hydrocephalus associated with vestibular schwannoma. J Neurosurg. 2003; 98(6):1188–1193

[17] Miyakoshi A, Kohno M, Nagata O, Sora S, Sato H. Hydrocephalus associated with vestibular schwannomas: perioperative changes in cerebrospinal fluid. Acta Neurochir (Wien). 2013; 155(7):1271–1276

[18] Gerganov VM, Pirayesh A, Nouri M, et al. Hydrocephalus associated with vestibular schwannomas: management options and factors predicting the outcome. J Neurosurg. 2011; 114(5):1209–1215

[19] Fukuda M, Oishi M, Kawaguchi T, et al. Etiopathological factors related to hydrocephalus associated with vestibular schwannoma. Neurosurgery. 2007; 61(6):1186–1192, discussion 1192–1193

[20] Hayhurst C, Javadpour M, O'Brien DF, Mallucci CL. The role of endoscopic third ventriculostomy in the management of hydrocephalus associated with cerebellopontine angle tumours. Acta Neurochir (Wien). 2006;148 (11):1147-1150; discussion 1150

47 Postoperative Cerebrospinal Fluid Leak, Pseudomeningocele, and Meningitis: Risks, Avoidance, and Treatment

Raghuram Sampath, Stephen P. Cass, and A. Samy Youssef

47.1 Introduction

Postoperative cerebrospinal fluid (CSF) leak is the second most common complication of vestibular schwannoma (VS) surgery, besides facial paralysis. Because postoperative CSF leak leads to prolonged hospitalization, additional procedures, and increased risk for meningitis, reducing the incidence of CSF is of utmost importance. In the 1960s, the introduction of the abdominal fat graft significantly reduced postoperative CSF leak rates in the translabyrinthine approach. Moreover, the introduction of muscle or fat grafts into the internal auditory canal (IAC) and bone wax obliteration of craniotomy and meatal air cells has reduced the incidence of CSF leaks in the retrosigmoid and middle fossa approaches as well. With greater attention to CSF leak prevention, the prevalence of this complication continues to decline but, nevertheless, the reported rates in the literature continue to range from 2 to 30%[1,2,3] with a realistic estimate of approximately 10%.[4] The objectives of this chapter are to (1) highlight risk factors and approach-based differences that affect the incidence of CSF leak; (2) review various techniques and principles of optimal surgical closure; (3) outline successful treatment strategies for CSF leak, pseudomeningocele, and/or meningitis.

47.2 Risk Factors

The risk of CSF leak has been investigated against tumor, patient, and surgical parameters. Patient characteristics including age, sex, and body mass index (BMI), as well as surgical parameters such as approach, specific closure techniques, length of surgery, use of lumbar drains, and even who performed closure (resident vs. attending) have been investigated. Although, comorbidities such as anemia, diabetes mellitus, renal failure, or malnourishment might be expected to have an important bearing on healing and CSF leak rates, none of these has been specifically studied to the authors' knowledge.

Of the aforementioned variables, none have been conclusively shown to affect risk of the postoperative CSF leak. However, for some factors, there is potential conflicting evidence. For example, several studies have shown an association between CSF leak risk and tumor size, with higher rates being reported with larger tumors,[5] others showing no association with size at all[4,6,7,8] and still others suggesting a higher rate of leak with smaller tumors.[9,10,11] Reoperation has also been suggested as a risk factor for CSF leak, where Stieglitz et al[11] reported leak rates escalating to 11.1% in revision cases as compared to 4.5% at primary surgery. Copeland et al demonstrated, in a series of greater than 450 patients, that increasing BMI is associated with an increase in postoperative CSF leak.[5] Other factors potentially associated with a postoperative CSF leak are degree of aeration of the petrous bone[10,12] with a greater risk in well-pneumatized temporal bones, closure with fat versus muscle,[9] and usage of perioperative lumbar drains.[6,13]

Regarding the influence of surgical approach, a systematic review of 35 studies by Ansari et al[14] found the incidence of CSF leak was significantly greater after the retrosigmoid approach than after either the middle cranial fossa or translabyrinthine approaches (10.3, 5.3, and 7.1%, respectively; $p = 0.001$). However, a large meta-analysis of 25 studies by Selesnick et al[4] showed no difference in leak rates among the different surgical approaches and another report by Mangus et al reached the same conclusion after evaluating more than 1,900 cases performed at a single center.[15] In contrast, Sughrue et al[8] found that rates of CSF leak were similar between middle fossa and retrosigmoid approaches and were higher with the translabyrinthine approach. The remaining literature is diverse in terms of the incidence of CSF leak rates comparing translabyrinthine and retrosigmoid approaches, with some reporting higher rates for translabyrinthine,[5,8] whereas others reporting no difference based on approach.[4,6,15] It is notable that the type of CSF leak may be different according to approach. For example, Mangus et al reported a higher rate of incision leak with translabyrinthine compared to retrosigmoid craniotomy and higher rates of CSF rhinorrhea with retrosigmoid and middle fossa approaches[15] (▶ Table 47.1).

47.3 General Principles of Closure

All surgeons agree on the need for a watertight multilayered closure. The five layers from deep to superficial include the dura, bone, muscle/fascia, subcutaneous tissue, and skin and attempts to reconstitute all these layers will reduce the risk of postoperative CSF leak. Particular to the retrosigmoid approach, watertight dural closure is key in preventing postoperative CSF leak and pseudomeningocele formation. In contrast, primary dural closure with the translabyrinthine approach is less feasible, and dural substitutes in addition to mastoid obliteration with fat may be useful.

Several allografts have been successfully developed and implemented over the years. For the retrosigmoid approach, if primary watertight dural closure cannot be achieved, the authors prefer a pericranial autograft. Alternatively, suturable collagen patches are used to achieve tight closure as tested by a Valsalva maneuver performed by anesthesia. Subsequently, we reinforce the dural closure with dural sealant and perform another Valsalva test. Rigid support of the dural closure using the craniotomy bone flap may act to decrease the differential pressure across the dura and resist breakdown against transmitted dural pulsations. Additionally, replacement of the bone flap may potentially reduce postoperative headache by preventing adhesions between the nuchal muscles and exposed dura.

For the retrosigmoid or translabyrinthine approaches, cranioplasty can be performed using titanium or resorbable plates/

Table 47.1 Selected publications reporting CSF leak rate after vestibular schwannoma resection according to surgical approach

Study (year)	CSF leak rate, approach			Comments
	RS	TL	MF	
Selesnick et al[4] (2004)	10.6%	9.5%	10.6%	Meta-analysis; 25 Medline indexed articles No difference was found based on approach
Sughrue et al[8] (2011)	6%	27%	7%	Medline search; 32,870 patients Similar rates for RS and MF; higher leak rate was associated with TL approach
Mangus et al[15] (2011)	12%	12%	13%	Retrospective review; 1,922 patients No difference was found based on approach
Ansari et al[14] (2012)	10.3%	7.1%	5.3%	Systematic review; 35 Medline-indexed articles Higher leak rate with RS approach compared to TL and MF
Nonaka et al[13] (2013)	7.9%	7.8%	0%	Retrospective review; 357 patients Similar leak rates for RS and TL approach
Copeland et al[5] (2015)	7%	15%	7%	Retrospective review; 457 patients Higher BMI was associated with higher leak rate Higher leak rate was seen with TL approach
Crowson et al[6] (2016)	9.2%	12.4%	6.5%	Retrospective review; 282 patients No difference was found based on approach

Abbreviations: BMI, body mass index; MF, middle fossa; RS, retrosigmoid; TL, translabyrinthine.

mesh and screws. For the retrosigmoid approach, the bone flap may be incorporated in this closure. Alternatively, hydroxyapatite (HA) bone cement can be used, which avoids hardware under the thin skin and provides a sealant effect of the mastoid air cells. Some surgeons use titanium mesh in combination with HA cement. For all approaches, it is paramount to thoroughly plug the perimeatal and mastoid air cells with bone wax in order to avoid CSF otorhinorrhea. It is a good habit to wax the craniotomy air cells "on the way in and the way out."

When possible, reapproximation of the musculoperiosteal layer should be performed. While this layer rarely achieves a truly watertight closure, it serves to buttress the replaced craniotomy plate or obliterating fat, depending on the approach. Reapproximation of the musculoperiosteal layer may also reduce the risk of plate or HA cement extrusion or exposure. Finally, watertight closure of the subcutaneous tissue and skin serve as the last line of defense against percutaneous CSF leakage. There is no evidence to suggest that staples or sutures are superior. Regardless of the final closure technique, generally sutures or staples are not removed until at least 2 weeks after surgery to reduce the risk of wound dehiscence and CSF leak, particularly if pseudomeningocele is present.

47.4 Surgical Approach–Specific Guidelines for CSF Leak Prevention

47.4.1 The Retrosigmoid Approach

The retrosigmoid approach is the workhorse for many posterior fossa lesions. It is particularly versatile for VS, and can be utilized to resect small tumors with attempted hearing preservation or large tumors even when hearing preservation is not a goal. The intracanalicular portion of the tumor is exposed after drilling of the posterior wall of the IAC. This step has been shown to increase the risk of CSF rhinorrhea but is almost always necessary for complete tumor removal.[16]

The degree of pneumatization of the petrous bone is a risk factor for CSF leak and opened perimeatal air cells provide a conduit for CSF leakage into the middle ear, and subsequently the nasopharynx through the eustachian tube.[10,11,12] Stieglitz et al suggested that a higher rate of CSF rhinorrhea occurs with smaller tumors due to less widening of the IAC, thus requiring more bone removal and exposure of more air cells.[10] Regardless, in all cases, all open air cells should be thoroughly waxed prior to dural closure of the posterior fossa. We have found that an angled 30-degree rigid endoscope is a useful adjunct to identify any remaining open meatal air cells that may be hidden from the line of sight of the microscope (▶ Fig. 47.1). After direct visualization and waxing of open air cells, a muscle or fat graft can be placed into the IAC. The authors employ a final layer of Surgicel (Johnson & Johnson Medical, Piscataway, NJ) that acts as a scaffold across the IAC, securing the graft in place. This technique provides another line of defense against the development of CSF leak. A second source for CSF rhinorrhea after a retrosigmoid approach is open mastoid air cells along the margin of the craniotomy. The golden rule of "wax in–wax out" should be applied in every case.

Watertight dural closure is key to preventing percutaneous CSF leak or the development of pseudomeningocele. If the dura cannot be primarily closed in a watertight fashion, several alternatives can be applied including autografts such as pericranium, fat, or muscle harvested from the same incision to supplement the dural closure. If closure with an autograft is not feasible, dural substitutes can be applied followed by dural sealant and Valsalva maneuver. Bony closure with the bone flap and HA cement has been a successful technique in our experience. Reinforcement with the bone flap or titanium mesh may act as a buttress against any potential development of high postoperative intracranial pressure. Other authors have used creative techniques such as Medpor mesh[17] or a HA–titanium combination[18] and noted a decrease in the incidence of CSF leak as well.

47.4.2 The Middle Fossa Approach

The subtemporal middle fossa craniotomy is a hearing preservation approach for accessing small tumors located primarily

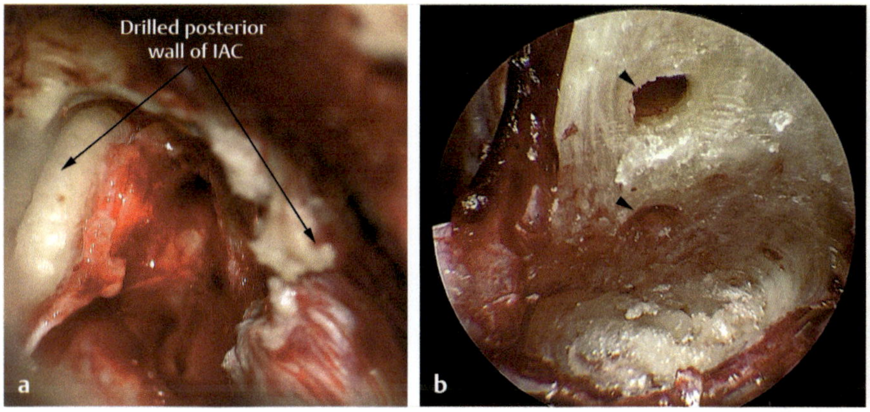

Fig. 47.1 (a) Microscopic view of the drilled posterior wall of the internal auditory canal after tumor resection. (**b**) The same drilled area now viewed with a 30-degree endoscope showing two prominent air cells (*arrow heads*) not visualized by the microscope as shown in **a**. These air cells can be occluded with bone wax under endoscopic view.

within the IAC. Some surgeons will utilize a lumbar drain prior to surgery for temporal lobe relaxation, particularly if under the dominant temporal lobe. With the middle fossa approach, the dural opening is usually limited to the IAC and primary watertight dural closure is generally not feasible. The resulting small dural defect is most commonly plugged with a fat or muscle graft along with tissue sealant. All air cells opened during drilling should be sealed with bone wax. Provided the temporal lobe dura has not been violated, the risk of CSF leak with the middle fossa approach is the lowest among all techniques in our experience. Closure is performed in layers starting with the bone flap, followed by the temporalis muscle, galea, and skin. In our practice, we use HA cement around the bone flap to avoid titanium hardware that may cause discomfort near the ear.

47.4.3 The Translabyrinthine Approach

The translabyrinthine craniotomy provides a more direct approach to the IAC and cerebellopontine angle through a wide mastoidectomy and labyrinthectomy. It is usually utilized in cases with poor preoperative hearing or larger tumors with a low probability of hearing preservation. The approach offers early identification of the facial nerve in the IAC, extradural drilling, in addition to minimal or no cerebellar retraction.

By necessity, the wide mastoidectomy and labyrinthectomy of the translabyrinthine approach leaves multiple air cell tracts, the middle ear, and the eustachian tube open to CSF egress, thereby increasing the potential for CSF leak. Moreover, since the dural opening of the IAC and posterior fossa cannot usually be closed primarily or watertight, closure must take into account all of these possible avenues of CSF leak. Many substances have been used to obliterate the eustachian tube orifice, middle ear, and mastoid cavity but use of autologous tissue is most common (e.g., dried periosteum, abdominal fat, temporalis fascia, muscle, bone pâté). First, all visible air cell tracts are meticulously occluded using bone wax. Next, the entrance to the middle ear space is opened via the antrum or facial recess to directly access the eustachian tube orifice. This may require removal of the incus and malleus head, taking care not to dislocate the stapes or tear the tympanic membrane. The eustachian tube orifice and middle ear cleft are then packed with autologous tissue such as fascia, periosteum, muscle, or fat.[19] Sanna and coworkers[7,19] described their experience with different graft materials used for such obliteration. In their experience, muscle graft tends to atrophy, whereas fat graft tends to dissolve on contact with air, which could lead to delayed rhinorrhea. Packing the middle ear cleft with periosteum collected at the beginning while drilling the mastoid appeared most successful.

The most common way to close the dural defect and obliterate the mastoid cavity is to apply strips of fat that extend into the cerebellopontine angle in a "cork-like" fashion.[7] Alternatively, a layer of dural substitute can be used to reconstruct the resected dura of the IAC and posterior fossa. Dural sealants may be applied; however, we believe these should be used judiciously as the sealants may interfere with the fat graft adhering to the walls of the drilled mastoid cavity. Additionally, if any bit of sealant is resorbed, a resulting conduit for CSF egress may result.

The general principles of multilayered closure are again key in order to reduce risk of CSF leak and pseudomeningocele. Different strategies have been applied to finalize closure after the translabyrinthine approach. Direct soft-tissue closure over the fat graft followed by a compressive mastoid dressing that is left in place for 3 to 5 days has been historically the most common practice. Alternatively, reconstructing the mastoid cortical bone with titanium mesh, resorbable mesh, bone cement, or even bone pâté is an increasingly common practice. Advocates of this technique reference the benefit of a long-lasting compressive effect over the fat graft, which may lower the risk of pseudomeningocele or percutaneous CSF leak. While HA bone cement has been associated with delayed extrusion and subsequent CSF fistula/infection in a small series,[20] this complication has not been reported in several other published series using this technique.[18,21] Some prefer the use of a resorbable mesh since this provides several months of support, but then resorbs, which may reduce the uncommon complication of hardware infection or pain that can occur with titanium mesh. The periosteum/soft-tissue layer is then primarily closed, followed by subcutaneous tissue and skin closure. In addition to closure techniques, other preventative postoperative maneuvers such as having the patient in a 30- to 45-degree head-up position, avoiding Valsalva maneuvers/straining, and stool softeners have been applied; however, no direct evidence is available to substantiate effectiveness (see Chapter 48).

47.5 Management of Cerebrospinal Fluid Leak

If an air cell tract is not obliterated during surgery or the surgical incision is not closed sufficiently, then CSF will flow from the relatively high intracranial pressure system (normal: 7–15 mm Hg) to the relatively low pressure systems of the eustachian tube, middle ear space, or a dehiscence in the periosteal or skin layers. This risk is theoretically higher in cases with elevated postoperative CSF pressure such as with aseptic meningitis or obesity for example. In most cases, a postoperative CSF leak will be obvious on physical examination, either with incisional leakage or clear unilateral rhinorrhea evident when leaning forward with or without Valsalva. As such, in many cases, a beta-2 transferrin test is not necessary to establish the diagnosis. However, for intermittent or questionable leaks, this laboratory assay may be very valuable. Less commonly, occult leaks may initially manifest with meningitis or headache with pneumocephalus. Pseudomeningocele may occur as a precursor to an incisional leak, particularly if tense. CSF otorrhea of course is very rare and only occurs when a hole or tear is present in the ear canal or tympanic membrane. This may inadvertently occur with any of the surgical approaches when raising the musculoperiosteal layer near the bony external auditory canal. It may also result from a tear in the tympanic membrane during eustachian tube and middle ear packing with the translabyrinthine approach. If a tear in the ear canal is identified during surgery, this must be repaired primarily, or alternatively the ear canal can be oversewn after removing the remaining ear canal skin and tympanic membrane.

47.5.1 Incisional Cerebrospinal Fluid Leak

For incisional leaks, many studies suggest treatment algorithms that start with a trial of conservative management and then escalate treatment to surgical intervention if conservative measures fail.[3,15] In the authors' opinion, it is valuable to obtain a head CT with any postoperative CSF leak to evaluate for hydrocephalus or concerning pneumocephalus. Most incisional leaks, regardless of the surgical approach used for tumor resection, respond to any combination of the following: oversewing the incision, elevation of the head of bed, bed rest, stool softeners and Diamox (acetazolamide). Lumbar drain for 3 to 5 days can be used either initially or if the aforementioned conservative measures fail to resolve the leak. The lumbar drain must be managed very carefully to avoid the dreaded complication of tension pneumocephalus that can occur with high-volume CSF leaks. Specifically, lumbar drain output should be carefully controlled, and any leak around the tubing or lumbar puncture site must be identified and addressed immediately. A "tap and wrap" (i.e., aspiration and application of a headwrap), performed in a sterile manner, should be considered in cases of a tense pseudomeningocele. Surgical repair is warranted when CSF leaks fail to respond to conservative measures. Surgical treatment includes reexploration of the surgical site following the general principles of multilayered watertight closure leaving a lumbar drain in place for 3 to 5 days. Subsequent recurrence of a CSF leak suggests the possibility of increased intracranial pressure and need for placement of a ventriculoperitoneal shunt. This should only be performed after ensuring no evidence of concurrent infection or meningitis is present.

47.5.2 Cerebrospinal Fluid Rhinorrhea

With CSF rhinorrhea, conservative management is usually attempted first particularly for low flow or intermittent leaks, but because there is an increased likelihood that surgical intervention will be needed, early surgical repair is often warranted.[15] Surgical repair of CSF rhinorrhea following a translabyrinthine approach entails wound exploration with obliteration of the mastoid air cells, middle ear, and the eustachian tube. This may be performed using the original surgical approach, or in combination with ear canal closure to assist with direct access to the eustachian tube orifice.

Surgical repair of CSF rhinorrhea following a retrosigmoid approach can be performed using a transmastoid approach if hearing has not been preserved. The original craniotomy incision can be used, or alternatively a separate smaller postauricular incision can be performed provided that the intervening soft-tissue segment is wide enough as not to become ischemic. With a transmastoid approach, leaking craniotomy or perilabyrinthine air cells can be directly sealed and the mastoid, middle ear, and eustachian tube can be obliterated using autologous grafts.

The management of CSF rhinorrhea after successful hearing preservation using the middle cranial fossa or retrosigmoid approach becomes more challenging. In these cases, an initial transmastoid approach is generally avoided, as packing and obliteration of the middle ear will result in substantial conductive hearing loss. In these situations, initial conservative measures should be first trialed. If surgical intervention is required, a CT scan may help determine the site of leak. Surgical treatment generally entails reopening the original incision and meticulous rewaxing of craniotomy and perimeatal air cells, with or without concomitant lumbar drain use. In some cases, exploration via a transmastoid approach can be successful if discrete culprit air cell tracts can be identified and directly occluded with bone wax.

Rarely, persistent CSF rhinorrhea may occur despite middle ear obliteration or other measures. In these cases, more proximal eustachian tube air cells may be the cause. These air cell tracks may be difficult to adequately access via a transmastoid approach. In such cases, reports of eustachian tube obliteration have been performed either via an external infratemporal approach or a transnasal approach. In the authors' experience, this is very rarely necessary.

47.5.3 Pseudomeningocele

Pseudomeningocele formation results from the combination of inadequate closure of the dura, musculoperiosteum, and subcutaneous tissue—the most important being watertight closure of the dura whenever possible. In the absence of hydrocephalus, conservative management is successful in the majority of cases. A lumbar puncture and CSF analysis with opening pressure may be useful as the pseudomeningocele may result from increased intracranial pressure associated with aseptic or bacterial meningitis. Distinguishing aseptic meningitis from bacterial meningitis may be challenging in some cases, particularly if antibiotics were given before CSF analysis. Aseptic meningitis is assumed when elevated cell counts and elevated protein are present; however, Gram stain and cultures return negative. If aseptic meningitis is identified as an underlying cause, an additional steroid taper may aid in pseudomeningocele resolution. Short-term use of Diamox (acetazolamide) may also be considered if elevated pressures are suspected. Lumbar drain or pseudomeningocele aspiration and compression may be utilized for tense pseudomeningoceles. Surgical repair is reserved for progressively growing, painful, or draining pseudomeningoceles or those that fail conservative treatment. In these cases, wound exploration is pursued with watertight dural closure with or without lumbar drain. Adjunctively, lumbar drains can be used for the initial 3 to 5 days in poor wound healers (e.g., medical comorbidities, prior surgery, or postradiation) or those with higher BMI, although practically this is rarely needed or utilized. Placement of a ventriculoperitoneal shunt may be indicated for persistent hydrocephalus. Of course, opening pressures may be falsely low in the setting of an active CSF leak, which must be taken into consideration. The interested reader may refer to Chapter 46 for a more detailed discussion of perioperative hydrocephalus management.

47.5.4 Meningitis

The risk of meningitis generally parallels rates of CSF leak, occurring in 1 to 8% of cases. Importantly, patients have a 10 times higher risk of meningitis if a CSF leak exists.[22] Meningitis can be bacterial or aseptic with the literature suggesting that aseptic meningitis is more common, and sometimes it is difficult to differentiate between the two types.[23] Aseptic meningitis is thought to result from an inflammatory reaction to blood products and bone dust in the postoperative surgical space and usually responds to a longer steroid taper. As reviewed earlier, bacterial meningitis can be definitively diagnosed when Gram stain and/or cultures reveal a causative organism. When associated with CSF leak, a lumbar drain will help monitor the response to tailored antibiotic therapy in addition to providing temporary CSF diversion.

47.6 Conclusion

Postoperative CSF leak following VS resection continues to be a significant source of morbidity and health care cost. The reported rate of CSF leak by surgical approach varies significantly between studies. Meticulous, multilayer, watertight surgical closure is the most important factor in preventing CSF leak. Thorough bone wax occlusion of all exposed perimeatal and craniotomy air cell tracts, use of autologous grafts, and meticulous soft-tissue closure are crucial. Use of a lumbar drain may be beneficial in the setting of an established CSF leak but not as a prophylactic measure. The treatment options for postoperative incisional CSF leaks include local reinforcement with sutures or wound revision, with or without concomitant lumbar drain. Low-flow or intermittent CSF rhinorrhea may be successfully managed with conservative measures in some cases; however, high-flow CSF rhinorrhea very frequently requires more definitive surgical intervention. Identifying certain risk factors such as elevated BMI, preexisting hydrocephalus, or excessive temporal bone pneumatization allows the surgeon to more accurately counsel patients as to the risk of postoperative CSF leak and manage accordingly.

References

[1] Fishman AJ, Hoffman RA, Roland JT, Jr, Lebowitz RA, Cohen NL. Cerebrospinal fluid drainage in the management of CSF leak following acoustic neuroma surgery. Laryngoscope. 1996; 106(8):1002–1004

[2] Glasscock ME, III, Kveton JF, Jackson CG, Levine SC, McKennan KX. A systematic approach to the surgical management of acoustic neuroma. Laryngoscope. 1986; 96(10):1088–1094

[3] Fishman AJ, Marrinan MS, Golfinos JG, Cohen NL, Roland JT, Jr. Prevention and management of cerebrospinal fluid leak following vestibular schwannoma surgery. Laryngoscope. 2004; 114(3):501–505

[4] Selesnick SH, Liu JC, Jen A, Newman J. The incidence of cerebrospinal fluid leak after vestibular schwannoma surgery. Otol Neurotol. 2004; 25(3):387–393

[5] Copeland WR, Mallory GW, Neff BA, Driscoll CL, Link MJ. Are there modifiable risk factors to prevent a cerebrospinal fluid leak following vestibular schwannoma surgery? J Neurosurg. 2015; 122(2):312–316

[6] Crowson MG, Cunningham CD, III, Moses H, Zomorodi AR, Kaylie DM. Preoperative lumbar drain use during acoustic neuroma surgery and effect on CSF leak incidence. Ann Otol Rhinol Laryngol. 2016; 125(1):63–68

[7] Merkus P, Taibah A, Sequino G, Sanna M. Less than 1% cerebrospinal fluid leakage in 1,803 translabyrinthine vestibular schwannoma surgery cases. Otol Neurotol. 2010; 31(2):276–283

[8] Sughrue ME, Yang I, Aranda D, et al. Beyond audiofacial morbidity after vestibular schwannoma surgery. J Neurosurg. 2011; 114(2):367–374

[9] Lüdemann WO, Stieglitz LH, Gerganov V, Samii A, Samii M. Fat implant is superior to muscle implant in vestibular schwannoma surgery for the prevention of cerebrospinal fluid fistulae. Neurosurgery. 2008; 63(1) Suppl 1: ONS38–ONS42, discussion 42–43

[10] Stieglitz LH, Giordano M, Gerganov VM, Samii A, Samii M, Lüdemann WO. How obliteration of petrosal air cells by vestibular schwannoma influences the risk of postoperative CSF fistula. Clin Neurol Neurosurg. 2011; 113(9): 746–751

[11] Stieglitz LH, Wrede KH, Gharabaghi A, et al. Factors affecting postoperative cerebrospinal fluid leaks after retrosigmoidal craniotomy for vestibular schwannomas. J Neurosurg. 2009; 111(4):874–883

[12] Stieglitz LH, Giordano M, Gerganov V, et al. Petrous bone pneumatization is a risk factor for cerebrospinal fluid fistula following vestibular schwannoma surgery. Neurosurgery. 2010; 67(2) Suppl Operative:509–515

[13] Nonaka Y, Fukushima T, Watanabe K, et al. Contemporary surgical management of vestibular schwannomas: analysis of complications and lessons learned over the past decade. Neurosurgery. 2013; 72(2) Suppl Operative: ons103–ons115, discussion ons115

[14] Ansari SF, Terry C, Cohen-Gadol AA. Surgery for vestibular schwannomas: a systematic review of complications by approach. Neurosurg Focus. 2012; 33 (3):E14

[15] Mangus BD, Rivas A, Yoo MJ, et al. Management of cerebrospinal fluid leaks after vestibular schwannoma surgery. Otol Neurotol. 2011; 32(9):1525–1529

[16] Hoffman RA. Cerebrospinal fluid leak following acoustic neuroma removal. Laryngoscope. 1994; 104(1, Pt 1):40–58

[17] Azad T, Mendelson ZS, Wong A, Jyung RW, Liu JK. Fat graft-assisted internal auditory canal closure after retrosigmoid transmeatal resection of acoustic neuroma: technique for prevention of cerebrospinal fluid leakage. J Clin Neurosci. 2016; 24:124–127

[18] Manjila S, Weidenbecher M, Semaan MT, Megerian CA, Bambakidis NC. Prevention of postoperative cerebrospinal fluid leaks with multilayered reconstruction using titanium mesh-hydroxyapatite cement cranioplasty after translabyrinthine resection of acoustic neuroma. J Neurosurg. 2013; 119 (1):113–120

[19] Ben Ammar M, Merkus P, Di Lella F, Sanna M. Management of CSF leak after vestibular schwannoma surgery. Otol Neurotol. 2012; 33(3):491–492

[20] Kerr RG, Hearst MJ, Samy RN, et al. Delayed extrusion of hydroxyapatite cement after transpetrosal reconstruction. Neurosurgery. 2009; 64(3):527–531, discussion 531–532

[21] Arriaga MA, Chen DA, Burke EL. Hydroxyapatite cement cranioplasty in translabyrinthine acoustic neuroma surgery-update. Otol Neurotol. 2007; 28 (4):538–540

[22] Allen KP, Isaacson B, Kutz JW, Purcell PL, Roland PS. The association of meningitis with postoperative cerebrospinal fluid fistula. J Neurol Surg B Skull Base. 2012; 73(6):401–404

[23] O'Malley MR, Haynes DS. Assessment and management of meningitis following cerebellopontine angle surgery. Curr Opin Otolaryngol Head Neck Surg. 2008; 16(5):427–433

48 Postoperative Counseling, Restrictions, and Care

David D. Walker and Michael B. Gluth

48.1 Introduction

Over the last 50 years, there have been a number of remarkable advancements in the surgical management of vestibular schwannomas. However, despite significant progress within the field, postoperative recovery following vestibular schwannoma surgery remains an arduous process for some patients. The immediate postoperative period can be plagued by headaches, vertigo, as well as the physical and psychological distress brought on by cranial nerve deficits. Even after many of these initial effects have been resolved, patients can face a lengthy road toward full rehabilitation. In a retrospective review by Wiegand and Fickel, 21% of patients reported that it took between 6 and 12 months before they regained their preoperative functional status.[1] More concerning still is that another 40% of patients felt that after 12 months, they had persistent postsurgical deficits.

Fortunately, there are measures that can be taken to promote a successful postoperative recovery. The principle objective during this phase of care is to support systemic and neurologic homeostasis while simultaneously preventing postsurgical complications. This is achieved by careful monitoring of vital signs, and serial physical examinations. While these measures are critical toward promoting successful recovery, additional prophylactic measures are often taken to prevent surgical complications. Unfortunately, even with appropriate preventive measures, some patients develop adverse outcomes. In these circumstances, early identification and intervention is critical to prevent further sequelae. Together, these measures can help limit perioperative morbidity and mortality while optimizing surgical outcome.

48.2 Support of Systemic and Neurologic Homeostasis

During the immediate postoperative period, patients are monitored closely for neurologic or systemic deterioration. This is performed in the neurosurgical intensive care unit (ICU) and includes vigilant monitoring of traditional physiologic markers. Similar to general postoperative care, alterations to normal vital signs may represent the downstream response of a systemic complication. However, skull base postoperative care is unique in that alterations to normal vitals can also reflect neurologic injury to central processing centers for respiration, and cardiovascular support.

48.2.1 Monitoring Physiologic Markers

Airway management following vestibular schwannoma surgery requires concise communication between the surgical team and the anesthesia provider. Ideally, the patient undergoes a nonstimulating emergence and uneventful extubation. In addition to allowing for prompt neurologic assessment, the removal of the endotracheal tube reduces coughing or bucking. These behaviors have been associated with various early postoperative intracranial complications including intracranial hemorrhage, cerebral edema, and tension pneumocephalus. However, indiscriminate extubation can put the airway in danger. In patients with larger tumors or neurofibromatosis type 2 (NF2), microsurgical dissection may encroach upon the lower cranial nerves. In rare cases where these nerves are damaged, or brainstem stroke has occurred, protective airway reflexes can be diminished or absent leading to poor airway protection and an increased risk of aspiration. In addition, if extubation is performed too early, the patient may require brief positive pressure mask ventilation, which potentially increases the risk of cerebrospinal fluid (CSF) leak and/or tension pneumocephalus. A final consideration during emergence from general anesthesia is the risk of significant tongue swelling and airway obstruction in the rare scenario where the prone or sitting position was used or inadequate bite block placement was performed.

After extubation, the airway and cardiovascular systems must continue to be monitored closely. This is in part because the brainstem plays a critical role in both systems. Thus, brainstem compression from hematoma can often manifest as subtle variations in the ventilatory status, most commonly hyperventilation, hypoventilation, and intermittent apnea. With significantly elevated intracranial pressure, the Cushing reflex may be observed, characterized by the triad of increased blood pressure, irregular breathing, and bradycardia. Strict arterial blood pressure parameters (systolic < 140; diastolic < 90) are also placed to decrease the possibility of intracranial hemorrhage. Routine daily labs including a complete blood cell count and basic metabolic profile may also be ordered at the discretion of the surgeon. Though electrolyte abnormalities are not common following vestibular schwannoma surgery, hyperglycemia can occur in the setting of postoperative corticosteroid administration.

48.3 Specific Complications: Education, Prevention, and Care

Prevention of postsurgical complications relies on the implementation of appropriate prophylactic measures. In addition, practitioners should engage in direct communication with both the patient and nurses regarding their expected role within the patient's recovery.

48.3.1 Intracranial Complications: Hemorrhage, CSF Leak, Meningitis, Hydrocephalus

A 2004 meta-analysis found the incidence of CSF leak following vestibular schwannoma surgery was between 9.5 and 10.6%.[2] Fortunately, careful postoperative care can decrease the likelihood of a leak occurring. Such measures include elevating the head of bed to ≥ 30 degrees, as well as the scheduled administration of prophylactic antiemetics, antitussives, and stool softeners. In addition to these measures, a conventional mastoid dressing or compression wrap is placed at the time of surgery and maintained for 3 days postoperatively. Once removed, the incision, forehead, and pinna are inspected for signs of wound breakdown or ulceration. If an incisional CSF leak is identified at this time, local management can be very effective, with published success rates between 63 and 71%.[3] In these cases, the surgical site should be sterilized with Betadine, and the incision oversewn with 2–0 Nylon suture. If a tense pseudomeningocele is present, sterile aspiration may be performed. The mastoid dressing is reapplied firmly, and bedrest is enforced for several days. In the setting of CSF rhinorrhea, local conservative measures are unlikely to be sufficient, with published success rates between 6 and 8%.[3] In these cases, as well as cases of CSF otorrhea, lumbar drain and/or surgical exploration is often required.[3] A complete discussion of CSF leak prevention and care can be found in Chapter 47.

Other intracranial complications include postsurgical hematoma and meningitis. Intracranial hematoma occurs in only 1 to 2% of surgical cases.[4] Intracranial hematomas are often identified on a postoperative CT scan obtained within 24 hours of surgery, or by changes in neurologic status. This underscores the importance of hourly neurological checks performed by nursing and at least daily examinations performed by the surgical team. The interested reader may refer to Chapter 45 for further discussion of hematoma prevention and management. Treatment is emergent surgical evacuation. In addition to the aforementioned measures, all patients receive 24 hours of antibiotic prophylaxis against gram-positive organisms to help protect against meningitis and superficial infections. Cephalosporins are generally preferred.

48.3.2 Vestibulopathy

Disequilibrium or vertigo is a common complaint following vestibular schwannoma microsurgery. In a retrospective review among pooled patients with varying surgical approaches, 45.5% of postoperative patients complained of vestibular disturbance.[5] The acute treatment of vertigo is divided into rehabilitation and medical vestibular suppression. Numerous studies have examined the utility of vestibular rehabilitation on postsurgical outcomes, with the majority advocating in favor of early rehabilitation efforts.[6] These studies and others are discussed in greater detail in Chapter 69. Vestibular suppressants can help ameliorate any acute vestibular disturbances, but should be used judiciously, with the caveat that they may result in mental status changes that could be mistaken for obtundation. In addition, they may retard central vestibular compensation, and prolong the duration of the vestibulopathy. For these reasons, vestibular suppressants should be discontinued once vertigo that is perceived while the patient is still at rest has ceased, and the patient's spontaneous nystagmus has started to resolve—ideally within 1 to 3 days from the time of surgery.

48.3.3 Headache and Pain

The incidence of postoperative headache within vestibular schwannoma patients may be as high as 75%.[7] For pain control in the immediate postoperative setting, codeine has long been favored given its ceiling on respiratory depression and the fact that it does not mask pupillary responses. However, Jellish et al demonstrated that morphine had even better analgesic control with no increased risk of respiratory depression at usual doses.[8] Nonsteroidal anti-inflammatory drugs are typically avoided given their well-known association with platelet dysfunction. For patients with pain refractory to opioid therapy, those with an opiate allergy, or those with a history of preoperative analgesia use, prompt consultation to the pain service can be extremely helpful.

48.3.4 Facial Nerve Paralysis

For many patients, learning to cope with a change in their appearance can be both challenging and devastating. Facial nerve paralysis can occur at varying times after surgery. In general, patients experience either immediate-onset facial nerve paralysis (IFP) or delayed-onset facial nerve paralysis (DFP). Not only do the two presentations have differing etiologies, they also have varying prognoses. Patients who present with IFP likely experience direct mechanical or thermal injury to the nerve at the time of surgery, and tend to have a more guarded clinical prognosis and prolonged recovery. In a study of 515 patients, the immediate postoperative House–Brackmann (HB) score was predictive of long-term facial nerve outcome. Of the patients with a good immediate function (HB I–II), 98% had acceptable (HB I–IV) long-term function. Meanwhile, in patients with poor immediate function (HB V–VI), only 69.8% had acceptable (HB I–IV) long-term function.[9] Delayed facial nerve paralysis is defined as any patient with a HB I–II immediately postoperatively who experiences a documented facial nerve decompensation at any time during the 4-week postoperative period. The pathogenesis of DFP is less well understood, and a definitive mechanism has yet to be identified. However, reactivation of latent herpes simplex virus remains the most popular and prevailing theory. The current literature suggests that DFP occurs in about 25% of vestibular schwannoma surgeries.[10] Patients generally have an excellent prognosis, with well over 90% of patients demonstrating HB I–II function at 1 year.[10] As a general rule of thumb, a longer delay in onset and a lower peak HB score portends a better long-term outcome in patients with DFP.

Regardless of timing or onset, there are two principle goals in the treatment of postsurgical facial nerve paralysis: (1) promote neural recovery and (2) limit morbidity. For patients with IFP, corticosteroids have been the historical mainstay of therapy, with typical regimens consisting of dexamethasone for a 5- to 7-day course followed by a taper. This practice persists despite a lack of data to support or discourage such measures. For the treatment of DFP, there are two main therapies within the literature: corticosteroids and antivirals. Much like IFP, there are limited data to support the utility of corticosteroids. In terms of antivirals, Brackmann et al examined the utility of broad-spectrum antiherpetic antivirals as a prophylactic agent against DFP.[11] The multi-institutional study demonstrated higher DFP rates in the nontreatment group of 29.8% compared to DFP rates of 19.9% in the famciclovir group.[11]

The second objective is the prevention of further complications that may stem from the facial paralysis itself. This is particularly applicable to patients with a postoperative HB ≥ IV. These patients typically demonstrate varying degrees of lagophthalmos, and should receive ocular precautions to prevent corneal drying and abrasion. However, even in patients with mild facial paralysis, concomitant dry eye or V1 hypoesthesia places the eye at significant risk and protective eye precautions should be considered. Options include ocular lubricants, protective eye shields, tarsorrhaphy, and taping the eye at night. In patients in whom the nerve has been sacrificed, early consideration for eyelid loading with a surgically placed weight is indicated. An in-depth discussion regarding care of the eye after facial paralysis is presented in Chapter 63.

48.3.5 Other Cranial Nerve Neuropathies

The facial and the vestibulocochlear nerves are by far the most frequently affected cranial nerves following vestibular schwannoma surgery, with compromise to other cranial nerves, being more rare. In a review of 390 cases by Darrouzet et al, trigeminal, abducens, and vagus/accessory nerve paresis occurred in only 2, 1, and 0.7% of patients, respectively.[5] The risk of concurrent cranial nerve injury is likely higher in NF2, where collision tumors may develop. Though rare, the dysfunction of these cranial nerves can have profound consequences on swallowing, airway protection, and corneal reflex. Thus, physicians should be aware of their possible occurrence. If nerve continuity is probable, corticosteroids may be of some benefit in these cases.

48.3.6 Postoperative Nausea and Vomiting

Vestibular schwannoma microsurgery has a well-established association with postoperative nausea and vomiting (PONV). The pathogenesis is multifactorial, but proposed mechanisms include vestibular irritation, irritation to the area postrema, and vagal stimulation. Regardless of its etiology, PONV can be a difficult-to-treat problem. Multiple treatment agents exist including corticosteroids such as dexamethasone, 5-HT3 antagonists such as ondansetron, and dopamine antagonists such as metoclopramide. Agents with vestibular suppressant effects such as scopolamine, prochlorperazine, or promethazine may be particularly useful immediately after surgery if nystagmus and vertigo are pronounced. While most of these agents have demonstrated promise, an evidence-based management algorithm does not exist. However, regardless of the initial agent chosen, consensus guidelines recommend that for patients who fail single-modality pharmacotherapy, an additional modality should be prescribed.[12] Since each agent has a unique mechanism of action, the effects are additive, leading to improved symptom control. Additional information regarding management of early PONV is provided in Chapter 26.

48.3.7 Depression/Anxiety

Despite several studies examining postoperative psychological well-being within vestibular schwannoma patients, depression and anxiety are not routinely discussed as potential complications of microsurgical resection.[1,13] However, in postoperative surveys, 40% of respondents report a permanent change in their self-image, with 15% indicating severe negative feelings about their posttreatment status.[1] Meanwhile, a retrospective analysis by Brooker et al demonstrated that as comorbidities relating to vestibular schwannoma increased, so did the incidence of anxiety and depression.[13] Treatment depends on the severity of symptoms, but resources include support groups, talk therapy, or pharmacotherapy. The patient should be made aware of their options, and empowered to design an appropriate action plan in coordination with their care team. The Acoustic Neuroma Association offers many valuable resources and tools available to the patient (Chapter 72).

48.3.8 Thromboembolic Events

Deep vein thrombosis (DVT) and pulmonary embolism (PE) are potentially devastating postsurgical complications. Prevention of these events is particularly challenging, as clinicians must balance the effects of anticoagulation with the risk of intracranial hemorrhage. For patients undergoing craniotomy for nonmalignant diseases such as vestibular schwannoma, the Evidenced-Based Practice Guidelines from the American College of Chest Physicians recommend intermittent pneumatic compression stockings without pharmacologic prophylaxis.[14] However, there are patients who have a preoperative indication for anticoagulant therapy, such as with mechanical heart valve, drug eluting stents, history of PE, atrial fibrillation, or hypercoagulopathy for example. Literature pertaining to discontinuation and reinstitution of these medications following craniotomy, including vestibular schwannoma, is scarce. However, authors have attempted to stratify these patients to guide therapy. Lazio and Simand created three risk stratification groups which are summarized in ▸ Table 48.1.[15] Preoperative consultation with a

Table 48.1 Postoperative anticoagulation and recommendations for reinstitution of maintenance therapy for neurosurgical patients[15]

Patient group	Therapeutic option
Group 1: high risk • DVT/PE ≤ 3 mo • Intracardiac thrombus ≤ 1 mo • CVA/TIA ≤ 1 mo • High-grade carotid stenosis or atrial fibrillation, high-risk peripheral bypass ≤ 9 mo ago • Other arterial thromboemboli ≤ 1 mo ago	Vena cava filter. If upper extremity, then subcutaneous heparin postoperatively, resume anticoagulation on POD 3–5 Subcutaneous heparin postoperatively. Resume anticoagulation on POD 3–5
Group 2: moderate risk • Intracardiac thrombus > 1 mo • Arterial thromboemboli > 1 mo • CVA/TIA with A fib 2 mo to 1 y since last event • High-grade carotid stenosis 2 mo to 1 y since last event • Any prosthetic valve with A fib • Mechanical mitral or combined valves • High-risk peripheral bypass 9 mo to 3 y ago • Carotid dissection	Subcutaneous heparin postoperatively. Resume anticoagulation on POD 5–7
Group 3: low risk • CVA/TIA with A fib > 1 y • Valvular disease without A fib • Mechanical aortic valves • Bioprosthetic valves • A fib • DVT/PE > 3 mo ago • Peripheral vascular disease	Subcutaneous heparin postoperatively. Resume anticoagulation on POD 7–14

Abbreviations: CVA, cerebrovascular accident; DVT, deep vein thrombosis; PE, pulmonary embolism; POD, postoperative day; TIA, transient ischemic attack.

medical team for guidance regarding temporary cessation of anticoagulation or pharmacological bridging is advisable. Regardless of the chosen regimen, early mobilization with fall precautions is encouraged. Furthermore, mechanical prophylaxis with graduated compression stockings and intermittent pneumatic compression should be used while the patient is in bed. While bedrest is typically recommended for at least 12 to 24 hours postoperatively, the physical therapy team should be consulted early in the recovery course.

48.4 Conclusion

The postoperative phase of care is critical to ensure optimal surgical outcomes. Careful support of clinical homeostasis, and the prevention of postsurgical complications, can position the patient for an excellent operative outcome.

References

[1] Wiegand DA, Fickel V. Acoustic neuroma–the patient's perspective: subjective assessment of symptoms, diagnosis, therapy, and outcome in 541 patients. Laryngoscope. 1989; 99(2):179–187

[2] Selesnick SH, Liu JC, Jen A, Newman J. The incidence of cerebrospinal fluid leak after vestibular schwannoma surgery. Otol Neurotol. 2004; 25(3): 387–393

[3] Selesnick SH, Liu JC, Jen A, Carew JF. Management options for cerebrospinal fluid leak after vestibular schwannoma surgery and introduction of an innovative treatment. Otol Neurotol. 2004; 25(4):580–586

[4] Sanna M, Taibah A, Russo A, Falcioni M, Agarwal M. Perioperative complications in acoustic neuroma (vestibular schwannoma) surgery. Otol Neurotol. 2004; 25(3):379–386

[5] Darrouzet V, Martel J, Enée V, Bébéar J-P, Guérin J. Vestibular schwannoma surgery outcomes: our multidisciplinary experience in 400 cases over 17 years. Laryngoscope. 2004; 114(4):681–688

[6] Enticott JC, O'leary SJ, Briggs RJS. Effects of vestibulo-ocular reflex exercises on vestibular compensation after vestibular schwannoma surgery. Otol Neurotol. 2005; 26(2):265–269

[7] de Gray LC, Matta BF. Acute and chronic pain following craniotomy: a review. Anaesthesia. 2005; 60(7):693–704

[8] Jellish WS, Murdoch J, Leonetti JP. Perioperative management of complex skull base surgery: the anesthesiologist's point of view. Neurosurg Focus. 2002; 12(5):e5

[9] Arriaga MA, Luxford WM, Atkins JS, Jr, Kwartler JA. Predicting long-term facial nerve outcome after acoustic neuroma surgery. Otolaryngol Head Neck Surg. 1993; 108(3):220–224

[10] Megerian CA, McKenna MJ, Ojemann RG. Delayed facial paralysis after acoustic neuroma surgery: factors influencing recovery. Am J Otol. 1996; 17(4):630–633

[11] Brackmann DE, Fisher LM, Hansen M, Halim A, Slattery WH. The effect of famciclovir on delayed facial paralysis after acoustic tumor resection. Laryngoscope. 2008; 118(9):1617–1620

[12] Gan TJ, Diemunsch P, Habib AS, et al. Society for Ambulatory Anesthesia. Consensus guidelines for the management of postoperative nausea and vomiting. Anesth Analg. 2014; 118(1):85–113

[13] Brooker JE, Fletcher JM, Dally MJ, et al. Factors associated with anxiety and depression in the management of acoustic neuroma patients. J Clin Neurosci. 2012; 19(2):246–251

[14] Gould MK, Garcia DA, Wren SM, et al. Prevention of VTE in nonorthopedic surgical patients. Antithrombotic therapy and prevention of thrombosis, 9th ed: American College of Chest Physicians Evidence-Based Clinical Practice Guidelines. Chest 2012;141(2, Suppl):e227S–e277S

[15] Lazio BE, Simard JM. Anticoagulation in neurosurgical patients. Neurosurgery. 1999; 45(4):838–847, discussion 847–848

49 Postoperative Imaging Surveillance Following Vestibular Schwannoma Resection

Alexander Sevy and Nikolas H. Blevins

49.1 Introduction

The approach to imaging for surveillance following resection of vestibular schwannoma (VS) varies based on the experience of the center, preoperative tumor size and geometry, intraoperative findings, evolution of symptoms, and other patient-specific factors. The frequency and modality of imaging can be effectively tailored to the particular clinical scenario. Postoperative imaging is used to establish the degree of tumor resection, assess for complications, and evaluate for tumor regrowth, which may necessitate additional therapy. Surveillance to assess the fate of a tumor remnant has become increasingly important with the trend toward more conservative VS surgical management and there has been additional focus on facial nerve functional outcomes.[1] With the advent of radiosurgery as an option to manage residual disease, and an increasing appreciation for the potential for tumor remnants to remain stable over time, surgeons are increasingly leaving some tumor behind to optimize postoperative function. With more conservative tumor resection comes additional need for ongoing vigilance. In this chapter, we will focus on imaging of VS following surgical resection, and will provide guidelines for its use, although there is no established paradigm and clinical practice varies widely. The topic of initial diagnostic imaging of VS is discussed separately in Chapter 8. In addition, the topic of VS surveillance following radiation treatment is discussed in Chapter 25.

49.2 Surveillance Modalities

Initial modes of detecting VS with imaging employed plain film radiography. It was common in the 1900s to obtain radiographs of the skull in the workup for brain tumors, but it was not until 1912 that dilation of the porus acusticus was noted to help localize VSs.[2] Cushing used preoperative plain films but did not mention the use of postoperative surveillance imaging in his seminal work, instead focusing on clinical signs and symptoms to indicate tumor growth. Intracranial tumor localization, and the potential to survey tumors postoperatively, became possible with contrast agents using angiography and cisternography. However, it was not until 1974 that posterior fossa cisternography was modified to become an outpatient procedure.[3] Commercial computed tomography (CT) first became available in 1974 which made possible axial cross-sectional visualization of bony changes of the temporal bone and in 1975 advances allowed visualization of soft-tissue intracranial structures. CT affords higher resolution of bone than magnetic resonance imaging (MRI), and excels when bony anatomic definition is helpful in surgical planning, but it is less useful in tumor surveillance. Both CT and MRI can provide useful complementing information for operative planning and intraoperative guidance. The limitations of CT in postoperative surveillance are similar to those seen in its application in the diagnosis of primary VS, where tumors are difficult to detect until they are of sufficient size to be seen with contrast administration, or they erode adjacent bone. There is also ionizing radiation with CTs, which can be detrimental, especially for use in serial exams in younger patients.[4] Current MRI sequences can provide excellent resolution of soft-tissue structures and have the ability to discriminate between different soft tissues, differentiating tumor from adjacent anatomic structures. MR has now become the primary surveillance modality replacing CT after first being proposed in 1985 by DeFilipp and Buchheit.[4]

49.3 MRI Protocols

Advances in MRI have revolutionized the imaging of VS for postoperative surveillance, just as it has for initial diagnosis. Contemporary MRI scanners with high-resolution sequences and gadolinium enhancement can diagnose intracranial tumors as small as 1 mm. Similar accuracy can be seen in postresection surveillance, and smallest detectable differences between serial scans can be made down to 21% of either linear difference or volume.[5] However, the presence of adjacent postoperative changes related to inflammation, scarring, and reconstructive materials can make identification of residual disease more challenging and can persist for years.[6] An internal auditory canal (IAC) MRI protocol is typically employed for postoperative surveillance, which includes contrast-enhanced thin (<5 mm) and often submillimeter (0.5–1 mm) slices through regions most affected by the tumor and resection (temporal bone, IAC, and cerebellopontine angle [CPA]). Additional whole head sequences can be included especially if there is any evidence of intracranial complications or concurrent lesions.[7,8] A standard protocol would include some variant of the following sequences:

1. T1-weighted, axial and coronal, pre- and postcontrast sequences for the detection of enhancement due to the relative vascularity of VS. It is essential to include precontrast T1 sequences to differentiate inherently bright signal from enhancement, such as from fat. Gadolinium uptake can also be increased by local inflammation, which can persist for 2 years postoperatively, and some enhancement may be permanent.[9,10,11] This is the gold standard for tumor detection and postoperative surveillance.
2. Fat-saturated T1-weighted postgadolinium sequences reduce the inherently bright signal of fat. Comparing these images with precontrast T1 sequences can help avoid the confusion of fat with enhancing tumor. It should be noted that muscle grafts, however, are isointense or hypointense on T1 and often take up gadolinium, making them difficult to distinguish from tumor based solely on signal characteristics.
3. Cisternography sequences with high-resolution slices (i.e., Constructive Interference in Steady State [CISS] or Fast Imaging Employing Steady-state Acquisition [FIESTA] from GE [General Electric, Milwaukee]) are heavily T2-weighted series that allow the visualization of low-signal

neurovascular anatomy in comparison with surrounding bright cerebrospinal fluid (CSF). By showing exclusion of CSF, these sequences can help differentiate between a true space-occupying structure such as residual tumor and inflammation. With submillimeter slice thickness, these sequences can provide adequate resolution for making fine measurements for comparing residual tumor size in sequential studies. This may offer a viable alternative to the need for sequential gadolinium administration when following selected patients.

4. Diffusion-weighted imaging (DWI)/Fluid-attenuated inversion recovery (FLAIR) sequences allow examination of central nervous system (CNS) changes. In particular, DWI excels at the detection of even subtle central ischemia. FLAIR sequences are sensitive in detecting edema, proteinaceous fluids, and demyelination. These sequences are more critical in perioperative imaging, especially with larger tumors, and cases in which CNS dysfunction is clinically apparent. These sequences may not be required in long-term surveillance of stable patients, but often are included in institutional protocols without additional cost, despite an increase in total scan time.
5. T2-weighted axial and coronal sequences can help provide additional information regarding central ischemia and edema with a higher resolution than DWI but a lower resolution than cisternography.

49.4 CT Protocols

CT can be highly effective in defining the extent of bone removal as well as in assessing the integrity of the inner ear in hearing-preservation attempts. When conducting CT for VS studies, it is typical to use submillimeter slices in a temporal bone/IAC protocol that can be later combined in thicker slices for decreased noise artifact. Contrast is not necessary to assess bony structures. However, for tumor detection in patients with adequate renal function, CT with contrast can be used to identify VS tumors down to 2 cm. With the use of gas cisternography CT, intracanalicular tumors can be detected but may lead to over diagnosis, with a 22% false-positive rate when described in the 1980s.[12] The role for cisternography in postresection surveillance has not been defined. CT becomes the surveillance modality of choice in patients unable to undergo MRI due to the presence of MRI-incompatible devices/prostheses or other ferromagnetic implants. This has additional significance as more VS patients are undergoing cochlear implantation (CI) or auditory brainstem implant (ABI), which may adversely affect the ability to image areas of interest with MRI (refer to Chapter 10 for further discussion).[13,14] Cone-beam CT, an increasingly popular in-office technology, can offer additional bone definition with less radiation, although these cannot be used with contrast, show little or no soft-tissue definition, and can be limited by the relatively small anatomic area covered.

49.5 Specific Considerations

Special considerations can be given for reconstructive materials, postoperative changes, metallic implants/prostheses, neurofibromatosis type 2 (NF2) patients, and reducing the risk of gadolinium exposure as reviewed later.

Tissue grafts used for CSF leak prevention have different imaging characteristics that can affect the appearance of postresection MRI, and may be a factor in selecting tissues used. Muscle grafts, for instance, can appear very similar on imaging sequences to residual tumor, including the uptake of gadolinium.[15] This has resulted in a reduction of the use of muscle grafts in anatomic areas where tumor recurrence may occur.[16] Adipose tissue is inherently bright on T1-weighted sequences, which can obscure adjacent enhancement with the administration of gadolinium, unless fat-saturated sequences are obtained. Often enhancement from postoperative scar and inflammation will be linear or diffuse, and can be differentiated from the nodular appearance of residual tumor.[17] However, these often cannot be definitively diagnosed without the benefit of serial studies that demonstrate either stability or growth.

The use of bone-anchored auditory prostheses, metallic mesh or plates, CIs, and ABIs can all introduce artifact that can make imaging of the ipsilateral skull base challenging.[13,14] Despite this, using a combination of sequences can usually yield sufficient diagnostic accuracy in most cases (▶ Fig. 49.1). There are now auditory prostheses with MRI-conditional magnets. The presence of such an internal magnet produces a significantly larger artifact than does the electronic device alone, and the implication of this potentially obscuring tumor recurrence/growth needs to be carefully considered in device selection and positioning.

Patients with NF2 also require special consideration since they typically require more frequent surveillance with the risk of bilateral VS, more aggressive growth patterns, and the potential for new and multifocal cranial and spinal neoplasms. There are some NF2 patients with relatively indolent disease that can be followed

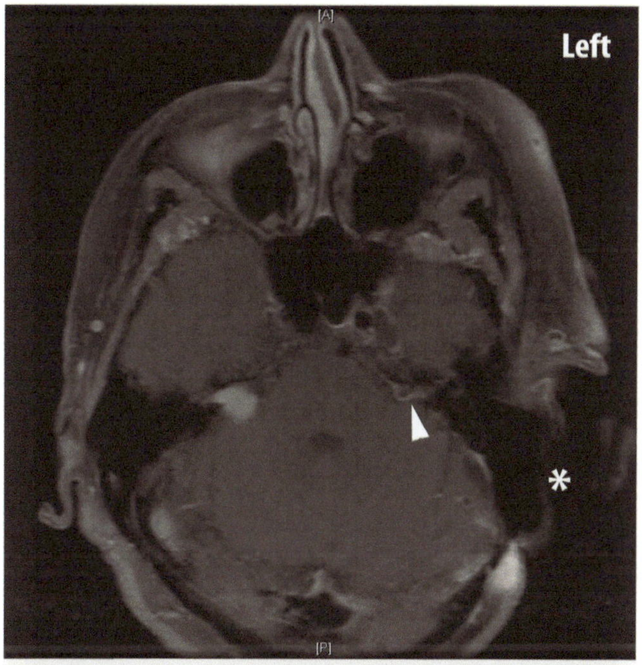

Fig. 49.1 Axial T1-weighted gadolinium-enhanced MRI of a patient with NF2. A female patient 12 years post–left retrosigmoid resection of a VS, being followed up for a small right-sided VS. She underwent successful cochlear implantation on the left without a magnet. Note the artifact (*) produced by the receiver stimulator. Ipsilateral postoperative changes including linear enhancement (*arrowhead*) and a contralateral untreated tumor can also be seen.

up in a manner similar to that for sporadic VSs, while more aggressive forms of the disease require more frequent imaging to guide intervention.[18] Surveillance MRI should not be limited to the temporal bone and CPA, but needs to include the entire head, and in most cases the spine as well. It is reasonable to anticipate the need for lifelong surveillance in patients with NF2.

The use of MRI cisternography sequences alone can be considered to avoid repeated contrast administration in stable patients. Gadolinium and other MRI contrast agents have been shown to deposit in the dentate nucleus and globus pallidus, even in patients with normal renal function—the clinical significance of which is not well known.[19] After baseline and serial images have demonstrated stability on both enhanced and cisternography sequences, it is reasonable to consider using noncontrast MRI cisternography alone in future studies.

49.6 Estimated Risk of Recurrence

Postoperative VS recurrence rates as defined by tumor regrowth have been reported over a wide range from 0.3 to 56%, with the most significant factor being the degree of resection.[20,21] Resections can be categorized as gross total, near total, or subtotal based on the degree of resection, which has implications for recurrence rates. Resections are considered to be gross total if there is no visible tumor remaining at the conclusion of surgery. While definitions vary between authors, we define near total as no more than a small residual tumor remnant remaining, less than 5 mm × 5 mm × 2 mm. Subtotal resection includes those with a greater volume of remaining tumor.[17,22] Surgeons are not always accurate in their assessment of the remaining tumor dimensions at the time of surgery, so some prefer to use the first baseline scan for these calculations. Studies have shown reduced rates of tumor recurrence with greater degrees of resection; subtotal resections carry a 3 to 12 times increased risk of recurrence than do more complete resections (▶ Fig. 49.2 and ▶ Fig. 49.3).[1,17,23] In a prospective multicenter cohort study, subtotal resections were three times more likely to have tumor regrowth compared to both near total and gross total resections.[1] In a retrospective study comparing recurrence rates after incomplete tumor resection, subtotal resections had a 12 times larger odds ratio for recurrence.[23] Following subtotal resection with a mean follow-up of 6.6 years, Rosenberg noted no growth in 47.4%, growth in 15.8%, and regression in 21.1% of patients, and only 6.1% required surgical revision.[24] In another study, the risk of recurrence was 9 times higher after subtotal resection than gross total resection, whereas nodular versus linear enhancement on postoperative imaging carried a 19 times higher risk of recurrence. When nodules are larger than 0.4 cm^3 or 15 mm (maximum dimension), there was a fivefold increased risk of recurrence.[17] Jacob et al evaluated 103 patients and, based on volumetric analysis of postoperative imaging, found subtotal VS resection to be 13 times more likely to recur than with near total resection.[25] Refer to Chapter 41 for further discussion regarding risk of regrowth following incomplete VS resection.

49.7 Surveillance Paradigms

There is a wide variation in practice for postoperative VS surveillance, highlighting the importance of specific surgeon

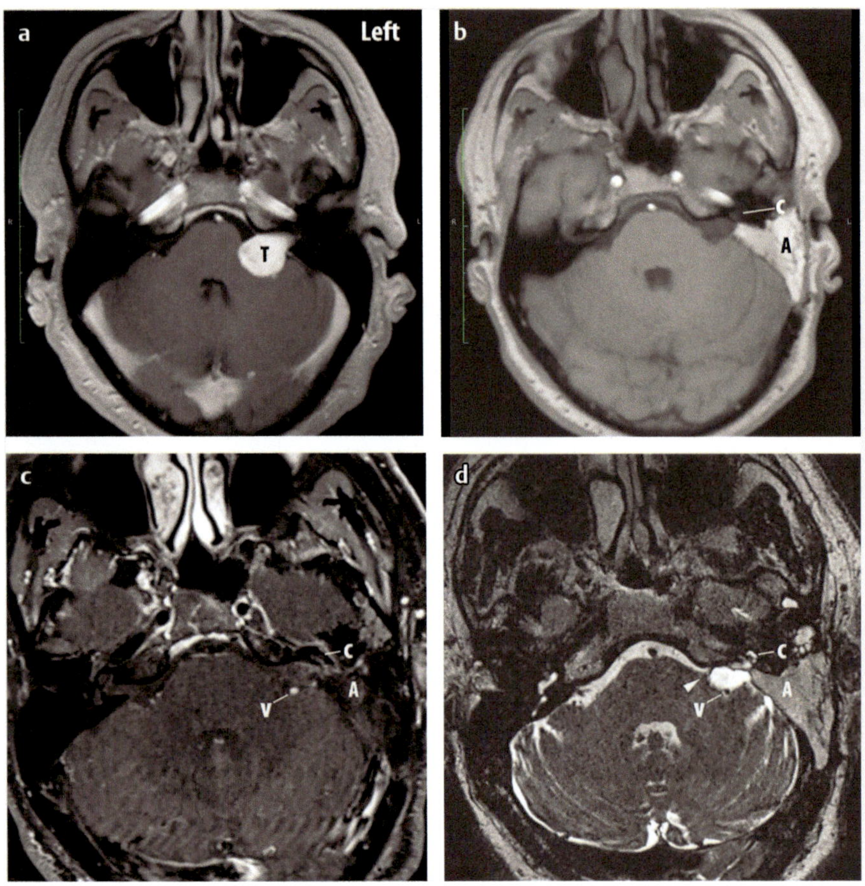

Fig. 49.2 Patient with a left-sided VS who underwent prior translabyrinthine gross total resection. **(a)** Preoperative gadolinium-enhanced axial T1-weighted image showing the enhancing tumor (T) filling the IAC and extending into the CPA. **(b)** Postoperative T1-weighted image without contrast. Note the bright signal of the adipose tissue graft (A), and cochlea (C). **(c)** Postoperative T1-weighted postgadolinium image with fat saturation. Note the suppression of signal in the adipose tissue, which allows for improved identification of regions of contrast uptake. There is some diffuse contrast uptake in the cochlea and IAC, consistent with postoperative changes. Enhancement in a vessel is seen (V). **(d)** Postoperative T2-weighted cisternography image demonstrating bright fluid in the resection cavity adjacent to the vessel (V), adipose tissue (A), cochlea (C), and root-entry zone of the facial nerve (*arrowhead*). There is no evidence of residual tumor after 4 years of follow-up.

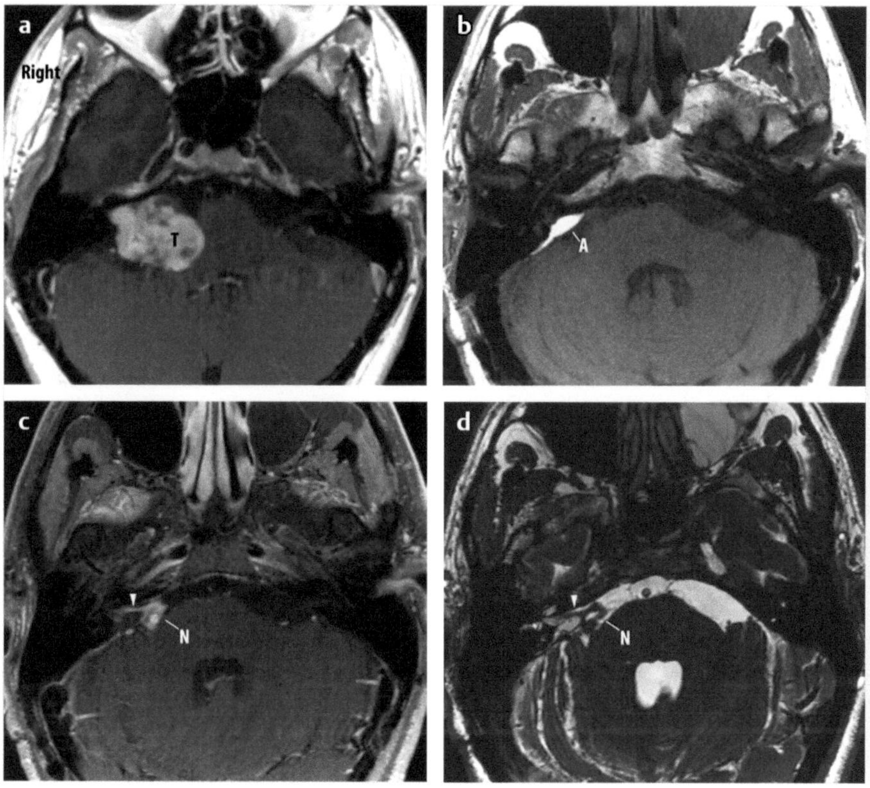

Fig. 49.3 Patient with a right-sided VS who underwent retrosigmoid near total resection. **(a)** Preoperative gadolinium-enhanced axial T1-weighted image showing a heterogenous enhancing tumor (T). **(b)** Postoperative T1-weighted image without contrast. There is a bright adipose tissue graft (A) present at the drilled edge of the IAC. Without additional fat-saturated images, this could be mistaken for residual tumor. **(c)** Postoperative T1-weighted postgadolinium image with fat saturation. Note the suppression of signal in the adipose tissue. There is a nodular-appearing region of contrast uptake (N) consistent with the known remnant of tumor left on the facial nerve. There is also adjacent linear enhancement (*arrowhead*) consistent with postoperative changes. **(d)** Postoperative T2-weighted cisternography image helping to further differentiate the nodular area of dark signal (N) representing residual tumor from the smooth appearance of the more normal tumor-free nerve (*arrowhead*).

preference and experience. Of significance, most surgeons agree that surveillance can be discontinued at some point for sporadic tumors that have undergone gross total resection or have remained stable over extended periods of time; yet, others contend that lifelong follow-up is needed given the low but possible risk of late or delayed recurrence. Lee and Isaacson conducted a survey of 135 neurotologists and neurosurgeons. The average planned follow-up was 5 years if there was no evidence of recurrent tumor growth at that time. The average number of postoperative MRIs obtained by neurotologists was 3.6 (range: 1–11) and neurosurgeons obtained an average of 5.6 (range: 1–13).[20] The average time to recurrence found by Bloch et al was 3 years.[23] Jacob et al found median time to recurrence with subtotal resection to be 32 versus 124 months with near total resection.[25] Shelton noted a 0.3% recurrence rate following translabyrinthine complete resection over a follow-up period of 10 years and proposed a conservative schedule, waiting postoperatively until 5 years for an MRI.[26] Some experienced centers recommend MRI as far out as 15 years or longer to ensure stability.[17] In patients for whom surveillance scans have been discontinued, additional scans should be obtained if new symptoms develop that may be indicative of tumor recurrence.

The timing of the initial postoperative scan is variable, and can be led by clinical grounds, with some centers routinely performing imaging on the first postoperative day, while others wait up to 5 years.[20] Ninety-eight percent of MRI scans performed 3 to 6 months postoperatively demonstrate inflammation that may obscure the early identification of a small residual tumor. While it may diminish over time, these findings often never completely resolved.[9,10,11] Therefore, the initial scan is not typically used to diagnose early recurrence, but rather to provide a baseline to compare future imaging. Carlson et al proposed obtaining a baseline scan at 3 to 6 months. If this shows linear enhancement and the surgeon reported gross total resection, the risk of recurrence is low, and they recommend repeat MRI at 7 and 15 years. However, if there is nodular enhancement on the initial postoperative MRI and the surgeon reported less-than-complete resection, the risk of recurrence is considerably higher. In these cases, they advocate repeat MRI at 3, 7, and 15 years after gross total or near total resections, and at 2, 5, 10, and 15 years after subtotal resections.[17]

Early postoperative imaging is indicated in patients with suspected intracranial complications, where early documentation of anatomy may alter the course of treatment. It should be noted that sending an immediate postoperative patient with altered mental status to an MRI scanner can carry some degree of risk, and its routine use may not be in the best interest of all patients. In patients with known residual tumor, or those in whom the degree of resection is uncertain, a scan at approximately 3 to 6 months postoperative is reasonable. This may provide a balance between providing an early baseline for subsequent studies, while also allowing for some of the most acute postoperative changes to resolve.[17] Patients having undergone gross total resection, in whom the surgeon is confident of complete tumor resection, obtaining the first study at 1 year postoperatively is reasonable. The frequency of subsequent imaging can be adjusted based on the surgeon's assessment of the extent of resection, and appearance and apparent stability of residual tumor (▶ Table 49.1).

Untreated sporadic VSs are typically slow growing and often do not grow for extended periods of observation. Growing tumors have an estimated rate of 1 to 2 mm growth per year, with a range of 0.6 to 2.9 mm/year in a large literature review of nonsurgical patients.[24] MRIs taken less than 6 months apart are unlikely to convincingly identify tumor growth versus variability related to MRI slice orientation through a tumor volume (▶ Fig. 49.4). For this reason, when reviewing serial scans during observation or following treatment, it is good practice to compare a new study not only to the most recent scan, but also to the earliest scans. Trends that may be difficult to discern over a year may become more readily apparent when scans taken over many years are compared. Given the expected slow growth of VSs, older patients and those developing comorbidities that may limit their life expectancy may not need as frequent surveillance imaging. Even if a tumor is growing in these patients, the clinician may choose not to act on the finding unless it presents imminent additional risk. Imaging after stereotactic radiosurgery carries its own set of challenges, in particular distinguishing true recurrence from early "pseudoprogression" related to transient tumor swell. This topic deserves special discussion and is reviewed separately in Chapters 25 and 44.

Table 49.1 Postoperative VS surveillance paradigm flowchart (a reasonable proposed follow-up paradigm in surveillance of sporadic VS based on the degree of resection)

	Gross total	Near or subtotal
3–6 mo		x
1 y	x	x
2 y		x
3 y	x	x
5 y		x
10 y	x[a]	x[a]
15 y	x[a]	x[a]

Abbreviation: VS, vestibular schwannoma.
[a]Beyond 5 years, consider obtaining MRI sequences without contrast if no growth has been detected on prior scans. This assumes stability of tumor and absence of new symptoms, which could require earlier imaging.

49.8 Imaging of Complications

In the event that concerning symptoms develop postoperatively, imaging may be employed outside of a chosen surveillance paradigm. The most common complications following resection of VS are CSF leak, wound infection, fat necrosis, pneumocephalus, venous sinus thrombosis, hemorrhage, and cerebral/cerebellar edema, infarction, or atrophy. CSF leaks have been reported at rates as high as 30% following VS resection, but more realistically occur in approximately 11% of cases regardless of surgical approach.[27] A CSF leak is a clinical diagnosis in the great majority of cases, without significant utility of imaging studies. MRI or CT may confirm the diagnosis by demonstrating pneumocephalus, and CT may on occasion identify open air cell tracts that may be targets for surgical closure. Tension pneumocephalus is a rare complication, seen in less than 1% of VS resections and, when present, can be rapidly detected on CT imaging.[28] CSF leaks can be detected clinically with further evidence noted on CT or MRI with fluid in the mastoid or middle ear or a pseudomeningocele often at the craniotomy site. Wound infections occur following resection in less than 4% of cases, and while the diagnosis can be made clinically, T1-weighted contrast MRI sequences can help delineate the extent of involvement and the presence of abscess.[29] The best sequence for acute changes in mentation is often a head CT, which can rapidly detect intracranial hemorrhage, infarction, and pneumocephalus. Arterial damage is rare, but can occur, especially in the management of large tumors. When this occurs, the anterior inferior cerebellar artery is most commonly affected, and MRI can show ischemia to the brainstem, cerebellum, or cerebellar peduncles. Venous sinus thrombosis occurs up to 5% of the time following VS resection and can be imaged with magnetic resonance venography sequences or CT venography.[30] The presence of intracranial complications may alter the clinician's recommendation for ongoing surveillance, with additional imaging studies to delineate the course of the complication in addition to the fate of the resected tumor.

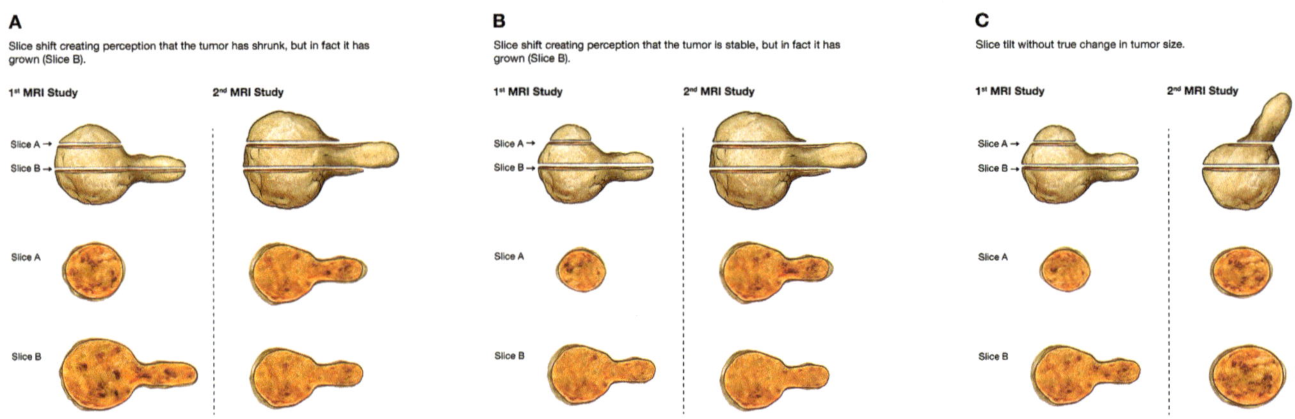

Fig. 49.4 Effect of MRI slice positioning. Slight changes in slice height or orientation can make it difficult to definitively determine small changes in tumor dimensions from the resulting serial two-dimensional slices. As tumor size increases relative to slice thickness (or with thinner absolute slice thickness), these effects are less pronounced.

References

[1] Monfared A, Corrales E, Theodosopoulos P, et al. Facial nerve outcome and tumor control rate as a function of degree of resection in treatment of large acoustic neuromas: preliminary report of the acoustic neuroma subtotal resection study. Neurosurgery. 2016; 79(2):194–203

[2] Cushing H. Tumors of the Nervus Acusticus and the Syndrome of the Cerebellopontile Angle. Philadelphia, PA: W. B. Saunders Company; 1917

[3] Gardner G. The early diagnosis of acoustic tumors using posterior fossa cisternography with iophendylate. Laryngoscope. 1980; 90(2):181–195

[4] DeFilipp GJ, Buchheit WA. Magnetic resonance imaging of acoustic neuromas. Neurosurgery. 1985; 16(6):763–765

[5] Lawson McLean AC, McLean AL, Rosahl SK. Evaluating vestibular schwannoma size and volume on magnetic resonance imaging: an inter- and intra-rater agreement study. Clin Neurol Neurosurg. 2016; 145:68–73

[6] Thedinger BA, Glasscock ME, III, Cueva RA, Jackson CG. Postoperative radiographic evaluation after acoustic neuroma and glomus jugulare tumor removal. Laryngoscope. 1992; 102(3):261–266

[7] Casselman JW, Kuhweide R, Deimling M, Ampe W, Dehaene I, Meeus L. Constructive interference in steady state-3DFT MR imaging of the inner ear and cerebellopontine angle. AJNR Am J Neuroradiol. 1993; 14(1):47–57

[8] Ginat DT, Martuza RL. Postoperative imaging of vestibular schwannomas. Neurosurg Focus. 2012; 33(3):E18

[9] Brors D, Schäfers M, Bodmer D, Draf W, Kahle G, Schick B. Postoperative magnetic resonance imaging findings after transtemporal and translabyrinthine vestibular schwannoma resection. Laryngoscope. 2003; 113(3):420–426

[10] Mueller DP, Gantz BJ, Dolan KD. Gadolinium-enhanced MR of the postoperative internal auditory canal following acoustic neuroma resection via the middle fossa approach. AJNR Am J Neuroradiol. 1992; 13(1):197–200

[11] Weissman JL, Hirsch BE, Fukui MB, Rudy TE. The evolving MR appearance of structures in the internal auditory canal after removal of an acoustic neuroma. AJNR Am J Neuroradiol. 1997; 18(2):313–323

[12] Barrs DM, Luxford WM, Becker TS, Brackmann DE. Computed tomography with gas cisternography for detection of small acoustic tumors. A study of five false-positive results. Arch Otolaryngol. 1984; 110(8):535–537

[13] Ramsden R, Khwaja S, Green K, O'Driscoll M, Mawman D. Vestibular schwannoma in the only hearing ear: cochlear implant or auditory brainstem implant? Otol Neurotol. 2005; 26(2):261–264

[14] Carlson ML, Neff BA, Link MJ, et al. Magnetic resonance imaging with cochlear implant magnet in place: safety and imaging quality. Otol Neurotol. 2015; 36 (6):965–971

[15] Umezu H, Seki Y. Postoperative magnetic resonance imaging after acoustic neuroma surgery: influence of packing materials in the drilled internal auditory canal on assessment of residual tumor. Neurol Med Chir (Tokyo). 1999; 39(2):141–147, discussion 147–149

[16] Lüdemann WO, Stieglitz LH, Gerganov V, Samii A, Samii M. Fat implant is superior to muscle implant in vestibular schwannoma surgery for the prevention of cerebrospinal fluid fistulae. Neurosurgery. 2008; 63(1) Suppl 1: ONS38–ONS42, discussion 42–43

[17] Carlson ML, Van Abel KM, Driscoll CL, et al. Magnetic resonance imaging surveillance following vestibular schwannoma resection. Laryngoscope. 2012; 122(2):378–388

[18] Peyre M, Goutagny S, Bah A, et al. Conservative management of bilateral vestibular schwannomas in neurofibromatosis type 2 patients: hearing and tumor growth results. Neurosurgery. 2013; 72(6):907–913, discussion 914, quiz 914

[19] Huckle JE, Altun E, Jay M, Semelka RC. Gadolinium deposition in humans: when did we learn that gadolinium was deposited in vivo? Invest Radiol. 2016; 51(4):236–240

[20] Lee WJ, Isaacson JE. Postoperative imaging and follow-up of vestibular schwannomas. Otol Neurotol. 2005; 26(1):102–104

[21] Roberson JB, Jr, Brackmann DE, Hitselberger WE. Acoustic neuroma recurrence after suboccipital resection: management with translabyrinthine resection. Am J Otol. 1996; 17(2):307–311

[22] Godefroy WP, van der Mey AG, de Bruine FT, Hoekstra ER, Malessy MJ. Surgery for large vestibular schwannoma: residual tumor and outcome. Otol Neurotol. 2009; 30(5):629–634

[23] Bloch DC, Oghalai JS, Jackler RK, Osofsky M, Pitts LH. The fate of the tumor remnant after less-than-complete acoustic neuroma resection. Otolaryngol Head Neck Surg. 2004; 130(1):104–112

[24] Rosenberg SI. Natural history of acoustic neuromas. Laryngoscope. 2000; 110 (4):497–508

[25] Jacob JT, Carlson ML, Driscoll CL, Link MJ. Volumetric analysis of tumor control following subtotal and near-total resection of vestibular schwannoma. Laryngoscope. 2016; 126(8):1877–1882

[26] Shelton C. Unilateral acoustic tumors: how often do they recur after translabyrinthine removal? Laryngoscope. 1995; 105(9, Pt 1):958–966

[27] Becker SS, Jackler RK, Pitts LH. Cerebrospinal fluid leak after acoustic neuroma surgery: a comparison of the translabyrinthine, middle fossa, and retrosigmoid approaches. Otol Neurotol. 2003; 24(1):107–112

[28] Ajalloveyan M, Doust B, Atlas MD, Fagan PA. Pneumocephalus after acoustic neuroma surgery. Am J Otol. 1998; 19(6):824–827

[29] Lee SH, Willcox TO, Buchheit WA. Current results of the surgical management of acoustic neuroma. Skull Base. 2002; 12(4):189–195

[30] Keiper GL, Jr, Sherman JD, Tomsick TA, Tew JM, Jr. Dural sinus thrombosis and pseudotumor cerebri: unexpected complications of suboccipital craniotomy and translabyrinthine craniectomy. J Neurosurg. 1999; 91(2):192–197

Part VII

Treatment Outcomes

VII

50 Reporting of Hearing Outcome Data for Vestibular Schwannoma

Christian A. Bowers and Richard K. Gurgel

50.1 Introduction

Hearing preservation is an important treatment goal for patients with vestibular schwannomas if they have serviceable hearing. The importance of hearing preservation is heightened in younger patients who have many years of potentially good hearing, with smaller tumors which are less technically challenging to treat than larger tumors, in patients with existing hearing loss in the contralateral ear, in patients with threatened hearing in the contralateral ear as with neurofibromatosis type 2, or in patients who depend upon binaural hearing and sound localization for occupational or recreational needs. Of the three primary surgical approaches used for the resection of vestibular schwannoma, only the translabyrinthine approach precludes an attempt at hearing preservation. Therefore, hearing preservation is a key focus for patients undergoing middle fossa or retrosigmoid approaches. Unfortunately, the historical use of various pre- and postoperative hearing measurements and classification schemes has made the comparison of hearing outcomes difficult and complicated.

Management of patients with vestibular schwannoma and serviceable hearing becomes quite complex. In addition to the middle fossa and retrosigmoid approaches, which can preserve inner ear structures and the integrity of the cochlear division of the eighth cranial nerve, nonsurgical management options—namely active surveillance and radiotherapy or radiosurgery—also preserve the anatomic structures critical for hearing. Deciding which of the various strategies to apply to any given patient with functional hearing requires an understanding of the techniques and existing data on the hearing preservation rates of these therapeutic options in addition to balancing other important outcome priorities such as tumor control and facial nerve outcome.

Pre- and postoperative assessment of hearing is fundamental to the diagnostic evaluation of patients with vestibular schwannoma. Hearing is measured by trained clinicians with a background in audiology and is graded according to published standards using calibrated equipment.[1,2] While conductive and sensorineural hearing loss are commonly measured, in the context of vestibular schwannoma, sensorineural hearing loss is the primary concern. Routine audiometry measures hearing thresholds (dB HL) using pure (single-frequency) tones at predetermined frequencies. At each frequency, the minimum loudness that the person can detect is recorded. Thus, behavioral pure-tone audiometry is a subjective test that requires patient cooperation. Representative frequencies for speech understanding (most commonly 0.5, 1, 2, and 3 or 4 kHz) are then averaged to provide one number that is representative of the average threshold of sound detection—the pure-tone average (PTA). Some studies have used the speech reception threshold (SRT), defined as the lowest intensity level (db HL) at which a patient can correctly identify 50% of common two-syllable words, in place of the PTA since these two measures should be within 5 dB of one another. Another critical component of hearing evaluation is the word recognition (or speech discrimination) score (WRS or SDS), which is a measurement of sound clarity at a volume well above the minimal threshold of hearing. The WRS gives information about the clarity of hearing for a patient, which is often diminished disproportionately more than the PTA in patients with vestibular schwannoma.[3] Of the two basic metrics—PTA and WRS—the WRS has more functional relevance for patients because WRS predicts whether hearing loss is amenable to amplification. Hearing aids can make sound louder, but they do not make sound clearer. Therefore, if patients experience marked WRS deterioration as a result of treatment or tumor progression, they will have functional hearing impairment that cannot be rectified by simply increasing the sound with a hearing aid.

Standardization in reporting hearing outcomes is imperative to comparing the efficacy of different treatment options and understanding the natural history of disease.[4] For example, an omission of either PTA or WRS can mislead a reader who is trying to interpret accurate hearing outcomes for a given therapeutic option. Thus, over the years, several hearing classification systems have been proposed. The objectives of this chapter are to (1) review the evolution and development of the various hearing classification systems used in vestibular schwannoma research and clinical care and (2) discuss unresolved issues and future directions.

50.2 Hearing Measurement and Classification Systems

50.2.1 Gardner–Robertson Scale (1988)

The first hearing metric widely adopted for measuring outcomes in vestibular schwannoma surgery was the Gardner–Robertson (GR) hearing scale derived from the seminal 1988 publication (▶ Table 50.1).[5] The goal of this report was to create a five-class scale that was simple, easy to remember, and clinically relevant.[5] Wade and House[6] had previously described the

Table 50.1 Gardner–Robertson classification for hearing preservation

Grade	PTA or SRT (dB HL)[a]	Speech discrimination (%)
I	0–30	70–100
II	31–50	50–69
II	51–90	5–49
IV	91 to max loss	1–4
V	No response	No response

Abbreviations: PTA, pure-tone average; SRT, speech reception threshold.
[a]Use better score. If PTA/SRT score and speech discrimination scores do not qualify for same class, use class appropriate for poorer of two scores.
Source: Used with permission from Gardner G, Robertson JH.. Hearing preservation in unilateral acoustic neuroma surgery. Ann Otol Rhinol Laryngol. 1988; 97(1):55 -66.[5]

"50/50 rule," which defined serviceable hearing as having a PTA of less than 50 dB HL with a SDS of 50% or better. The GR scale arose from the notion that the "50/50" rule did not provide the important useful clinical information necessary to differentiate and classify the potential variety of hearing outcomes. Therefore, Gardner and Robertson modified a classification system scale of hearing preservation in vestibular schwannoma surgery initially proposed by Silverstein et al.[7] Their modification became the widely standardized hearing scale used for reporting hearing outcomes in vestibular schwannoma surgery for most of the following decade.[5]

50.2.2 1995 American Academy of Otolaryngology–Head and Neck Surgery Guidelines

In 1995, the American Academy of Otolaryngology–Head and Neck Surgery (AAO–HNS) Committee on Hearing and Equilibrium established their own specialty-specific guidelines for reporting hearing outcomes after hearing preservation surgery for vestibular schwannoma resection.[8] In the 1995 AAO–HNS guidelines, hearing thresholds were to be reported as the average of the pure-tone hearing thresholds by air conduction at 0.5, 1, 2, and 3 kHz. The best WRS/SDS at presentation levels of up to 40-dB sensation or maximum comfortable loudness (whichever is less) was to be recorded before and after treatment. Investigators were to report pretreatment and posttreatment pure-tone hearing thresholds, best WRS/SDS, and hearing class. The hearing class was also to be reported as unchanged, improved, or worse.

This standardization of reporting hearing preservation outcomes was an important step in the development of modern vestibular schwannoma hearing preservation reporting that it established a simple nomogram of hearing classes that was based on SDS and PTA (▶ Table 50.2). The guidelines simplified hearing preservation classification by creating just four classes of hearing —designated as A, B, C, and D—from the previous five grades in the GR system (▶ Fig. 50.1). For example, using the GR system, a patient with a SDS of less than 50% could have one of three classes of hearing depending on his or her PTA. The 1995 AAO–HNS update was an improvement over the GR system because it provided more granularities for describing postoperative hearing outcomes, particularly as they applied to SDS. This system was recognized as the standard method for reporting vestibular schwannoma hearing outcomes for more than 15 years.

50.2.3 Modified or "Simplified" Word Recognition Score Hearing Classification

Word recognition is arguably the most important metric of routine audiometry in determining a patient's functional hearing.

Table 50.2 AAO–HNS 1995 hearing classification system

Class	Pure-tone thresholds (dB HL)	Speech discrimination (%)
A	≤ 30 dB and	≥ 70
B	> 30 dB, ≤ 50 dB and	≥ 50
C	> 50 dB and	≥ 50
D	Any level	< 50

Source: Data from Committee on Hearing and Equilibrium guidelines for the evaluation of hearing preservation in acoustic neuroma (vestibular schwannoma). American Academy of Otolaryngology-Head and Neck Surgery Foundation, Inc. Otolaryngol Head Neck Surg. 1995; 113 (3):179 -180.[8]

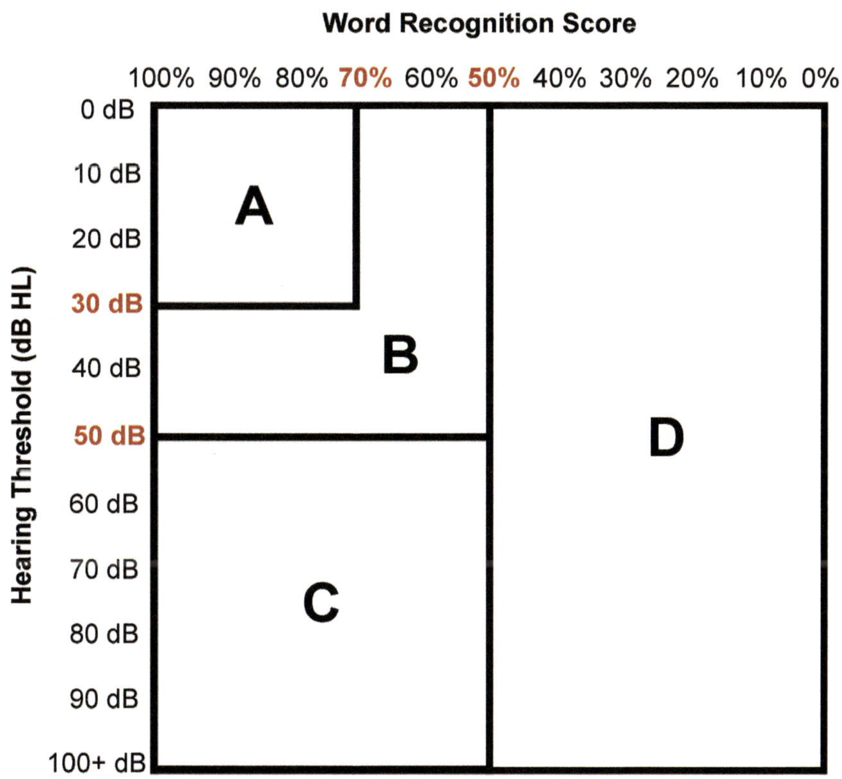

Fig. 50.1 The nomogram of hearing classification from the 1995 American Academy of Otolaryngology – Head and Neck Surgery guidelines for the evaluation of hearing preservation in vestibular schwannoma. Pure-tone averages are represented on the *y*-axis and word recognition scores are represented on the *x*-axis. (Adapted from *Otolaryngol Head Neck Surg* 1995;113[3]:179–180.)

As Meyer et al. wrote, "A reporting strategy based on word recognition scores may be more useful than one incorporating pure tone averages." In their 2006 article, they proposed a simplified classification of hearing status based solely on a patient's word recognition score: class I = 100 to 70% WRS; class II = 69 to 50% WRS; class III = 49 to 1% WRS; class IV = 0%.[9] This simplified classification effectively modified the WRS boundaries from the 1995 AAO–HNS standards and used them exclusively to determine hearing class. This system relies solely on data from WRS to the exclusion of pure tone thresholds because WRS likely has the best predictive value when determining whether an ear will benefit from amplification. For example, a patient with a PTA of 55 dB HL and 90% WRS qualifies for nonserviceable hearing (AAO–HNS class C) according to the 1995 AAO–HNS classification system, but class I hearing according to the simplified word recognition score hearing classification. This patient would likely do much better with a hearing aid than someone with a PTA of 40 dB HL and a WRS of 55% (AAO–HNS class B). This simplified schema has been utilized in numerous publications reporting hearing outcomes.[9,10,11,12]

50.2.4 2012 AAO–HNS Guidelines

The Hearing and Equilibrium Committee of the AAO–HNS made significant modifications to the 1995 guidelines in their 2012 update for minimal requirements for reporting hearing outcomes after vestibular schwannoma treatment.[13] These new guidelines were meant to be inclusive of any intervention in which hearing outcomes are recorded (i.e., surgery, stereotactic radiation, observation, etc.).[13] Perhaps the most striking change from the 1995 guidelines is that patients are no longer classified into one of four hearing classifications of A, B, C, or D.[13] The key limitation of the 1995 guidelines classification schema was that patients could be classified into the same group and yet have very different functional hearing, thus making it extremely difficult to report and interpret the actual functional hearing outcomes. For example, under the 1995 classification, consider two patients with a PTA in the 30- to 50-dB range, one with a WRS of 51% and the other with a WRS of 100%. Both patients would be classified as having class B hearing despite significant differences in the functional hearing outcomes.[13] Raw hearing data are also cumbersome to report and interpret. Therefore, the GR and 1995 AAO–HNS classification systems attempted to classify heterogeneous populations into categories, although these can potentially include very disparate patient groups that can be clinically misleading and ineffective for reporting outcomes for research.

In an attempt to improve upon the existing guidelines, the 2012 AAO–HNS guidelines recommended the creation of a scattergram method that would allow readers to quickly interpret hearing outcomes for multiple patients in one clear concise figure.[13] The guidelines require a pre- and postintervention scattergram to more accurately demonstrate the true hearing results from the attempted hearing preservation intervention (▶ Fig. 50.2a).[13] The preoperative scattergram contains the WRS and PTA on the *x*- and *y*-axis, respectively. Like the 1995 AAO–HNS standard, the 2102 guidelines describe a standardized way of testing and recording these values.[13] Pure-tone hearing thresholds by air conduction are measured at 0.5, 1, 2, and 3 kHz. Since 3 kHz is not always measured in routine audiometry, researchers can derive this value by averaging the 2- and 4-kHz values.[14] The postoperative or postintervention scattergram only records the number of changes in response to the intervention and quantifies the extent of those changes.[13] For example, a postoperative scattergram after vestibular schwannoma surgery (▶ Fig. 50.2b) shows that no patients had improved hearing, as expected, but also quantifies how many had complete hearing preservation (i.e., no change in hearing)

a

Word Recognition Score (%)

Pure-Tone Average (dB)	100 - 90	89 - 80	79 - 70	69 - 60	59 - 50	49 - 40	39 - 30	29 - 20	19 - 10	9 - 0
0 - 10	12									
11 - 20		3	1							
21 - 30		2	8			1				
31 - 40			3	3						
41 - 50			2	6	10	8		1		
51 - 60					11	3	6	2		
61 - 70			2		2		4	9		
71 - 80				1		9			1	
81 - 90								3		3
>91										13

b

← Improved — Word Recognition Score (%) — Worse →

Pure-Tone Average (dB)	≥50	40	30	20	10	No Change	10	20	30	40	≥50
Improved ≥50											
40											
30											
20											
10											
No Change						16	1		1		
10							1	1			
20							1		1	1	
30								2	2	2	
40									1	2	
Worse ≥50											25

Fig. 50.2 (a) Scattergram of pretreatment hearing results in a hypothetical sample of patients. Pure-tone averages are represented on the *y*-axis and word recognition scores are represented on the *x*-axis. Each number represents the number of patients whose audiometric data place them into a certain square. (Adapted from Gurgel et al.[13]) (b) An example of a posttreatment scattergram for patients with vestibular schwannoma. As hearing improvement would be unlikely, this hypothetical example shows 16 patients with complete hearing preservation (i.e., unchanged word recognition scores and pure-tone averages). The number of patients who had a decrease in hearing in WRS, PTA, or both is represented in the boxes of the right lower quadrant. (Reproduced with permission from Gurgel et al.[13])

or loss of serviceable hearing and visually displays how the majority of patients fall somewhere along that spectrum.[13] The changes are recorded in intervals of 10% WRS and 10 dB PTA and the percentage change for WRS is an absolute change such that a pretreatment WRS of 60% and posttreatment WRS of 30% would be reported as a −30% change.[13]

This scattergram reporting method is completely different from the previous 4- and 5-grade classification schemes of the 1995 AAO–HNS and GR systems and avoids a less granular hearing outcome scale.[13] The 2012 AAO–HNS guidelines are the first universal standard for reporting hearing outcomes in clinical trials and will hopefully allow for future meta-analyses and a more clear comparison of results of hearing preservation attempts.[13] A free online tool for generating scattergrams to report clinical hearing data that meets the 2012 AAO–HNS minimum reporting standards can be found at http://hearingoutcomes.stanford.edu.

50.3 Future Directions

The way in which we report hearing outcomes after treatment for vestibular schwannoma has evolved over time. Original standards including the GR and 1995 AAO–HNS classification systems, which relied on broad categories to classify hearing loss, may be replaced by newer models requiring more specific data sets to compare pre- and posttreatment hearing outcomes. The major questions of hearing preservation with vestibular schwannoma management will need to be reexamined or studied more closely within the framework of the new guidelines. Some of these questions include the natural history of vestibular schwannoma growth and its effects on hearing, the rates of hearing preservation with radiosurgery versus those achieved with the middle fossa and retrosigmoid approaches stratified by tumor size, and long-term follow-up.

Still needed are evidence-based guidelines that define different categories of hearing quality based on patient-reported feedback. Previous classification systems have relied on relatively arbitrary boundaries to distinguish different types of functional hearing. An ideal reporting standard would be able to classify patients based on data-driven boundaries to distinguish one patient's quality of hearing from another's. There may also be different ways to measure hearing that are not included in the standard audiogram but that may be informative about a patient's "real-world" hearing acuity. For example, hearing in noise tests is not part of the routine audiologic battery but may be a more accurate way to assess a patient's functional hearing before and after vestibular schwannoma treatment. Such measures may give us further insight into how hearing outcomes should be classified.

References

[1] American National Standards Institute. Maximum permissible ambient noise levels for audiometric test rooms. ANSI/ASA S3 1-1999 (R2008). Available at: http://webstore.ansi.org. Accessed September 20, 2018

[2] Walker JJ, Cleveland LM, Davis JL, Seales JS.. Audiometry screening and interpretation. Am Fam Physician. 2013; 87(1):41–47

[3] Goycoolea M, Guzmán H, Levy R, Orellana V, Ernst J. Basic audiology. In: Goycoolea M, ed. Atlas of Otologic Surgery and Magic Otology. Vol 1. New Delhi, India: Jaypee Brothers Medical Pub; 2012:289–298

[4] Jackler RK.. Comparability in reporting outcomes: a scientific imperative. Otol Neurotol. 1996; 17(6):811

[5] Gardner G, Robertson JH.. Hearing preservation in unilateral acoustic neuroma surgery. Ann Otol Rhinol Laryngol. 1988; 97(1):55–66

[6] Wade PJ, House W.. Hearing preservation in patients with acoustic neuromas via the middle fossa approach. Otolaryngol Head Neck Surg. 1984; 92(2): 184–193

[7] Silverstein H, McDaniel A, Norrell H, Haberkamp T.. Hearing preservation after acoustic neuroma surgery with intraoperative direct eighth cranial nerve monitoring: Part II. A classification of results. Otolaryngol Head Neck Surg. 1986; 95(3, Pt 1):285–291

[8] Committee on Hearing and Equilibrium guidelines for the evaluation of hearing preservation in acoustic neuroma (vestibular schwannoma). American Academy of Otolaryngology-Head and Neck Surgery Foundation, INC. Otolaryngol Head Neck Surg. 1995; 113(3):179–180

[9] Meyer TA, Canty PA, Wilkinson EP, Hansen MR, Rubinstein JT, Gantz BJ.. Small acoustic neuromas: surgical outcomes versus observation or radiation. Otol Neurotol. 2006; 27(3):380–392

[10] Woodson EA, Dempewolf RD, Gubbels SP, Porter AT, Oleson JJ, Hansen MR, et al. Long-term hearing preservation after microsurgical excision of vestibular schwannoma. Otol Neurotol. 2010; 31(7):1144–1152

[11] Stangerup SE, Tos M, Thomsen J, Caye-Thomasen P.. Hearing outcomes of vestibular schwannoma patients managed with 'wait and scan': predictive value of hearing level at diagnosis. J Laryngol Otol. 2010; 124(5): 490–494

[12] Stangerup SE, Caye-Thomasen P, Tos M, Thomsen J.. Change in hearing during 'wait and scan' management of patients with vestibular schwannoma. J Laryngol Otol. 2008; 122(7):673–681

[13] Gurgel RK, Jackler RK, Dobie RA, Popelka GR.. A new standardized format for reporting hearing outcome in clinical trials. Otolaryngol Head Neck Surg. 2012; 147(5):803–807

[14] Gurgel RK, Popelka GR, Oghalai JS, Blevins NH, Chang KW, Jackler RK.. Is it valid to calculate the 3-kilohertz threshold by averaging 2 and 4 kilohertz? Otolaryngol Head Neck Surg. 2012; 147(1):102–104

51 Natural History of Hearing and Vestibular Function in Untreated Sporadic Vestibular Schwannoma

Matthew L. Kircher, Dennis M. Moore, Sam J. Marzo, and John P. Leonetti

51.1 Introduction

Over the last century, advances in treatment of vestibular schwannoma (VS) have paralleled refinements in diagnostic capability.[1,2] In particular, improvements in audiometric screening protocols and the widespread availability of contrast-enhanced magnetic resonance imaging (MRI) have led to an increasing number of small to medium size tumors being diagnosed in patients with minimal symptoms.[3,4] Less tolerance of treatment-associated morbidity and a better understanding of VS growth patterns—particularly the realization that many tumors remain stable or may even involute—has led to greater acceptance of observation as an initial management strategy.[5,6,7,8,9] In fact, according to recent national trends in the United States, it is estimated that by 2026, half of all cases of VS will be managed initially with observation.[10]

Ultimately, most patients who elect initial observation of their VS will experience gradual deterioration of hearing and vestibular function over time.[11,12,13] However, there is substantial variability in audiovestibular loss between patients at the time of diagnosis, and the rate of decline is inconsistent. Unfortunately, the exact mechanism(s) and factors that drive loss of inner ear function remain unclear. With the recent paradigm shift toward conservative observation, understanding the natural history of hearing and vestibular function has become ever more relevant. Such information may be used to guide patient counseling and provides a context to compare the advantages and drawbacks of radiation therapy and microsurgery.

51.2 Mechanisms of Hearing Loss and Vestibular Dysfunction

Potential mechanisms of hearing loss and vestibular dysfunction in sporadic VS include neural compression, vascular compression, VIIIth nerve infiltration, invasion of the inner ear, and accumulation of toxic metabolites or proteins in the fundus and inner ear from poor CSF recirculation. Our knowledge of vestibular dysfunction in observed VS patients is very limited compared with the rather extensive knowledge gathered on hearing deterioration and tumor growth,[14] but presumably many of these factors that influence hearing decline will also result in vestibular loss.

VS-associated hearing loss is thought to occur due to both cochlear and retrocochlear degenerative changes. Supporting evidence for retrocochlear dysfunction include abnormalities on auditory brainstem response measurements[15,16] and histopathologic data demonstrating atrophy of the cochlear nerve.[17,18] Evidence for cochlear dysfunction comes from clinical data showing abnormalities in otoacoustic emissions in VS[19,20,21] and histopathologic data in patients with VS showing pathologic changes within the cochlea such as degeneration of the organ of Corti and the stria vascularis, occurrence of endolymphatic hydrops, and an acidophilic-staining precipitate.[17,22,23,24,25] This inner ear precipitate reflects higher protein content present in ears with VS[26,27] that may interfere with labyrinthine biochemical homeostasis.[24,28] Proposed mechanisms of hearing loss attributed to this protein include blockage of cochlear nerve protein transport, an immune response to VS, or an alteration in the blood–labyrinthine barrier.

Perilymphatic protein accumulation is also being evaluated using fluid-attenuated inversion recovery (FLAIR) MRI sequences. Increased inner ear signal on FLAIR sequences is thought to represent elevated perilymphatic protein, and several authors have found a positive association between FLAIR intensity within the cochlea and hearing deterioration in patients with VS.[29,30,31,32,33]

In cases of cochlear nerve atrophy or neuron loss, speech discrimination is often disproportionately affected over pure-tone hearing thresholds—a pattern classically termed "retrocochlear pattern loss."[34,35,36] Studies have shown that pure-tone threshold shifts occur only after losses of more than 80 to 90% of cochlear nerve fibers[37]; however, clinical data have also demonstrated preserved speech discrimination with mild-to-moderate sensorineural hearing loss (SNHL) in many cases.[24] If retrocochlear mechanisms alone lead to hearing loss in VS, then pure-tone shifts should always be accompanied by severe decrement in speech discrimination, but this is clearly not always the case. Therefore, hearing loss in VS is multifactorial and likely results from a combination of cochlear and retrocochlear mechanisms with pure-tone hearing most affected by cochlear pathology and speech discrimination most affected by retrocochlear mechanisms.

It has also been shown that labyrinthine as well as "retrolabyrinthine" pathology contributes to tumor-related vestibular dysfunction. Hizli et al discovered that findings of labyrinthine pathology, including hair cell loss, hydrops, and inner ear fluid precipitate, are analogous to findings in the cochleae of ears with VS.[23,24,28] Moller et al demonstrated peripheral nerve atrophy and degeneration of Scarpa's ganglion and vestibular neuroepithelia in cases of observed VS.[14] Histopathologic changes were localized to the nerve of tumor origin, and the degree of peripheral nerve fiber and vestibular end-organ degeneration was related to the degree of vestibular ganglion degeneration. The authors described a tumor-induced anterograde progression of vestibular nerve atrophy, and degeneration of Scarpa's ganglion and vestibular neuroepithelia.

51.3 Interpreting the Literature

When reviewing the relevant VS literature, there are several significant biases and limitations that should be acknowledged. Today, common indications for electing initial observation include small to medium tumor size (generally ≤ 1.5 cm in the cerebellopontine angle [CPA]), the presence of serviceable hearing, minimal attributable symptoms at the time of diagnosis, poor surgical candidacy, advanced age or limited life expectancy, and patient preference. Despite trends toward greater use of observation in recent years, it is still important to realize that many patients who could be safely observed may ultimately undergo upfront treatment due to patient or treating physician preference. Thus, the pools of subjects analyzed in natural history studies often represent biased heterogeneous populations at baseline.

In addition to selection bias, disparities in outcome reporting render pooled data analyses and comparison between studies challenging. Hearing loss may be reported using several classification schemes including the 1995 American Academy of Otolaryngology–Head and Neck Surgery (AAO–HNS) guidelines,[38] the Gardner-Robertson classification,[39] the word recognition score (WRS),[40] the modified word recognition score (mWRS)[41] systems, and the more recent 2012 AAO–HNS hearing reporting guidelines.[42] Even with a broad range of grading systems available, many publications merely report the presence of any detectable hearing or patient subjective report (refer to Chapter 50 for further discussion). Lastly, because hearing loss is expected to decline over time, it is critical that similar time points are examined between studies and, ideally, loss of serviceable hearing should be examined using time-to-event analysis, such as the Kaplan–Meier survival curve.

51.4 Pattern(s) of Sensorineural Hearing Loss in Untreated Sporadic Vestibular Schwannoma

Asymmetric SNHL is the most common symptom experienced by patients with sporadic VS, present in over 90% of subjects at the time of diagnosis. In most patients, ipsilateral SNHL occurs at a slow rate, and is often only brought to the patient's attention after experiencing difficulty with telephone use, for example. The published rate of pure-tone threshold and WRS deterioration varies between studies. Fayad et al found that after 4.8 years of follow-up, patients experienced a mean pure-tone average (PTA) deterioration of 20.7 dB HL to a mean of 58.1 dB and an average WRS decrease of 23.3% to a mean of 55.5%.[43]

Among VS patients electing initial wait-and-scan management, unilateral SNHL usually occurs most rapidly over the first 4 to 5 years of observation after which a more indolent loss is typically observed (▶ Fig. 51.1).[12] Authors have reported a wide range of hearing preservation in conservatively managed VS over time. The results of recent large published series are summarized in ▶ Table 51.1 and select publications are discussed further here.[12,13,43,44,45,46,47]

To date, the largest published series of VS managed with a wait-and-scan approach comes from Denmark, where centralized VS care is performed, and a national prospective database has been maintained since 1976.[48] In a large series of 932 patients with audiometric follow-up data, 491 patients (53%) presented with good hearing with speech discrimination better than 70%. After a mean of 4.7 years of observation, 59% of these patients maintained good hearing. In the subgroup of 159 patients (17%) with 100% speech discrimination at diagnosis (mWRS class 0), 138 (87%) maintained good hearing. In the 116 patients with even a minor loss in speech discrimination at diagnosis (1–10%), 63 (54%) maintained good hearing. In the group with a loss of speech discrimination of 21 to 30% at diagnosis, only 28 (33%) of 84 patients maintained good hearing.[12]

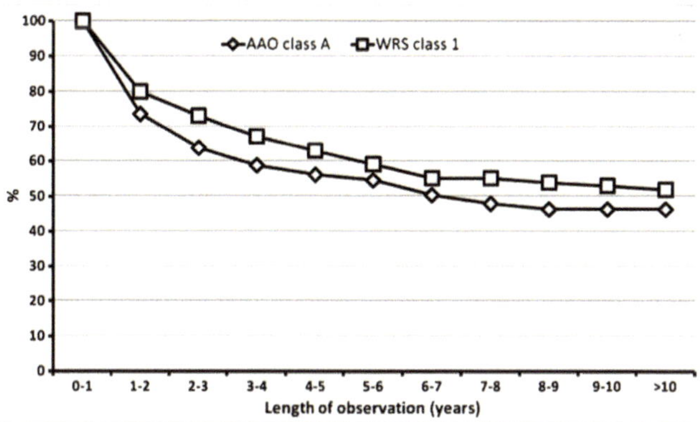

Fig. 51.1 Hearing preservation during observation in patients presenting with good hearing (AAO class A or WRS class 0/I) at diagnosis ($n = 932$).[12] (Used with permission from Stangerup et al.[12])

Table 51.1 Serviceable hearing in patients with untreated sporadic vestibular schwannoma

Author (year)	N	SH initial	SH at last follow-up	Follow-up
Series				
Jethanamest et al (2015); AAO–HNS A/B	75	49%	37%	2.9 y
Fayad et al (2014); mWRS 0/I	44	68%	43%	6.4 y
Stangerup et al (2010); mWRS 0/I	932	53%	31%	4.7 y
Godefroy et al (2009); AAO–HNS A/B	41	40%	23%	3.9 y
Lin et al (2005); WRS I/II	86	77%	33%	6.8 y
Literature review				
Sughrue et al (2010); < 2.5 mm annual growth rate, AAO–HNS A/B or WRS I/II	151		75%	26–52 mo
Sughrue et al (2010); > 2.5 mm annual growth rate, AAO–HNS A/B or WRS I/II	461		32%	26–52 mo
Smouha et al (2005); not defined	347		49%	2.2–5 y

Abbreviations: AAO–HNS, American Academy of Otolaryngology–Head and Neck Surgery; SH, serviceable hearing; WRS, word recognition score.

Overall, it is estimated that between 1 and 4% of patients with VS experience sudden SNHL as a presenting symptom or during the course of observation.[49,50,51,52] Curiously, several reports had documented that in some instances these patients may experience partial or complete recovery of their hearing loss either spontaneously or after steroid therapy.[50,51] Thus, successful treatment of "idiopathic sudden SNHL" with glucocorticoids does not exclude the possibility of an underlying VS—all patients experiencing this symptom should be evaluated with imaging. This also suggests that patients with VS who are being observed and experience sudden SNHL may potentially gain benefit from steroid therapy.[53,54,55]

51.5 Predictors of Hearing Loss in Untreated Sporadic Vestibular Schwannoma

Much attention has been given to elucidating factors that predict future loss of serviceable hearing during observation. Not only would this be helpful toward guiding patient expectations during observation, but such information could be used to guide decision making regarding upfront treatment. While many factors have been analyzed, few have been found reliable. Hearing can still decline in nongrowing tumors, and demographic factors such as age and gender are not predictive of future hearing decline.[13,48]

One of the strongest predictors of long-term serviceable hearing preservation during observation is speech discrimination score at diagnosis. Stangerup et al found that of patients with 100% speech discrimination at diagnosis ($n = 159$), only 3% had lost class I hearing after 1 year, 12% had lost class I after 5 years, and 31% had lost class I hearing after 10 years. Of patients with only a small discrimination loss at diagnosis ($n = 116$), only 38% maintained good hearing at 10 years (▶ Fig. 51.2).[12] Based on these data, strong consideration should be given to observation in appropriate patients who present with 100% speech discrimination at diagnosis as the probability of retaining good hearing in the long term is favorable.[56]

Sughrue et al performed a comprehensive review of the literature to assess the impact of initial tumor size and tumor growth rate on hearing decline in patients being observed over a period of 26 to 52 months.[13] Patients with slow growing tumors (≤2.5 mm/year) had markedly better rates of hearing preservation compared to patients with higher rates of tumor growth. In addition, patients with preserved hearing had a statistically significantly larger average initial tumor size than those whose hearing declined during the observation period, suggesting that growth rate rather than tumor size is a better predictor of hearing loss.

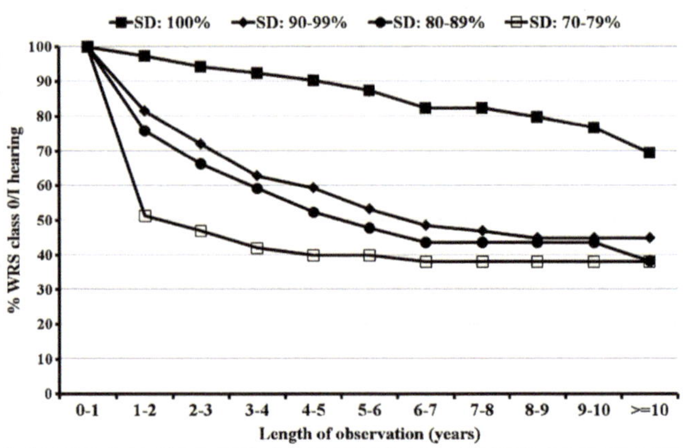

Fig. 51.2 Preservation of good hearing (WRS class I) during observation according to categories of speech discrimination at diagnosis ($n = 932$).[12] (Used with permission from Stangerup et al.[12])

51.6 Vestibular Function and Balance in Untreated Sporadic Vestibular Schwannoma

Among VS patients electing initial observation, between 40 and 65% will report dizziness or vestibular complaints (▶ Table 51.2).[31,44,57,58,59] In a broader sense, there are three methods that can be employed to assess vestibular and balance function in VS: (1) objective measures of vestibular function and balance such as videonystagmography, rotatory chair, and posturography; (3) physician-reported assessment of patient dizziness according to reported symptoms and physical examination findings; and (3) patient-reported assessment utilizing validated self-reporting measures such as the dizziness handicap inventory (DHI).[60]

In 2006, Myrseth et al evaluated 91 Norwegian patients with conservatively managed VS and demonstrated, via sway magnetometry, more pronounced unsteadiness in tumor patients versus controls.[58] Collins et al similarly confirmed increased sway patterns in roughly half of 51 VS patients tested preoperatively as compared to controls.[61]

Blödow et al conducted a retrospective study of 69 participants with untreated unilateral VS.[62] They found an abnormal ipsilateral video head impulse testing (vHIT) gain in 36% of participants, an abnormal vHIT gain asymmetry in 44%, and abnormal caloric results in 72%. Batuecas-Caletrio et al performed a retrospective study of 50 patients with unilateral VS and found that the caloric test was abnormal in 31 of 50 (62%) cases, while the vHIT to the ipsilateral side was abnormal in 27 of 50 (54%).[63] The caloric and vHIT gain asymmetry results were both significantly related to tumor size.

Andersen et al performed vestibular testing on over 400 untreated VS and found patient-reported visual analog scale (VAS) scores depicting none, mild, moderate, and severe dizziness in 35, 34, 22, and 9% of patients, respectively.[59] Dynamic posturography correlated with both tumor size and canal paresis in this study, but less than 10% of variance in VAS could be

Table 51.2 Vestibular complaints in patients with untreated sporadic vestibular schwannoma

Author (year)	N	Vestibular complaint	Follow-up (y)
Andersen et al (2015)	303	65%	None
Lloyd et al (2010)	165	46%	5.7
Godefroy et al (2009)	41	46%	3.9
Myrseth et al (2006)	91	40%	4.2
Driscoll et al (1998)	202	63%	Preoperative

predicted reliably based on postural sway. It has been postulated that central compensation explains the potential disparity between dizzy complaints and vestibular testing results.[64] Using MRI, caloric testing, vHIT, and the DHI, Tranter-Entwistle et al showed that tumor size could be predicted from vHIT gain and canal paresis.[64] In contrast, however, degree of canal paresis, vHIT gain, and MRI measures did not correlate with DHI scores, again demonstrating that central compensation can ameliorate the perceived effects of a slow-growing vestibular tumor.

Using the DHI and a separate VS symptom questionnaire, Carlson et al found that 61% of VS patients endorsed varying severities of dizziness at a mean of 7.7 years following treatment regardless of management modality.[11] In 538 respondents surveyed via a postal questionnaire, the prevalence of vertigo was highest in the observation group (12.0%), compared to SRS (6.8%) and microsurgery (6.4%). In this study, the authors found that pretreatment dizziness and ongoing posttreatment headaches were the strongest predictors of poor long-term dizziness outcomes. This link between headache and dizziness in VS patients regardless of treatment is interesting given the increasing recognition of migraine-associated vertigo in the general population.

51.7 Summary

In recent years, an increasing proportion of patients with small sporadic VS undergo an initial trial of observation, understanding that a significant number of tumors do not grow for extended periods of time. Although this option avoids potential upfront morbidity from treatment, we still must anticipate progressive hearing loss even with a nongrowing tumor. Factors including speech discrimination at diagnosis and tumor growth rate can be used to predict the likelihood of maintaining long-term serviceable hearing. Varying degrees of ongoing dizziness occur in approximately half of observed VS patients and headache may be a contributing factor for some.

References

[1] Ramsden RT. The bloody angle: 100 years of acoustic neuroma surgery. J R Soc Med. 1995; 88(8):464P–468P

[2] Carlson ML, Tveiten OV, Driscoll CL, et al. Long-term quality of life in patients with vestibular schwannoma: an international multicenter cross-sectional study comparing microsurgery, stereotactic radiosurgery, observation, and nontumor controls. J Neurosurg. 2015; 122(4):833–842

[3] Glasscock ME, III, Levine SC, McKennan KX. The changing characteristics of acoustic neuroma patients over the last 10 years. Laryngoscope. 1987; 97 (10):1164–1167

[4] Stangerup SE, Tos M, Caye-Thomasen P, Tos T, Klokker M, Thomsen J. Increasing annual incidence of vestibular schwannoma and age at diagnosis. J Laryngol Otol. 2004; 118(8):622–627

[5] Ferri GG, Modugno GC, Pirodda A, Fioravanti A, Calbucci F, Ceroni AR. Conservative management of vestibular schwannomas: an effective strategy. Laryngoscope. 2008; 118(6):951–957

[6] Fucci MJ, Buchman CA, Brackmann DE, Berliner KI. Acoustic tumor growth: implications for treatment choices. Am J Otol. 1999; 20(4):495–499

[7] Mohyuddin A, Vokurka EA, Evans DG, Ramsden RT, Jackson A. Is clinical growth index a reliable predictor of tumour growth in vestibular schwannomas? Clin Otolaryngol Allied Sci. 2003; 28(2):85–90

[8] Solares CA, Panizza B. Vestibular schwannoma: an understanding of growth should influence management decisions. Otol Neurotol. 2008; 29(6):829–834

[9] Tan M, Myrie OA, Lin FR, et al. Trends in the management of vestibular schwannomas at Johns Hopkins 1997–2007. Laryngoscope. 2010; 120(1): 144–149

[10] Carlson ML, Habermann EB, Wagie AE, et al. The changing landscape of vestibular schwannoma management in the United States–a shift toward conservatism. Otolaryngol Head Neck Surg. 2015; 153(3):440–446

[11] Carlson ML, Tveiten OV, Driscoll CL, et al. Long-term dizziness handicap in patients with vestibular schwannoma: a multicenter cross-sectional study. Otolaryngol Head Neck Surg. 2014; 151(6):1028–1037

[12] Stangerup SE, Thomsen J, Tos M, Caye-Thomasen P. Long-term hearing preservation in vestibular schwannoma. Otol Neurotol. 2010; 31(2):271–275

[13] Sughrue ME, Yang I, Aranda D, et al. The natural history of untreated sporadic vestibular schwannomas: a comprehensive review of hearing outcomes. J Neurosurg. 2010; 112(1):163–167

[14] Moller MN, Hansen S, Caye-Thomasen P. Peripheral vestibular system disease in vestibular schwannomas: a human temporal bone study. Otol Neurotol. 2015; 36(9):1547–1553

[15] Bozorg Grayeli A, Refass A, Smail M, et al. Diagnostic value of auditory brainstem responses in cerebellopontine angle tumours. Acta Otolaryngol. 2008; 128(10):1096–1100

[16] Selters WA, Brackmann DE. Acoustic tumor detection with brain stem electric response audiometry. Arch Otolaryngol. 1977; 103(4):181–187

[17] Eckermeier L, Pirsig W, Mueller D. Histopathology of 30 non-operated acoustic schwannomas. Arch Otorhinolaryngol. 1979; 222(1):1–9

[18] Johnsson LG, Hawkins JE, Jr, Rouse RC. Sensorineural and vascular changes in an ear with acoustic neurinoma. Am J Otolaryngol. 1984; 5(1):49–59

[19] Gouveris HT, Victor A, Mann WJ. Cochlear origin of early hearing loss in vestibular schwannoma. Laryngoscope. 2007; 117(4):680–683

[20] Prasher DK, Tun T, Brookes GB, Luxon LM. Mechanisms of hearing loss in acoustic neuroma: an otoacoustic emission study. Acta Otolaryngol. 1995; 115(3):375–381

[21] Telischi F. An objective method of analyzing cochlear versus noncochlear patterns of distortion-product otoacoustic emissions in patients with acoustic neuromas. Laryngoscope. 2000; 110(4):553–562

[22] Dix MR, Hallpike CS. Observations on the pathological mechanism of conductive deafness in certain cases of neuroma of the VIII nerve. Proc R Soc Med. 1950; 43(4):291–298

[23] Mahmud MR, Khan AM, Nadol JB, Jr. Histopathology of the inner ear in unoperated acoustic neuroma. Ann Otol Rhinol Laryngol. 2003; 112(11):979–986

[24] Roosli C, Linthicum FH, Jr, Cureoglu S, Merchant SN. Dysfunction of the cochlea contributing to hearing loss in acoustic neuromas: an underappreciated entity. Otol Neurotol. 2012; 33(3):473–480

[25] Schuknecht HF, McNeill RA. Light microscopic observations on the pathology of endolymph. J Laryngol Otol. 1966; 80(1):1–10

[26] Lysaght AC, Kao SY, Paulo JA, Merchant SN, Steen H, Stankovic KM. Proteome of human perilymph. J Proteome Res. 2011; 10(9):3845–3851

[27] Silverstein H, Schuknecht HF. Biochemical studies of inner ear fluid in man. Changes in otosclerosis, Meniere's disease, and acoustic neuroma. Arch Otolaryngol. 1966; 84(4):395–402

[28] Hizli O, Cureoglu S, Kaya S, Schachern PA, Paparella MM, Adams ME. Quantitative vestibular labyrinthine otopathology in temporal bones with vestibular schwannoma. Head Neck Surg. 2016; 154(1):150–156

[29] Bhadelia RA, Tedesco KL, Hwang S, et al. Increased cochlear fluid-attenuated inversion recovery signal in patients with vestibular schwannoma. AJNR Am J Neuroradiol. 2008; 29(4):720–723

[30] Lee IH, Kim HJ, Chung WH, et al. Signal intensity change of the labyrinth in patients with surgically confirmed or radiologically diagnosed vestibular schwannoma on isotropic 3D fluid-attenuated inversion recovery MR imaging at 3 T. Eur Radiol. 2010; 20(4):949–957

[31] Lloyd SK, Kasbekar AV, Baguley DM, Moffat DA. Audiovestibular factors influencing quality of life in patients with conservatively managed sporadic vestibular schwannoma. Otol Neurotol. 2010; 31(6):968–976

[32] Yamazaki M, Naganawa S, Kawai H, Nihashi T, Fukatsu H, Nakashima T. Increased signal intensity of the cochlea on pre- and post-contrast enhanced 3D-FLAIR in patients with vestibular schwannoma. Neuroradiology. 2009; 51 (12):855–863

[33] Miller ME, Mafee MF, Bykowski J, et al. Hearing preservation and vestibular schwannoma: intracochlear FLAIR signal relates to hearing level. Otol Neurotol. 2014; 35(2):348–352

[34] Otte J, Schunknecht HF, Kerr AG. Ganglion cell populations in normal and pathological human cochleae. Implications for cochlear implantation. Laryngoscope. 1978; 88(8, Pt 1):1231–1246

[35] Pauler M, Schuknecht HF, Thornton AR. Correlative studies of cochlear neuronal loss with speech discrimination and pure-tone thresholds. Arch Otorhinolaryngol. 1986; 243(3):200–206

[36] Schuknecht HF. Auditory and cytocochlear correlates of inner ear disorders. Head Neck Surg. 1994; 110(6):530–538

[37] Schuknecht HF, Woellner RC. An experimental and clinical study of deafness from lesions of the cochlear nerve. J Laryngol Otol. 1955; 69(2):75–97

[38] Committee on Hearing and Equilibrium guidelines for the evaluation of hearing preservation in acoustic neuroma (vestibular schwannoma). American Academy of Otolaryngology-Head and Neck Surgery Foundation, INC. Head Neck Surg. 1995; 113(3):179–180

[39] Gardner G, Robertson JH. Hearing preservation in unilateral acoustic neuroma surgery. Ann Otol Rhinol Laryngol. 1988; 97(1):55–66

[40] Meyer TA, Canty PA, Wilkinson EP, Hansen MR, Rubinstein JT, Gantz BJ. Small acoustic neuromas: surgical outcomes versus observation or radiation. Otol Neurotol. 2006; 27(3):380–392

[41] Stangerup SE, Caye-Thomasen P, Tos M, Thomsen J. Change in hearing during 'wait and scan' management of patients with vestibular schwannoma. J Laryngol Otol. 2008; 122(7):673–681

[42] Gurgel RK, Jackler RK, Dobie RA, Popelka GR. A new standardized format for reporting hearing outcome in clinical trials. Head Neck Surg. 2012; 147(5): 803–807

[43] Fayad JN, Semaan MT, Lin J, Berliner KI, Brackmann DE. Conservative management of vestibular schwannoma: expectations based on the length of the observation period. Otol Neurotol. 2014; 35(7):1258–1265

[44] Godefroy WP, Kaptein AA, Vogel JJ, van der Mey AG. Conservative treatment of vestibular schwannoma: a follow-up study on clinical and quality-of-life outcome. Otol Neurotol. 2009; 30(7):968–974

[45] Jethanamest D, Rivera AM, Ji H, Chokkalingam V, Telischi FF, Angeli SI. Conservative management of vestibular schwannoma: predictors of growth and hearing. Laryngoscope. 2015; 125(9):2163–2168

[46] Lin VY, Stewart C, Grebenyuk J, et al. Unilateral acoustic neuromas: long-term hearing results in patients managed with fractionated stereotactic radiotherapy, hearing preservation surgery, and expectantly. Laryngoscope. 2005; 115 (2):292–296

[47] Smouha EE, Yoo M, Mohr K, Davis RP. Conservative management of acoustic neuroma: a meta-analysis and proposed treatment algorithm. Laryngoscope. 2005; 115(3):450–454

[48] Stangerup SE, Caye-Thomasen P. Epidemiology and natural history of vestibular schwannomas. Otolaryngol Clin North Am. 2012; 45(2):257–268, vii

[49] Gong QL, Zhou AD, Lin C. [A clinical analysis for sudden sensorineural hearing loss with acoustic neurinoma]. Zhonghua Er Bi Yan Hou Tou Jing Wai Ke Za Zhi. 2013; 48(4):270–273

[50] Lee JD, Lee BD, Hwang SC. Vestibular schwannoma in patients with sudden sensorineural hearing loss. Skull Base. 2011; 21(2):75–78

[51] Lin C, Gong Q, Zuo W, Zhang R, Zhou A. The clinical characteristics and treatment for sudden sensorineural hearing loss with vestibular schwannoma. Eur Arch Otorhinolaryngol. 2015; 272(4):839–842

[52] Saunders JE, Luxford WM, Devgan KK, Fetterman BL. Sudden hearing loss in acoustic neuroma patients. Head Neck Surg. 1995; 113(1):23–31

[53] Aronzon A, Ruckenstein MJ, Bigelow DC. The efficacy of corticosteroids in restoring hearing in patients undergoing conservative management of acoustic neuromas. Otol Neurotol. 2003; 24(3):465–468

[54] Berg HM, Cohen NL, Hammerschlag PE, Waltzman SB. Acoustic neuroma presenting as sudden hearing loss with recovery. Head Neck Surg. 1986; 94 (1):15–22

[55] Nageris BI, Popovtzer A. Acoustic neuroma in patients with completely resolved sudden hearing loss. Ann Otol Rhinol Laryngol. 2003; 112(5):395–397

[56] Kirchmann M, Karnov K, Hansen S, Dethloff T, Stangerup SE, Caye-Thomasen P. Ten-year follow-up on tumor growth and hearing in patients observed with an intracanalicular vestibular schwannoma. Neurosurgery. 2017; 80(1): 49–56

[57] Driscoll CL, Lynn SG, Harner SG, Beatty CW, Atkinson EJ. Preoperative identification of patients at risk of developing persistent dysequilibrium after acoustic neuroma removal. Am J Otol. 1998; 19(4):491–495

[58] Myrseth E, Møller P, Wentzel-Larsen T, Goplen F, Lund-Johansen M. Untreated vestibular schwannomas: vertigo is a powerful predictor for health-related quality of life. Neurosurgery. 2006; 59(1):67–76, discussion 67–76

[59] Andersen JF, Nilsen KS, Vassbotn FS, et al. Predictors of vertigo in patients with untreated vestibular schwannoma. Otol Neurotol. 2015; 36 (4):647–652

[60] Jacobson GP, Newman CW. The development of the Dizziness Handicap Inventory. Arch Otolaryngol Head Neck Surg. 1990; 116(4):424–427

[61] Collins MM, Johnson IJ, Clifford E, Birchall JP, O'Donoghue GM. Postural stability of preoperative acoustic neuroma patients assessed by sway magnetometry: are they unsteady? Laryngoscope. 2003; 113(4):640–642

[62] Blödow A, Blödow J, Bloching MB, Helbig R, Walther LE. Horizontal VOR function shows frequency dynamics in vestibular schwannoma. Eur Arch Otorhinolaryngol. 2015; 272(9):2143–2148

[63] Batuecas-Caletrio A, Santa Cruz-Ruiz S, Muñoz-Herrera A, Perez-Fernandez N. The map of dizziness in vestibular schwannoma. Laryngoscope. 2015; 125 (12):2784–2789

[64] Tranter-Entwistle I, Dawes P, Darlington CL, Smith PF, Cutfield N. Video head impulse in comparison to caloric testing in unilateral vestibular schwannoma. Acta Otolaryngol. 2016; 136(11):1110–1114

52 Hearing and Vestibular Function Loss After Radiation Treatment of Sporadic Vestibular Schwannoma

Cameron C. Wick, Brandon Isaacson, and J. Walter Kutz Jr.

52.1 Introduction

Long-term audiometric and vestibular outcomes after stereotactic radiosurgery (SRS) or stereotactic radiotherapy (SRT) for vestibular schwannoma (VS) remain a contentious issue. The primary challenges are to distinguish treatment effect from the natural history of disease and to decipher which factors best predict outcomes and how those factors interact (▶ Table 52.1). The current literature pertaining to this topic is frequently mired by heterogeneity in outcome reporting and imperfect methodology, making data interpretation and inter-study comparison difficult.

The primary objective of the current chapter is to review factors that influence hearing and balance after SRS for VS. Priority is given to the most recent and relevant data and only those studies that present data using standard reporting guidelines including the American Academy of Otolaryngology–Head and Neck Surgery (AAO–HNS) and Gardner–Robertson (GR) hearing classification systems—both designating serviceable hearing as greater than 50% on word recognition testing and less than a 50-dB pure-tone average (PTA; ▶ Table 52.2).[1,2]

52.2 Patient-Related Factors

Patients with normal or mild hearing loss prior to treatment tend to retain functional hearing longer following radiation treatment than patients with greater degrees of hearing loss. Hasegawa et al. found that 64% of patients with GR class I hearing retained serviceable at 5 years following treatment, compared to only 24% in patients who started with GR class II hearing.[3] Furthermore, even among patients with GR class I or AAO–HNS class A hearing, even mild hearing loss and subtle asymmetry predicts poorer long-term audiologic outcome compared to those with normal hearing.[4,5] Mousavi et al. classified 68 patients with pretreatment GR class I hearing into groups, with or without subjective hearing loss. At 3-year follow-up, the patients without subjective hearing loss had 100% maintenance of serviceable hearing, compared to 57% in patients with subjective hearing loss.[4] In a follow-up study, the authors divided 166 patients with GR class I hearing into three groups based on the level of PTA asymmetry: no asymmetry, less than 10 dB difference, and more than 10 dB difference. After 5-year posttreatment, follow-up serviceable hearing was maintained in 98, 73, and 33% of patients, respectively.[5] Carlson et al. proposed that each 10-dB increase in pretreatment PTA results in a twofold increased risk of posttreatment hearing loss.[6] The correlation between pretreatment hearing thresholds and posttreatment time to nonserviceable hearing has also been supported by multivariate analyses.[6,7]

Paralleling the aforementioned data, studies on the natural history of hearing loss with VS also report different trajectories for maintenance of serviceable hearing once hearing loss has started, even if that loss is mild. In a study by Stangerup et al., audiometric data were available for 932 patients managed with a "wait-and-scan" approach. Patients with an initial speech discrimination score (SDS) of 100% had a significantly higher rate of long-term hearing preservation than patients with an initial SDS between 99 and 90% (87 vs. 54%).[8] These data further support that subdivisions may exist within patients classified as "good" according to either the GR or AAO–HNS scales. Whether discussing the natural disease history or treatment outcomes, the early signs of hearing loss predict eventual hearing decline in all treatment cohorts. The specific role of radiation effect versus natural history remains undetermined.

Patient age has also been identified as a potential predictor for hearing preservation after SRS. Kano et al. demonstrated that age less than 60 years was associated with better hearing preservation.[9] Franzin et al. showed that age less than 54 years predicts better hearing preservation, while Tamura et al. reported that age less than 50 years was the statistical cutoff

Table 52.1 Factors that can affect audiovestibular outcomes in vestibular schwannoma research

Influences on audiovestibular outcomes			
Patient factors	**Tumor factors**	**Radiation factors**	**Publication factors**
Hearing status Age Comorbidities NF2 Status Prior treatments Patient preference	Size (dimension) Size (volume) Growth rate Location Edema Secretions Natural history	Marginal dose Maximum dose Cochlear dose Fractionation Modality Isocenters	Quality of evidence Publication bias Statistical method Clinical vs. statistical significance

Table 52.2 Two commonly cited classification systems for assessment of vestibular schwannoma audiometric outcomes

Hearing Classification Schemes		
	Pure-tone average (dB)	**Speech discrimination (%)**
AAO–HNS		
A	≤ 30	> 70
B	> 30 and ≤ 50	≥ 50
C	> 50	≥ 50
D	Any level	< 50
Gardner–Robertson		
I	0–30	70–100
II	31–50	50–69
III	51–90	5–49
IV	> 91	1–4
V	Not testable	0

Notes: American Academy of Otolaryngology–Head and Neck Surgery (AAO–HNS) class A and Gardner–Robertson (GR) class I represent good hearing. Serviceable hearing is equal or better to AAO–HNS class B and GR class II.

point distinguishing hearing outcomes.[7,10] Other studies showed no correlation between age and hearing preservation.[11,12,13] The selection of a specific cutoff age is often arbitrary and use of appropriate statistical methodology is critical to control for other confounding variables. The study by Franzin et al. highlights this issue. Their age cutoff of 54 years was statistically significant on univariate analysis but not with multivariate regression. Age-related hearing loss, with or without the added complexity of the presence of a VS, incorporates many variables that are ideally analyzed with multivariate analysis. When reviewing the VS treatment literature, it is crucial to consider these subtleties, particularly if inferences are made regarding causality or clinical significance.

Data regarding vestibular function after SRS are less robust than reports on hearing outcomes. Vestibular outcomes, like hearing outcomes, must be compared against the natural history of disease and changes associated with aging.[14,15,16] Wackym et al. compared pre- and posttreatment vestibular function in 54 patients managed with SRS. All patients had at least 6-month follow-up and 27 patients were followed up for longer than 60 months. The majority of patients did not experience long-term change in vestibular function as measured by electronystagmography or the dizziness handicap inventory (DHI). The mean pretreatment DHI was 15.5 compared to the mean posttreatment DHI of 13.5. A subset of patients older than 65 years were more likely to have improvement in their DHI scores. Vestibular function fluctuated the most after the first 6 months of treatment. This early posttreatment window may represent a critical period for vestibular rehabilitation.[17] Another study identified severe headaches as predictive of severe dizziness (DHI > 26). This association was maintained among cohorts of patients treated with observation, microsurgery, and SRS. After a mean follow-up of 7.7 years, nearly 60% of patients experienced some degree of dizziness, although the majority had only mild symptoms. Multivariate analysis found an association between poor DHI scores and increasing age, tumors greater than 20 mm, pretreatment dizziness, frequent headaches, and severe headaches. Migraine features were significant in univariate analysis only.[16]

52.3 Tumor-Related Factors

Hearing preservation after SRS may be affected by tumor-related factors such as VS size, tumor location in relationship to the cochlear nucleus or cochlea, tumor enlargement after treatment, growth rate, cytokine secretions, or cystic characteristics.

Although decreased rates of hearing preservation would be suspected with larger tumors, the effect of tumor size alone on hearing preservation is inconclusive. Interpretation of the data regarding tumor size is often difficult because of the variability in measurement techniques. Multiple reports demonstrate total tumor size has no effect on hearing preservation.[11,12,18] However, other studies have demonstrated tumor size predicts hearing preservation after SRS.[6,9,19] Carlson et al. showed a 2.4-fold increased risk of progression to nonserviceable hearing in tumors that contacted the brainstem compared to smaller tumors.[6]

Hearing decline after SRS is strongly associated with radiation dose delivered to the cochlea. As a result, the volume and location of tumor within the internal auditory canal (IAC) will largely determine the amount of radiation the cochlea will receive. Massager et al. evaluated the effects of intracanalicular tumor volume on hearing preservation in 82 patients treated with 12 Gy at the 50% isodose line. The authors demonstrated that intracanalicular tumor volume and radiation dose were predictive of hearing preservation. Patients with preserved hearing had a mean tumor volume of 136.16 mm^3 (range of 0–556 mm^3) compared to a mean tumor volume of 220.01 mm^3 (range of 46.5–555 mm^3) in patients who demonstrated hearing decline. The authors conclude SRS delivered with an intracanalicular volume of greater than 100 mm^3 has a 3.5-fold rate of hearing degradation when compared to tumor volumes less than 100 mm^3. In this study, total tumor volume did not predict hearing preservation.[18]

Niranjan et al. analyzed hearing preservation in 15 patients with purely intracanalicular tumors and serviceable hearing, with a median follow-up of 33 months (range, 9–65 months). At last follow-up, 73% maintained serviceable hearing after SRS. Use of 4-mm collimators and a tumor diameter less than 4 mm was associated with improved hearing preservation. Position of the tumor within the IAC and tumor length did not correlate with maintenance of hearing. Patients who received ≤ 14 Gy to the tumor margin also had better hearing outcomes.[20]

The natural history of hearing loss in relation to tumor growth is controversial. Hajioff et al. followed up 72 patients for a median of 10 years. The majority of patients had tumor growth of less than 1 mm/year. Forty patients had audiometric data and all showed some degree of hearing decline with no correlation to tumor growth.[21] In contrast, an institutional review and a systematic analysis by Sughrue et al. showed that tumor growth rate was inversely correlated with hearing preservation. Specifically, 75% of patients with tumor growth less than 2.5 mm/year maintained functional hearing at the time of last follow-up, while only 32% of patients with tumor growth greater than 2.5 mm/year had preserved hearing.[22,23] The poor correlation between tumor growth and hearing status implies that other factors may be involved. One factor is whether or not tumors secrete cytokines that may influence the health of the cochlea or cochlear nerve. Using a cytokine microarray from surgically excised tumor specimens, high levels of fibroblast growth factor 2 (FGF2) corresponded to a 3.5-fold higher rate of better hearing.[24] Biomarkers, like FGF2, may someday help us predict the natural course of hearing. Another factor for hearing loss may be the buildup of proteinaceous material within the cochlea or CSF fundal cap. Three-dimensional fluid-attenuated inversion recovery (FLAIR) magnetic resonance imaging has the ability to detect increased protein concentrations within the cochlea perilymph. An increased FLAIR signal within the cochlea has been correlated with worse hearing in VS, as well as other disease processes such as sudden idiopathic sensorineural hearing loss, Ramsay Hunt syndrome, and radiation toxicity.[25,26,27,28,29]

Tumor swelling after radiation treatment may also have an effect on hearing decline. Nearly 50% of VS will have at least 1 mm of mean diameter expansion after radiation and 17% will have greater than 2 mm of expansion.[30] This posttreatment edema is often transient, although delayed cyst formation may have a more refractory course.[30,31] Kim et al. showed more hearing deterioration in patients who demonstrated ≥ 20% tumor enlargement after radiosurgery.[32] It is unclear whether

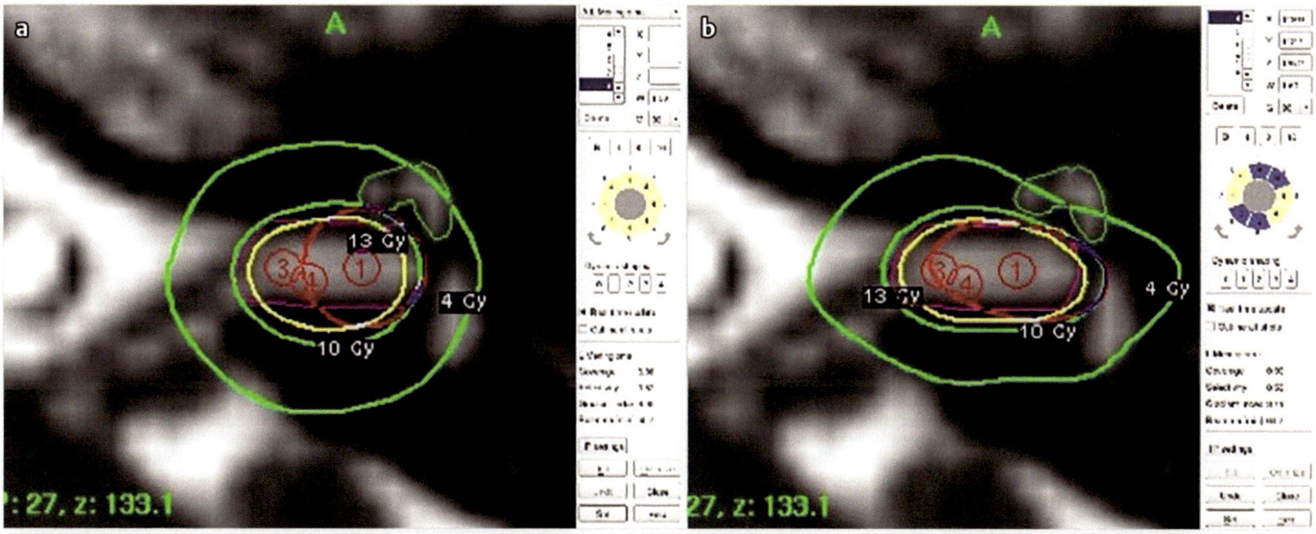

Fig. 52.1 Cochlear shield technique limits cochlear radiation dose during treatment of a left vestibular schwannoma of the internal auditory canal (IAC). In these axial MRI images, the cochlea is highlighted in green anterior to the IAC. (**a**) Gamma Knife treatment plan prior to cochlear shielding shows the majority of the cochlea receiving greater than 4 Gy of radiation. The inset shows no blockage of the Gamma Knife beams. (**b**) Gamma Knife treatment plan after cochlear shielding with the majority of the cochlea receiving less than 4 Gy of radiation. The inset shows blockage of the beams that would pass through the cochlea.

transient tumoral edema causes hearing deterioration through acute compression or traction of the cochlear nerve or its blood supply, from tumor cytokine release or other unknown factors.

52.4 Radiation-Associated Factors

Ewald initially described the detrimental effects of radiation to the otic capsule on pigeons in 1905.[33,34] As the utilization of external beam radiation for the management of head and neck cancers increased, two patterns of hearing loss became apparent. The early manifestation is serous otitis media with its incipient conductive hearing loss. The later manifestation is progressive sensorineural hearing loss starting 1 to 5 years after treatment, particularly in patients who received higher doses for nasopharyngeal carcinoma.[13,35] Injury to the stria vascularis, hair cells, cochlear nerve cell bodies (spiral ganglion neurons), cochlear nucleus, and the labyrinthine artery are all potential mechanisms for radiation-induced cochleovestibular dysfunction.[36,37] A number of variables have been examined with respect to radiation-induced ototoxicity including dose, fractionation, and method of radiation delivery.

52.4.1 Cochlear Dose

A number of studies have demonstrated that cochlear dose is a significant factor in hearing preservation with SRS, while other studies have refuted this claim. Hasegawa and colleagues demonstrated that 5-year post–Gamma Knife treatment hearing preservation was significantly improved from 15 to 50% when cochlear dose was less than 6 Gy.[3] Tamura and colleagues provided an in-depth analysis of 74 patients with pretreatment GR class I hearing. This study demonstrated that doses less than 4 Gy to the modiolus of the cochlea had a statistically significant effect on improved functional hearing preservation. Meanwhile, the mean dose to the total tumor, the mean dose to the intracanalicular tumor, and the number of isocenters had no significant effect on hearing preservation.[10] Kano et al. evaluated the hearing preservation results in 77 patients who had GR class I or II hearing prior to treatment and demonstrated a better outcome when the dose to the central cochlea was less than 4.2 Gy.[9] Several other centers have demonstrated either a statistically significant relationship or trend between cochlear dose and hearing preservation.[11,18,38,39,40,41] Techniques that limit the amount of radiation passing through the cochlea are useful adjuncts to keep the cochlear dose as low as possible (▶ Fig. 52.1).[41] One area of debate is whether one should consider undertreating the lateral tumor margin within the IAC in order to effectively reduce the cochlear dose, a strategy that potentially compromises tumor control with the goal of improved hearing preservation.[41] This approach has been considered because, even with optimal dose planning, the cochlear dose cannot be lowered below 4 Gy in cases that extend to the fundus of the IAC given the properties of SRS dose fall-off.

In contrast to the aforementioned studies, Kim and colleagues did not find evidence that cochlear dose had a statistically significant effect on hearing preservation in 27 patients.[42] Similarly, Mousavi et al. examined 68 patients with GR class I hearing and found that cochlear dose had no significant effect on hearing preservation.[4] Despite an abundance of data that implies causation between cochlear dose and hearing results, some centers continue to dispute the significance of this effect.[32] One possible explanation for differences in conclusions between studies regarding the significance of cochlear dose is the divergent methodology. For example, some studies measure dose to the modiolus, while others evaluate mean or maximum dose to the cochlear volume. Notably, cochlear point dose may exhibit high interobserver variability.[41]

Data on radiation dose to the vestibule are limited. Stavas et al. analyzed 10 patients who underwent treatment with a

Table 52.3 Selected publications documenting hearing preservation outcomes following stereotactic radiosurgery or stereotactic radiotherapy for vestibular schwannoma

Hearing preservation rates after stereotactic radiation								
Author (year)	**Patients**	**Hearing status**	**Radiation modality**	**Marginal dose (Gy)**	**3 y**	**5 y**	**Long term**	**Notes**
Tamura et al. (2009)[10]	74	GR I	SRS	12.0	78%	-	70% (7 y)	Cochlear dose < 4 Gy improved 5-y outcome to 90.9%
Hasegawa et al. (2011)[3]	117	GR I, II	SRS	12.0	55%	43%	34% (8 y)	Cochlear dose < 6 Gy improved 5-y outcome to 50% GR I status improved 3-y (71%) and 5-y (64%) outcomes
Hansasuta et al. (2011)[19]	200	GR I, II	SRT (3 fractions)	18.0	76%	-	-	Tumor volume < 3 cm^3 improved 3-y outcome to 80%
Carlson et al. (2013)[6]	44	AAO–HNS A, B	SRS	12–13	55%	48%	23% (10 y)	Each 10-dB increase in pretreatment hearing loss led to a twofold increase in nonserviceable hearing
Kano et al. (2013)[9]	77	GR I, II	SRS	12.5	71%*	-	-	Cochlear dose <4.2 Gy and GR I predicted better outcome (median follow-up was 20 months)
Kim et al. (2013)[32]	60	GR I, II	SRS	12.2	63%	55%	-	Transient volume expansion > 20% led to a 7.6-fold increase in nonserviceable hearing
Vivas et al. (2013)[54]	28	AAO–HNS A, B	SRT (3 fractions)	18.0	54%	-	-	AAO–HNS class A status improved 3-y outcome to 77%
Mousavi et al. (2016)[5]	166	GR I	SRS	12.5	75%	72%	68% (10 y)	Variations exist even within GR I pretreatment hearing status. No subjective hearing asymmetry or < 10-dB difference improved 5-y outcomes to 100 and 77%, respectively

Abbreviations: AAO–HNS, American Academy of Otolaryngology–Head and Neck Surgery hearing classification (classes A and B represent serviceable hearing); GR, Gardner–Robertson hearing classification (classes I and II represent serviceable hearing); SRS, stereotactic radiosurgery (i.e., Gamma Knife); SRT, stereotactic radiotherapy (i.e., CyberKnife).

linear-accelerator–based system. The mean radiation dose to the vestibule was 10.5 Gy (range, 2.3–19.9 Gy) and was not found to be predictive of posttreatment vestibular function as measured with DHI and electronystagmography.[43]

52.4.2 Type of Radiation Delivery Mechanism (Gamma Knife vs. Linear Accelerator)

Radiation delivery mechanisms can be divided into two categories: (1) a mobile linear accelerator that pivots around a stable target (i.e., BrainLab or CyberKnife) or (2) an immobile radiation source where the patient's position is adjusted on a treatment table relative to the radiation source (i.e., Gamma Knife).

Dutta and colleagues compared treatment plans in seven VS patients using the BrainLab LINAC system and the Cyberknife robotic radiosurgery system. The Cyberknife appeared to have a statistically significantly lower cochlear dose when compared to the BrainLab system (5.4 vs. 6.9 Gy, $p = 0.001$).[44] Gevaert and colleagues compared dosimetry of Gamma Knife Perfexion, CyberKnife, and Novalis in five patients with VS. Conformity and reduced dose to healthy surrounding tissues was best achieved with the Gamma Knife but at the cost of significant dose heterogeneity within the lesion (i.e., hot spots). CyberKnife and Novalis achieved improved dose homogeneity with the use of inverse planning.[45]

52.4.3 Single Dose versus Fractionation

A number of radiation treatment schedules have been used for the management of VS. These schedules can be divided into three broad categories: (1) single fraction treatment (SRS), (2) hypofractionated treatment (SRT), and (3) standard fractionated treatment. Patients undergoing SRT are typically treated in 3 to 10 sessions as opposed to 15 to 30 sessions with standard fractionation. Hearing preservation with radiation treatment for VS was rare with initial introduction of SRS. Advances in treatment planning software, hardware, medical imaging, and most importantly radiation dose reduction have all contributed to improved hearing preservation.

A number of centers have reported improved hearing outcomes using SRT compared to SRS. Movsas et al. summarized six studies that compared SRS to SRT with respect to hearing outcomes.[46] Three of the six studies demonstrated statistically significant improved hearing preservation with standard fractionated radiation as compared to SRS. One study demonstrated a trend toward improved hearing preservation with standard fractionated radiation compared to SRS. The two remaining studies showed no difference. A number of confounding factors were present in each of the six studies including lack of randomization and none were controlled for tumor size, patient age, radiation dose, and fractionation schedule.[47,48,49,50,51,52] One of the studies, which showed no difference in hearing outcomes, used a single question of whether the patient could still use the telephone as a means of assessing hearing.[52] Combs and colleagues analyzed the results of SRS versus SRT in 207 VS patients with serviceable hearing across three centers and demonstrated no difference in hearing preservation between the two techniques according to the GR classification.[53]

A shorter 3-day SRT treatment was reported by Vivas et al. and demonstrated 53.5% hearing preservation rate among 28 patients after 3 years of follow-up.[54] Hansasuta et al. reported serviceable hearing preservation after a median follow-up of 3 years in 151 of 200 (76%) patients treated with a hypofractionated 3-day SRS plan with a total of 18 Gy.[19]

At present, there are no randomized controlled trials comparing SRS to SRT. Study heterogeneity and methodological weaknesses limit any definitive statement on whether SRS or SRT is superior for hearing preservation or tumor control. Hearing preservation data among patients with pretreatment serviceable hearing has been summarized in ▶ Table 52.3.

52.5 Conclusion

The existent literature on audiometric and vestibular outcomes after SRS is fraught with heterogeneity in reporting, variable follow-up, publication bias, and numerous other confounding factors that may influence outcome. Despite these limitations, some predictive factors have been elucidated.

Good pretreatment hearing portends longer retention of serviceable hearing. Mild hearing loss, even if still classified as good hearing, predicts eventual hearing decline. In general, when hearing loss has declined to GR class II or AAO–HNS class B, eventual progression to nonserviceable hearing is anticipated regardless of intervention. The role of radiation versus natural disease course in subsequent hearing decline remains controversial. Tumor burden in the IAC and radiation dose to the cochlea show strong predictive value. The significance of other factors such as age, overall tumor volume, tumor edema after treatment, growth rate, cytokine secretion, and radiation modality are more complex and will require further investigation before summary statements can be made.

References

[1] Committee on Hearing and Equilibrium guidelines for the evaluation of hearing preservation in acoustic neuroma (vestibular schwannoma). American Academy of Otolaryngology-Head and Neck Surgery Foundation, INC. Otolaryngol Head Neck Surg. 1995; 113(3):179–180

[2] Gardner G, Robertson JH. Hearing preservation in unilateral acoustic neuroma surgery. Ann Otol Rhinol Laryngol. 1988; 97(1):55–66

[3] Hasegawa T, Kida Y, Kato T, Iizuka H, Yamamoto T. Factors associated with hearing preservation after Gamma Knife surgery for vestibular schwannomas in patients who retain serviceable hearing. J Neurosurg. 2011; 115(6):1078–1086

[4] Mousavi SH, Kano H, Faraji AH, et al. Hearing preservation up to 3 years after gamma knife radiosurgery for Gardner-Robertson class I patients with vestibular Schwannomas. Neurosurgery. 2015; 76(5):584–590, discussion 590–591

[5] Mousavi SH, Niranjan A, Akpinar B, et al. Hearing subclassification may predict long-term auditory outcomes after radiosurgery for vestibular schwannoma patients with good hearing. J Neurosurg. 2016; 125(4):845–852

[6] Carlson ML, Jacob JT, Pollock BE, et al. Long-term hearing outcomes following stereotactic radiosurgery for vestibular schwannoma: patterns of hearing loss and variables influencing audiometric decline. J Neurosurg. 2013; 118 (3):579–587

[7] Franzin A, Spatola G, Serra C, et al. Evaluation of hearing function after Gamma Knife surgery of vestibular schwannomas. Neurosurg Focus. 2009; 27 (6):E3

[8] Stangerup SE, Thomsen J, Tos M, Cayé-Thomasen P. Long-term hearing preservation in vestibular schwannoma. Otol Neurotol. 2010; 31(2):271–275

[9] Kano H, Kondziolka D, Khan A, Flickinger JC, Lunsford LD. Predictors of hearing preservation after stereotactic radiosurgery for acoustic neuroma: clinical article. J Neurosurg. 2013; 119 Suppl:863–873

[10] Tamura M, Carron R, Yomo S, et al. Hearing preservation after gamma knife radiosurgery for vestibular schwannomas presenting with high-level hearing. Neurosurgery. 2009; 64(2):289–296, discussion 296

[11] Baschnagel AM, Chen PY, Bojrab D, et al. Hearing preservation in patients with vestibular schwannoma treated with Gamma Knife surgery. J Neurosurg. 2013; 118(3):571–578

[12] Yang I, Sughrue ME, Han SJ, et al. A comprehensive analysis of hearing preservation after radiosurgery for vestibular schwannoma. J Neurosurg. 2010; 112 (4):851–859

[13] Thomas C, Di Maio S, Ma R, et al. Hearing preservation following fractionated stereotactic radiotherapy for vestibular schwannomas: prognostic implications of cochlear dose. J Neurosurg. 2007; 107(5):917–926

[14] Agrawal Y, Carey JP, Della Santina CC, Schubert MC, Minor LB. Disorders of balance and vestibular function in US adults: data from the National Health and Nutrition Examination Survey, 2001–2004. Arch Intern Med. 2009; 169 (10):938–944

[15] Bigelow RT, Semenov YR, Trevino C, et al. Association between visuospatial ability and vestibular function in the Baltimore longitudinal study of aging. J Am Geriatr Soc. 2015; 63(9):1837–1844

[16] Carlson ML, Tveiten OV, Driscoll CL, et al. Long-term dizziness handicap in patients with vestibular schwannoma: a multicenter cross-sectional study. Otolaryngol Head Neck Surg. 2014; 151(6):1028–1037

[17] Wackym PA, Hannley MT, Runge-Samuelson CL, Jensen J, Zhu YR. Gamma Knife surgery of vestibular schwannomas: longitudinal changes in vestibular function and measurement of the Dizziness Handicap Inventory. J Neurosurg. 2008; 109 Suppl:137–143

[18] Massager N, Nissim O, Delbrouck C, et al. Role of intracanalicular volumetric and dosimetric parameters on hearing preservation after vestibular schwannoma radiosurgery. Int J Radiat Oncol Biol Phys. 2006; 64(5):1331–1340

[19] Hansasuta A, Choi CYH, Gibbs IC, et al. Multisession stereotactic radiosurgery for vestibular schwannomas: single-institution experience with 383 cases. Neurosurgery. 2011; 69(6):1200–1209

[20] Niranjan A, Mathieu D, Flickinger JC, Kondziolka D, Lunsford LD. Hearing preservation after intracanalicular vestibular schwannoma radiosurgery. Neurosurgery. 2008; 63(6):1054–1062, discussion 1062–1063

[21] Hajioff D, Raut VV, Walsh RM, et al. Conservative management of vestibular schwannomas: third review of a 10-year prospective study. Clin Otolaryngol. 2008; 33(3):255–259

[22] Sughrue ME, Yang I, Aranda D, et al. The natural history of untreated sporadic vestibular schwannomas: a comprehensive review of hearing outcomes. J Neurosurg. 2010; 112(1):163–167

[23] Sughrue ME, Kane AJ, Kaur R, et al. A prospective study of hearing preservation in untreated vestibular schwannomas. J Neurosurg. 2011; 114(2):381–385

[24] Dilwali S, Lysaght A, Roberts D, Barker FG, II, McKenna MJ, Stankovic KM. Sporadic vestibular schwannomas associated with good hearing secrete higher levels of fibroblast growth factor 2 than those associated with poor hearing irrespective of tumor size. Otol Neurotol. 2013; 34(4):748–754

[25] Kim DY, Lee JH, Goh MJ, et al. Clinical significance of an increased cochlear 3D fluid-attenuated inversion recovery signal intensity on an MR imaging examination in patients with acoustic neuroma. AJNR Am J Neuroradiol. 2014; 35(9):1825–1829

[26] Miller ME, Mafee MF, Bykowski J, et al. Hearing preservation and vestibular schwannoma: intracochlear FLAIR signal relates to hearing level. Otol Neurotol. 2014; 35(2):348–352

[27] Yoshida T, Sugiura M, Naganawa S, Teranishi M, Nakata S, Nakashima T. Three-dimensional fluid-attenuated inversion recovery magnetic resonance imaging findings and prognosis in sudden sensorineural hearing loss. Laryngoscope. 2008; 118(8):1433–1437

[28] Sugiura M, Naganawa S, Nakata S, Kojima S, Nakashima T. 3D-FLAIR MRI findings in a patient with Ramsay Hunt syndrome. Acta Otolaryngol. 2007; 127 (5):547–549

[29] Hegarty JL, Patel S, Fischbein N, Jackler RK, Lalwani AK. The value of enhanced magnetic resonance imaging in the evaluation of endocochlear disease. Laryngoscope. 2002; 112(1):8–17

[30] Hasegawa T, Kida Y, Yoshimoto M, Koike J, Goto K. Evaluation of tumor expansion after stereotactic radiosurgery in patients harboring vestibular schwannomas. Neurosurgery. 2006; 58(6):1119–1128, discussion 1119–1128

[31] Hasegawa T, Kida Y, Kato T, Iizuka H, Kuramitsu S, Yamamoto T. Long-term safety and efficacy of stereotactic radiosurgery for vestibular schwannomas: evaluation of 440 patients more than 10 years after treatment with Gamma Knife surgery. J Neurosurg. 2013; 118(3):557–565

[32] Kim YH, Kim DG, Han JH, et al. Hearing outcomes after stereotactic radiosurgery for unilateral intracanalicular vestibular schwannomas: implication of transient volume expansion. Int J Radiat Oncol Biol Phys. 2013; 85(1):61–67

[33] Borsanyi SJ. The effects of radiation therapy on the ear: with particular reference to radiation otitis media. South Med J. 1962; 55:740–743

[34] Borsanyi SJ, Blanchard CL. Ionizing radiation and the ear. JAMA. 1962; 181: 958–961

[35] Kwong DL, Wei WI, Sham JS, et al. Sensorineural hearing loss in patients treated for nasopharyngeal carcinoma: a prospective study of the effect of radiation and cisplatin treatment. Int J Radiat Oncol Biol Phys. 1996; 36(2): 281–289

[36] Gasser Rutledge KL, Prasad KG, Emery KR, Mikulec AA, Varvares M, Gratton MA. Short-term peripheral auditory effects of cranial irradiation: a mouse model. Ann Otol Rhinol Laryngol. 2015; 124(11):903–910

[37] Wackym PA, Runge-Samuelson CL, Nash JJ, et al. Gamma knife surgery of vestibular schwannomas: volumetric dosimetry correlations to hearing loss suggest stria vascularis devascularization as the mechanism of early hearing loss. Otol Neurotol. 2010; 31(9):1480–1487

[38] Timmer FC, Hanssens PE, van Haren AE, et al. Gamma knife radiosurgery for vestibular schwannomas: results of hearing preservation in relation to the cochlear radiation dose. Laryngoscope. 2009; 119(6):1076–1081

[39] Lasak JM, Klish D, Kryzer TC, Hearn C, Gorecki JP, Rine GP. Gamma knife radiosurgery for vestibular schwannoma: early hearing outcomes and evaluation of the cochlear dose. Otol Neurotol. 2008; 29(8):1179–1186

[40] Hayden Gephart MG, Hansasuta A, Balise RR, et al. Cochlea radiation dose correlates with hearing loss after stereotactic radiosurgery of vestibular schwannoma. World Neurosurg. 2013; 80(3–4):359–363

[41] Jacob JT, Carlson ML, Schiefer TK, Pollock BE, Driscoll CL, Link MJ. Significance of cochlear dose in the radiosurgical treatment of vestibular schwannoma: controversies and unanswered questions. Neurosurgery. 2014; 74(5):466–474, discussion 474

[42] Kim CH, Chung KW, Kong DS, et al. Prognostic factors of hearing preservation after gamma knife radiosurgery for vestibular schwannoma. J Clin Neurosci. 2010; 17(2):214–218

[43] Stavas MJ, Carlson ML, Attia A. Does radiation does to the vestibular predict change in balance function and patient perceived dizziness following stereotactic radiotherapy for vestibular schwannoma. Am J Otolaryngol Head Neck Surg. 2014; 35:565–571

[44] Dutta D, Balaji Subramanian S, Murli V, Sudahar H, Gopalakrishna Kurup PG, Potharaju M. Dosimetric comparison of Linac-based (BrainLAB®) and robotic radiosurgery (CyberKnife ®) stereotactic system plans for acoustic schwannoma. J Neurooncol. 2012; 106(3):637–642

[45] Gevaert T, Levivier M, Lacornerie T, et al. Dosimetric comparison of different treatment modalities for stereotactic radiosurgery of arteriovenous malformations and acoustic neuromas. Radiother Oncol. 2013; 106(2):192–197

[46] Movsas S, Hefferly M, Movsas B, Shafiro V. An audiological analysis of stereotactic radiation strategies to preserve hearing in patients with vestibular schwannomas. J Radiosurg SBRT. 2014; 3(1):13–20

[47] Fong BM, Pezeshkian P, Nagasawa DT, De Salles A, Gopen Q, Yang I. Hearing preservation after LINAC radiosurgery and LINAC radiotherapy for vestibular schwannoma. J Clin Neurosci. 2012; 19(8):1065–1070

[48] Andrews DW, Suarez O, Goldman HW, et al. Stereotactic radiosurgery and fractionated stereotactic radiotherapy for the treatment of acoustic schwannomas: comparative observations of 125 patients treated at one institution. Int J Radiat Oncol Biol Phys. 2001; 50(5):1265–1278

[49] Collen C, Ampe B, Gevaert T, et al. Single fraction versus fractionated Linac-based stereotactic radiotherapy for vestibular schwannoma: a single-institution experience. Int J Radiat Oncol Biol Phys. 2011; 81(4):e503–e509

[50] Combs SE, Welzel T, Kessel K, et al. Hearing preservation after radiotherapy for vestibular schwannomas is comparable to hearing deterioration in healthy adults and is accompanied by local tumor control and a highly preserved quality of life (QOL) as patients' self-reported outcome. Radiother Oncol. 2013; 106(2):175–180

[51] Kopp C, Fauser C, Müller A, et al. Stereotactic fractionated radiotherapy and LINAC radiosurgery in the treatment of vestibular schwannoma-report about both stereotactic methods from a single institution. Int J Radiat Oncol Biol Phys. 2011; 80(5):1485–1491

[52] Meijer OW, Vandertop WP, Baayen JC, Slotman BJ. Single-fraction vs. fractionated Linac-based stereotactic radiosurgery for vestibular schwannoma: a single-institution study. Int J Radiat Oncol Biol Phys. 2003; 56(5):1390–1396

[53] Combs SE, Engelhard C, Kopp C, et al. Long-term outcome after highly advanced single-dose or fractionated radiotherapy in patients with vestibular schwannomas - pooled results from 3 large German centers. Radiother Oncol. 2015; 114(3):378–383

[54] Vivas EX, Wegner R, Conley G, et al. Treatment outcomes in patients treated with CyberKnife radiosurgery for vestibular schwannoma. Otol Neurotol. 2014; 35(1):162–170

53 Results of Hearing Preservation Microsurgery for Sporadic Vestibular Schwannoma

Sameer Ahmed and H. Alexander Arts

53.1 Introduction

The three main benchmarks for evaluating treatment outcomes for vestibular schwannoma (VS) are facial nerve function, tumor control, and hearing preservation. The first two outcomes take precedence and are discussed elsewhere in this book. Of the three classic approaches to VS microsurgery, the retrosigmoid/suboccipital (RS/SO) and middle cranial fossa approaches (MCF) are the two that confer the possibility of hearing preservation while the translabyrinthine approach inherently eliminates this possibility. The widespread use of magnetic resonance imaging (MRI) has resulted in the diagnosis of VS much earlier than in the past, and now patients with excellent hearing routinely present for treatment. In these cases—patients with smaller tumors and good hearing—hearing preservation has become a realistic treatment goal.

A critical analysis of the hearing preservation literature is challenged by inconsistent reporting of pre- and postoperative hearing levels, tumor size, variable inclusion criteria, treatment selection biases, heterogeneous study populations, and limited or inconsistent follow-up. The Committee on Hearing and Equilibrium from the American Academy of Otolaryngology—Head and Neck Surgery (AAO–HNS) adopted a standard for reporting hearing outcomes in 1995, but there were obvious shortcomings even with this original consensus guideline which ultimately led to the latest modification by the academy in 2012.[1,2] Although this recently modified standard for reporting should help provide uniformity in future clinical studies, it cannot be readily applied to the older literature since the raw data on individual subjects are typically unavailable in most of these studies. Thus, for the purpose of comparing literature in this chapter, the AAO–HNS classification scheme from 1995 will be utilized as often as possible when discussing the results of prior studies.

The primary objective of the current chapter is to review hearing preservation outcomes—short-term and long-term—in patients who have undergone attempted hearing preservation microsurgery with either the RS/SO or MCF approach for sporadic VS. The secondary objective is to examine preoperative and intraoperative factors that influence hearing outcomes in hearing preservation surgery. Hearing outcomes with conservative management and radiation therapy are described separately, in Chapters 51 and 52, respectively.

53.2 Terminology in Hearing Outcome Data

Patients may have unchanged, worse, or, rarely, better hearing after microsurgical resection. One of the confusing aspects in the hearing preservation literature is the usage of different phrases to describe the hearing status of patients. It is not uncommon in the literature for hearing outcomes to be described by ambiguous terms, such as “good hearing,” “useful hearing,” or “functional hearing,” with definitions that vary according to different authors. In 1984, Wade and House described “serviceable hearing” as a pure-tone average (PTA) less than or equal to 50 dB and a word recognition score (WRS) as greater than or equal to 50%.[3] This became known as the “50/50 rule” when assessing the hearing status of patients prior to pursuing a hearing preservation surgical intervention. As the name “serviceable hearing” suggests, patients within this category could potentially benefit from amplification. In 1995, the AAO–HNS took this into account when creating a four-tiered classification scheme for evaluating hearing status in patients with VSs.[1] Specifically, the 1995 AAO-HNS VS reporting guidelines divided hearing status into the following four classes:

- *Class A*: PTA ≤ 30 dB and WRS ≥ 70%.
- *Class B*: PTA > 30 dB and ≤ 50 dB and WRS ≥ 50%.
- *Class C*: PTA > 50 dB and WRS ≥ 50%.
- *Class D*: PTA any level and WRS < 50%.

Thus, patients with class A or class B hearing are considered to have “serviceable hearing” and patients in classes C and D have “nonserviceable hearing.” However, it is conceivable that patients in class C could also benefit from amplification if their word recognition scores are high enough. Clearly, the value of any retained hearing is also strongly influenced by the status of the hearing in the contralateral ear.

The phrase “measurable hearing” is also vague and is defined differently by different authors.[4,5] In most settings, “measurable hearing” entails nonserviceable hearing with PTA scores that are quantifiable according to the upper output limits of commercial audiometers (i.e., < 125 dB HL), along with a word recognition score of any value. In particular situations, “measurable hearing” that is not serviceable may still be very valuable to the patient, for example, preservation of class D hearing in the only hearing ear.

The degree of hearing preservation is exceedingly important to decipher from each study. Some studies are cleverly worded to embellish results and conclusions. For example, the percentage of patients who obtained “serviceable hearing” postoperatively reflects a different degree of hearing preservation when compared to a study that examined “measurable hearing” as its criterion for hearing preservation. Thus, the phrase “hearing preservation” must be analyzed carefully before drawing conclusions. In this chapter, the focus is on preserving *serviceable hearing*, which is categorized as class A or B hearing according to the 1995 AAO–HNS scale. This method of categorization was used to summarize the existent literature, since the 2012 AAO–HNS guidelines have only been in place for the last 6 years. This cut point is essentially equivalent to grade I or II hearing in the Gardner–Robertson scale. Further discussion regarding hearing outcome reporting guidelines can be found in Chapter 50.

53.3 Short-Term Hearing Results after the Middle Cranial Fossa Approach

In 1961, William F. House presented the middle fossa craniotomy technique to expose the contents of the internal auditory canal as his thesis to the Triologic Society.[6] Since then, multiple surgical groups have employed the MCF approach to resect VSs and preserve hearing. Successful hearing preservation using this approach has varied widely from 20 to 85%.[5,7,8,9,10,11,12,13,14,15,16,17] However, inconsistent study parameters in these reports make it incredibly challenging to compare hearing outcome data from one study to that of the next. The relevant studies along with key study criteria have been listed in ▶ Table 53.1. Some of these studies have been discussed further below.

Wade and House published their experience with the MCF technique from 1975 to 1979.[3] Out of approximately 300 patients operated for VS resection, 20 patients underwent a MCF approach with the intent of hearing preservation. In this article, the authors proposed the "50/50 rule" as the definition of serviceable hearing. From their experience, they also identified the ideal candidate as one who has a PTA of ≤ 30 dB and a WRS ≥ 70% (i.e., AAO–HNS class A) along with a tumor that is less than 1.5 cm in its maximal dimension. All 20 patients in their study had "serviceable hearing" (class A or B) preoperatively and 17 of the 20 met the proposed ideal criteria. The average tumor size was 13 mm. Of these 20 patients, 6 patients retained serviceable hearing postoperatively (30%). One patient had class C hearing postoperatively and the other 13 patients had no measurable hearing postoperatively.

In 1998, Irving et al compared the hearing results for patients who underwent either the MCF approach or RS approach for similar size VSs over a 9-year period of time.[18] In addition to being divided by surgical approach, hearing outcome data were stratified by tumor size into the following categories: intracanalicular, 1 to 10 mm of cerebellopontine angle (CPA) extension, and 11 to 20 mm of CPA extension. The CPA component was determined from the axial MRI that demonstrated the tumor's maximum diameter parallel to the petrous ridge and the maximum diameter perpendicular to the petrous ridge. Most of the patients in both surgical groups had serviceable hearing (class

Table 53.1 Hearing results after middle cranial fossa approach for vestibular schwannoma resection

Authors (year)	Study time range	No. of patients	Average tumor size	Serviceable hearing preservation rate (%)
Wade and House (1984)	1975–1979	20	13 mm	30
Dornhoffer et al (1995)	1987–1992	93	Not disclosed[a]	58
Weber and Gantz, 1996	1986–1993	43	Not disclosed[b]	50
Arriaga et al (1997)	1989–1996	34	7.2 mm	73[c]
Hecht et al (1997)	1981–1995	18	7.4 mm	39
Slattery et al (1997)	1993–1995	135	12 mm	55
Ishikawa et al (1998)	Not disclosed	39	Not disclosed	44[d]
Irving et al (1998)	1989–1996	48	Intracanalicular CPA ext. 1–10 mm CPA ext. 10–20 mm	46 70 20
Kanzaki et al (1998)	1992–1998	94	6.9 mm[e]	24
Staecker et al (2000)	1996–1998	17	11 mm	65
Kumon et al (2000)	1988–1997	36	Not disclosed	53[d]
Brackmann et al (2000)	1992–1998	333	11.2 mm	63
Gjurić et al (2001)	1975–1998	735	Intracanalicular CPA ext. 1–10 mm CPA ext. 10–20 mm CPA ext. > 20 mm	61 49 28 20
Meyer et al (2006)	1993–2004	162	< 10 mm 10–14 mm > 15 mm	66 46 44
Arts et al (2006)	1999–2005	73	8.9 mm[f] > 10 mm	73 58
Kutz et al (2012)	1998–2008	46	8.3 mm > 10 mm	63[g] 25

Notes: The results are not directly comparable because of variations in tumor size, tumor measurements, and levels of preoperative hearing.
[a]Most patients in this study had tumors with less than 5 mm of extrameatal extension.
[b]Average tumor size not disclosed in this study. The majority of their patients had intracanalicular tumors or tumors with less than 5 mm of extrameatal extension. This study also used speech-reception threshold (SRT) instead of pure-tone average (PTA).
[c]Arriaga et al did not use PTA in their analysis of AAO–HNS classification. They used SRT, which is often lower/better than PTA.
[d]Ishikawa et al and Kumon et al had significantly poor facial nerve outcomes, in relation to other studies.
[e]Kanzaki et al defined intracanalicular tumors as being 0 mm in size; they essentially measured extrameatal extension.
[f]Overall average tumor size was 8.9 mm and overall serviceable hearing preservation rate was 73%.
[g]The overall average tumor size was 8.3 mm with an associated serviceable hearing preservation rate of 63%. When tumors were noted to be greater than 10 mm in size, the serviceable hearing preservation rate was 25%.

A or B) preoperatively. In the intracanalicular group, 46% of the MCF patients preserved serviceable hearing, while only 13% of the RS patients preserved serviceable hearing. In the group with minimal CPA extension (1–10 mm), 70% of the MCF patients preserved serviceable hearing, while only 27% of the RS cohort preserved serviceable hearing. In the group with larger CPA extension (11–20 mm), 20% of the MCF patients preserved serviceable hearing and 13% of the RS patients preserved serviceable hearing. However, the sample size in this "larger CPA extension" group was too small to make meaningful conclusions. The authors supported using the MCF approach over the RS approach for intracanalicular tumors and for tumors with a CPA component measuring 10 mm or less. Of note, facial nerve function was noticeably worse in the MCF group immediately after surgery. However, after 1 year, the facial nerve function results were similar for both groups.

Brackmann et al published a more extensive dataset in 2000 that reviewed 333 patients operated via a MCF approach at the House Ear Institute from 1992 to 1998.[4] In this study, patients with neurofibromatosis type 2 (NF2) were excluded. The mean tumor size was 11.2 mm. One important classification they clarified in their study was the difference between "measurable hearing" and "no measurable hearing." "Measurable hearing" was defined as a PTA ≤ 90 dB and any WRS. "No measurable hearing" was defined as a PTA greater than 90 dB and any WRS. Three-hundred of the 333 patients had class A or B hearing preoperatively. Postoperatively, 188 patients preserved class A or B hearing, providing a 63% overall rate of serviceable hearing preservation. Fifty percent of patients preserved their hearing at or near their preoperative baseline levels, which was defined as a change within 15 dB of their preoperative PTA and within 15% of their preoperative WRS. Eight patients improved from class C or D to class A or B. Overall, 5% improved their hearing classification, which included patients who improved from classes D to C and those who improved from classes B to A. Seventy-six percent of patients had some degree of measurable hearing postoperatively.

In 2001, Gjurić et al from Germany published their experience with the MCF approach over a 23-year period (1975–1998).[13] Seven hundred thirty-five patients were included in this study. Twenty-two percent had intracanalicular tumors, 42% had tumors with less than 1 cm of extension into the CPA, 29% had tumors with 1 to 1.9 cm of extension into the CPA, and 7% had greater than 2 cm of extension into the CPA. Of the patients with preoperative serviceable hearing and intracanalicular tumors, 61% maintained serviceable hearing after surgery. Two patients improved from class C or D to class A or B. The authors demonstrated that as tumor size increases, the rate of serviceable hearing preservation decreases (see ▶ Table 53.1). In addition, none of their patients with tumors that extended 1.0 cm or greater into the CPA demonstrated improvement of hearing from the class C or D stage to class A or B. The authors advocated for early diagnosis and treatment because the best outcomes are seen in patients with smaller tumors and better preoperative hearing status.

In 2006, Meyer et al published their results on 162 patients who underwent the MCF approach for VS resection with the intent of hearing preservation.[19] These surgeries were performed over the course of 11 years (1993–2004); the latter portion of their study involved direct cochlear nerve action potential (CAP) monitoring. Patients with NF2 were excluded. The majority of their patients had serviceable hearing preoperatively, and after surgery 57% maintained serviceable hearing. One of the important features of this study was the analysis of hearing outcome data as a function of tumor size, as shown in ▶ Table 53.1. Their data demonstrated improved hearing preservation results with CAP monitoring and smaller tumors.

In 2006, Arts et al reported their results on 73 consecutive patients who underwent the MCF approach for VS resection over a span of 6 years (1999–2005), including three patients with NF2.[20] The mean tumor size was 8.9 mm with a range between 3 and 18 mm and the vast majority of patients had serviceable hearing preoperatively. Postoperatively, 73% of patients maintained serviceable hearing. Interestingly, none of their patients improved their hearing status from class C or D to class A or B and as tumor size increased beyond 8 mm, hearing outcomes noticeably declined.

53.4 Short-Term Hearing Results after the Retrosigmoid Approach

In 1954, Elliott and McKissock were the first to report successful hearing preservation after VS surgery in three patients, all performed via a RS/SO approach.[21] Although they did not describe the level of hearing pre- or postoperatively, this marked the inauguration of hearing preservation surgery. Since this time, reported hearing preservation rates utilizing the retrosigmoid approach have ranged between 0 and 58%.[8,22,23,24,25,26,27,28,29] However, as with the MCF literature, there is great variability in outcome reporting and in what constitutes hearing preservation. ▶ Table 53.2 summarizes the pertinent studies that investigated hearing preservation via the RS approach. A few of these studies have been selected for more detailed discussion.

In 1984, Harner et al reported their results on 149 patients (151 ears) with the RS approach including 119 patients who had at least measurable hearing preoperatively.[22] Postoperatively, 7% of their patients had serviceable hearing. Their study does not allow one to make a comment on hearing preservation success, as the preoperative hearing status for the 119 patients was not detailed. In 1984, Ojemann et al examined 22 patients who underwent the RS approach for tumor resection and hearing preservation. Of the 20 patients with serviceable hearing preoperatively, 6 retained serviceable hearing following surgery, providing a 30% rate of serviceable hearing preservation. Of note, this study utilized only WRS and did not include PTA in evaluating hearing outcomes.[30] Gardner and Robertson performed a thorough literature search in the late 1980s and discovered 17 articles that reviewed a total of 621 operated cases.[31] However, there were only 394 patients for whom pre- and postoperative audiometry was documented. Of these, 131 patients had preserved hearing after surgery, providing a 33% rate of measurable hearing preservation.

In 1990, Kemink et al reported their results on 20 patients who underwent hearing preservation RS surgery. One of their patients underwent planned subtotal resection, one had non-serviceable hearing prior to surgery, and three other patients had NF2. Of the remaining 15 sporadic VS with preoperative serviceable, 9 retained serviceable hearing postoperatively

Table 53.2 Hearing results after retrosigmoid approach for vestibular schwannoma resection

Authors (year)	Study time range	No. of patients	Average tumor size	Serviceable hearing preservation rate (%)
Janetta et al (1984)	Not disclosed	9	15 mm	33[a]
Ojemann et al (1984)	1977–1982	22	19.5 mm	30[b]
Palva et al (1985)	1978–1982	30	Not disclosed	30[a]
Sanna et al (1987)	1975–1986	14	Not disclosed	0
Kemink et al (1990)	1985–1989	15[c]	14 mm	60
Fischer et al (1992)	1970–1989	99	20–29 mm[d]	5
			≥ 30 mm	10
			Overall	12
Cohen et al (1993)	1974–1991	146	15–19 mm[e]	19
			20–24 mm	0
			25–29 mm	0
			≥ 30 mm	8
			Overall	21
Post et al (1995)	Not disclosed	46[f]	< 10 mm[e]	83
			10–20 mm	44
			20–30 mm	20
			> 30 mm	25
			Overall	39
Arriaga et al (1997)	1989–1996	26	15–19 mm[d]	70
			20–24 mm	25
			25–29 mm	50 (*n* = 1)
			≥ 30 mm	50 (*n* = 1)
Samii and Matthies (1997)[g]	1978–1993	880 patients (1,000 ears/tumors)	T1[h]	29
			T2	37
			T3	25
			T4	5
Irving et al (1998)	1987–1995	50	Intracanalicular	13
			CPA ext. 1–10 mm	27
			CPA ext. 10–20 mm	13
Moffat et al (1999)	Not disclosed	50	5–24 mm[d]	5
			25–34 mm	17
			35–44 mm	0
			≥ 45 mm	0
			Overall	8
Kumon et al (2000)	1988–1997	14	Not disclosed	57
Yates et al (2003)	1984–2001	64	15–19 mm[e]	18
			20–24 mm	4
			25–29 mm	0
			≥ 30 mm	0
			Overall	6
Danner et al (2004)	1992–2002	86	≤ 10 mm	45
			> 10 to < 15 mm	45
			≥ 15 to < 20 mm	18
			≥ 20 to ≤ 25 mm	11
			> 25 mm	0

Note: The results are not directly comparable because of variations in tumor size, tumor measurements, and levels of preoperative hearing.

[a]The hearing preservation rates for these studies actually refer to the percentages of patients who the authors believed had "useful hearing" preserved. However, no definition of "useful hearing" was provided in these studies.

[b]The word recognition score was used in classifying the hearing status for these patients. Pure-tone average was not calculated.

[c]In the study of Kemink et al, 20 patients were included in their study, but 3 of them had NF2; 1 patient underwent a planned subtotal resection; and 1 patient had measurable hearing that was not serviceable preoperatively. This left 15 patients with serviceable hearing who underwent RS surgery with the intention of hearing preservation and total tumor resection for sporadic vestibular schwannoma.

[d]These studies reported tumor size in terms of the CPA component and intracanalicular component added together.

[e]These studies reported tumor size in terms of the CPA component only. Thus, these tumor dimensions do not include the intracanalicular component.

[f]In this study, 46 patients had serviceable hearing preoperatively and 10 patients had measurable hearing that was not serviceable preoperatively.

[g]This study has significant limitations in terms of audiometric workup of patients preoperatively and postoperatively (refer to the chapter text for more detail).

[h]New Hannover classification for tumor extension: T1, purely intrameatal; T2, intrameatal and extrameatal; T3a, filling the cerebellopontine cistern; T3b, reaching the brain stem; T4a, compressing the brain stem; T4b, severely dislocating the brain stem and compressing the fourth ventricle.

[i]At times, the rate of serviceable hearing preservation appears high simply because of the low sample size in a particular patient distribution. For these instances, we have included the number of patients next to the percentage in the serviceable hearing preservation column. For example, in the study of Arriaga et al, 50% of the patients with tumors ≥ 30 mm had serviceable hearing preservation. However, the data demonstrate that this occurred in only one of two patients.

providing a 60% rate of serviceable hearing preservation. They noticed that neither serviceable nor measurable hearing was preserved in patients with tumors 1.5 cm or larger.[25]

In 1995, Post et al reported their results on 56 patients who underwent the RS approach with the intention of total tumor resection and hearing preservation.[27] Tumors were measured in terms of their extrameatal extension into the CPA and the intracanalicular portion of the tumor was intentionally not measured. Forty-six patients had serviceable hearing preoperatively and 41% retained serviceable hearing after surgery. Notably, in patients who had serviceable hearing and tumors smaller than 1 cm, the rate of serviceable hearing preservation was 83% (5 out of 6 patients). If the tumor was less than 2 cm, the authors maintained serviceable hearing in 52% of patients (16 out of 31 patients). Finally, when the extrameatal component was greater than 2 cm, the rate of serviceable hearing preservation was 21% (3 out of 14 patients).

In 1997, Samii and Matthies published their results using the RS approach in 1,000 VS resections including 880 patients with sporadic VSs and 82 with NF2.[29] Of these 1,000 tumors, 268 ears were profoundly deaf prior to surgery and 732 ears had at least some measurable hearing preoperatively. Of these 732 ears, 289 had some degree of measurable hearing preserved postoperatively (40% rate of measurable hearing preservation). Of these 289 ears with measurable hearing postoperatively, 140 had enough hearing data to be classified by the 1995 AAO–HNS criteria. Within this subgroup, 56 retained class A or B postoperatively, conferring a 40% rate of serviceable hearing. Although this study has one of the largest patient populations in the hearing preservation literature, its lack of thoroughly evaluating pre- and postoperative hearing status of patients makes it very difficult to utilize and compare their results to those of other studies. In particular, the single most obvious deficiency is the lack of adequate WRS data. Only 76% of patients had preoperative WRS reported. Postoperatively, WRS data were available in only 50% of patients who had "some hearing" after surgery.

To investigate the chance of preserving hearing in patients who have serviceable hearing but also have medium to large tumors, Yates et al performed at retrospective study in 2003. They examined 64 of their patients who had serviceable hearing and underwent the RS approach to resect tumors that were at least 15 mm in size in the CPA. Overall, they had a 6% rate of serviceable hearing preservation. Tumors in which the CPA component measured 15 to 19 mm in size had a 17.6% chance of serviceable hearing preservation. As tumor size increased, the rate of serviceable hearing preservation declined and was 0% for patients who had tumors 25 mm and larger.[32]

53.5 Long-Term Hearing Results after Hearing Preservation Microsurgery

Patients who undergo microsurgery and successfully preserve their hearing immediately postoperatively are at risk for losing residual hearing over time. This phenomenon, known as delayed hearing loss, occurs in patients who undergo the MCF or RS approach and must be separated from progressive sensorineural hearing loss, which can be seen in the nonoperated ear in some patients from presbycusis or other causes. Although the pattern of delayed hearing loss can be in the form of a sudden stepwise loss, the pattern is usually a gradual decline of auditory function. In 1990, Shelton et al described this in detail for a patient who demonstrated gradual hearing loss in the operated ear on serial audiograms while maintaining normal hearing in her nonoperated ear over the course of follow-up.[33]

The exact mechanism driving delayed hearing loss remains unknown; however, several hypotheses have been put forward. Tumor recurrence with compression or invasion of the cochlear nerve is an obvious cause of delayed hearing loss. Temporal bone histopathologic analysis by Linthicum et al and Neely demonstrated rests of tumor cells in the internal auditory canals and cochlear nerves in patients who had previously undergone the MCF approach.[34,35] Scar formation in the internal auditory canal is another possible explanation for delayed hearing loss.[33] Some authors attribute better long-term hearing outcomes with packing the internal auditory canal with adipose tissue as opposed to temporalis muscle, which is thought to be more reactive.[36] Belal et al performed a temporal bone study on a patient who had previously undergone successful hearing preservation with a MCF approach. They found increased intracochlear fibrosis and significantly fewer spiral ganglion neurons in the operated ear. Their findings lent credence to the possibility of a vascular insult as the cause for delayed hearing loss.[37] Endolymphatic hydrops could be another cause for delayed hearing loss, as has been previously suggested in patients who undergo the retrosigmoid approach and have their endolymphatic structures traumatized.[38] The data on long-term hearing outcomes with each surgical approach are summarized below.

53.6 Long-Term Hearing Results after the Middle Cranial Fossa Approach

In 1990, Shelton et al reported on the long-term hearing results in 25 patients who underwent the MCF approach at the House Ear Institute, with a mean follow-up duration of 8 years.[36] Immediately after surgery, 17 of their patients had serviceable hearing, which they defined as a WRS ≥ 50% and speech-reception threshold (SRT) ≤ 50 dB; they did not use PTA in the classification of "serviceable hearing." Fourteen of these 17 patients maintained "serviceable hearing" throughout the follow-up period, which gave them an 82% rate of maintaining long-term serviceable hearing. "Significant" hearing loss was defined as an increase in PTA of ≥ 15 dB or a reduction in the WRS of 20% or more. With these criteria, they identified a 56% chance of "significant" delayed hearing loss.[33] In 2003, Friedman et al updated the House Ear Institute experience on long-term hearing results after the MCF approach. Of the 38 patients who had 5-year follow-up audiometric data, 23 were noted to have serviceable hearing immediately after surgery. Of these 23 patients, 16 maintained serviceable hearing after 5 years, providing a 70% rate of maintaining long-term serviceable hearing.[39] In 2010, Woodson et al examined the University of Iowa series of 49 patients who underwent the MCF approach for VS resection and had at least 2 years of postoperative audiometric data.[40] Forty-three patients retained serviceable hearing immediately postoperatively. Of these who had initial successful hearing preservation, 38 (88%) maintained serviceable hearing at last follow-up. Of note, the authors corrected for changes in the contralateral ear to account for patients with progressive sensorineural hearing loss. The authors advocated for placing greater emphasis on WRS instead of PTA, given its greater contribution to functional hearing. They found that progressive bilateral sensorineural hearing loss observed in many of their long-term subjects affected the AAO–HNS score by elevating the PTA. The WRS, however, was preserved until quite late. Thus, they concluded that WRS was less affected by aging and more accurately represented the hearing outcome related to the surgical intervention.[40]

In 2015, Quist et al examined 27 patients who had serviceable hearing immediately after undergoing the MCF approach for tumor resection.[36] Of these 27 patients, 16 had 5-year follow-up audiometric data. Of these 16 patients, 12 (75%) patients maintained durable serviceable hearing at last follow-up. "Significant" hearing loss, as defined by Shelton et al, was seen in five (31%) patients. In this study, the authors did not correct for loss of hearing in the nonoperated ear.

53.7 Long-Term Hearing Results after the Retrosigmoid Approach

In 1992, McKenna et al examined 18 patients who underwent RS hearing preservation surgery who were followed up for an average of 5.4 years. Notably, the contralateral ear was also considered to control for the possibility of progressive sensorineural hearing loss unrelated to surgery.[41] Fourteen of the 18 patients (78%) did not experience a significant decline in hearing during follow-up, while 4 patients did. The phrase "significant decline in hearing" was defined as ≥ 15 dB PTA or as a significant change in speech discrimination. In 1994, Tucci et al reported 17 patients who had some measurable hearing after RS surgery and had follow-up audiometric data ranging from 1.5 to 8 years.[42] Over this period of time, the PTA worsened by 6 dB on average when compared to the immediate postoperative PTA; however, the WRS remained stable in 15 of 17 patients and the hearing in the contralateral ear remained the same throughout the follow-up period. Of note, three of their patients developed a tumor recurrence and only one of them had a significant change in speech audiometry during follow-up.

In 2003, Chee et al reported their outcomes on patients who underwent the RS approach for tumors ≤ 2 cm within the CPA.[43] Twenty-nine patients had serviceable hearing immediately after surgery and were followed up for an average of approximately 9 years. Hearing changes in the operated ear were compared to hearing changes in the unoperated ear to control for progressive sensorineural hearing loss. None of their patients experienced tumor recurrence. Over the follow-up course, they discovered a 44% rate of delayed hearing loss in their patients, defined as a ≥ 15 dB loss in the PTA or SRT or a "significant" change in the WRS. Their data demonstrated that most cases of delayed hearing loss involved deterioration in PTA or SRT, but only half (6 of 12) of these patients experienced a significant decline in WRS.

53.8 Factors Associated with Hearing Preservation

Several studies within the MCF and RS bodies of literature have examined pre- and intraoperative factors that potentially influence hearing preservation postoperatively. Although conceptually promising, the results have varied significantly for many of the criteria.

Tumor size is most often predictive of the hearing preservation outcome.[18,19,20,32,44,45,46,47,48] Although some studies showed no correlation between tumor size and hearing preservation,[4,11,41] the vast majority of the literature suggests that as tumor size increases (especially around the range of 15 mm and larger), the rate of hearing preservation decreases.

The surgical approach has also been heavily investigated. Although the overall results for the RS approach may seem worse than the MCF approach, one must recall that the RS studies often include significantly larger tumors, which probably is the main reason for the difference in hearing outcomes between the two approaches. Irving et al demonstrated that patients with intracanalicular tumors and tumors with less than 10 mm of extension into the CPA have better hearing outcomes with the MCF approach than with the RS approach.[18] They theorized that disrupting the eighth cranial nerve at the glial–Schwann sheath junction by retracting the cerebellum might be the cause of worsened hearing outcomes with the RS approach.[18,49] Additionally, tumors that extend to the fundus are better visualized with the MCF approach, which improves development of the tumor-arachnoid plane at the fundus. Tumors with lateral extension that are approached via the RS route could necessitate "blind dissection" in the fundus, leading to disruption of the fine filaments of the cochlear nerve within the modiolus, violation of the inner ear (particularly, the posterior semicircular canal), or injury of the distal labyrinthine artery.[14,18] However, those who advocate the RS approach have important counter arguments to consider. Nguyen et al demonstrated that the RS approach achieves excellent and comparable hearing outcome results for patients with serviceable hearing who have intracanalicular tumors.[50] In fact, they obtained better hearing results in patients whose tumors extended to the fundus than in patients whose tumors did not extend to the fundus. They highlight the work of Driscoll et al who analyzed the anatomic limitations of the MCF approach. In particular, the transverse crest and immobility of the facial nerve at the meatal foramen can block a significant portion of the inferior half of the fundus.[51] In the setting of a tumor originating from the inferior vestibular nerve, total tumor resection could very well necessitate "blind dissection" in the inferior fundus with the MCF approach.[50]

Better preoperative hearing (PTA and WRS) has been associated with better postoperative hearing outcomes in some studies[4,19,29,44,47,52] but is unrelated in other studies.[18,41,45,53,54] Brackmann et al pointed out that although there was a statistically significant difference in the preoperative hearing levels in patients who had hearing preserved versus those who lost their hearing, the mean preoperative hearing levels in those patients who lost their hearing was well within the "50/50 rule."[4] Along these lines, preoperative ABR testing has also been thoroughly examined but with mixed results. Slattery et al showed that a preoperative ABR had no responses correlated with a poor hearing outcome. However, a normal ABR did not predict hearing preservation in their study.[11] Brackmann et al demonstrated that intra-aural wave V latencies were significantly lower (0.51 ms) in patients who retained hearing compared to those who did not (0.70 ms). They also demonstrated that the absolute wave V latency was significantly worse in patients who lost hearing (5.96 ms) compared to those who had serviceable hearing (5.41 ms) postoperatively.[4] Dornhoffer et al and Glasscock et al have also shown that a good preoperative ABR confers a favorable hearing outcome.[45,55] However, multiple other studies have not demonstrated any correlation with preoperative ABR results and postoperative hearing outcomes.[47,56] Likewise, preoperative otoacoustic emission testing has been shown to prognosticate hearing outcomes in some studies[57,58,59] but not in others.[4]

Advanced age has been investigated as a potential factor that could influence hearing preservation, but the results have been mixed. The average age of patients who lost hearing postoperatively was not significantly higher than those who retained hearing in some studies.[4,44,56] However, Oghalai et al found that older patients did have a significantly lower chance of serviceable hearing preservation even after accounting for tumor size as a confounding variable. They discovered that the odds of hearing preservation decreases by 4.4% per year over the age of 60 years.[60]

Some studies have demonstrated that hearing is more likely preserved when tumors originate from the superior vestibular nerve.[4,44,54] Tumors that originate from the superior vestibular nerve require less dissection near the cochlear nerve and invade the cochlear nerve at a later stage. In contrast, tumors that originate from the inferior vestibular nerve are in close proximity to the cochlear nerve and are associated with a higher risk of cochlear nerve injury during tumor resection. Identifying the nerve of origin is usually accomplished intraoperatively, but this is often difficult to distinguish with a high degree of accuracy, particularly with larger tumor size. Caloric testing has served as a preoperative test for superior vestibular nerve function, as this nerve supplies the ampulla of the lateral semicircular canal. A hypoactive caloric response may indicate a tumor originating from the superior vestibular nerve or a larger tumor originating from the inferior vestibular nerve. A reduced caloric response has shown to be predictive of a good outcome in some studies[11,54,55] but unrelated in others.[4,45] Other researchers have examined the ability of ocular and cervical vestibular evoked myogenic potential (oVEMP and cVEMP, respectively) testing to predict the nerve of origin. oVEMP testing is thought to assess the utricle and thus serves as a marker for the superior vestibular nerve. cVEMP testing analyzes the saccule, and thus serves as a marker for the inferior vestibular nerve. Although conceptually promising, the data utilizing VEMP testing have not reliably predicted the nerve of origin in VS surgeries.[61,62]

Aside from measuring tumor dimensions, the radiographic evaluation of VS is an important factor when discussing probability of hearing preservation. Regardless of the surgical approach, tumor extension into the fundus is generally regarded by most to be a poor prognostic factor for hearing preservation.[18,47,63] In contrast, Nguyen et al and Phillips et al did not find a relationship with hearing preservation and the extent of tumor involvement within the IAC.[50,64] Overall, however, there is general agreement that tumors in the fundus are harder to resect without putting excessive shearing forces on the cochlear nerve fibers within the modiolus or disrupting the cochlear nerve blood supply. Goddard et al analyzed their MCF data and found that postoperative measurable hearing was obtained more often in patients who had CSF present in the fundus as opposed to tumor impacting the fundus.[65] As for serviceable hearing, their data showed a trend favoring higher serviceable hearing preservation rates in patients who had fundal fluid ("CSF cap"), but their numbers did not reach statistical significance.[65] Other radiographic factors that have demonstrated poorer hearing outcomes include direct tumor extension into the cochlea and a greater degree of extracanalicular contact between the tumor and cochlear nerve.[66,67]

Intraoperative factors associated with hearing preservation have also been examined. As expected, hearing is lost if the cochlear nerve is severed. However, the converse is not necessarily true, as many studies have shown hearing is often lost even when the cochlear nerve is anatomically preserved. In these scenarios, although the cochlear nerve appears grossly intact, there could be intraneural disruption anywhere along the nerve's path, trauma to the fine cochlear nerve filaments within the modiolus, vascular compromise to the inner ear, or violation of the inner ear structures. With regard to vascular compromise, the distal labyrinthine artery is particularly sensitive at its foraminal end, where it has less elasticity and is more susceptible to a traction injury.[18] In addition, manipulation of this artery during dissection can induce vasospasm and result in cochlear ischemia.[68] In an effort to reverse this vasospastic response, Brackmann et al began applying papaverine-soaked Gelfoam pledgets on to the cochlear nerve and modiolus.[69] They attributed improved hearing preservation rates in part to the use of papaverine, which is a potent vasodilator. However, undiluted papaverine has been associated with facial palsy in multiple cases.[20,70,71] The underlying mechanism for this neuropraxic effect is likely from a temporary conduction block affecting the facial nerve.[70,71] In light of this, other authors have advocated the use of diluted papaverine.[11]

Intraoperative ABR is used by many surgical teams utilizing either surgical approach (MCF or RS) for monitoring of hearing function. This is a far-field technique that necessitates averaging of several hundred to several thousand sweeps, which can take minutes to accomplish, and thus does not provide the surgeon with real-time feedback. Kemink et al demonstrated that loss of wave 5 intraoperatively correlated with significant hearing loss postoperatively, whereas persistence of wave V (with a latency prolongation not exceeding 3.00 ms) was predictive of successful hearing preservation.[25] Phillips et al showed that preserving an intraoperative wave V response after tumor resection correlated well to maintaining serviceable hearing preservation. However, they noted that 40% of their patients still had hearing preserved despite losing wave V intraoperatively.[64] Due to the limitations with ABR, some surgical groups routinely utilize direct monitoring of the CAP in order to provide near instantaneous responses and large action potential amplitudes (refer to Chapter 28 for additional details). Their experience and data demonstrate improved hearing outcomes after implementing this form of monitoring.[19,72]

53.9 Conclusion

In the case of sporadic VS, hearing preservation should remain the third rung in the ladder of priorities, with facial nerve function and tumor resection status remaining as the top two priorities. There are numerous studies investigating hearing preservation results with the MCF and RS approaches. The early absence of standards, and more recent inconsistency in adhering to standards with regard to assessing hearing status (pre- and postoperatively) and calculating tumor dimensions significantly, limits the ability to make meaningful comparative statements. Hearing preservation is a loaded term, and we have intentionally focused on "serviceable" hearing preservation in this chapter, as this is generally the minimum useful level for patients. Serviceable hearing preservation is an achievable goal in many patients with the RS or MCF approach. Although some studies have shown hearing improvement after resection of VS, this is quite rare and should not be considered a realistic expectation when counseling patients preoperatively. Multiple preoperative factors and the surgical team's experience should be taken into account when selecting the best hearing preservation approach. Although there are some exceptions, tumor size remains the single most important criterion in assessing the chance for hearing preservation. The large collection of hearing preservation factors is important for the neurotologist and neurosurgeon to understand prior to recommending a hearing preservation endeavor. In addition, understanding the nuances with multiple hearing preservation factors can help counsel patients about the likelihood of realistically preserving their hearing with microsurgery. Surgical teams should be open to utilizing either the MCF or the RS approach, as each approach has distinct advantages and disadvantages, which should be taken into account for the individual patient. Some patients will develop delayed hearing loss after successful hearing preservation surgery, and this phenomenon should be discussed with patients prior to surgery.

References

[1] Committee on Hearing and Equilibrium guidelines for the evaluation of hearing preservation in acoustic neuroma (vestibular schwannoma). American Academy of Otolaryngology-Head and Neck Surgery Foundation, INC. Otolaryngol Head Neck Surg. 1995; 113(3):179–180

[2] Gurgel RK, Jackler RK, Dobie RA, Popelka GR. A new standardized format for reporting hearing outcome in clinical trials. Otolaryngol Head Neck Surg. 2012; 147(5):803–807

[3] Wade PJ, House W. Hearing preservation in patients with acoustic neuromas via the middle fossa approach. Otolaryngol Head Neck Surg. 1984; 92(2): 184–193

[4] Brackmann DE, Owens RM, Friedman RA, et al. Prognostic factors for hearing preservation in vestibular schwannoma surgery. Am J Otol. 2000; 21(3):417–424

[5] Holsinger FC, Coker NJ, Jenkins HA. Hearing preservation in conservation surgery for vestibular schwannoma. Am J Otol. 2000; 21(5):695–700

[6] House WF. Surgical exposure of the internal auditory canal and its contents through the middle, cranial fossa. Laryngoscope. 1961; 71:1363–1385

[7] Hecht CS, Honrubia VF, Wiet RJ, Sims HS. Hearing preservation after acoustic neuroma resection with tumor size used as a clinical prognosticator. Laryngoscope. 1997; 107(8):1122–1126

[8] Sanna M, Zini C, Mazzoni A, et al. Hearing preservation in acoustic neuroma surgery. Middle fossa versus suboccipital approach. Am J Otol. 1987; 8(6): 500–506

[9] Betchen SA, Walsh J, Post KD. Long-term hearing preservation after surgery for vestibular schwannoma. J Neurosurg. 2005; 102(1):6–9

[10] Arriaga MA, Chen DA, Fukushima T. Individualizing hearing preservation in acoustic neuroma surgery. Laryngoscope. 1997; 107(8):1043–1047

[11] Slattery WH, III, Brackmann DE, Hitselberger W. Middle fossa approach for hearing preservation with acoustic neuromas. [erratum appears in Am J Otol 1997 Nov;18(6):796]. Am J Otol. 1997; 18(5):596–601

[12] Staecker H, Nadol JB, Jr, Ojeman R, Ronner S, McKenna MJ. Hearing preservation in acoustic neuroma surgery: middle fossa versus retrosigmoid approach. Am J Otol. 2000; 21(3):399–404

[13] Gjurić M, Wigand ME, Wolf SR. Enlarged middle fossa vestibular schwannoma surgery: experience with 735 cases. Otol Neurotol. 2001; 22(2):223–230, discussion 230–231

[14] Mohr G, Sade B, Dufour JJ, Rappaport JM. Preservation of hearing in patients undergoing microsurgery for vestibular schwannoma: degree of meatal filling. J Neurosurg. 2005; 102(1):1–5

[15] Sanna M, Khrais T, Russo A, Piccirillo E, Augurio A. Hearing preservation surgery in vestibular schwannoma: the hidden truth. Ann Otol Rhinol Laryngol. 2004; 113(2):156–163

[16] Weber PC, Gantz BJ. Results and complications from acoustic neuroma excision via middle cranial fossa approach. Am J Otol. 1996; 17(4):669–675

[17] Colletti V, Fiorino F. Is the middle fossa approach the treatment of choice for intracanalicular vestibular schwannoma? Otolaryngol Head Neck Surg. 2005; 132(3):459–466

[18] Irving RM, Jackler RK, Pitts LH. Hearing preservation in patients undergoing vestibular schwannoma surgery: comparison of middle fossa and retrosigmoid approaches. J Neurosurg. 1998; 88(5):840–845

[19] Meyer TA, Canty PA, Wilkinson EP, Hansen MR, Rubinstein JT, Gantz BJ. Small acoustic neuromas: surgical outcomes versus observation or radiation. Otol Neurotol. 2006; 27(3):380–392

[20] Arts HA, Telian SA, El-Kashlan H, Thompson BG. Hearing preservation and facial nerve outcomes in vestibular schwannoma surgery: results using the middle cranial fossa approach. Otol Neurotol. 2006; 27(2):234–241

[21] Elliott FA, McKissock W. Acoustic neuroma; early diagnosis. Lancet. 1954; 267(6850):1189–1191

[22] Harner SG, Laws ER, Jr, Onofrio BM. Hearing preservation after removal of acoustic neurinoma. Laryngoscope. 1984; 94(11, Pt 1):1431–1434

[23] Glasscock ME, McKennan KX, Levine SC. Acoustic neuroma surgery: the results of hearing conservation surgery. Laryngoscope. 1989

[24] Nadol JB, Jr, Levine R, Ojemann RG, Martuza RL, Montgomery WW, de Sandoval PK. Preservation of hearing in surgical removal of acoustic neuromas of the internal auditory canal and cerebellar pontine angle. Laryngoscope. 1987; 97(11):1287–1294

[25] Kemink JL, LaRouere MJ, Kileny PR, Telian SA, Hoff JT. Hearing preservation following suboccipital removal of acoustic neuromas. Laryngoscope. 1990; 100(6):597–602

[26] Sterkers J-M, Morrison GAJ, Sterkers O, El-Dine MM. Preservation of facial, cochlear, and other nerve functions in acoustic neuroma treatment. Otolaryngol Head Neck Surg. 1994; 110(2):146–155

[27] Post KD, Eisenberg MB, Catalano PJ. Hearing preservation in vestibular schwannoma surgery: what factors influence outcome? J Neurosurg. 1995; 83(2):191–196

[28] Gormley WB, Sekhar LN, Wright DC, Kamerer D, Schessel D. Acoustic neuromas: results of current surgical management. Neurosurgery. 1997; 41(1):50–58, discussion 58–60

[29] Samii M, Matthies C. Management of 1000 vestibular schwannomas (acoustic neuromas): hearing function in 1000 tumor resections. Neurosurgery. 1997; 40(2):248–260, discussion 260–262

[30] Ojemann RG, Levine RA, Montgomery WM, McGaffigan P. Use of intraoperative auditory evoked potentials to preserve hearing in unilateral acoustic neuroma removal. J Neurosurg. 1984; 61(5):938–948

[31] Gardner G, Robertson JH. Hearing preservation in unilateral acoustic neuroma surgery. Ann Otol Rhinol Laryngol. 1988; 97(1):55–66

[32] Yates PD, Jackler RK, Satar B, Pitts LH, Oghalai JS. Is it worthwhile to attempt hearing preservation in larger acoustic neuromas? Otol Neurotol. 2003; 24 (3):460–464

[33] Shelton C, Hitselberger WE, House WF, Brackmann DE. Hearing preservation after acoustic tumor removal: long-term results. Laryngoscope. 1990; 100(2, Pt 1):115–119

[34] Linthicum FH, Jr, Saleh ES, Hitselberger WE, Brackmann DE, Hung G. Growth of postoperative remnants of unilateral vestibular nerve schwannoma: role of the vestibular ganglion. ORL J Otorhinolaryngol Relat Spec. 2002; 64(2): 138–142

[35] Neely JG. Is it possible to totally resect an acoustic tumor and conserve hearing? Otolaryngol Head Neck Surg. 1984; 92(2):162–167

[36] Quist TS, Givens DJ, Gurgel RK, Chamoun R, Shelton C. Hearing preservation after middle fossa vestibular schwannoma removal: are the results durable? Otolaryngol Head Neck Surg. 2015; 152(4):706–711

[37] Belal A, Jr, Linthicum FH, Jr, House WF. Acoustic tumor surgery with preservation of hearing. A histopathologic report. Am J Otol. 1982; 4(1):9–16

[38] Clemis JD, Mastricola PG, Schuler-Vogler M. The contralateral ear in acoustic tumors and hearing conservation. Laryngoscope. 1981; 91(11):1792–1800

[39] Friedman RA, Kesser B, Brackmann DE, Fisher LM, Slattery WH, Hitselberger WE. Long-term hearing preservation after middle fossa removal of vestibular schwannoma. Otolaryngol Head Neck Surg. 2003; 129(6):660–665

[40] Woodson EA, Dempewolf RD, Gubbels SP, et al. Long-term hearing preservation after microsurgical excision of vestibular schwannoma. Otol Neurotol. 2010; 31(7):1144–1152

[41] McKenna MJ, Halpin C, Ojemann RG, et al. Long-term hearing results in patients after surgical removal of acoustic tumors with hearing preservation. Am J Otol. 1992; 13(2):134–136

[42] Tucci DL, Telian SA, Kileny PR, Hoff JT, Kemink JL. Stability of hearing preservation following acoustic neuroma surgery. Am J Otol. 1994; 15(2):183–188

[43] Chee GH, Nedzelski JM, Rowed D. Acoustic neuroma surgery: the results of long-term hearing preservation. Otol Neurotol. 2003; 24(4):672–676

[44] Cohen NL, Lewis WS, Ransohoff J. Hearing preservation in cerebellopontine angle tumor surgery: the NYU experience 1974–1991. Am J Otol. 1993; 14(5):423–433

[45] Dornhoffer JL, Helms J, Hoehmann DH. Hearing preservation in acoustic tumor surgery: results and prognostic factors. Laryngoscope. 1995; 105(2):184–187

[46] Mangham CA, Skalabrin TA. Indications for hearing preservation in acoustic tumor surgery. Am J Otol. 1992; 13(2):137–140

[47] Nadol JB, Jr, Chiong CM, Ojemann RG, et al. Preservation of hearing and facial nerve function in resection of acoustic neuroma. Laryngoscope. 1992; 102 (10):1153–1158

[48] Shelton C. Hearing preservation in acoustic tumor surgery. Otolaryngol Clin North Am. 1992; 25(3):609–621

[49] Sekiya T, Møller AR, Jannetta PJ. Pathophysiological mechanisms of intraoperative and postoperative hearing deficits in cerebellopontine angle surgery: an experimental study. Acta Neurochir (Wien). 1986; 81(3–4):142–151

[50] Nguyen QT, Wu AP, Mastrodimos BJ, Cueva RA. Impact of fundal extension on hearing after surgery for vestibular schwannomas. Otol Neurotol. 2012; 33 (3):455–458

[51] Driscoll CL, Jackler RK, Pitts LH, Banthia V. Is the entire fundus of the internal auditory canal visible during the middle fossa approach for acoustic neuroma? Am J Otol. 2000; 21(3):382–388

[52] Neely JG. Hearing conservation surgery for acoustic tumors–a clinical-pathologic correlative study. Am J Otol. 1985; 6 Suppl:143–146

[53] Josey AF, Glasscock ME, III, Jackson CG. Preservation of hearing in acoustic tumor surgery: audiologic indicators. Ann Otol Rhinol Laryngol. 1988; 97(6, Pt 1):626–630

[54] Shelton C, Brackmann DE, House WF, Hitselberger WE. Acoustic tumor surgery. Prognostic factors in hearing conversation. Arch Otolaryngol Head Neck Surg. 1989; 115(10):1213–1216

[55] Glasscock ME, III, Hays JW, Minor LB, Haynes DS, Carrasco VN. Preservation of hearing in surgery for acoustic neuromas. J Neurosurg. 1993; 78(6):864–870

[56] Fischer G, Fischer C, Rémond J. Hearing preservation in acoustic neurinoma surgery. J Neurosurg. 1992; 76(6):910–917

[57] Telischi FF, Roth J, Stagner BB, Lonsbury-Martin BL, Balkany TJ. Patterns of evoked otoacoustic emissions associated with acoustic neuromas. Laryngoscope. 1995; 105(7, Pt 1):675–682

[58] Ferber-Viart C, Colleaux B, Laoust L, Dubreuil C, Duclaux R. Is the presence of transient evoked otoacoustic emissions in ears with acoustic neuroma significant? Laryngoscope. 1998; 108(4, Pt 1):605–609

[59] Kim AH, Edwards BM, Telian SA, Kileny PR, Arts HA. Transient evoked otoacoustic emissions pattern as a prognostic indicator for hearing preservation in acoustic neuroma surgery. Otol Neurotol. 2006; 27(3): 372–379

[60] Oghalai JS, Buxbaum JL, Pitts LH, Jackler RK. The effect of age on acoustic neuroma surgery outcomes. Otol Neurotol. 2003; 24(3):473–477

[61] Iwasaki S, Murofushi T, Chihara Y, et al. Ocular vestibular evoked myogenic potentials to bone-conducted vibration in vestibular schwannomas. Otol Neurotol. 2010; 31(1):147–152

[62] Ushio M, Iwasaki S, Chihara Y, et al. Is the nerve origin of the vestibular schwannoma correlated with vestibular evoked myogenic potential, caloric test, and auditory brainstem response? Acta Otolaryngol. 2009; 129(10): 1095–1100

[63] MacDonald CB, Hirsch BE, Kamerer DB, Sekhar L. Acoustic neuroma surgery: predictive criteria for hearing preservation. Otolaryngol Head Neck Surg. 1991; 104(1):128

[64] Phillips DJ, Kobylarz EJ, De Peralta ET, Stieg PE, Selesnick SH. Predictive factors of hearing preservation after surgical resection of small vestibular schwannomas. Otol Neurotol. 2010; 31(9):1463–1468

[65] Goddard JC, Schwartz MS, Friedman RA. Fundal fluid as a predictor of hearing preservation in the middle cranial fossa approach for vestibular schwannoma. Otol Neurotol. 2010; 31(7):1128–1134

[66] Somers T, Casselman J, de Ceulaer G, Govaerts P, Offeciers E. Prognostic value of magnetic resonance imaging findings in hearing preservation surgery for vestibular schwannoma. Otol Neurotol. 2001; 22(1):87–94

[67] Yong RL, Westerberg BD, Dong C, Akagami R. Length of tumor-cochlear nerve contact and hearing outcome after surgery for vestibular schwannoma. J Neurosurg. 2008; 108(1):105–110

[68] Ren T, Brown NJ, Zhang M, Nuttall AL, Miller JM. A reversible ischemia model in gerbil cochlea. Hear Res. 1995; 92(1–2):30–37

[69] Brackmann DE, House JR, III, Hitselberger WE. Technical modifications to the middle fossa craniotomy approach in removal of acoustic neuromas. Am J Otol. 1994; 15(5):614–619

[70] Eisenman DJ, Digoy GP, Victor JD, Selesnick SH. Topical papaverine and facial nerve dysfunction in cerebellopontine angle surgery. Am J Otol. 1999; 20(1): 77–80

[71] Liu JK, Sayama CM, Shelton C, MacDonald JD. Transient facial nerve palsy after topical papaverine application during vestibular schwannoma surgery. Case report. J Neurosurg. 2007; 107(5):1039–1042

[72] Danner C, Mastrodimos B, Cueva RA. A comparison of direct eighth nerve monitoring and auditory brainstem response in hearing preservation surgery for vestibular schwannoma. Otol Neurotol. 2004; 25(5):826–832

[73] Kutz JW Jr, Scoresby T, Isaacson B, et al. Hearing preservation using the middle fossa approach for the treatment of vestibular schwannoma. Neurosurgery. 2012;70:334-341

[74] Kumon Y, Sakaki S, Kohno K, et al. Selection of surgical approaches for small acoustic neurinomas. Surg Neurol 2000; 53:52-9

[75] Palva T, Troupp H, Jauhiainen T. Hearing preservation in acoustic neurinoma surgery. Acta Otolaryngol. 1985 Jan-Feb;99(1-2):1-7

[76] Moffat DA, da Cruz MJ, Baguley DM, Beynon GJ, Hardy DG. Hearing preservation in solitary vestibular schwannoma surgery using the retrosigmoid approach. Otolaryngol Head Neck Surg. 1999 Dec;121(6):781-8

54 Reporting of Facial Nerve Outcome Data for Vestibular Schwannoma

Matthew L. Carlson, John P. Marinelli, and Neil S. Patel

54.1 Introduction

In the modern era, facial nerve function, hearing status, and tumor control remain the three primary benchmarks used to assess vestibular schwannoma (VS) outcome. Facial nerve paralysis is associated with significant psychological and functional impairment and reduction in quality of life. The widespread acceptance of a convenient, easily reproducible, and accurate facial nerve grading system is critical to facilitate uniform interpretation and clinical outcome reporting. There have been a number of unique instruments that have been developed; however, the House–Brackmann (HB) facial nerve grading scale stands as the most universally accepted system for reporting facial nerve function following VS treatment and has been invaluable toward standardization of facial nerve outcome reporting in the literature.[1,2] Despite its advantages, several limitations exist and the ideal facial nerve grading system continues to elude clinicians and researchers alike. The observation that at least 19 unique systems have been developed over the last seven decades underscores the importance, complexity, and great difficulty of this task.[3] The objectives of the current chapter are to: (1) provide an overview of functional impairment associated with facial nerve injury; (2) outline the ideal attributes of a facial nerve grading instrument; (3) review the most commonly utilized facial grading systems today including the HB, Facial Nerve Grading Scale 2.0 (FNGS 2.0), and Sunnybrook (SB) systems; and (4) discuss unresolved issues and future direction.

54.2 Facial Nerve Dysfunction following Injury

To understand the workings of facial nerve assessment, it is critical to first review the relevant functions derived from the seventh cranial nerve and the unique set of impairments associated with facial nerve injury (▶ Fig. 54.1). Chiefly, the facial nerve is responsible for special visceral efferent innervation of the 20 ipsilateral muscles of facial expression. In addition, special visceral afferent fibers convey taste from the anterior two-thirds of the tongue, and general visceral efferent pathways supply parasympathetic innervation to the lacrimal, submandibular, and sublingual glands, both via the nervus intermedius. From a practical standpoint, the main categories of impairment following facial nerve injury include early and late motor dysfunction and parasympathetic dysfunction. Within these groupings, "early" refers to immediate loss of function from axonal injury such as reduced facial tone and strength or dry eye, while "late" refers to secondary sequelae associated with aberrant axonal regeneration, such as synkinesis, contracture, or gustatory lacrimation (i.e., crocodile tears). The potential for primary and late sequelae of varying severities, the frequent differential involvement of the five motor divisions of the facial nerve, and varying possibilities of parasympathetic deficits provides an infinite number of permutations a patient may experience. In addition, even between patients with a similar severity of facial nerve injury, there is often tremendous variability in perceived disability. For example, mild motor dysfunction may be career ending for a film actor, but may go nearly unnoticed by others.

54.3 Attributes of the Ideal Facial Nerve Grading System

54.3.1 General Principles of Instrument Scoring

With regard to summarizing data, an instrument that utilizes a continuous score and results in a relatively normal distribution

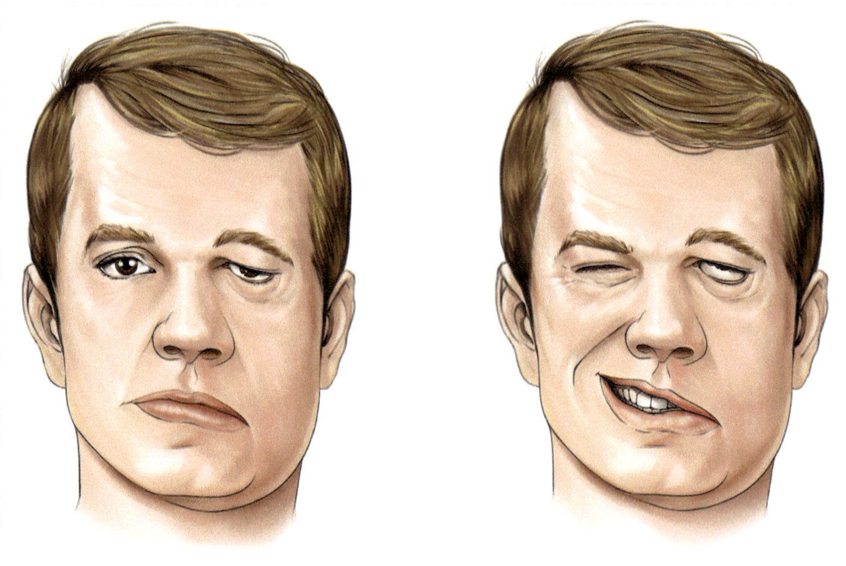

Fig. 54.1 Patient with severe left facial nerve paralysis during rest and maximal effort. Note the loss of forehead rhytids, brow ptosis, lateral eyelid hooding, lower eyelid ectropion, flattening of the nasolabial fold, and drooping of the corner of mouth. During attempted eye closure with maximum effort, upward and outward movement of the eye is noted, termed "Bell's phenomenon."

of outcomes is more conducive to statistical analysis than an ordinal scale utilizing arbitrary levels. For example, the HB scale includes six levels where incremental differences between levels are not necessarily equal—the difference in severity of facial nerve paralysis between HB grades II and III may be significantly greater than the difference between grades V and VI. In this setting, nonparametric analyses may be needed and medians rather than means should be reported. Additionally, the possible number of discrete scores for the instrument should be large enough to capture small changes that may occur longitudinally or with intervention, without being needlessly excessive. Since reliability in reporting for many of these subjective instruments is limited by observer bias, a larger number of scores is not necessarily better—that is, a large point spread assumes a level of precision that is not substantiated.[4] For example, a grading system that only incorporates three levels of motor dysfunction—"normal," "partial paralysis," and "complete paralysis"—could fail to detect changes with one of those three broad levels that could potentially be clinically significant. Conversely, a scale with 20 levels may be overly detailed and outside the range of what we can dependably interpret or would consider clinically significant. Finally, the scoring system should offer clinically meaningful information relevant to daily patient care. For example, a single composite score from multiple subdomains, if reported alone, may not convey information that is critical toward patient care, such as status of eye closure to prevent risk of exposure keratopathy.

54.3.2 Reliability and Validity

Reliability and validity are two technical properties of a clinical assessment tool that indicate the quality and usefulness of the measure. The reliability of an instrument describes the consistency in scoring between repeated measures on the same subject. After brief orientation, an ideal facial grading scale should demonstrate good inter-rater reliability between healthcare professionals, independent of experience or level of training. Additionally, there should be minimal test–retest variability within a single observer at two separate points in time. An ideal assessment tool should also have good validity—it must succeed in quantifying that which it was designed to measure. Because there is currently no gold standard to correlate with, criterion-related validity cannot be assessed; however, expert assessment can assist with determining if the measure appears logical (face validity) and if the items assessed adequately represent all important aspects of the condition (content validity). Most publications emphasize the importance of assessing both static and dynamic facial motor function of various regions compared to the normal side, "nervus intermedius dysfunction" including dysgeusia and dry eye, as well as late sequelae such as synkinesis, contracture, spasm, and gustatory lacrimation.

54.3.3 Convenience and Simplicity

While it is evident that many of the aforementioned attributes drive an instrument toward increasing complexity, the environment of the "end user" must also be strongly considered. For a system to become widely adopted, it must be brief and simple to administer in the office setting without requiring an elaborate setup. The methodology must be easy to learn by all levels of the healthcare team and understood by patients. In the fast-paced clinical setting where the majority of time is given toward patient counseling, an onerous or complex system will likely never be adopted.[5] This issue is demonstrated by the fact that gross scales, such as the HB grading system of facial function, the Glasgow Coma Scale for communicating level of consciousness, and the Hunt-Hess score for assessing patients after subarachnoid hemorrhage, remain the most widely utilized scales today.

54.4 Current Facial Nerve Grading Systems

54.4.1 Classifications

There are several different categories by which facial nerve assessment tools can be classified. Broadly, the method of analysis may be objective or subjective and may include gross, regional, or specific scales.[4,6] Objective instruments incorporate precisely measurable observations such as distance of oral commissure excursion or linear distance between lateral canthus and angle of mouth at rest and maximal effort. Such measures may include fully automated, semiautomated, or manual determination, depending on the degree of reliance on a computer-based system. Subjective assessment tools can be further divided into provider reported or patient reported. Provider-reported scales commonly interrogate tone at rest, voluntary movement, and synkinesis, while patient-reported outcomes often additionally incorporate questions pertaining to symptomatology and social function in order to determine how facial nerve injury has impacted daily life. Finally, gross, regional, and specific scales refer to instruments that evaluate global function, individual divisions of the face separately, or specific areas of the face with "yes" or "no" responses, respectively.[4,6] Regional scales may be further subclassified into weighted and non-weighted scales based on whether a particular division is prioritized over another. For example, some systems consider strength of eye closure and oral competence over brow function. Currently, the most widely adopted scales are subjective provider-reported gross and regional systems, which will be the focus of the remaining section. These include the HB (1983 and 1985), modified HB (2003), Sunnybrook (1996), and FNGS 2.0 (2009).[1,7,8,9] It should be acknowledged that several other quality facial grading systems have been proposed, including the Yanagihara (1976), Fisch-Burrow, and Nottingham systems; however, a detailed review of these less frequently used scales is beyond the scope of this chapter.[10,11,12]

54.5 House–Brackmann and Modified House–Brackmann System

Building upon previous gross ordinal scales, the HB system was initially proposed by John House in 1983 and was subsequently revised by John House and Derald Brackmann.[1,4,13] The HB system is a subjective gross scale that incorporates six levels evaluating resting and dynamic motor function and synkinesis (▶ Table 54.1). The primary advantages of

Table 54.1 The House–Brackmann grading system

Grade	Description	Characteristics
I	Normal	Normal facial function in all areas
II	Mild dysfunction	Gross: slight weakness noticeable on close inspection; may have very slight synkinesis At rest: normal symmetry and tone Motion Forehead: moderate to good function Eye: complete closure with minimum effort Mouth: slight asymmetry
III	Moderate dysfunction	Gross: obvious but not disfiguring difference between two sides; noticeable but not severe synkinesis, contracture, and/or hemifacial spasm At rest: normal symmetry and tone Motion Forehead: slight to moderate movement Eye: complete closure with effort Mouth: slightly weak with maximum effort
IV	Moderately severe dysfunction	Gross: obvious weakness and/or disfiguring asymmetry At rest: normal symmetry and tone Motion Forehead: none Eye: incomplete closure Mouth: asymmetric with maximal effort
V	Severe dysfunction	Gross: only barely perceptible motion At rest: asymmetry Motion Forehead: none Eye: incomplete closure Mouth: slight movement
VI	Total paralysis	No movement

Source: Used with permission from House JW, Brackmann DE. Facial nerve grading system. Otolaryngol Head Neck Surg. 1985; 93(2):146–147.

this system include ease of use and general good reliability between observers compared to previous systems. Related to its predecessor scales, the HB scale adds one additional category (grade IV, moderately severe) to further differentiate intermediate paralysis and more clearly defines each level to reduce interobserver variability. The HB scale was the first facial grading system to be endorsed by the Facial Nerve Disorders Committee of the American Academy of Otolaryngology in 1985 and was reaffirmed by the 1995 Committee on Hearing and Equilibrium for specific use with VS outcome reporting.[1,14] To date, the HB scale has made the most headway toward standardized interpretation and universal reporting of facial nerve outcomes following VS surgery.

Despite these contributions, several important limitations of the HB scale have been identified. First, by nature of gross assessment, regional differences are not distinguished, which is problematic as differential facial function often occurs. In studying this limitation, Yen et al found that most clinicians prioritized eye function when discrepancies between regions were present.[15] A second limitation is related to interobserver variability with relatively poor agreement between HB grades III and IV in particular, secondary to subjectivity of level descriptions and the difficulty in separating intermediate dysfunction.[9,16] Finally, the original HB system failed to quantify "nervus intermedius dysfunction," which has been shown to significantly impact patient quality of life.

These limitations have led to a modified reporting system by the 2003 Consensus Meeting on Systems for Reporting Results in Vestibular Schwannoma.[7] The major proposed changes included the division of grade III into IIIA and IIIB, separated by the degree of synkinesis and "eye comfortable and in good condition with or without lubricants" versus "eye dry and uncomfortable with evidence of exposure keratitis, requiring lubricants and possibly tarsorrhaphy." In addition, the presence or absence of crocodile tears (C0 vs. C1), metallic or aberrant taste (T0 vs. T1), and dry eye (E0 vs. E1) became separately documented. At this consensus meeting, it was also recommended that the Iowa Repaired Facial Nerve Recovery Scale supplant the HB scale for assessing outcomes following facial nerve repair.[17]

54.5.1 Sunnybrook Facial Grading System

The SB grading system is a subjective regional weighted instrument proposed by Ross and colleagues in 1996.[8] The SB scale analyzes resting symmetry of the eye, cheek, and mouth, as well as voluntary excursion and synkinesis evaluated during five standard facial expressions to achieve a maximum composite score of 100 (▶ Fig. 54.2). The larger number of discrete scores with the SB instrument confers greater capacity to detect change with time or intervention without significantly compromising reliability. Additionally, the greater range of scores may allow for more flexibility during statistical analysis. Similar to the HB scale, the SB system does not integrate other secondary deficits such as dysgeusia, dry eye, and crocodile tears. Additionally, while the SB evaluation form fits on a single page, it still requires more time and preparation than the HB score, which undoubtedly remains an obstacle toward adoption by surgeons.

54.5.2 Facial Nerve Grading Scale 2.0

The FNGS 2.0 was proposed by the Facial Nerve Disorders Committee in 2009 to address many criticisms and misinterpretations of the original Facial Nerve Grading Scale developed by House and Brackmann, while retaining much of its simplicity.[9] The FNGS 2.0 incorporates two separate domains (▶ Table 54.2). The first is a regional scale evaluating resting symmetry and voluntary motor function of the brow, eye, nasolabial fold, and oral region. Reminiscent of the original HB scale, a 1 to 6 score is assigned to each region, permitting a minimum overall score of 4 (best) and maximum score of 24 points (worst). The second scale is a global assessment of secondary movement including synkinesis and contracture—a score of 0 to 3 is applied for no synkinesis or contracture to disfiguring synkinesis and severe contracture, respectively. In this way, secondary movement is disentangled from the grading of primary motor dysfunction, and deemphasized with a maximum contribution of 3 points to the overall scale. The stricter descriptions of each grade permit greater differentiation between mild and moderate dysfunction, grades II through IV in the original HB scale.

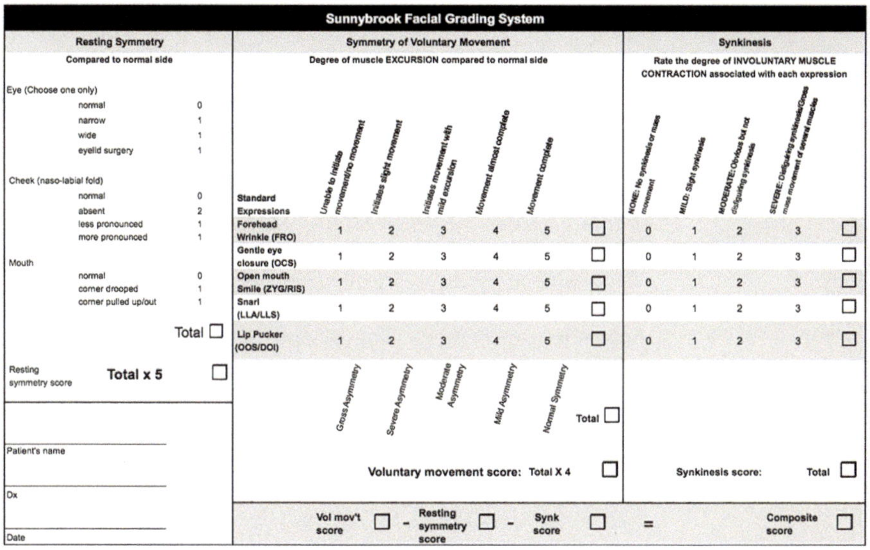

Fig. 54.2 Sunnybrook Facial Grading System. (Reproduced with permission from Ross, Fradet and Nedzelski[8]).

Table 54.2 Facial Nerve Grading Scale 2.0

	Region			
Score	**Brow**	**Eye**	**Nasolabial fold**	**Oral**
1	Normal	Normal	Normal	Normal
2	Slight weakness >75% of normal	Slight weakness >75% of normal Complete closure with mild effort	Slight weakness >75% of normal	Slight weakness >75% of normal
3	Obvious weakness >50% of normal Resting symmetry	Obvious weakness >50% of normal Complete closure with maximal effort	Obvious weakness >50% of normal Resting symmetry	Obvious weakness >50% of normal Resting symmetry
4	Asymmetry at rest <50% of normal	Asymmetry at rest <50% of normal Cannot close completely	Asymmetry at rest <50% of normal	Asymmetry at rest <50% of normal
5	Trace movement	Trace movement	Trace movement	Trace movement
6	No movement	No movement	No movement	No movement
Secondary movement (global assessment)				
Score	Degree of movement			
0	None			
1	Slight synkinesis; minimal contracture			
2	Obvious synkinesis; mild to moderate contracture			
3	Disfiguring synkinesis; severe contracture			
Reporting: sum scores for each region and secondary movement				
Grade	Total score			
I	4			
II	5–9			
III	10–14			
IV	15–19			
V	20–23			
VI	24			

Source: Used with permission from Vrabec JT, Backous DD, Djalilian HR, et al. Facial Nerve Disorders Committee. Facial Nerve Grading System 2.0. Otolaryngol Head Neck Surg. 2009; 140(4):445–450.

54.6 Unresolved Issues and Future Directions

54.6.1 Are We Forcing a Single System with Competing Goals?

The benefits of a single universal facial nerve grading system include ease of communication across specialties and centers, and facilitation of interstudy comparison. However, are we forcing the impossible—a single system that satisfies the competing priorities of different specialty groups or purposes? For example, neurotologists and neurosurgeons commonly emphasize the importance of a practical and efficient instrument, favoring gross scales such as the HB system. In a busy clinical practice where a large volume of patients are evaluated on a regular basis, a system that requires any amount of equipment (even a calculator) or more than several seconds to complete may never be adopted. In contrast, those involved in facial nerve rehabilitation are keenly interested in detecting very subtle changes with treatment, and often have more individual time with the patient. Under these conditions, systems such as the SB system or objective linear measurement scales are often preferred. Even further is the observation that facial nerve reanimation procedures, particularly nerve substitution, muscle transposition, and free muscle transfer techniques, inherently alter facial function; for these conditions, the current systems designed to evaluate facial nerve injury are grossly inadequate. In these cases, natural initiation of movement is lost and the best outcome that can be achieved in proximal nerve repair is good tone with mass movement. Instead of forcing a single compromised system, perhaps it would be more fitting to improve several specialized instruments, where scores can be grossly converted between studies for comparison when needed. The obvious limitation of this would be the conversion of a gross scale with a narrow score range to a more comprehensive regional scale, as detail cannot be gained with point conversion.

54.6.2 Are We Forgetting to Ask the Patient?

One of the glaring inadequacies of most contemporary facial nerve grading systems is the failure to critically evaluate the priorities of the patient. In recent years, there has been increasing importance placed on patient-reported outcome measures, understanding that there is often disparity between what we as healthcare professionals prioritize and what patients value. It may be possible to incorporate responses from several important patient questions during facial nerve assessment, or alternatively patient-reported outcome data could be indirectly implemented. An example of indirect application could include refinement of scale weighting. Specifically, many instruments arbitrarily weight the scoring of certain domains greater than others, which may profoundly alter the final composite score. By ascertaining the categories of dysfunction that most significantly influence patient quality of life, we may be able to weigh different aspects of the scale in a more meaningful way.[18] For example, perhaps symptoms of dry eye are associated with a two times greater reduction in quality of life than moderate synkinesis. A second application of patient-reported metrics may be the calculation of the minimally clinically important difference, defined as "the smallest difference in score in the domain of interest that patients perceive as important, either beneficial or harmful, and that would lead the clinician to consider a change in the patient's management."[19] Such information may discourage efforts to produce overly detailed or complex scales, recognizing that a several point difference on a 100-point scale is well beyond the perception of patients and clinicians. Finally, patient-reported data may help us further refine how study outcomes are presented. Currently, it is very common to group HB grades I to II or I to III as satisfactory; however, it is evident from previous studies that the greatest reduction in quality of life occurs between normal (HB I) and any degree of facial paralysis (HB II–VI).[18]

54.6.3 The Development of Objective Facial Function Assessment Tools

One of the primary limitations of most contemporary facial grading systems is subjectivity in data interpretation. Objective measures are appealing as they mitigate the impact of observer bias. The primary drawback of objective manual tests such as the Burres-Fisch and Nottingham systems that incorporate linear measurement is the time-consuming nature of handheld caliper measurements and the complexity of calculations.[10,11] Computer-assisted methods commonly incorporate photographic documentation or videography with pixel subtraction and landmark-based systems that evaluate resting symmetry and range of motion compared to the normal side.[6] Despite several advantages, the complex setup and need for specialized proprietary software remains a significant barrier. It could be argued that the only truly objective measure of facial nerve injury is resting and evoked electromyography (i.e., electroneuronography), as electrophysiological testing does not rely on active patient participation. However, such methods are impractical and have appeared only in a limited number of facial grading systems. Furthermore, strict use of electrophysiological testing does not consider important differences of intrinsic facial tone. For example, young patients with greater skin elasticity commonly exhibit better resting symmetry with less brow ptosis, ectropion, and facial sag than elderly patients, despite similar electromyographic findings. It is likely that the ideal system will utilize a combination of objective and subjective measures to provide a more comprehensive assessment of facial function.

54.7 Conclusion

The development of an accurate, reliable, and pragmatic measure of facial nerve injury remains critical toward standardized assessment and reporting of VS outcomes. Currently, the HB scale remains the most widely adopted system in North America and Europe; however, other quality measures such as the FNGS 2.0 and SB systems overcome several limitations of the original HB system. Future improvements may include adoption of a limited number of specialty-specific scales according to practice needs, greater inclusion of patient-reported outcome data, and refinements in more objective computer-assisted measures.

References

[1] House JW, Brackmann DE. Facial nerve grading system. Otolaryngol Head Neck Surg. 1985; 93(2):146–147

[2] Fattah AY, Gavilan J, Hadlock TA, et al. Survey of methods of facial palsy documentation in use by members of the Sir Charles Bell Society. Laryngoscope. 2014; 124(10):2247–2251

[3] Fattah AY, Gurusinghe AD, Gavilan J, et al. Sir Charles Bell Society. Facial nerve grading instruments: systematic review of the literature and suggestion for uniformity. Plast Reconstr Surg. 2015; 135(2):569–579

[4] House JW. Facial nerve grading systems. Laryngoscope. 1983; 93(8):1056–1069

[5] Alicandri-Ciufelli M, Pavesi G, Presutti L. Facial nerve grading scales: systematic review of the literature and suggestion for uniformity. Plast Reconstr Surg. 2015; 135(5):929e–930e

[6] Brenner MJ, Neely JG. Approaches to grading facial nerve function. Semin Plast Surg. 2004; 18(1):13–22

[7] Kanzaki J, Tos M, Sanna M, Moffat DA, Monsell EM, Berliner KI. New and modified reporting systems from the consensus meeting on systems for reporting results in vestibular schwannoma. Otol Neurotol. 2003; 24(4):642–648, discussion 648–649

[8] Ross BG, Fradet G, Nedzelski JM. Development of a sensitive clinical facial grading system. Otolaryngol Head Neck Surg. 1996; 114(3):380–386

[9] Vrabec JT, Backous DD, Djalilian HR, et al. Facial Nerve Disorders Committee. Facial Nerve Grading System 2.0. Otolaryngol Head Neck Surg. 2009; 140(4): 445–450

[10] Burres S, Fisch U. The comparison of facial grading systems. Arch Otolaryngol Head Neck Surg. 1986; 112(7):755–758

[11] Murty GE, Diver JP, Kelly PJ, O'Donoghue GM, Bradley PJ. The Nottingham system: objective assessment of facial nerve function in the clinic. Otolaryngol Head Neck Surg. 1994; 110(2):156–161

[12] Yanagihara N. Grading of facial palsy. Proceedings of the Third International Symposium on Facial Nerve Surgery, Zurich, 1976. In: Fisch U, ed. Facial Nerve Surgery. Amstelveen, The Netherlands: Kugler Medical Publications; 1977:533–535

[13] Brackmann DE, Barrs DM. Assessing recovery of facial function following acoustic neuroma surgery. Otolaryngol Head Neck Surg. 1984; 92(1):88–93

[14] Committee on Hearing and Equilibrium guidelines for the evaluation of hearing preservation in acoustic neuroma (vestibular schwannoma). American Academy of Otolaryngology-Head and Neck Surgery Foundation, INC. Otolaryngol Head Neck Surg. 1995; 113(3):179–180

[15] Yen TL, Driscoll CL, Lalwani AK. Significance of House-Brackmann facial nerve grading global score in the setting of differential facial nerve function. Otol Neurotol. 2003; 24(1):118–122

[16] Kang TS, Vrabec JT, Giddings N, Terris DJ. Facial nerve grading systems (1985–2002): beyond the House-Brackmann scale. Otol Neurotol. 2002; 23(5):767–771

[17] Gidley PW, Gantz BJ, Rubinstein JT. Facial nerve grafts: from cerebellopontine angle and beyond. Am J Otol. 1999; 20(6):781–788

[18] Carlson ML, Tveiten OV, Driscoll CL, et al. What drives quality of life in patients with sporadic vestibular schwannoma? Laryngoscope. 2015; 125(7): 1697–1702

[19] Carlson ML, Tveiten OV, Yost KJ, Lohse CM, Lund-Johansen M, Link MJ. The minimal clinically important difference in vestibular schwannoma quality-of-life assessment: an important step beyond P<. 05. Otolaryngol Head Neck Surg. 2015; 153(2):202–208

55 Facial Nerve Injury in Sporadic Vestibular Schwannoma: Mechanisms, Predictors, and Outcomes

Philip V. Theodosopoulos

55.1 Introduction

In the modern era, facial nerve function and tumor control are the primary benchmarks used to assess treatment outcome in vestibular schwannoma (VS). In most scenarios, these two goals are competing at least to some degree. That is, treatments that provide the most definitive tumor control, such as gross total microsurgical resection, usually place the facial nerve at greater risk. Conversely, management strategies that are more conservative by nature (e.g., low-dose radiosurgery, observation, subtotal resection [STR]) have a lower risk of facial paresis, but are also less definitive in terms of "cure." While there are numerous variables considered by the patient when navigating treatment options, in many cases, the choice can be distilled down to a balance of priority between facial nerve outcome and tumor control.[1]

At the time of diagnosis, facial nerve paresis or spasm is highly unusual even for very large tumors, and therefore, these symptoms should raise suspicion for a primary facial nerve tumor or malignancy.[2] As opposed to the impact VSs have on eighth nerve function, the facial nerve is highly resistant to the indolent growth and compression imposed by most VS. With rare exceptions such as rapid cystic growth or intratumoral hemorrhage where abrupt tumor expansion occurs, gross facial nerve impairment is generally only affected by treatment rather than progression of the underlying disease process.[3,4] This chapter reviews the mechanisms of facial nerve injury, reviews predictors of facial nerve outcome, and summarizes published facial nerve outcomes according to modality. An in-depth discussion regarding intraoperative facial nerve monitoring and facial nerve dissection technique is presented separately in Chapters 27 and 32, respectively. In addition, the interested reader may refer to the individual chapters on separate treatment modalities for detailed summaries of facial nerve outcomes for each.

55.2 Facial Nerve Injury

The facial nerve is composed of approximately 10,000 axons, encompassing 7,000 motor fibers that primarily innervate ipsilateral facial musculature and 3,000 fibers that convey gustatory afferents from the oral tongue in addition to parasympathetic efferents to the ipsilateral lacrimal, submandibular, and sublingual glands. Within the CPA and IAC, parasympathetic fibers are carried in the nervus intermedius of Wrisberg, aptly named as it exits the brainstem between the facial motor root and the eighth cranial nerve, before converging with the facial motor fibers proximal to the meatal foramen. As a result, acute facial nerve injury may result in partial or complete facial paralysis, dysgeusia, and parasympathetic dysfunction, including dry eye. Delayed sequela resulting from faulty or incomplete axonal regeneration includes ipsilateral synkinesis, spasm, hypertonicity, or contracture, in addition to gustatory hyperlacrimation (also known as crocodile tears).[5] Synkinesis, or mass muscle movement, primarily results from splitting of regenerating axons and cross reinnervation after endoneurial disruption and faulty myelination. Spasm is thought to result from ephaptic coupling, ectopic discharges, and lateral spread of excitation along nerve fibers.[6] Gustatory hyperlacrimation is derived from misdirection of regenerating gustatory fibers to the lacrimal gland. Treatment for hypertonicity, spasm, and synkinesis include biofeedback and muscle retraining, botulinum toxin (Botox) therapy, selective neurectomy, and selective myectomy, as discussed further in Chapter 62. Details regarding facial nerve grading is discussed separately in Chapter 54.

It is notable that normal gross facial movement and resting tone does not imply that all facial nerve fibers are functioning. The facial nerve has a moderate degree of innate reserve, such that normal function may be retained even after a significant proportion of axons are lost, up to 50% by some reports.[7,8] Thus, the degree of clinical facial weakness is proportional to the number of functioning fibers after this threshold is surpassed. This observation may, to a limited degree, contribute to why facial nerve outcomes following salvage microsurgery may be poorer than after primary microsurgery, or why the risk of worsening facial nerve function after radiosurgery is greater when there is an existing facial nerve deficit or if the patient previously underwent microsurgical resection.

In the context of VS, facial nerve paresis most commonly results from microsurgical manipulation causing mechanical injury (i.e., stretch or sharp cutting), thermal injury (i.e., bipolar coagulation), or vascular compromise. However, abrupt facial nerve paralysis can also occur without prior treatment in the setting of rapid cystic growth or gross intratumoral hemorrhage.[3,4] Similarly, facial nerve paralysis may occur in a delayed fashion after stereotactic radiosurgery or fractionated radiotherapy. It is presumed that early post-SRS facial nerve dysfunction, most commonly occurring between 3 and 12 months, is related to peritumoral edema and tumor swell, while delayed dysfunction is caused by progressive microvascular ischemia from endothelial injury, intimal thickening, and vessel obliteration with hyalinization.[9,10,11,12]

The two most common classification systems used to describe nerve injury include Seddon's 1943 description of neuropraxia, axonotmesis, and neurotmesis and Sunderland's 1951 classification of types 1 to 5 (▶ Fig. 55.1).[13,14] First-degree neural injury (i.e., neuropraxia) represents a simple reversible conduction block and is associated with increased intraneural pressure without disruption of axoplasmic flow. In this condition, full continuity of the axon is maintained and Wallerian degeneration does not develop. Full recovery occurs within days to several months. Second-degree injury (i.e., axonotmesis) occurs when the axon is disrupted, but the endoneurium remains intact. In this setting, Wallerian degeneration results; however, recovery is still complete since the endoneurial tubules serve to guide individual regenerating axons thereby

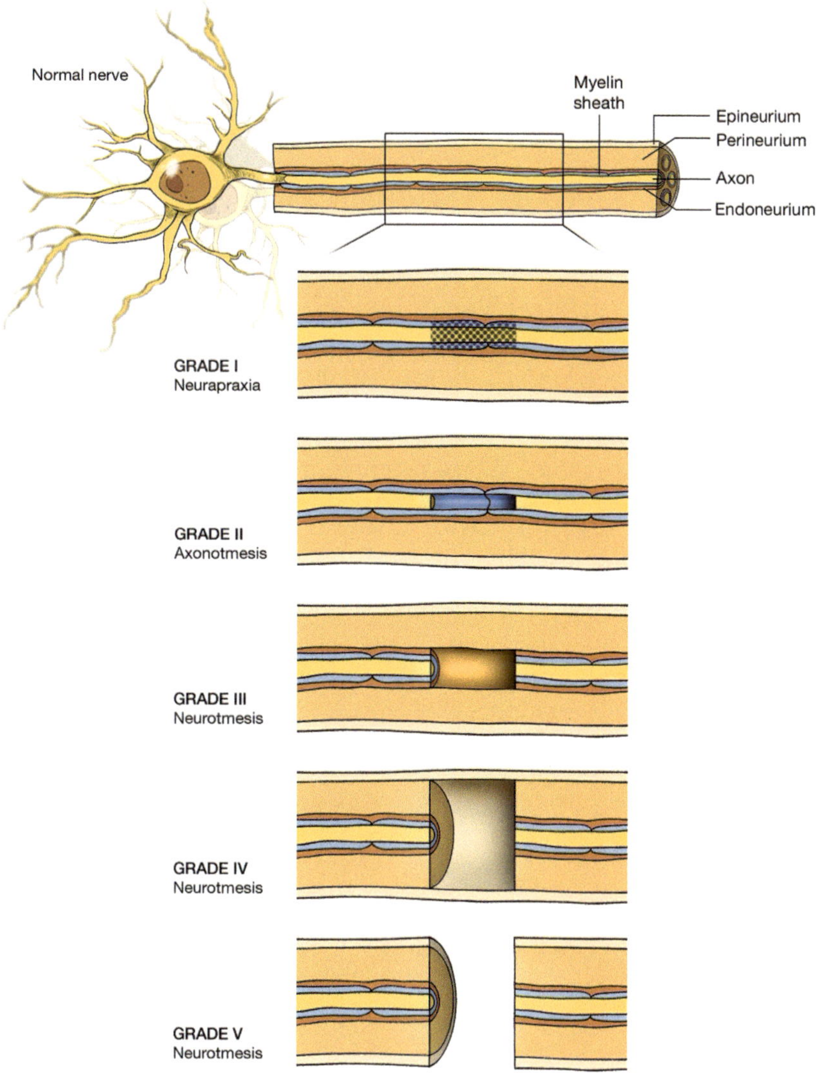

Fig. 55.1 Seddon's (neuropraxia, axonotmesis, neurotmesis) and Sunderland's (grades I–V) classifications of neural injury.

mitigating synkinesis. The time to full recovery for second-degree injury is longer than for first-degree neural injury. Seddon's classification of neurotmesis was expanded upon by Sunderland to encompass third-, fourth-, and fifth-degree injuries, corresponding to disruption of the endoneurium, perineurium, and epineurium (i.e., nerve division), respectively. In each, partial recovery is expected as a result of incomplete and haphazard axonal regeneration and motor end-plate reinnervation. While these classification systems suggest a uniform pattern of injury across all nerve fibers, it can be assumed that most injuries are truly mixed—some axons may remain healthy, while others sustain varying levels of injury. In the acute setting, the amplitude of the compound motor action potential (CMAP) is proportional to the number of intact axons, which serves as the basis for electroprognostic testing of the facial nerve (Chapter 27).

Proceeding distal to the site of axonal injury, Wallerian degeneration begins at 12 to 24 hours after injury and peaks within 3 days. This delay explains why the distal facial nerve segment remains stimulatable for 48 to 72 hours following even complete transection, with normal latency and CMAPs. As a result, during microsurgery the site of severe facial nerve injury can be estimated as immediately proximal to where the nerve first reliably stimulates. This time course also explains a vital limitation of intraoperative facial nerve electroprognostic testing—in the case where facial nerve stimulation is lost but the nerve remains anatomically intact, intraoperative proximal stimulation cannot definitively distinguish a simple neuropraxia from more severe injury[15] (see Chapter 27 for further discussion).

Coinciding with the timing of Wallerian degeneration, retrograde axonal sprouting develops approximately 72 hours after injury. Regenerating axons grow at a rate of approximately 1 mm per day and myelination is generally complete 1 month after axonal growth. Following injury, the critical period for motor end-plate reinnervation is approximately 1 year, but this timing is variable and should be looked at as a continuum rather than assigning a strict cut-point. Beyond the practical value of patient counseling regarding long-term expectations of facial nerve recovery, the timing and rate of neural regeneration is important when considering nerve transfer procedures. In patients with postoperative House–Brackmann (HB) grade VI paralysis and an anatomically intact nerve, the surgeon must wait and evaluate for spontaneous recovery as this may ultimately provide the best possible outcome.[15,16] However, reinnervation procedures should not be delayed too long as to compromise recipient motor end plates—"time is muscle." Historically, most authors advocate waiting a minimum of 1 year to ascertain final outcome before pursuing donor nerve procedures that require division of the facial nerve. However, Rivas et al determined that for patients with postoperative HB grades V to VI facial weakness, the rate of early facial nerve improvement can predict final recovery.[16] The issue of timing before donor nerve transfer in patients with complete paralysis is discussed further in Chapters 64 through 67.

55.3 Facial Nerve Injury with Microsurgery

55.3.1 Anatomical Considerations

The facial nerve lies in direct anatomical apposition to the tumor capsule in all cases regardless of tumor size. Small tumors typically interface the facial nerve along its intracanalicular course, with the nerve located along the anterior and superior aspect in most cases. As tumors enlarge and extend out of the internal auditory canal (IAC), the facial nerve invariably has more extensive length of contact with the tumor capsule. In part, this relationship between tumor size and length of facial nerve contact explains the greater risk of facial neuropathy when resecting or radiating larger tumors.

In the context of VS microsurgery, there are only two locations where the facial nerve position is constant: the facial nerve departs the brainstem at the pontomedullary junction, just anteroinferior to the cochlear nerve, and the facial nerve enters the temporal bone at the meatal foramen at the fundus of the IAC. Apart from this, significant variability arises with larger tumors with respect to the location of the facial nerve along the tumor capsule. In most VS, the facial nerve follows a course along the ventral aspect of the tumor in the cerebellopontine angle (CPA); however, not uncommonly it may be encountered along the superior or inferior aspect of the tumor and rarely along the dorsal capsule.[17,18] Another curious observation is that with larger tumors, the facial nerve does not always take the shortest route from the brainstem to the fundus. For example, in some cases, the facial nerve may follow a meandering course over the superior pole of the tumor in the cistern before acquiring a more ventral position at the porus acusticus. As a general rule, the risk of facial nerve injury or need for less than gross total resection (GTR) is greater in cases where the facial nerve courses over the dorsal side of the tumor, over the superior pole, or has significant redundancy.[17,18,19]

A final important consideration is the organization and microscopic anatomy of the facial nerve. True fascicular organization of the facial nerve with perineurium and epineurium begins at the geniculate ganglion.[20,21] The perineurium provides tensile strength to the nerve and resists mechanical stretch, while the epineurium contains the vasa nervorum of the nerve and is important for nutrient delivery. Together, the perineurium and epineurium support bundling of facial nerve axons. Medial to the geniculate ganglion, the facial nerve is more vulnerable to mechanical or ischemic injury during dissection and more susceptible to splay. In the CPA and IAC, the facial nerve is without epineurium and is covered by pia mater and bathed in CSF.[21] The proximal cisternal facial nerve receives its blood supply from the anterior inferior cerebellar artery, while a branch of the middle meningeal artery feeds the perigeniculate nerve.[22,23,24] During tumor dissection, parasitized tumor feeders are systematically coagulated and divided, while every attempt is made to preserve brainstem perforators. Few anastomotic connections exist along the course of the subarachnoid segment of the facial nerve and as a result, varying degrees of devascularization inevitably occur.

The facial nerve can be injured at any point along its course from the brainstem to the fundus of the IAC. Of particular importance is the area of the facial nerve just proximal to the porus acusticus. Given the abrupt change in direction as the nerve transitions from the CPA to the IAC in addition to the compressive force of the cisternal component of the tumor as it enters the IAC, the nerve fibers can be splayed making safe dissection of the tumor capsule away from the nerve difficult. This is the most common site where the facial nerve is injured and the most frequent location to leave residual tumor should STR be performed. Early identification of the facial nerve at the brainstem or fundus, as well as frequent low threshold stimulation during tumor dissection, is imperative for optimal postoperative facial function. Chapters 30 and 32 offer further discussion on facial nerve anatomy and course. The interested reader is encouraged to review Chapters 27, 32, and 41 for further discussion relevant to intraoperative facial nerve monitoring and intraoperative decision making as it pertains to optimizing facial nerve function.

55.3.2 Preoperative Predictors of Facial Nerve Outcome

One of the most intensely studied topics in the VS literature is pre- and intraoperative prognosticators of facial nerve outcome. Many candidate predictors have been extensively evaluated including age, sex, tumor size, degree of ventral tumor extension, degree of fundal obliteration, surgical approach, tumor cystic quality, tumor vascularity, facial nerve course, prior treatment, preoperative electromyography, intraoperative facial nerve stimulation testing, and extent of resection.[7,25,26,27,28,29,30]

Of all baseline predictive factors, tumor size remains the most consistent predictor of early and long-term facial nerve function following microsurgical resection.[25,27] This relationship is most obvious when comparing the extremes: the risk of facial paralysis after resection of an intracanalicular tumor or one with minimal cisternal growth is approximately 5 to 10%, while the risk of facial paralysis with GTR of large tumors approaches 65%, according to a recent systematic review.[31] Larger tumors have a lengthier nerve–capsule interface for dissection, in addition to a higher likelihood of acquiring an unfavorable nerve course, nerve adherence, nerve splay, and peritumoral edema.[27,31,32] Related to tumor extent is the degree of fundus obliteration. The literature suggests that hearing preservation is more feasible in cases of a large lateral CSF cap, that is, greater distance between the lateral tumor margin and the fundus.[33] Paralleling this, Rompaey et al found that fundus obliteration is associated with poorer early postoperative facial nerve outcome.[34] Specifically, among patients with fundal obliteration, 30% had HB III or worse, compared to only 13% without fundal obliteration at 1 month following surgery. However, this significant difference was lost at 1 year.

A more recent factor that parallels tumor size is volume of tumor located anterior to the axis of the IAC.[28,30,35] While most tumors are more or less centered on the porus acusticus, some medium- and large-size tumors acquire eccentric growth. Tumors that grow disproportionately more ventral have a greater risk of facial nerve paralysis for the same reasons a large tumor might. Wong et al reported that tumors extending greater than 1.5 cm anterior to the IAC were three times more likely to have postoperative HB grade III function or higher.[35] Similarly, Grahnke et al found that after controlling for tumor size, there was a 3.8 times greater likelihood of higher HB score for every 1 standard deviation increase in the anterior-to-posterior tumor extension ratio.[28]

Tumor consistency and tumor vascularity are two associated factors that have been studied in several recent publications. In 2013, Copeland et al examined MRI signal intensities to predict intraoperative tumor consistency and facial nerve outcome.[26] Firm and soft tumors were equally hypointense on T1 sequences; however, soft VSs were more likely to be hyperintense on T2 sequences (88 vs. 14%, $p < 0.005$). This finding parallels the meningioma literature.[36] In contrast, Rizk et al found that T2 signal was not predictive of tumor consistency, but rather widening of the IAC was.[37] Specifically, the mean widening of the IAC in relation to the nontumor side was 1.9 mm for soft tumors and 3.6 mm for firm tumors. Both authors found better facial nerve outcomes in softer tumors. Recently, Patel et al found that tumors exhibiting prominent dural enhancement, reminiscent of dural tails in meningioma, at the porus acusticus had greater facial nerve tumor adhesion and were more likely to undergo STR compared to those without (31 vs. 3%, $p = 0.01$).[38] While still under investigation, magnetic resonance elastography, slip interface imaging, and diffusion tensor imaging tractography may be used in the future to predict intraoperative VS tumor consistency, adhesion, and facial nerve course, respectively.[39,40,41] This aspect is covered in greater detail in Chapter 9.

The association between facial nerve outcome and presence of prominent cystic growth has also been extensively examined. As reviewed in Chapter 76, one of the primary obstacles in characterizing this association is a lack of consensus of what constitutes a "cystic VS," and the varying classification of intratumoral thick-walled cysts versus peripheral thin-walled cysts. The latter type, in particular, has been linked to poorer facial nerve outcome or increased need for STR.[42] The mechanisms to explain the greater risk of facial nerve injury with macrocystic VS are twofold: first, many cystic tumors undergo periods of rapid expansion, which may result in peritumoral edema, facial nerve splay, or tumor adhesion. Second, dissection of a flimsy, thin-walled, adherent tumor capsule from the nerve can be challenging with less substance to work with when applying countertraction.[42,43]

A final area of discussion relates to preoperative subclinical facial nerve involvement. As discussed previously, HB grade I function does not inherently indicate a completely healthy nerve. Indeed, a substantial portion of facial nerve fibers may be compromised before gross motor weakness is seen.[7,8,44] In line with this, several authors have correlated preoperative electroneurography (ENoG) amplitude testing with postoperative facial nerve outcome. They hypothesized that a tumor with a presurgical compromised nerve is more likely to develop a significant injury during microsurgical resection compared to a nerve that is not compromised at baseline. Kartush et al found that 8 of 10 patients with VS exhibited reduced ENoG amplitude on preoperative testing.[7] The authors subsequently found that preoperative ENoG amplitude data inversely correlated with tumor size.[44] While intriguing, most subsequent studies did not find a consistent association between preoperative reduction in ENoG amplitude and postoperative facial function.[44,45] As a result, most centers do not employ preoperative EMG testing given the added expense and uncertain overall predictive value.

55.3.3 Facial Nerve Outcome by Surgical Approach

Despite the increasing use of radiosurgery and observation within the last two decades for small- and medium-sized VS, microsurgery remains the most prevalent management strategy for VS worldwide.[46] Various surgical approaches have been described; however, the retrosigmoid, translabyrinthine, and middle fossa approaches are used almost exclusively today. Controversy over which surgical approach is best for VS resection dates back over 100 years and is beautifully described in Chapter 1. Suffice it to say, no consensus has been reached.

The primary obstacles that impede objective comparison of surgical approaches include inherent selection biases, inconsistent reporting, confounding variables such as completeness of resection, and other less tangible aspects such as skill and experience of the surgical team. These challenges are well illustrated in the age-long debate comparing the middle fossa and retrosigmoid approaches for hearing preservation. Inherently, the average tumor size among middle cranial fossa cases is much smaller than retrosigmoid cases, since most surgeons will not use the former for tumors greater than 0.5 cm in the CPA. Additionally, the average pure-tone threshold and word recognition score is likely better for most middle fossa cases. Without accounting for tumor size and baseline hearing levels, one might prematurely conclude that facial nerve and hearing preservation outcomes are superior with the middle cranial fossa approach. However, when comparing comparable tumors, several studies have demonstrated superior facial nerve outcomes with the retrosigmoid approach and equivalent hearing preservation rates.[29,47]

In 2012, Gurgel et al published a systematic review of the literature examining facial nerve outcome according to surgical approach for large VS, defined as ≥ 2.5 cm in the CPA.[31] Pooled data from 30 eligible studies and 1,688 tumor resections demonstrated that good facial nerve outcomes (HB I–II) were achieved in 62.5% of translabyrinthine cases and 65.2% of retrosigmoid approaches, a difference that was not statistically significant. The same year, Ansari et al published a systematic review analyzing facial nerve outcomes according to surgical approach, after stratifying according to tumor size. In total, 35 studies encompassing 5,064 patients were included.[29] For intracanalicular tumors, the middle cranial fossa approach was associated with a higher risk of facial nerve injury compared to the retrosigmoid approach; however, both were not statistically different from the translabyrinthine approach (16.7, 4, 0%, respectively, $p < 0.001$). The middle cranial fossa approach exhibited poorer facial nerve outcomes compared to the translabyrinthine approach for tumors smaller than 1.5 cm, whereas neither differed from the retrosigmoid approach (11.5, 3.3, and 7.2%, respectively, $p = 0.001$). The retrosigmoid approach exhibited less facial nerve paresis than the middle cranial fossa or translabyrinthine approaches for tumors 1.5 to 3.0 cm (6.1, 17.3, and 15.8, respectively; $p < 0.001$). In contrast to the findings of Gurgel et al, Ansari and colleagues reported that facial nerve outcome with the retrosigmoid approach was superior to the translabyrinthine approach for tumors greater than 3.0 cm (30.2 vs. 42.5%, respectively, $p < 0.001$). In evaluating the current literature, and based on personal experience, it is fair to conclude that in many cases, more than one surgical approach is reasonable, and the best surgical approach in one surgeon's hands may be different for another. It is also true that tumor-related factors, such as size, degree of ventral extension, course of the facial nerve, and tumor consistency, and other factors invariably impact tumor control and cranial nerve outcomes more than approach selection in many cases. Chapter 31 provides a detailed summary of select large clinical series comparing facial nerve and hearing preservation outcomes according to surgical approach.

55.3.4 Facial Nerve Outcome by Extent of Resection

When considering all factors, large tumors pose the greatest risk to the facial nerve.[25,27] Postoperative facial nerve paralysis following attempted GTR ranges from 20 to 50% in several large surgical series.[31,48] Recognizing this significant limitation, in 2005 Raftopoulos et al proposed an alternate surgical strategy of prioritizing facial nerve function over complete tumor removal.[48] The authors advocated for maximizing tumor resection, but intentionally leaving small adherent tumor remnants along the course of the facial nerve to protect neural integrity. Utilizing this strategy, they reported much improved facial nerve outcomes, with HB grades I to II function in all 15 tumors ≥ 3 cm included in their study. The surgical strategy conferring primacy of facial nerve function over extent of resection has since been used with greater frequency, particularly in light of refined radiosurgery techniques for the management of residual progressive disease. Observed reduction in facial nerve response to intraoperative stimulation, increasing neurotonic firing, and intraoperative appreciation of tumor capsule adherence are examples of indications for termination of tumor dissection according to such a surgical strategy. The predictive value of intraoperative facial nerve stimulation for postoperative facial nerve outcome is reviewed further in Chapter 27.

A similar strategy of less than GTR has been used by others reporting comparable outcomes. A series by Haque et al reported good facial nerve outcomes (HB I–II) in 97% of 96 patients with sporadic VS treated with a strategy that allowed intentional incomplete resection.[49] Twenty patients showed progression of their tumors and required radiosurgery following microsurgery. Overall 80% of those patients who required salvage radiosurgery treatment retained or improved their postoperative facial nerve function. Similarly, a study by the author's group of 52 patients with Koos grades III and IV VS revealed good facial nerve outcomes in 91% of patients who underwent STR (> 5 mm thick residual) and 92% in patients undergoing near total resection (NTR; < 5 mm thick residual).[50] Tumor remnants were observed with serial imaging with progression confirmed in 4 of the 19 patients following STR and 1 of 11 patients in the NTR group. Radiotherapy was used to treat those five patients with residual progressive disease, as well as five other cases before any radiographic evidence of tumor progression was evident, for an overall tumor control rate of 90% at an average follow-up of 33 months. Chapter 21 further discusses salvage radiosurgery for residual progressive or recurrent VS.

Based on these earlier data, a multicenter prospective trial was designed to study the question of optimal treatment of residual tumor.[51] The Acoustic Neuroma Subtotal Resection Study (ANSRS) involved patients treated at eight institutions with tumors ≥ 2.5 cm undergoing surgical resection. The intent of the resection was to maximize tumor removal; however, STR or NTR was permitted in order to reduce the risk of permanent facial paresis. The aim of the study was to assess, in a systematic prospective fashion, whether more conservative surgical resection confers an advantage in optimizing facial nerve outcome. Tumor remnants were followed up with serial imaging, and in the face of progression, they were treated with radiosurgery. The results for 77 patients with more than a year of follow-up indicate a significant improvement in facial nerve outcome for patients with less than GTR compared to those who received GTR. Additionally, the data suggest that NTR has similar facial nerve outcomes to STR, indicating that maximal tumor resection should be pursued when feasible in order to optimize tumor control. Rate of residual progressive or recurrent disease was 19% with an association between extent of resection and progression. Specifically, the overall failure rate was 8.3% for GTR, 9.1% for NTR, and 28.2% for STR, with an average time to regrowth of 35 months (4–74 months). The trial is ongoing and longer-term outcomes, particularly with respect to tumor remnant progression and the need for further treatment, will be important to further compile and analyze.

Although there are data to suggest that less than complete resection confers improved postoperative facial nerve outcomes, the reported increased rates of tumor remnant progression and need for subsequent treatment raises valid concerns for overall long-term patient outcomes. The relatively limited available length of follow-up regarding tumor control after adjuvant and salvage treatment of tumor remnants poses uncertainty regarding the merit of conservative resection followed by radiosurgery and warrants continued study. The topic of STR for facial nerve preservation is reviewed further in Chapter 41.

55.3.5 Delayed Facial Nerve Paresis

Within the first couple of days to a month following surgery, delayed deterioration of facial nerve function may develop. Currently, there is no consensus definition of what constitutes delayed facial nerve paralysis (DFP). Some authors include cases with any incremental decline in function after the first postoperative examination, while others only count those cases that develop after a time interval of days to a week after surgery.[8,52,53,54,55] Sargent et al identified a bimodal distribution of DFP latency, in which one population experienced deterioration within hours to 2 days after surgery and a second population experienced delayed deterioration up to 17 days after surgery.[56] The incidence of DFP varies significantly in published reports, ranging from 2% to as high as 41%.[57,58] This wide variation likely reflects the differences in how DFP is defined in each study, and how closely patients are followed up. It is likely that the true incidence is underreported in most series as DFP commonly occurs after hospital discharge and may resolve within weeks thereafter.

The exact cause of DFP is unknown. Reactivation of dormant herpes virus in the geniculate ganglion, vasospasm of nerve microvasculature, delayed neural swelling at the meatal foramen and labyrinthine segment, and aseptic subarachnoid inflammation have all been postulated as potential causes.[52,53,55,56] Gianoli found that mean HSV-1, HSV-2, and VZV IgM titers rose 92, 70, and 495%, respectively, in patients who experienced DFP, compared to no titer change or even decline in patients without DFP.[53] In a prospective study, Brackmann et al identified a reduction in DFP, from 25 to 20%, when famciclovir was given prophylactically.[59] This benefit was most noticeable in the translabyrinthine group compared to the middle fossa group. Using multivariate modeling, Carlstrom et al identified that GTR (odds ratio [OR] = 2.03, 95% confidence interval [CI] = 1.00–4.18; $p = 0.05$) and the retrosigmoid approach (OR = 2.31, 95% CI = 1.26–4.22, $p < 0.01$) were associated with the development of DFP in 16% of cases, while sex, tumor size, operative duration, body mass index, postoperative complications, preoperative HB grade, or intraoperative facial nerve monitoring results did not.[52] However, others have not found surgical approach to predict DFP development.[8,58] Several groups have retrospectively reported that decompression of the labyrinthine segment of the facial nerve, during either middle cranial fossa or the translabyrinthine approach, reduces the risk of DFP.[56,57] Finally, Scheller et al identified a subset of patients who experienced DFP that developed as soon as hydroxyethyl starch and nimodipine were discontinued and improved after reinitiating these medications.[60] The authors concluded that this observation supports a vasoactive mechanism to explain the phenomenon of delayed deterioration of facial nerve function.

Despite the lack of certainty as to the cause, DFP is almost always a temporary phenomenon resolving to normal or near normal (HB I–II) in the great majority of patients within weeks or months with or without treatment. Steroids and antiviral medications have been used in the setting of DFP with varied success.[52,59,61] Some authors have not advocated for prophylactic measures or treatment of DFP as the majority recover normal facial nerve function. Furthermore, some treatments, such as labyrinthine segment decompression, carry some inherent risk. A summary of the literature pertaining to DFP following microsurgical resection can be found in ▶ Table 55.1.

55.4 Facial Nerve Injury with Radiation

55.4.1 Predictors of Facial Nerve Injury after Radiation

Uncommonly, fractionated and single-fraction radiosurgery dosing may cause facial neuropathy from direct axonal damage, brainstem parenchymal injury, ischemia from microvascular damage, or transient abrupt tumor swelling.[9,10,62] In most cases, onset of facial weakness is between 3 and 18 months after treatment, with approximately half of cases resolving within 3 to 6 months after onset. Only very rarely does facial nerve paralysis develop within the immediate posttreatment period.[63,64] Uncommonly, patients may also develop transient facial nerve spasm associated with tumor swelling approximately 6 to 12 months after treatment, which nearly always resolves spontaneously within 6 months after onset. However, even in cases where overt facial nerve symptoms do not occur, experience with microsurgical resection following failed radiation suggests that subclinical facial nerve injury is common. In these cases, facial nerve electromyography frequently demonstrates greater excitability and exceedingly high train-time values with any degree of surgical manipulation.[65]

Histological studies in animal models evaluating peripheral nerve injury after high-dose radiation demonstrate loss and fragmentation of axons, fragmentation of myelin sheaths, and an increase in neural fibrosis.[10] Assessment of supporting microvasculature demonstrates evidence of ischemic neuropathy from inflammatory cell infiltration of vessel walls, thrombosis of small vessels, and hyalinization of the tunica media within arterioles. Moreover, Schwann cells may have reduced proliferative capacity following radiation thereby encumbering recovery. In 2003, Watanabe et al reported a case of a patient who received repeat low-dose radiosurgery (marginal dose of 12 Gy twice, cumulative dose of 24 Gy) for progressive tumor growth 33 months after primary radiosurgery.[9] This 63-year-old man developed facial paralysis 25 months after the second radiation treatment and ultimately underwent microsurgical resection for persistent growth. Histopathology reveled loss of axons, demyelination, proliferation of Schwann cells, and microvasculitis supporting the results of previous animal studies, despite a lower cumulative dose.

Although rare today, facial paralysis following radiation appears to correlate to maximal dose to the tumor margin, maximum dose to the brainstem,[66] tumor volume, and history of prior treatment.[12,66,67,68,69] In sporadic VS, the facial nerve is invariably located along the tumor periphery, and therefore, the dose received by the nerve approximates the marginal dose. This is in contrast to severe phenotype neurofibromatosis type-2, where the facial nerve may be engulfed by lobules of colliding tumor. Contemporary single-fraction dosing of 12 to 13 Gy to the margin is associated with less than 1% risk of facial nerve paralysis, while marginal doses of 18 to 20 Gy are used in the early Gamma Knife studies–reported rates of facial nerve injury of ≥ 30%.[70,71] In 1999, Miller et al compared rates of cranial neuropathy among patients who received a standard-dose protocol of 16 to 20 Gy depending on tumor size, and those who received a reduced-dose protocol of 12 to 16 Gy.[72] The Kaplan–Meier estimate of facial neuropathy at 2 years was 38% for the standard-dose protocol versus 8% (95% CI, 0–17%) for the reduced-dose protocol ($p = 0.006$). After controlling for baseline factors, the only factor associated with increased risk of posttreatment facial neuropathy was a tumor margin dose greater than 18 Gy. Subsequently, in 2004, Flickinger et al published the outcomes of 313 sporadic VS treated with 12 to 13 Gy, reporting a 100% rate of facial nerve preservation at 6 years following treatment.[73] In 2009, Yang et al performed a systematic review of the literature including 23 publications, encompassing 2,204

Table 55.1 Summary of literature pertaining to delayed facial nerve paralysis following microsurgical resection of vestibular schwannoma.

Study	Center	Design	Dates	Definition of delayed facial paralysis	Incidence rates	Latency	Predictors	Outcome
Lalwani et al (1995)	University of California, San Francisco, CA	Retrospective	1986–1990	Deterioration of function from normal to abnormal or increase in the severity of weakness compared to the immediate postoperative period	41%, 38 of 93	Mean or median and range NR	Not correlated with tumor size, approach, or age	34 of 38 had HB I–II and 97% had HB I–III at 1 y
Megerian et al (1996)	Massachusetts Eye and Ear Infirmary, Boston, MA	Retrospective	1986–1992	Only patients with immediate post-op HB I–II were included in the study. Any deterioration of function compared to the immediate postoperative period	24%, 62 of 255	Mean: 3.6 d after surgery, range: 1–16 d	Not correlated with age, sex, or tumor size. Only retrosigmoid cases evaluated. Early onset of paralysis (<48 h) resulted in shorter average recovery time. Less severe change resulted in shorter average recovery time	90% recovered to their initial post-op HB grade and 98.3% to within HB grade of their initial score
Magliulo et al (1998)	University La Sapienza, Rome, Italy	Retrospective	1990–1995	Deterioration of function from normal to abnormal or increase in the severity of weakness compared to the immediate postoperative period	25%, 15 of 60	Mean or median and range NR	Not correlated with age, sex, or tumor size	80% returned to HB I–II
Sampath et al (1998)	Johns Hopkins Hospital, Baltimore, MD	Retrospective	1973–1994	Profound deterioration in facial nerve function (HB V or VI) that occurred 1 wk or more after surgery in patients with normal or nearly normal facial function in the immediate postoperative period	2%, 13 of 611	Mean or median NR, range: 1–4 wk after surgery	NR	None regained HB I function, 77% recovered to HB II, 15% recovered to HB III, and 8% to HB IV at 1 y
Fenton et al (2001)	St. Vincent's Hospital, Sydney, NSW 2010, Australia	Prospective	1994–1995	Any deterioration of function compared to the immediate postoperative period	14%, 8 of 57	Mean or median NR, range: 1–14 d	NR	Five patients with normal immediate function recovered within 1 mo of onset and one patient with normal function initially deteriorated to HB VI but recovered to HB III at 2 y. The two patients with abnormal initial postoperative function recovered to an ultimate HB III and normal function, respectively

Table 55.1 (Continued)

Study	Center	Design	Dates	Definition of delayed facial paralysis	Incidence rates	Latency	Predictors	Outcome
Gianoli (2002)	The Ear and Balance Institute, Baton Rouge, Louisiana	Prospective	NR	Initially normal facial nerve function immediately postoperatively with subsequent deterioration of facial nerve function	35%, 7 of 20	Mean or median and range NR	Correlated with elevated HSV-1 and VZV IgM titers	All patients had return of normal facial function by 7 wk after onset of the palsy
Grant et al (2002)	University of Washington, Seattle, WA	Retrospective	1988–2000	A deterioration of facial nerve function from HB I–II more than 3 d postoperatively	5%, 15 of 314	Mean: 10.9 d, range: 4–30 d	Smaller tumor size correlated with greater recovery of facial nerve function. There was no correlation between the latency or severity of recovery and age, sex, surgical approach, tumor course, neurotonic discharges during surgery, history of tobacco use, or cardiovascular disease	In six patients (40%) minor deterioration (2 HB grades) had occurred at a mean of 10.2 d postsurgery, whereas in nine patients (60%) moderate deterioration (3 HB grades) had occurred at a mean of 11.8 d postoperatively. Five (33%) of 15 patients recovered to grade I or II function within 6 wk of DFP onset. Of the 15 patients with DFP, 14 had completed 1 y of follow-up at the time of this study. Twelve (80%) of these 15 patients recovered to grade I or II function within 3 mo, and 13 (93%) of 14 patients recovered within 1 y
Magliulo et al (2003)	University La Sapienza, Rome, Italy	Retrospective	1990–2000	Any deterioration of function compared to the immediate postoperative period	26%, 25 of 98	Mean or median and range NR	Not correlated with age, sex, tumor size, or surgical approach	20 of 25 (80%) recovered HB I–II function
Morton et al (2011)	Loyola University Medical Center, Chicago, IL	Retrospective	2005–2007	Any subsequent worsening of normal or near-normal facial function (HB I–II) during the 4-wk postoperative period	25%, 26 of 104	Mean: 3 d, range: 1–28 d	Patients with DFP presented with significantly smaller tumor sizes than patients with IFP. This IFP group averaged significantly smaller intraoperative facial nerve responses than patients without facial palsy, and larger tumor sizes than both the DFP and no facial palsy groups. Within the DFP	96% recovered HB I–II at last follow-up

Table 55.1 (*Continued*)

Study	Center	Design	Dates	Definition of delayed facial paralysis	Incidence rates	Latency	Predictors	Outcome
							group, patients with late-onset DFP showed diminished intraoperative facial nerve responses when compared with the total DFP patient population	
Carlstrom et al (2016)	Mayo Clinic, Rochester, MN	Retrospective	2000–2014	Deterioration in facial function of at least 2 HB grades between postoperative days 5 and 30. Only patients with a HB grades I to III by postoperative day 5 were eligible for study inclusion	16%, 60 of 368	Mean: 12 d, range: 5–25 d	Correlated with GTR (83 vs. 71%, $p = 0.05$) and retrosigmoid approaches (72 vs. 52%, $p = 0.01$). There was no difference in recovery time between patients who received treatment with steroids, steroids with antivirals, or no treatment at all ($p = 0.530$). Patients with delayed facial paralysis and no facial paralysis did not differ significantly between sex, tumor size, operative duration, body mass index, postoperative complications, preoperative HB grade, or intraoperative facial nerve monitoring results	All patients recovered HB I–II by a mean of 33 d (range: 7–86 d)

Abbreviations: DFP, delayed facial paresis; GTR, gross total resection; HB, House–Brackmann; IFP, immediate facial paralysis; NR, not reported.

VSs and found that patients receiving a marginal dose of ≤ 13 Gy had better facial nerve function than those who received greater than 13 Gy (≤ 13 Gy = 98.5% HB I vs. > 13 Gy = 94.7% HB I; $p = 0.0001$).[68] In 2001, Foote et al demonstrated that with linear accelerator-based (LINAC) radiosurgery, dose to the brainstem was the strongest multivariate predictor of facial neuropathy.[11] In line with these results, Ganz et al found that radiation-induced facial nerve deficits following Gamma Knife radiosurgery were always associated with posttreatment increased T2 signal in the adjacent brainstem parenchyma.[62]

Second to marginal dose, history of prior treatment is an important predictor of facial nerve injury following radiosurgery. Even when normal facial nerve function exists, it is assumed that prior treatment results in some degree of subclinical nerve injury that lowers the threshold for facial paralysis with subsequent radiosurgery.[8,44] On multivariate analysis, Foote et al found that a history of prior microsurgical resection conferred a four fold increased risk of developing facial neuropathy after LINAC radiosurgery (Relative Risk: 3.9, $p = 0.009$).[11] In 1998, Pollock et al reported a 23% (11/47) rate of worsening facial nerve function with radiosurgery after failed microsurgery; however, stratified by dose, the rates of facial nerve dysfunction for ≥18 Gy, 15-17 Gy, and 12-14 Gy was 57%, 22% and 14%, respectively.[12] In a more recent study, Huang et al evaluated 173 Gamma Knife radiosurgery procedures in patients who had one or multiple prior microsurgical resections. Among patients with any degree of preexisting facial nerve dysfunction (HB II–VI), 19% had improvement in this condition after radiosurgery, and 5.5% with some facial function (HB I–V) developed new or worsening facial weakness.[74] Thus, it would appear that modern, low-dose planning effectively reduces the risk of facial neuropathy following radiosurgery for post-microsurgery tumor remnants.

A final risk factor for paralysis after radiosurgery is baseline tumor volume. Larger tumors may already impose some degree of subclinical facial nerve deficit, may exhibit greater transient tumor swelling with resultant facial nerve traction, have a greater length of the nerve that will receive radiation, and receive a larger dose to the brainstem.[10,11,12,44,68,75] Flickinger et al developed diameter–response curves at different doses to predict temporary or permanent facial neuropathy.[75] When using a marginal dose of 12 to 14 Gy, they found that the risk of facial nerve dysfunction increased significantly for tumors exceeding 2.5 to 3 cm CPA diameter. Milligan et al published a recent study evaluating radiosurgery for large VS (> 2.5 cm) and found that new permanent facial paralysis occurred in 14% of cases and new temporary hemifacial spasm occurred in 4%.[76] In 2013, Williams et al performed a retrospective case-matched comparison of large VS (> 3 cm) to small VS (≤ 3 cm) to assess the effect of lesion size on outcome.[67] Among patients with large tumors and good baseline facial function (HB I–II), 30% experienced worsening function. In contrast, among patients with smaller tumors and good baseline facial nerve function, only one patient experienced worsening function after treatment ($p = 0.003$). Corroborating these studies, a systematic review by Yang et al found that patients with a tumor volume ≤ 1.5 cm^3 experienced greater facial nerve preservation than patients with tumors > 1.5 cm^3 (≤ 1.5 cm^3 = 99.5% vs. > 1.5 cm^3 = 95.5%, $p = 0.0001$).[68]

55.5 Conclusion

Preservation of facial nerve function remains a high priority for both VS patients and surgeons. The mechanism, timing, incidence, and severity of facial nerve injury vary significantly according to tumor size and treatment. Increasingly utilized strategies, including STR with or without adjuvant radiation, and low-dose radiosurgery have effectively reduced the incidence of facial nerve paralysis. Large prospective studies with long-term follow-up will be required to validate the utility of these more conservative approaches to ensure we are not simply trading long-term success for short-term benefit.

References

[1] Carlson ML, Link MJ, Wanna GB, Driscoll CL. Management of sporadic vestibular schwannoma. Otolaryngol Clin North Am. 2015; 48(3):407–422

[2] Espahbodi M, Carlson ML, Fang TY, Thompson RC, Haynes DS. Small vestibular schwannomas presenting with facial nerve palsy. Otol Neurotol. 2014; 35(5): 895–898

[3] Carlson ML, Tombers NM, Driscoll CLW, et al. Clinically significant intratumoral hemorrhage in patients with vestibular schwannoma. Laryngoscope. 2017; 127(6):1420–1426

[4] Paldor I, Chen AS, Kaye AH. Growth rate of vestibular schwannoma. J Clin Neurosci. 2016; 32:1–8

[5] Axelsson A, Laage-Hellman JE. The gusto-lachrymal reflex. The syndrome of crocodile tears. Acta Otolaryngol. 1962; 54:239–254

[6] Nielsen VK. Electrophysiology of the facial nerve in hemifacial spasm: ectopic/ephaptic excitation. Muscle Nerve. 1985; 8(7):545–555

[7] Kartush JM, Graham MD, Kemink JL. Electroneurography: preoperative facial nerve assessment in acoustic neuroma surgery: a preliminary study. Am J Otol. 1986; 7(5):322–325

[8] Fenton JE, Chin RY, Kalamarides M, Sterkers O, Sterkers JM, Fagan PA. Delayed facial palsy after vestibular schwannoma surgery. Auris Nasus Larynx. 2001; 28(2):113–116

[9] Watanabe T, Saito N, Hirato J, Shimaguchi H, Fujimaki H, Sasaki T. Facial neuropathy due to axonal degeneration and microvasculitis following gamma knife surgery for vestibular schwannoma: a histological analysis. Case report. J Neurosurg. 2003; 99(5):916–920

[10] Linskey ME, Flickinger JC, Lunsford LD. Cranial nerve length predicts the risk of delayed facial and trigeminal neuropathies after acoustic tumor stereotactic radiosurgery. Int J Radiat Oncol Biol Phys. 1993; 25(2):227–233

[11] Foote KD, Friedman WA, Buatti JM, Meeks SL, Bova FJ, Kubilis PS. Analysis of risk factors associated with radiosurgery for vestibular schwannoma. J Neurosurg. 2001; 95(3):440–449

[12] Pollock BE, Lunsford LD, Flickinger JC, Clyde BL, Kondziolka D. Vestibular schwannoma management. Part I. Failed microsurgery and the role of delayed stereotactic radiosurgery. J Neurosurg. 1998; 89(6):944–948

[13] Three types of nerve injuries. Brain. 1943(66):237

[14] Sunderland S. A classification of peripheral nerve injuries producing loss of function. Brain. 1951; 74(4):491–516

[15] Carlson ML, Van Abel KM, Schmitt WR, Driscoll CL, Neff BA, Link MJ. The anatomically intact but electrically unresponsive facial nerve in vestibular schwannoma surgery. Neurosurgery. 2012; 71(6):1125–1130, discussion 1130

[16] Rivas A, Boahene KD, Bravo HC, Tan M, Tamargo RJ, Francis HW. A model for early prediction of facial nerve recovery after vestibular schwannoma surgery. Otol Neurotol. 2011; 32(5):826–833

[17] Sameshima T, Morita A, Tanikawa R, et al. Evaluation of variation in the course of the facial nerve, nerve adhesion to tumors, and postoperative facial palsy in acoustic neuroma. J Neurol Surg B Skull Base. 2013; 74(1):39–43

[18] Nejo T, Kohno M, Nagata O, Sora S, Sato H. Dorsal displacement of the facial nerve in acoustic neuroma surgery: clinical features and surgical outcomes of 21 consecutive dorsal pattern cases. Neurosurg Rev. 2016; 39(2):277–288, discussion 288

[19] Mastronardi L, Cacciotti G, Roperto R, Di Scipio E, Tonelli MP, Carpineta E. Position and course of facial nerve and postoperative facial nerve results in vestibular schwannoma microsurgery. World Neurosurg. 2016; 94:174–180

[20] Captier G, Canovas F, Bonnel F, Seignarbieux F. Organization and microscopic anatomy of the adult human facial nerve: anatomical and histological basis for surgery. Plast Reconstr Surg. 2005; 115(6):1457–1465
[21] May M. Anatomy for the clinician. In: May M, Schaitkin BM, eds. The Facial Nerve. New York, NY: Thieme Medical; 2000:19–57
[22] Minatogawa T, Kumoi T, Hosomi H, Kokan T. The blood supply of the facial nerve in the human temporal bone. Auris Nasus Larynx. 1980; 7(1):7–18
[23] Blunt MJ. The blood supply of the facial nerve. J Anat. 1954; 88(4):520–526
[24] Martin RG, Grant JL, Peace D, Theiss C, Rhoton AL, Jr. Microsurgical relationships of the anterior inferior cerebellar artery and the facial-vestibulocochlear nerve complex. Neurosurgery. 1980; 6(5):483–507
[25] Bloch O, Sughrue ME, Kaur R, et al. Factors associated with preservation of facial nerve function after surgical resection of vestibular schwannoma. J Neurooncol. 2011; 102(2):281–286
[26] Copeland WR, Van Gompel JJ, Giannini C, Eckel LJ, Koeller KK, Link MJ. Can preoperative imaging predict tumor involvement of the anterior clinoid in clinoid region meningiomas? Neurosurgery. 2015; 77(4):525–529, discussion 530
[27] Falcioni M, Fois P, Taibah A, Sanna M. Facial nerve function after vestibular schwannoma surgery. J Neurosurg. 2011; 115(4):820–826
[28] Grahnke K, Garst JR, Martin B, Leonetti JP, Anderson DE. Prognostic indices for predicting facial nerve outcome following the resection of large acoustic neuromas. J Neurol Surg B Skull Base. 2017; 78(6):454–460
[29] Ansari SF, Terry C, Cohen-Gadol AA. Surgery for vestibular schwannomas: a systematic review of complications by approach. Neurosurg Focus. 2012; 33 (3):E14
[30] Gerganov VM, Klinge PM, Nouri M, Stieglitz L, Samii M, Samii A. Prognostic clinical and radiological parameters for immediate facial nerve function following vestibular schwannoma surgery. Acta Neurochir (Wien). 2009; 151 (6):581–587, discussion 587
[31] Gurgel RK, Dogru S, Amdur RL, Monfared A. Facial nerve outcomes after surgery for large vestibular schwannomas: do surgical approach and extent of resection matter? Neurosurg Focus. 2012; 33(3):E16
[32] Samii M, Gerganov V, Samii A. Improved preservation of hearing and facial nerve function in vestibular schwannoma surgery via the retrosigmoid approach in a series of 200 patients. J Neurosurg. 2006; 105(4):527–535
[33] Tringali S, Ferber-Viart C, Fuchsmann C, Buiret G, Zaouche S, Dubreuil C. Hearing preservation in retrosigmoid approach of small vestibular schwannomas: prognostic value of the degree of internal auditory canal filling. Otol Neurotol. 2010; 31(9):1469–1472
[34] Rompaey VV, Dinther Jv, Zarowski A, Offeciers E, Somers T. Fundus obliteration and facial nerve outcome in vestibular schwannoma surgery. Skull Base. 2011; 21(2):99–102
[35] Wong RH, Copeland WR, Jacob JT, et al. Anterior extension of tumor is as important as tumor size to facial nerve outcome and extent of resection for vestibular schwannomas. J Neurol Surg B Skull Base. 2017; 78(6):473–480
[36] Hoover JM, Morris JM, Meyer FB. Use of preoperative magnetic resonance imaging T1 and T2 sequences to determine intraoperative meningioma consistency. Surg Neurol Int. 2011; 2:142
[37] Rizk AR, Adam A, Gugel I, Schittenhelm J, Tatagiba M, Ebner FH. Implications of vestibular schwannoma consistency: analysis of 140 cases regarding radiologic and clinical features. World Neurosurg. 2017; 99:159–163
[38] Patel NS, Van Abel KM, Link MJ, et al. Prevalence and surgical implications of dural enhancement at the porus acusticus in vestibular schwannomas. Otolaryngol Head Neck Surg. 2016; 155(6):1021–1027
[39] Ung N, Mathur M, Chung LK, et al. A systematic analysis of the reliability of diffusion tensor imaging tractography for facial nerve imaging in patients with vestibular schwannoma. J Neurol Surg B Skull Base. 2016; 77(4):314–318
[40] Hughes JD, Fattahi N, Van Gompel J, et al. Higher-resolution magnetic resonance elastography in meningiomas to determine intratumoral consistency. Neurosurgery. 2015; 77(4):653–658, discussion 658–659
[41] Yin Z, Glaser KJ, Manduca A, et al. Slip interface imaging predicts tumor-brain adhesion in vestibular schwannomas. Radiology. 2015; 277(2):507–517
[42] Piccirillo E, Wiet MR, Flanagan S, et al. Cystic vestibular schwannoma: classification, management, and facial nerve outcomes. Otol Neurotol. 2009; 30(6): 826–834
[43] Metwali H, Samii M, Samii A, Gerganov V. The peculiar cystic vestibular schwannoma: a single-center experience. World Neurosurg. 2014; 82(6): 1271–1275
[44] Kartush JM, Niparko JK, Graham MD, Kemink JL. Electroneurography: preoperative facial nerve assessment for tumors of the temporal bone. Otolaryngol Head Neck Surg. 1987; 97(3):257–261
[45] Syms CA, III, House JR, III, Luxford WM, Brackmann DE. Preoperative electroneuronography and facial nerve outcome in acoustic neuroma surgery. Am J Otol. 1997; 18(3):401–403
[46] Carlson ML, Habermann EB, Wagie AE, et al. The changing landscape of vestibular schwannoma management in the United States–a shift toward conservatism. Otolaryngol Head Neck Surg. 2015; 153(3):440–446
[47] Rabelo de Freitas M, Russo A, Sequino G, Piccirillo E, Sanna M. Analysis of hearing preservation and facial nerve function for patients undergoing vestibular schwannoma surgery: the middle cranial fossa approach versus the retrosigmoid approach–personal experience and literature review. Audiol Neurootol. 2012; 17(2):71–81
[48] Raftopoulos C, Abu Serieh B, Duprez T, Docquier MA, Guérit JM. Microsurgical results with large vestibular schwannomas with preservation of facial and cochlear nerve function as the primary aim. Acta Neurochir (Wien). 2005; 147(7):697–706, discussion 706
[49] Haque R, Wojtasiewicz TJ, Gigante PR, et al. Efficacy of facial nerve-sparing approach in patients with vestibular schwannomas. J Neurosurg. 2011; 115 (5):917–923
[50] Anaizi AN, Gantwerker EA, Pensak ML, Theodosopoulos PV. Facial nerve preservation surgery for KOOS grade 3 and 4 vestibular schwannomas. Neurosurgery. 2014; 75(6):671–675, discussion 676–677, quiz 677
[51] Monfared A, Corrales E, Theodosopoulos P, et al. Facial nerve outcome and tumor control rate as a function of degree of resection in treatment of large acoustic neuromas: preliminary report of the Acoustic Neuroma Subtotal Resection Study. Neurosurgery. 2015
[52] Carlstrom LP, Copeland WR, III, Neff BA, Castner ML, Driscoll CL, Link MJ. Incidence and risk factors of delayed facial palsy after vestibular schwannoma resection. Neurosurgery. 2016; 78(2):251–255
[53] Gianoli GJ. Viral titers and delayed facial palsy after acoustic neuroma surgery. Otolaryngol Head Neck Surg. 2002; 127(5):427–431
[54] Grant GA, Rostomily RR, Kim DK, et al. Delayed facial palsy after resection of vestibular schwannoma. J Neurosurg. 2002; 97(1):93–96
[55] Sampath P, Rhines LD, Holliday MJ, Brem H, Long DM. Late-onset facial nerve degeneration after vestibular schwannoma surgery: incidence, putative mechanisms, and prevention. Neurosurg Focus. 1998; 5(3):e6
[56] Sargent EW, Kartush JM, Graham MD. Meatal facial nerve decompression in acoustic neuroma resection. Am J Otol. 1995; 16(4):457–464
[57] Holliday MJ, Sampath P. Decompression of the labyrinthine segment of the facial nerve in acoustic neuroma surgery: a consideration for minimizing postoperative delayed facial nerve dysfunction. Neurosurg Focus. 1998; 5(3): e7
[58] Lalwani AK, Butt FY, Jackler RK, Pitts LH, Yingling CD. Delayed onset facial nerve dysfunction following acoustic neuroma surgery. Am J Otol. 1995; 16 (6):758–764
[59] Brackmann DE, Fisher LM, Hansen M, Halim A, Slattery WH. The effect of famciclovir on delayed facial paralysis after acoustic tumor resection. Laryngoscope. 2008; 118(9):1617–1620
[60] Scheller C, Strauss C, Fahlbusch R, Romstöck J. Delayed facial nerve paresis following acoustic neuroma resection and postoperative vasoactive treatment. Zentralbl Neurochir. 2004; 65(3):103–107
[61] Franco-Vidal V, Nguyen DQ, Guerin J, Darrouzet V. Delayed facial paralysis after vestibular schwannoma surgery: role of herpes viruses reactivation–our experience in eight cases. Otol Neurotol. 2004; 25(5):805–810
[62] Ganz JC, Reda WA, Abdelkarim K. Adverse radiation effects after Gamma Knife Surgery in relation to dose and volume. Acta Neurochir (Wien). 2009; 151(1):9–19
[63] Pollack AG, Marymont MH, Kalapurakal JA, Kepka A, Sathiaseelan V, Chandler JP. Acute neurological complications following gamma knife surgery for vestibular schwannoma: case report. J Neurosurg. 2013; 119 Suppl:546–551
[64] Tago M, Terahara A, Nakagawa K, et al. Immediate neurological deterioration after gamma knife radiosurgery for acoustic neuroma: case report. J Neurosurg. 2013; 119 Suppl:78–81
[65] Rampp S, Strauss C, Scheller C, Rachinger J, Prell J. A-trains for intraoperative monitoring in patients with recurrent vestibular schwannoma. Acta Neurochir (Wien). 2013; 155(12):2273–2279, discussion 2279
[66] Meeks SL, Buatti JM, Foote KD, Friedman WA, Bova FJ. Calculation of cranial nerve complication probability for acoustic neuroma radiosurgery. Int J Radiat Oncol Biol Phys. 2000; 47(3):597–602
[67] Williams BJ, Xu Z, Salvetti DJ, McNeill IT, Larner J, Sheehan JP. Gamma Knife surgery for large vestibular schwannomas: a single-center retrospective case-matched comparison assessing the effect of lesion size. J Neurosurg. 2013; 119(2):463–471

[68] Yang I, Sughrue ME, Han SJ, et al. Facial nerve preservation after vestibular schwannoma Gamma Knife radiosurgery. J Neurooncol. 2009; 93(1):41–48
[69] Murphy ES, Suh JH. Radiotherapy for vestibular schwannomas: a critical review. Int J Radiat Oncol Biol Phys. 2011; 79(4):985–997
[70] Foote RL, Coffey RJ, Swanson JW, et al. Stereotactic radiosurgery using the gamma knife for acoustic neuromas. Int J Radiat Oncol Biol Phys. 1995; 32(4): 1153–1160
[71] Lunsford LD, Niranjan A, Flickinger JC, Maitz A, Kondziolka D. Radiosurgery of vestibular schwannomas: summary of experience in 829 cases. J Neurosurg. 2013; 119 Suppl:195–199
[72] Miller RC, Foote RL, Coffey RJ, et al. Decrease in cranial nerve complications after radiosurgery for acoustic neuromas: a prospective study of dose and volume. Int J Radiat Oncol Biol Phys. 1999; 43(2):305–311
[73] Flickinger JC, Kondziolka D, Niranjan A, Maitz A, Voynov G, Lunsford LD. Acoustic neuroma radiosurgery with marginal tumor doses of 12 to 13 Gy. Int J Radiat Oncol Biol Phys. 2004; 60(1):225–230
[74] Huang MJ, Kano H, Mousavi SH, et al. Stereotactic radiosurgery for recurrent vestibular schwannoma after previous resection. J Neurosurg. 2017; 126(5): 1506–1513
[75] Flickinger JC, Kondziolka D, Lunsford LD. Dose and diameter relationships for facial, trigeminal, and acoustic neuropathies following acoustic neuroma radiosurgery. Radiother Oncol. 1996; 41(3):215–219
[76] Milligan BD, Pollock BE, Foote RL, Link MJ. Long-term tumor control and cranial nerve outcomes following γ knife surgery for larger-volume vestibular schwannomas. J Neurosurg. 2012; 116(3):598–604
[77] Magliulo G, Sepe C, Varacalli S, Crupi J. Acoustic neuroma surgery and delayed facial palsy. Eur Arch Otorhinolaryngol. 1998;255(3):124-6
[78] Megerian CA, McKenna MJ, Ojemann RG. Delayed facial paralysis after acoustic neuroma surgery: factors influencing recovery. Am J Otol. 1996 Jul;17 (4):630-3
[79] Magliulo G, D'Amico R, Di Cello P. Delayed facial palsy after vestibular schwannoma resection: clinical data and prognosis. J Otolaryngol. 2003 Dec;32(6):400-4
[80] Morton RP, Ackerman PD, Pisansky MT, Krezalek M, Leonetti JP, Raffin MJ, Anderson DE. Prognostic factors for the incidence and recovery of delayed facial nerve palsy after vestibular schwannoma resection. J Neurosurg. 2011 Feb;114(2):375-80

56 Patient Self-Assessment of Symptom Disability and Handicap in Vestibular Schwannoma

Matthew L. Carlson, John P. Marinelli, and Theodore McRackan

56.1 Introduction

In recent years, there has been growing interest within the medical community to examine patient-reported outcome measures (PROMs) in order to move beyond the provider's viewpoint and assess health care experience from the patient's perspective. While traditional outcome measures such as morbidity and mortality provide useful benchmarks for quality of care assessment, they sideline the patient's perception of health care and their experience with system structure, the care process, and other less tangible outcomes.[1,2] The use of PROMs is particularly relevant to vestibular schwannoma (VS) and other benign diseases, where current care is directed toward treatment of symptoms, maintenance or improvement of function, and prevention of disease-related complications, rather than mortality reduction.[3,4,5]

Under the heading of PROM are common constructs including health status, functional status, symptom experience, patient satisfaction, health-related quality of life, and well-being.[1,6] Broadly, individual PROM questionnaires can be categorized as generic versus disease specific and unidimensional (i.e., examining a single construct such as dizziness alone) versus multidimensional (i.e., examining multiple constructs, such as an instrument analyzing energy, anxiety, facial function, and dizziness domains).

This chapter focuses on reviewing validated instruments pertaining to symptom experience and functional status, while health-related quality of life assessment using multidimensional, generic, and disease-specific measures is discussed further in Chapter 60. As a foundation for this chapter, it is critical to review the differences between impairments, disabilities, and handicaps—terms that are often used incorrectly and interchangeably within health literature. Defined by the World Health Organization in 1980, impairment refers to "any loss or abnormality of psychological, physiological, or anatomical structure or function"; disability is defined as "any restriction or lack of ability to perform an activity in the manner or within the range considered normal for a human being"; and handicap is defined as "the result when an individual with an impairment cannot fulfill a normal life role."[7] To draw from an example relevant to the VS population, unilateral deafness is an impairment, the inability to localize sound is a disability, and the failure to secure a position in a particular occupation because of this impairment and disability is a handicap.

The benefit of utilizing patient self-assessment of disability and handicap for conditions such as tinnitus and headache is obvious; these are disorders that can significantly affect patient well-being, yet cannot be objectively quantified or outwardly observed. However, PROMs for conditions that can be examined and empirically quantified—facial nerve function, vestibular function, and hearing for example—still provide valuable and complementing information. For example, the Hearing Handicap Inventory (HHI) was developed because of the poor association that exists between pure-tone and speech audiometry with everyday communication and psychosocial function.[8] Similarly, the Dizziness Handicap Inventory (DHI) was developed because results of vestibular testing do not adequately quantify or predict the impact of dizziness on daily life.[9]

56.2 Disability and Handicap Inventories Relevant to Vestibular Schwannoma

The most common symptom-specific self-assessment inventories of disability and handicap in the VS literature pertain to hearing loss, tinnitus, dizziness, facial nerve dysfunction, and headache (▶ Table 56.1).[8,9,10,11,12,13,14,15,16,17,18] While individual instruments vary, most contain between 15 and 30 questions, with closed set 1 to 5 Likert scale responses. In most cases, the instrument is recorded such that the score is transformed to a 0- to 100-point scale, where a higher score indicates more severe disability or more severe handicap.

56.3 Summary of Literature Evaluating Disability and Handicap in Vestibular Schwannoma

56.3.1 Hearing

Most of the VS literature examining hearing outcomes has focused on pure-tone audiometry and word recognition scores, while less than 10 studies have examined hearing handicap using validated self-report measures.[19,20,21,22,23,24,25,26]

In 2004, Humphriss et al examined 119 patients who underwent translabyrinthine surgery and compared the preoperative HHI score to the 3- and 12-month postoperative HHI scores.[21] Remarkably, they found that 58% of subjects had no significant change in hearing handicap comparing preoperative and 12-month postoperative HHI scores, while 25% had worsening and 17% had improvement in their HHI score. The most plausible explanation for these findings is that most patients in this study (74%) already had nonserviceable hearing before surgery and progression to profound SNHL following surgery did not have a significant impact. In 2011, Park et al administered serial HHI questionnaires to 59 patients treated with radiosurgery.[20] Prior to intervention, half of patients had serviceable hearing, and at 12 months following radiation serviceable hearing was retained in 47% of patients. The mean baseline pure-tone average and speech discrimination scores were 44 dB and 65%, respectively, compared to 56 dB and 51% postradiosurgery. Despite progressive hearing loss, the HHI scores were not statistically significantly different following treatment. The lack of score decline seen in this study may reflect the limited amount of hearing loss (mean loss of 12 dB and 14%) seen during the short-term follow-up interval.

Table 56.1 Patient self-reported disability and handicap measures relevant to vestibular schwannoma

Metric	No. of questions	Domains	Scale	Pros	Cons
Dizziness					
DHI[9]	25	Functional; emotional; physical	0–100	Length; ease of use; long publication history	Developed over 30 y ago; structure validity not established
VSS[10]	27	Acute attack of vertigo; vertigo of short duration; somatization; autonomic symptoms	0–136	Short form available; can help differentiate pathology	Very symptom specific; less generalizable
VDI[11]	36	Symptoms; QOL	0–100	High internal consistency and reproducibility; balance of symptoms and impact on life	Low responsiveness to change in symptoms
Facial nerve function					
FDI[12]	10	Physical function; social/ well-being	0–55	Length; balance of symptoms and impact on life	Reproducibility not established
FaCE[13]	15	Facial movement; facial comfort; oral function; eye comfort; lacrimal control; social function	0–100	Length; correlates well with House–Brackmann scale	Uses combination of Likert and visual analog scale
Tinnitus					
THI[14]	25	Functional; emotional; catastrophic	0–100	Ease of use; long publication history	Less responsive than TFI
TFI[15]	25	Intrusive, sense of control; cognitive; sleep; auditory; relaxation; quality of life; emotional	0–00	Length; highly responsive	No overall score given—only calculate scores for each subscale
Headache[a]					
HDI[16]	25	Emotional; functional	0–100	Generalizable	May not correlate with specific AN patient complaints
HIT[17]	6	n/a	36–78	Length; gives data on frequency and severity of headache	Validated on migraine patients
Hearing					
Speech, spatial, and qualities of hearing scale[18]	49	Speech hearing; spatial hearing; qualities of hearing	0–10	Focused on hearing quality	Length; no emotional or social domains
Hearing handicap inventory in adults[8]	25	Emotional; social/ situational	0–100	Length; long publication history	Only two domains

Abbreviations: DHI, Dizziness Handicap Inventory; VSS, Vertigo Symptoms Score; VDI, Vertigo, Dizziness, Imbalance questionnaire; FDI, Facial Disability Index; FaCE, facial clinimetric evaluation; THI, Tinnitus Handicap Inventory; TFI, Tinnitus Functional Index; HDI, Headache Disability Inventory; HIT, Headache Impact Test.
[a]Excluding instruments assessing migraine.

In 2007, Douglas et al compared 44 subjects with profound unilateral SNHL following VS microsurgery and 127 control subjects using the Speech, Spatial, and Quality (SSQ) of hearing scale.[24] Despite having good hearing in the contralateral ear, VS subjects scored poorer than controls in the presence of competing background noise, with spatial hearing including direction, distance, and movement components, and reported poorer sound quality and impaired ease of listening. These findings mirror other studies examining handicap in patients with unilateral hearing loss.[27]

In 2015, Tveiten et al found that among 539 patients with unilateral VS, the contribution of hearing from the contralateral ear significantly affected overall HHI score.[22] For example, a patient with class A hearing bilaterally scored substantially better than a subject with class A hearing in one ear and nonserviceable hearing in the contralateral ear. This finding underscores the importance of considering hearing status in both ears when determining optimal treatment for each individual patient. In a follow-up study, Tveiten and colleagues also found that among VS patients with bilateral American Academy of Otolaryngology—Head and Neck Surgery (AAO–HNS) class A hearing, approximately 15% experienced "significant hearing handicap," and the mean HHI score was three times greater for VS patients with bilateral class A hearing compared to normal control subjects.[28]

56.3.2 Tinnitus

The use of self-reported measures for assessment of tinnitus is valuable because currently there are no other widely available or agreed upon methods to empirically quantify this outwardly invisible symptom. Summarized below are key findings reported in the literature pertaining to tinnitus disability in patients with VS.[19,20,21,26,29,30,31,32,33] Tinnitus handicap outcome between VS treatment modalities do not clearly demonstrate an advantage of one particular modality over others.[22] Furthermore, even between surgical approaches, the impact of treatment on tinnitus is unpredictable.[22,29] By most accounts, tinnitus frequently remains unchanged following treatment—those who are bothered by tinnitus before intervention are more likely to be bothered after, and vice versa.[20,30,31] Examining other predictive factors, two studies found a negative correlation between patient age and THI score—older patients reported lower (better) tinnitus handicap scores.[22,29] With few exceptions, most studies have not found a strong association between tinnitus and tumor size, hearing status, cochlear nerve preservation, or patient sex.[22,29] A more in-depth discussion of tinnitus in patients with VS can be found in Chapter 57.

56.3.3 Dizziness

Perhaps out of all disease-specific symptoms, dizziness remains one of the most complex to study. The symptom of dizziness can be caused by many common conditions including vestibular dysfunction, impaired vision, peripheral neuropathy, vestibular migraine, and heart conditions, among many other causes. Furthermore, the end symptom of dizziness may be influenced by other comorbid conditions such as anxiety and depression. It is now well established that results of vestibulometric testing and patient-reported dizziness handicap are often disparate—some patients with complete loss of unilateral vestibular function may report minimal daily impact, while others with even mild loss may be disabled.[9,34,35,36] With these complexities, the use of validated self-reported measures has significantly enhanced our ability to study this complex and multifaceted condition.[34,35,37,38,39,40,41,42,43,44]

One interesting and reproducible finding from several studies is that among all VS symptoms, dizziness is the primary driver of quality of life reduction.[4,19,26,39] Several authors have identified predictors of posttreatment dizziness handicap. In 2014, Carlson et al found that female sex, older age, larger tumor size, preexisting diagnosis of headache or migraine, and symptoms of dizziness predating treatment predicted poorer DHI scores following treatment.[43] In this study, it was found that at a mean of approximately 8 years following treatment, management strategy (i.e., radiosurgery, microsurgery, or observation) did not influence long-term dizziness handicap on multivariable analysis. Additionally, surgical approach does not appear to have any bearing on dizziness handicap outcome.[43] In contrast, other studies have demonstrated that microsurgery is associated with poorer DHI outcome compared to radiosurgery.[37] Differences in baseline dizziness symptoms that may influence treatment choice and duration of follow-up may explain contrasting conclusions.

Two studies have examined the benefit of surgery on dizziness handicap in a very selected cohort of subjects presenting with severe disabling vestibular symptoms.[41,44] Samii et al[44] examined 19 subjects with a mean preoperative DHI score of 66, and Godefroy et al[41] examined 18 patients presenting with a mean preoperative DHI score of 51. Both studies found that microsurgical resection resulted in a substantial improvement of over 30 points on the DHI at 12 months.

In 2003, Humphriss et al examined 100 consecutive *unselected* patients who underwent translabyrinthine surgery and found that DHI scores remained largely unchanged 1 year following surgery.[38] When defining 18 points as a minimum cutoff to designate change within an individual subject, 81 patients experienced no change in DHI score following surgery, 11 were significantly better, and 8 were significantly worse. In 2008, Wackym et al examined serial DHI scores in 55 patients with sporadic VS who were treated with Gamma Knife radiosurgery.[42] The authors found that after a mean follow-up of 55 months, there was no significant change in DHI score following treatment (15.5 vs. 13.5). Similarly, Park et al examined 59 subjects who underwent Gamma Knife radiosurgery for VS management, and at a mean of 15 months of follow-up, there was no significant change in DHI score (16.1 vs. 14.5).[20]

56.3.4 Facial Nerve Function

To the authors' knowledge, only two studies to date have utilized validated PROMs to assess facial nerve disability in patients with sporadic VS.[45,46] In 2009, Lin et al examined 25 VS patients who underwent facial nerve reinnervation for treatment of complete facial nerve paralysis using the facial disability index (FDI) among other measures.[45] This study is not discussed further as these patients do not represent the general VS population.

More recently, Tveiten et al performed a cross-sectional survey utilizing the FDI examining subjects with VS treated with microsurgery, radiosurgery, or observation.[46] In this study, several notable observations were made. First, paralleling House–Brackmann (HB) reporting, subjects who underwent microsurgery had a higher incidence of poorer FDI scores compared to radiosurgery or observation cohorts. Second, the largest FDI score reduction is seen between HB grades I and II, while the differences in FDI scores between HB grades II and IV were small by comparison. This highlights the importance of collecting and reporting PROM data as the VS literature tends to label "good" or "satisfactory" facial nerve outcomes according to HB grades I to II or HB grades I to III, respectively. Finally, the FDI questionnaire item that evaluated "excessive tearing and drying of the eye" explained most of the poorer scores seen in the surgery group—a condition that is generally not factored into facial nerve grading systems.

56.3.5 Headache

Based on our review of the current literature, there has been only one study that has utilized a validated headache disability questionnaire to assess self-reported headache outcome in patients with sporadic VS. In 2015, Carlson et al examined a total of 538 patients with VS and an additional 103 control subjects without tumors in a cross-sectional survey study.[47] At a mean of approximately 8 years following treatment, multivariable regression demonstrated no difference in headache disability inventory (HDI) score between treatment modalities, surgical approaches, or tumor size. The primary drivers of poor HDI were younger age, greater anxiety and depression, and pre-existing diagnosis of headache. Additional discussion regarding headache in patients with VS can be reviewed in Chapters 59 and 71.

56.4 Conclusion

This chapter outlines self-assessment inventories of disability and handicap that are most frequently employed in the VS literature. Validated self-reported measures provide valuable information that complement traditional, physician-defined endpoints. When feasible, PROM questionnaires should be incorporated in clinical outcome assessment to provide a more comprehensive understanding of how individual patients are impacted by a particular disease process or intervention.

References

[1] Chow A, Mayer EK, Darzi AW, Athanasiou T. Patient-reported outcome measures: the importance of patient satisfaction in surgery. Surgery. 2009; 146(3):435–443

[2] Marshall S, Haywood K, Fitzpatrick R. Impact of patient-reported outcome measures on routine practice: a structured review. J Eval Clin Pract. 2006; 12 (5):559–568

[3] Carlson ML, Tveiten OV, Driscoll CL, et al. Long-term quality of life in patients with vestibular schwannoma: an international multicenter cross-sectional study comparing microsurgery, stereotactic radiosurgery, observation, and nontumor controls. J Neurosurg. 2015; 122(4):833–842

[4] Carlson ML, Tveiten OV, Driscoll CL, et al. What drives quality of life in patients with sporadic vestibular schwannoma? Laryngoscope. 2015; 125(7): 1697–1702

[5] Gauden A, Weir P, Hawthorne G, Kaye A. Systematic review of quality of life in the management of vestibular schwannoma. J Clin Neurosci. 2011; 18(12): 1573–1584

[6] Meadows KA. Patient-reported outcome measures: an overview. Br J Community Nurs. 2011; 16(3):146–151

[7] World Health Organization (1980) International classification of impairments, disabilities, and handicaps (ICIDH), manual of classification relating to the consequences of disease. WHO, Geneva. Available at: http://apps.who.int/iris/bitstream/handle/10665/41003/9241541261_eng.pdf?sequence=1

[8] Newman CW, Weinstein BE, Jacobson GP, Hug GA. The Hearing Handicap Inventory for Adults: psychometric adequacy and audiometric correlates. Ear Hear. 1990; 11(6):430–433

[9] Jacobson GP, Newman CW. The development of the Dizziness Handicap Inventory. Arch Otolaryngol Head Neck Surg. 1990; 116(4):424–427

[10] Yardley L, Masson E, Verschuur C, Haacke N, Luxon L. Symptoms, anxiety and handicap in dizzy patients: development of the vertigo symptom scale. J Psychosom Res. 1992; 36(8):731–741

[11] Prieto L, Santed R, Cobo E, Alonso J. A new measure for assessing the health-related quality of life of patients with vertigo, dizziness or imbalance: the VDI questionnaire. Qual Life Res. 1999; 8(1–2):131–139

[12] VanSwearingen JM, Brach JS. The Facial Disability Index: reliability and validity of a disability assessment instrument for disorders of the facial neuromuscular system. Phys Ther. 1996; 76(12):1288–1298, discussion 1298–1300

[13] Kahn JB, Gliklich RE, Boyev KP, Stewart MG, Metson RB, McKenna MJ. Validation of a patient-graded instrument for facial nerve paralysis: the FaCE scale. Laryngoscope. 2001; 111(3):387–398

[14] Newman CW, Jacobson GP, Spitzer JB. Development of the Tinnitus Handicap Inventory. Arch Otolaryngol Head Neck Surg. 1996; 122(2):143–148

[15] Meikle MB, Henry JA, Griest SE, et al. The tinnitus functional index: development of a new clinical measure for chronic, intrusive tinnitus. Ear Hear. 2012; 33(2):153–176

[16] Jacobson GP, Ramadan NM, Aggarwal SK, Newman CW. The Henry Ford Hospital Headache Disability Inventory (HDI). Neurology. 1994; 44(5):837–842

[17] Yang M, Rendas-Baum R, Varon SF, Kosinski M. Validation of the Headache Impact Test (HIT-6™) across episodic and chronic migraine. Cephalalgia. 2011; 31(3):357–367

[18] Gatehouse S, Noble W. The Speech, Spatial and Qualities of Hearing Scale (SSQ). Int J Audiol. 2004; 43(2):85–99

[19] Lloyd SK, Kasbekar AV, Baguley DM, Moffat DA. Audiovestibular factors influencing quality of life in patients with conservatively managed sporadic vestibular schwannoma. Otol Neurotol. 2010; 31:968–976

[20] Park SS, Grills IS, Bojrab D, et al. Longitudinal assessment of quality of life and audiometric test outcomes in vestibular schwannoma patients treated with gamma knife surgery. Otol Neurotol. 2011; 32:676–679

[21] Humphriss RL, Baguley DM, Axon PR, Moffat DA. Change in hearing handicap after translabyrinthine vestibular schwannoma excision. Otol Neurotol. 2004; 25:371–378

[22] Tveiten OV, Carlson ML, Goplen F, Vassbotn F, Link MJ, Lund-Johansen M. Long-term auditory symptoms in patients with sporadic vestibular schwannoma: an international cross-sectional study. Neurosurgery. 2015; 77(2): 218–227, discussion 227

[23] Humphriss RL, Baguley DM, Axon PR, Moffat DA. Preoperative audiovestibular handicap in patients with vestibular schwannoma. Skull Base. 2006; 16(4): 193–199

[24] Douglas SA, Yeung P, Daudia A, Gatehouse S, O'Donoghue GM. Spatial hearing disability after acoustic neuroma removal. Laryngoscope. 2007; 117(9): 1648–1651

[25] Andersen HT, Schroder SA, Bonding P. Unilateral deafness after acoustic neuroma surgery: subjective hearing handicap and the effect of the bone-anchored hearing aid. Otol Neurotol. 2006; 27:809–814

[26] Jufas N, Flanagan S, Biggs N, Chang P, Fagan P. Quality of life in vestibular schwannoma patients managed by surgical or conservative approaches. Otol Neurotol. 2015; 36:1245–1254

[27] Noble W, Gatehouse S. Interaural asymmetry of hearing loss, Speech, Spatial and Qualities of Hearing Scale (SSQ) disabilities, and handicap. Int J Audiol. 2004; 43(2):100–114

[28] Tveiten OV, Carlson ML, Link MJ, Lund-Johansen M. Audiovestibular Handicap and Quality of Life in Patients With Vestibular Schwannoma and "Excellent" Hearing. Neurosurgery. 2017 Mar 1;80(3):386-392

[29] Bell JR, Anderson-Kim SJ, Low C, Leonetti JP. The persistence of tinnitus after acoustic neuroma surgery. Otolaryngol Head Neck Surg. 2016; 155:317–323

[30] Baguley DM, Humphriss RL, Axon PR, Moffat DA. Change in tinnitus handicap after translabyrinthine vestibular schwannoma excision. Otol Neurotol. 2005; 26:1061–1063

[31] Vivas EX, Wegner R, Conley G, et al. Treatment outcomes in patients treated with CyberKnife radiosurgery for vestibular schwannoma. Otol Neurotol. 2014; 35:162–170

[32] Baguley DM, Andersson G. Factor analysis of the Tinnitus Handicap Inventory. Am J Audiol. 2003; 12(1):31–34

[33] Park SH, Oh HS, Jeon JH, Lee YJ, Moon IS, Lee WS. Change in tinnitus after treatment of vestibular schwannoma: microsurgery vs. gamma knife radiosurgery. Yonsei Med J. 2014; 55(1):19–24

[34] El-Kashlan HK, Shepard NT, Arts HA, Telian SA. Disability from vestibular symptoms after acoustic neuroma resection. Am J Otol. 1998; 19(1):104–111

[35] Thomeer H, Bonnard D, Franco-Vidal V, et al. Prognostic factors of balance quality after transpetrosal vestibular schwannoma microsurgery: an instrumentally and DHI-based prospective cohort study of 48 patients. Otol Neurotol. 2015; 36:886–891

[36] Wagner JN, Glaser M, Wowra B, et al. Vestibular function and quality of life in vestibular schwannoma: does size matter? Front Neurol. 2011; 2:55

[37] Pollock BE, Driscoll CL, Foote RL, et al. Patient outcomes after vestibular schwannoma management: a prospective comparison of microsurgical resection and stereotactic radiosurgery. Neurosurgery. 2006; 59(1):77–85, discussion 77–85

[38] Humphriss RL, Baguley DM, Moffat DA. Change in dizziness handicap after vestibular schwannoma excision. Otol Neurotol. 2003; 24:661–665

[39] Tufarelli D, Meli A, Alesii A, et al. Quality of life after acoustic neuroma surgery. Otol Neurotol. 2006; 27:403–409

[40] Low Choy NL, Lucey MM, Lewandowski SL, Panizza BJ. Impacts of small vestibular schwannoma on community ambulation, postural, and ocular control. Laryngoscope. 2017; 127(5):1147–1152

[41] Godefroy WP, Hastan D, van der Mey AG. Translabyrinthine surgery for disabling vertigo in vestibular schwannoma patients. Clin Otolaryngol. 2007; 32(3):167–172

[42] Wackym PA, Hannley MT, Runge-Samuelson CL, Jensen J, Zhu YR. Gamma Knife surgery of vestibular schwannomas: longitudinal changes in vestibular

function and measurement of the Dizziness Handicap Inventory. J Neurosurg. 2008; 109 Suppl:137–143

[43] Carlson ML, Tveiten OV, Driscoll CL, et al. Long-term dizziness handicap in patients with vestibular schwannoma: a multicenter cross-sectional study. Otolaryngol Head Neck Surg. 2014; 151:1028–1037

[44] Samii M, Metwali H, Gerganov V. Efficacy of microsurgical tumor removal for treatment of patients with intracanalicular vestibular schwannoma presenting with disabling vestibular symptoms. J Neurosurg. 2017 May;126 (5):1514-1519

[45] Lin V, Jacobson M, Dorion J, Chen J, Nedzelski J. Global assessment of outcomes after varying reinnervation techniques for patients with facial paralysis subsequent to acoustic neuroma excision. Otol Neurotol. 2009; 30:408–413

[46] Tveiten OV, Carlson ML, Goplen F, et al. Patient- versus physician-reported facial disability in vestibular schwannoma: an international cross-sectional study. J Neurosurg. 2016:1–10

[47] Carlson ML, Tveiten OV, Driscoll CL, et al. Risk factors and analysis of long-term headache in sporadic vestibular schwannoma: a multicenter cross-sectional study. J Neurosurg. 2015; 123(5):1276–1286

57 Tinnitus in Sporadic Vestibular Schwannoma

Jamie J. Van Gompel and Matthew L. Carlson

57.1 Introduction

Tonal tinnitus is the phantom perception of sound when no external generating stimulus is present. In the general U.S. population, 15% of adults experience tinnitus.[1,2] However, with vestibular schwannoma (VS), it can be a presenting symptom in up to 70 to 80% of patients.[3] For some, subjective tinnitus is merely a fleeting annoyance; however, a significant subset of individuals experience audiological, neurological, and/or cognitive impairment resulting in poor attention, increased distractibility, anxiety, sleep deprivation, depression, and even suicide.[2] It appears that factors beyond tinnitus pitch, loudness, and quality of noise influence tinnitus handicap, as some patients appear greatly distressed by what they describe as relatively quiet or intermittent noise, while other seem to tolerate constant loud ringing. Unfortunately, most publications in the VS literature detail whether tinnitus was simply present or absent without attempting to ascertain the perceived severity or impact on the patient's well-being. Furthermore, it still remains unclear whether one treatment strategy demonstrates a clear benefit over another with mitigating or preventing severe tinnitus.

57.2 Mechanism of Tinnitus

The primary mechanisms underlying the development and persistence of tinnitus remain largely unknown. However, one can imagine any of the following as potential underlying causes: ephaptic coupling of cochlear nerve fibers by compression, cochlear dysfunction by ischemia or by biochemical degradation (protein or ionic changes), and cortical reorganization following hearing loss or surgical deafferentation. A leading hypothesis holds that tinnitus occurs as a result of detrimental cortical reorganization following an injury to the peripheral auditory pathway that disrupts the equilibrium between afferent and efferent signaling.[4] The theory of cochlear deafferentation as a cause for tinnitus parallels phantom limb pain, where cortical maladaptation develops in response to loss of sensory input.

Curiously, some patients with VS present with normal hearing by all objective criteria and still report tinnitus, thus making ephaptic transmission (i.e., abnormal cochlear nerve firing) a possible origin of tinnitus in these patients.[5] In other cases, tinnitus may worsen following surgical tumor resection including division of the cochleovestibular nerve, suggesting that in these cases cortical reorganization after deafferentation may be causative. Lastly, vascular compression as a source of tinnitus is perhaps the most understudied possibility. Paralleling this hypothesis, a limited population of patients with VS present with trigeminal neuralgia, in which circumstance the authors will commonly recommend surgical removal with formal microvascular decompression (MVD) for relief. In the general neurosurgical literature, there is evidence that MVD may be effective for some forms of tinnitus.[6] While only speculative, it may be possible that formal MVD of the eighth cranial nerve at the root exit zone following hearing preservation microsurgical resection provides an advantage for tinnitus outcome in a select population over simple tumor resection alone. This topic is explored further later in the chapter.

57.3 Outcome of Tinnitus after Vestibular Schwannoma Treatment

There are a number of validated self-report inventories for tinnitus assessment that VS surgeons should be aware of (▶ Table 57.1). Symptom-specific and disease-specific instruments are critical in characterizing outcomes in diseases such as VS, since other generic measures such as the SF36 lack the sensitivity required to detect longitudinal changes within an individual or between treatment strategies. In addition, the absolute scores help ascertain the degree to which the symptom is affecting patient well-being.

Table 57.1 Patient-reported outcome measures for assessment of tinnitus

Questionnaire	Author (year)	Number of items	Response tiers	Validated languages
Tinnitus Questionnaire	Hallam et al[7] (1988)	52	3: true, partly true, not true	English, German, Dutch, French, Chinese
Tinnitus Handicap Questionnaire	Kuk et al[8] (1990)	27	100: 100 = strongly agree, 0 = strongly disagree	English, French
Subjective Tinnitus Severity Scale	Halford and Anderson[9] (1991)	16	2: yes, no	English, Dutch, French
Tinnitus Reaction Questionnaire	Wilson et al[10] (1991)	26	not at all; a little of the time; a good deal of the time; almost all the time	English, French
Tinnitus Handicap Inventory	Newman et al[11] (1996)	25	3: yes, sometimes, no	English, French, Danish, Spanish, Korean, Portuguese
Mini TQ	Hiller and Goebel[12] (2004)	12	3: true, partly true, not true	German, Portuguese
Tinnitus Functional Index	Meikle et al[13] (2012)	25	10	English

Table 57.2 Published tinnitus outcomes in patients with vestibular schwannoma following treatment

Author(year)	Study type	N	Treatment	Tinnitus (%)				Notes
				Resolved	Improved	No change	Worse	
Henrich et al[14] (1995)	Retrospective	160	Surgery	45	17	30	8	
Kameda et al[15] (2010)	Retrospective	242	Surgery	25.2	33.3	31.6	9.9	No difference in tinnitus outcome with cochlear nerve sectioning
Kohno et al[16] (2014)	Retrospective	367	Surgery	20	22	45	14	22% new onset in those that did not have pre-op tinnitus
Chovanec et al[17] (2015)	Prospective	89	Surgery	66	9	11	14	
Kano et al (2009)	Retrospective	77	Radiation	0	12	79	9	Margin dose 12.5 Gy, follow-up median 20 mo (maybe too early to see effect)

A summary of published studies with reported tinnitus outcomes in VS is presented in ▶ Table 57.2. In 2014, Kohno et al reported that of 290 patients with preoperative tinnitus who were treated with retrosigmoid craniotomy for VS resection, tinnitus resolved in 20%, improved in 22%, was unchanged in 35%, and worsened in 14%. In addition, among 77 patients without preoperative tinnitus, 22% developed new-onset tinnitus following the operation.[16] Therefore, this study found that among subjects with preoperative tinnitus, microsurgical treatment was associated with improvement in just over 40% of cases.[16] Interestingly, it was found that younger age, better preoperative hearing, and smaller tumor size demonstrated worse tinnitus outcomes postoperatively.[16] Furthermore, the prognosis of tinnitus was significantly worse in the group of patients left with an anatomically preserved cochlear nerve without useful hearing compared to the group with a surgically divided cochlear nerve. In a more recent study, Bell et al found that among 53 patients who underwent microsurgical resection of VS, 17% reported that their tinnitus resolved, 9% reported improvement, 23% reported no change, 43% reported worsening, and 8% were unsure. Sex, tumor size, surgical approach, hearing preservation, and cochlear nerve status did not correlate with the prognosis of tinnitus after surgery. However, the prognosis of tinnitus was worse for younger respondents, those with serviceable hearing preoperatively, and those with residual tumor postoperatively.[18] Henrich and colleagues published their experience with 160 VS cases treated by translabyrinthine approach between 1980 and 1991. Data regarding the presence and severity of tinnitus after treatment were obtained via telephone correspondence. Overall, among patients with tinnitus preoperatively, the condition was absent postoperatively in 45%, lessened in 17%, was unchanged in 30%, and worsened in 8%.[14] These results appear to be similar to the retrosigmoid cohort reviewed earlier.

Currently, there is a paucity of published data reporting tinnitus outcomes in the stereotactic radiosurgery (SRS) literature for VS. In 2009, Kano et al reported tinnitus improvement in only approximately 10% of patients. Although this appears poor, the SRS literature focuses less on this symptom. One prospective study comparing SRS to a smaller number of microsurgical patients reported stable to worsening tinnitus in the patients treated with stereotactic radiation and a reduction in tinnitus in those treated with microsurgery.[19]

Van Gompel et al previously explored the symptom of tinnitus and its relationship with treatment utilizing the Acoustic Neuroma Association (ANA) 2007–2008 annual survey which included 2,004 respondents.[20] In this survey, tinnitus severity was recorded as a continuous variable, asking respondents at initial presentation and presently to grade their tinnitus on a 10-point scale, from 1 (least severe/mild) to 10 (most severe/disabling).[21] Overall, there were 1,138 patients who received treatment and 289 patients who received no treatment or observation in this study.[21] Overall, the average presentation score and most recent tinnitus score were 4.3 ± 0.1 and 3.8 ± 0.1, respectively ($p < 0.001$).[21] Tinnitus scores worsened over time among patients who did not receive active intervention (3.7 ± 0.1 to 4.1 ± 0.2; $p = 0.018$).[21] When evaluating tinnitus improvement by microsurgical approach, the cohort of patients who underwent translabyrinthine and retrosigmoid craniotomy both demonstrated an improvement in score. However, the middle fossa approach did not appear to impact tinnitus.[21] SRS was performed in 221 patients as primary treatment and further appeared to improve postoperative tinnitus at last follow-up.[21] The authors conclude that those undergoing observation have a greater risk of experiencing worsening tinnitus, while intervention (microsurgery or radiation) has a higher likelihood of tinnitus stabilization or improvement.[21] Future studies will be necessary to examine tinnitus outcomes according to treatment modality. As with hearing preservation, tinnitus outcomes will require very long-term follow-up as delayed audiovestibular symptoms are common.

57.3.1 Treatment of Tinnitus after Vestibular Schwannoma Resection: Present Day

Currently, there are no Food and Drug Administration (FDA)-approved pharmacological therapies or surgical devices available for the treatment of tinnitus.[2,22] The 2014 Clinical Practice Guideline on tinnitus from the American Academy of Otolaryngology—Head and Neck Surgery (AAO-HNS) summarized the state of tinnitus management by stating, "A cure for primary tinnitus does not yet exist, and despite claims to the contrary, no method has been proven to provide long-term suppression of tinnitus."[2] Existing treatment methods focus on counseling, cognitive behavioral therapy, masking, and sound therapy—strategies that may render tinnitus more tolerable but do not permanently reduce the intensity of tinnitus and do not reverse the pathological changes underlying the development and persistence of disease.

The interested reader is encouraged to review the 2014 AAO-HNS tinnitus clinical practice guideline for in-depth discussion.[2] The executive summary of the guideline action statement specifies that clinicians ***should*** (1) distinguish patients with bothersome tinnitus from patients with nonbothersome tinnitus; (2) recommend a hearing aid evaluation for patients with hearing loss and persistent bothersome tinnitus; and (3) recommend cognitive-behavioral therapy for patients with persistent bothersome tinnitus. Clinicians ***may*** recommend sound therapy to patients with persistent bothersome tinnitus. Clinicians ***should not*** (1) routinely recommend antidepressants, anticonvulsants, anxiolytics, or intratympanic medications for a primary indication of treating persistent bothersome tinnitus; (2) recommend Gingko biloba, melatonin, zinc, or other dietary supplements for treating patients with persistent bothersome tinnitus; or (3) recommend transcranial magnetic stimulation for the routine treatment of patients with persist bothersome tinnitus. Finally, *no recommendations* could be made regarding the effect of acupuncture based on insufficient data. Of course, in the setting of profound sensorineural hearing loss, an ipsilateral hearing aid or masking device will not provide benefit.

57.3.2 Treatment of Tinnitus after Vestibular Schwannoma Resection: New Frontiers

Cochlear implantation: Cochlear implantation is not currently approved by the FDA for implantation in patients with unilateral or asymmetrical sensorineural hearing loss. Furthermore, the presence of retrocochlear pathology has long been considered a relative contraindication to implantation. However, growing data have demonstrated the efficacy of cochlear implantation for auditory rehabilitation in patients with sporadic unilateral VS and in NF2—either in untreated VS or following radiation treatment or microsurgical resection when the cochlear nerve is anatomically preserved. In addition to enhanced speech understanding, particularly in noise, and improved sound localization, cochlear implantation provides an effective means of tinnitus suppression in many cases. In fact, a 2012 systematic review of cochlear implantation for treatment of intractable tinnitus in patients with single-sided deafness revealed that more than 90% of patients experienced improvement or resolution of tinnitus during implant use.[23] The benefit of tinnitus reduction from cochlear implantation in patients with VS is not yet known. Paralleling these findings, a recent study also demonstrated similar benefits of tinnitus suppression with auditory brainstem implantation.[24] Of course, these strategies present a unique set of challenges in the VS population, including MRI tumor surveillance with a retained internal device magnet. Further discussion on cochlear implantation and auditory brainstem implantation for aural rehabilitation and tinnitus suppression in VS can be found in Chapters 61 and 84.

Central pathway stimulation: Cortical or central auditory pathway stimulation for treatment of tinnitus is not FDA approved; however, there are several studies demonstrating the potential benefits of cortical stimulation for medically intractable tinnitus. Although many central targets exist, such as the cochlear nuclei,[25] follicular stimulation,[25] medial geniculate body,[26] and the dorsolateral prefrontal cortex,[27] the most logical target is the primary auditory cortex (Heschl's gyrus).[28,29,30,31] Currently, most implants incorporate epidural paddle electrodes; however, given the configuration of Heschl's gyrus, intraparenchymal electrodes similar to those used for deep brain stimulation may prove most effective (▶ Fig. 57.1).[31]

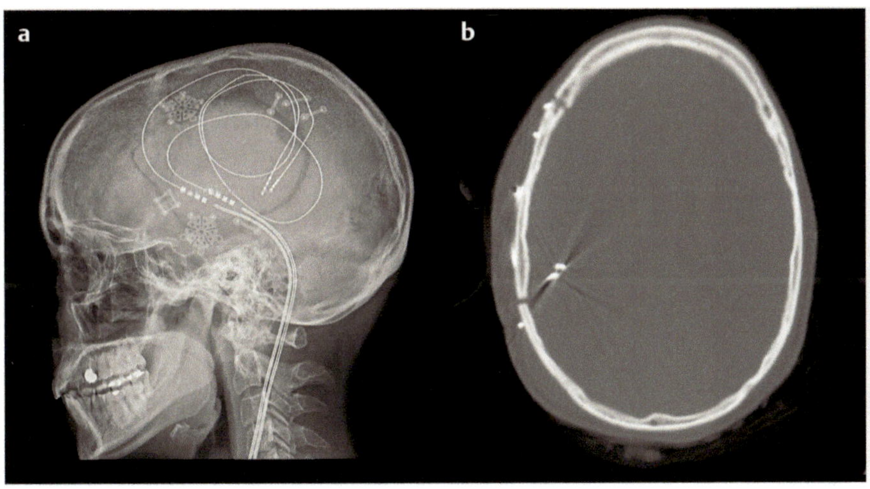

Fig. 57.1 Direct electrical stimulation of Heschl's gyrus for epilepsy with aura of tinnitus.

MVD in tinnitus: Although not currently considered during VS tumor resection, MVD of the brainstem after tumor resection could be a potential treatment option in those patients with preoperative tinnitus. The first reported MVD for tinnitus was reported in 1975 by Jannetta.[32] We recently completed a systematic review evaluating outcomes of MVD for intractable tinnitus, including 43 unique cases.[33,34,35,36,37,38,39] On average, patients experienced tinnitus symptoms for 4 years prior to MVD. Nine patients experienced complete resolution of their tinnitus following MVD, 17 patients experienced improvement of their tinnitus symptoms (60% positive response), 16 patients experienced no change in symptoms, and one patient experienced a worsening of tinnitus symptoms.[33,34,35,36,37,38,39] Admittedly it is difficult to ascertain the long-term efficacy of this treatment.

Paralleling this, trigeminal neuralgia in the setting of VS is often associated with a compressing vessel—most commonly the superior cerebellar artery. In these cases, it is hypothesized that a growing tumor displaces the fifth nerve toward a culprit vessel or a culprit vessel into the fifth nerve. In such cases, we have been most successful at alleviating facial pain when MVD is performed concurrently with tumor resection. Perhaps in the same way, in patients presenting with tinnitus, one should examine the brainstem for associated vascular conflict and, if present, pad the adjacent vessel from the brainstem in cases where microsurgical resection is pursued.

References

[1] Centers for Disease Control and Prevention (CDC). National Center for Health Statistics (NCHS). National Health and Nutrition Examination Survey Data. Hyattsville, MD: U.S. Department of Health and Human Services, Centers for Disease Control and Prevention, 2011–2012 Survey. Available at: https://wwwn.cdc.gov/nchs/nhanes/2011-2012/AUQ_G.htm. Accessed September 20, 2018

[2] Tunkel DE, Bauer CA, Sun GH, et al. Clinical practice guideline: tinnitus. Otolaryngol Head Neck Surg. 2014; 151(2) Suppl:S1–S40

[3] Wiegand DA, Ojemann RG, Fickel V. Surgical treatment of acoustic neuroma (vestibular schwannoma) in the United States: report from the Acoustic Neuroma Registry. Laryngoscope. 1996; 106(1, Pt 1):58–66

[4] Tyler RS, Rubinstein J, Pan T, et al. Electrical stimulation of the cochlea to reduce tinnitus. Semin Hear. 2008; 29(4):326–332

[5] Weisz N, Hartmann T, Dohrmann K, Schlee W, Norena A. High-frequency tinnitus without hearing loss does not mean absence of deafferentation. Hear Res. 2006; 222(1–2):108–114

[6] Nash B, Carlson ML, Van Gompel JJ. Microvascular decompression for tinnitus: systematic review. J Neurosurg. 2017; 126(4):1148–1157

[7] Hallam RS, Jakes SC, Hinchcliffe R. Cognitive variables in tinnitus annoyance. Br J Clin Psychol. 1988; 27(Pt 3):213–222

[8] Kuk FK, Tyler RS, Russell D, Jordan H. The psychometric properties of a tinnitus handicap questionnaire. Ear Hear. 1990; 11(6):434–445

[9] Halford JB, Anderson SD. Tinnitus severity measured by a subjective scale, audiometry and clinical judgement. J Laryngol Otol. 1991; 105(2):89–93

[10] Wilson PH, Henry J, Bowen M, Haralambous G. Tinnitus reaction questionnaire: psychometric properties of a measure of distress associated with tinnitus. J Speech Hear Res. 1991; 34(1):197–201

[11] Newman CW, Jacobson GP, Spitzer JB. Development of the tinnitus handicap inventory. Arch Otolaryngol Head Neck Surg. 1996; 122(2):143–148

[12] Hiller W, Goebel G. Rapid assessment of tinnitus-related psychological distress using the Mini-TQ. Int J Audiol. 2004; 43(10):600–604

[13] Meikle MB, Henry JA, Griest SE, et al. The tinnitus functional index: development of a new clinical measure for chronic, intrusive tinnitus. Ear Hear. 2012; 33(2):153–176

[14] Henrich DE, McCabe BF, Gantz BJ. Tinnitus and acoustic neuromas: analysis of the effect of surgical excision on postoperative tinnitus. Ear Nose Throat J. 1995; 74(7):462–466

[15] Kameda K, Shono T, Hashiguchi K, Yoshida F, Sasaki T. Effect of tumor removal on tinnitus in patients with vestibular schwannoma. J Neurosurg. 2010; 112 (1):152–157

[16] Kohno M, Shinogami M, Yoneyama H, Nagata O, Sora S, Sato H. Prognosis of tinnitus after acoustic neuroma surgery—surgical management of postoperative tinnitus. World Neurosurg. 2014; 81(2):357–367

[17] Chovanec M, Zvěřina E, Profant O, et al. Does attempt at hearing preservation microsurgery of vestibular schwannoma affect postoperative tinnitus? BioMed Res Int. 2015; 2015:783169

[18] Bell JR, Anderson-Kim SJ, Low C, Leonetti JP. The persistence of tinnitus after acoustic neuroma surgery. Otolaryngol Head Neck Surg. 2016; 155(2):317–323

[19] Myrseth E, Møller P, Pedersen P-H, Lund-Johansen M. Vestibular schwannoma: surgery or gamma knife radiosurgery? A prospective, nonrandomized study. Neurosurgery. 2009; 64(4):654–661, discussion 661–663

[20] Acoustic Neuroma Association. Available at: http://anausa.org/index.php/patient-surveys. Accessed September 21, 2012

[21] Van Gompel JJ, Patel J, Danner C, et al. Acoustic neuroma observation associated with an increase in symptomatic tinnitus: results of the 2007–2008 Acoustic Neuroma Association survey. J Neurosurg. 2013; 119(4):864–868

[22] Henry JA, Zaugg TL, Myers PJ, Schmidt CJ, Ribbe C, Edmonds K. Adult Tinnitus Management Clinical Practice Recommendation. Portland, OR: Department of Veterans Affairs; 2015

[23] Arts RA, George EL, Stokroos RJ, Vermeire K. Review: cochlear implants as a treatment of tinnitus in single-sided deafness. Curr Opin Otolaryngol Head Neck Surg. 2012; 20(5):398–403

[24] Roberts DS, Otto S, Chen B, et al. Tinnitus suppression after auditory brainstem implantation in patients with neurofibromatosis type-2. Otol Neurotol. 2017; 38(1):118–122

[25] Soussi T, Otto SR. Effects of electrical brainstem stimulation on tinnitus. Acta Otolaryngol. 1994; 114(2):135–140

[26] Barry KM, Paolini AG, Robertson D, Mulders WH. Modulation of medial geniculate nucleus neuronal activity by electrical stimulation of the nucleus accumbens. Neuroscience. 2015; 308:1–10

[27] De Ridder D, Vanneste S, Plazier M, et al. Dorsolateral prefrontal cortex transcranial magnetic stimulation and electrode implant for intractable tinnitus. World Neurosurg. 2012; 77(5–6):778–784

[28] De Ridder D, De Mulder G, Menovsky T, Sunaert S, Kovacs S. Electrical stimulation of auditory and somatosensory cortices for treatment of tinnitus and pain. Prog Brain Res. 2007; 166:377–388

[29] De Ridder D, De Mulder G, Verstraeten E, et al. Primary and secondary auditory cortex stimulation for intractable tinnitus. ORL J Otorhinolaryngol Relat Spec. 2006; 68(1):48–54, discussion 54–55

[30] Langguth B, De Ridder D. Tinnitus: therapeutic use of superficial brain stimulation. Handb Clin Neurol. 2013; 116:441–467

[31] Seidman MD, Ridder DD, Elisevich K, et al. Direct electrical stimulation of Heschl's gyrus for tinnitus treatment. Laryngoscope. 2008; 118(3):491–500

[32] Jannetta PJ. Neurovascular cross-compression in patients with hyperactive dysfunction symptoms of the eighth cranial nerve. Surg Forum. 1975; 26:467–469

[33] Borghei-Razavi H, Darvish O, Schick U. Disabling vertigo and tinnitus caused by intrameatal compression of the anterior inferior cerebellar artery on the vestibulocochlear nerve: a case report, surgical considerations, and review of the literature. J Neurol Surg Rep. 2014; 75(1):e47–e51

[34] De Ridder D, Ryu H, Møller AR, Nowé V, Van de Heyning P, Verlooy J. Functional anatomy of the human cochlear nerve and its role in microvascular decompressions for tinnitus. Neurosurgery. 2004; 54(2):381–388, discussion 388–390

[35] De Ridder D, Vanneste S, Adriaensens I, Lee AP, van de Heyning P, Möller A. Vascular compression of the cochlear nerve and tinnitus: a pathophysiological investigation. Acta Neurochir (Wien). 2012; 154(5):807–813

[36] De Ridder D, Vanneste S, Adriaenssens I, et al. Microvascular decompression for tinnitus: significant improvement for tinnitus intensity without improvement for distress. A 4-year limit. Neurosurgery. 2010; 66(4):656–660

[37] Pirayesh Islamian A, Lütjens G, Krauss JK. Microvascular decompression of the eighth cranial nerve for unilateral pulsatile tinnitus. Clin Neurol Neurosurg. 2014; 117:102–106

[38] Vasama JP, Moller MB, Moller AR. Microvascular decompression of the cochlear nerve in patients with severe tinnitus. Preoperative findings and operative outcome in 22 patients. Neurol Res. 1998; 20(3):242–248

[39] Yap L, Pothula VB, Lesser T. Microvascular decompression of cochleovestibular nerve. Eur Arch Otorhinolaryngol. 2008; 265(8):861–869

[40] Kano H, Kondziolka D, Khan A, Flickinger JC, Lunsford LD. Predictors of hearing preservation after stereotactic radiosurgery for acoustic neuroma. J Neurosurg. 2009 Oct;111(4):863-73

[41] Kano H, Kondziolka D, Khan A, Flickinger JC, Lunsford LD. Predictors of hearing preservation after stereotactic radiosurgery for acoustic neuroma. J Neurosurg. 2009 Oct;111(4):863-73

58 Dizziness in Sporadic Vestibular Schwannoma

Jeffrey D. Sharon and Yuri Agrawal

58.1 Introduction

One curious feature of vestibular schwannoma (VS) is that despite arising from the vestibular nerve, most patients do not present with imbalance or vertigo as a primary complaint. Instead, dysfunction of the cochlear nerve, manifesting as hearing loss or tinnitus, is the most common presentation. Theoretically, this phenomenon could be explained by either subclinical damage to the vestibular nerve (as occurs with the facial nerve), such that gross function is preserved, or alternatively that many patients are able to effectively compensate for a slowly evolving loss of function. Vestibular testing in patients with VS prior to treatment shows that the latter explanation accounts for most cases—caloric hypofunction, absent cervical vestibular evoked myogenic potentials (cVEMPs), and abnormal subjective visual vertical testing occur in many patients.[1] While it would seem intuitive that the nerve of origin could be predicted by the pattern of loss on vestibular testing (i.e., caloric tests and ocular VEMPs for superior nerve tumors, and cVEMPs for inferior nerve tumors), this has not been shown to be the case in most studies.[2] Furthermore, on questioning, many patients with VS do endorse imbalance and dizziness as a secondary complaint. In patients with a VS that is being observed, balance dysfunction has been found to be a significant predictor of quality of life.[3,4] Furthermore, in a large cross-sectional survey of patients treated with all modalities, dizziness was found to have the greatest impact on quality of life when present.[5] Interestingly, Saman et al compared the severity of vertigo symptoms, as measured by the Vertigo Symptom Scale, and found that patients with observed VS had higher scores (mean: 0.46, SD: 0.51) than control patients (mean: 0.07, SD: 0.09), but lower scores than patients with migrainous vertigo (mean: 1.61, SD: 0.86).[6]

58.2 Overview of the Vestibular System

58.2.1 Vestibular Physiology

In order to understand how loss of vestibular function and how the treatment of vestibular rehabilitation assists with functional recovery, it will be helpful to briefly review the normal physiology of the vestibular system.[7] There are five end organs housed within the inner ear: the utricle, saccule, horizontal (lateral), superior (anterior), and posterior semicircular canals. The otolith organs (utricle and saccule) sense linear acceleration in the horizontal and vertical planes, respectively, and head tilt (utricle). The semicircular canals sense angular head acceleration. The utricle, superior canal, and horizontal canal are innervated by the superior vestibular nerve. The inferior vestibular nerve innervates the saccule and posterior canal ampulla. One primary function of the vestibular system is maintaining objects of interest steady on the fovea during head movements via the vestibulo-ocular reflex (VOR). As this reflex must be quick and sensitive to keep the visual world in focus during demanding tasks (e.g., running on uneven ground), the system maintains a fast and constant neural firing rate, which is then increased or decreased depending on the direction of head acceleration. This cardinal feature of the system allows the VOR to function on the order of 7 ms.

The non-zero resting firing rate of the vestibular nerve has implications for the expected outcome from nerve dysfunction. A unilateral sudden loss of function will be transmitted to the brain as an asymmetry in peripheral firing rates. This asymmetry is then interpreted as an intense and sustained head acceleration toward the healthy ear. We will use the horizontal canal as an example, and assume that the normal firing rate of the vestibular nerve is 100 spikes per second, which increases up to 400 spikes per second for an ipsilateral head turn, and decreases to 0 spikes per second for a contralateral head turn. Therefore, if one horizontal canal ceases firing, the resting firing rate of the contralateral side, 100 spikes per second, will appear to the brain as a head turn toward the functioning side. This will cause the VOR to drive the eyes toward the nonfunctioning side, and nystagmus will result, with the fast phase (central repositioning of the eye due to a physical limit on rotation of the globe) directed toward the functioning side. As nystagmus is named for the fast phase, the nystagmus driven by the horizontal canal will beat toward the healthy ear. The effects of a sudden loss of vestibular function are summarized in ▶ Table 58.1.

Loss of unilateral utricular function results in peripheral asymmetry in perception of head tilt. This is because the utricle, which is horizontally oriented, encodes information about the tilt of the head with respect to gravity. Loss of functionality causes a characteristic triad of behavioral responses called the "ocular tilt reaction": head tilt (to the ipsilateral side), ocular tilt (superior poles of the eyes rotate toward the ipsilateral side), and skew deviation (ipsilateral eye depresses, and contralateral eye elevates). This response occurs because of perceived tilt of the head to the contralateral side. This functionally can result in vertical diplopia.[8]

Bilateral loss of vestibular function, which can occur as a result of bilateral VS in neurofibromatosis type 2, will not cause the sensation of rapid head acceleration. As the peripheral input is symmetrically diminished or absent, there is no percept of vertigo. Instead, bilateral loss manifests with loss of the normal functionality of the vestibular system. Loss of the VOR causes movement of visual objects of interest with head movement; this bobbing of the visual world is termed "oscillopsia."

Loss of the vestibulospinal reflex results in difficulty in maintaining posture, and the effect is magnified with decreased visual and lower extremity proprioceptive input. Postural instability and ataxia can occur, and the subject typically falls toward the side of the lesion. However, it should be noted that the vestibular system projects to multiple areas of the central nervous system, including the brainstem, cerebellum, reticular formation, thalamus, and cortex; therefore, the effects of vestibular dysfunction can affect not just gaze and posture but also spatial orientation, reasoning, alertness, autonomic function, and mood.

Table 58.1 Effects of sudden unilateral loss of vestibular function

	Perception	Clinical findings	Duration of findings	Compensation	Treatment
Asymmetry in firing rate from semicircular canals	Head being turned to contralateral side	Horizontal/rotary nystagmus with fast phase to the contralateral side	Typically lasts 3–5 d; however, with IR goggles spontaneous nystagmus can be seen in long term	Static	Usually self resolves, needs visual input, vestibular suppressants and brainstem/ cerebellar injury can delay recovery
Asymmetry in utricular firing	Head being tilted to contralateral side	Ocular tilt reaction (see text for details), vertical diplopia	Typically 1–2 d	Static	Usually none required
Loss of VOR	Visual world moving or blurry vision with rapid head movement	Catch-up saccade on head impulse test	Variable, overt catch-up saccade may resolve over time, covert catch-up saccades usually persist	Dynamic	Vestibular physical therapy aimed at improving VOR gain and compensatory saccades
Loss of vestibular-spinal reflex	Falling toward side of lesion, unsteadiness	Ataxia	Days to weeks		Physical therapy aimed at postural control and gait

Abbreviation: VOR, vestibulo-ocular reflex.

58.2.2 Vestibular Compensation after Unilateral Loss of Function

After a unilateral loss of function, central mechanisms initiate a series of steps aimed at adaptation.[9] The resting asymmetry in firing rates between the vestibular nerves is addressed through the process of static compensation. First, cerebellar clamping occurs, which decreases the resting firing rate on the contralateral (normal) side. This occurs within a few hours of tonic firing of the vestibular nerve, and reduces the asymmetry in firing rates. In order to eliminate the asymmetry, a second stage of compensation occurs in which the ipsilateral firing rate increases (thought to be from commissural fibers from the intact side), and the clamping is further increased on the contralateral side, until the resting asymmetry is either gone or reduced to a subclinical threshold. This ipsilateral increase in firing accounts for "recovery nystagmus," which is sometimes observed as a peripheral nystagmus with the fast phase directed toward the damaged side. Over time, the cerebellar clamping is tapered off, and the resting firing rate of the ipsilateral side is restored to prelesion levels. Once static compensation is achieved, spontaneous nystagmus is absent, and the percept of resting head rotation is eliminated.

Dynamic compensation is aimed at improving the vestibular response to rapid head movements. VOR gain (ratio of eye movement to head movement) is decreased after unilateral loss of function. This is because only the intact labyrinth can respond to head movement, and with a resting firing rate around 100 spikes per second, there is a floor in the reduction in firing rate that can occur with ipsilateral head turns. Improvements in gaze stability can be achieved through improvements in VOR gain on the ipsilateral side, and with compensatory saccades. Vestibular physical therapy plays an important role in promoting dynamic compensation.

58.3 Vestibular Pathophysiology in Vestibular Schwannoma

As indicated in the introduction, conventional wisdom indicates that it is not typical for a patient to report dizziness as a symptom associated with sporadic VS. In a study of 81 histologically confirmed VSs, only 53% reported any dizziness symptoms prior to surgery and yet 71% of the patients had indications of peripheral vestibular damage on the side of the schwannoma.[10] Of the 53% of patients reporting symptoms of dizziness, only 19% reported that these interfered with their activities of daily living and 4% indicated that the symptoms interfered with work. In other studies of 48 and 64 patients, they found 77% with unsteadiness and 40% with vertigo, respectively.[1,11] After microsurgical resection, the two latter studies reported dizziness in the postoperative group of 71% with stable or improved symptoms and 28% with vertigo, respectively.[1,11] It is suggested in a recent publication that after treatment with microsurgery resection, radiation or conservative management with observation dizziness was a common complaint. In this study, quality of life was quantified in 247 patients who underwent stereotactic radiosurgery, in 143 patients with microsurgery, and in 148 patients with observation in a retrospective manner.[5] It was found that the principle driving force behind a lower quality of life was that of dizziness, followed by headaches. This was found to be independent of the treatment modality. In another large retrospective study that quantified quality of life in a total of 223 patients, 78 patients had microsurgery for their VS with the remaining 145 managed conservatively with observation.[12] Their results also showed dizziness as the primary symptom leading to poorer quality of life, but in this study the effect was greater for the surgery group compared to the nonsurgery group.

58.3.1 Character of the Symptoms of Dizziness

While dizziness takes on many forms in VS, the most common is that of general unsteadiness with exacerbation to mild vertigo for seconds to minutes provoked by head movement. As would be expected, the variation in symptoms posttreatment depends on the status of vestibular function prior to surgical treatment as well as the size of the tumor.[10] Preoperative positional nystagmus and abnormal rotary chair were correlated with lower Dizziness Handicap Inventory (DHI) scores and a shorter time to independent walking after surgery, possibly because vestibular loss preoperatively was already compensated for by the time surgery occurred. The magnitude of the caloric asymmetry was mildly negatively correlated with postoperative measures of symptom intensity.

In a study of 64 patients,[7] the specific symptom of a vertiginous sensation decreased from 40% preoperatively to 28% postoperatively, while there was no significant change in the complaints of unsteadiness. Of these 64 patients, 80% showed postoperative reduced vestibular response by caloric irrigations, while indications from nystagmus or asymmetries on rotary chair showed that lack of central compensation was associated with increased postoperative unsteadiness. In those with indications of normal rotary chair or compensated status, there was no change in the complaints of unsteadiness pre- to postoperatively.

There are no studies that compare the modality of treatments for sporadic VS to characterize the nature of the postoperative symptoms, vertigo, unsteadiness, etc. As reported earlier, there are comparisons for the overall quality of life posttreatment and the two principle studies[5,12] disagree as to the impact of microsurgery versus the other two modalities of stereotactic radiation and observation.

58.4 Treatment of Dizziness in Vestibular Schwannoma

58.4.1 Pharmacologic Ablation of Vestibular Function

Use of aminoglycoside antibiotics for selective pharmacologic ablation of the vestibular system was first described by Fowler in 1948, and soon popularized by Schuknecht. Since then, it has gained acceptance as a treatment modality for Ménière's disease, and placebo-controlled trials have demonstrated its efficacy.[13] More recently, aminoglycosides have been investigated to ablate residual function in VS. Usage generally falls into two categories: to reduce vertigo symptoms in patients being treated nonsurgically or to ablate function preoperatively in surgical patients to help with postoperative recovery.

In patients with nonsurgically managed VS, vertigo has been shown to have a significant negative impact on quality of life. Giannuzzi et al described four cases of elderly patients being managed with observation for small VS, who developed disabling vertigo.[14] After treatment with intratympanic gentamicin, all four experienced subjective improvement in vertigo, although developed unsteadiness that was treated with vestibular physical therapy. Brantberg et al reported similar success in one patient with a medium-sized tumor.[15] Preoperative administration of gentamicin will be covered later in the chapter.

58.4.2 Microsurgical Resection

While most patients with VS present with hearing loss or tinnitus, dizziness is present in a subset of patients, and is a very strong predictor of quality of life. In one study of 199 consecutive patients, Myrseth et al found that vertigo was present in 15% of patients during the initial assessment, unsteadiness in 7%, hearing impairment in 64%, and tinnitus in 37%.[4] In regression analysis, vertigo was significantly associated with decreased quality of life in all domains in the short form 36 (SF-36), which was the largest effect seen for any presenting symptom. Fortunately, surgery can be quite effective at reducing or eliminating dizziness from VS in select cases. Godefroy et al studied 18 patients with severe dizziness who underwent translabyrinthine resections, and found significant reductions in the DHI and improvements in the SF-36 at 12 months after surgery.[16] While the mechanism of dizziness is unknown in these patients, it is presumed that the tumor causes unpredictable interruptions in the firing rate of the vestibular nerve, resulting in episodic asymmetry and vertigo. This may occur from mass effect or edema, vascular compromise, or demyelination. In larger tumors, obstructive hydrocephalus can occur, which can cause a variety of symptoms through elevated intracranial pressure, including dizziness, ataxia, nausea, diplopia, lethargy, confusion, blurred vision, and headaches. Finally, in some larger tumors, cerebellar compression can cause dysfunction, resulting in saccadic dysmetria, impaired motor control, and ataxia.

58.4.3 Vestibular Rehabilitation after Surgery

Vestibular physical therapy was first introduced by Cawthorne in the 1940s as a treatment for postconcussive dizziness (see Chapter 69 for detailed discussion of this treatment method).[17] Exercises were designed to stimulate the semicircular canals through movements of the eyes and head. Some features of these early exercises, including the need for frequent repetition and escalating difficulty, are still in use today. Over time, these exercises have evolved with an increased understanding of the neurophysiology and compensatory mechanisms of the vestibular system. Currently, the use of vestibular physical therapy for various forms of dizziness, especially after unilateral loss of function as occurs with sporadic VS, has been studied extensively and is well supported by the literature.[18]

Immediately after unilateral loss of vestibular function, the VOR gain is decreased from the normal value of 1 (equal rotation of the eyes and head in opposite directions) to approximately 0.3 for the ipsilateral side, and approximately 0.8 for the contralateral ear (▶ Fig. 58.1).[19] Therefore, with quick head motions, overt catch-up saccades, occurring at a latency of approximately 200 ms, are too slow, and the visual world moves and bobs with head motion. Improvements in dynamic visual acuity can be made by both improving the VOR gain and by increasing the speed and accuracy of saccades when VOR gain is deficient.[20] Compensatory saccades become more covert over time (i.e., more difficult to see because they occur during head rotation, on the order of ~100 ms), and can contribute significantly to the reduction in gaze error.[21] Interestingly, data suggest that these saccades are more effective for predictable head movements, rather than random movements.[21] This makes sense, as these saccades occur too quickly to be driven by visual errors, and must therefore be preprogrammed to occur.

Vestibular rehabilitation has been shown to be effective for gaze stability, and static and dynamic balance following VS resection. The gain of the VOR is plastic, and changes to gain are driven by error signals.[22] The primary error signal is retinal slip, which refers to image motion on the retina during head motion. Therefore, exercises focused on providing an error signal to the

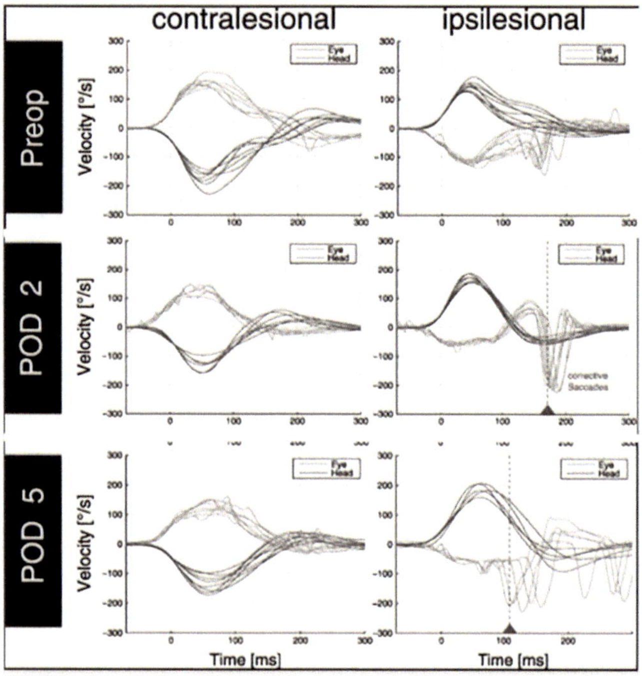

Fig. 58.1 Head impulses were performed preoperatively and postoperatively (POD 2 and 5) on the ipsilateral and contralesional side in a patient who underwent resection of a vestibular schwannoma. *Black traces* indicate head velocity; *grey traces* indicate eye velocity. *Black dotted lines* mark the time of the first appearance of a corrective saccade. Note that over time the corrective saccades begin to appear earlier, during the head motion, reflecting a transition from overt to covert saccades. (Adapted with permission from Mantokoudis et al.[9])

patient in terms of retinal slip are effective at restoring VOR gain. Because of the unilateral loss of function, head motion is primarily encoded through the contralateral vestibular system, although neck proprioception may play a role as well (cervico-ocular reflex). Furthermore, much of adaptation occurs in the brainstem and cerebellum, and particularly in the vestibular nuclei, superior colliculus, vermis, flocculus, and vestigial nuclei.[23] However, despite successful rehabilitation, the VOR system can never return to completely normal function, and subtle vestibular deficits will persist. Vestibular therapy has also been shown to improve postural stability and decrease subjective perception of disequilibrium after VS resection.[24]

Exercises are generally performed several times per day, and should increase in difficulty as the patient adapts to provide a constant challenge. Gaze stability exercises are aimed at improving the ability of the eyes to maintain fixation on a visual target during head movement.[23] Typically, patients will concentrate on a point in space, and keep that point in focus during progressively quicker horizontal and vertical head motions. Variations exist in terms of the distance of the target from the eyes (closer is more difficult), the number of targets, the background (a busy background such as a geometric pattern can make the task more difficult), and the standing surface (e.g., foam vs. hard floor). Another variant exists where the patient is instructed to first fixate on an eccentric target, without head movement, and then to quickly turn the head to the target. This exercise can be used with two or more targets. A third variant involves movement of the visual target in the opposite direction of head movement; this is a more difficult task.

Balance exercises are aimed at improving both static and dynamic postural control. One exercise mimics the Romberg test by having the subject stand on hard ground or foam with arms crossed and eyes closed. Another involves swaying in the anteroposterior and side-to-side direction to improve balance and center of gravity control. The swaying should be directed from the ankles. In dynamic exercises, patients are asked to walk while performing additional tasks, such as turning their head side to side, or turning 180 degrees. Lower extremity strength training exercises can be quite helpful as well.

Vestibular rehabilitation has been shown to be effective for improving balance function after VS resection. Vereeck et al randomized 53 patients to general rehabilitation instructions or customized vestibular rehabilitation after VS resection. They found that in patients over the age of 50 years, the group receiving customized vestibular therapy did significantly better at both 3 and 12 months in several balance assessments, including standing balance sum, tandem gait, and dynamic gait index.[24]

58.4.4 Vestibular Prehabilitation Prior to Surgery

Vestibular "prehab," or rehabilitation prior to a planned ablation of the vestibular system, was introduced by Magnusson et al for Ménière's disease.[25] It was later expanded to include patients with a planned resection of a cerebellopontine angle tumor.[23] They identified two reasons to ablate and habilitate the vestibular system prior to surgery. First, by shifting the loss of function to before surgery, patients are spared from trying to compensate from the vestibular loss while also trying to recover from a craniotomy. Second, since compensation depends on intact cerebellar function, if the cerebellum is impaired postoperatively (e.g., swelling from retraction, or infarction due to impaired vascularity), compensation will be much more difficult. Therefore, it may be beneficial to undergo compensation while the cerebellar function is normal.

Magnusson et al studied a cohort of 12 patients with normal preoperative vestibular function.[25] They were treated with intratympanic gentamicin and vestibular therapy prior to surgery. Loss of labyrinthine reactivity was confirmed with caloric testing. After surgery, no spontaneous nystagmus was observed, patients did not complain of dizziness, and they had an expedited hospital course.

58.5 Conclusion

To date, there are no compelling data to suggest that one treatment modality (surgery, radiation, or observation) leads to less symptoms of dizziness in sporadic VS patients. Dizziness, and specifically unsteadiness, continues to present as a leading cause of reduced quality of life after treatment for VS. Rehabilitation following complete unilateral loss of vestibular function results in improved gaze stability, balance, and dizziness handicap and therefore should be considered in all patients following treatment.

References

[1] Thomeer H, Bonnard D, Franco-Vidal V, et al. Prognostic factors of balance quality after transpetrosal vestibular schwannoma microsurgery: an instrumentally and DHI-based prospective cohort study of 48 patients. Otol Neurotol. 2015; 36(5):886–891

[2] Suzuki M, Yamada C, Inoue R, Kashio A, Saito Y, Nakanishi W. Analysis of vestibular testing in patients with vestibular schwannoma based on the nerve of origin, the localization, and the size of the tumor. Otol Neurotol. 2008; 29(7): 1029–1033

[3] Lloyd SK, Kasbekar AV, Baguley DM, Moffat DA. Audiovestibular factors influencing quality of life in patients with conservatively managed sporadic vestibular schwannoma. Otol Neurotol. 2010; 31(6):968–976

[4] Myrseth E, Møller P, Wentzel-Larsen T, Goplen F, Lund-Johansen M. Untreated vestibular schwannomas: vertigo is a powerful predictor for health-related quality of life. Neurosurgery. 2006; 59(1):67–76, discussion 67–76

[5] Carlson ML, Tveiten OV, Driscoll CL, et al. What drives quality of life in patients with sporadic vestibular schwannoma? Laryngoscope. 2015; 125(7): 1697–1702

[6] Saman Y, Bamiou DE, Murdin L, et al. Balance, falls risk, and related disability in untreated vestibular schwannoma patients. J Neurol Surg B Skull Base. 2014; 75(5):332–338

[7] Angelaki DE, Cullen KE. Vestibular system: the many facets of a multimodal sense. Annu Rev Neurosci. 2008; 31:125–150

[8] Cosetti MK, Tawfik K, Fouladvand M, Roland JT, Jr, Lalwani AK. Diplopia due to skew deviation following neurotologic procedures. Otol Neurotol. 2012; 33 (5):840–842

[9] Mantokoudis G, Schubert MC, Tehrani AS, Wong AL, Agrawal Y. Early adaptation and compensation of clinical vestibular responses after unilateral vestibular deafferentation surgery. Otol Neurotol. 2014; 35(1):148–154

[10] El-Kashlan HK, Shepard NT, Arts HA, Telian SA. Disability from vestibular symptoms after acoustic neuroma resection. Am J Otol. 1998; 19(1):104–111

[11] Abboud T, Regelsberger J, Matschke J, Jowett N, Westphal M, Dalchow C. Long-term vestibulocochlear functional outcome following retro-sigmoid approach to resection of vestibular schwannoma. Eur Arch Otorhinolaryngol. 2016; 273(3):719–725

[12] Jufas N, Flanagan S, Biggs N, Chang P, Fagan P. Quality of life in vestibular schwannoma patients managed by surgical or conservative approaches. Otol Neurotol. 2015; 36(7):1245–1254

[13] Postema RJ, Kingma CM, Wit HP, Albers FW, Van Der Laan BF. Intratympanic gentamicin therapy for control of vertigo in unilateral Menire's disease: a prospective, double-blind, randomized, placebo-controlled trial. Acta Otolaryngol. 2008; 128(8):876–880

[14] Giannuzzi AL, Merkus P, Falcioni M. The use of intratympanic gentamicin in patients with vestibular schwannoma and disabling vertigo. Otol Neurotol. 2013; 34(6):1096–1098

[15] Brantberg K, Bergenius J, Tribukait A. Gentamicin treatment in peripheral vestibular disorders other than Ménière's disease. ORL J Otorhinolaryngol Relat Spec. 1996; 58(5):277–279

[16] Godefroy WP, Hastan D, van der Mey AG. Translabyrinthine surgery for disabling vertigo in vestibular schwannoma patients. Clin Otolaryngol. 2007; 32(3):167–172

[17] Cawthorne T. The physiological basis for head movements. Journal of the Chartered Society of Physiotherapy. 1944; 3:106–107

[18] McDonnell MN, Hillier SL. Vestibular rehabilitation for unilateral peripheral vestibular dysfunction. Cochrane Database Syst Rev. 2015; 1:CD005397

[19] Macdougall HG, Curthoys IS. Plasticity during vestibular compensation: the role of saccades. Front Neurol. 2012; 3:21

[20] Schubert MC, Migliaccio AA, Clendaniel RA, Allak A, Carey JP. Mechanism of dynamic visual acuity recovery with vestibular rehabilitation. Arch Phys Med Rehabil. 2008; 89(3):500–507

[21] Schubert MC, Zee DS. Saccade and vestibular ocular motor adaptation. Restor Neurol Neurosci. 2010; 28(1):9–18

[22] Herdman SJ, Clendaniel RA, Mattox DE, Holliday MJ, Niparko JK. Vestibular adaptation exercises and recovery: acute stage after acoustic neuroma resection. Otolaryngol Head Neck Surg. 1995; 113(1):77–87

[23] Snapp HA, Schubert MC. Habilitation of auditory and vestibular dysfunction. Otolaryngol Clin North Am. 2012; 45(2):487–511, x–xi

[24] Vereeck L, Wuyts FL, Truijen S, De Valck C, Van de Heyning PH. The effect of early customized vestibular rehabilitation on balance after acoustic neuroma resection. Clin Rehabil. 2008; 22(8):698–713

[25] Magnusson M, Kahlon B, Karlberg M, Lindberg S, Siesjö P. Preoperative vestibular ablation with gentamicin and vestibular 'prehab' enhance postoperative recovery after surgery for pontine angle tumours–first report. Acta Otolaryngol. 2007; 127(12):1236–1240

59 Epidemiology and Pathogenesis of Headache in Patients with Vestibular Schwannoma

Stanley Pelosi and Christopher J. Farrell

59.1 Introduction

As vestibular schwannoma (VS) management strategies have evolved over the years, significant advances have been achieved with regard to disease-associated morbidity and mortality. In an effort to further improve upon this progress, greater attention is now being paid to assessment of patient-reported quality-of-life (QOL) measures. Headache disability is one such measure that is associated with substantial health-related QOL reduction in the VS population.[1] This chapter will explore the frequency of headaches in VS patients and the mechanisms underlying their development. Clinical evaluation and treatment is presented separately in Chapter 71.

59.2 Epidemiology

59.2.1 Pretreatment Headache Prevalence

Pretreatment, there is a wide variability in the prevalence of headache in patients presenting with VS. Studies suggest that 6 to 60% of patients with VS will complain of headache, paralleling the general population.[2,3] The largest series of 1,657 patients with VS reported approximately one-third have preoperative headache.[4] Whether the presence of headache is directly attributable to the tumor or other preexisting headache disorders has not been clarified. The coexistence of headache disorders with VSs has been frequently observed. In a study of 192 patients with VS, Rimaaja and colleagues indicated 24% of patients met International Headache Criteria for migraine, while 9% patients had tension-type headaches.[5]

59.2.2 Postsurgical Headache Prevalence and Risk Factors

The prevalence of headaches postoperatively in patients undergoing craniotomy for VS has been more difficult to study. Retrospective studies often underestimate the prevalence of headache based on what clinical features were recorded in the medical record. Prospective studies may be hindered by recall bias depending on when a patient is assessed relative to the time of surgery (in some studies, up to 15 years postoperatively). Studies also vary in regards to inclusion criteria, with some studies reporting headache outcomes in all patients undergoing VS surgery regardless of the approach and others reporting outcomes only after specific approaches and surgical techniques. In addition, studies vary in their definitions of headache type with few using International Classification of Headache Disorders (ICHD) criteria.

With the limitations noted earlier, postcraniotomy headaches are present in 0 to 75% of patients undergoing surgery for VS (▶ Table 59.1). In about 90% of patients, the headache is noted immediately postoperatively.[3] Many patients improve within 1 to 2 months.[6] About 20 to 30% of these patients have headaches that begin postoperatively, but persist beyond 6 months.[3,6,7] By 1 to 2 years, the prevalence of headache diminishes.[3,8] The persistence of headaches after the retrosigmoid approach for VS has been estimated to be 63% at 6 months, falling to 24% by 1 year and to 12% by 2 years.[3]

In patients undergoing surgery for VS, risk factors for postoperative headache or headache severity include preoperative headache,[2,7,9] retrosigmoid approach,[4,17] craniectomy rather than craniotomy,[13] coexisting anxiety and depression,[2] perioperative complications,[18] and younger age.[2,4] Tumor size was not associated with postoperative headache[2,3,4,7] in some studies, but others[5,12,19] suggest a small tumor size is associated with higher risk of postoperative headache. Similarly, there is conflicting results on the influence of gender, with some suggesting female sex as a risk factor[4,5] and others not. There seems to be no clear correlation of postoperative headache with complete versus partial resection and whether or not the facial or cochlear nerve is preserved.[3]

The prevalence of headache based on surgical approach has also been compared. Early series suggested that the retrosigmoid approach is associated with a higher prevalence of postsurgical headache. In one large meta-analysis of 5,064 patients from 35 studies, complications of VS microsurgery were assessed by approach. In this study, the incidence of postoperative headache was noted in 17.3% who underwent the retrosigmoid approach, 8% in the middle cranial fossa approach, and 0% for the translabyrinthine approach.[17] The study was limited by variable length of follow-up and lack of specific headache definitions. Similarly other studies have reported that the retrosigmoid approach is associated with a higher risk of postoperative headache and/or a higher risk of severe headache.[4,16,17,20] Schessel and colleagues[16] reported a 64% incidence of headache for the retrosigmoid approach, in comparison to 0% for the translabyrinthine approach.

However, studies have not uniformly suggested that surgical approach is a major risk factor for long-term headache.[2,7] The latter results may be due to the timing and manner of surveying patients for these types of studies. Ruckenstein and colleagues evaluated 52 patients for postoperative headache, some of who underwent a suboccipital craniotomy and some of who underwent a translabyrinthine approach.[10] At 1 and 6 months, patients undergoing the suboccipital craniotomy had more severe pain than those who had undergone a translabyrinthine approach. By 1 year, however, there was no difference in the headache severity among these patients. Similarly, Carlson and colleagues did not find a significant difference in long-term headache disability at a mean of approximately 7 years following treatment, when comparing amongst 143 patients who underwent retrosigmoid, translabyrinthine, or middle fossa microsurgical approaches.[2] While it appears that the retrosigmoid approach is associated with more frequent and severe headaches in the early postoperative period, the relationship between surgical approach and long-term headache outcome remains controversial.

Table 59.1 Variability in reported headache prevalence in vestibular schwannoma patients based on treatment

Treatment	Author (Year)	Headache prevalence	Length of follow-up
Microsurgery (all cases, not approach specific)	Levo et al (2001)[9]	37%	Not specified
	Rimaaja et al (2007)[5]	55%	5 y (mean)
	Carlson et al (2015)[2]	60%	7.7 y (mean)
	Vijayan et al (1995)	75%	Not specified
Retrosigmoid	Schaller and Baumann (2003)[3]	6%	2 y
	Harner et al (1993)[8]	16%	12 mo
	Ruckenstein et al (1996)[10]	17%	12 mo
	Jackson et al (2000)[11]	21%	2 y
	Glasscock et al (1993)[12]	22%	3 mo
	Mosek et al (1999)[6]	23%	4 mo
	Schankin et al (2009)[7]	32%	6 mo
	Wazen et al (2000)[13]	43%	3 mo
	Koperer et al (1999)[14]	48%	1 y
	Catalano et al (1996)[15]	51%	3 mo
	Hanson et al (1998)	54%	25 mo (mean)
	Schessel et al (1992)[16]	64%	3 mo
	Ryzenman et al (2005)[4]	66%	3 y
	Pedrosa et al (1994)	73%	3 mo
Translabyrinthine	Schessel et al (1992)[16]	0%	3 mo
	Ruckenstein et al (1996)[10]	13%	12 mo
	Parving et al (1992)	14%	3 mo
	Andersson et al (1997)	22%	3.3 y (mean)
	Pedrosa et al (1994)	53%	3 mo
	Ryzenman et al (2005)[4]	64%	3 y
Middle fossa	Glasscock et al (1993)	0%	3 mo
	Weber et al (1996)	1%	3 mo
	Ryzenman et al (2005)[4]	50%	3 y
Stereotactic radiation	Carlson et al (2015)[2]	49%	7.7 y (mean)
Observation	Carlson et al (2015)[2]	45%	7.7 y (mean)

59.2.3 Prevalence of Headache after Radiosurgery and during Conservative Observation

The majority of studies evaluating headache in VS patients have focused on the development of new or worsening headache following surgical intervention. The incidence of new headaches in patients undergoing observation or following radiation therapy has not been well studied (▶ Table 59.1). In a cross-sectional survey, one study reported the percentage of patients who complained of long-term headaches, many years after treatment, did not significantly differ between patients undergoing surgery, radiation, or observation.[2] Interestingly, 14% of patients experienced improvement in their headaches following intervention with no statistical difference among the groups.

59.3 Postcraniotomy Headache: Criteria and Pathogenesis

59.3.1 Criteria for Postcraniotomy Headache

Discussion of postoperative and postcraniotomy headache largely began to appear in the literature in the 1980s. Many of these studies were related to surgery for VS.[21] Criteria for postcraniotomy headache by the ICHD first appeared in the ICHD2 publication in 2004 and was subsequently updated in the ICHD3 publication in *Cephalalgia* (▶ Table 59.2).[22]

59.3.2 Pathogenesis of Postcraniotomy Headache in Vestibular Schwannoma

There are several theories as to the mechanism of pain in postoperative headache in patients with VS not found to have a secondary cause (e.g., intracerebral hemorrhage, venous thrombosis; ▶ Fig. 59.1). It is likely that the cause of postcraniotomy headache is multifactorial with contributions from many of the proposed theories. The clinical phenotype of the headache is likely dependent on the underlying factors proposed to be playing a role in the pathogenesis of the headache, which may vary from patient to patient. These theories are reviewed later and include muscle/soft-tissue injury, aseptic meningitis due to bone dust debris, muscle-dural adhesion, dural traction, cranial or spinal nerve entrapment, cervical spondylosis, exacerbation of underlying migrainous phenomenon, and central sensitization.

59.3.3 Muscle/Soft-Tissue Injury

Because many patients complain of "superficial" pain around the incision, some feel this is more attributable to pain from soft tissue and muscle rather than meningeal irritation.[21] Injury to muscles or nuchal attachments, wound retraction, or positioning of the patient during surgery could all contribute. The

Table 59.2 ICHD3 criteria for postcraniotomy headache

	Acute headache attributed to craniotomy	Persistent headache attributed to craniotomy
Description	Headache of less than 3-mo duration caused by surgical craniotomy	Headache of more than 3-mo duration caused by surgical craniotomy
Criteria	A. Any headache fulfilling C and D B. Surgical craniotomy performed for something other than head trauma C. Headache is reported to have developed within 7 d of the following: 1. Craniotomy 2. Regaining consciousness from craniotomy 3. Discontinuation of medication(s) that impair ability to sense or report headache following craniotomy D. Either of the following: 1. Headache has resolved within 3 mo after craniotomy 2. Headache not yet resolved but 3 mo has not yet passed since craniotomy E. Not better accounted for by another ICHD-3 diagnosis	A. Any headache fulfilling criteria C and D B. Surgical craniotomy performed for something other than head trauma C. Headache is reported to have developed within 7 d after one of the following: 1. Craniotomy 2. Regaining consciousness following craniotomy 3. Discontinuation of medication(s) that impairs ability to sense or report headache following the craniotomy D. Headache persists for > 3 mo after the craniotomy E. Not better accounted for by another ICHD-3 diagnosis

Abbreviation: ICHD, International Classification of Headache Disorders.
Source: Data from Headache Classification Committee of the International Headache Society (IHS). The International Classification of Headache Disorders. 3rd ed. (beta version). Cephalalgia 2013;33:629–808.

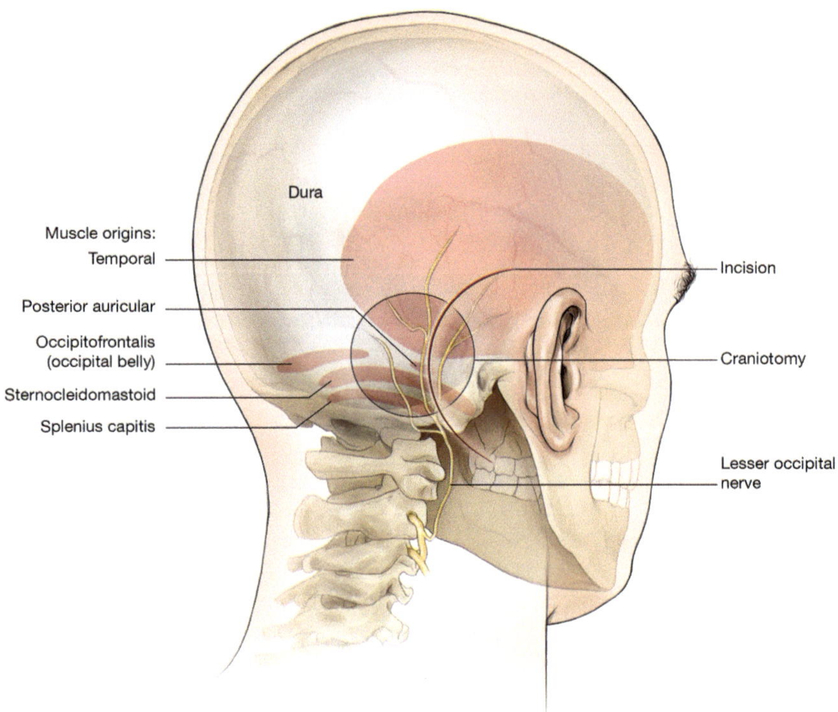

Fig. 59.1 Postulated mechanisms of postoperative headache following retrosigmoid craniotomy.

duration of pain observed with incisional pain from surgery correlates with the different stages of wound healing.[6] This theory of muscle and/or soft-tissue injury is further supported by studies suggesting that temporal and retrosigmoid craniotomies, where substantial muscle bulk is commonly divided, have higher risk of postoperative pain.[21] In the retrosigmoid approach, significant extension of the patient's neck is often required to expose the internal auditory canal (IAC).[23] In addition, some studies, but not all, have suggested that the size of the incision directly correlates with postoperative pain.[24] Further support to this theory comes from data suggesting that one of the common postcraniotomy subtypes of headache after the retrosigmoid approach for VS is a cervicogenic type of headache,[18] where pain begins in the neck and is often exacerbated by head and neck position changes.

59.3.4 Bone Dust, Blood Products, and Fibrin Glue in the Subarachnoid Space

Another proposed mechanism for postoperative headache following the retrosigmoid approach is bone debris.[3,11,15] In contrast to the translabyrinthine and middle cranial fossa approaches where extradural drilling is performed, the retrosigmoid transmeatal approach requires intradural drilling and the potential for subarachnoid bone dust dissemination. Bone debris or fibrin glue may result in an inflammatory reaction resulting in aseptic meningitis. Support of this theory comes from data showing laboratory-proven aseptic meningitis in patients with postoperative headache compared to patients without headache.[3] In one study,[11] investigators compared the risk of postoperative headaches in patients undergoing VS surgery via the retrosigmoid approach versus patients undergoing vestibular nerve section by the same approach. The main difference between these two operations is the need for IAC bone drilling in VS surgery. In this study, 54% of those undergoing VS surgery had headache compared to only 5% of those undergoing vestibular nerve section only. Such a mechanism was also supported by Schaller and Baumann who found in their series that patients who experienced headache were significantly more likely to have undergone IAC drilling.[3] Another study supported the concept of aseptic meningitis causing dural nociceptor sensitization when describing an "exaggerated intracranial mechanosensitivity" that exists in many VS patients.[5] Adding further evidence to this theory, Catalano and colleagues showed a reduction of headaches with meticulous bone dust removal.[15]

Large tumor size, somewhat surprisingly, has not been consistently associated with an increased incidence of long-term headache following VS surgery.[2,3,8,15] In fact, several series have actually reported an inverse relationship between tumor size and headache.[3,8] Hypotheses for this observation again relate to intradural drilling with large tumors potentially reducing the widespread disbursement of bone–dust. Furthermore, larger tumors may require less drilling as there is often greater bony expansion of the IAC.[3] One study found increased tumor size to be associated with more preoperative, but not postoperative, headache.[4]

59.3.5 Dural-Muscle Adhesion and Traction

Headache has been found to be more common in patients with infratentorial tumors,[25] and posterior fossa surgery is associated with a higher incidence of postoperative headache than other craniotomy locations.[26] Schessel and colleagues proposed that headaches following retrosigmoid VS removal resulted from adherence of exposed dura to the nuchal musculature, causing excessive traction.[20] Adhesion of muscles to the pain-sensitive dura is further supported as the cause of ongoing head pain by a number of studies.[3,13,14,21,27] Histologically, adherence of nuchal muscle to the dura was shown in one patient who suffered from ongoing, severe headache after retrosigmoid VS resection.[20] One retrospective study found patients undergoing duraplasty had no headaches after retrosigmoid surgery for VS.[3] Further supporting this theory, studies have suggested that if the bone flap is replaced or alloplastic material is used to separate the dura from the muscle, the risk of postoperative headache and/or severity of headache is diminished.[3,13,14] One retrospective study[28] found less postoperative headaches in those undergoing retrosigmoid craniotomy with cranioplasty for cerebellopontine angle tumors compared to those without cranioplasty. However, some patients have headache despite cranioplasty; so, this is unlikely to be the only explanation in many cases.[27] Furthermore, this mechanism would not explain postoperative headache after the middle cranial fossa or translabyrinthine approach.

59.3.6 Cranial or Spinal Nerve Injury

Injury to cranial or spinal nerves and the formation of traumatic neuromas may be the cause of postcraniotomy pain in some patients undergoing VS surgery. Injury, entrapment, or neuroma formation of the occipital, trigeminal, or intermedius nerve has been described.

The retrosigmoid incision line may cause injury to the greater or lesser occipital nerves. Mosek and colleagues reported that pain or tenderness at the incision site was experienced by 82% of patients following surgical resection at an average time of 12 months, although only 19% of patients described this as a problem.[6] Another study suggested that injury to these nerves contributed to postoperative headache in a small number of their patients.[9] It was postulated that nerve severing might cause subsequent development of a painful neuroma, or the nerve could become entrapped in scar and cause traction-related pain. Some have advocated a high arching or curved skin incision to reduce damage to the occipital nerve. Interestingly, however, another recent study challenged this hypothesis with the finding that preservation of the greater occipital nerve was actually an independent risk factor for postoperative debilitating headache.

59.3.7 Cervical Spondylosis

A cervicogenic-like headache can develop in some patients undergoing the retrosigmoid approach. In addition to soft-tissue injury, patient positioning during the operation can provoke or exacerbate pain related to degenerative cervical osteoarthritis. The most commonly treated cause of cervicogenic headache is related to cervical facet arthritis.[18,29] The disruption of the soft tissue and bone from surgery likely results in added stress on cervical spine, which is a phenomenon seen in cervical spine fusions.[30]

59.3.8 Migraine and Central Sensitization

Patients with a history of migraine headache are more likely to develop a postcraniotomy headache and often postcraniotomy headaches present with migrainous features.[5] A full discussion of migraine pathophysiology is beyond the scope of this discussion, but migraine is thought to be initiated by sensitization of meningeal nociceptors within the trigeminal ganglion along with central trigeminovascular pathways.[31] It is conceivable, then, that posterior fossa surgery may exacerbate the preexisting sensitization of these nociceptors through mechanisms described earlier, thus leading to persistence or worsening of headache in the postoperative period. Another study found that 15 of 122 patients with postoperative headache met International Headache Society criteria for migraine.[5]

Central sensitization is another potential contributor to headache in the postoperative setting. In central sensitization, peripheral cranial nerve injury may result in chronic nociceptive afferent input ultimately causing increased excitability of central nociceptive pathways.[32]

59.4 Future Directions

Headache represents a significant source of disability in the VS population. In order to better assess this important condition, future studies evaluating headache outcomes in VS patients should include the use of validated assessment measures to characterize headache both before and after any treatment and should classify headache patterns in accord with ICHD3 criteria. With more well-designed studies, patients at highest risk for headache-related morbidity following treatment can be identified and treatment can be tailored accordingly. Refinement of existing therapies, and the development of new medical and surgical strategies to prevent and treat headache in order to improve the well-being and QOL for patients with VS, is imperative.

References

[1] Betchen SA, Walsh J, Post KD. Self-assessed quality of life after acoustic neuroma surgery. J Neurosurg. 2003; 99(5):818–823

[2] Carlson ML, Tveiten OV, Driscoll CL, et al. Risk factors and analysis of long-term headache in sporadic vestibular schwannoma: a multicenter cross-sectional study. J Neurosurg. 2015; 123(5):1276–1286

[3] Schaller B, Baumann A. Headache after removal of vestibular schwannoma via the retrosigmoid approach: a long-term follow-up-study. Head Neck Surg. 2003; 128:387–395

[4] Ryzenman JM, Pensak ML, Tew JM, Jr. Headache: a quality of life analysis in a cohort of 1,657 patients undergoing acoustic neuroma surgery, results from the acoustic neuroma association. Laryngoscope. 2005; 115(4):703–711

[5] Rimaaja T, Haanpaa M, Blomstedt G, Farkkila M. Headaches after acoustic neuroma surgery. Cephalalgia. 2007; 27:1128–1135

[6] Mosek AC, Dodick DW, Ebersold MJ, Swanson JW. Headache after resection of acoustic neuroma. Headache. 1999; 39(2):89–94

[7] Schankin CJ, Gall C, Straube A. Headache syndromes after acoustic neuroma surgery and their implications for quality of life. Cephalalgia. 2009; 29:760–771

[8] Harner SG, Beatty CW, Ebersold MJ. Headache after acoustic neuroma excision. Am J Otol. 1993; 14(6):552–555

[9] Levo H, Blomstedt G, Hirvonen T, Pyykkö I. Causes of persistent postoperative headache after surgery for vestibular schwannoma. Clin Otolaryngol Allied Sci. 2001; 26(5):401–406

[10] Ruckenstein MJ, Harris JP, Cueva RA, Prioleau G, Alksne J. Pain subsequent to resection of acoustic neuromas via suboccipital and translabyrinthine approaches. Am J Otol. 1996; 17(4):620–624

[11] Jackson CG, McGrew BM, Forest JA, et al. Comparison of postoperative headache after retrosigmoid approach: vestibular nerve section versus vestibular schwannoma resection. Am J Otol. 2000; 21(3):412–416

[12] Tos T, Cayé-Thomasen P, Stangerup SE, Tos M, Thomsen J. Patients' fears, expectations and satisfaction in relation to management of vestibular schwannoma: a comparison of surgery and observation. Acta Otolaryngol. 2003; 123(5):600–605

[13] Wazen JJ, Sisti M, Lam SM. Cranioplasty in acoustic neuroma surgery. Laryngoscope. 2000; 110(8):1294–1297

[14] Koperer H, Deinsberger W, Jödicke A, Böker DK. Postoperative headache after the lateral suboccipital approach: craniotomy versus craniectomy. Minim Invasive Neurosurg. 1999; 42(4):175–178

[15] Catalano PJ, Jacobowitz O, Post KD. Prevention of headache after retrosigmoid removal of acoustic tumors. Am J Otol. 1996; 17(6):904–908

[16] Schessel DA, Nedzelski JM, Kassel EE, Rowed DW. Recurrence rates of acoustic neuroma in hearing preservation surgery. Am J Otol. 1992; 13(3):233–235

[17] Ansari SF, Terry C, Cohen-Gadol AA. Surgery for vestibular schwannomas: a systematic review of complications by approach. Neurosurg Focus. 2012; 33 (3):E14

[18] Boswell MV, Colson JD, Sehgal N, Dunbar EE, Epter R. A systematic review of therapeutic facet joint interventions in chronic spinal pain. Pain Physician. 2007; 10(1):229–253

[19] Tos T, Caye-Thomasen P, Stangerup SE, Tos M, Thomsen J. Long-term socio-economic impact of vestibular schwannoma for patients under observation and after surgery. J Laryngol Otol. 2003; 117(12):955–964

[20] Schessel DA, Nedzelski JM, Rowed D, Feghali JG. Pain after surgery for acoustic neuroma. Otolaryngol Head Neck Surg. 1992; 107:424–429

[21] Rocha-Filho PA. Post-craniotomy headache: a clinical view with a focus on the persistent form. Headache. 2015; 55(5):733–738

[22] Headache Classification Committee of the International Headache Society (IHS). The International Classification of Headache Disorders. 3rd ed. (beta version). Cephalalgia 2013;33:629–808

[23] Acoustic Neuroma Association. Headache associated with acoustic neuroma treatment. 2015. https://acusticusneurinom.dk/wp-content/uploads/2015/10/booklet_-_headache.2012_-_final.pdf

[24] Santarius T, D'Sousa AR, Zeitoun HM, Cruickshank G, Morgan DW. Audit of headache following resection of acoustic neuroma using three different techniques of suboccipital approach. Rev Laryngol Otol Rhinol (Bord). 2000; 121 (2):75–78

[25] Suwanwela N, Phanthumchinda K, Kaoropthum S. Headache in brain tumor: a cross-sectional study. Headache. 1994; 34(7):435–438

[26] de Gray LC, Matta BF. Acute and chronic pain following craniotomy: a review. Anaesthesia. 2005; 60:693–704

[27] Schessel DA, Rowed DW, Nedzelski JM, Feghali JG. Postoperative pain following excision of acoustic neuroma by the suboccipital approach: observations on possible cause and potential amelioration. Am J Otol. 1993; 14(5):491–494

[28] Soumekh B, Levine SC, Haines SJ, Wulf JA. Retrospective study of postcraniotomy headaches in suboccipital approach: diagnosis and management. Am J Otol. 1996; 17(4):617–619

[29] Cooper G, Bailey B, Bogduk N. Cervical zygapophysial joint pain maps. Pain Med. 2007; 8(4):344–353

[30] Virk SS, Niedermeier S, Yu E, Khan SN. Adjacent segment disease. Orthopedics. 2014; 37(8):547–555

[31] Levy D, Jakubowski M, Burstein R. Disruption of communication between peripheral and central trigeminovascular neurons mediates the antimigraine action of 5HT 1B/1D receptor agonists. Proc Natl Acad Sci U S A. 2004; 101 (12):4274–4279

[32] Woolf CJ. Central sensitization: implications for the diagnosis and treatment of pain. Pain. 2011; 152(3) Suppl:S2–S15

[33] Garzon-Muvdi, T., Jackson, C., See, A. P., Woodworth, G. F. & Tamargo, R. J. Preservation of the greater occipital nerve during suboccipital craniectomy results in a paradoxical increase in postoperative headaches. Neurosurgery 76, 435440; discussion 440 (2015)

[34] Vijayan, N. Postoperative headache in acoustic neuroma. Headache 35, 98100 (1995)

[35] Hanson, M. B., Glasscock, M. E., Brandes, J. L. & Jackson, C. G. Medical treatment of headache after suboccipital acoustic tumor removal. The Laryngoscope 108, 11111114 (1998)

[36] Pedrosa, C. A., Ahern, D. K., McKenna, M. J., Ojemann, R. G. & Acquadro, M. A. Determinants and impact of headache after acoustic neuroma surgery. Am. J. Otol. 15, 793797 (1994)

[37] Parving, A., Tos, M., Thomsen, J., Møller, H. & Buchwald, C. Some aspects of life quality after surgery for acoustic neuroma. Arch. Otolaryngol. Head Neck Surg. 118, 10611064 (1992)

[38] Andersson, G., Ekvall, L., Kinnefors, A., Nyberg, G. & Rask-Andersen, H. Evaluation of quality of life and symptoms after translabyrinthine acoustic neuroma surgery. Am. J. Otol. 18, 421426 (1997)

[39] Glasscock, M. E., Hays, J. W., Minor, L. B., Haynes, D. S. & Carrasco, V. N. Preservation of hearing in surgery for acoustic neuromas. J. Neurosurg. 78, 864870 (1993)

[40] Weber, P. C. & Gantz, B. J. Results and complications from acoustic neuroma excision via middle cranial fossa approach. Am. J. Otol. 17, 669675 (1996)

60 Quality-of-Life Outcomes in Sporadic Vestibular Schwannoma

Matthew L. Carlson and Kathleen J. Yost

60.1 Introduction

In the early 20th century, the focus of vestibular schwannoma (VS) treatment was mortality reduction.[1,2] In the last five decades, advances in surgical technique, radiation delivery, and a better understanding of the natural history of disease have led to a substantial reduction in disease- and treatment-related mortality. Accordingly, we have witnessed a shift in outcome priorities from life preservation to cranial nerve preservation—namely, facial nerve function and serviceable hearing.[1,2,3] With a relative plateau in cranial nerve outcomes and the understanding that there are many other less tangible factors that significantly affect patient's well-being, many groups have begun exploring quality-of-life (QoL) outcomes. The growing priority of QoL outcomes in VS is evidenced by a fourfold increase in publications on this topic in the decade after the year 2000, compared to the decade prior.[4]

In 1995, the World Health Organization defined QoL as "an individual's perception of their position in life in the context of the culture and value system in which they live and in relation to their goals, expectations, standards, and concerns."[5] When QoL is assessed in the context of overall health and disease, the term health-related quality of life (HRQoL) is commonly applied. HRQoL is a broad, multidimensional concept that looks beyond morbidity and mortality and assesses domains related to physical, mental, emotional, and social functioning in the setting of one's social environment.[6] Where traditional physician-defined outcome measures such as hearing loss of facial paresis only assess impairment, a temporary or permanent loss of physiological function, QoL assessment moves several steps beyond this to ascertain the impact on overall well-being.

The study of HRQoL is particularly germane to sporadic VS and other benign skull base tumors, where normal life expectancy is anticipated, and treatment remains controversial with multiple viable management options available.[3,7] The objectives of this chapter are to (1) provide an overview of HRQoL as it pertains to VS; (2) review the most commonly utilized HRQoL measures used in the VS literature; (3) explore the concept of the minimum clinically important difference (MCID) in HRQoL measures; (4) examine the impact of diagnosis and treatment on HRQoL; and (5) to discuss future direction of HRQoL research.

60.2 Overview of Health-Related Quality-of-Life Assessment in Vestibular Schwannoma

Broadly, HRQoL assessment tools can be classified into generic or disease-specific measures. Generic, multipurpose instruments are useful for understanding various disease processes in the context of global health and for comparing HRQoL across conditions; however, these instruments commonly lack the sensitivity required to detect subtle changes that may arise from the disease process over time or as a result of treatment.[3] For example, common questions utilized by generic measures may be asked about one's ability to carry groceries or climb one flight of stairs—inquiries that are not specific to the concerns faced by a VS population.

To date, the great majority of the VS HRQoL literature has utilized the multipurpose 36-Item Short-Form (SF-36) Health Survey and Glasgow Benefit Inventory (GBI).[8,9,10] However, in 2010, Shaffer et al introduced the first disease-specific HRQoL measure, the Penn Acoustic Neuroma Quality of Life (PANQOL) scale.[9] Several recent studies have demonstrated important advantages of the PANQOL over the SF-36 and GBI.[3,9] In 2015, after reviewing HRQoL questionnaire survey data from 642 respondents, Carlson et al found that the PANQOL was far more sensitive toward detecting differences between treatment groups compared to the SF-36, GBI, and the Patient-Reported Outcomes Measurement Information System Global 10 (PROMIS-10) short form.[3]

60.3 Health-Related Quality-of-Life Instruments

The following are the disease-specific and generic measures that are commonly employed in VS HRQoL assessment. While this chapter is focused on HRQoL in sporadic VS, it is notable that there is currently only one validated disease-specific measure for this population with sporadic tumors, while there are three instruments that have been developed for patients with neurofibromatosis type 2.[11,12,13]

60.3.1 Disease-Specific Quality-of-Life Assessment

Penn Acoustic Neuroma Quality-of-Life Scale (PANQOL)

The PANQOL scale was developed by Shaffer et al in 2010 and consists of 26 questions with responses ranging from 1 to 5: 1 denoting strong disagreement through 5 indicating strong agreement.[9] Domain scores for facial function, balance, hearing, pain, anxiety, energy, and general health are obtained by averaging the responses of items assigned to the domain. A total score is calculated as the equal average of the seven domain scores. As such, the domain scores and the total score can range from 0 to 100, with higher scores indicating better HRQOL. The PANQOL was originally validated in U.S. patients, and subsequently in the Dutch population, and was shown to discriminate VS patients from nontumor controls better than the SF-36 and other generic measures.[3,9,14]

60.3.2 Generic Quality-of-Life Assessment

Short-Form 36 (SF-36) Health Survey

The SF-36 is a generic, 36-item instrument that assesses HRQoL status across eight scales including physical functioning, role limitations secondary to physical problems, bodily pain, general health, vitality, social functioning, role limitations secondary to emotional problems, and mental health.[15] Scores for each domain are calculated based on the weighted sum of corresponding responses and are transformed to a 0- to 100-point scale, with higher scores indicating more favorable HRQoL. Finally, individual scales can be combined to form physical and mental health component summary scores that are standardized using a linear T-score transformation to have a mean of 50 and a standard deviation of 10 in the general U.S. population.[15] The SF-36 remains one the most widely used multipurpose QoL instruments today, having been validated in many countries worldwide, with established normative data available for reference.

Patient-Reported Outcomes Measurement Information System Global 10 (PROMIS-10)

The PROMIS-10 is a validated 10-item generic global health scale designed to assess physical, mental, and social health, as well as pain, fatigue, and overall QoL in adults. First available in 2004, the PROMIS-10 covers similar content as several other well-established measures including the SF-36 and EQ5D.[16] Reminiscent of the SF-36, 8 of the 10 PROMIS-10 items can be combined to yield mental and physical health summary scores.[17] Each item uses a five-point response scale with the exception of an 11-point pain scale; a higher score once again indicates better HRQOL. Normative data for the U.S. general population are available, and raw scores from the PROMIS-10 can be converted to T-scores that have a mean of 50 and a standard deviation of 10 in the general U.S. population.

Glasgow Benefit Inventory (GBI)

The GBI is an 18-point postintervention questionnaire used to assess change in health status as a result of treatment, developed especially for otolaryngological interventions.[18] Each item contains five responses ranging from a large deterioration in HRQoL to a large improvement following treatment. A total score is generated from general, social support and physical health subscale scores. The GBI total and subdomain scores range from −100 to + 100 with a score of zero indicating no change in health status as a result of treatment, and scores of −100 and + 100 denoting a maximum decline and improvement, respectively.

60.4 The Minimal Clinically Important Difference

Several studies assessing HRQoL in VS have demonstrated small, but statistically significant differences between treatment modalities. The question remains whether a several point difference on a 100-point scale really matters clinically. First conceived by Guyatt et al in 1987 and later refined by Jaeschke and colleagues in 1989, the concept of the minimal clinically important difference (MCID) was developed to answer this critical question.[19,20] Today, the MCID is defined as the smallest point difference in HRQOL scores that patients perceive as important, either beneficial or harmful, and that could lead to change in management.[21]

MCID values are established according to a specific disease of interest, using one particular instrument. For example, the MCID for the SF-36 in patients with rheumatoid arthritis will likely be different from the MCID for the SF-36 in patients with VS. Furthermore, the MCID may vary according to study population and clinical context even within a disease. For these reasons, the MCID is often presented with a range, in addition to the point estimate. The methodology behind establishing the MCID is beyond the scope of this chapter; however, two valuable summary articles by King as well as Yost and Eton are available for the interested reader.[21,22]

In a recent publication, anchor- and distribution-based methods were used to determine the MCID for the PANQOL and the SF-36 in patients with sporadic VS.[7] In this study, the median (interquartile range) MCID for the PANQOL total score was 11 points (10–12); and the MCIDs for individual PANQOL domains were as follows: hearing, 6 (5–8); balance, 16 (14–19); facial, 10 (no interquartile range); pain, 11 (10–13); energy, 13 (10–17); anxiety, 11 (5–22); and general, 15 (11–19; ▶ Fig. 60.1). The MCID was 7 points (6–11) for the SF-36 Mental Health Summary Scale and 8 (6–10) for the Physical Health Summary Scale (▶ Fig. 60.2). To the authors' knowledge, no other study to date has determined MCID values for these instruments in VS.

60.5 Impact of Disease on Health-Related Quality of Life

The emphasis in HRQoL assessment is usually placed on determining the impact of treatment, or comparison between available modalities; however, understanding the influence of the disease itself on HRQoL also provides valuable insight into the

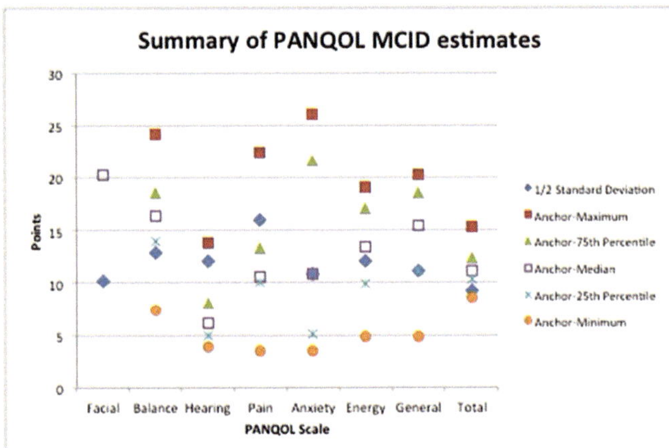

Fig. 60.1 Minimal clinically important difference estimates for the Penn Acoustic Neuroma Quality of Life scale. (Reproduced with permission from Carlson et al.[7])

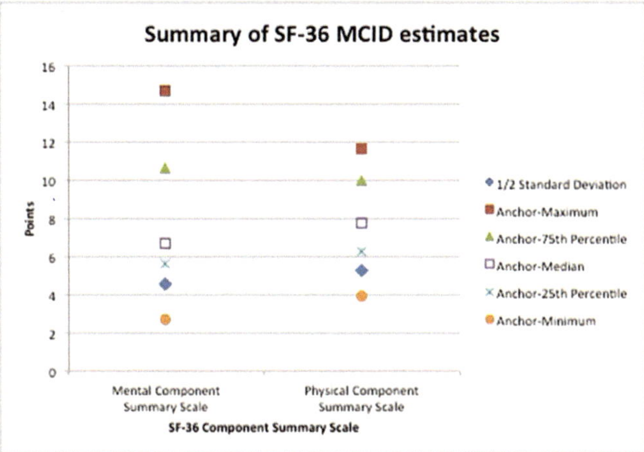

Fig. 60.2 Minimal clinically important difference estimates for the 36-Item Short-Form Health Survey mental- and physical-health component summary scores. (Reproduced with permission from Carlson et al.[7])

psychosocial impact of the disease, and potential motivations behind treatment decisions. For the patient, simply being diagnosed with a brain tumor, albeit benign, may render significant psychological repercussions. For example, this may be a primary motivating factor to select microsurgical resection for some patients, where the tumor is physically removed, instead of radiation or observation, where the tumor remains.

How does the mere diagnosis of VS impact patient well-being? Since patients are generally not surveyed before a diagnosis is established, this question is most directly answered by comparing HRQoL scores between patients with previously untreated VS and normative data for the general, nontumor population. When answering this question, it is critical to exclude studies that only examine HRQoL after radiation or surgery since the added impact of treatment confounds data interpretation. In 2008, Vogel et al surveyed 90 consecutive patients upon diagnosis, to assess illness perceptions, coping, and HRQoL using the SF-36.[23] They found that HRQoL was significantly reduced for nearly all SF-36 subscales in VS patients compared to normal population controls. However, even more remarkable, SF-36 scores were worse compared to reference populations with head and neck cancer, and deaf patients. Furthermore, men with VS had significantly poorer SF-36 scores in most subscales, compared to male reference populations with benign prostatic hypertrophy and chronic obstructive pulmonary disease. Notably, in most of these comparisons, the differences between subscale scores exceeded 10 points—well above the established MCID. More recently, Carlson et al compared outcomes between patients who underwent surgery, radiosurgery, conservative observation, and nontumor controls—the latter composed of normal U.S. population controls.[3] When analyzing differences between conservatively managed VS and controls, the observation cohort had statistically significantly worse scores on the PROMIS-10 mental summary score, PANQOL total score, as well as the PANQOL energy, hearing, balance, general, and facial subscales. Notably, the differences in HRQoL between normal controls and patients with observed VS, in most cases, were greater than the differences seen between management modalities, suggesting that the diagnosis itself has a greater impact on HRQoL than treatment.

This subject also potentially carries important implications for patients undergoing microsurgical resection. Recently, Link et al explored differences in HRQoL in a cohort of 143 patients with sporadic (< 3 cm) VS who received surgical resection—122 receiving gross total resection and 21 receiving subtotal resection.[24] After adjusting for differences between groups with regard to hearing and facial nerve outcomes, subjects who received gross total tumor removal had better SF-36 physical and mental scores, PROMIS-10 physical and mental scores, and PANQOL total, facial, energy, and general health scores compared to patients receiving less-than-complete resection. The authors surmise that in this selected patient population, there was a significant psychological benefit to patients who were radiographically cured of their VS, and this may translate into overall better HRQoL.

60.6 Comparison of Health-Related Quality of Life Between Treatment Modalities

60.6.1 Prospective Studies Utilizing Generic Health-Related Quality-of-Life Measures

While there have been a number of published studies providing valuable information toward understanding various aspects of HRQoL in patients with VS, our ultimate ability to develop evidence-based consensus regarding optimal treatment has been mired by frequent methodological limitations including short-term follow-up, small study populations, lack of control subjects, use of generic instruments, and the presence of significant selection biases. Currently, only a limited number of prospective, nonrandomized studies comparing treatment modalities have been published and no level 1 evidence exists.[25,26,27,28] To the best of our knowledge, there is only one prospective randomized study that is underway, in Bergen Norway, comparing radiosurgery and conservative observation, but not a microsurgical arm. It is unlikely that a multicenter prospective study incorporating all three treatment modalities will ever materialize, given challenges with patient recruitment, number of subjects required to detect statistically and clinically significant differences, as well as notable biases and disparities in treatment practices between centers.[3]

Details regarding four important prospective cohort studies comparing HRQoL in sporadic VS are outlined in ▶ Table 60.1 and are further described here.[25,26,27,28] Pollock and colleagues published the first nonrandomized prospective study in 2006 including 82 patients with primary sporadic, small- to medium-sized (< 3 cm) VS who underwent microsurgery or stereotactic radiosurgery (SRS).[27] The average duration of follow-up was 42 months, and the generic Health Status Questionnaire (modification of the SF-36) was utilized to quantify change in HRQoL over time.[27] The SRS cohort did not experience any deterioration in HRQoL, while the microsurgical arm exhibited decline in the physical component score at 3 months following treatment, which subsequently returned to near baseline. At

Table 60.1 Major prospective, nonrandomized observational studies comparing treatment modalities in patients with sporadic vestibular schwannoma using generic QoL measures

Study	Setting	Design	Subjects and treatment	Follow-up	QoL measures utilized	Reporting description
Pollock et al[27]	Mayo Clinic, Minnesota	Prospective cohort, < 3 cm size tumors	82 total Microsurgery = 36 Radiosurgery = 46	Mean: 42 mo	Health status questionnaire (modified SF-36)	Baseline, 3 mo, 1 y, last follow-up
Myrseth et al[26]	Haukeland University Hospital, Bergen, Norway	Prospective cohort, < 2.5 cm size tumors	88 total Microsurgery = 28 Radiosurgery = 60	2 y	SF-36, GBI	Baseline, 1 y, 2 y
Di Maio and Akagami[25]	Vancouver General Hospital, University of British Columbia	Prospective cohort, separated ≤ 3 cm and > 3 cm size tumors	229 total Observation = 47 Radiation = 48 Surgery = 134	Mean: 31.8 mo	SF-36	Surgery: baseline, 6 wk, 3 mo, yearly observation or radiosurgery: Baseline, 6 mo, yearly
Breivik et al[28]	Haukeland University Hospital, Bergen, Norway	Prospective cohort, < 2.5 cm size tumors	237 total Observation = 124 Radiosurgery = 113	Mean: 55.0 mo	SF-36	Baseline, 1 y, 2 y, 5 y

Abbreviations: GBI, Glasgow Benefit Inventory; QoL, quality of life; SF-36, Short-Form 36 Health Survey.

last follow-up, the net change for the physical and mental summary scores for both treatment groups was very similar; there was a net decrease of 3.1 and 3.6 points in the physical component scores and a net improvement of 4.5 and 3.7 points in the mental component score for the SRS and microsurgery groups, respectively. These small differences are not likely to be considered clinically meaningful to patients or clinicians as they fall below MCID thresholds, as discussed earlier.[7]

In 2009, Myrseth et al published the second nonrandomized prospective study comparing microsurgery and SRS in a cohort of 91 patients using the SF-36 and GBI to evaluate changes in HRQoL at baseline, 1 year, and 2 years following treatment.[26] At last follow-up, there were no statistical differences between treatment groups on individual or summary scores for the SF-36. Similarly, using the GBI, there were no differences between groups at 1 year after treatment. However, at 2 years, there was a statistically significant decline in the GBI total score, and the general and physical subdomain scores for the microsurgery cohort. At last follow-up, there were no statistically significant differences in sick leave status or job disability between groups.

In 2009, Di Maio and Akagami presented a nonrandomized prospective study examining 47 patients who underwent observation, 48 who received linear accelerator–based radiotherapy, and 97 who underwent microsurgical resection of VS smaller than 3 cm in size.[25] At a mean follow-up of 31.8 months, there were no statistically significant differences between groups on either the SF-36 physical or mental health summary score—all three groups were within approximately 4 points of baseline. Notably, HRQoL remained unchanged for the observation and radiotherapy cohorts throughout follow-up, while the surgical group experienced an improvement in mental health at 24 months, which subsequently returned to baseline at last follow-up.

In 2013, Breivik and colleagues published the most recent prospective study, including 237 patients with sporadic VS with extrameatal tumor (i.e., intracanalicular VSs were excluded) extension who either received SRS ($n = 113$) or conservative management ($n = 124$).[28] The primary objective of the study was to compare growth rates and hearing loss between modalities, with a secondary objective of HRQoL comparison utilizing the SF-36 instrument. Aside from the SRS cohort having larger tumors and greater incidence of facial numbness, there were no noteworthy baseline differences between groups. At a mean of 55 months of follow-up, no statistically significant differences in HRQoL scores were seen between SRS and conservatively managed groups. Furthermore, patients who received SRS were less likely to experience tumor growth and less frequently required additional treatment.

60.6.2 Cross-Sectional Studies Utilizing the PANQOL

Given the recent availability of the PANQOL, there have not yet been any published prospective studies comparing treatment modalities using this instrument. However, given the potential advantages of the disease-specific PANQOL over generic measures, the few recent cross-sectional studies involving the PANQOL are reviewed later.[3,29,30] The first cross-sectional study comparing treatment modalities utilizing the PANQOL survey was published by Robinett et al in 2014. Six hundred patients who were evaluated and managed by the authors' center were surveyed and a 49% response rate was obtained. Overall, the mean time interval between initial management and survey was 7.9 years.[29] Comparing baseline differences, tumor size at diagnosis was largest in the surgical cohort and smallest in the stereotactic radiotherapy group ($p = 0.012$); presenting symptoms of vertigo/imbalance were most common in the microsurgery arm, compared to the observation and radiation therapy cohorts ($p = 0.019$), and the mean duration of follow-up was shortest for the radiation arm ($p = 0.002$). When dividing patient follow-up into three discrete time intervals, 0 to 5 years, 6 to 10 years, and more than 10 years, the only difference in total PANQOL score was stereotactic radiotherapy having a higher score than microsurgery and observation at the 0- to 5-year interval; however, no differences in composite HRQoL scores were detected between treatment groups at 6 to 10 years, or more than 10-year intervals. When examining subscale scores, hearing domain scores were highest for stereotactic radiotherapy and lowest for surgery at all intervals, balance domain scores were highest for stereotactic radiotherapy and observation and lowest for surgery at 0 to 5 years, and facial domain scores were highest for observation at 0 to 5 years.

Later in 2014, McLaughlin et al published a cross-sectional survey of 186 patients utilizing the PANQOL—98 conservatively managed subjects, 49 received SRS, and 39 underwent surgery.[30] Details regarding survey response rate were not provided. Several notable baseline differences were present, including a younger age in the surgical cohort, smallest tumor size in the observation group and largest in the microsurgical arm, and better speech recognition threshold and speech discrimination percentage in the conservative group (all, $p < 0.001$). The mean follow-up time, determined by the time interval between diagnosis and completing the PANQOL survey, was 2.6 years. PANQOL subscale and total scores were presented; however, statistical analyses were not performed given intrinsic differences between groups. Overall, the conservative group had the highest total score and the microsurgical cohort had the highest general score. The authors remark that differences between the microsurgery and SRS cohorts were less dramatic than the differences between the microsurgery and conservative groups.

Most recently, in 2015, Carlson et al published a cross-sectional study utilizing the PANQOL, SF-36, GBI, and PROMIS-10, including 642 respondents with a survey response rate of 79%.[3] This study included patients who were evaluated at the Mayo Clinic, Rochester, MN, and Haukeland University in Bergen, Norway—247 received SRS, 148 were under observation, and 144 received microsurgery, in addition to 103 nontumor normal U. S. population control subjects. The mean time interval between initial management and the HRQOL surveys was 7.7 years. Several notable baseline differences were present including younger age at the time of treatment for the microsurgery arm, poorer pretreatment hearing in the SRS arm, and larger tumor size in the microsurgery cohort. A multivariate model accounting for baseline differences between groups demonstrated that overall PANQOL total score was lowest for surgery and not significantly different between SRS and observation. Regarding subscale scores, there were no differences between groups with respect to anxiety, general hearing, or energy domains; however, surgery had lower scores compared to SRS and observation for PANQOL pain, facial, and balance subscales.

Collectively, the results of these two study groups—prospective comparisons utilizing generic measures and cross sectional studies utilizing the disease-specific PANQOL—do not show that one treatment modality is superior over others. Perhaps most notably, the differences in these studies, even when achieving statistically significant values, generally did not exceed the MCID for their respective instruments. Thus, at least based on the current evidence, no consensus guidelines can be established currently. Without conclusive high-level evidence, treatment should be individualized according to tumor- and patient-specific factors. Dogmatic statements regarding the categorical superiority of a given treatment modality are misguided.

60.7 Future Directions

In this section, two important remaining discussion points are highlighted: (1) opportunities for improvement in VS HRQoL assessment (2)and methodology of future studies, balancing what is ideal and what is feasible. Despite being the preferred instrument for VS HRQoL assessment, several limitations in the PANQOL have recently been discussed. First, PANQOL scoring weights the seven individual subscales equally when calculating the total score. However, there is strong evidence that factors such as pain and dizziness impact HRQoL greater than other conditions, such as unilateral hearing loss, for example.[31] Thus, one consideration would be preferential weighting of subscales to more accurately account for these differences. Taking this concept one step further, it may be valuable to weight specific questions within a domain when there is evidence that one aspect has a greater impact on HRQoL than others. For example, Tveiten et al utilized the Facial Disability Index and found that symptoms of intermedius nerve dysfunction (i.e., excessive tearing and "drying of the eye") explained most of the increased disability in a surgical cohort, compared to other sequelae.[32] A final consideration is for expansion of certain subscale question sets, such as the pain scale, where only the single question exists: "I have problems with head pain on the side of my acoustic neuroma tumor."

Although considered the "gold standard," prospective randomized controlled studies assessing HRQoL may not be entirely feasible for reasons outlined earlier. In a recent study by Myrseth et al., an initial plan of patient randomization was abandoned given patient reluctance to submit their treatment to chance.[26] Short of this, well-designed cohort studies remain an achievable goal, and still afford impactful data in the hierarchy of evidence. Understanding that survey response rates may suffer from laborious questionnaires, a priority should be placed on utilizing disease-specific measures (e.g., PANQOL), over multiple generic measures (e.g., SF-36, GBI, PROMIS-10) when there are survey length considerations. Every effort should be made to include longitudinal data from point of diagnosis through treatment, and an absolute minimum of 2 years of follow-up is a requisite. Long-term follow-up is particularly germane to patients with VS, as the average person is expected to live decades after initial diagnosis and treatment, and the effects of surgery are upfront, whereas the sequelae of observation or radiation are generally protracted. In other words, short follow-up often unfairly favors observation or radiation over surgery. Finally, when interpreting the results of studies, we must look beyond statistical differences, and ensure that differences between treatment arms are also clinically meaningful to patients and clinicians.

References

[1] Carlson ML, Link MJ, Wanna GB, Driscoll CL. Management of sporadic vestibular schwannoma. Otolaryngol Clin North Am. 2015; 48(3):407–422

[2] Ramsden RT. The bloody angle: 100 years of acoustic neuroma surgery. J R Soc Med. 1995; 88(8):464P–468P

[3] Carlson ML, Tveiten OV, Driscoll CL, et al. Long-term quality of life in patients with vestibular schwannoma: an international multicenter cross-sectional study comparing microsurgery, stereotactic radiosurgery, observation, and nontumor controls. J Neurosurg. 2015; 122(4):833–842

[4] Carlson ML, Tveiten OV, Driscoll CL, Lund-Johansen M, Link MJ. Long-Term Quality of Life in Vestibular Schwannoma: Impact of Disease and Treatment. Tampa, FL: North American Skull Base Society; 2015

[5] The World Health Organization Quality of Life assessment (WHOQOL): position paper from the World Health Organization. Soc Sci Med. 1995; 41(10): 1403–1409

[6] Ferrans F. Definitions and conceptual models of quality of life. In: Lipscomb J, Gotay CC, Snyder C, eds. Outcomes Assessment in Cancer. Cambridge, England: Cambridge University; 2005:14–30

[7] Carlson ML, Tveiten OV, Yost KJ, Lohse CM, Lund-Johansen M, Link MJ. The minimal clinically important difference in vestibular schwannoma quality-of-life assessment: an important step beyond p < . 05. Otolaryngol Head Neck Surg. 2015; 153(2):202–208

[8] Gauden A, Weir P, Hawthorne G, Kaye A. Systematic review of quality of life in the management of vestibular schwannoma. J Clin Neurosci. 2011; 18(12): 1573–1584

[9] Shaffer BT, Cohen MS, Bigelow DC, Ruckenstein MJ. Validation of a disease-specific quality-of-life instrument for acoustic neuroma: the Penn Acoustic Neuroma Quality-of-Life Scale. Laryngoscope. 2010; 120(8):1646–1654

[10] Gouveris HT, Mann WJ. Quality of life in sporadic vestibular schwannoma: a review. ORL J Otorhinolaryngol Relat Spec. 2010; 72(2):69–74

[11] Cosetti MK, Golfinos JG, Roland JT, Jr. Quality of life (QoL) assessment in patients with neurofibromatosis type 2 (NF2). Otolaryngol Head Neck Surg. 2015; 153(4):599–605

[12] Hornigold RE, Golding JF, Leschziner G, et al. The NFTI-QOL: a disease-specific quality of life questionnaire for neurofibromatosis 2. J Neurol Surg B Skull Base. 2012; 73(2):104–111

[13] Neary WJ, Hillier VF, Flute T, Stephens SD, Ramsden RT, Evans DG. The relationship between patients' perception of the effects of neurofibromatosis type 2 and the domains of the Short Form-36. Clin Otolaryngol. 2010; 35(4): 291–299

[14] van Leeuwen BM, Herruer JM, Putter H, Jansen JC, van der Mey AG, Kaptein AA. Validating the Penn Acoustic Neuroma Quality of Life Scale in a sample of Dutch patients recently diagnosed with vestibular schwannoma. Otol Neurotol. 2013; 34(5):952–957

[15] Ware JE, Jr, Sherbourne CD. The MOS 36-item short-form health survey (SF-36). I. Conceptual framework and item selection. Med Care. 1992; 30(6): 473–483

[16] Rabin R, de Charro F. EQ-5D: a measure of health status from the EuroQol Group. Ann Med. 2001; 33(5):337–343

[17] Hays RD, Bjorner JB, Revicki DA, Spritzer KL, Cella D. Development of physical and mental health summary scores from the patient-reported outcomes measurement information system (PROMIS) global items. Qual Life Res. 2009; 18(7):873–880

[18] Robinson K, Gatehouse S, Browning GG. Measuring patient benefit from otorhinolaryngological surgery and therapy. Ann Otol Rhinol Laryngol. 1996; 105(6):415–422

[19] Guyatt G, Walter S, Norman G. Measuring change over time: assessing the usefulness of evaluative instruments. J Chronic Dis. 1987; 40(2):171–178

[20] Jaeschke R, Singer J, Guyatt GH. Measurement of health status. Ascertaining the minimal clinically important difference. Control Clin Trials. 1989; 10(4): 407–415

[21] King MT. A point of minimal important difference (MID): a critique of terminology and methods. Expert Rev Pharmacoecon Outcomes Res. 2011; 11(2): 171–184

[22] Yost KJ, Eton DT. Combining distribution- and anchor-based approaches to determine minimally important differences: the FACIT experience. Eval Health Prof. 2005; 28(2):172–191

[23] Vogel JJ, Godefroy WP, van der Mey AG, le Cessie S, Kaptein AA. Illness perceptions, coping, and quality of life in vestibular schwannoma patients at diagnosis. Otol Neurotol. 2008; 29(6):839–845

[24] Link MJ, Carlson ML, Lund-Johansen M, et al. Quality of life analysis in vestibular schwannoma patients: to leave or not to leave...gross total vs. less than gross total resection in an international cohort of patients. Oral presentation, North American Skull Base Society Annual Meeting, Scottsdale Arizona, February 2016

[25] Di Maio S, Akagami R. Prospective comparison of quality of life before and after observation, radiation, or surgery for vestibular schwannomas. J Neurosurg. 2009; 111(4):855–862

[26] Myrseth E, Møller P, Pedersen PH, Lund-Johansen M. Vestibular schwannoma: surgery or gamma knife radiosurgery? A prospective, nonrandomized study. Neurosurgery. 2009; 64(4):654–661, discussion 661–663

[27] Pollock BE, Driscoll CL, Foote RL, et al. Patient outcomes after vestibular schwannoma management: a prospective comparison of microsurgical resection and stereotactic radiosurgery. Neurosurgery. 2006; 59(1):77–85, discussion 77–85

[28] Breivik CN, Nilsen RM, Myrseth E, et al. Conservative management or gamma knife radiosurgery for vestibular schwannoma: tumor growth, symptoms, and quality of life. Neurosurgery. 2013; 73(1):48–56, discussion 56–57

[29] Robinett ZN, Walz PC, Miles-Markley B, Moberly AC, Welling DB. Comparison of long-term quality-of-life outcomes in vestibular schwannoma patients. Otolaryngol Head Neck Surg. 2014; 150(6):1024–1032

[30] McLaughlin EJ, Bigelow DC, Lee JY, Ruckenstein MJ. Quality of life in acoustic neuroma patients. Otol Neurotol. 2015; 36(4):653–656

[31] Carlson ML, Tveiten OV, Driscoll CL, et al. What drives quality of life in patients with sporadic vestibular schwannoma? Laryngoscope. 2015; 125(7): 1697–1702

[32] Tveiten ØV, Carlson ML, Goplen F, Myrseth E, Driscoll CLW, Mahesparan R, Link MJ, Lund-Johansen M. Patient- versus physician-reported facial disability in vestibular schwannoma: an international cross-sectional study. J Neurosurg. 2017 Nov;127(5):1015-1024

Part VIII

Medical and Surgical Rehabilitation

VIII

61 Auditory Rehabilitation in Sporadic Vestibular Schwannoma

Brendan P. O'Connell, David S. Haynes, and George B. Wanna

61.1 Introduction

Hearing loss in patients with sporadic vestibular schwannoma (VS) can occur either as part of the natural history of the disease or secondary to intervention by way of surgery or stereotactic radiation. Patients with minimal or no hearing loss in the tumor ear and good hearing in the contralateral ear generally fair well and do no pursue amplification. For patients with greater degrees of hearing loss, conventional hearing amplification is successful in most patients with a word recognition score greater than 60% and pure-tone thresholds better than 80 dB HL.

In patients with more advanced unilateral hearing loss, or single-sided deafness (SSD), the loss of binaural hearing can have the following audiologic consequences: decreased perception of sound coming from the affected side, reduced ability to localize sound, difficulty with speech perception in noise, and increased listening effort. The level of hearing loss, of course, must be evaluated in the context of the patient. For example, a person who works in a quiet office may be only minimally impacted by SSD, while a police officer that relies heavily on accurate sound localization or a waitress who works in a noisy restaurant may encounter significant difficulty. Furthermore, many patients are more bothered by their hearing loss if lost abruptly from sudden hearing loss or immediately following surgery. In these cases, we generally advise that the patient not pursue surgical treatments until at least 6 months, as a significant number of patients adjust to the loss and ultimately do not pursue additional treatments.

Depending on the patient and their daily environment, advanced unilateral hearing loss can cause psychological and social impairment; therefore, it is important for clinicians to be cognizant of the potential quality-of-life implications that profound unilateral hearing loss can have on patients with VS. Furthermore, specialists caring for patients with VS should be knowledgeable about the available auditory rehabilitation options.

61.2 Impact of Hearing Loss on Patients with Sporadic Vestibular Schwannoma

Despite our best efforts at hearing preservation, the majority of patients eventually experience significant unilateral hearing loss following diagnosis and/or treatment.[1] Studies that retrospectively survey patients after VS treatment demonstrate that hearing loss is indeed bothersome, albeit to variable degrees. In patients with unilateral deafness after translabyrinthine VS removal, 80% of individuals endorsed a subjective hearing handicap of varying severity.[2,3,4,5] When asked to report one's most disabling symptom, hearing loss is cited by 10 to 61% of patients. Furthermore, when using the World Health Organization (WHO) classification of functional deficits, reported disabilities were attributed to auditory impairment in the majority of cases.[6] Patients with good hearing in the nontumor ear report far less hearing handicap than patients with bilateral hearing impairment.[1]

Studies have also looked at changes in hearing handicap comparing pre- and postoperative time points. While 58% of patients demonstrated no change in their hearing handicap between preoperative and 12-month postoperative follow-up, 25% of patients had significant worsening in their hearing handicap.[7] Not surprisingly, the patients who noted worsening disability were those with a better hearing class preoperatively.

Studies have also assessed the association between hearing loss and overall quality of life using validated health-related quality-of-life instruments. While poor hearing has been shown to be predictive of decreased quality of life when using the validated Penn Acoustic Neuroma Quality of Life Scale (PANQOL), surprisingly no relation between hearing loss and other global measures of health-related quality of life has been demonstrated.[8,9,10,11] Although instruments used in these studies have been validated and are well-established measures, perhaps they are not sensitive enough to detect more subtle changes in hearing handicap that are associated with SSD.

61.3 Auditory Rehabilitation in Cases of Functional Residual Hearing

Amplification with a conventional hearing aid is an option for patients with either treated or untreated VSs so long as hearing remains functional. In most cases, conventional hearing aids provide benefit if ipsilateral word recognition scores are greater than 60% and pure-tone thresholds are better than 80 dB HL. This threshold varies between patients and may also be influenced by hearing status in the opposite ear. Several unique considerations regarding sensorineural hearing loss and hearing aid fitting in patients with VS deserve review. First, patients with retrocochlear hearing loss may experience rollover effects in which speech recognition decreases as presentation level increases. Second, patients often have disproportionally poorer word recognition scores than would be expected from pure-tone levels and may experience abnormal loudness growth functions with reduced dynamic ranges. Finally, patients have a much greater probability of accelerated deterioration of hearing than the average population, which may require more frequent hearing aid adjustments and upgrades. The latter has cost implications, particularly in cases of either untreated or previously radiated tumors that may demonstrate progressive hearing loss over time. Given the aforementioned points, the degree of durable benefit from traditional amplification in patients with VS is less predictable than the general population. Nevertheless, conventional hearing aids may be worthwhile in select patients with benefits including improved word recognition, enhanced sound localization, and perhaps even tinnitus masking.

61.4 Auditory Rehabilitation of Single-Sided Deafness in Vestibular Schwannoma

Traditionally, audiologic rehabilitation of SSD was limited to devices that allow for routing of sound from the affected ear to the hearing ear, thus overcoming the head shadow effect. More recently, cochlear implantation (CI) has emerged as an option for sound restoration in the deaf ear. Both surgical and nonsurgical options for contralateral routing of sound (CROS) are available to patients, and are discussed later.

61.4.1 Contralateral Routing of Sound Hearing Aids

CROS hearing aids collect sound through a microphone placed in the hearing-impaired ear, transferring the signal wirelessly to a receiver placed in the contralateral normal hearing ear. Patients who have aidable hearing loss in the better hearing ear should be fitted with a bilateral contralateral routing of signals (BiCROS) system. In addition to transferring sound from the deaf ear, the BiCROS system delivers amplified sound from both sides to the better hearing ear. Available data support that CROS aids provide modest improvement in speech discrimination in noise when compared to the unaided condition.[12,13] Historically, CROS hearing aids were not universally accepted, as patients complained of sound distortion, the need to wear devices in both ears with occlusion effect, and discomfort related to occlusion of the better hearing ear.[14] Long-term usage rates in patients treated for VS have been reported to be as low as 32%.[2] With recent advances in hearing aid technology, in particular digital noise reduction and directional microphones, there appears to be an increased acceptance rate of newer generation CROS and BiCROS systems.[15,16,17]

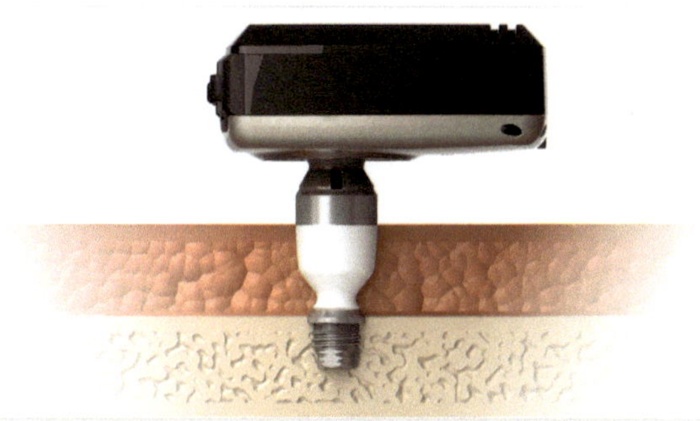

Fig. 61.1 Schematic of a percutaneous bone-anchored implant. (Image courtesy of Cochlear Americas, © 2016.)

61.4.2 Bone-Anchored Implants

Bone-anchored implants (BAIs) are surgically implanted systems that were initially approved for conductive or mixed bilateral hearing loss, but in recent years have been popularized as transcranial cochlear stimulators for rehabilitation of SSD. Currently available BAIs include Baha Attract (Cochlear Corporation, Centennial, CO), Baha Connect (Cochlear Corporation), Ponto (Oticon Medical, Somerset, NJ), and Sophono (Sophono Inc, Boulder, CO). The Baha Connect and Ponto devices are percutaneous bone-conduction hearing implants (▶ Fig. 61.1). Specifically, an osseointegrated screw is implanted into the skull and an abutment is attached that protrudes through the skin. Allowing time for osseointegration, a sound processor is then connected to the abutment weeks to months after surgery. The Baha Attract and Sophono are transcutaneous implants without abutments (▶ Fig. 61.2). Although the design of these particular devices differs slightly, an internal magnet is implanted into the skull beneath the skin. The processor then couples to the internal device via an external magnet. Both percutaneous and transcutaneous devices allow for transmission of sound through bone to the contralateral cochlea (▶ Fig. 61.3). While transcutaneous devices decrease the risk of postoperative crusting and skin overgrowth, cases of pressure necrosis have been reported. In addition, signal gain is reduced secondary to the intervening soft tissue between magnets and the audiologic outcomes remain unclear in the setting of SSD. For this reason,

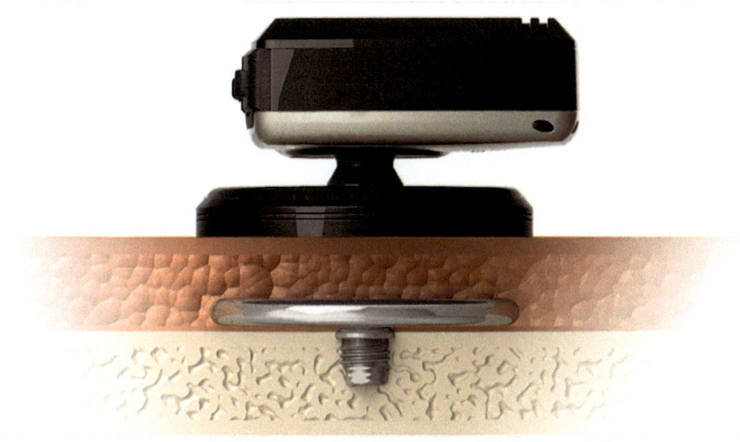

Fig. 61.2 Schematic of a transcutaneous bone-anchored implant. (Image courtesy of Cochlear Americas, ©2016.)

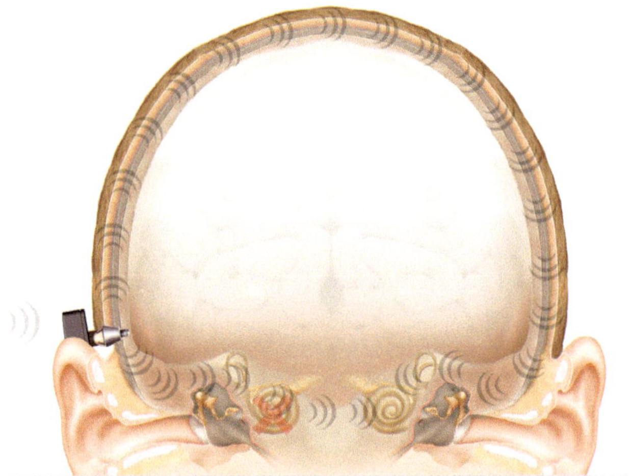

Fig. 61.3 In patients with right-sided deafness, a bone-anchored implant placed on the right can transmit sound via bone conduction to the contralateral cochlea. (Image courtesy of Cochlear Americas, ©2016.)

further discussion regarding BAIs will be largely limited to the use of percutaneous devices.

Strong evidence supports that BAIs are associated with improved speech recognition in noise in patients with SSD.[2,12,18,19] In addition, the majority of BAI users report satisfaction and improved hearing-related quality of life with their device, which has been shown to persist at long-term follow-up.[2,12,18,20,21,22] Long-term usage rates are generally reported to be around 80 and 95%.[19,20,23] Postoperative healing issues should be discussed when counseling patients about implantable bone-conductive devices as the rate of skin reactions around the abutment site with BAIs has been reported to range between 5 and 38%.[12,20,24,25] Of course, it is critical that the patient understands that BAIs will not improve sound localization. In addition, all patients should trial a bone conduction hearing aid for several days before proceeding with BAI placement. Proper patient selection is key to long-term consistent use.

61.4.3 CROS versus BAI for Rehabilitation of Single-Sided Deafness in Nontumor Patients

Traditionally, studies comparing CROS and BAI devices for SSD demonstrated superior audiologic outcomes and better patient satisfaction with BAIs.[12,19,26] In patients undergoing a trial with a CROS aid who subsequently were implanted with a BAI, improved speech discrimination scores and quality-of-life measures were noted with BAIs.[19,26] A multi-institutional prospective study further confirmed these findings by showing that BAIs provided greater improvement in speech intelligibility in noise and greater perceived benefit when compared to the CROS aid.[12] As discussed earlier, neither BAIs nor CROS aids improve sound localization.[12,13] There have been considerable technological advancements with both BAI and CROS devices in recent years. Current studies suggest that performance between devices may not differ as much as previously thought.[16]

61.4.4 CROS and BAI in Patients with Vestibular Schwannoma

The benefit of CROS aids and BAIs in patients with VS is not well studied. Fifty-nine patients undergoing translabyrinthine resection of VS were prospectively studied in regards to subjective hearing handicap.[2] At 2 to 3 years postoperatively, roughly half of the patients (53%) reported trialing a CROS hearing aid, but none felt that it was satisfactory. Furthermore, only 32% of the patients who initially pursued a CROS hearing aid still used the device at last follow-up. Others have prospectively studied outcomes of both CROS and BAI devices in patients with VS.[13] Better performance was again noted for BAIs when compared to conventional CROS aids. Hearing-specific quality-of-life questionnaires demonstrated the greatest improvement within the BAI group. Long-term device satisfaction with BAIs has been reported in 95% of select VS patients.[24]

61.4.5 Surgical Considerations Pertinent to BAI Placement after Treatment of Vestibular Schwannoma

Implantation of BAIs can be performed either at the time of VS surgery or at some point after tumor removal. The former is potentially advantageous, as it shortens the period without acoustic stimulation from the deafened side and avoids a second operation. Patients with poor preoperative hearing can undergo a device trial and make an informed decision about proceeding with BAI placement in conjunction with tumor removal. Patients with good preoperative hearing may be better served by going through tumor removal and a period of recovery and adaptation prior to trialing a device. A significant percentage of patients will forego any further intervention, presumably due to limited perceived deficit. In patients undergoing BAI implantation at the time of VS removal, overall complication rates did not differ from generally published BAI complication rates.[24] In one specific case, a patient did develop a cerebrospinal fluid leak through the implant site, leading the authors to emphasize the importance of avoiding any connection between the BAI and craniotomy site. Less invasive BAI techniques with minimal skin undermining are likely best if implantation is to be performed concurrent with tumor removal.

To summarize, both CROS hearing aids and BAIs are viable options for rehabilitation of SSD in patients with VS. Both options provide improved access to sound and relief from head shadow effect, but neither can overcome the inability to localize sound. Despite the lack of randomized control trials comparing BAIs to CROS aids, available data suggest that superior outcomes are achieved with bone-anchored devices.

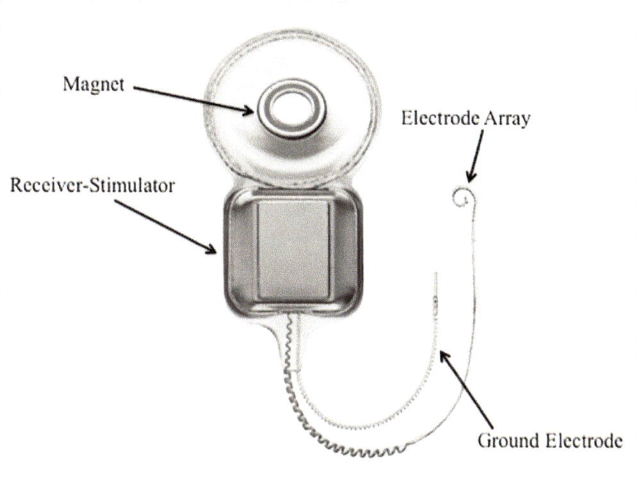

Fig. 61.4 The internal portion of a cochlear implant is depicted. The magnet and receiver-stimulator rest on the lateral surface of the skull, while the electrode array is inserted into the cochlea. (Image courtesy of Cochlear Americas, ©2016.)

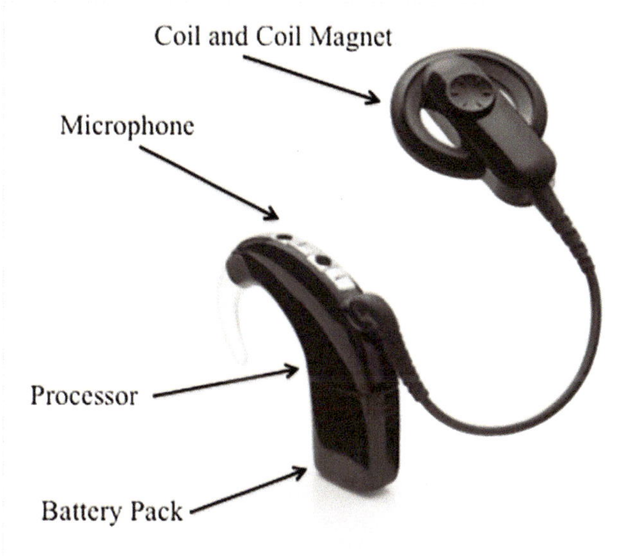

Fig. 61.5 The external processor of a cochlear implant is depicted. (Image courtesy of Cochlear Americas, ©2016.)

61.5 Restoration of Binaural Hearing with Cochlear Implantation

In recent years, treatment options for rehabilitation of SSD have expanded to include CI (▶ Fig. 61.4 and ▶ Fig. 61.5). Aside from auditory brainstem implants (ABI), which are not currently used for unilateral VS or SSD, CI is the only rehabilitative option that potentially restores binaural hearing. In the United States, CI for SSD is not currently approved by the Food and Drug Administration (FDA). As such, insurance approval commonly presents a major barrier. In patients with SSD and without cerebellopontine angle tumors, studies have demonstrated that CI results in better speech understanding in noise, enhanced sound localization, and improved quality of life. In patients with VS, the use of a CI is predicated on the presence of an anatomically intact cochlear nerve.

61.5.1 Determining CI Candidacy and Electrophysiologic Testing

In the case of an observed VS or one that has received radiosurgery, the anatomical continuity of the nerve can be assured. However, following microsurgical resection, particularly for a large tumor, the viability of the cochlear nerve may be difficult to ascertain. Among patients who have undergone microsurgical resection, ideal CI candidates are those with small tumors who underwent unsuccessful hearing preservation surgery but are known to have an anatomically intact cochlear nerve. In these cases, hearing may have been lost because of vascular spasm or cochlear ischemia. Because of the somewhat unreliable nature of intraoperative eighth nerve monitoring, concurrent CI placement should not be performed if the auditory brainstem response is lost during hearing preservation microsurgery. Rather, the patient should undergo reliable behavioral testing after surgery to determine hearing status. In another scenario, concurrent CI with translabyrinthine surgery has been reported, when the cochlear nerve can be anatomically preserved. This strategy is logical because all patients will not have functional hearing after this approach, concurrent access to the cochlea is available, and delayed implantation after the translabyrinthine approach risks cochlear ossification.

The ability of promontory testing to predict outcomes with CI has been investigated in hopes of predicting CI outcomes when the viability of the cochlear nerve is unknown. The principle behind promontory testing is that measuring responses to electrical stimulation of the spiral ganglion cells at the origin of the cochlear nerve should provide information regarding the functional integrity of both the nerve and the cochlea. This is accomplished by placing an electrode on the promontory near the round window niche that delivers electrical stimulation to the cochlea. While a positive promontory stimulation test has been shown to predict a favorable outcome following CI, a negative response does not exclude the possibility of achieving a good result.[27] False-negative results with promontory testing may occur more commonly in the early postoperative period.[27,28] For these reasons, the authors generally do not use promontory testing to help determine CI candidacy. Rather, a close review of the surgical notes may provide important clues regarding anatomical eighth nerve preservation. In addition, detectable hearing in the operated ear assures anatomical continuity. Finally, as discussed earlier, anatomical continuity should be assumed in VS that has been managed with observation or radiation treatment.

61.5.2 Surgical Consideration of Cochlear Implantation in an Ear with a Vestibular Schwannoma

The timing and technique of CI placement in an ear that has been surgically treated for a VS varies according to the approach used. With a translabyrinthine approach, CI can be placed either at the time of tumor extirpation or at a second surgery. If implanted concurrent to tumor removal, a posterior tympanotomy can be performed and the implant can be inserted in typical fashion through the facial recess. Modified translabyrinthine approaches have also been described, in which the external auditory canal skin is closed and the posterior ear canal is removed.[29] In translabyrinthine resections in which CI is planned for a later date, some authors advocate placement of a placeholder or dummy electrode in the cochlea to improve the likelihood of successful electrode insertion in the setting of cochlear ossification.[30] Progressive cochlear ossification has been demonstrated at various time points after translabyrinthine tumor removal.[31] If the tumor is removed through a middle fossa or retrosigmoid approach, staged implantation is more commonly described.[32,33] Simultaneous implantation in these approaches would require otherwise unnecessary exposure of the mastoid air cells and could potentially increase the risk of postoperative spinal fluid leak. In addition, as discussed earlier, CI should be pursued only after nonserviceable hearing is demonstrated on postoperative behavioral testing.

61.5.3 Cochlear Implant Outcomes in Vestibular Schwannoma

To our knowledge, only two studies report CI outcomes for SSD after the treatment of sporadic VS, totaling five patients. Of these patients, the majority benefited from acquisition of sound awareness and most obtained open-set discrimination ability.[29,30] Improvement in sound localization and marked tinnitus suppression was also reported by a few patients.[30] The benefits of CI in sporadic VS can also be inferred from reports of implantation in the neurofibromatosis type 2 (NF2) population, which is more common. While only speculative, one can assume that the outcomes in sporadic patients would be as good or perhaps better, since sporadic tumors are generally less aggressive, unifocal, and are less likely to invade the cochlear nerve. CI outcomes in NF2 are further summarized in Chapter 84.

61.5.4 Imaging Considerations with Cochlear Implants

Historically, magnetic resonance imaging (MRI) in patients with CI was contraindicated given concerns over patient safety and device malfunction. For patients to receive an MRI scan, the internal magnet had to be removed. MED-EL devices were the first to receive FDA approval for use with 1.5 T MRI without magnet removal, with the SYNCHRONY implant recently getting approval for 3.0 T scans.[34] More recently, Advanced Bionics has also introduced a CI device with a rotating, self-aligning magnet that is FDA approved for use in 1.5 and 3.0T MRI without magnet removal. Studies assessing the safety of imaging patients with 1.5 T MRI have demonstrated that after tight head-wrap application, the procedure is well tolerated by most patients and the risk of device malfunction is exceedingly low.[34,35,36] In addition, imaging artifact is unlikely to impede the evaluation of the ipsilateral skull base.[34] Pain and magnet displacement can nonetheless occur in up to 15% of cases, and should be discussed with patients who are considering CI. Chapter 10 provides a more in-depth discussion regarding MRI tumor surveillance after CI.

61.6 Auditory Rehabilitation of Sporadic Vestibular Schwannoma in an Only Hearing Ear

Sporadic VS in an only hearing ear is a rare but challenging clinical scenario. While decision making in regards to tumor management is beyond the scope of this chapter, hearing rehabilitation strategies that reduce the chance of total bilateral deafness are paramount.

Assuming the contralateral (nontumor) ear has an intact cochlear nerve, CI can be performed in that ear before or after treatment of the tumor. A few studies report favorable results after placing a CI in the nontumor ear prior to VS treatment. Specifically, the majority of patients achieve open-set speech discrimination, report subjective benefit of the CI, and continue to regularly use the device after treatment of the contralateral tumor.[37,38,39] Interestingly, some patients experience significant improvement in CI performance as hearing loss progresses on the tumor side.[37] Contralateral CI placement following tumor removal has also been reported in three patients, with mean word and sentence recognition scores of 90 and 80%, respectively.[37] As with CI in the general population, the etiology of hearing loss and duration of deafness are important considerations when implanting the nontumor ear. In patients with congenital deafness on one side and VS in the contralateral only hearing ear, performance with CI in the congenitally deaf ear may be poor.[40]

Cochlear implantation in the tumor ear, whether the tumor has been treated or not, is also possible as long as the cochlear nerve is intact. Outcome data regarding CI on the same side of a treated VS with poor hearing in the contralateral nontumor ear are limited to small series of patients with varying results.[37,41,42,43] In the largest series to date of seven patients with sporadic VS undergoing simultaneous CI at the time of translabyrinthine resection, 71% of patients achieved open set speech recognition with a mean score of 56%; 71% of patients were CI users at last follow-up.[41] In a smaller report of two patients who underwent surgery for VS in an only hearing ear, CI on the tumor side allowed sound detection in one patient.[37] CI has also been reported in the tumor ear of three patients in which no treatment for the tumor was prescribed; an objective increase in speech perception scores was reported.[44,45]

Given that patients with bilateral profound hearing loss and a unilateral sporadic VS likely will have at least one intact cochlear nerve, the role of ABI is limited. Placement of ABI has been reported after treatment of three patients affected by VS in their only hearing ear, two of who had previously undergone contralateral CI.[46] Performance with the ABI was poor, and only one patient was a daily ABI user.

While CI appears to confer benefit when placed in the nontumor ear either before or after tumor removal, the results obtained with CI on the tumor side are variable. As such, CI should be encouraged in the nontumor ear before tumor removal if surgery is expected to result in bilateral deafness. This approach maximizes time to get accustomed to a CI in the nontumor ear prior to VS treatment.

61.7 Conclusion

The majority of patients with sporadic VS report some degree of hearing handicap related to unilateral hearing loss; for certain individuals, it can be very disabling. Auditory rehabilitation becomes even more important in patients with bilateral hearing loss. Decisions regarding the need to pursue auditory rehabilitation and the rehabilitative approach should be individualized to each patient in the context of their daily needs and preferences.

References

[1] Tveiten OV, Carlson ML, Goplen F, Vassbotn F, Link MJ, Lund-Johansen M. Long-term auditory symptoms in patients with sporadic vestibular schwannoma: an international cross-sectional study. Neurosurgery. 2015; 77(2): 218–227, discussion 227

[2] Andersen HT, Schrøder SA, Bonding P. Unilateral deafness after acoustic neuroma surgery: subjective hearing handicap and the effect of the bone-anchored hearing aid. Otol Neurotol. 2006; 27(6):809–814

[3] Rigby PL, Shah SB, Jackler RK, Chung JH, Cooke DD. Acoustic neuroma surgery: outcome analysis of patient-perceived disability. Am J Otol. 1997; 18(4):427–435

[4] Tufarelli D, Meli A, Alesii A, et al. Quality of life after acoustic neuroma surgery. Otol Neurotol. 2006; 27(3):403–409

[5] Ryzenman JM, Pensak ML, Tew JM, Jr. Patient perception of comorbid conditions after acoustic neuroma management: survey results from the acoustic neuroma association. Laryngoscope. 2004; 114(5):814–820

[6] Bateman N, Nikolopoulos TP, Robinson K, O'Donoghue GM. Impairments, disabilities, and handicaps after acoustic neuroma surgery. Clin Otolaryngol Allied Sci. 2000; 25(1):62–65

[7] Humphriss RL, Baguley DM, Axon PR, Moffat DA. Change in hearing handicap after translabyrinthine vestibular schwannoma excision. Otol Neurotol. 2004; 25(3):371–378

[8] Lassaletta L, Alfonso C, Del Rio L, Roda JM, Gavilan J. Impact of facial dysfunction on quality of life after vestibular schwannoma surgery. Ann Otol Rhinol Laryngol. 2006; 115(9):694–698

[9] Betchen SA, Walsh J, Post KD. Self-assessed quality of life after acoustic neuroma surgery. J Neurosurg. 2003; 99(5):818–823

[10] Lloyd SK, Kasbekar AV, Baguley DM, Moffat DA. Audiovestibular factors influencing quality of life in patients with conservatively managed sporadic vestibular schwannoma. Otol Neurotol. 2010; 31(6):968–976

[11] Carlson ML, Tveiten OV, Driscoll CL, et al. What drives quality of life in patients with sporadic vestibular schwannoma? Laryngoscope. 2015; 125(7): 1697–1702

[12] Wazen JJ, Spitzer JB, Ghossaini SN, et al. Transcranial contralateral cochlear stimulation in unilateral deafness. Otolaryngol Head Neck Surg. 2003; 129 (3):248–254

[13] Hol MK, Bosman AJ, Snik AF, Mylanus EA, Cremers CW. Bone-anchored hearing aids in unilateral inner ear deafness: an evaluation of audiometric and patient outcome measurements. Otol Neurotol. 2005; 26(5):999–1006

[14] Bishop CE, Eby TL. The current status of audiologic rehabilitation for profound unilateral sensorineural hearing loss. Laryngoscope. 2010; 120(3):552–556

[15] Hill SL, III, Marcus A, Digges EN, Gillman N, Silverstein H. Assessment of patient satisfaction with various configurations of digital CROS and BiCROS hearing aids. Ear Nose Throat J. 2006; 85(7):427–430, 442

[16] Finbow J, Bance M, Aiken S, Gulliver M, Verge J, Caissie R. A comparison between wireless CROS and bone-anchored hearing devices for single-sided deafness: a pilot study. Otol Neurotol. 2015; 36(5):819–825

[17] Williams VA, McArdle RA, Chisolm TH. Subjective and objective outcomes from new BiCROS technology in a veteran sample. J Am Acad Audiol. 2012; 23(10):789–806

[18] Linstrom CJ, Silverman CA, Yu GP. Efficacy of the bone-anchored hearing aid for single-sided deafness. Laryngoscope. 2009; 119(4):713–720

[19] Lin LM, Bowditch S, Anderson MJ, May B, Cox KM, Niparko JK. Amplification in the rehabilitation of unilateral deafness: speech in noise and directional hearing effects with bone-anchored hearing and contralateral routing of signal amplification. Otol Neurotol. 2006; 27(2):172–182

[20] Gluth MB, Eager KM, Eikelboom RH, Atlas MD. Long-term benefit perception, complications, and device malfunction rate of bone-anchored hearing aid implantation for profound unilateral sensorineural hearing loss. Otol Neurotol. 2010; 31(9):1427–1434

[21] Faber HT, Nelissen RC, Kramer SE, Cremers CW, Snik AF, Hol MK. Bone-anchored hearing implants in single-sided deafness patients: long-term use and satisfaction by gender. Laryngoscope. 2015; 125(12):2790–2795

[22] House JW, Kutz JW, Jr, Chung J, Fisher LM. Bone-anchored hearing aid subjective benefit for unilateral deafness. Laryngoscope. 2010; 120(3):601–607

[23] Martin TP, Lowther R, Cooper H, et al. The bone-anchored hearing aid in the rehabilitation of single-sided deafness: experience with 58 patients. Clin Otolaryngol. 2010; 35(4):284–290

[24] McRackan TR, Goddard JC, Wilkinson EP, Slattery WH, Brackmann DE. Bone-anchored hearing device placement with translabyrinthine tumor removal. Otolaryngol Head Neck Surg. 2015; 152(2):314–318

[25] Kiringoda R, Lustig LR. A meta-analysis of the complications associated with osseointegrated hearing aids. Otol Neurotol. 2013; 34(5):790–794

[26] Niparko JK, Cox KM, Lustig LR. Comparison of the bone anchored hearing aid implantable hearing device with contralateral routing of offside signal amplification in the rehabilitation of unilateral deafness. Otol Neurotol. 2003; 24(1):73–78

[27] Neff BA, Wiet RM, Lasak JM, et al. Cochlear implantation in the neurofibromatosis type 2 patient: long-term follow-up. Laryngoscope. 2007; 117(6):1069–1072

[28] Hoffman RA, Kohan D, Cohen NL. Cochlear implants in the management of bilateral acoustic neuromas. Am J Otol. 1992; 13(6):525–528

[29] Arriaga MA, Marks S. Simultaneous cochlear implantation and acoustic neuroma resection: imaging considerations, technique, and functional outcome. Otolaryngol Head Neck Surg. 1995; 112(2):325–328

[30] Hassepass F, Arndt S, Aschendorff A, Laszig R, Wesarg T. Cochlear implantation for hearing rehabilitation in single-sided deafness after translabyrinthine vestibular schwannoma surgery. Eur Arch Otorhinolaryngol. 201 6; 273(9): 2373–2383

[31] Belal A. Is cochlear implantation possible after acoustic tumor removal? Otol Neurotol. 2001; 22(4):497–500

[32] Hulka GF, Bernard EJ, Pillsbury HC. Cochlear implantation in a patient after removal of an acoustic neuroma. The implications of magnetic resonance imaging with gadolinium on patient management. Arch Otolaryngol Head Neck Surg. 1995; 121(4):465–468

[33] Temple RH, Axon PR, Ramsden RT, Keles N, Deger K, Yücel E. Auditory rehabilitation in neurofibromatosis type 2: a case for cochlear implantation. J Laryngol Otol. 1999; 113(2):161–163

[34] Carlson ML, Neff BA, Link MJ, et al. Magnetic resonance imaging with cochlear implant magnet in place: safety and imaging quality. Otol Neurotol. 2015; 36 (6):965–971

[35] Walton J, Donnelly NP, Tam YC, et al. MRI without magnet removal in neurofibromatosis type 2 patients with cochlear and auditory brainstem implants. Otol Neurotol. 2014; 35(5):821–825

[36] Crane BT, Gottschalk B, Kraut M, Aygun N, Niparko JK. Magnetic resonance imaging at 1.5 T after cochlear implantation. Otol Neurotol. 2010; 31(8):1215–1220

[37] Di Lella F, Merkus P, Di Trapani G, Taibah A, Guida M, Sanna M. Vestibular schwannoma in the only hearing ear: role of cochlear implants. Ann Otol Rhinol Laryngol. 2013; 122(2):91–99

[38] Thedinger BA, Cueva RA, Glasscock ME, III. Treatment of an acoustic neuroma in an only-hearing ear: case reports and considerations for the future. Laryngoscope. 1993; 103(9):976–980

[39] Shin YJ, Fraysse B, Sterkers O, Bouccara D, Rey A, Lazorthes Y. Hearing restoration in posterior fossa tumors. Am J Otol. 1998; 19(5):649–653

[40] Ramsden R, Khwaja S, Green K, O'Driscoll M, Mawman D. Vestibular schwannoma in the only hearing ear: cochlear implant or auditory brainstem implant? Otol Neurotol. 2005; 26(2):261–264

[41] Lassaletta L, Aristegui M, Medina M, et al. Ipsilateral cochlear implantation in patients with sporadic vestibular schwannoma in the only or best hearing ear and in patients with NF2. Eur Arch Otorhinolaryngol. 2016; 273(1):27–35

[42] Arístegui M, Denia A. Simultaneous cochlear implantation and translabyrinthine removal of vestibular schwannoma in an only hearing ear: report of two cases (neurofibromatosis type 2 and unilateral vestibular schwannoma). Otol Neurotol. 2005; 26(2):205–210

[43] Pensak ML, Tew JM, Keith RW, Vanloveren HR. Management of the acoustic neuroma in an only hearing ear. Skull Base Surg. 1991; 1(2):93–96

[44] Mukherjee P, Ramsden JD, Donnelly N, et al. Cochlear implants to treat deafness caused by vestibular schwannomas. Otol Neurotol. 2013; 34(7): 1291–1298

[45] Helbig S, Rader T, Bahmer A, Baumann U. A case of bilateral cochlear implantation in single-sided untreated acoustic neurinoma. Acta Otolaryngol. 2009; 129(6):694–696

[46] Grayeli AB, Kalamarides M, Bouccara D, Ambert-Dahan E, Sterkers O. Auditory brainstem implant in neurofibromatosis type 2 and non-neurofibromatosis type 2 patients. Otol Neurotol. 2008; 29(8):1140–1146

62 Nonoperative Facial Rehabilitation in Vestibular Schwannoma: Facial Neuromuscular Retraining

Jacqueline Diels

62.1 Introduction

Patients consistently report facial paralysis as one of the most debilitating complications after vestibular schwannoma resection.[1,2] Far from being a simple cosmetic issue, facial paralysis can result in significant functional and psychological consequences, substantially decreasing quality of life. Facial muscles play a unique role in the human body. Simply stated, their purpose is to move the facial skin in various directions, producing a wide variety of movement patterns used primarily for nonverbal communication, eye closure, and oral motor functions. The subtleties of human expression require a delicate balance of activity among multiple facial muscles. Acutely, injury to the facial nerve causes a readily recognizable flaccid paralysis. In delayed recovery, this may be followed by aberrant neural reinnervation causing inappropriate movement. Termed "synkinesis," this condition is less common and can go unrecognized by patients as well as medical professionals. What can deceptively appear to be weakness in the synkinetic face may in fact be abnormal cocontraction of opposing musculature limiting normal movement patterns.

For the patient with incomplete recovery, facial neuromuscular retraining (fNMR) offers a nonsurgical approach to rehabilitation for restoring and refining functional facial expression.

The objectives of this chapter are to (1) provide an overview of fNMR, highlighting the differences between fNMR and traditional therapy methods; (2) explain specific therapeutic approaches for treating flaccidity, paresis, and synkinesis with timelines for referral; (3) discuss the adjunct of Botulinum toxin (Botox) to fNMR to optimize outcomes in synkinesis.

62.2 Facial Neuromuscular Retraining

Facial neuromuscular retraining is a specific subset of occupational and physical therapy created for improving functional outcomes in patients with facial paralysis, paresis, and/or synkinesis after facial nerve injury. This comprehensive clinical program was first described by Balliet and colleagues in 1982, who reported improved function in patients more than 2 years after facial nerve injury.[3] Acquisition of new motor behaviors was attributed to brain plasticity, the capacity of the central nervous system to modify its organization, resulting in lasting functional change.[3]

Current programs are based largely on the works of Balliet et al,[3,4] Diels,[5] Beurskens,[6] Ross et al,[7] and Coulson,[8] the most salient features being detailed patient education, individualized program development using a wide variety of motor learning techniques, and active patient participation.

To address the complexities of facial movement, the fNMR process identifies neuromuscular firing and sequencing abnormalities and treats them by focusing on improving coordination between muscles as opposed to simply increasing their strength. The ability to create a myriad of expressions requires subtlety, accuracy, and precise control of the 20 plus pairs of facial muscles. fNMR employs modalities such as surface electromyography and proprioceptive, sensory, and mirror feedback to teach subtle, precise, coordinated movement patterns to achieve that aim. Techniques are based on characteristics unique to the facial neuromuscular system: lack of muscle spindles,[9] resistance to fatigue and atrophy,[10] small motor units,[11] and the presence of emotional as well as volitional, neural inputs.[12] These attributes distinguish facial muscles from other skeletal muscles and are the basis for the distinct techniques that make fNMR effective.

Facial paralysis is rare in the practice of rehabilitation medicine, one of few peripheral nerve (lower motor neuron) injuries requiring intervention. There is little training in its effective management. In contrast to the precise, functional patterns that exemplify fNMR, general therapy techniques may include generic exercises and/or electrical stimulation, both of which may be contraindicated in treating this population.[13]

Acutely after vestibular schwannoma resection, the absence of muscle contraction is due to lack of neural signal. Like flipping a switch to light the bulb on a lamp that is unplugged, no amount of exercise will trigger the facial muscles to contract without a functional electrical circuit.

Electrical stimulation continues to be widely used despite evidence suggesting it may interfere with neural regeneration after peripheral nerve injury.[14,15] Clinical experience suggests that patients who receive it acutely may have more synkinesis and mass action than those who do not. Because its application coincides with the spontaneous recovery period, improvements can erroneously be attributed to the stimulation rather than the natural course of recovery. In the synkinetic face, electrical stimulation and maximum effort exercises can reinforce abnormal movements.

Typical duration of fNMR is 18 months to 3 years. Treatment schedules vary widely depending on multiple factors. Local patients may be scheduled once a month, while those traveling a distance might return every 6 months. Home practice hours between clinic visits far exceed billed-therapy hours resulting in a cost-effective program that greatly amplifies the effect of treatment. This process empowers patients to assume control of their own recovery.

62.3 Patient Selection and Evaluation

Criteria for patient selection include neural supply or reanimation, motivation, and adequate cognition. Elements of patient evaluation include:

- Medical history.
- Detailed motion analysis during clinical observation.
- House–Brackmann facial grading scale.
- Sunnybrook facial grading system.

- Synkinesis Assessment Questionnaire (SAQ).
- Facial Clinimetric Evaluation (FaCE) scale.
- Standardized video and photographic evaluations.

Evaluation results, prognosis, and course of treatment are discussed with the patient and used to develop goals and a comprehensive treatment plan.

62.4 Functional Progression and Timeline for Referral to Facial Neuromuscular Retraining

Recovery progresses acutely from flaccid paralysis to paresis, with return of tone and minimal movement indicating reinnervation. If recovery is delayed with persistent flaccidity beyond 5 to 6 months postoperatively, synkinesis will most likely follow. This timeline is highly variable and dependent on many factors as discussed in Chapter 55. Patients should be referred for fNMR when visible signs of functional return are evident (e.g., increasing facial tone, minimal motion) or as soon as synkinesis is noted.

62.5 Patient Education

Patient education is an essential component of the fNMR program. It provides the foundation for learning the selective movement patterns that will improve motor control. It is the key to comprehending the difference between a deficiency of muscle activity resulting in no movement (flaccidity) and aberrant muscle activity resulting in inappropriate movement (synkinesis). Training includes basic facial anatomy and kinematics pertinent to each individual. No two faces are the same; so every treatment program is unique. There are no generic lists of exercises. The value of patient education, though time consuming, cannot be overstated to facilitate mindful analysis of what is typically automatic expression. ▶ Fig. 62.1 acquaints patients with the facial muscles and corresponding angles of pull to gain insight into which muscles flex to produce specific movements and which muscles contracting abnormally are implicated in synkinesis. Armed with this new knowledge, a simple instruction such as "smile with the cheeks (zygomaticus) instead of the mouth" can immediately improve expressive movement.

62.6 Facial Neuromuscular Retraining for Flaccid Paralysis

Given an intact facial nerve, most cases of flaccid paralysis will resolve over time, to some degree. fNMR is not indicated for the patient with neurotmesis without surgical repair. For the patient with axonotmesis, fNMR is deferred until signs of reinnervation are present. Early fNMR does not appear to accelerate recovery of flaccid paralysis; however, a one-time consult can be beneficial to (1) establish care, (2) help the patient cope with life-altering postoperative changes, (3) review eye care, (4) instruct in gentle stroking to maintain sensory cortex representation.[16] If flaccidity persists at 9 months, an evaluation is warranted to assess functional status. Beyond 12 months, retraining is unlikely to be effective in a completely flaccid face.

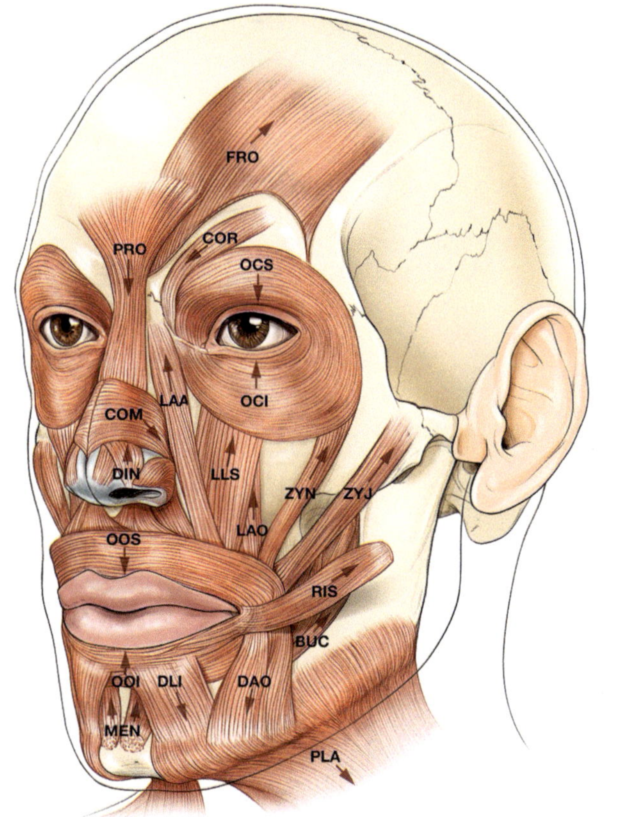

Fig. 62.1 Facial neuromuscular retraining teaching diagram representing the muscles of facial expression and corresponding angles of pull as indicated by *arrows*. (Adapted with permission from Diels and Beurskens.[13])

62.7 Facial Neuromuscular Retraining for Paresis

Commonly, paretic patients exaggerate movements attempting to strengthen muscles. In contrast, fNMR teaches small symmetrical patterns to mimic functional expressions, reducing abnormal cocontraction. Performed slowly, this strategy trains accuracy and proper technique for controlling synkinesis should it occur.

62.8 Facial Neuromuscular Retraining for Synkinesis

Synkinesis is the most common condition treated by the fNMR therapist. Since it does not occur in other areas of the body, there is no precedent for identifying, understanding, or treating it. The evaluation and interpretation of movement patterns in the synkinetic face can be challenging due to simultaneous activation of opposing musculature which limits excursion of the facial skin, sometimes to the extent that little dynamic motion is observed. Synkinesis varies in location and severity, from mild to severe (mass action), which can result in gross

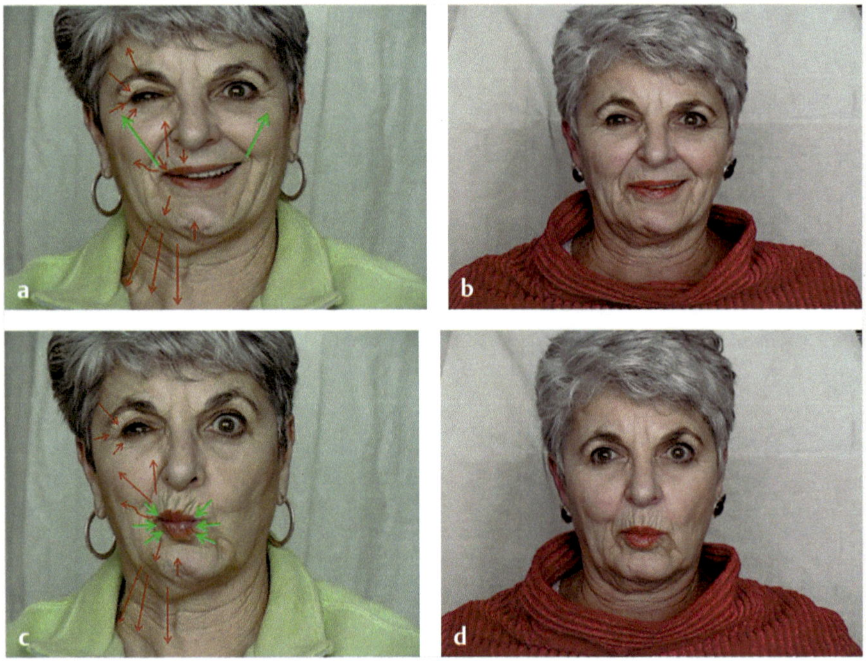

Fig. 62.2 Photographic evaluation of a 69-year-old female 2 years post–right facial paralysis with synkinesis. Initial facial neuromuscular retraining (fNMR) evaluation, January 2008. Smile (**a**), pucker (**c**). Primary movement indicated by *green arrows*; synkinetic movements indicated by *red arrows*. Reevaluation after 12 months of fNMR, January 2009. Smile (**b**), pucker (**d**). Note decreased synkinesis with improved range of motion and symmetry. (Adapted with permission from Diels and Beurskens.[13])

deformity during facial movements. Appropriate intervention focuses on coordinating viable, albeit synkinetic, muscles rather than stimulating flaccid ones. The practitioner must be intimately familiar with the functional anatomy (i.e., know how to activate muscles separately and in combination with others) to decipher the synkinetic patterns observed in patients.

Treatment begins by (1) establishing the viability of the primary mover for a particular expression, (2) identifying erroneous movements, and (3) instructing the patient in specific techniques that inhibit (dissociate) synkinetic activity while simultaneously activating the primary mover. This practice of selective inhibition is counterintuitive and challenging in both concept and practice. Essentially, the patient learns what *not* to move. As control improves, range of motion gradually extends, increasing excursion and improving expression[3] (▶ Fig. 62.2). Although synkinesis is never entirely eliminated, with skilled training and consistent home practice over time, it is possible to improve movement patterns and expression even many years after synkinesis develops.[3,4,5,17,18] Specialized techniques have been developed for patients who have undergone surgical reanimation procedures.[13,19] These are beyond the scope of this chapter.

Contracture and spasm often accompany synkinesis and further decrease mobility, range of motion, and expressiveness. At rest, a deepened nasolabial fold, decreased palpebral fissure, retracted angle of the mouth, or banding of the platysma indicate increased tone. The affected midface may appear thick, immobile, and contracted. Trigger points may be present. Patients frequently complain of tightness, spasms, and persistent discomfort throughout the affected side. Soft-tissue mobilization, heat, and massage techniques specific to facial musculature effectively decrease contracture and improve suppleness, mobility, and comfort.[8,13,18]

62.9 Facial Neuromuscular Retraining and Botox

When used in conjunction with fNMR, Botox injected into targeted synkinetic muscles provides a "window of opportunity" during which the patient can practice coordinated movement patterns with decreased synkinetic constraint. Within the multidisciplinary team, the fNMR therapist precisely identifies the synkinetic muscles which, when injected, should allow greater freedom of movement without additional morbidity. The most common injection sites include the orbicularis oculi, corrugator, platysma, and mentalis.[20] The midfacial muscles are rarely injected to avoid creating weakness in areas targeted during the fNMR process, such as smile (zygomaticus). Recently, minimal dose injections to the synkinetic buccinator have proven to be beneficial.[20] fNMR follow-up 1 to 2 weeks after Botox administration incorporates injection effects into new practice patterns to capitalize on increased range of motion and to refine the home program. As with any new motor learning, accurate repetition of new patterns results in new skill acquisition.

62.10 Conclusion

For the patient with postoperative facial paralysis, fNMR provides continuity of care through delivery of a cost-effective, individualized, patient-centered rehabilitation program founded on the unique properties of the facial neuromuscular system. It is a small but important discipline, still in its infancy that shows great promise for improving patient satisfaction and quality of life after vestibular schwannoma surgery. To date, few randomized clinical trials have proven its effectiveness.[21] Procedures require standardization, therapists require training, and additional randomized clinical trials are needed to mature this growing and much needed field.

References

[1] Acoustic Neuroma Association. 2014 Report on ANA Patient Database. Patient Survey Report Idleman & Associates; Acoustic Neuroma Association, 600 Peachtree Parkway, Suite 108, Cumming, GA 30041

[2] Leong SC, Lesser TH. A national survey of facial paralysis on the quality of life of patients with acoustic neuroma. Otol Neurotol. 2015; 36(3):503–509

[3] Balliet R, Shinn JB, Bach-y-Rita P. Facial paralysis rehabilitation: retraining selective muscle control. Int Rehabil Med. 1982; 4(2):67–74

[4] Balliet R. Motor control strategies in the retraining of facial paralysis. In: Portmann M, ed. Facial Nerve. New York, NY: Masson Publishing; 1985:465–469

[5] Diels HJ. New concepts in nonsurgical facial nerve rehabilitation. In: Myers E, Bluestone C, eds. Advances in Otolaryngology-Head and Neck Surgery. Chicago, IL: Mosby-Year Book; 1995:289–315

[6] Beurskens CHG. Mime Therapy: Rehabilitation of Facial Expression. Thesis. Nijmegen: KUN; 2003

[7] Ross B, Nedzelski JM, McLean JA. Efficacy of feedback training in long-standing facial nerve paresis. Laryngoscope. 1991; 101(7, Pt 1):744–750

[8] Coulson SE. Physiotherapy rehabilitation following facial nerve paresis. In: Beurskens CHG, Van Gelder RS, Heymans PG, Manni JJ, Nicolai JPA, eds. The Facial Palsies. Utrecht, The Netherlands: Lemma; 2005:263–274

[9] Basmajian JV, DeLuca CJ. Muscles Alive: Their Functions Revealed by Electromyography. Baltimore, MD: Williams & Wilkins; 1985

[10] May M. Microanatomy and pathophysiology of the facial nerve. In: May M, Shaitkin BM, eds. The Facial Nerve. New York, NY: Thieme; 2000:57–65

[11] Belal A. Structure of human muscle in facial paralysis: role of muscle biopsy. In: May M, ed. The Facial Nerve. New York, NY: Thieme; 1986:99–106

[12] Rinn WE. The neuropsychology of facial expression: a review of the neurological and psychological mechanisms for producing facial expressions. Psychol Bull. 1984; 95(1):52–77

[13] Diels HJ, Beurskens C. Neuromuscular retraining: non-surgical therapy for facial palsy. In: Slattery W, Azizzadeh B, eds. The Facial Nerve. New York, NY: Thieme; 2014:205–212

[14] Cohan CS, Kater SB. Suppression of neurite elongation and growth cone motility by electrical activity. Science. 1986; 232(4758):1638–1640

[15] Brown MC, Holland RL. A central role for denervated tissues in causing nerve sprouting. Nature. 1979; 282(5740):724–726

[16] Angelov DN, Ceynowa M, Guntinas-Lichius O, et al. Mechanical stimulation of paralyzed vibrissal muscles following facial nerve injury in adult rat promotes full recovery of whisking. Neurobiol Dis. 2007; 26(1):229–242

[17] Diels HJ. Facial paralysis: is there a role for a therapist? Facial Plast Surg. 2000; 16(4):361–364

[18] Lindsay RW, Robinson M, Hadlock TA. Comprehensive facial rehabilitation improves function in people with facial paralysis: a 5-year experience at the Massachusetts Eye and Ear Infirmary. Phys Ther. 2010; 90(3):391–397

[19] Hadlock TA, Greenfield LJ, Wernick-Robinson M, Cheney ML. Multimodality approach to management of the paralyzed face. Laryngoscope. 2006; 116(8): 1385–1389

[20] Wei LA, Diels J, Lucarelli MJ. Treating buccinator with botulinum toxin in patients with facial synkinesis: a previously overlooked target. Ophthal Plast Reconstr Surg. 2015

[21] Pereira LM, Obara K, Dias JM, Menacho MO, Lavado EL, Cardoso JR. Facial exercise therapy for facial palsy: systematic review and meta-analysis. Clin Rehabil. 2011; 25(7):649–658

63 Medical and Surgical Care of the Eye in Facial Paralysis

Scott Owen and Doug Henstrom

63.1 Introduction

Perhaps the most immediate and debilitating complication resulting from facial paralysis is the loss of complete eye closure. Impaired lid function may result in pain and irritation of the eye, and in severe untreated cases, corneal disease, exposure keratitis, and potentially vision loss.[1] Synkinesis and gustatory lacrimation add to the potential long-term morbidity of aberrant facial nerve regeneration.

Management of the eye is challenging. Prognosis varies widely depending on etiology, patient demographic, and other medical comorbidities. No reliable method of prognosticating recovery exists[2] and many protective interventions interfere with the potential for spontaneous recovery.

63.2 Presentation and Etiology

Lid dysfunction in the setting of facial nerve paralysis results from loss of orbicularis oculi function, which normally opposes the levator palpebrae superioris muscle. The balance of these two opposing muscles allows the eye to remain open for light collection, while maintaining the protective and restorative function of the blink reflex and eye closure.

Blinking is primarily an upper lid function, with only 1 to 2 mm of the palpebral aperture traversed by the lower lid. Resting tone keeps the lid against the globe and in good position to oppose the superior lid, and to assist in the natural lateral-to-medial tear flow. Closure of the superior lid sweeps debris from the cornea into the inferior lid trough, and lacrimal fluids along with protective balanced salts and antibodies are collected along the sill of the lower lid to be spread across the cornea in a thin film. Lacrimation is stimulated by parasympathetic impulses through the greater superficial petrosal branch of the facial nerve.

Levine and Shapiro summarize three primary responsibilities of the functioning lid[3]:

- Function 1: Define the limits of the palpebral aperture, limiting surface area of the globe exposed to evaporation.
- Function 2: Close the palpebral aperture voluntarily to protect the cornea against potential injury and keep the cornea covered during sleep.
- Function 3: Distribute tear film across the eye, and clear debris.

Facial nerve paralysis impairs all three functions of the eyelid, and restoration of these should be the focus of any intervention (▶ Fig. 63.1).

63.3 Decision Making

Many reanimation interventions may wait for a patient's final degree of recovery, but protection of the cornea cannot. Immediate intervention is warranted to prevent permanent corneal damage, particularly in the setting of concomitant trigeminal neuropathy which may occur with large vestibular schwannoma.

63.4 Nonsurgical Treatment Options

Noninvasive eye care should be initiated as soon as paralysis is detected. Maintaining ocular lubrication with methylcellulose drops multiple times daily is a mainstay of treatment. Nighttime use of petroleum or mineral oil-based ointment will provide a longer-lasting lubricant, but may obscure vision during daytime function.

Many of the initial issues may be addressed temporarily by using medical tape on the lid while sleeping. Tape can be

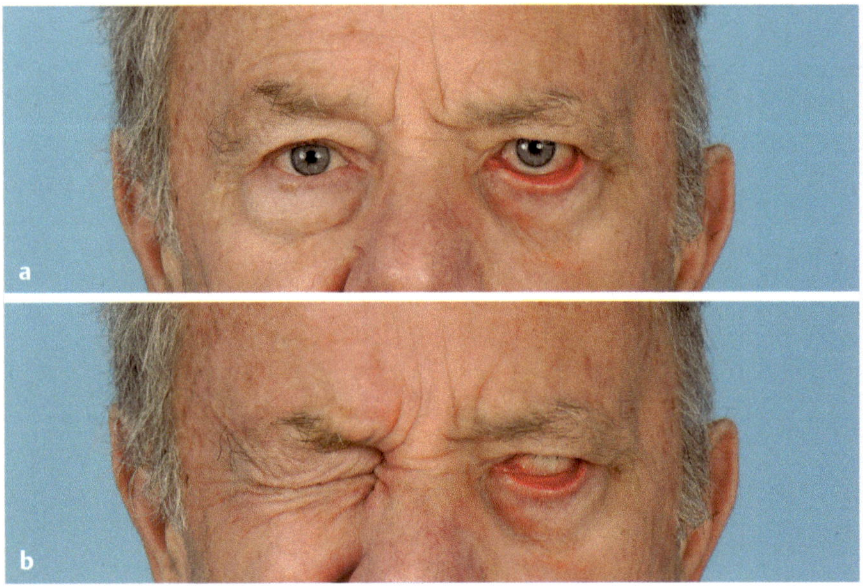

Fig. 63.1 Patient with recent facial paralysis demonstrating lagophthalmos, ectropion, and corneal exposure. **(a)** Face at rest. **(b)** Attempted tight eye closure. Possible negative consequences of the exposed/paralyzed eye include corneal abrasion and exposure keratitis and may ultimately lead to permanent blindness.

applied to the lower lid/lateral canthus to improve ectropion, or along the superior lid lash line to assist with mild lagophthalmos during the day. A moisture chamber fashioned from petroleum jelly to the orbital rim and cellophane is useful in patients who fail lid taping due to tape sensitivity or technique.

Scleral contact lenses have been described as a good long-term solution for corneal protection in paralytic lagophthalmos.[4] Consideration warrants an ophthalmologic evaluation, and involves a large transparent scleral shield applied to the eye with a reservoir of saline that ensures corneal protection and prevents desiccation. Shields are usually well tolerated by patients, and provide better visual acuity over ocular lubricants, though application takes practice.[5]

63.5 Surgical Treatment Options

Failure of nonsurgical treatment options, or an expectation of long-term paralysis, warrants consideration for surgical intervention. Improvement in patient-reported quality-of-life FaCE survey scores has been well demonstrated after proper surgical management of the eye by Henstrom et al.[6]

Levine[7] listed criteria for surgery as follows:

- Symptomatic patients with signs of conjunctival or corneal injury despite maximal medical therapy.
- Patients who require rapid ocular rehabilitation to resume their livelihood.
- Patients with a stable ocular status, but at high risk for corneal complications (concomitant cranial nerves V and VII palsy, poor Bell's phenomenon).

Exposure of the patient to surgical risk, or interference with spontaneous nerve recovery, warrants careful consideration before any operative intervention.

63.5.1 Upper Lid Alloplasts

Recreation of an oppositional force to the levator muscle remains a mainstay in paralytic lagophthalmos. Generally, lid alloplasts are reversible, and should not interfere with the spontaneous recovery of lid function. All bear the possible complication of infection and extrusion, and may cause varying degrees of pseudoptosis at rest. Lid alloplasts are easily implanted under local anesthesia allowing for intraoperative adjustments (if needed) depending on each individual's loading need.

63.5.2 Lid Loading

Loading of the upper lid involves placement of a dense material, such as gold or platinum weights, that uses gravity to oppose the levator muscle and improve eye closure. They work best during waking hours when a patient is upright, maximizing the effect of gravity on the implant. At night, patients may still need to manually pull the upper lid closed, sleep with their head elevated, or continue with eye taping to prevent corneal exposure when lying supine.

Weight/size is determined preoperatively by securing non-sterile sizers to the patient's upper lid skin with adhesive. A weight is chosen that allows for maximal lid closure that still allows the patient minimal pseudoptosis at rest.

Gold weights have long been the standard of treatment of paralytic lagophthalmos. Gold has several advantages as an alloplast, including a high specific gravity, minimal tissue reactivity in its pure form (99.99% for 24k), and a color similar to fat. It is a nonferrous metal and is MRI compatible. Gold is malleable, and can be either purchased or custom made for an individual. Implantation technique is straightforward and usually does not require additional manipulation. They can be removed or exchanged in the setting of spontaneous recovery or patient preference.[3]

Rates of adequate eye closure with gold are cited between 22 and 91%,[8,9] with closure sufficient to cover the cornea in 78% of cases,[8] and improvement in visual acuity and complete resolution of exposure keratitis in 62 to 100% of cases.[8] The most commonly reported complication is extrusion of the implant, resulting from infection, tight skin closure, injury, or allergic reaction to Neosporin.[3] Weights are also reported to occasionally shift position, the incidence of which is decreased significantly by suturing the weight to the tarsal plate.[8]

Platinum has emerged as a viable alternative to gold. The authors advocate the use of platinum for the increased density (platinum 21.5 g/cm^3 vs. gold 19.4 g/cm^3) allowing for a similar weight with less foreign material. Platinum has also been observed histologically to cause less tissue inflammation than gold.[10] The platinum chain is also available, which has been reported to conform more closely to the patient's globe.[10] An additional alternative to solid implantable weights include external taping of weights[11] or the injection of hyaluronic acid to the upper eyelid[12] (▶ Fig. 63.2).

63.5.3 Palpebral Spring

The palpebral spring is an alternative to upper lid weighting that provides opposition to the levator muscle in facial paralysis. A custom-shaped 0.011-in stainless steel dental wire is anchored to the orbital rim, while the other limb is secured to the tarsal plate. A tension loop is tucked laterally, providing a constant oppositional force inferiorly.

Advocates of the spring cite multiple advantages over lid weights. The spring's force is independent of gravity, allowing patients freedom from lid taping while supine. While theoretical blink speed with a weight is limited to terminal velocity, the spring is limited only by the strength of the levator muscle, and may be increased to more closely match physiologic speed. The levator may even be tightened to allow for implantation of a stronger spring.[7]

Rates of complete eye closure are reported between 79 and 95%,[13,14] with wires removed for device malfunction, tension adjustment, or extrusion. Improved results have been attributed to the use of a 0.011-in stainless steel wire, placement of the palpebral limb in a protective sleeve, or securing the palpebral limb to the tarsus with a suture.[13,14] Implantation of a spring is more complicated than the relatively straightforward placement of a weight, and extrusion, symptomatic pseudoptosis, and spring failure are commonly cited complications among weight advocates.

63.5.4 Lower Lid

The lower lid falls away from the globe as it loses support from the orbicularis oculi, interfering with its reservoir function for

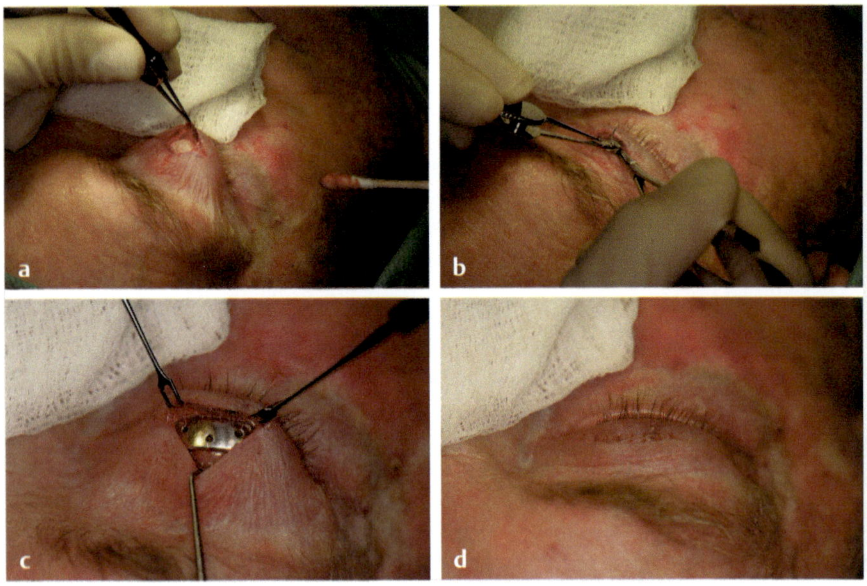

Fig. 63.2 Placement of a platinum eyelid weight: (**a**) Exposure of the tarsal plate. (**b**) Suture fixation of weight. (**c**) Weight in place with 3-point suture fixation. (**d**) Eyelid closed with weight in place.

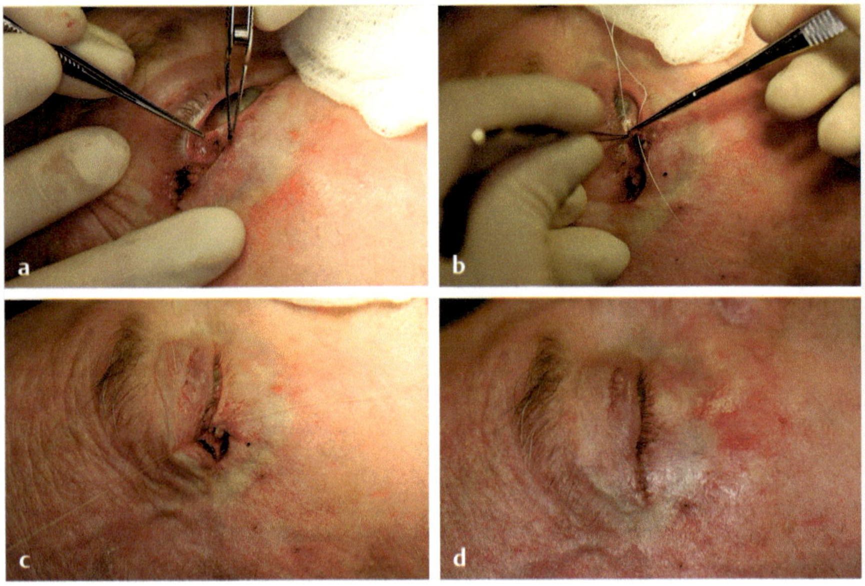

Fig. 63.3 Lateral tarsal strip procedure: (**a**) Separation of lower tarsal plate from anterior muscle, skin, and canthal attachment. (**b**) Double-armed Mersilene suture used to refixate canthal attachment after appropriate shortening of tarsal plate. (**c**) Reattachment to superior/ medial orbital rim, lifting lid appropriately. (**d**) Incision closed.

tear film. This prevents lid opposition, and the proper windshield-wiper function resulting in ectropion, epiphora, and corneal exposure. In many patients, the lateral tarsal strip procedure is adequate, involving division of the inferior limb of the lateral canthus, repositioning the lateral tarsus and tightening of the lower lid (▶ Fig. 63.3).

In patients with excess laxity, absorbing this laterally may shift the punctum. This can be addressed by simultaneous mobilization of the medial canthus to maintain adequate lacrimal drainage.

Lower lid adjustment may be performed under local anesthesia, and in repositioning the affected eyelid, lower limbus position in the unaffected eye should be used as a guide. The correctly positioned lower lid should sit tangential to the iris in neutral gaze.

A suspension technique or other grafting may be required with a lid that sags anteriorly off of the globe. Fascia lata, conchal cartilage, and hard palate mucosal/spacer grafts have all been described.[7]

63.5.5 Brow

Periorbital tissue may obstruct visual fields in the setting of decreased frontalis tone. Older patients with tissue laxity may have functionally or cosmetically problematic brow ptosis. Generally, approaches for correcting a paralytic brow are similar to other brow-lift approaches. Coronal, trichophytic, and endoscopic brow lifting techniques remain valid, well-supported methods.

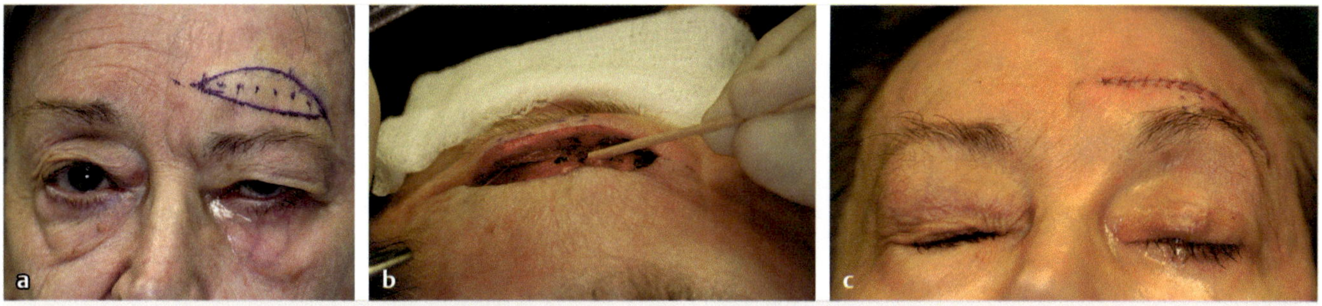

Fig. 63.4 The midforehead brow lift technique: (**a**) Midforehead skin marked for excision. (**b**) Suspension of superior aspect of orbicularis oculi muscle. (**c**) Postoperative brow lift allowing for adequate eye closure.

Direct and midforehead approaches to the brow are useful in older patients with less concern for cosmesis and the presence of deeper forehead wrinkles. The appeal of a shorter recovery, immediate results, and a procedure that can be easily performed under local anesthesia is advantageous in patients with poor health who may not tolerate general anesthesia (▶ Fig. 63.4).

An approach to the distinction between a cosmetic brow lift and a patient with facial paralysis is lid function. In the setting of lid weakness, a ptotic brow may be an important component of lid closure. An extensive physical exam with simulated brow placement should be performed preoperatively to prevent granting a patient visual field expansion at the expense of corneal protection.

63.5.6 Long-Term Management of Sequelae

Facial nerve recovery is unpredictable, and patients benefit from strategies to manage long-term sequelae from aberrant nerve regeneration, surgically altered anatomy, or incomplete recovery. Effective management requires a multimodality approach, composed of physical therapy, chemodenervation, and surgical intervention, when indicated.[2]

Involvement of a physical therapist specializing in facial paralysis is essential. Improvement in facial symmetry, synkinesis, and control can be provided through prescribed exercises geared toward retraining of facial musculature, and grants the patient an active role in his or her recovery (also see Chapter 62). A study from Hadlock et al prescribed physical therapy to patients with chronic facial paralysis.[2] Of the 111 patients studied, 66% followed through with therapy. Of these, 82.4% reported subjective improvement in facial function, and 97.3% improved subjectively on provider's facial grading scale.[2]

Paradoxically, aberrant regeneration of axonal fibers after facial palsy may lead to several unwanted effects such as hypertonicity and synkinesis between orbicularis oculi and oris muscles, commonly manifesting as narrowing of the palpebral fissure during talking, smiling, or chewing.[15] Collateral axonal sprouting reestablishes accidental connections between 3 and 5 months after injury[16,17] with resulting morbidity. Before the introduction of chemodenervation agents, no effective therapy for these symptoms existed.

Botulinum toxin type A (BTX A) is the most widely used chemodenervation agent. Synthesized from naturally occurring botulinum toxin, it irreversibly binds and blocks the presynaptic release of acetylcholine and causes a functional denervation of neuromuscular endplates, which must be replaced by the cell to reactivate the synapse. In facial musculature, onset of therapeutic weakness averages 4 to 7 days and lasts approximately 3 months.[18]

Targeting specific areas of the orbicularis oculi by visualizing and palpating contraction bands during a voluntary smile will allow precise delivery of chemodenervation agents to the most symptomatic muscle fibers, and careful dose titration up to the desired result prevents worsening of any paralytic lagophthalmos.

Gustatory lacrimation, or "crocodile tears," is caused by reinnervation of the lacrimal gland by aberrant efferent fibers from the superior salivary nucleus. The responsible lacrimal gland responds well to 5 units (U) of BTX A injected directly into the gland, and can be performed transconjunctivally or transcutaneously into the palpebral lobe.[11]

Patients who will no longer tolerate botulinum toxin injections may be considered for a highly selective neurectomy, which is beyond the scope of this chapter and only used in unique circumstances.[19]

63.5.7 Future Directions

The last 50 years has seen several large advances in the study and treatment of facial paralysis. The evolution of static slings and microsurgical techniques with dynamic muscle transfer has transformed the way we manage chronic facial paralysis, and the discovery of chemodenervation agents has yielded tools to fine-tune paralytic sequelae.[20] Future possibilities for improving management of the eye following paralysis include the use of artificial muscle to create an eyelid blink[21] as well as blink-detecting glasses for facial pacing[22] (▶ Fig. 63.5).

Advancements in basic science research continue to aim toward improvement of nerve regeneration and bridging large graft gaps, thus improving axon repair in oncologically sacrificed nerves and cross-face grafts.[9]

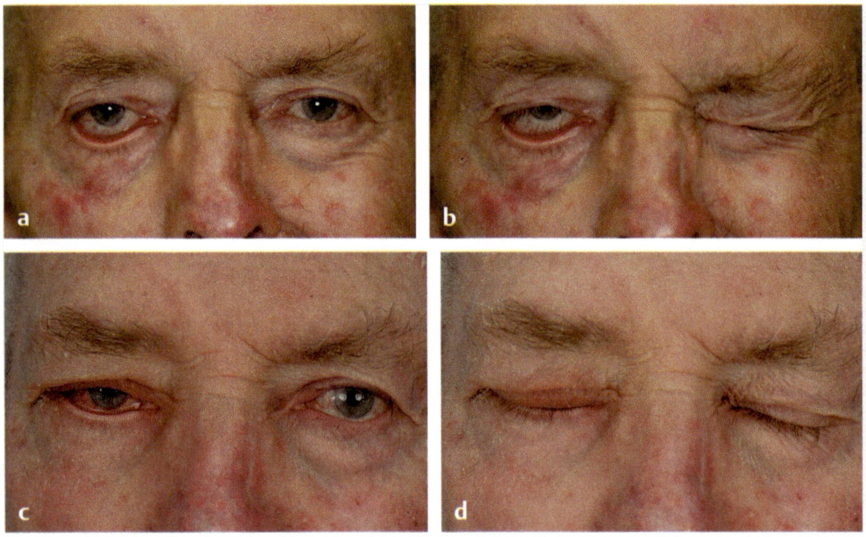

Fig. 63.5 Patient with paralytic lagophthalmos and ectropion. (**a**) Preoperative eye open. (**b**) Preoperative tight eye closure. (**c**) 10 days postoperative eye open. (**d**) 10 days postoperative tight eye closure.

References

[1] Clarke JC, Owen SR, Henstrom DK. Surgical rehabilitation of the paralyzed face. Otolaryngol Head Neck Surg 2014:155–175

[2] Hadlock TA, Greenfield LJ, Wernick-Robinson M, Cheney ML. Multimodality approach to management of the paralyzed face. Laryngoscope. 2006; 116(8): 1385–1389

[3] Levine RE, Shapiro JP. Reanimation of the paralyzed eyelid with the enhanced palpebral spring or the gold weight: modern replacements for tarsorrhaphy. Facial Plast Surg. 2000; 16(4):325–336

[4] Weyns M, Koppen C, Tassignon MJ. Scleral contact lenses as an alternative to tarsorrhaphy for the long-term management of combined exposure and neurotrophic keratopathy. Cornea. 2013; 32(3):359–361

[5] Gire A, Kwok A, Marx DP. PROSE treatment for lagophthalmos and exposure keratopathy. Ophthal Plast Reconstr Surg. 2013; 29(2):e38–e40

[6] Henstrom DK, Lindsay RW, Cheney ML, Hadlock TA. Surgical treatment of the periocular complex and improvement of quality of life in patients with facial paralysis. Arch Facial Plast Surg. 2011; 13(2):125–128

[7] Levine RE. Care of the eye in facial paralysis. In: Brackmann DE, Shelton C, Arriaga MA, eds. Otologic Surgery, Philadelphia, PA: WB Saunders; 1994:717–740

[8] May M, MM. Gold weight and wire spring implants as alternatives to tarsorrhaphy. Arch Otolaryngol Head Neck Surg. 1987; 113(6):656–660

[9] Hadlock T. Facial paralysis: research and future directions. Facial Plast Surg. 2008; 24(2):260–267

[10] Berghaus A, Neumann K, Schrom T. The platinum chain: a new upper-lid implant for facial palsy. Arch Facial Plast Surg. 2003; 5(2):166–170

[11] Sohrab M, Abugo U, Grant M, Merbs S. Management of the eye in facial paralysis. Facial Plast Surg. 2015; 31(2):140–144

[12] Martín-Oviedo C, García I, Lowy A, Scola E, Aristegui M, Scola B. Hyaluronic acid gel weight: a nonsurgical option for the management of paralytic lagophthalmos. Laryngoscope. 2013; 123(12):E91–E96

[13] May M. Gold weight and wire spring implants as alternatives to tarsorrhaphy. Arch Otolaryngol Head Neck Surg. 1987; 113(6):656–660

[14] Demirci H, Frueh BR. Palpebral spring in the management of lagophthalmos and exposure keratopathy secondary to facial nerve palsy. Ophthal Plast Reconstr Surg. 2009; 25(4):270–275

[15] Stennert E. Das Autoparalytische Syndrom–ein Leitsymptom der postparetischen Fazialisfunktion. Arch Otorhinolaryngol. 1982; 236(1):97–114

[16] Jankovic J, Brin MF. Therapeutic uses of botulinum toxin. N Engl J Med. 1991; 324(17):1186–1194

[17] Comella JX, Molgo J, Faille L. Sprouting of mammalian motor nerve terminals induced by in vivo injection of botulinum type-D toxin and the functional recovery of paralysed neuromuscular junctions. Neurosci Lett. 1993; 153(1): 61–64

[18] Bikhazi NB, Maas CS. Refinement in the rehabilitation of the paralyzed face using botulinum toxin. Otolaryngol Head Neck Surg. 1997; 117(4):303–307

[19] Hohman MH, Lee LN, Hadlock TA. Two-step highly selective neurectomy for refractory periocular synkinesis. Laryngoscope. 2013; 123(6):1385–1388

[20] Tate JR, Jr, Tollefson TT. Advances in facial reanimation. Curr Opin Otolaryngol Head Neck Surg. 2006; 14(4):242–248

[21] Tollefson TT, Senders CW. Restoration of eyelid closure in facial paralysis using artificial muscle: preliminary cadaveric analysis. Laryngoscope. 2007; 117(11):1907–1911

[22] Frigerio A, Hadlock TA, Murray EH, Heaton JT. Infrared-based blink-detecting glasses for facial pacing: toward a bionic blink. JAMA Facial Plast Surg. 2014; 16(3):211–218

64 Interposition Cable Nerve Graft of the Facial Nerve After Resection of Vestibular Schwannoma

Sampath Chandra Prasad, Alessandra Russo, Abdelkader Taibah, Enrico Pasanisi, Francesco Galletti, and Mario Sanna

64.1 Introduction

The facial nerve (FN) is one of the most important structures in the skull base and its tortuous transtemporal course poses a formidable challenge to a lateral skull base surgeon. Saving or salvaging the FN is often as important as tumor clearance itself, if not more, because of the social, emotional, and psychological consequences of a damaged nerve, especially in young patients. The FN is intimately involved with the vestibular schwannoma (VS) capsule and in most cases is found adherent to the tumor. There is a small but significant number of patients in whom the goals of total tumor removal and FN preservation are not compatible. In some situations, the surgeon may decide in favor of total tumor removal, as the possibility and consequences of an aggressive growing residual tumor are more hazardous than a compromised FN. In other circumstances, the FN may be accidentally sectioned during tumor removal. Once the nerve is interrupted, reconstruction must be performed immediately to obtain the best results, either by means of a primary end-to-end anastomosis or by a cable nerve graft interposition.[1] The results of immediately establishing continuity of the FN have been found to be superior to alternatives such as facial–hypoglossal anastomosis, with a significant number achieving House–Brackmann (HB) grade III function in the long term, not to mention the obvious benefit of avoiding a subsequent additional procedure.[2,3] In 2009, we reported our experience with intracranial cable nerve grafting for VS in 33 cases and found that approximately 75% of patients achieve HB grade III function at 1 year (▸ Table 64.1).[4] We recently updated our series and found similar results in a larger cohort of patients with VS and other pathologies.[5] It is generally unacceptable that in the event of FN interruption during VS surgery, no intraoperative attempt is made to reestablish continuity of the FN.[2,6] In this chapter, we will discuss the techniques and results of FN grafting after VS excision.

64.2 Preoperative Protocols

Pre- and postoperative FN function should be recorded according to the HB grading system.[3] To precisely evaluate FN function, color photographs are taken of the face in a minimum of four positions (facial muscles at rest, tight closure of eyes, raised eyebrows, and smiling and pouting lips) during the preoperative workup and postoperatively, when FN paresis is apparent.[7] All cases are evaluated with thin slice magnetic resonance imaging with contrast enhancement.

64.3 Indications for Cable Nerve Graft Interposition of the Facial Nerve

- Grafting is considered when there is a definite and complete interruption of the FN during tumor removal and when a proximal stump of the FN is available at the brainstem that is long enough for the anastomosis.
- If there is no tension and retraction of the two nerve ends (proximal and distal) and the apposition can be self-maintained without the help of any instrument, an end-to-end anastomosis is indicated.
- If the proximal stump of the FN is unavailable, too short, or severely injured, FN reinnervation using a donor nerve, such as the hypoglossal or masseteric branch of V3, should be considered.
- When anatomical continuity of the nerve is confirmed but the nerve shows no response during electrical stimulation, it is advisable to leave the nerve undisturbed and consider reinnervation procedures at a later stage if satisfactory spontaneous recovery does not occur. In most cases, postoperative total paralysis of the anatomically intact nerve recovers considerably over 12 months.[8] The rate of recovery may provide the surgeon with important information regarding ultimate prognosis as discussed further in Chapter 66.

Table 64.1 Results of FN repair following vestibular schwannoma resection using cable graft interposition with microsuture and fibrin glue coaptation techniques

Group	Preoperative	Immediate postoperative	3 mo	6 mo	9 mo	1-y follow-up
Microsuture	7 (I)	8 (VI)	8 (VI	6 (V)	1 (III)	6 (III)
	1 (III)			2 (VI)	5 (IV)	1 (IV)
					1 (V)	1 (VI)
					1 (VI)	
Fibrin glue	24 (I)	25 (VI)	25 (VI)	3 (III)	11 (III)	19 (III)
	1 (VI)			4 (IV)	10 (IV)	5 (IV)
				9 (V)	2 (V)	1 (V)
				9 (VI)	2 (VI)	

Source: Adapted from Used with permission from Bacciu A, Falcioni M, Pasanisi E, et al. Intracranial facial nerve grafting after removal of vestibular schwannoma. Am J Otolaryngol 2009; 30:83-88.[8]

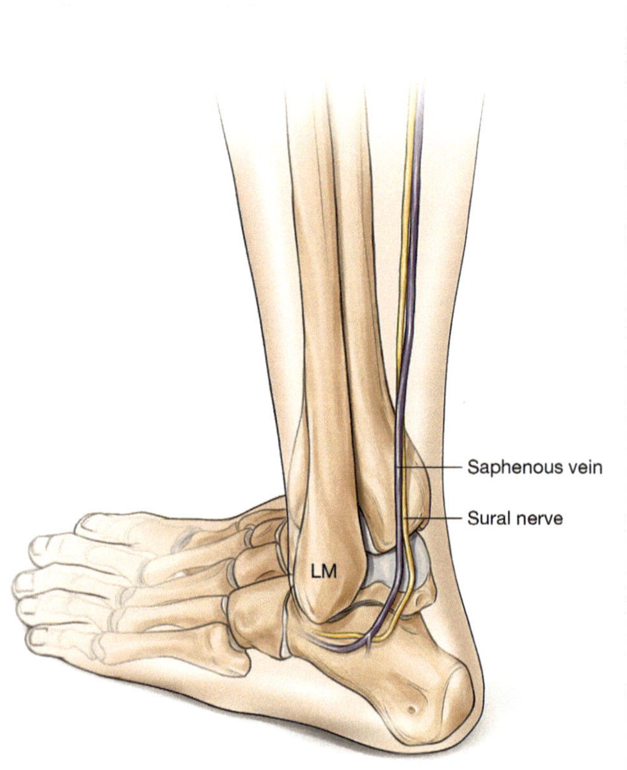

Fig. 64.1 Anatomy of the sural nerve. The relationship between the saphenous vein and the sural nerve is illustrated. LM, lateral malleolus.

64.4 Preferred Cable Nerve Grafts

The two nerves most commonly used for FN grafting are the great auricular nerve and the sural nerve (SN). Both nerves are suitable for use because of their comparable size to the FN and because their loss produces minimal sensory loss that is generally acceptable to patients. In our practice, we prefer the use of the SN (▶ Fig. 64.1) because a longer graft can be harvested if needed and because the harvest of the nerve can be done by an assistant while the surgeon continues working on the tumor. Over the years, the SN cable graft interposition has developed as a standard procedure for FN repair. In 1885, Albert Einige performed the first two cases of SN reconstruction for a 3-cm median and a 10-cm ulnar nerve defect, respectively.[9] Seventy years later, in 1955, John Conley performed the first case of great auricular nerve interposition of the FN after total parotidectomy.[10] Recent studies have shown that cable nerve graft interpositioning has the potential to provide as good a result as a primary end-to-end anastomosis.[2,11,12,13] However, the best possible postoperative outcome is HB grade III regardless of the graft material used or the technique employed, because frontal muscle function rarely recovers and a certain degree of synkinesis is unavoidable after grafting.[2,3,14,15]

64.5 Types of Cable Nerve Graft Interposition Anastomosis

The site of anastomosis is based on the proximal and distal sites where the nerve is involved. According to this, three groups can be described: (1) *intradural anastomosis*, wherein the proximal anastomosis is at the brainstem and the distal site is in the internal auditory canal (IAC; ▶ Fig. 64.2a); (2)

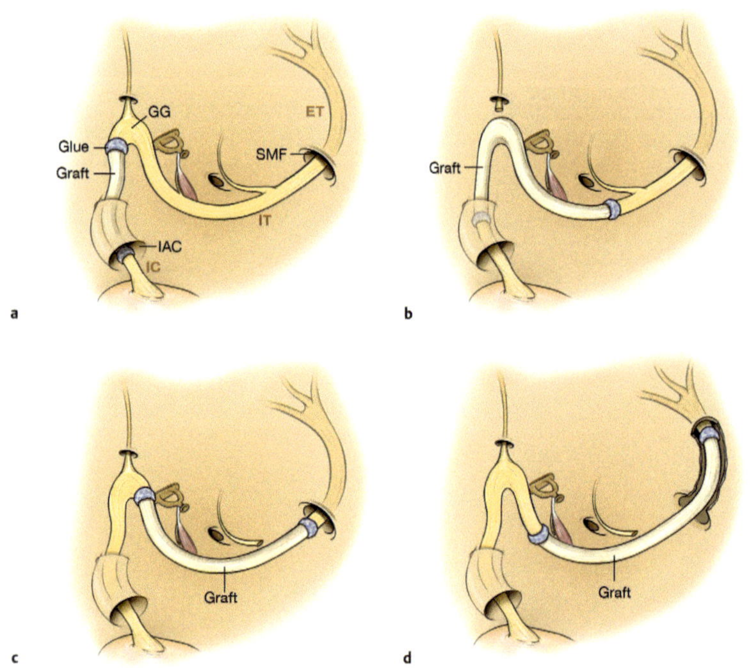

Fig. 64.2 **(a)** Intradural anastomosis; **(b)** transdural anastomosis; **(c)** extradural anastomosis limited to the temporal bone; **(d)** extradural anastomosis with involvement of the extratemporal facial nerve. GG, geniculate ganglion; IAC, internal auditory canal; IC, intracranial; IT, intratemporal; SMF, stylomastoid foramen.

transdural anastomosis, wherein the proximal site is in the cerebellopontine angle (CPA) or the IAC and the distal site is in the part of the temporal bone that remained after excision of the lesion (▸ Fig. 64.2b); and (3) *extradural anastomosis*, wherein both the proximal and distal sites of anastomosis are in the temporal bone or extratemporally (pre-parotid and parotid parts of the FN; ▸ Fig. 64.2c,d). In case of FN reconstruction after VS resection, the anastomoses are usually intradural.

64.6 Stitch versus Stitchless Techniques

Delicate maneuvers of nerve approximation such as perineurial, group funicular, and epineurial suturing are very difficult to perform in the depths of a pulsating CPA and even more so in the setting of a tired surgeon subsequent to a long and frequently laborious procedure.[3] Furthermore, the FN lacks a true fascicular organization until the geniculate ganglion, and this makes it practically impossible to perform any kind of epi- or perineurial suturing intradurally.[2,10,16,17] Hence, we prefer to use the stitchless fibrin glue technique for intradural and transdural anastomoses (▸ Fig. 64.3).[18] The success of this technique has been researched and replicated by other authors.[15,19,20,21] Suturing is reserved only for extradural anastomosis.

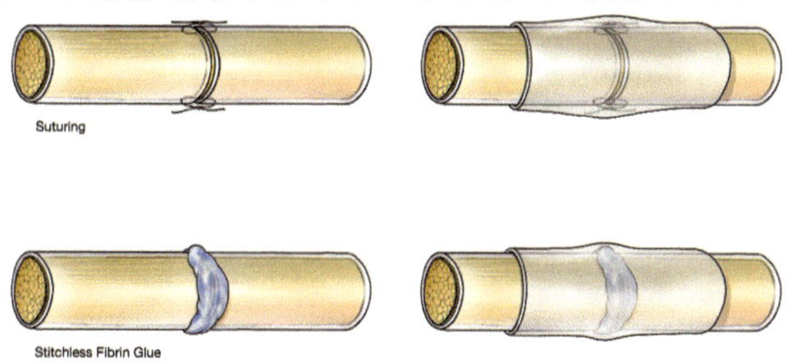

Fig. 64.3 Stitch versus stitchless fibrin glue technique for anastomosis of the FN.

64.7 Technique of Harvesting the Sural Nerve Graft and Anastomosis

Frequently, the site of interruption of the FN in VS surgery is at the porus of the IAC. In this situation, the distal segment is longer than the bony remnant of the IAC and should always be trimmed so as to occupy approximately a little less than half the length of the available bone (▸ Fig. 64.4). This provides a stable supporting surface for the ensuing anastomosis. The distal segment of the nerve in the vicinity of the IAC generally does not pose any particular difficulty and is easily visualized and often readily stimulates with a FN stimulating probe. However, the proximal segment can often be difficult to locate. Furthermore, its identity proximally cannot be confirmed with FN stimulation.

64.7.1 Harvesting the Sural Nerve Graft

When the need for the graft is confirmed, sterilizing and draping the selected foot and leg are carried out. An assisting surgeon harvests the graft after the main surgeon has completed tumor removal and while hemostasis is being achieved. An incision is made starting from behind the lower border of the lateral malleolus extending superiorly up to a distance of 8 to 10 cm; this distance can be increased if a greater length of the nerve is needed (▸ Fig. 64.5). The incision is extended superiorly for a thicker portion of the nerve and inferiorly to obtain a bifurcated nerve (the SN branches into two or more branches anteroinferior to the malleolus) that may be needed for anastomosis at the parotid bifurcation of the FN. Of course, a bifurcated nerve graft is not required for intradural anastomosis, but is mainly used in extratemporal repairs.

After incising the skin and the fascia, blunt dissection is carried out in the area located between the Achilles tendon and

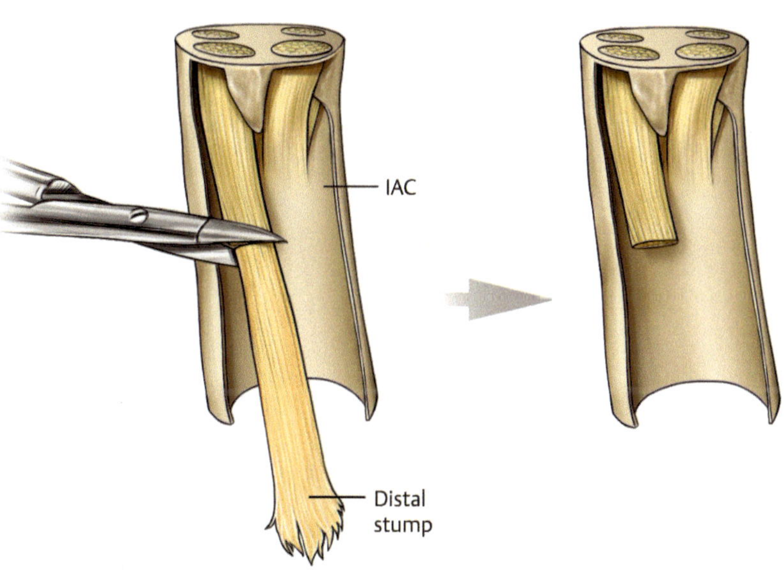

Fig. 64.4 If distal stump of the facial nerve is longer than the length of the remaining internal auditory canal (IAC), the excess length is trimmed to fit well inside the bony remnant so as to be able to place the anastomosis on a supporting surface.

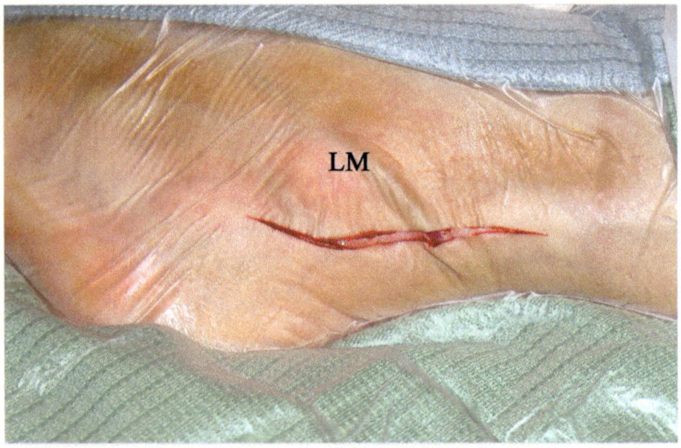

Fig. 64.5 An incision is started from behind the lower border of the lateral malleolus extending superiorly up to a distance of 8 to 10 cm.

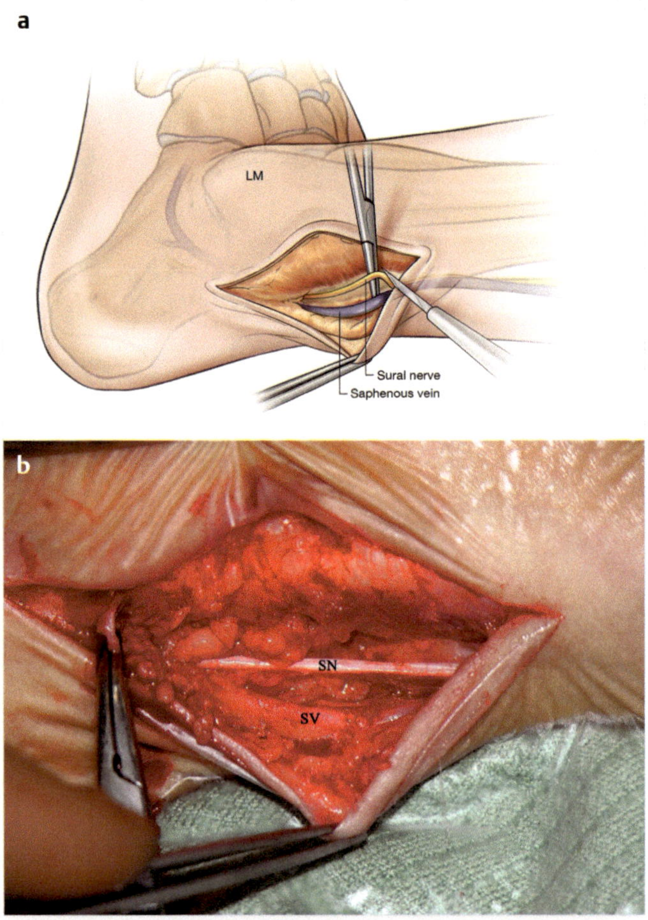

Fig. 64.6 **(a)** The sural nerve (SN) can be found located anterior to the saphenous vein (SV). **(b)** The nerve is harvested using a sharp Beaver blade.

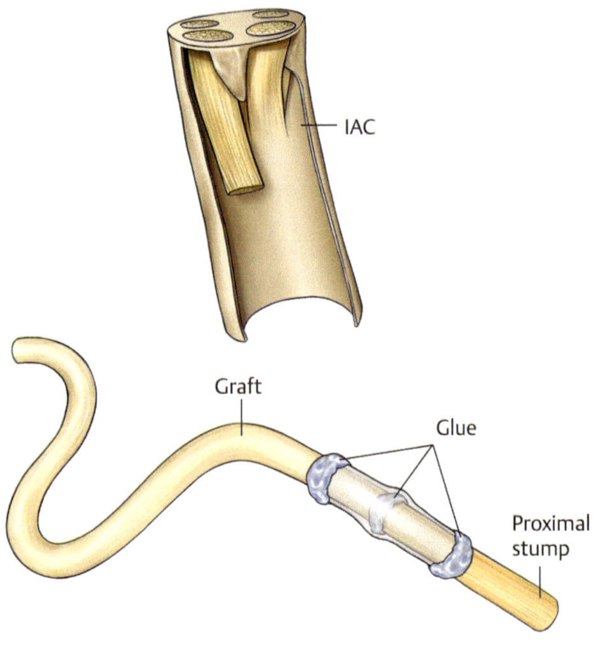

Fig. 64.7 A piece of temporalis fascia is wrapped around the anastomosis and the entire facial nerve stump–cable graft–temporalis fascia complex is secured to underlying brainstem with fibrin glue. IAC, internal auditory canal.

the lateral malleolus parallel to the expected course of the nerve in order to avoid injury. The saphenous vein also serves as an important landmark for the nerve, which is located just posterior to the nerve (▶ Fig. 64.6). The length of the nerve exposed should be adequate to bridge the gap between the FN ends; generally, extra length of the nerve is harvested. The length of the actual nerve deficit is measured by placing a suture thread between the proximal and distal ends of the sectioned nerve. The nerve is carefully dissected with minimal trauma and always handled minimally with a non-toothed forceps. The required length of the nerve is cut using sharp scissors. Care is taken to select parts of the nerve that match the diameter of the cut ends of the nerves. The nerve is then aligned on a tongue depressor wherein the nerve is cleaned of its nerve sheath and its edges are beveled at both ends by cutting it sharply with a knife. The proximal and the distal cut ends of the nerve are also cut sharply and beveled using a sharp scissor. If the thickness of the graft is less than that of the FN, the graft's end can be incised obliquely to optimize the contact surface.

The proximal end is anastomosed first. The anastomoses at both the proximal and distal ends are achieved by placing the beveled ends of the nerve and the graft together in apposition over a small piece of harvested temporalis fascia that is used to wrap and secure the anastomoses. Fibrin glue is applied after the anastomosis and once again after wrapping the fascia over the anastomosis (▶ Fig. 64.7). At the proximal anastomosis in the CPA, care is taken to position the length of the graft along the brainstem surface against the fifth cranial nerve root for support (▶ Fig. 64.8).

The distal end is anastomosed in any remaining bone of the IAC or by making a channel in the temporal bone (▶ Fig. 64.9). Fibrin glue is also applied at various points, wherever possible along the length of the graft, to further secure the graft. 9–0 monofilament sutures are used only for extratemporal epineurial anastomosis. Sutures are not routinely used in anastomosis in the intracranial

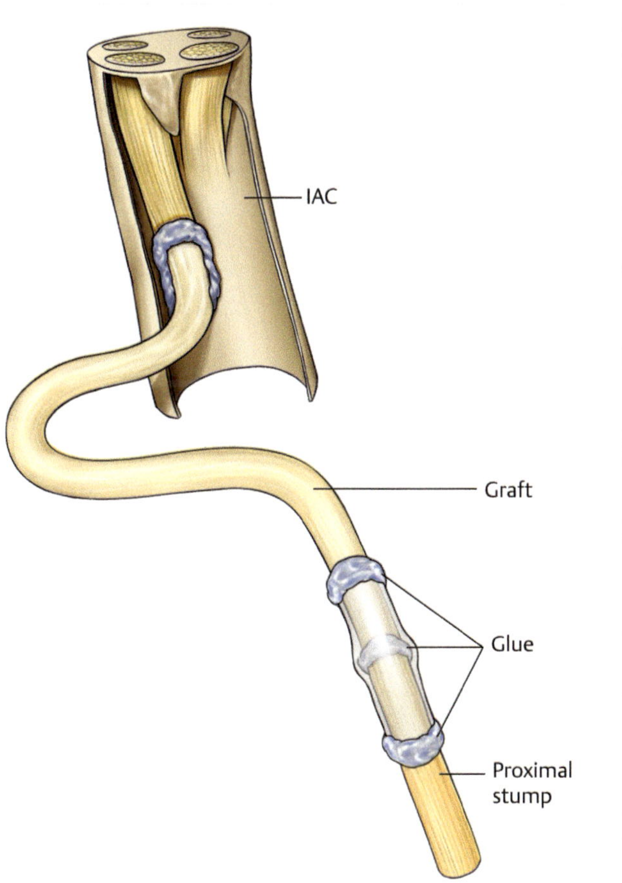

Fig. 64.8 Cable graft placed on brainstem surface and anterior wall of internal auditory canal (IAC) en route to the distal stump of the facial nerve. Application of fibrin glue to the distal anastomosis.

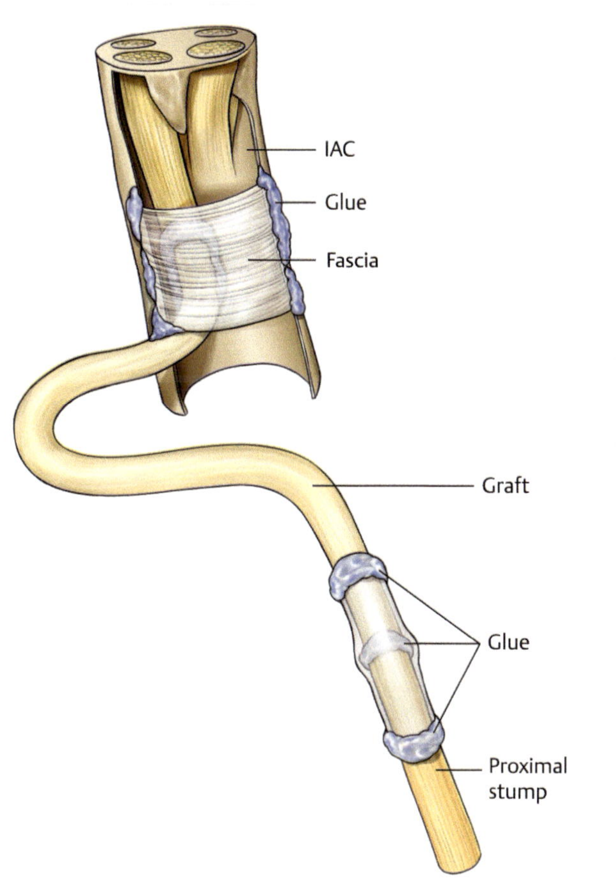

Fig. 64.9 Fascia placed on the distal anastomosis and secured with fibrin glue. IAC, internal auditory canal.

and temporal parts of the skull base, as the epineurium is not adequately developed in these segments of the FN. The CPA is sealed in the usual fashion, using long, thin strips of fat and ensuring a meticulous multilayered closure of the incision.

64.8 Pearls

1. Restoration of FN continuity is considered to be the most effective way of FN reconstruction and the only way that can restore natural facial mimetic movements.
2. An adequate length of fresh healthy FN ends should be available to allow for successful reconstruction.
3. Any degree of tension in the anastomosis can lead to its disruption and should be avoided by creating a gentle S-shaped curve in the graft.
4. The sural nerve is suitable for the grafting of the FN because (1) its diameter is equal to the FN; (2) the loss of the nerve produces minimal sensory loss in the donor site; (3) a long graft can be harvested; and (4) it can be harvested while the surgeon continues work on the tumor.
5. To ensure better contact between the anastomotic surfaces of the graft and the stumps of the FN, the edges of the graft are cut in an oblique manner.
6. It is very important to place the anastomosed portion of the nerve and, if possible, the entire graft on some supporting surface. We use the surface of the brainstem, the fifth cranial nerve, and the anterior bony wall of the IAC for this purpose. The graft is fixed to these structures using fibrin glue. At the end of the procedure, the graft is found lying in the CPA coursing through a gentle curve resting on the brainstem surface, the fifth cranial nerve, and any remaining bone, frequently the anterior wall of the IAC.
7. It is important to ensure that the length of the graft is sufficient to allow a tension-free anastomosis and to allow its placement on the various surfaces for support as described previously. At the same time, the length should not be so excessive as to leave a freely floating segment in the CPA that could be subsequently subjected to tension or torsion.

64.9 Pitfalls

1. The nerve ends must be held extremely delicately without causing undue trauma to the nerve bundles, especially the proximal FN stump, which is devoid of epineurium in this segment.

2. It is very difficult to suture nerve segments in the CPA due to the fact that the FN does not have an epineurium in this segment. The pulsating cerebellum also makes it difficult to apply sutures. Hence, we prefer to wrap the anastomosis with a small piece of temporalis fascia that not only secures the anastomosis but also provides a channel for neuronal regeneration. The fascia is wrapped all around the proximal anastomosis, but at the distal junction, which is usually at the anterior bony wall of IAC, merely draping the fascia over the union of the two ends usually suffices.

64.10 Clinical Case Example: Cable Graft Interposition using the SN for an Interrupted FN after VS surgery (Right Ear). ▶ Fig. 64.10– ▶ Fig. 64.23

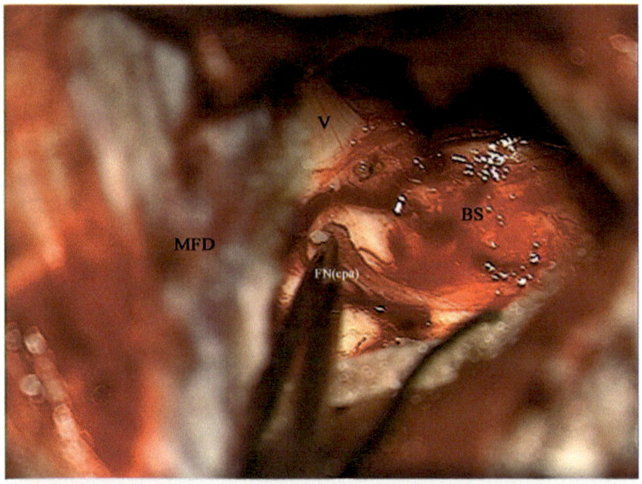

Fig. 64.10 The proximal stump of the facial nerve is identified near its origin from the brainstem. FN(cpa), facial nerve at the cerebellopontine angle; BS, brainstem; MFD, middle fossa dura; V, trigeminal nerve.

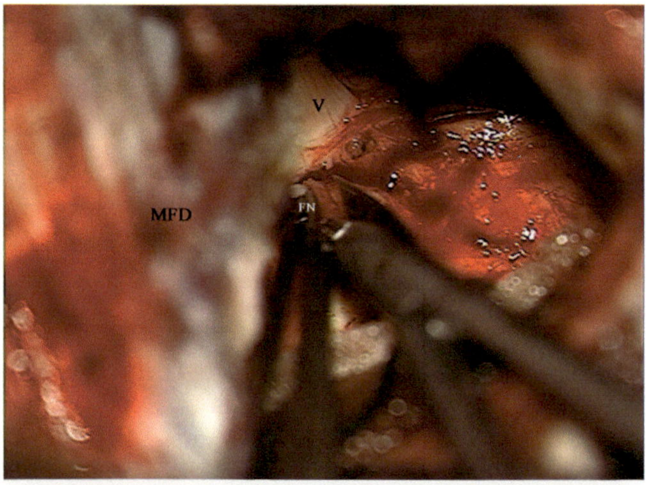

Fig. 64.11 Microscissors are used to refresh the ends of the facial nerve. FN, facial nerve; MFD, middle fossa dura; V, trigeminal nerve.

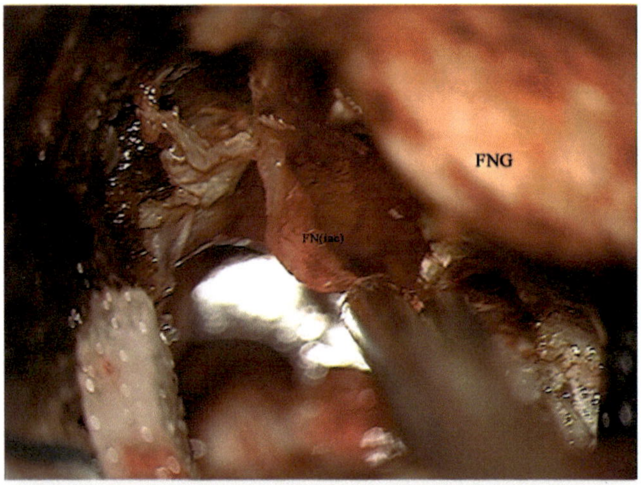

Fig. 64.12 The distal end of the facial nerve within the internal auditory canal [FN(iac)] is identified. FNG, facial nerve genu.

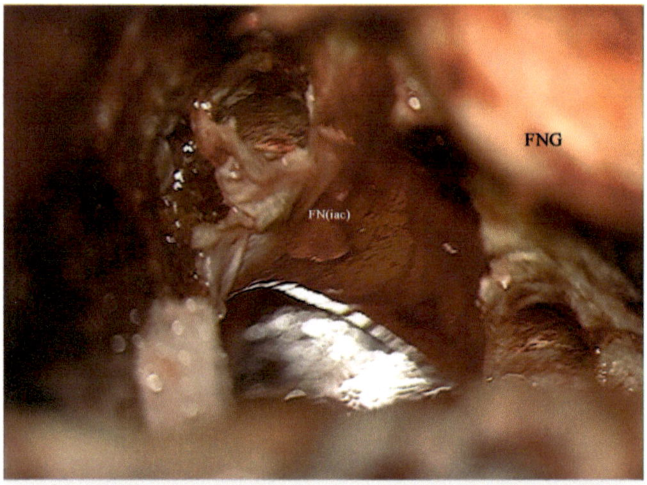

Fig. 64.13 The distal part of the facial nerve, in the internal auditory canal [FN(iac)], is refreshed by sharply cutting its end. This segment of the nerve should be cut in such a way that the remaining part occupies approximately only the distal half of the internal auditory canal, leaving the proximal half free as a bed for the graft. FNG, facial nerve genu.

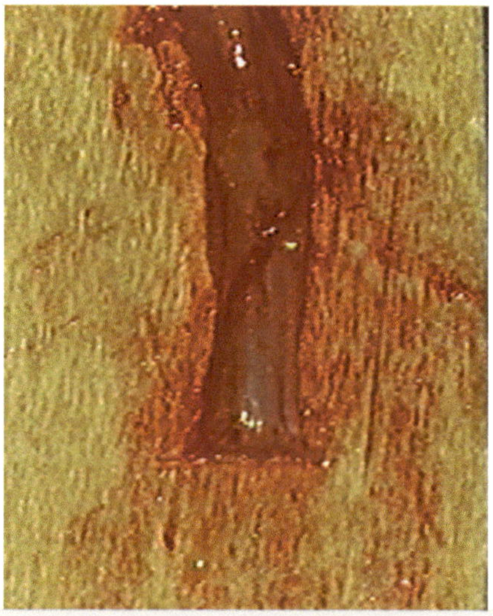

Fig. 64.14 The harvested sural nerve is prepared for grafting. The thicker end of the sural is to be laid against the distal end of the facial nerve. Since the internal auditory canal supplies a stable bed for the fixation of this part of the anastomosis, the diameter of the apposed nerves should be approximately equal; thus the cut performed at this end of the nerve should be at right angles, as shown.

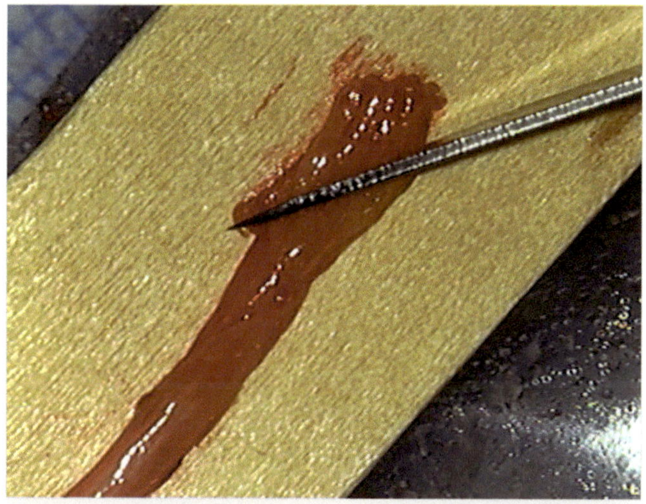

Fig. 64.15 Preparing the opposite end of the sural nerve. Note here that the cut end of the nerve has been fashioned in an oblique manner to achieve a wide contact area between the graft and the thinner proximal stump of the facial nerve. Also, this part of the anastomosis lies on the brainstem, lacking a fixed bed and rendering it less stable than the distal anastomosis. Thus the wide surface area will provide a greater opportunity for contact between neurons.

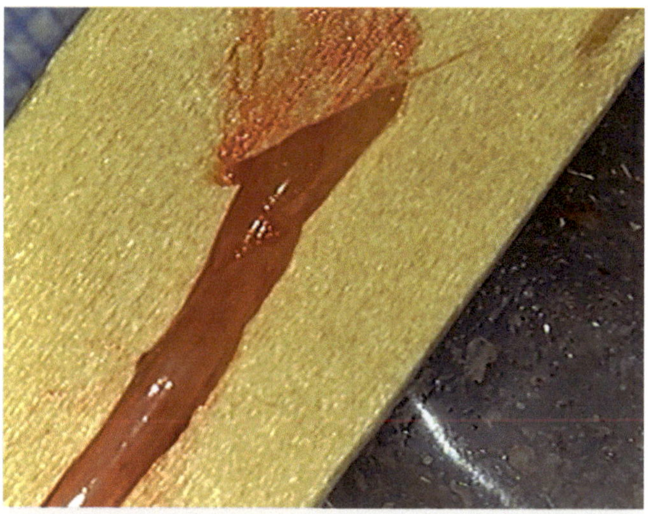

Fig. 64.16 The oblique end of the graft.

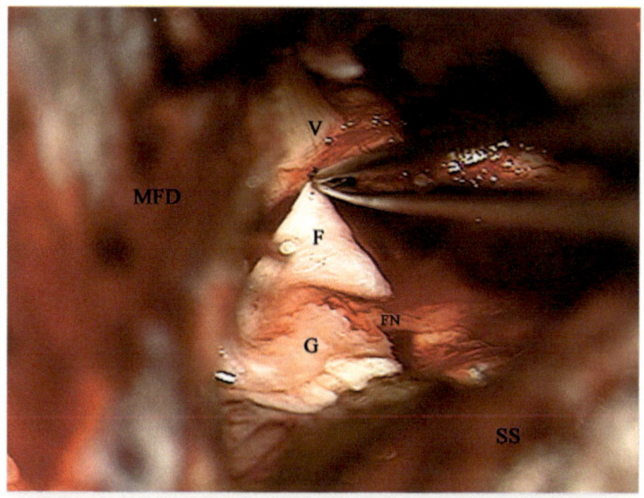

Fig. 64.17 The facia (F) is being folded around the already glued nerve ends. G, sural nerve graft; FN, facial nerve; MFD, middle fossa dura; V, trigeminal nerve; SS, sigmoid sinus.

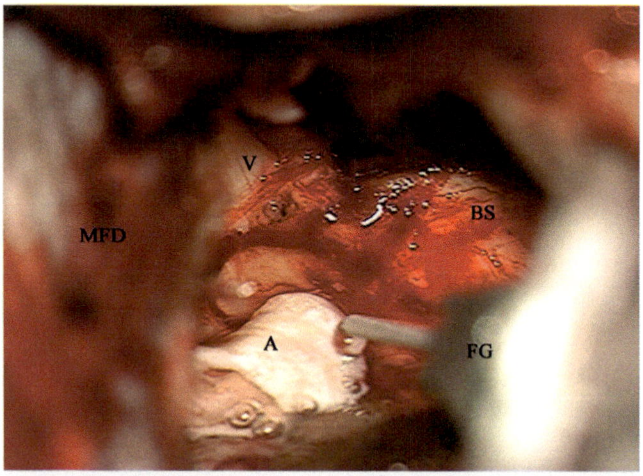

Fig. 64.18 Fibrin glue (FG) is used once again to secure the anastomosis (A) after folding the fascia over the nerve ends. BS, brainstem; V, trigeminal nerve; MFD, middle fossa dura.

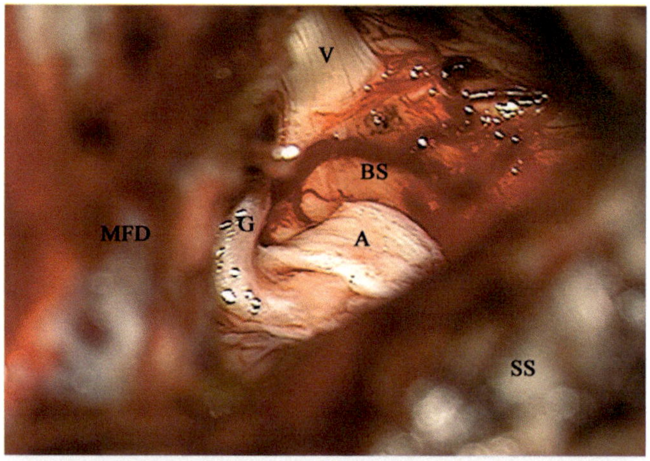

Fig. 64.19 The sural nerve graft (G) is directed anteriorly to be laid on the trigeminal nerve root (V). This maneuver will support the weight of the sural nerve, thus reducing any tension in the distal anastomosis. A, anastomosis; BS, brainstem; MFD, middle fossa dura, SS, sigmoid sinus.

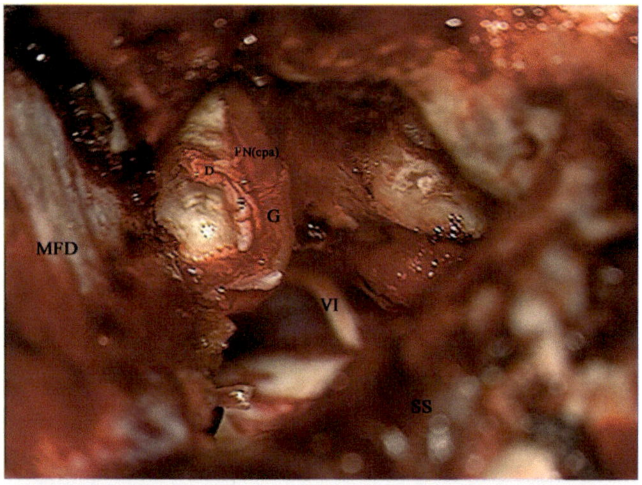

Fig. 64.20 The contralateral end of the sural graft (G) has been approximated to the distal end of the facial nerve in the cerebellopontine angle [FN(cpa)]. Note the exact apposition and contact between the nerve ends. D, dura of the IAC; MFD, middle fossa dura; VI, abducent nerve; SS, sigmoid sinus.

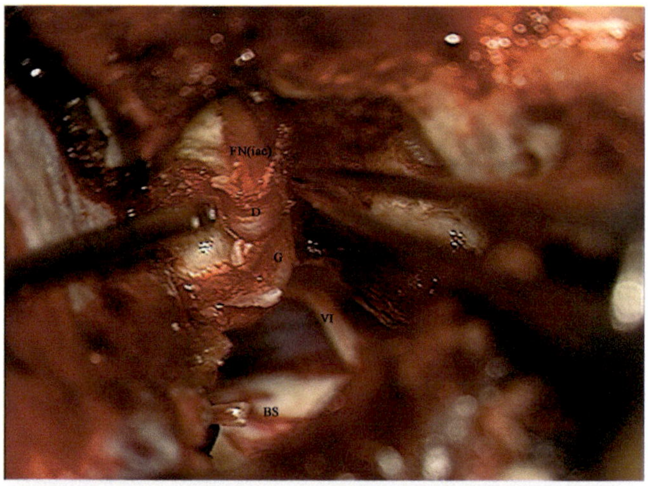

Fig. 64.21 The dura of the internal auditory canal has been folded around the anastomosis. G, sural nerve graft; FN(iac), the FN end within the IAC; VI, abducens nerve; BS, brainstem.

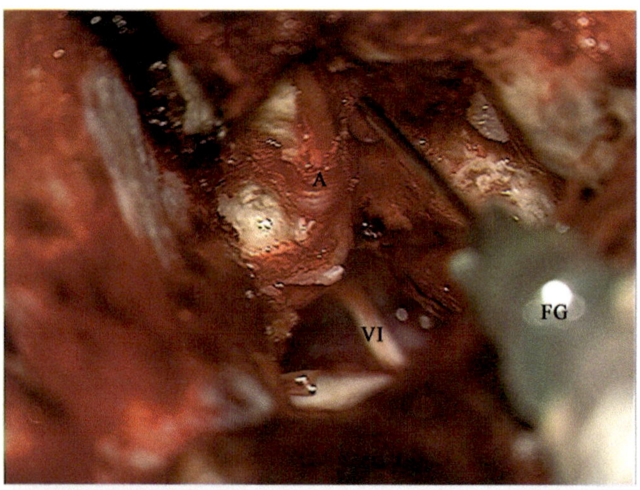

Fig. 64.22 Fibrin glue (FG) is used to reinforce the distal anastomosis (A). VI, abducens nerve.

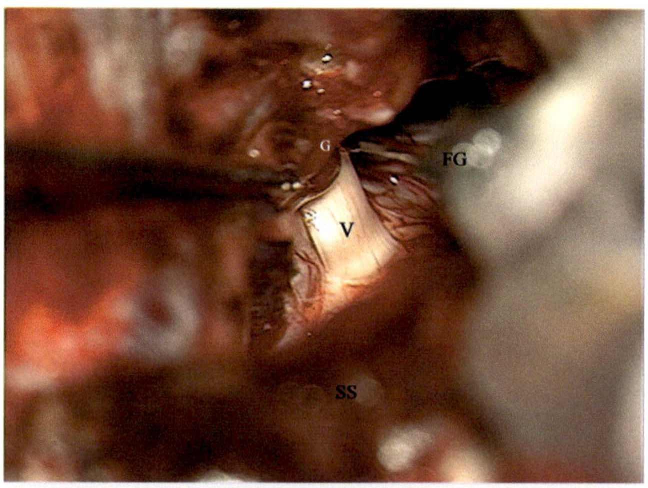

Fig. 64.23 Fibrin glue (FG) is used to fix the middle part of the graft (G) on the trigeminal nerve (V). SS, sigmoid sinus.

References

[1] Ozmen OA, Falcioni M, Lauda L, Sanna M. Outcomes of facial nerve grafting in 155 cases: predictive value of history and preoperative function. Otol Neurotol. 2011; 32:1341–1346

[2] Arriaga MA, Brackmann DE. Facial nerve repair techniques in cerebellopontine angle tumor surgery. Am J Otol. 1992; 13(4):356–359

[3] House JW, Brackmann DE. Facial nerve grading system. Otolaryngol Head Neck Surg. 1985; 93(2):146–147

[4] Bacciu A, Falcioni M, Pasanisi E, et al. Intracranial facial nerve grafting after removal of vestibular schwannoma. Am J Otolaryngol. 2009; 30(2):83–88

[5] Prasad SC, Balasubramanian K, Piccirillo E. Surgical technique and results of cable graft interpositioning of the facial nerve in lateral skull base surgeries: experience with 213 consecutive cases. J Neurosurg. 2018; 128:631–638

[6] Brackmann DE, Hitselberger WE, Robinson JV. Facial nerve repair in cerebellopontine angle surgery. Ann Otol Rhinol Laryngol. 1978; 87(6, Pt 1): 772–777

[7] Sanna M, Khrais T, Mancini F, Russo A, Taibah A. Facial nerve management in middle ear and external auditory canal carcinoma. In: The Facial Nerve in the Temporal Bone and Lateral Skull Base Microsurgery. Stuttgart: Georg Thieme Verlag; 2006:270–271

[8] Sanna MMF, Russo A, Taibah A, Falcioni M, Di Trapani G. Atlas of Acoustic Neurinoma Microsurgery. Stuttgart: Georg Thieme Verlag; 2008

[9] Einige AE. Operationen an Nerven. Wied Med Presse. 1885; 26:1285–1288

[10] Conley JJ. Facial nerve grafting in treatment of parotid gland tumors; new technique. AMA Arch Surg. 1955; 70(3):359–366

[11] Hohman MH, Kleiss IJ, Knox CJ, Weinberg JS, Heaton JT, Hadlock TA. Functional recovery after facial nerve cable grafting in a rodent model. JAMA Facial Plast Surg. 2014; 16(1):20–24

[12] Wang Z, Zhang Z, Huang Q, Yang J, Wu H. Long-term facial nerve function following facial reanimation after translabyrinthine vestibular schwannoma surgery: a comparison between sural grafting and VII-XII anastomosis. Exp Ther Med. 2013; 6(1):101–104

[13] Slutsky DJ. A practical approach to nerve grafting in the upper extremity. Atlas Hand Clin. 2005; 10:73–92

[14] Lee MC, Kim DH, Jeon YR, et al. Functional outcomes of multiple sural nerve grafts for facial nerve defects after tumor-ablative surgery. Arch Plast Surg. 2015; 42(4):461–468

[15] Ramos DS, Bonnard D, Franco-Vidal V, Liguoro D, Darrouzet V. Stitchless fibrin glue-aided facial nerve grafting after cerebellopontine angle schwannoma removal: technique and results in 15 cases. Otol Neurotol. 2015; 36: 498–502

[16] Captier G, Canovas F, Bonnel F, Seignarbieux F. Organization and microscopic anatomy of the adult human facial nerve: anatomical and histological basis for surgery. Plast Reconstr Surg. 2005; 115(6):1457–1465

[17] Lacombe H. [Functional anatomy of the facial nerve]. Neurochirurgie. 2009; 55(2):113–119

[18] Sanna M, Jain Y, Falcioni M, Mancini F, Romano G. Facial nerve grafting in the cerebellopontine angle. Laryngoscope. 2004; 114(4):782–785

[19] Attar BM, Zalzali H, Razavi M, Ghoreishian M, Rezaei M. Effectiveness of fibrin adhesive in facial nerve anastomosis in dogs compared with standard microsuturing technique. J Oral Maxillofac Surg. 2012; 70(10):2427–2432

[20] Wang Q, Hua Q, Wang S. [Application of fibrin glue in facial nerve repair]. J Biomed Eng. 2007; 24:612–614

[21] Bozorg Grayeli A, Mosnier I, Julien N, El Garem H, Bouccara D, Sterkers O. Long-term functional outcome in facial nerve graft by fibrin glue in the temporal bone and cerebellopontine angle. Eur Arch Otorhinolaryngol. 2005; 262(5):404–407

65 Hypoglossal-to-Facial Nerve Transfer with Parotid Release for Rehabilitation of the Paralyzed Face in Vestibular Schwannoma

David R. Friedmann and J. Thomas Roland Jr.

65.1 Introduction

Facial reanimation after paralysis is an important tool in the armamentarium of any skull base surgical practice and may be carried out by neurotologists, neurosurgeons, and microvascular-trained head and neck or facial plastic surgeons. A comprehensive facial nerve center often encompasses some or all of these members to assist in selecting the best treatment for a given patient. In cases where possible, an end-to-end anastomosis or interposition graft bridging the two ends of the facial nerve is preferred for dynamic reanimation.

When the proximal facial nerve is not available for use, the distal facial nerve may be anastomosed to a separate motor nerve, traditionally the hypoglossal nerve and more recently the masseteric branch of the trigeminal nerve (see Chapter 66), with the goals of providing facial tone, symmetry, and volitional dynamic movement. Our center has modified prior techniques of hypoglossal-to-facial (12–7) nerve transfer through a parotid release maneuver to facilitate a single tension-free anastomosis with minimal or no tongue morbidity.

65.2 History and Overview of the Procedure

Hypoglossal-to-facial anastomosis was first performed in 1901 by Korte in end-to-end fashion.[1] As this report indicated, transection of the hypoglossal nerve to allow for end-to-end anastomosis results in ipsilateral paralysis and atrophy of the tongue musculature, which can lead to dysphagia and dysarthria. This can be of even greater functional consequence in patients with preexisting facial weakness and/or lower cranial neuropathies as in neurofibromatosis type 2 patients. Subsequently, May et al introduced a modification involving end-to-side coaptation using an interposition graft, hence preserving ipsilateral tongue function.[2] This technique has also been termed "jump interposition graft hypoglossal-facial anastomosis" (JIGFA). Subsequent reports of a split hypoglossal-facial nerve anastomosis have been published, where a part of the hypoglossal nerve is left in its anatomic position with subsequent end-to-end anastomosis.

In 1997, Atlas and Sawamura independently reported on a facial nerve transposition technique in which the facial nerve is freed from its intratemporal location and transposed and anastomosed to the hypoglossal nerve in an end-to-side fashion without use of an interposition graft.[3,4] In 2006, our group first published our modification of the facial nerve transposition technique by including a parotid release maneuver to ensure consistent tension-free anastomoses.[5] In a subsequent publication, Slattery et al and members of the House Clinic described a similar technique that they termed *a hypoglossal-to-facial anastomosis "swingdown" technique*.[6]

65.3 Advantages and Limitations

This technique allows for a single tension-free anastomosis without associated tongue morbidity. The JIGFA technique also spares tongue morbidity, but still requires harvest of a separate nerve jump graft with associated donor site morbidity, and also incorporates two anastomotic sites. The parotid release maneuver, to aid in direct anastomosis, takes advantage of the intratemporal facial nerve in the temporal bone.

Primary facial nerve pathology involving the tympanic or mastoid segments of the facial nerve (i.e., schwannoma, glomus faciale, hemangioma) precludes its use for this technique. Additionally, the parotid release maneuver bears the risk of postoperative sialocele, which often resolves with conservative measures. Finally, the released portion of the parotid gland may protrude in the preauricular region, but this generally resolves during the postoperative period.

65.4 Patient Evaluation and Selection

This procedure is appropriate for patients with intact facial musculature and an intact distal course of the facial nerve. Pathology of the tympanic or mastoid segments of the facial nerve precludes use of the parotid release technique, but may still be amenable to 12–7 anastomosis with an interposition graft of sufficient length.

Optimally, this procedure is performed as early as possible after nerve transection and not beyond 12 to 16 months because of concern for atrophy of facial musculature and loss of motor end plates prohibiting reinnervation. In cases where facial nerve sacrifice is anticipated or preoperative facial function is poor, the reanimation procedure may be performed in the same operative procedure as tumor resection. In our experience, if no movement is seen 6 months after original vestibular schwannoma resection and the facial nerve is confidently anatomically intact, there is a role for electromyography to confirm the absence of reinnervation potentials. If none are present, the patient may be offered a dynamic facial reanimation procedure.

65.5 Relevant Anatomy, Surgical Technique, and Outcomes

A C-shaped postauricular-cervical incision is made beginning at the temporal scalp, curving posteriorly and inferiorly behind the mastoid, to a natural neck crease 3 cm inferior to the angle of the mandible. At the superior extent of the incision, the temporalis fascia is exposed. At the level of the mastoid, the incision proceeds deeper to expose the periosteum. In the neck and face, dissection is performed in the subplatysmal and sub-SMAS plane, respectively. The external auditory canal remains intact and efforts are made to include prior postauricular incisions. The intratemporal facial nerve is then skeletonized via mastoidectomy, from the immediate postgeniculate region to the stylomastoid foramen. If the patient has serviceable hearing, the incus is often removed via a facial recess exposure to facilitate dissection of the tympanic segment of the facial nerve. The incus is replaced as an interposition at the conclusion of the case. We have also performed this without incus removal in some cases. The facial nerve is transected distal to the geniculate ganglion, is elevated from the fallopian canal, and is completely mobilized from the stylomastoid foramen in order to freely move the proximal end to the upper neck (▶ Fig. 65.1 and ▶ Fig. 65.2). Care is taken to avoid cerebrospinal fluid leakage, especially in a patient who has undergone prior skull base surgery.

The superficial lobe of the parotid, the facial nerve, and a cuff of deep parotid tissue are elevated and rotated inferiorly to provide additional facial nerve length. This maneuver is performed by separating the parotid gland from the cartilaginous external auditory canal and by undercutting the parotid tail, medial to the facial nerve. The parotid-release maneuver provides an additional 3 to 5 cm of inferior extension to the mobilized facial nerve, thereby affording a tension-free anastomosis to the hypoglossal nerve distal to the origin of the ansa hypoglossi. The mobilized parotid tail is secured inferiorly with absorbable sutures to maintain a tension-free facial nerve segment. A nerve graft (sural or greater auricular nerve) may also be harvested if needed to allow for tension-free anastomosis.

With the sternocleidomastoid muscle retracted posteriorly, the denervated posterior belly of the digastric is reflected to expose the hypoglossal nerve. Dissection proceeds medially until the hypoglossal nerve is located. The hypoglossal nerve is followed anterograde to a point where the facial nerve can be transposed to rest on the hypoglossal nerve without tension (▶ Fig. 65.3).

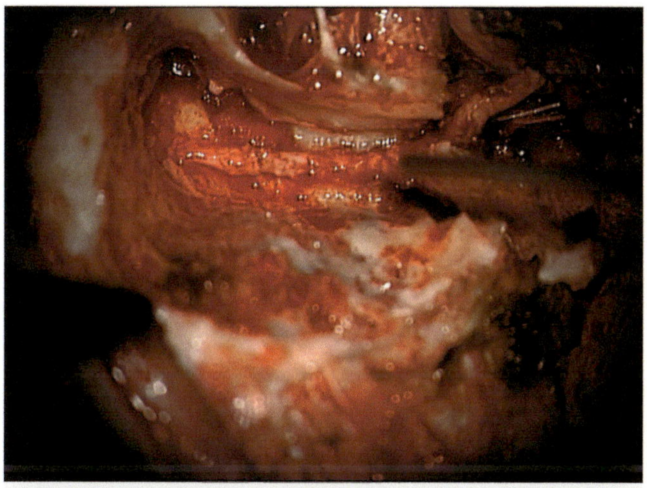

Fig. 65.1 The facial nerve has been divided lateral to the geniculum and elevated from the fallopian canal.

Under the operating microscope, a wedge incision, no more than half the diameter of the hypoglossal nerve, is made distal to the ansa hypoglossi. The distal end of the facial nerve is revised with a fine knife. Three or four interrupted 9–0 monofilament nylon sutures are used to approximate the epineurium of the facial nerve stump to the wedge incision on the proximal aspect of the hypoglossal nerve. The nerve endings should be approximated without any tension (▶ Fig. 65.4). The wound is then closed in anatomical layers. A nonsuction drain is placed at the end of the procedure and removed after 24 hours. A summary of published outcomes is reported in ▶ Table 65.1.

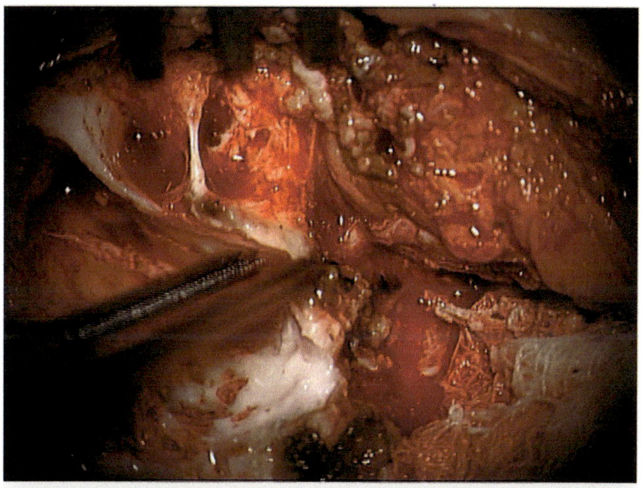

Fig. 65.2 After removal of the mastoid tip, the facial nerve is mobilized from the stylomastoid foramen while the parotid is retracted anteriorly. The facial nerve and a cuff of parotid tissue are rotated inferiorly into the neck, gaining an additional 3 to 5 cm of length for anastomosis to the hypoglossal nerve.

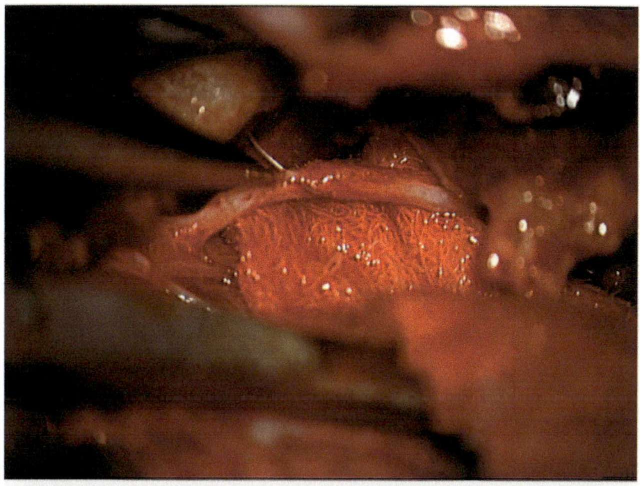

Fig. 65.3 The hypoglossal nerve is identified in the neck and a wedge of the nerve is identified and resected distal to the ansa take off to facilitate the end-to-side anastomosis.

Table 65.1 Outcomes using hypoglossal-to-facial nerve transfer

Study	No. of cases	Duration from paralysis to repair	Mean follow-up period	Outcomes	Complications
Roland et al[5]	10			9 pts score of C or better (GG scale)	
Franco-Vidal[7]	15		57 mo	73% HB III, 20% HB IV, 7% HB V	
Martins et al[8]	24			17 (70%) HB III, 6 (25%) HB IV, 1 HB V	7 patients tongue atrophy
Venail et al[9]	12			6 HB III, 6 HB IV	
Jacobson et al[10]	21	12.1 mo (range: 0–36 mo)	55 mo	18 pts score B/C (GG scale)	
Slattery et al[6]	19	Best outcomes < 6 mo from paralysis	48 mo	7 (36.8%) HB III, 9 (47.4%) HB IV, 3 (15.8%) HB V	

Abbreviations: HB, House–Brackmann facial nerve grading scale; GG, Gidley–Gantz facial nerve grading scale: appropriate for assessing outcomes after facial nerve reanimation (the Repaired Facial Nerve Recovery Scale).[11]
Notes: Description of outcomes using inherently subjective grading systems, often evaluated by the operating surgeon, may hamper interpretation. However, a number of studies utilizing the techniques described here are included. Of note, some reported improvement beyond 12 months, as late as 24 months, after repair.

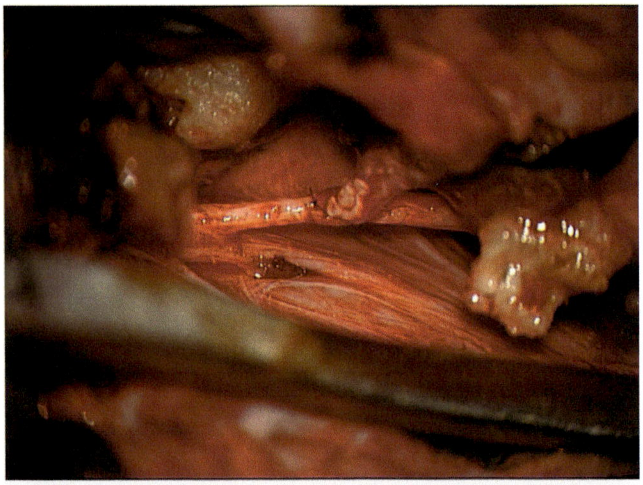

Fig. 65.4 The hypoglossal nerve is left in its normal anatomic location and the end-to-side anastomosis to the facial nerve is completed.

References

[1] Korte W. Ein Fal von Nerven Fropfung: des Nervus facialis auf den Nervus hypoglossus. Dtsch Med Wochenschr. 1903;29:293

[2] May M, Sobol SM, Mester SJ. Hypoglossal-facial nerve interpositional-jump graft for facial reanimation without tongue atrophy. Otolaryngol Head Neck Surg. 1991; 104(6):818–825

[3] Atlas MD, Lowinger DS. A new technique for hypoglossal-facial nerve repair. Laryngoscope. 1997; 107(7):984–991

[4] Sawamura Y, Abe H. Hypoglossal-facial nerve side-to-end anastomosis for preservation of hypoglossal function: results of delayed treatment with a new technique. J Neurosurg. 1997; 86(2):203–206

[5] Roland JT, Jr, Lin K, Klausner LM, Miller PJ. Direct facial-to-hypoglossal neurorrhaphy with parotid release. Skull Base. 2006; 16(2):101–108

[6] Slattery WH, III, Cassis AM, Wilkinson EP, Santos F, Berliner K. Side-to-end hypoglossal to facial anastomosis with transposition of the intratemporal facial nerve. Otol Neurotol. 2014; 35(3):509–513

[7] Franco-Vidal V, Blanchet H, Liguoro D, Darrouzet V. Side-to-end hypoglossal-facial nerve anastomosis with intratemporal facial nerve translocation. Long-term results and indications in 15 cases over 10 years. Rev Laryngol Otol Rhinol (Bord). 2006; 127(1–2):97–102

[8] Martins RS, Socolovsky M, Siqueira MG, Campero A. Hemihypoglossal-facial neurorrhaphy after mastoid dissection of the facial nerve: results in 24 patients and comparison with the classic technique. Neurosurgery. 2008; 63 (2):310–316, discussion 317

[9] Venail F, Sabatier P, Mondain M, Segniarbieux F, Leipp C, Uziel A. Outcomes and complications of direct end-to-side facial-hypoglossal nerve anastomosis according to the modified May technique. J Neurosurg. 2009; 110(4):786–791

[10] Jacobson J, Rihani J, Lin K, Miller PJ, Roland JT, Jr. Outcomes of direct facial-to-hypoglossal neurorrhaphy with parotid release. Skull Base. 2011; 21(1):7–12

[11] Gidley PW, Gantz BJ, Rubinstein JT. Facial nerve grafts: from cerebellopontine angle and beyond. Am J Otol. 1999; 20(6):781–788

66 V3 Masseteric Branch Reinnervation for Rehabilitation of the Paralyzed Face in Vestibular Schwannoma

James A. Owusu and Kofi O. Boahene

66.1 Introduction

Advanced techniques in microsurgery, high-resolution magnification, and sensitive intraoperative electrophysiologic monitoring have all contributed to a high percentage of facial nerve preservation following resection of vestibular schwannoma (VS). An anatomically preserved facial nerve, however, does not always result in normal facial function. Depending on the degree of facial nerve manipulation and tumor effect, postoperative facial function may be completely normal, partially weak, or totally paralyzed. Fortunately, a high percentage of patients with facial nerve paresis and some with complete paralysis after VS resection recover spontaneously and regain satisfactory facial movement. However, some patients do not spontaneously recover facial muscle function and require surgical intervention to restore facial tone and animation. For these patients, timely intervention is critical in minimizing irreversible degeneration of the facial muscles and poor functional outcome after reanimation surgery. In a small set of patients, the anatomical continuity of the facial nerve is lost during tumor dissection and a suitable proximal stump at the brainstem is not available for interposition nerve grafting. These patients have no chance of recovering dynamic facial function without timely reanimation surgery.

The goal of facial reanimation surgery is to restore resting facial symmetry, spontaneous and voluntary facial motion, as well as emotional facial expression. The facial nerve and facial nucleus is unique in its ability to provide normal synchronized facial animation and cannot be adequately replaced by any other cranial nerve. When interrupted, the proximal end of the facial nerve from the brainstem may be coapted either directly or with an interposition graft. When the proximal facial nerve is unavailable for reanimation, alternative donor cranial nerves may be substituted to power the facial muscles. Potential donor sources include the hypoglossal, trigeminal, contralateral facial, spinal accessory, and phrenic nerves. For several years, the hypoglossal nerve was considered the go-to donor nerve for facial reanimation surgery.[1] In the classical description, the hypoglossal nerve is completely sectioned in the neck and coapted to the main facial nerve branch. Coaptation of the entire hypoglossal nerve to the facial nerve effectively restores facial tone and some volitional movement, but is also associated with severe tongue hemiatrophy and dysfunction leading to difficulties with speech, mastication, and swallowing. Modifications to the classic total hypoglossal nerve transfer procedure including the use of the split hypoglossal technique, interposition jump grafts, and transfer of the facial nerve for an end-to-side coaptation to an intact hypoglossal nerve have minimized morbidity of the tongue. Hypoglossal-to-facial nerve transfer is discussed further in Chapter 65.

The masseteric nerve, as a substitute donor source in facial reanimation, is increasing in popularity. As a substitute nerve for facial reanimation, Escat and Viela first reported the use of the masseteric nerve in 1925.[2] Spira wrote a similar report in 1978.[3] Several factors make the masseteric nerve an attractive donor source. These include its anatomic proximity to the facial nerve and mimetic muscles, its axonal density, low morbidity when sacrificed, and potential neurophysiologic and functional synergy with the facial nerve for facial expression.[4,5]

66.2 Anatomy of the Masseteric Nerve

The masseteric nerve is a branch of the trigeminal nerve originating from its motor root in the lateral aspects of the pons. On exiting the cranium through the foramen ovale, V3 divides into anterior and posterior divisions. The masseteric nerve arises from the anterior division of V3 together with the deep temporal, buccal, and the lateral pterygoid nerves. It passes through the posterior aspect of the sigmoid notch accompanied by the masseteric artery posterior to the insertion of the temporalis muscle on the coronoid process.[6] The masseteric neurovascular bundle enters the deep surface of the masseter muscle and arborizes in an anteroinferior trajectory to innervate the muscle (▶ Fig. 66.1). The average diameter of the masseteric nerve is

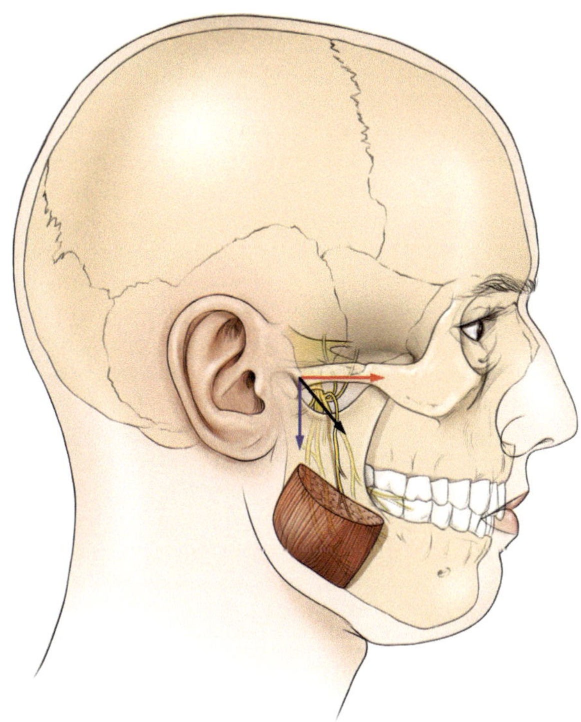

Fig. 66.1 Illustration showing the anatomy of the masseteric nerve and its relation to the masseter muscle, the temporomandibular joint, and the zygomatic arch.

2 mm at the level of the sigmoid notch. The nerve can be traced inferiorly for an average length of 27 mm before it divides into smaller caliber branches, less than 0.6 mm wide.[7] Direct electrical stimulation of the trigeminal nerve in the retrogasserian region shows a motor conduction velocity of the masseteric nerve of about 54 m/s,[8] which compares favorably to a velocity of 45 to 60 m/s in facial nerves.

66.3 Advantages of the Masseteric Nerve

The close proximity of the masseteric nerve to the facial nerve is a unique advantage, as it allows for mobilization of both nerves in a single surgical field for tension-free coaptation. The masseteric nerve may be coapted to the main trunk of the facial nerve or selected branches without the need for an interposition graft. Direct coaptation allows faster onset of recovery as the regenerating axons have a single barrier to cross to innervate the muscles. The masseteric nerve has a high fiber density which translates to strong neural input when coapted to facial nerve branches. Histologic studies have recorded an average myelinated fiber count from 1,500 to 2,700.[6,9] By comparison, the numbers of axons in normal hypoglossal and facial nerves were estimated at 9,778 ± 1,516 and 7,228 ± 950, respectively.[10] A cross-facial nerve graft has been reported to have 100 to 200 fiber counts.[11] The functional morbidity associated with the sacrifice of the masseteric nerve and subsequent denervation of the masseter muscle is usually minimal due to the overlapping function of the temporalis and medial pterygoid muscles. Additionally, anatomic studies have shown proximal branches of the masseteric nerve that can be preserved during nerve transfer preventing total denervation of the masseter muscle.[6,12] A major drawback that applies to the use of alternative cranial nerves for facial reanimation is the lack of spontaneous and emotional facial movement. Masseteric nerve transfer initially requires teeth clenching for activation; however, several studies have reported development of spontaneous facial motion with time. Manktelow et al reported 85% of patients were able to smile without biting in a review of 45 patients who underwent smile restoration with free flap innervated by masseteric nerve.[13] In a similar study, Wang et al reported an effortless smile in 81% of their 16 patients at 12 months postoperatively.[14] There are several reasons behind this potential cerebral adaptation. Electromyography (EMG) of the masseter muscle during normal smile has shown concurrent electrical activity in a subset of patients, suggesting a connection between the masseteric nucleus and the facial nucleus.[15] Embryologic studies have also demonstrated the presence of trigeminal nerve fibers within the facial nerve branches.[16] This potential connection between the masseteric and facial nerves most likely accounts for the potential to develop effortless smile.

Disadvantages of using the masseteric nerve for facial reanimation are relatively few. Wang et al reported masseter muscle atrophy following nerve transfer in 25% of their series of patients resulting in a concavity of the face.[14] There are also reports of involuntary movements of the face during mastication following masseter nerve substitution.[17] These reports are few and appear to have minimal impact on the patient's quality of life. ▶ Table 66.1 summarizes the pros and cons of the masseteric nerve and alternative cranial nerves commonly considered for facial reanimation.[4]

Table 66.1 Summary of the pros and cons of available donor nerves for substitution in facial reanimation

Nerve	Pros	Cons
Masseteric	• Close proximity to facial nerve • High axonal density • Potential for cerebral adaptation • Minimal donor site morbidity	• Potential masseter atrophy • Potential unwanted movements with mastication
Hypoglossal	• Close proximity to the facial nerve • High axonal density • Potential for cerebral adaptation	• Donor site morbidity (tongue atrophy, speech impairment) • Potential for mass movement • Unwanted facial movements
Spinal accessory	• Used when the masseteric nerve or hypoglossal nerve are contraindicated	• Unwanted facial movement with shoulder movement • Donor site morbidity (shoulder weakness) • Minimal to no potential for cerebral adaptation
Cross facial	• Potential for mimetic facial animation	• Low axonal density • Two-stage procedure • Increased denervation time
Phrenic	• Used when more suitable nerves are not available or contraindicated	• Unwanted facial movement with respiration • Donor site morbidity (hemidiaphragm paralysis) • No potential for cerebral adaptation

66.4 Patient Evaluation

Facial paralysis following VS resection can be classified as reversible or irreversible based on the status of the facial muscles.[5] Reversible paralysis implies the presence of electrophysiological and mechanically viable facial muscle fibers that will respond to reinnervation. In the absence of longstanding preoperative paralysis, most patients who developed facial paralysis after VS resection will have reversible paralysis. Patients who have prolonged preoperative paralysis or prolonged periods of denervation following tumor resection may be classified as having irreversible paralysis as the facial muscles become fibrotic and lose the ability to accept axonal ingrowth. In patients with incomplete paralysis or partial recovery, the facial muscles may remain electrophysiologically viable for many years and respond to further innervation. EMG studies may be helpful in determining the status of the facial muscles. The presence of fibrillation potentials indicates a physiological intact facial muscle despite denervation, whereas electrical silence represents irreversibly paralyzed facial muscles.[18]

Patients deemed to have a reversible paralysis should undergo reinnervation as early as possible using the selected donor nerve or nerves. Patients with irreversible paralysis can only achieve dynamic facial movement after undergoing functional muscle tendon unit transfer or free functional muscle transfer procedures. Given the unique features of the facial muscles, all effort must be made to reestablish innervation to denervated facial muscles long before they become irreversibly paralyzed.

66.5 Timing of Intervention

The duration of denervation of the facial muscle following VS is the most important factor that determines the ultimate success of any reinnervation procedure. With prolonged denervation, degenerative changes in facial muscles and connected nerves as well as mechanical barriers from scarring impair the ingrowth of axons and mechanical response of the contractile components.

The status of the facial nerve following tumor resection may be used as a guide when deciding how to time further management of the paralyzed face.

66.5.1 Management When Facial Nerve Continuity is Interrupted During Tumor Removal

In humans, the intricate network of nerve fibers connecting the motor cortex, limbic system, facial nucleus, and muscles is unique in projecting individual identities by maintaining facial form, characteristic animation, and emotional expression. Injury to the facial nerve results in changes to all components of this delicate network that cannot be adequately restored with any other cranial nerve. Therefore, whenever feasible, continuity of the facial nerve should be restored either by direct coaptation or via an interposition graft (see Chapter 64). This is usually performed at the time of tumor resection. The neurosurgeon and neurotologist should convey their confidence in the quality of nerve repair to the reconstructive team and in their operative report, as this information can influence the timing and type of any subsequent reconstruction. When there is expressed confidence in the quality of facial nerve repair, one may choose to wait for at least 6 months before offering further reanimation options if the outcome is not satisfactory. If, for various reasons, confidence in the quality of the repair is questionable, early nerve grafting with the masseteric nerve, or alternative donor nerves, connected to a single buccal branch may be performed keeping the main facial nerve uninterrupted. This allows early reinnervation of the facial muscles by masseteric axons and late reinnervation from the repaired facial nerve.

When intracranial coaptation of the facial nerve is not feasible, the facial muscles should be reinnervated using substitute cranial nerves as soon as possible, preferably within 3 months (▶ Fig. 66.2). The masseteric nerve can be transposed and coapted to the main facial nerve or a selected distal branch. A more proximal coaptation allows axonal growth through multiple buccal and zygomatic branches. To channel axonal growth into desired areas, unwanted side branches can be selectively sectioned to prevent axonal escape. With this approach, facial tone and excursion is restored within 3 to 6 months mostly to the upper lip elevators and eyelid. Simultaneously, single-stage cross-facial nerve grafting using a sural nerve can be performed to recruit facial nerve axons from the intact side allowing for emotional and spontaneous facial movement in addition to the motor input from the masseteric nerve.

66.5.2 Management When the Facial Nerve is Anatomically Intact following Tumor Resection

Advanced techniques in microsurgery have contributed to a high percentage (> 90%) of facial nerve preservation after cerebellopontine angle (CPA) tumor resection. Unfortunately, anatomic preservation of the facial nerve after tumor resection does not always result in acceptable facial function. In a study by Falcioni et al, 65% of patients who underwent CPA tumor resection regained normal, or near normal, facial nerve function (House–Brackmann [HB] I and II), and 29% reported a satisfactory facial nerve recovery (HB III) at 12 months.[19] However, in a subgroup of patients with preserved facial nerve

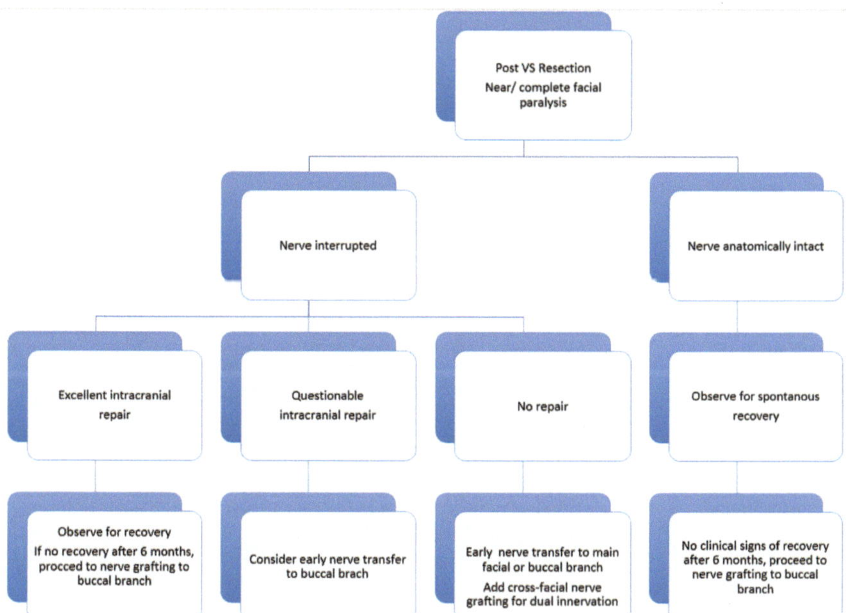

Fig. 66.2 Algorithm for facial rehabilitation following VS resection.

continuity, early postoperative facial nerve function is poor. In the study by Falcioni et al, poor functional recovery (HB IV, V, and VI) was reported in 6% of the study population.[19]

The patient who has complete or near-complete facial paralysis but an intact nerve presents a clinical conundrum. It is often recommended to observe for a period of 1 year for spontaneous recovery before intervening. This approach delays the timely intervention of a subset of patients who ultimately will not recover spontaneously. Prognosticating the pattern of facial nerve recovery has been the subject of many studies because of the quality-of-life implications and time-sensitive nature of any potential intervention. Several studies have failed to show strong correlation between long-term facial nerve recovery and tumor size, intraoperative response to nerve stimulation, intraoperative stimulation thresholds, and patient age, gender, and postoperative EMG findings.[20] In a study of 184 patients with facial paralysis after VS, Axon and Ramsden concluded that the severity of immediate postoperative clinical facial function was the most accurate predictor of long-term outcome.[21] In a review of 281 patients with an anatomically intact facial nerve following VS resection, Rivas et al found that for patients starting with a HB grade V or VI facial paralysis, the recovery rate was the most reliable predictor of poor outcome after 1 year. The resulting predictive model using rate of functional improvement as the independent variable was found to anticipate poor outcome before 1 year in more than 50% of cases with 97% sensitivity and 97% specificity. Based on this model, when a patient with an anatomically intact facial nerve and a HB V or worse facial paralysis shows no improvement of at least one HB grade after 6 months of observation, plans for nerve repair can be entertained.[22] Using this predictive model in selecting patients for early intervention, one study recorded zero premature surgical interventions based on the absence of EMG response to direct intraoperative stimulation of the intraparotid facial nerve at the time of nerve exploration for nerve grafting.[22] The same study also showed that without surgical intervention, facial nerve recovery in patients with postoperative HB V or VI will likely remain poor (best recovery HB V) even after a prolong period of observation when there was no clinical improvement over the first postoperative 6 months.

Other factors may influence the timing of reinnervation surgery in patients with facial paralysis after VS resection when facial nerve continuity is preserved. The presence of any degree of longstanding facial weakness prior to the VS resection should prompt consideration for early intervention. Preoperative facial weakness suggests prolonged facial nerve compression enough to result in clinically evident muscle denervation. Extended postoperative observation periods in such cases may irreversibly establish the effects of denervation.

66.6 Surgical Technique

66.6.1 Patient Positioning and Preparation

Patients are positioned and draped as is typical for parotid surgery. Electrodes are placed for EMG monitoring and all long-acting paralytic agents are strictly avoided. A preauricular incision is planned extending from the helical root to the infralobular region. Infiltration of 1:100,000 epinephrine only solution allows for local vasoconstriction without nerve blockade.

66.6.2 Identifying the Masseteric Nerve

Several reports have published landmarks for identifying the masseteric nerve. Borschel et al described the nerve to be located at the intersection of a vertical line 3 cm anterior to the tragus and a horizontal line 1 cm inferior to the zygomatic arch.[6] While this surface landmark is helpful in most cases, it may not be applicable in patients with distorted anatomy, course facial features, or in children. Recently, Collar et al described the subzygomatic triangle as a guide for identifying the masseteric nerve.[23] The subzygomatic triangle is demarcated by the inferior border of the zygomatic arch, a vertical line through the anterior margin of the temporomandibular joint (TMJ) and the temporal branch of the facial nerve (▶ Fig. 66.3, ▶ Fig. 66.4). A line bisecting the angle between the TMJ line and the zygomatic arch corresponds to the course of the masseteric nerve. The subzygomatic triangle relies on reproducible anatomic structures that overlie the sigmoid notch of the mandible through which the masseteric nerve leaves the infratemporal fossa to enter the deep aspects of the masseter muscle. The subzygomatic triangle is a reliable landmark that remains reproducible in children and adults of various ethnicities and facial dimensions.

The masseteric nerve is approached through a preauricular incision and SMAS flap elevated off the parotid capsule. Blunt dissection is used to identify and preserve branches of the facial nerve. Identifying the frontal and zygomatic branches of the facial nerve allows their safe mobilization and retraction to expose the subzygomatic triangle. Palpation of the soft-tissue depression over the sigmoid notch focuses the surgeon to the deep location of the masseteric nerve. To confirm that one is over the sigmoid notch, the surgeon can insert a needle directly in the outlined triangle. If the needle encounters bone, then one is either too anterior (coronoid), too posterior (condyle), or too inferior (mandibular ramus). The needle passes freely into the infratemporal fossa when one is over the sigmoid notch. Using a fine tip hemostat and dissecting layer by layer, fibers of the

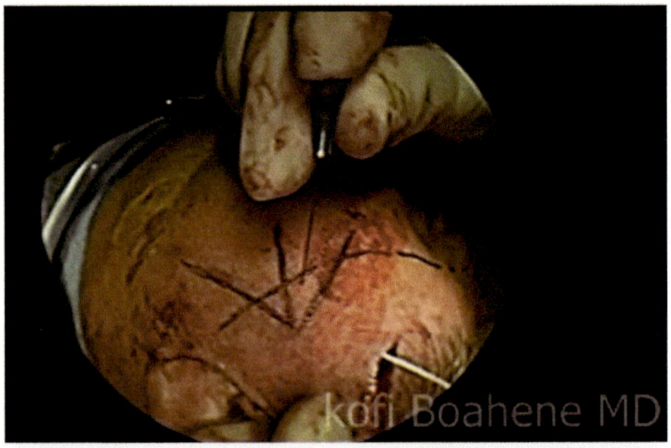

Fig. 66.3 Surface landmarks to the subzygomatic triangle for identifying the masseteric nerve. The inferior border of the zygomatic arch, the anterior margin of the temporomandibular joint, and the temporal branch of the facial nerve form the subzygomatic triangle.

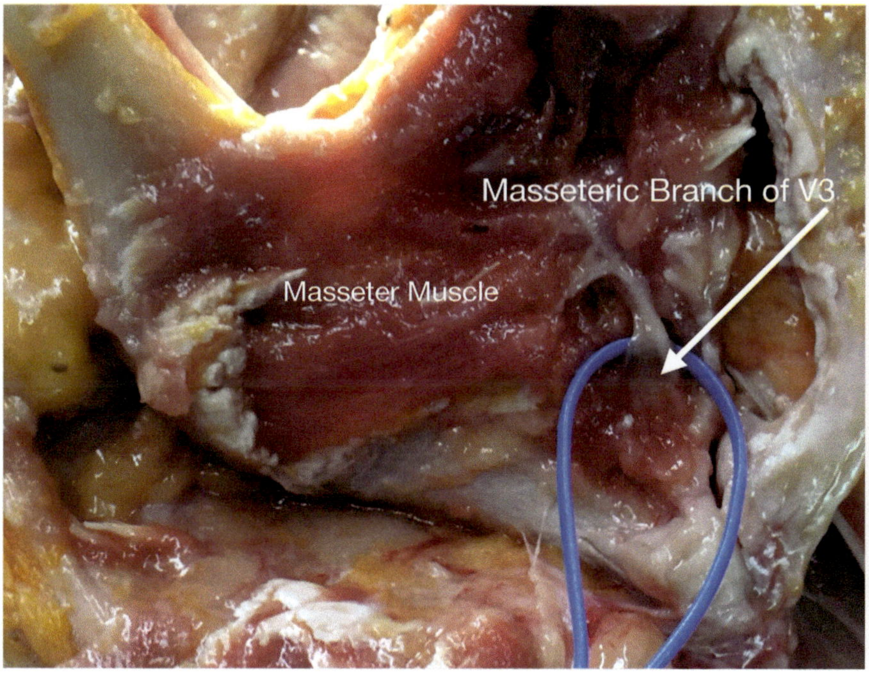

Fig. 66.4 Anatomy of the masseteric nerve and its relation to the temporomandibular joint and the zygomatic arch.

masseter muscle are carefully elevated and retracted. A narrow S-shaped retractor is ideal for this aspect of the dissection. As the dissection approaches the middle aspect of the masseter muscle, a shiny intramuscular tendon is exposed. The nerve is usually found just deep to this structure. At this level, a nerve stimulator may be used to confirm the location of the nerve. With this approach, it is unnecessary to broadly disrupt the parotid or a large segment of the masseter, as this can only complicate identification of the nerve. Limiting the dissection to the confines of the subzygomatic triangle narrows the search field. As one approaches the nerve, vessels accompanying the nerve may be encountered. Bleeding from these vessels will significantly obscure the surgical field and infiltration of epinephrine solution into the masseter muscle may assist in hemostasis. Should one encounter bleeding, it is preferable to achieve control with vasoconstrictor-soaked pledgets instead of cauterization, as the latter may cause thermal nerve injury. Once identified, a vessel loop is passed around the nerve for gentle retraction. The nerve can then be traced inferiorly until an adequate length is mobilized to allow direct coaptation to the intended target nerve. The nerve stimulator should be used at low settings (0.5 mA) to minimize early nerve conduction block, and the masseteric nerve should be kept intact and divided only when the surgeon is ready for coaptation to the facial nerve. Dividing the masseteric nerve too early can lead to frustrating minutes searching through a bloodied field should the nerve become displaced or retract.

66.6.3 Masseteric to Facial Nerve Coaptation

Once mobilized, the masseteric nerve is coapted to the facial nerve in an end-to-end configuration. The site of coaptation to the facial nerve is selected based on the branching pattern and desired outcome. For restoration of tone and dynamic contraction of the orbicularis oculi and upper lip elevator muscles, the zygomatic and buccal branches are the main targets for coaptation. Reinnervation of temporal and marginal branches is usually not clinically evident even when coaptation is performed to the main facial nerve branch. Excluding the cervical, marginal, and frontal branches helps concentrate the axons to the orbicularis oris and upper lip elevators.

66.7 Signal Upgrading with Masseteric Nerve Grafts

A subset of patients undergoing VS resection recover only partial facial nerve function and display inadequate eyelid closure, asymmetric commissure tone, and decreased lip excursion when smiling. These patients may be candidates for signal upgrading innervation using the masseteric nerve to increase the axonal input into the facial muscles. The concept of signal upgrading or supercharging relies on the presence of viable facial muscles with unoccupied neuromuscular receptors. Clinically, such patients show some muscle tone and contraction at rest but have increased resting muscle length (zygomaticus major) and hypotonus. Patients with hypertonicity (shortened zygomaticus major resting muscle length) but inadequate excursion are not good candidates for signal upgrading procedures (▸ Fig. 66.5).

66.8 Masseteric Nerve in Free Functional Muscle Transfer

In irreversible paralysis where the facial muscles have lost their contractile ability, the masseteric nerve can also be used to power a free functional muscle flap, such as the gracilis, for facial reanimation (see Chapter 67).[24,25,26,27,28,29] As a sole source of innervation, the masseteric nerve is reliable in powering a gracilis flap.

The masseteric nerve can also be combined with another nerve for dual innervation of the facial muscles or a transplanted

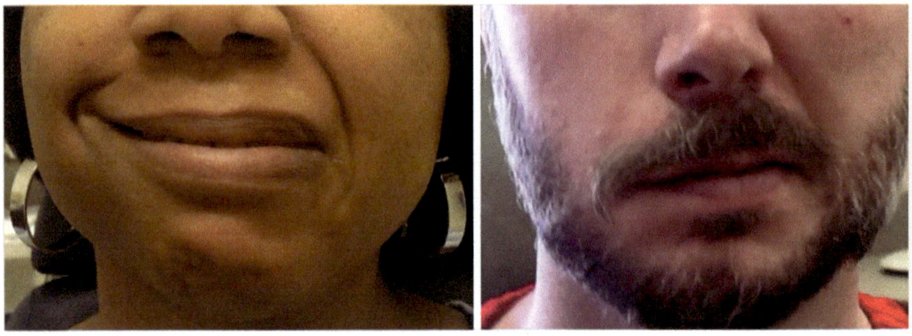

Fig. 66.5 Patients with partial facial nerve recovery and hypotonic muscles are candidates for signal upgrade nerve grafting (right photo). Signal upgrade nerve transfer is ineffective in patients with incomplete recovery and hypertonic muscle contracture (left photo).

gracilis muscle. When combined with a cross-facial nerve graft, the masseteric nerve provides reliable muscle tone and excursion, while the cross-facial nerve provides coordinated spontaneous movement with the unaffected side of the face.[30]

The dual use of the masseteric nerve together with a cross-facial nerve is somewhat similar to the "babysitter" concept described by Terzis in 1984. In the original "babysitter" procedure, an interposition graft from the hypoglossal nerve to the facial nerve is used to provide rapid neural input to the paralyzed facial muscle while waiting for axons to grow through a cross-facial nerve graft. The neural input from the hypoglossal nerve reduces the scaring and fibrosis that occurs in denervated muscles over time. The cross-facial nerve is then connected to the facial nerve at a second-stage procedure.[18] The masseter nerve can be used as a babysitter in conjunction with a cross-facial nerve graft in a two-stage procedure.[31] Single-stage cross-facial and masseteric nerve transfers performed simultaneously have also shown success.

66.9 Complications Related to the Use of the Masseteric Nerve in Facial Reanimation

The use of the masseteric nerve in facial reanimation is generally well tolerated even in cases of bilateral nerve sacrifice, and jaw function is rarely affected. Complete denervation of the masseter muscle may, however, result in facial asymmetry that may be obvious in thin-faced patients. Such asymmetries may be treated with fat grafting or use of facial fillers. Some patients complain of synkinetic eyelid contraction when chewing. This unwanted movement may be treated with selective chemodenervation or myectomy of the orbicularis oculi muscles.

66.10 Outcomes

Compared to the commonly used alternatives, such as the hypoglossal nerve and cross-facial nerve graft, the masseteric nerve provides a more rapid reinnervation and stronger axonal input resulting in better excursion. Hontanilla and Marré compared smile rehabilitation using the masseteric nerve to the hypoglossal nerve and reported stronger commissure excursion and faster onset of movement (62 vs. 132 days) with masseteric nerve transfer.[32] A similar study comparing facial rehabilitation using a gracilis muscle neurotized by the masseteric nerve versus cross-facial nerve graft showed that better commissure displacement was achieved with the masseteric nerve transfer.[33] A review of 60 patients by Bianchi et al using masseteric nerve for facial reanimation reported successful reinnervation in all cases.[34]

Physical therapy plays an important role in the eventual outcome following reanimation surgery. It provides a means of actively involving patients in their care and can improve symmetry and development of spontaneous smile.

66.11 Conclusion

Facial expression is a complex activity resulting from a delicate and complex symphony of communication between the brain and brainstem, transmitted to the facial muscle through the facial nucleus and facial nerve. Facial nerve injury resulting from VS resection cannot be completely corrected by any other cranial nerve. However, when performed in a timely fashion, the masseteric nerve provides an effective and reliable means of restoring both tone and voluntary facial motion to the paralyzed face.

References

[1] Conley J, Baker DC. Hypoglossal-facial nerve anastomosis for reinnervation of the paralyzed face. Plast Reconstr Surg. 1979; 63(1):63–72

[2] Escat E, Viela A. Manuel operatoire de l'anastomose du nerf facial avec le nerf masserterin. Ann Mal Oreille Larynx. 1925; 77:1149–1159

[3] Spira M. Anastomosis of masseteric nerve to lower division of facial nerve for correction of lower facial paralysis. Preliminary report. Plast Reconstr Surg. 1978; 61(3):330–334

[4] Klebuc M, Shenaq SM. Donor nerve selection in facial reanimation surgery. Semin Plast Surg. 2004; 18(1):53–60

[5] Boahene K. Facial reanimation after acoustic neuroma resection: options and timing of intervention. Facial Plast Surg. 2015; 31(2):103–109

[6] Borschel GH, Kawamura DH, Kasukurthi R, Hunter DA, Zuker RM, Woo AS. The motor nerve to the masseter muscle: an anatomic and histomorphometric study to facilitate its use in facial reanimation. J Plast Reconstr Aesthet Surg. 2012; 65(3):363–366

[7] Cotrufo S, Hart A, Payne AP, Sjogren A, Lorenzo A, Morley S. Topographic anatomy of the nerve to masseter: an anatomical and clinical study. J Plast Reconstr Aesthet Surg. 2011; 64(11):1424–1429

[8] Cruccu G. Intracranial stimulation of the trigeminal nerve in man. I. Direct motor responses. J Neurol Neurosurg Psychiatry. 1986; 49(4):411–418

[9] Coombs CJ, Ek EW, Wu T, Cleland H, Leung MK. Masseteric-facial nerve coaptation—an alternative technique for facial nerve reinnervation. J Plast Reconstr Aesthet Surg. 2009; 62(12):1580–1588

[10] Asaoka K, Sawamura Y, Nagashima M, Fukushima T. Surgical anatomy for direct hypoglossal-facial nerve side-to-end "anastomosis.". J Neurosurg. 1999; 91(2):268–275

[11] Frey M, Happak W, Girsch W, Bittner RE, Gruber H. Histomorphometric studies in patients with facial palsy treated by functional muscle transplantation: new aspects for the surgical concept. Ann Plast Surg. 1991; 26(4):370–379

[12] Brenner E, Schoeller T. Masseteric nerve: a possible donor for facial nerve anastomosis? Clin Anat. 1998; 11(6):396–400

[13] Manktelow RT, Tomat LR, Zuker RM, Chang M. Smile reconstruction in adults with free muscle transfer innervated by the masseter motor nerve: effectiveness and cerebral adaptation. Plast Reconstr Surg. 2006; 118(4):885–899
[14] Wang W, Yang C, Li Q, Li W, Yang X, Zhang YX. Masseter-to-facial nerve transfer: a highly effective technique for facial reanimation after acoustic neuroma resection. Ann Plast Surg. 2014; 73 Suppl 1:S63–S69
[15] Schaverien M, Moran G, Stewart K, Addison P. Activation of the masseter muscle during normal smile production and the implications for dynamic reanimation surgery for facial paralysis. J Plast Reconstr Aesthet Surg. 2011; 64(12):1585–1588
[16] Gasser RF. The development of the facial nerve in man. Ann Otol Rhinol Laryngol. 1967; 76(1):37–56
[17] Rozen S, Harrison B. Involuntary movement during mastication in patients with long-term facial paralysis reanimated with a partial gracilis free neuromuscular flap innervated by the masseteric nerve. Plast Reconstr Surg. 2013; 132(1):110e–116e
[18] Terzis JK, Tzafetta K. The "babysitter" procedure: minihypoglossal to facial nerve transfer and cross-facial nerve grafting. Plast Reconstr Surg. 2009; 123 (3):865–876
[19] Falcioni M, Fois P, Taibah A, Sanna M. Facial nerve function after vestibular schwannoma surgery. J Neurosurg. 2011; 115(4):820–826
[20] Silverstein H, Willcox TO, Jr, Rosenberg SI, Seidman MD. Prediction of facial nerve function following acoustic neuroma resection using intraoperative facial nerve stimulation. Laryngoscope. 1994; 104(5, Pt 1):539–544
[21] Axon PR, Ramsden RT. Intraoperative electromyography for predicting facial function in vestibular schwannoma surgery. Laryngoscope. 1999; 109(6): 922–926
[22] Rivas A, Boahene KD, Bravo HC, Tan M, Tamargo RJ, Francis HW. A model for early prediction of facial nerve recovery after vestibular schwannoma surgery. Otol Neurotol. 2011; 32(5):826–833
[23] Collar RM, Byrne PJ, Boahene KD. The subzygomatic triangle: rapid, minimally invasive identification of the masseteric nerve for facial reanimation. Plast Reconstr Surg. 2013; 132(1):183–188
[24] Henstrom DK. Masseteric nerve use in facial reanimation. Curr Opin Otolaryngol Head Neck Surg. 2014; 22(4):284–290
[25] Bermudez LE, Nieto LE. Masseteric-facial nerve anastomosis: case report. J Reconstr Microsurg. 2004; 20(1):25–30
[26] Biglioli F, Frigerio A, Colombo V, et al. Masseteric-facial nerve anastomosis for early facial reanimation. J Craniomaxillofac Surg. 2012; 40 (2):149–155
[27] Sforza C, Frigerio A, Mapelli A, et al. Facial movement before and after masseteric-facial nerves anastomosis: a three-dimensional optoelectronic pilot study. J Craniomaxillofac Surg. 2012; 40(5):473–479
[28] Alam DS, Haffey T, Vakharia K, et al. Sternohyoid flap for facial reanimation: a comprehensive preclinical evaluation of a novel technique. JAMA Facial Plast Surg. 2013; 15(4):305–313
[29] Harrison DH, Grobbelaar AO. Pectoralis minor muscle transfer for unilateral facial palsy reanimation: an experience of 35 years and 637 cases. J Plast Reconstr Aesthet Surg. 2012; 65(7):845–850
[30] Biglioli F, Colombo V, Tarabbia F, et al. Double innervation in free-flap surgery for long-standing facial paralysis. J Plast Reconstr Aesthet Surg. 2012; 65(10): 1343–1349
[31] Faria JC, Scopel GP, Ferreira MC. Facial reanimation with masseteric nerve: babysitter or permanent procedure? Preliminary results. Ann Plast Surg. 2010; 64(1):31–34
[32] Hontanilla B, Marré D. Comparison of hemihypoglossal nerve versus masseteric nerve transpositions in the rehabilitation of short-term facial paralysis using the Facial Clima evaluating system. Plast Reconstr Surg. 2012; 130(5): 662e–672e
[33] Hontanilla B, Marre D, Cabello A. Facial reanimation with gracilis muscle transfer neurotized to cross-facial nerve graft versus masseteric nerve: a comparative study using the FACIAL CLIMA evaluating system. Plast Reconstr Surg. 2013; 131(6):1241–1252
[34] Bianchi B, Ferri A, Ferrari S, Copelli C, Salvagni L, Sesenna E. The masseteric nerve: a versatile power source in facial animation techniques. Br J Oral Maxillofac Surg. 2014; 52(3):264–269

67 Gracilis Free Flap Rehabilitation of the Paralyzed Face in Vestibular Schwannoma

Samir Mardini and Marissa A. Suchyta

67.1 Introduction

In patients with vestibular schwannoma (VS), facial paralysis can be caused by compression of the facial nerve, traction or transection of the nerve during tumor resection, or as a rare complication of stereotactic radiosurgery (SRS). Temporary and permanent facial paralysis imparts significant social and psychological consequences. Facial expression is an integral aspect of social integration and communication, leading healthy individuals to state that they would be willing to sacrifice eight years of life to correct unilateral facial paralysis.[1] Free gracilis muscle transfer is one surgical approach to restore dynamic and spontaneous facial expression when salvaging native facial muscles is not possible or when the results of nerve transfers or cross-face nerve grafting have yielded suboptimal outcomes.

Gracilis free muscle transfer was first utilized by Pickrell et al in 1952 for rectal sphincter reconstruction.[2] In 1976, Harii and colleagues utilized the gracilis muscle to restore facial animation, coapting the muscle to the deep temporal branch of the trigeminal nerve so that a smile was elicited upon biting.[3] Reanimating the smile using a one-stage procedure has been performed, commonly utilizing the motor branch to the masseter to innervate the gracilis, and continues to have a role when cross-face nerve grafting is likely to yield poor outcomes. Mostly, this is true for older patients where reinnervation from the contralateral side is slower and less optimal,[4] in patients with bilateral facial paralysis for whom cross-face nerve grafting is not possible, or in patients who may develop paralysis on the contralateral side due to neurofibromatosis type 2 or other causes.[5]

In 1990, the two-stage cross-face nerve graft technique was pioneered by Thompson and Gustavson.[6] A cross-face nerve graft utilizing the sural nerve is coapted to branches of the contralateral functional facial nerve. The sural nerve graft is tunneled under the skin of the upper lip, and buried in the subcutaneous tissue for 6 to 12 months followed by the second stage, where the gracilis muscle is transferred to restore smile function through upper lip elevation and lateral and upward movement of the oral commissure. Cross-face nerve grafting enables axonal fibers from the facial nerve to traverse the nerve graft to the nonfunctional side of the face. In the second stage of the procedure, a free muscle flap is harvested and inset into the paralyzed face and coapted to the previously placed cross-face nerve graft. The initial report of the cross-face nerve graft utilized an extensor digitorum free flap.[7] Terzis described the pectoralis minor as a favorable muscle for facial reanimation,[8] particularly in children, and later Harrison and Grobbelaar published a large series on the use of this muscle for reanimating the paralyzed face.[9] In 1990, O'Brien and colleagues pioneered utilizing the gracilis free muscle transfer in the second stage of the procedure.[10] Pairing a cross-face nerve graft procedure with gracilis free muscle transfer enables restoration of dynamic and spontaneous facial animation. Despite the advantages of the pectoralis minor, the gracilis free muscle transfer is more commonly used due to the ease of harvest and the ability to easily work in two teams.

In patients younger than 60 years with unilateral facial paralysis who are willing to undergo a two-stage procedure, the authors recommend cross-face nerve grafting followed by a gracilis muscle transfer in a second stage, as the spontaneity is clearly better than the one-stage procedure utilizing the branch to the masseter. More recently, we have been performing cross-face nerve grafting and, in the second stage, when the gracilis muscle transfer is performed, we transfer the branch to the masseter to the cross-face nerve graft in an end-to-side fashion to improve strength (see Chapter 66).[11]

67.2 Advantages and Limitations of This Surgical Approach and Rationale for Use

The gracilis free flap has several distinct advantages when utilized for facial reanimation. The muscle has consistent anatomy with a reliably located neurovascular pedicle. Following some debulking, its size and volume are ideal for use in the face. Furthermore, two teams can work simultaneously to harvest the flap and prepare the recipient site, thus reducing operative time. Flap harvest does not create a functional deficit and the donor site is closed primarily leaving a discrete scar on the medial thigh.[12] The proximal attachment of the fascia to the pubic bone can be harvested with the flap and utilized to anchor to the upper lip as described by Terzis and Karypidis.[13] This provides thin tissue at the upper lip and solid tissue capable of suture retention (▶ Fig. 67.1). A skin island can be harvested with the flap and utilized to augment an external or intraoral soft-tissue defect.[14] These positive aspects of gracilis transfer have made it most surgeons' preference for free muscle transfer for facial reanimation.

67.3 Patient Evaluation and Selection

The timing and approach of facial reanimation intervention following VS resection is critical. There are three distinct clinical subgroups of patients presenting with facial palsy following VS resection: the first has completely reversible facial paralysis, with viable facial muscle fibers that will respond to reinnervation by ingrowing nerve axons. These patients have polyphasic action potentials on needle electromyogram (EMG), demonstrating active facial nerve regeneration and the presence of healthy facial muscles.[15] If the facial nerve is anatomically disrupted in these patients, nerve repair, supplementary nerve grafting, or cross-face nerve grafting should be performed as soon as possible to minimize muscle denervation time. If the facial nerve is anatomically intact, the patient should first be observed for spontaneous recovery.

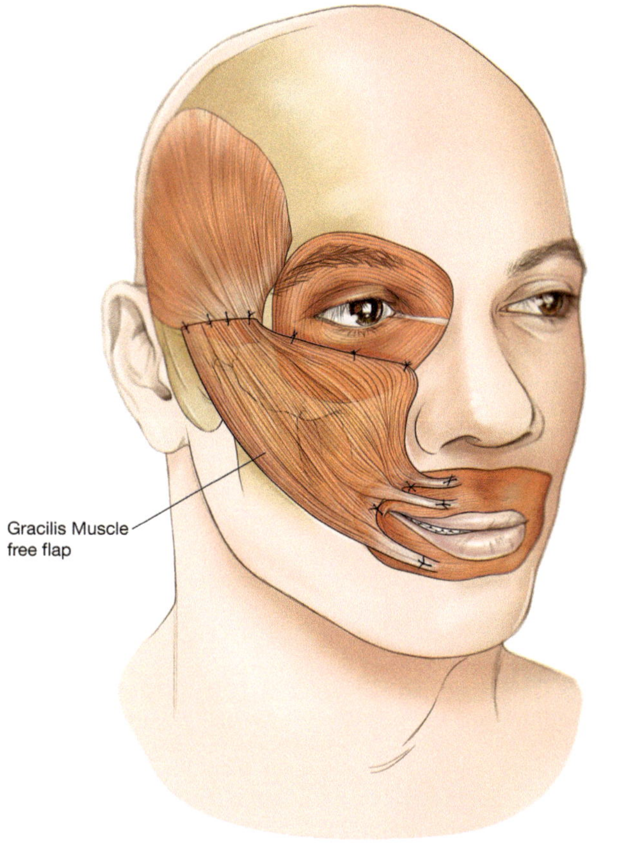

Fig. 67.1 Illustration of the inset of a gracilis muscle used to reanimate smile function.

The timing of facial nerve reanimation is a controversial issue. The most common recommendation is to wait for 1 year for spontaneous recovery in cases of facial paralysis with an intact facial nerve. This decision is based on many reports that intraoperative and postoperative electrodiagnostic tests are not reliable enough to predict facial nerve functional status 1 year after VS surgery. However, one disadvantage of this standard approach is that a long waiting period delays nerve grafting and often yields inadequate functional outcomes, ultimately requiring further procedures to achieve the desired final outcome. Long delays lead to loss of motor endplate function of facial muscles.[16] A different approach has been proffered which utilizes a predictive model introduced by Rivas and colleagues, based on an outcomes review of 281 patients. They recommended determining the intervention timeline based on the rate of recovery during the 6 months following VS resection.[17] This model recommends planning for nerve repair at 6 months for patients with anatomically intact facial nerves and a House–Brackmann (HB) grade V or worse who show no improvement of at least one grade at 6 months. This model is also supported by Albathi et al, who advocated for intervention at 6 months should there be no clinical sign of reinnervation.[18] Neither of these most recent studies advocating intervention at 6 months incorporate postoperative EMG findings, but rather are solely based on clinical recovery rates.

The second clinical subgroup of patients presents with completely irreversible damage to the facial muscles as a result of long-standing denervation. Many of these patients had intact facial nerves following resection, with the expectation of spontaneous muscle function recovery. Patients in this subgroup likely have dysfunctional facial muscle contractile units, atrophic muscle fibers, and loss of muscle satellite cells, and thus would be unresponsive to reinnervation attempts.[19] These patients show no EMG potentials, yielding what is commonly called a "silent EMG." This subgroup is best treated with a free-muscle transfer or a regional muscle transfer to replace the nonfunctional muscles. In this subgroup, the timing of intervention depends on convenience to the patients. There is no true urgency to performing the surgery, as the denervation of the facial muscles is permanent. This subgroup is the focus of this chapter. Smile restoration with a gracilis muscle transfer,[20] in a two-stage procedure, innervated by a cross-face nerve graft, is our preferred method of reconstruction. We also perform, in select patients, a gracilis free muscle transfer in one stage innervated by the branch to the masseter.

The third clinical subgroup of patients are those who present with partial recovery of facial nerve function, which leads to a more complex decision regarding intervention. These patients have muscle function but weakness that can be addressed through additional innervation via nerve grafting or through functional muscle transfer. Additional reinnervation procedures, through supplementary nerve grafting or cross-face nerve grafting, may be considered in this subgroup of patients who present with poorly defined melolabial folds, droopy oral commissure and eyelids, but some evidence of muscle movement upon attempted facial expression.[21] For nerve transfers to be considered, fibrillations on EMG should be present. Nevertheless, even in patients with the above-mentioned criteria, it is not clear which patients will do well enough with nerve transfers that they will not require further reconstruction. Muscle transfer, alternatively, should be performed when patients present with a stable result for over 1 year and in patients without evidence of fibrillations on EMG. Rarely, muscle transfer could also be considered in patients with severe spastic muscle function or synkinesis. These patients have hypercontracted levator and zygomatic muscles, manifesting as exaggerated melolabial folds, and no excursion upon attempted smile.[21]

Functional muscle transfer, including gracilis free muscle transfer, is indicated in patients who present with complete irreversible facial paralysis from long-term muscle denervation and in patients with partial recovery of facial nerve function, for whom nerve grafting is not expected to yield improvement.

67.4 Relevant Anatomy Specific to Approach

Gracilis, derived from the Latin word *gracile*, meaning slender, is a thin, strap-like muscle located most superficially in the thigh adductor group. The muscle's origin is at the pubic symphysis, medial and posterior to the adductor longus muscle tendon. The adductor longus tendon can be palpated in the medial thigh in front of the pubis when the patient is in the frog leg position. The gracilis has a wide origin, from the inferior ramus of the pubis to the lower symphysis. It lies posterior to the sartorius and anterior to the semitendinosus in its lower half. Its insertion onto the medial tibial condyle is immediately posterior to the sartorius muscle. The gracilis muscle size is dependent on the size and build of the patient and averages 30 cm long, 5 to 8 cm wide proximally (3–4 cm in children), and 3 cm thick.[22] The muscle tapers superiorly to inferiorly.

The dominant vascular pedicle of the gracilis muscle flap is the branch of the medial femoral circumflex artery or a direct branch from the profunda femoris artery.[23,24] This dominant pedicle enters the medial aspect of the muscle between the adductor longus and adductor magnus at approximately 10 cm inferior to the pubic tubercle. The gracilis muscle also has a minor pedicle in the distal half of the muscle, which is a branch from the superficial femoral artery (▶ Fig. 67.2), and in 10% of cases a branch from the descending genicular artery also supplies this flap.[25] The dominant pedicle has two vena comitantes that are located alongside the artery, draining into the profunda femoris vein either separately or by converging into a common vein.[26]

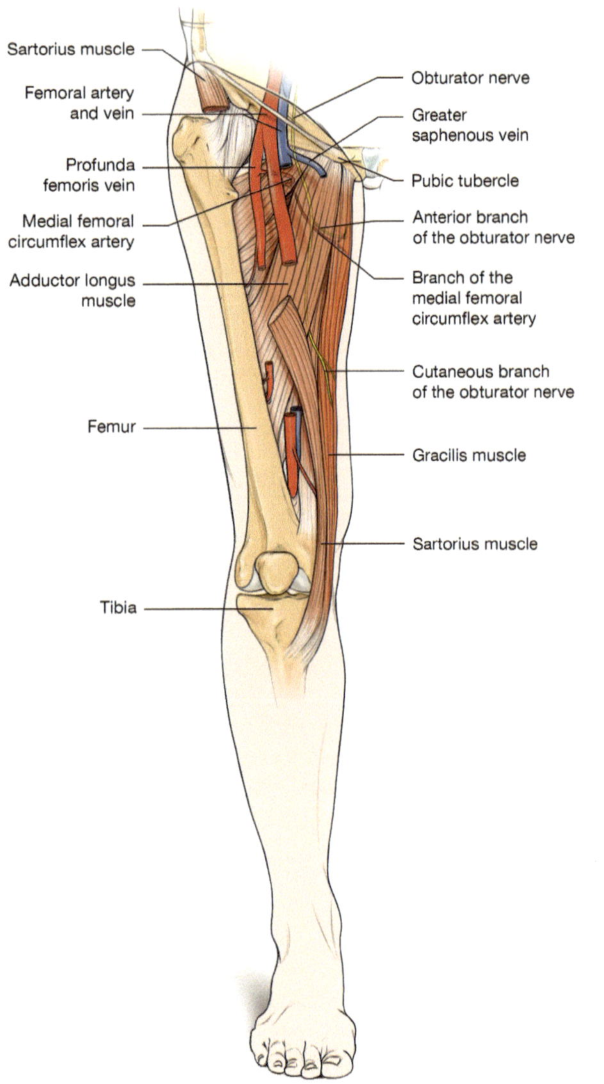

Fig. 67.2 Anatomy of the gracilis muscle.

The single motor nerve of the gracilis is the anterior branch of the obturator nerve. This enters the gracilis on the medial surface 1 to 2 cm superior to the vascular pedicle (6–7 cm from the pubic tubercle). The nerve has an average of three fascicles, and often divides into two branches that supply the superior and inferior muscle.[27] The bifurcation of the nerve is located, on average, 2 cm proximal to the vascular bifurcation. The superior branch is usually the larger branch, and runs first transverse then inferior and posterior. The inferior branch runs parallel to the anterior muscle border, with a mean distance of 2 cm from this edge.[28] This anatomical bifurcation has been utilized to divide the gracilis into two separate motor units upon free muscle transfer.[29]

The gracilis muscle functions to flex the knee and adduct the thigh. However, there is no functional deficit noticed clinically following removal of the muscle. The scar is usually around 10 to 15 cm and inconspicuously placed on the medial aspect of the thigh. By performing meticulous reapproximation of the superficial fascia of the thigh as well and by taking breaks from retracting the skin during the harvest, excellent scar healing can be expected.

67.5 Surgical Technique

67.5.1 Gracilis Muscle Flap Harvest

Preoperatively, the patient is photographed in repose and while smiling, so that the vector of the smile on the functional side of the face can be mirror imaged onto the affected side. In the sitting position, prior to being put under anesthesia, the nasolabial crease and the vector of the smile are marked on the normal side. On the affected side, the vector of the smile is marked based on the normal side. The harvest and inset procedures are performed with the patient under general anesthesia via orotracheal intubation. The endotracheal tube is sutured to one of the lower teeth on the nonaffected side so that the lips are not distorted and access can be gained to the midline of the upper and lower lips. The patient is placed in the supine position and prepped and draped widely. We use the contralateral thigh, and the gracilis is rotated 180 degrees after harvest so that the proximal fascia of the gracilis is attached to the upper and lower lips and the distal part of the gracilis is sutured to the deep temporal fascia and preauricular region (▶ Fig. 67.1). The leg to be used is placed in the "frog-leg" position and the surgeon stands on the contralateral side. A line is drawn marking the course of the adductor longus. The gracilis lies posterior to the adductor longus. Therefore, a parallel line is marked 2 to 3 cm posterior to the posterior margin of the adductor muscle (▶ Fig. 67.3). The incision starts 5 cm distal to the pubic crease and is extended approximately 10 to 15 cm, depending on the size of the patient and the gracilis to be harvested. We like to be able to access the public bone to get the entire length on the fascia of the gracilis, yet we do not want to place an incision close to the crease.

The incision is made through the skin and subcutaneous tissue down to the fascia lata, avoiding injury to the greater saphenous vein, which lies anterior to the incision. The fascia lata is incised over the adductor longus muscle, and the dissection is then continued posteriorly until the septum between the adductor and the gracilis is reached. This septum must be included in the flap if a skin island is to be harvested. The

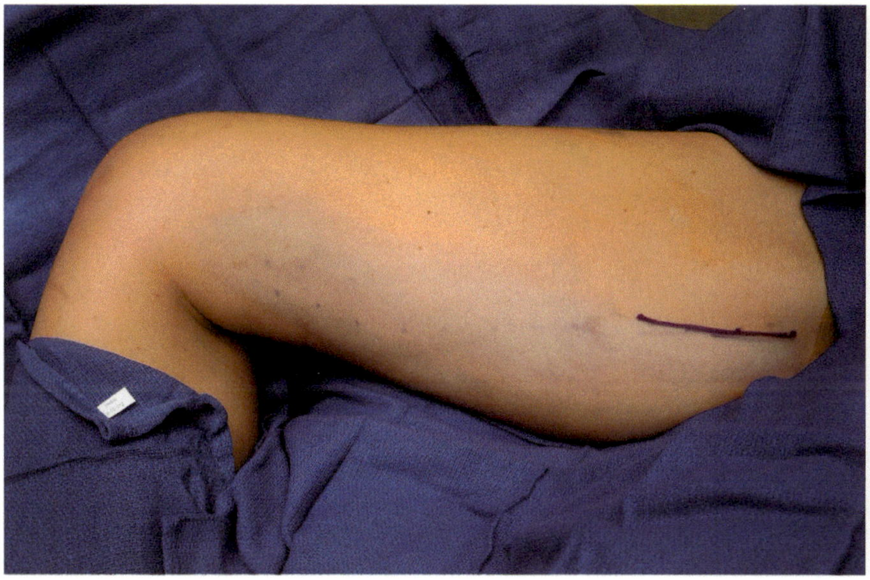

Fig. 67.3 The incision is marked 2 to 3 cm posterior to the posterior edge of the adductor longus muscle. The incision starts 5 cm distal to the groin crease and extends 10 to 15 cm distally.

adductor longus muscle is retracted anteriorly and the pedicle of the gracilis muscle is exposed. In adults, the vascular pedicle enters the muscle at a 90-degree angle 8 to 10 cm inferior to the pubic tubercle. The plane between the adductor longus and gracilis is created and as the dissection is carried deeper, the plane between the adductor longus and magnus is created and the pedicle as well as the branch of the obturator nerve is exposed. A second pedicle is visualized distally if the dissection is carried out beyond the middle of the thigh. Exposure of the gracilis muscle is performed to the pubic tubercle proximally and approximately 15 to 20 cm distally depending on the size of the gracilis needed for the reconstruction. The muscle is dissected circumferentially throughout this length taking care not to injure the epimysium of the muscle. Interfering with the epimysium may lead to pitting of the skin if a thin skin flap in the cheek becomes tethered to the muscle fibers. We prefer not to thin the muscle on its anterior surface to avoid this tethering. If the facial skin flaps are thick, this becomes less of a concern. Next, the muscle is circumferentially dissected, and the vascular pedicle is dissected proximally until adequate length is achieved. In our experience, harvesting the full length of the vessels is preferable to avoid issues during the inset. Usually, the vascular pedicle is dissected proximally until its takeoff from the deep femoral artery and vein. The obturator nerve is dissected proximally until the obturator foramen. Interfascicular dissection is required to separate the branch to the gracilis from the obturator nerve's other anterior branches to adductor longus and brevis. The nerve can be stimulated to elicit contraction of the gracilis muscle.

Several 4–0 absorbable sutures are placed in two rows on the superficial aspect of the muscle—one row at the anterior border and another row 2 to 3 cm posterior (▶ Fig. 67.4). This will allow accurate restoration of *in situ* tension and length during inset in the face. The pedicle, nerve, and muscle body are then divided. Two-thirds of the muscle circumference is harvested to help avoid bulk in the cheek. When the branch to the masseter is used to innervate the gracilis, less muscle can create stronger

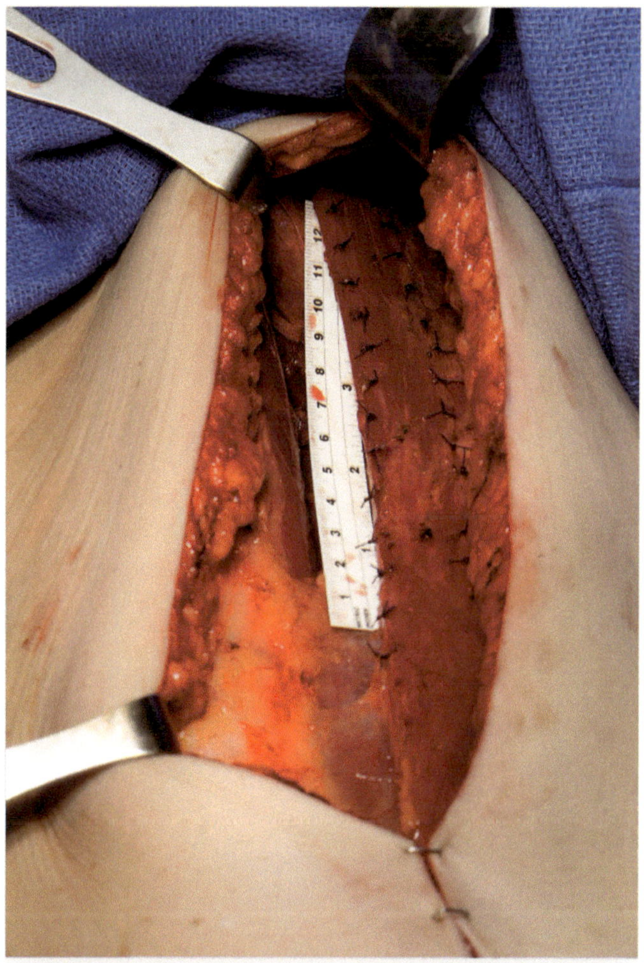

Fig. 67.4 After exposure and dissection of the gracilis muscle, absorbable sutures are placed in two rows at the anterior surface of the gracilis muscle, one row at the superior border and another row 2 to 3 cm posterior to the anterior border.

excursion; therefore, we are more comfortable using less muscle in that situation. The template created in the face (*explained in the following section on recipient site preparation*) is used to mark the size of the gracilis to be taken (▶ Fig. 67.5). The proximal end of the muscle is removed from the bone using electrocautery. The distal end is transected using a gastrointestinal stapler. This allows for hemostasis as well as a solid structure to suture around during the inset. The muscle is transferred to the face. If a stapler is not available, a running locking suture with a 4–0 permanent monofilament suture can be performed. This distal end of the muscle is inset into the lateral aspect of the face, and the staples are deep and unlikely to create problems with extrusion or palpability.

67.5.2 Donor Site Management

Taking the anterior two-thirds of the muscle leads to an ideal harvested gracilis weight of 10 to 30 g depending on the size of the patient. The muscle is ideally sculpted in situ to minimize ischemia time. When the face has been fully dissected, the nerve is cut and the vessels are ligated and transected. After hemostasis is achieved, a drain is placed, and the fascia lata is loosely approximated, followed by approximation of the superficial fascia of the thigh. The skin is closed using interrupted dermal sutures followed by a running subcuticular suture.

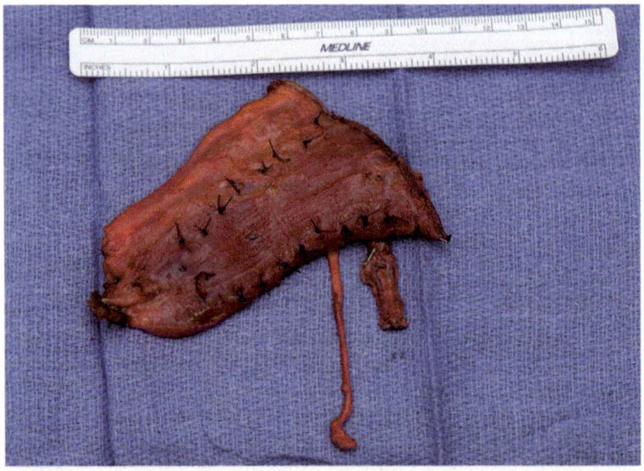

Fig. 67.5 The gracilis muscle is sculpted according to the template created using a sterile towel. In this image, the gracilis muscle has been rotated 180 degrees and oriented the way it will be inset. The thin proximal fascia can be seen on the left of the image.

67.5.3 Recipient Site Preparation

A modified Blair incision is extended to immediately below the mandible (▶ Fig. 67.6). A deep subcutaneous flap is elevated to the anterior border of the parotid, and then the SMAS is incised. The dissection continues in this plane until the oral commissure and nasolabial fold are reached, exposing the zygomatic arch and malar eminence as well as, medially, the orbicularis oris. We perform the dissection medially to the philtral column of the upper lip and the midline of the lower lip. The fascia of the gracilis muscle is inset at those points to centralize the midline of the upper and lower lips. Buccal fat is removed as needed to make room for the added bulk of the muscle flap, thereby creating the pocket where the muscle will be inset. In the case of a two-stage procedure, the cross-face nerve graft stump is identified where it was anchored in the first stage of the procedure (▶ Fig. 67.7). If a one-stage procedure is being performed, the masseteric nerve is identified under the zygomatic arch.

Mersilene sutures of 2.0 are used for the anchoring medially and laterally. Zuker and Bains used 0–0 Vicryl sutures for the same purpose with excellent results.[22] The sutures are placed in the lower lip, commissure, upper lip, philtrum, alar base, and inferior to the medial and lower canthi along the infraorbital rim and zygoma body (▶ Fig. 67.8). Proper suture placement is crucial to achieving good outcomes, as placement of these sutures determines the subsequent smile vectors and successful facial symmetry. Tension is placed on the sutures to mimic the contralateral smile (▶ Fig. 67.9). We spend as much time as needed replacing these sutures until we are completely satisfied with the smile achieved. Care is taken to avoid eversion or inversion of the lip as well as notching. A smooth pull and con-

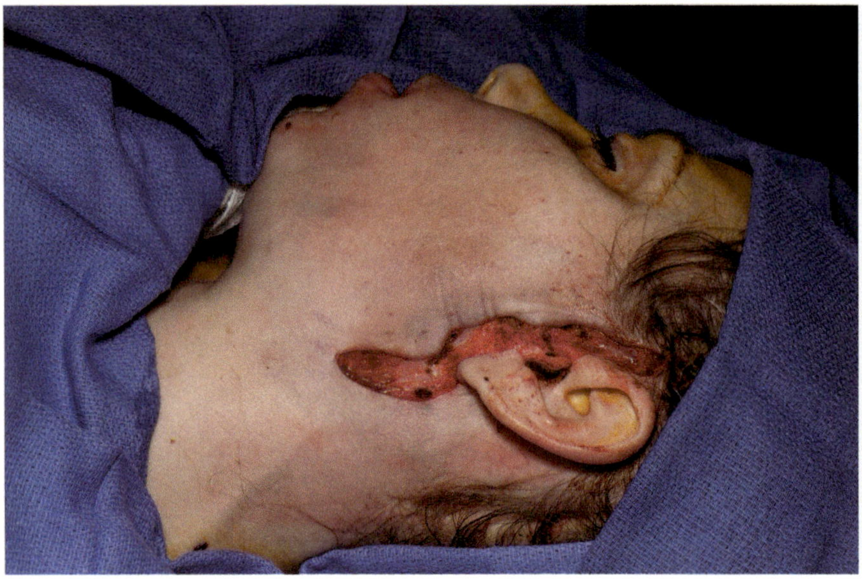

Fig. 67.6 On the paralyzed side of the face, a modified Blair incision is extended below the mandible.

tour as well as proper vector is needed for optimal results. On validation that suture placement provides the ideal smile, the measurements for the gracilis muscle are made with the commissure and lips in the proper position to match the contralateral normal side in repose. Using these measurements, a template of the desired muscle shape in the face is created from a sterile operative towel to guide tailoring of the gracilis muscle and the muscle is harvested (▸ Fig. 67.10). In order to avoid muscle bulk over the zygoma, we expose the bone through an incision in the periosteum 1 cm anterior to the root of the helix, elevating the periosteum, and burring the arch and zygoma body to create symmetry.

The tailored muscle is brought into the field, and the previously placed sutures are anchored to the muscle fascia and tied down (▸ Fig. 67.1). The lateral aspect of the gracilis is then retracted laterally until the previously placed tension-adjusting

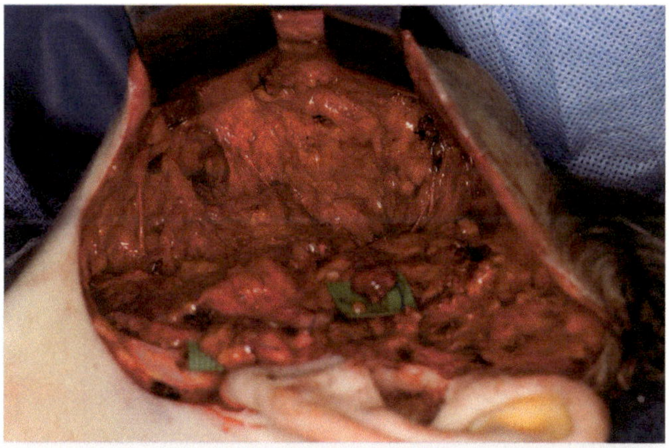

Fig. 67.7 The facial flaps are elevated in a deep plane. The cross-face nerve graft has been identified and protected, see *green* backgrounds. We have two cross-face nerve grafts: the upper one on the right is for smile animation and the lower one on the left of this image will be used in the future for lower lip animation (not discussed in this chapter).

sutures are restored to 1 cm apart (▸ Fig. 67.11). Once the muscle is restored to the appropriate length, it is sutured to the deep temporal fascia superior to the zygomatic arch and to the SMAS anterior to the upper part of the ear. The vector determines the location of the anchoring of the muscle laterally. The oral commissure and nasolabial fold should be slightly overexaggerated, as slight relaxation is expected to occur postoperatively.

The vascular pedicle is passed toward the lower border of the mandible and the microvascular anastomoses are then performed. The arterial anastomosis is performed with 10–0 nylon suture, and the venous anastomosis is completed with a Synovis Coupler. The obturator branch is approximated to the cross-face nerve graft or the branch to the masseter. Previously, we placed the cross-face nerve graft in the gingivobuccal sulcus and performed the neurorrhaphy in the sulcus through a gingivobuccal sulcus incision. Over the last 3 years, we have been passing the cross-face nerve graft all the way to the preauricular region to be able to use the branch to the masseter in an end-to-side fashion to the cross-face nerve graft when needed. The neurorrhaphy is performed close to the muscle to minimize denervation time.

Once the muscle is reperfused, microstimulation of the obturator nerve is performed. This stimulation helps determine whether the position of the muscle is optimal. Hemostasis is achieved and a Penrose drain is placed at the most dependent portion of the wound lateral to the pedicle. The incision is closed with interrupted dermal sutures followed by simple interrupted 4–0 nylon sutures (▸ Fig. 67.12).

67.6 Complications of the Gracilis Free Flap and Management

Complications are uncommon in gracilis free flap muscle transfers for facial reanimation. The most common complication is a hematoma presenting in a small percentage of patients. When swelling in the cheek is detected, this is managed in a couple of

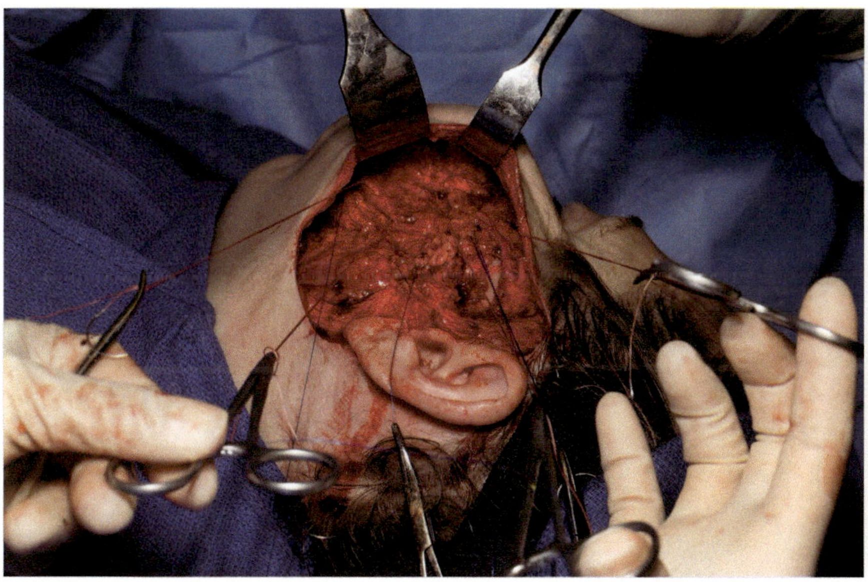

Fig. 67.8 Sutures are placed in the lower lip, commissure, upper lip, philtrum, alar base, and inferior to the medial and lower canthi along the infraorbital rim and zygoma body.

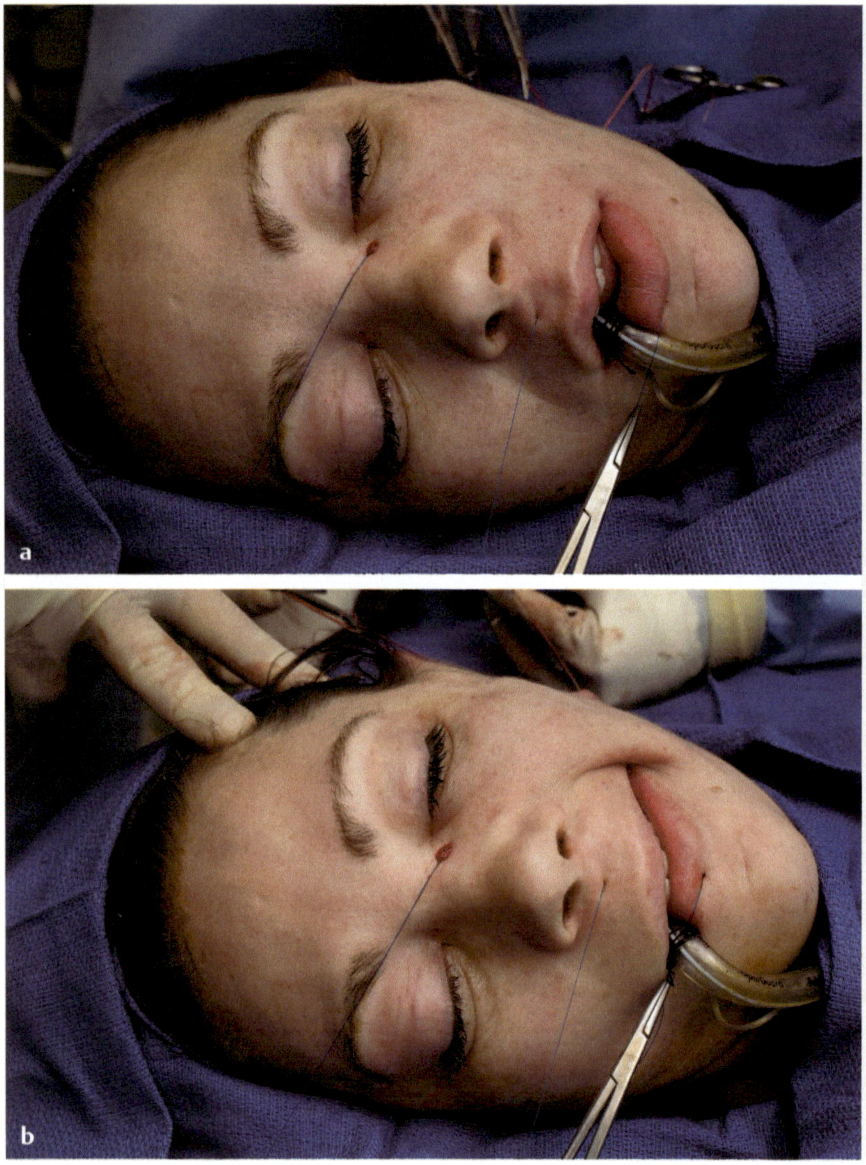

Fig. 67.9 (a, b) Tension is placed on the sutures to mimic the contralateral smile. The Prolene sutures seen in this image are used to anchor a component of the fascia to the center of the upper and lower lips and the upper suture is used to help provide lip elevation by bringing a part of the muscle medially.

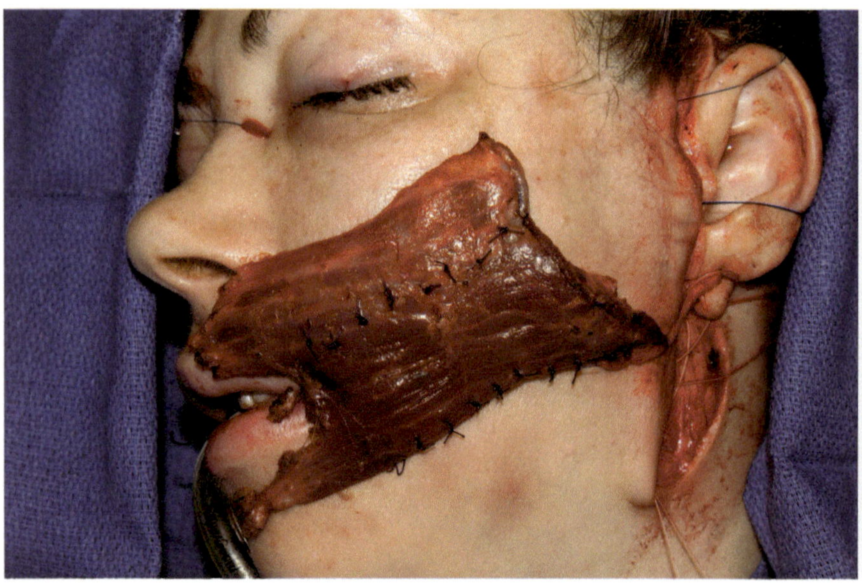

Fig. 67.10 The muscle is tailored to the desired shape. A smooth contour and optimal vector are needed for this procedure to yield the optimal outcome. The tailoring occurs in the leg prior to harvest. This image demonstrates the inset for easier visualization.

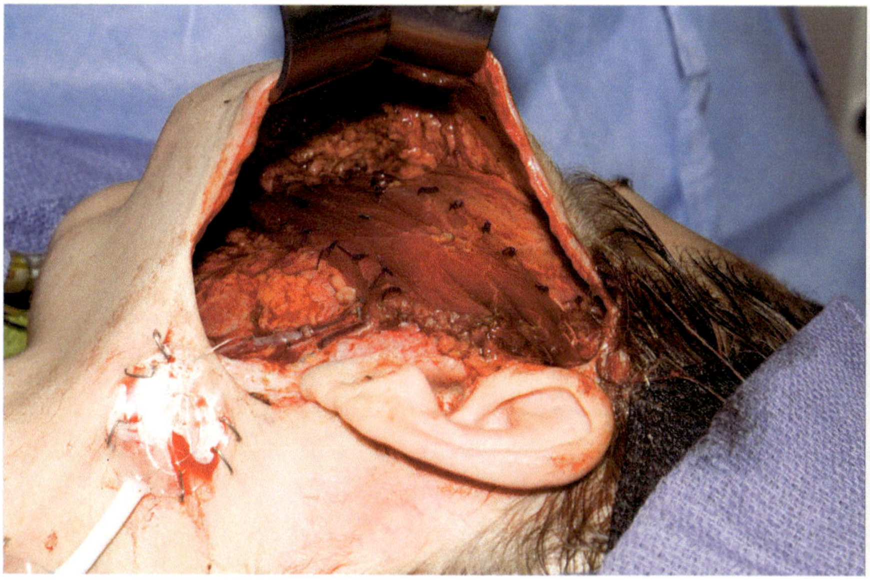

Fig. 67.11 The gracilis muscle after inset and microvascular anastomosis of the artery and vein. A cook Schwartz implantable Doppler is placed for postoperative monitoring.

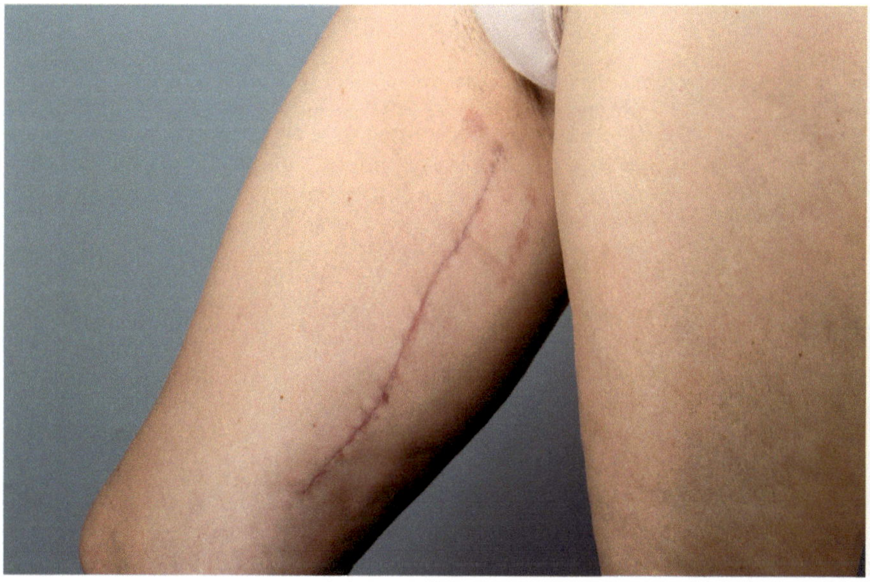

Fig. 67.12 Donor site at 7 months post-gracilis free muscle transfer. The incision in this patient was extended beyond what is necessary to harvest the flap.

ways depending on the clinical signs. If the cheek size is rapidly expanding and/or there is vascular compromise detected by Doppler examination, operative intervention is required immediately. If the cheek size is stable, and the artery and vein of the flap are patent, we obtain an ultrasound urgently and evaluate the cheek with a radiologist to make the best decision. A member of the surgical team is present during the ultrasound evaluation to determine the exact location and volume of the hematoma and its effect on the vessels. This has helped avoid reexplorations in cases where the clinical swelling is due more to tissue edema than a hematoma. This also allows an attempt at ultrasound-guided drainage when feasible. When surgical evacuation is deemed necessary, evacuation is performed without delay and with extreme caution to avoid compression of the pedicle, which could lead to thrombosis, as well as to avoid compromise of the overlying skin. There should be no hesitation in performing reexploration if there is any doubt about vessel patency or flap viability. It is critical to identify problems early, as flap salvage can be successful in more than 80% of patients. Hematomas can also occur at the thigh harvest site, which also require prompt drainage. Hematomas following gracilis free muscle transfer for facial reanimation were estimated to occur at an average rate of 3.6% by systematic review of the literature.[30]

Microvascular failure of the transferred gracilis muscle is not common; however, vascular spasm can occur. Although it is a rare complication, venous insufficiency is generally a greater concern than arterial thrombosis. This can be identified by swelling and firmness of the muscle before a Doppler signal change occurs.[31] Vascular compromise is estimated to occur at an average rate of 1.4%.[32]

Infections are rare, and all patients are given perioperative antibiotics which are continued for 5 days. Studies have demonstrated an average infection rate of 3.5% requiring debridement or further antibiotic treatment. Lee and colleagues reported six infections in a cohort of 107 patients undergoing gracilis free muscle transfer.[32] All of these patients were on prophylactic clindamycin or a clindamycin combination therapy, which indicates that clindamycin may not provide sufficient antimicrobial coverage in this case. None of the patients on ampicillin–sulbactam in this study had postoperative infections, suggesting that utilizing ampicillin–sulbactam as a perioperative single agent may provide necessary broader coverage and be the most effective first-line prophylaxis.

67.7 Revision Surgery

Some patients require debulking procedures, revision of the inset (changing the vector), repositioning of the oral commissure and lip sutures, and correction of rippling in the skin. The most common revision needed is for patients with lateralization of the nasolabial fold and for removal of excessive bulk. An estimated 10 to 20% of patients require a subsequent surgery to debulk the flap or reposition the nasolabial fold.[25] Facial swelling resolves over the first 6 to 12 weeks. Over time, the muscle atrophies because of its limited muscle load, moving the lips and not the leg. Therefore, further reduction in cheek bulk occurs over the first year following surgery. The most common cause of lack of function is inadequate donor nerve due to a poor first-stage cross-face nerve grafting procedure.

67.8 Technical Pearls and Pitfalls

67.8.1 Gracilis flap harvest:

- Keep the skin incision at least 3 to 5 cm away from the groin crease.
- Preserve the epimysium of the gracilis muscle to avoid ripples in the facial skin after inset.
- Harvest the entire length of the vascular pedicle even when you think you have enough recipient vessel length.
- During the process of dissecting the pedicle, you should visualize a large branch supplying the adductor muscle. Prior to placing a clip on the branch and cutting, make sure you can see the other side of the gracilis pedicle.
- Harvest two-thirds of the muscle leaving behind the posterior one-third. Nerve branches supplying the posterior third of the muscle can be placed into the anterior two-thirds of the muscle as a direct neurotization.
- Occasionally, during the harvest, relax skin and muscle retraction to reperfuse the tissues.

67.8.2 Recipient site preparation and flap inset:

- Raise thick skin flaps in the face to avoid contour issues and visible ripples that can occur from abnormal attachment of the muscle to the skin.
- To decrease muscle bulk over the zygoma, the bone can be reduced by burring. If the patient has absent function of the frontal and zygomatic branches of the facial nerve, soft tissue overlying the zygomatic arch can be removed. If the patient has function of the frontal and zygomatic branches, the zygoma arch can be approached through a subperiosteal dissection from lateral to medial and then burring of the bone can ensue.
- Dissect the facial artery and facial vein distally up to the level of the oral commissure. This will allow for the pedicle of the flap to reach the facial vessels. When the proximal fascia of the gracilis is used to anchor to the lips (as we describe in this chapter), the pedicle of the gracilis may end up more lateral than desired which could create a situation where the pedicle cannot reach the facial vessels. In that situation, the superficial temporal vessels are used as recipient vessels.
- During recipient site preparation, do not damage the superficial temporal vessels in case they may be needed for microvascular anastomoses.

67.9 Clinical Case Example

A 36-year-old woman presented 7 years following initial diagnosis of a left-sided VS (▸ Fig. 67.13). She underwent her first resection shortly after diagnosis, which resulted in a mild left facial paresis followed by near-complete recovery. Due to residual tumor, she then had a subsequent resection the following year, which resulted in a complete left facial paralysis. A gold weight was placed in her left eyelid prior to presentation to our center. She presented with further enlargement of the residual tumor at the fundus of the internal auditory canal, which was treated with Gamma Knife radiosurgery.

An EMG study was performed, which demonstrated electrophysiological evidence of severe left facial neuropathy with unobtainable left compound action potentials. Needle examination demonstrated atrophic facial nerve innervated muscles with some, though minimal, reinnervation of only the mentalis muscle.

Due to the long-standing nature of her facial paralysis, we performed cross-face nerve grafting followed by a gracilis muscle transfer. The obturator nerve was anastomosed to the cross-face nerve graft. We used an additional nonvascularized nerve graft to connect the branch to the masseter to the cross-face nerve graft. The branch to the masseter provides nerve fibers to augment the function of the gracilis. During the first stage of cross-face nerve grafting, the patient also underwent a left canthopexy with the use of a mini-palmaris tendon as described by Terzis and Kyere.[33]

At 6 months, the patient began to have a spontaneous smile and 3 weeks later she felt she had movement with biting. The patient had excellent function and symmetry of the smile. However, she had significant asymmetry of the lower lip function and was not interested in Botox injections.

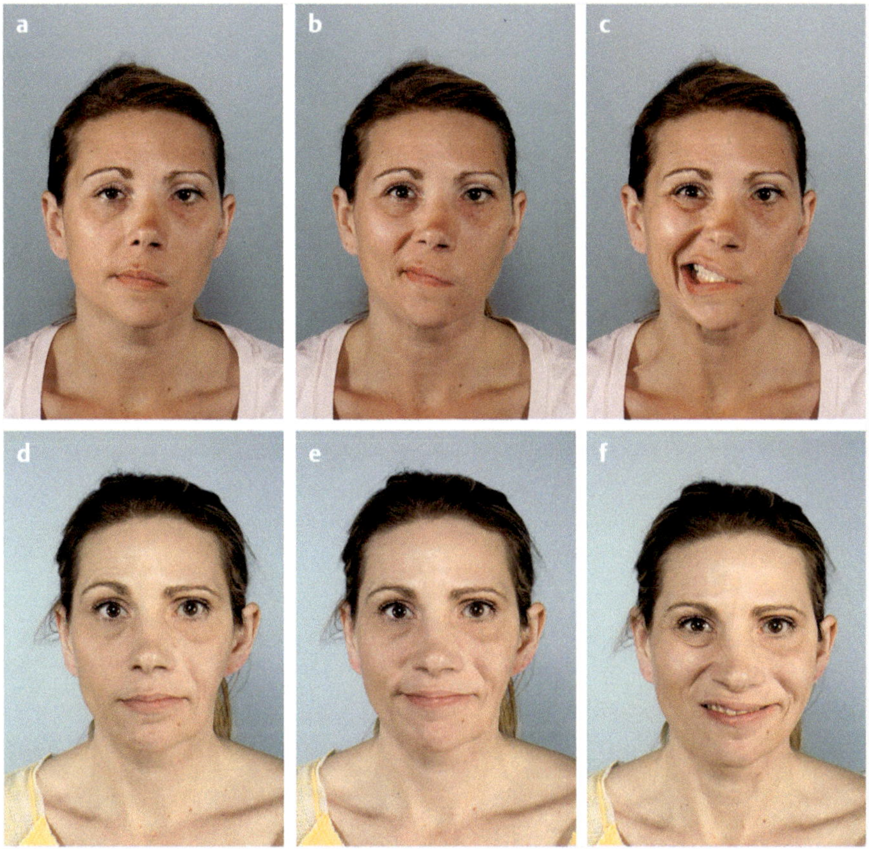

Fig. 67.13 Preoperative views of the patient (**a**) in repose, (**b**) soft smile, and (**c**) a full smile. Postoperative result at 15 months showing the patient (**d**) in repose, with (**e**) a soft smile and (**f**) a full smile.

References

[1] Sinno H, Thibaudeau S, Izadpanah A, et al. Utility outcome scores for unilateral facial paralysis. Ann Plast Surg. 2012; 69(4):435–438

[2] Pickrell KL, Broadbent TR, Masters FW, Metzger JT. Construction of a rectal sphingter and restoration of anal continence by transplanting the gracilis muscle. Ann Surg. 1952; 135(6):853–862

[3] Harii K, Ohmori K, Torii S, Harii K. Free gracilis muscle transplantation, with microneurovascular anastomoses for the treatment of facial paralysis. A preliminary report. Plast Reconstr Surg. 1976; 57(2):133–143

[4] Verdú E, Ceballos D, Vilches JJ, Navarro X. Influence of aging on peripheral nerve function and regeneration. J Peripher Nerv Syst. 2000; 5(4):191–208

[5] Evans DGR, Lye R, Neary W, et al. Probability of bilateral disease in people presenting with a unilateral vestibular schwannoma. J Neurol Neurosurg Psychiatry. 1999; 66(6):764–767

[6] Thompson N, Gustavson EH. The use of neuromuscular free autografts with microneural anastomosis to restore elevation to the paralysed angle of the mouth in cases of unilateral facial paralysis. Chir Plastica Chirurgia Plastica. 1976; 3(3):165–174

[7] Vedung S, Hakelius L, Stålberg E. Cross-face nerve grafting followed by free muscle transplantation in young patients with long-standing facial paralysis. Reanimation of the cheek and the angle of the mouth. Scand J Plast Reconstr Surg. 1984; 18(2):201–208

[8] Terzis JK. Pectoralis minor: a unique muscle for correction of facial palsy. Plast Reconstr Surg. 1989; 83(5):767–776

[9] Harrison DH, Grobbelaar AO. Pectoralis minor muscle transfer for unilateral facial palsy reanimation: an experience of 35 years and 637 cases. J Plast Reconstr Aesthet Surg. 2012; 65(7):845–850

[10] O'Brien BM, Pederson WC, Khazanchi RK, Morrison WA, MacLeod AM, Kumar V. Results of management of facial palsy with microvascular free-muscle transfer. Plast Reconstr Surg. 1990; 86(1):12–22, discussion 23–24

[11] Mardini S. Dual innervation of the Gracilis muscle for facial reanimation. To be submitted

[12] Carr MM, Manktelow RT, Zuker RM. Gracilis donor site morbidity. Microsurgery. 1995; 16(9):598–600

[13] Terzis J, Karypidis D. Facial reanimation: evolution and refinements. In: Wei FC, Mardini S, eds. Flaps and Reconstructive Surgery. Elsevier; 2016:162–192

[14] Chuang DC, Mardini S, Lin SH, Chen HC. Free proximal gracilis muscle and its skin paddle compound flap transplantation for complex facial paralysis. Plast Reconstr Surg. 2004; 113(1):126–132, discussion 133–135

[15] Cannaday S, Wax M, Friedman O. Facial nerve paresis and paralysis. In: Wax MK, ed. Facial Paralysis: A Comprehensive Rehabilitative Approach. San Diego, CA: Plural Publishing; 2015:11–26

[16] Knott PD. A facial nerve anniversary—twelve months of treatment time saved. JAMA Facial Plast Surg. 2016; 18(1):60–61

[17] Rivas A, Boahene KD, Bravo HC, Tan M, Tamargo RJ, Francis HW. A model for early prediction of facial nerve recovery after vestibular schwannoma surgery. Otol Neurotol. 2011; 32(5):826–833

[18] Albathi M, Oyer S, Ishii LE, Byrne P, Ishii M, Boahene KO. Early nerve grafting for facial paralysis after cerebellopontine angle tumor resection with preserved facial nerve continuity. JAMA Facial Plast Surg. 2016; 18 (1):54–60

[19] Boahene K. Reanimating the paralyzed face. F1000Prime Rep. 2013 Nov 1;5:49

[20] Lindsay RW, Bhama P, Weinberg J, Hadlock TA. The success of free gracilis muscle transfer to restore smile in patients with nonflaccid facial paralysis. Ann Plast Surg. 2014; 73(2):177–182

[21] Boahene K. Facial reanimation after acoustic neuroma resection: options and timing of intervention. Facial Plast Surg. 2015; 31(2):103–109

[22] Fu SY, Gordon T. Contributing factors to poor functional recovery after delayed nerve repair: prolonged denervation. J Neurosci. 1995 May;15(5 Pt 2):3886-95

[23] Juricic M, Vaysse P, Guitard J, Moscovici J, Becue J, Juskiewenski S. Anatomic basis for use of a gracilis muscle flap. Surg Radiol Anat. 1993; 15(3):163–168

[24] Magden O, Tayfur V, Edizer M, Atabey A. Anatomy of gracilis muscle flap. J Craniofac Surg. 2010; 21(6):1948–1950

[25] Azizzadeh B, Pettijohn KJ. The gracilis free flap. Facial Plast Surg Clin North Am. 2016; 24(1):47–60

[26] Papadopoulos O, Georgiou P, Christopoulos A, Sandris P. The gracilis flap revisited. Eur J Plast Surg. 2000; 23(8):413–418

[27] Mckee NH, Fish JS, Manktelow RT, Mcavoy GV, Young S, Zuker RM. Gracilis muscle anatomy as related to function of a free functioning muscle transplant. Clin Anat Clinical Anatomy. 1990; 3(2):87–92

[28] Hassan KM, El-Moghazy AE, Mahmoud MA, El-Oteify M. Study of Neurovascular Anatomy of the Split Gracilis Muscle for the Purpose of Facial Reanimation. Egypt J Plast Reconstr Surg. 2009; 33(2):261-269

[29] Rodríguez Lorenzo A, Morley S, Payne AP, Tollan CJ, Soutar DS. Anatomy of the motor nerve to the gracilis muscle and its implications in a one-stage microneurovascular gracilis transfer for facial reanimation. J Plast Reconstr Aesthet Surg. 2010; 63(1):54–58

[30] Garcia RM, Gosain AK, Zenn MR, Marcus JR. Early postoperative complications following gracilis free muscle transfer for facial reanimation: a systematic review and pooled data analysis. J Reconstr Microsurg. 2015; 31(8):558–564

[31] Banks CA, Hadlock TA. Pediatric facial nerve rehabilitation. Facial Plast Surg Clin North Am. 2014; 22(4):487–502

[32] Lee LN, Susarla SM, Henstrom DK, et al. Surgical site infections after gracilis free flap reconstruction for facial paralysis. Otolaryngol Head Neck Surg. 2012; 147(2):245–248

[33] Terzis JK, Kyere SA. Minitendon graft transfer for suspension of the paralyzed lower eyelid: our experience. Plast Reconstr Surg. 2008; 121(4):1206–1216

68 Static Procedures for Rehabilitation of the Paralyzed Face in Vestibular Schwannoma

Daniel L. Price

68.1 Introduction

Static procedures, once the mainstay of rehabilitation of the paralyzed face, have been relegated to the back seat in the era of dynamic gracilis free flaps and nerve transfer. Despite the measurable benefit of dynamic procedures, static procedures represent a critical and often central element in the rehabilitation of the paralyzed face. Static procedures can be used in patients who are not candidates for dynamic reconstruction, whether they are unfit for more involved surgical procedures, the lack of adequate patient resources for dynamic reconstruction, or the experience of the surgeon. They can also be used as adjuncts to dynamic procedures, particularly dynamic temporalis procedures or gracilis free flaps, which provide a unidirectional vector of excursion, and do not address the complex features of facial expression. Finally, they can provide resting symmetry and immediate functional benefit during the lengthy process of recovery and regeneration from procedures requiring neural regeneration and retraining.

The primary goals of facial reanimation are three-fold: (1) to restore facial symmetry, (2) to replace deficient facial volume due to atrophy and loss of static suspension of facial structures, and (3) most importantly to restore facial function necessary for vision, globe protection, nasal breathing, and oral function for competence and articulation. Management of the eye after facial paralysis is discussed in Chapter 63, gracilis free muscle transfer in Chapter 67, and nerve substitution techniques in Chapters 65 and 66. The focus of this chapter will be procedures designed to restore form and function to the mid and lower face.

68.2 Anatomy

The nasalis muscle is the most developed of the nasal muscles (▶ Fig. 68.1). It consists of the compressor naris (transverse) and dilator naris (alar). The compressor naris runs vertically from the canine eminence to pair with the same muscle of the contralateral side and extends to an aponeurosis of the procerus muscle. The paired contraction results in the depression of the cartilaginous portion of the nose and contraction of the ala toward the septum. The dilator naris muscle originates in the subnasal fossa and inserts in the cartilaginous ala of the nose.

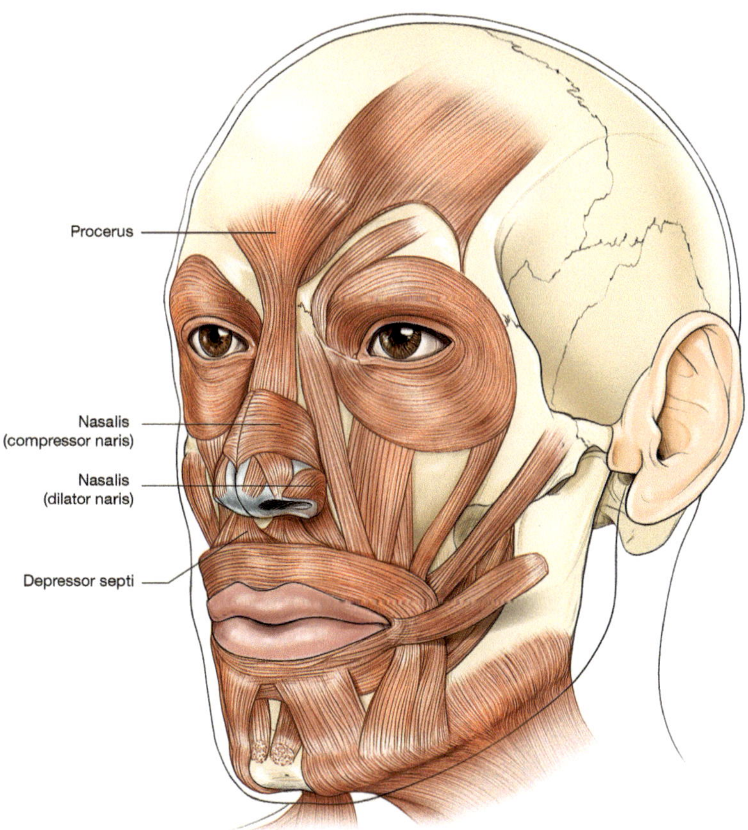

Fig. 68.1 The nasal muscles of facial expression.

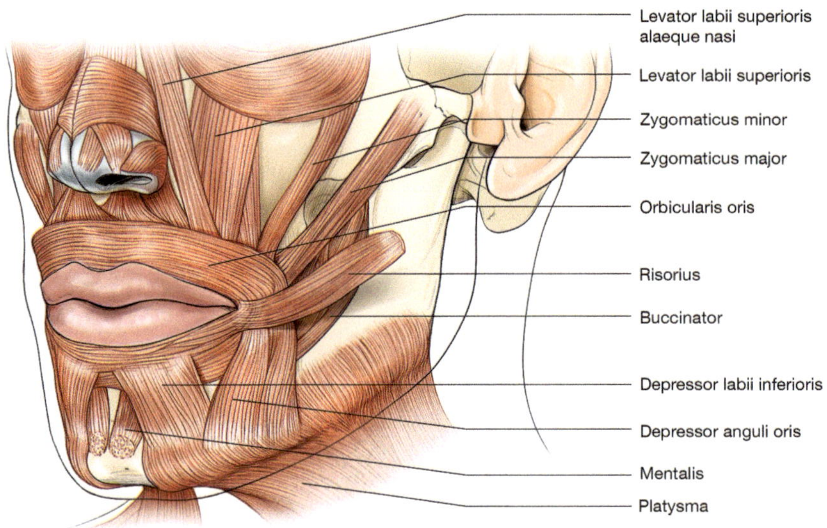

Fig. 68.2 Muscles of facial expression, mid and lower face.

The nasal slip of the levator labii superioris alaeque nasi serves as a dilator of the nares, originating on the frontal process of the maxilla. In flaccid facial paralysis, nasal asymmetry and functional collapse also occur secondary to the absence of tone and the effects of gravity resulting in medial and inferior displacement of the alar base. Notably no muscles insert directly into the alar base with an oblique lateral trajectory, and maneuvers to correct this portion of facial deformity should be tailored with this in mind.[1]

Progressing clockwise around the mouth are the five upper lip elevators (levator labii superioris alaeque nasi, levator labii superioris, zygomaticus minor, levator anguli oris, and zygomaticus major); the risorius, which laterally retracts the commissure; three depressors (platysma, depressor anguli oris, and depressor labii inferioris); and the mentalis muscle, which elevates the lower lip (▶ Fig. 68.2). The orbicularis oris muscle forms a circumferential sphincter around the mouth. The two levator labii muscles act primarily to elevate and evert the upper lip. The levator anguli oris originates on the canine fossa of the maxilla just below the infraorbital foramen, deepening the nasolabial fold. The zygomaticus major originates on the medial zygoma and inserts into the skin and mucosa of the corner of the mouth as part of the modiolus, drawing it upward and laterally, and with the levator anguli oris, raises the angle of the mouth to form the nasolabial fold. The zygomaticus minor muscle originates just medial to the major muscle, and is not part of the modiolus, and elevates and everts the lip.[1]

The depressor anguli oris and depressor labii inferioris depress the angle of the mouth and lower lip, respectively, along with the platysma muscle. The mentalis muscle has the paradoxical function of raising and everting the lower lip, as well as elevating the skin of the chin.[1]

68.3 Materials

A wide variety of tissues and materials have been described for static facial slings, including autologous fascia lata or palmaris longus tendon, cadaveric fascia lata, suture suspension, acellular dermis products, expanded polytetrafluoroethylene (Gore-Tex), crystalline polypropylene and high-density polyethylene (Marlex), and silicone rods. Each option has its advantages and disadvantages. The issue of relaxation or stretching is frequently cited as an advantage of one material over another over time, though it would appear that this issue exists for all materials, and no side-by-side comparisons have clearly demonstrated one to be superior over another with regard to this aspect.[3,4]

Autologous tendon has the distinct advantage of lower risk of infection, rejection, or reaction. Tensor fascia lata (TFL) can be easily harvested in sufficient quantity from one side to provide for several reconstructive needs. The incisions can be minimized to limit deformity at the donor site.[5] It has the disadvantage of the time for harvest and the donor site is frequently complicated by seroma formation. In a radiated field, TFL or palmaris longus tendon should be used. The TFL originates from the lateral surface of the lateral iliac crest and inserts on the condyle of the tibia. It serves as a minor hip flexor and abductor.[2] The palmaris longus tendon is a small tendon arising from the medial epicondyle of the humerus and inserts on the flexor retinaculum, and is variably absent in approximately 14% of the population.[6]

Acellular dermis has the advantage of being readily available with no donor-site morbidity. It is less likely to result in infection, but still carries the risk of local reaction or infection.[7] A weakness but potential utility of acellular dermis is that it will frequently reabsorb, and can therefore be used for temporary suspension when neural recover is anticipated.[8]

Gore-Tex and Marlex also share the advantage of being off-the-shelf products with no associated donor-site morbidity. Gore-Tex has been noted to relax significantly over time, and carries a risk of infection, granulation formation, and extrusion, and should be avoided in patients with poor wound healing potential or in radiated tissue.[9]

68.4 Goals of Static Reconstruction

The goals for static mid and lower face reconstruction are to: (1) restore nasal external valve dimensions, alar height, and lateral position; (2) restore the nasolabial fold, philtral position, and oral commissure symmetry and oral competence; (3) provide lower lip bulk and symmetric position; (4) and improve symmetric facial tone with rhytidectomy.

68.5 Timing of Static Reconstruction

Timing of static reconstruction has much greater flexibility than neural coaptation procedures that may become less successful with increasing time. Correction of the nasal valve and alar position can be done at any time after onset of facial paralysis without significant risk of permanent injury or need for reversal. Static lower face resuspension carries both the risk of facial nerve injury and the need for reversal should normal function return. It is therefore typically reserved for patients in whom permanent paralysis is confirmed or expected.

68.6 External Nasal Valve Correction and Alar Position

External valve restoration can be managed with the use of alar batten grafts with or without the concomitant use of spreader grafts using septal cartilage, conchal cartilage, or other sources of autologous or cadaveric cartilage. While these maneuvers will improve nasal airflow, they will not correct the inferomedial displacement of the alar base associated with flaccid facial paralysis.[10] This displacement can be addressed with the use of suspension sutures or fascial grafts. If fascia is being used for other purposes, this is our preferred material. A 1-cm alar incision and temporal incisions are fashioned and connected via a subcutaneous tunnel. A 5-mm strip of fascia is first secured to the alar cartilage at the lateral base with nonabsorbable monofilament suture and the alar incision is closed. The strip is then tunneled laterally where it is secured. This tension should be gentle—minor changes will improve nasal breathing, and major changes will lead to nasal flattening. Lindsay et al described improved quality-of-life outcomes with securing the fascia to the true temporalis fascia.[10] The author prefers a more medial securing stitch to the malar eminence 2 cm lateral to the infraorbital foramen. This more superiorly oriented vector closely recreates the natural alar forces generated by the levator muscles, and prevents flattening of the ala. Concomitant use of alar batten grafts can mitigate this deformity as well. Alternatively, a bone-anchored suture provides a reliable, straightforward technique for external valve correction. Mitek bone-anchored sutures (1.3 mm Micro Quick Anchor, Ethicon) come in a variety of sizes with nonabsorbable suture attached to a small anchor, which is easily implanted into bone. Small (3–5 mm) incisions are made at the ala and implant site, and a subcutaneous tunnel between them fashioned. The anchor hole is drilled 2 cm lateral to the infraorbital foramen and the anchor inserted flush with the bone surface. The suture should be pulled up from the bone to ensure solid placement, and a dislocated anchor should be discarded and a new implant placed securely. One suture is then passed to the alar incision, passed through the alar cartilage, and back to the implant, where the sutures are tied to the appropriate tension.

68.7 Nasolabial Fold and Oral Commissure Repositioning and Restoration

Static and semidynamic options exist for the management of the oral commissure and nasolabial fold when nerve reanimation or dynamic reconstruction is not an option. Static procedures can also be used to improve immediate asymmetry and prevent stretching while waiting for recovery after reinnervation or dynamic reconstruction. Again, while many materials are available for reconstruction, fascia lata is available in abundance, has very low risk of infection, can be used for a variety of issues associated with facial paralysis, and can provide a lasting reconstruction. Temporalis muscle and fascia have been used in both the antidromic (temporal origin transferred to commissure)[11] and orthodromic (coronoid insertion transferred to oral commissure),[12] as well as a lengthening temporalis myoplasty (Labbé Procedure)[13] and can provide an immediate dynamic result in some cases. Both the antidromic temporalis transfer and lengthening temporalis myoplasty involve significant mobilization of the temporalis muscle, often resulting in temporary paresis of the muscle. The antidromic temporalis transfer until very recently was the most popular technique for reanimation. It has several drawbacks, however, including nonanatomical orientation of the muscle, fullness over the zygoma as the muscle was delivered over it, and hollowing of the temporal defect. Because superior options now exist, it has little role currently. Orthodromic temporalis transfer was originally described by McLaughlin in 1952, once again demonstrating that there is nothing new under the sun.[14] The procedure involves removal of the coronoid process with the temporalis insertion and transfer to the modiolus of the oral commissure. This can provide immediate postoperative dynamic function for patients and with training can result in a spontaneous smile.[15] The coronoid can be approached via a parotid/face lift incision, via a nasolabial incision, or transorally.[14,15] Division of the anterior masseter fibers or removal of the zygoma can facilitate exposure, but is rarely required. The nasolabial incision provides direct access to the muscle with minimal disruption of normal tissue. When the nasolabial crease is not prominent, a buccal sulcus incision is made. Through this incision, dissection is made through the buccal fat to the coronoid process. Caution is exercised to avoid penetration of the oral mucosa. Manipulation of the mandible and palpation with a right angle clamp identifies the mandibular notch. Deep retractors are placed medial and lateral to the coronoid process (▶ Fig. 68.3). The coronoid process is divided as low as possible with a reciprocating sagittal saw. The cut is angled obliquely superior to detach maximal tendon and finish the osteotomy at the inferior aspect of the notch. Prior to the completion of the cut, the tendon and bone are grasped with an Allis clamp to prevent retraction and facilitate distraction to the site of inset.[16] The tendon can then be directly inset into the modiolus, though this does not give the ideal smile contour, as it stretches the paralyzed lip, creating an elongated, thin lip. When insetting to the modiolus, two holes are either drilled through the coronoid process with a wire-passing bur, or the bone is removed and the tendon sutured directly to the modiolus. 2–0 nonabsorbable monofilament sutures are used to secure the temporalis to the modiolus

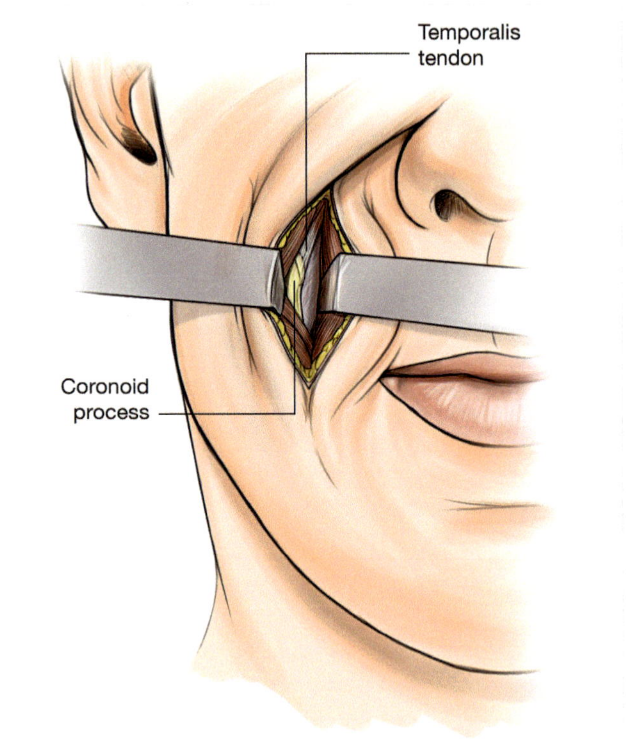

Fig. 68.3 Access to the coronoid process and temporalis tendon for orthodromic temporalis tendon transfer (coronoid insertion transferred to oral commissure) via melolabial incision.

with a horizontal mattress suture through the holes or directly to the tendon.

As described by Sherris, direct suturing to the modiolus creates an elongated thin lip, but leaves the philtrum and midline of the lower lip distracted toward the nonparalyzed side.[11] This can be overcome by attaching the sling to the midline of the upper and lower lips, as well as to the modiolus. In this technique, 1-cm incisions are made in the vermillion at the midline of the upper and lower lips. A tunnel is then fashioned from these incisions over the orbicularis to the cheek tunnel. Fascia lata, or other appropriate reconstructive material, is then secured to the temporalis tendon and the orbicularis at the modiolus and the superior and inferior orbicularis in the midline using 2–0 nonabsorbable monofilament horizontal mattress stitches (▶ Fig. 68.4).[11]

The orthodromic temporalis procedure and similar procedures provide a moderate degree of movement of the oral commissure. The patient benefits from formal training to produce a symmetric spontaneous smile, which requires retraining the nonparalyzed side to mimic the reconstructed side.

If the temporalis tendon is not available due to temporalis paralysis or atrophy, static reanimation of the midface can be performed with any of the appropriate materials discussed earlier. The graft is secured to the midline of the upper and lower lip and modiolus, as described earlier, and then tunneled subcutaneously to the zygomatic arch. The graft is then secured to the zygomatic arch periosteum, or around the zygomatic arch, with multiple nonabsorbable 2–0 monofilament sutures.

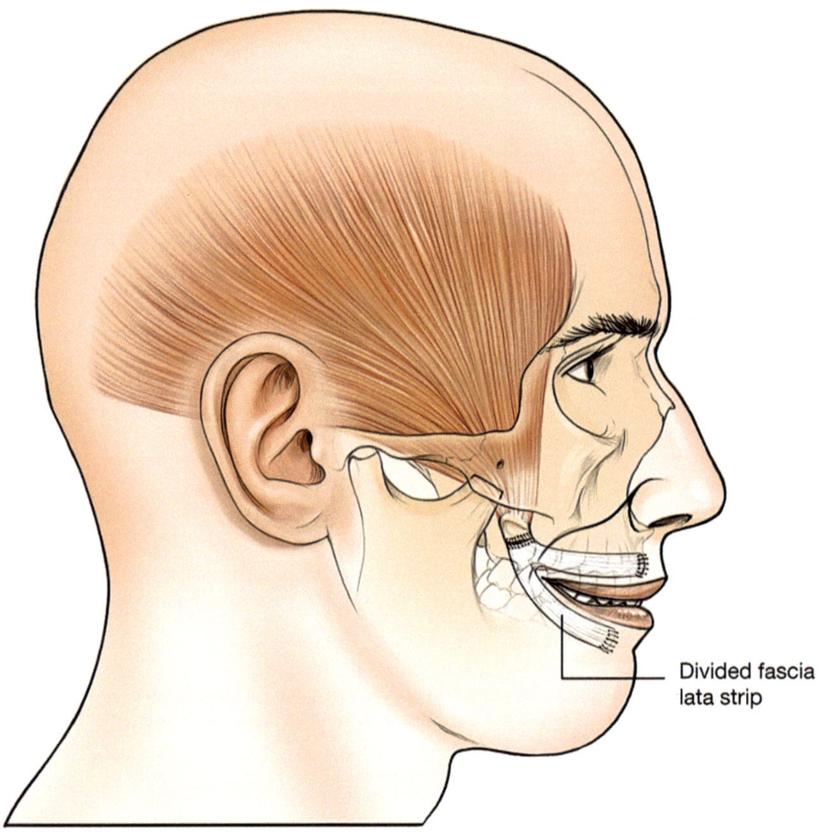

Fig. 68.4 Attachment of fascia sling to connect orthodromic temporalis transfer to the midline of the upper and lower lip. This technique works to mitigate distraction of the upper and lower lip toward the non-paralyzed side and an elongated thin lip.

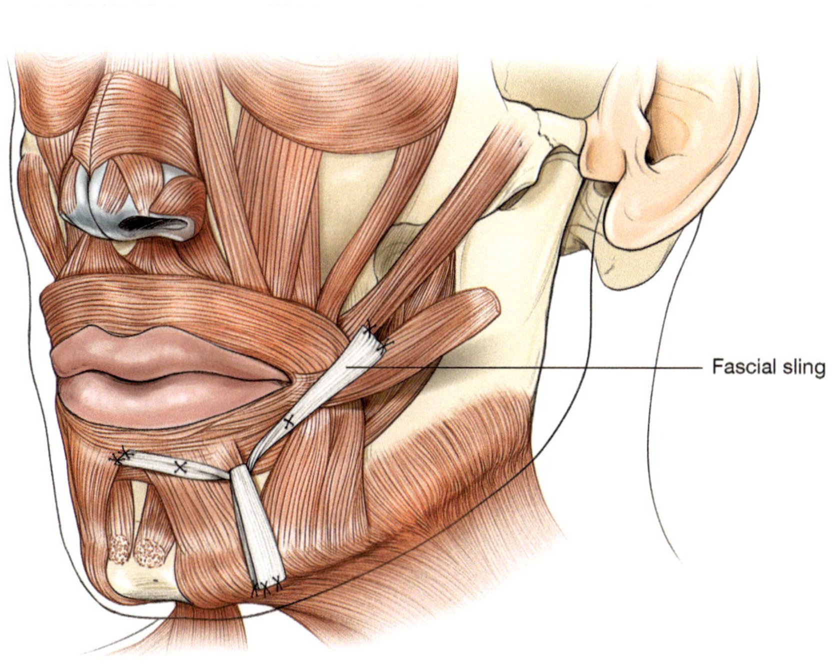

Fig. 68.5 Fascial sling for dynamic reanimation of the lower lip depressors.

Perhaps the greatest challenge of midface suspension is determining the correct degree of tension to apply. Too much tension will give a highly unnatural distorted appearance; too little tension will relax quickly and provide no benefit. Preoperative photographs should be performed with the patient at rest and smiling. Marking and measuring of the degree of displacement of the nonparalyzed side should be performed with the patient awake. Nasal intubation, if appropriate, will allow undistorted intraoperative assessment of both sides of the oral cavity. With the tendon secured to the perioral sites, the tendon is distracted laterally until the desired appearance is achieved. An additional 3 to 6 mm of displacement is added to compensate for relaxation, avoiding overdisplacement, and the tendon secured in place to the temporalis tendon or zygomatic arch.

As relaxation is expected overtime, the patient should be counseled regarding the potential need for modification or revision in the future. Placement into the midline of the lip facilitates revision, and this can often be done under local anesthesia with incisions made at the vermillion only, the tendon identified, advanced, secured, and the excess trimmed.

Prolonged paralysis will lead to atrophy and thinning of the lips. Excessively long lips can be treated with wedge excision to match the length of the normal side. The orbicularis can be divided, but not removed, and plicated to provide bulk, or the lips augmented.

The paralyzed lower lip is the most difficult aspect to manage, and no widely accepted technique has been developed. During natural smile and eating, the depressors pull inferiorly. The paralyzed lower lip is pulled inward and upward by the contralateral nonparalyzed side or by a dynamic reconstruction on the paralyzed side with activation. This appears unnatural, and can cause the patient to bite the lower lip. Various techniques have been reported, though often extensive with inconsistent results.[17] Watanabe et al[17] recently described a technique, which may provide some benefit. A fascial sling is secured to the mentum, through which the lower limb of a dynamic midface sling is passed, such that a downward vector of movement is created with lateral pull (▶ Fig. 68.5). This technique has no benefit in a purely static reanimation, but bears consideration and further investigation.

68.8 Conclusion

Static procedures are a vital component to the management of mid and lower facial paralysis. They can be used as adjuncts to dynamic procedures or in isolation when dynamic procedures are not an option. Reconstructive materials should be selected based on biocompatibility, availability, cost, and morbidity. Reconstruction should be performed with normal muscle vectors in mind, and with the understanding that current technology and procedures cannot match the complexity of natural facial expression and function. Relaxation should be anticipated over time, and slight overcorrection used to mitigate this, but minimal revision should be favored over gross overcorrection whenever possible.

References

[1] Gassner HG, Brissett AE, Otley CC, et al. Botulinum toxin to improve facial wound healing: a prospective, blinded, placebo-controlled study. Mayo Clin Proc. 2006; 81(8):1023–1028

[2] Livi L, Isidori AM, Sherris D, Gravina GL. Advances in prostate cancer research and treatment. BioMed Res Int. 2014; 2014:708383

[3] Ponikau JU, Sherris DA, Kern EB. Immunologic response to fungus is not universally associated with chronic rhinosinusitis. Otolaryngol Head Neck Surg. 2010; 143(5):607–610

[4] Liu YM, Sherris DA. Static procedures for the management of the midface and lower face. Facial Plast Surg. 2008; 24(2):211–215

[5] Kern EB, Sherris D, Stergiou AM, Katz LM, Rosenblatt LC, Ponikau J. Diagnosis and treatment of chronic rhinosinusitis: focus on intranasal Amphotericin B. Ther Clin Risk Manag. 2007; 3(2):319–325

[6] Sebastin SJ, Puhaindran ME, Lim AY, Lim IJ, Bee WH. The prevalence of absence of the palmaris longus—a study in a Chinese population and a review of the literature. J Hand Surg [Br]. 2005; 30(5):525–527
[7] Govindaraj S, Cohen M, Genden EM, Costantino PD, Urken ML. The use of acellular dermis in the prevention of Frey's syndrome. Laryngoscope. 2001; 111(11, Pt 1):1993–1998
[8] Frodel JL. Facial suspension with acellular human dermal allograft. Arch Facial Plast Surg. 2011; 13(1):60–61
[9] Constantinides M, Galli SK, Miller PJ. Complications of static facial suspensions with expanded polytetrafluoroethylene (ePTFE). Laryngoscope. 2001; 111(12):2114–2121
[10] Lindsay RW, Bhama P, Hohman M, Hadlock TA. Prospective evaluation of quality-of-life improvement after correction of the alar base in the flaccidly paralyzed face. JAMA Facial Plast Surg. 2015 Mar-Apr;17(2):108-12
[11] Sherris DA. Refinement in reanimation of the lower face. Arch Facial Plast Surg. 2004; 6(1):49–53
[12] Byrne PJ, Kim M, Boahene K, Millar J, Moe K. Temporalis tendon transfer as part of a comprehensive approach to facial reanimation. Arch Facial Plast Surg. 2007; 9(4):234–241
[13] Ponikau JU, Sherris DA, Weaver A, Kita H. Treatment of chronic rhinosinusitis with intranasal amphotericin B: a randomized, placebo-controlled, double-blind pilot trial. J Allergy Clin Immunol. 2005; 115(1):125–131
[14] Ponikau JU, Sherris DA, Kephart GM, et al. Features of airway remodeling and eosinophilic inflammation in chronic rhinosinusitis: is the histopathology similar to asthma? J Allergy Clin Immunol. 2003; 112(5):877–882
[15] Moore EJ, Strome SA, Kasperbauer JL, Sherris DA, Manning LA. Vascularized radial forearm free tissue transfer for lining in nasal reconstruction. Laryngoscope. 2003; 113(12):2078–2085
[16] Boahene KD, Farrag TY, Ishii L, Byrne PJ. Minimally invasive temporalis tendon transposition. Arch Facial Plast Surg. 2011; 13(1):8–13
[17] Watanabe Y, Sasaki R, Agawa K, Akizuki T. Bidirectional/double fascia grafting for simple and semi-dynamic reconstruction of lower lip deformity in facial paralysis. J Plast Reconstr Aesthet Surg. 2015; 68(3):321–328

69 Vestibular Rehabilitation and “PreHab” in Sporadic Vestibular Schwannoma

Susan J. Herdman and Neil T. Shepard

69.1 Introduction

This chapter provides an overview of vestibular rehabilitation in the context of acute or subacute unilateral vestibular hypofunction, which commonly occurs after vestibular schwannoma (VS) resection. Fundamental principles including theory, exercise strategies, and evidence for treatment efficacy are reviewed. The interested reader is also encouraged to reference Chapter 58 for further discussion regarding the underling pathophysiology, evaluation, management, and outcomes of dizziness in sporadic VS.

The sudden loss of vestibular function caused by the resection of a VS typically causes vertigo, nausea, oscillopsia, dysequilibrium, and unsteadiness of standing balance and gait. Although vertigo, nausea, and the accompanying spontaneous nystagmus usually subside within hours to a few days, imbalance and the sensations of dysequilibrium and oscillopsia, especially during head movement, may endure for many months and can result in extensive time away from work and decreased quality of life.

In recent years, vestibular rehabilitation has been used to help patients make an earlier and more thorough recovery following loss of vestibular function. The use of exercises to improve balance and decrease symptoms specifically in patients with acute loss of vestibular function following VS resection is relatively new. There is, however, clear evidence indicating that vestibular rehabilitation provides substantial benefits to these patients when initiated during the acute or subacute stage following surgery. Following VS surgery, vestibular rehabilitation should be offered to patients who are experiencing symptoms (e.g., dizziness, dysequilibrium, motion sensitivity, oscillopsia) or imbalance due to unilateral vestibular hypofunction during the acute and subacute stage. The goals of early intervention are to (1) decrease the patient's dysequilibrium (sense of being off-balance); (2) improve the patient's balance while walking, especially during head movements or turning, thus decreasing the risk for falls; (3) improve the patient's ability to see clearly during head movements; and (4) enable the patient to resume normal activities more quickly.

The first study to examine whether vestibular rehabilitation would be beneficial for patients following VS resection was published in 1995.[1] The study followed up a group of patients performing simple head movement exercises (see discussion on gaze stabilization exercises later) from postoperative day 3 through postoperative day 6 (day of discharge from the hospital). Balance function and symptom scores of patients performing the exercises were compared to a group of similar patients performing control exercises. The study showed that patients performing the exercises had significantly less dysequilibrium and significant improvement in balance in some posturography measures on the day of discharge. Additionally, more patients in the vestibular exercise group (50%) were able to walk with head turns without staggering than in the control group (0%), suggesting that they would be safer while walking. However, the number of subjects was small ($n = 19$). Studies that followed this initial paper all found substantial benefits for initiating exercises during the acute stage following VS microsurgery.[2,3,4]

69.2 Exercise Approaches

Standard vestibular rehabilitation for the patient with acute vestibular hypofunction typically includes combinations of several different exercises to address the impairments and functional limitations identified during initial evaluation. The goals of the exercises are to (1) foster gaze stability (gaze stability exercises), (2) decrease symptoms (habituation and adaptation exercises), (3) improve standing balance and gait, and (4) improve endurance. Additional treatment approaches that will be discussed include the use of exercise, activity, or chemical ablation of vestibular function prior to surgery (prehab).

Management of patients during the acute stage following resection of VS typically includes medications, such as vestibular suppressants or antiemetics. Several authors have suggested that vestibular suppressant medications such as diazepam may delay or slow recovery by slowing central compensation; however, few studies have examined the influence of medication on the level of recovery when given during the acute stage after surgery.[15,31]

Patient age should not be considered a deterrent to the use of the exercises. Results from numerous studies have found that age is not a factor in attaining improvement in intensity of subjective complaints, visual acuity during head movement, fall risk, and gait speed in patients performing vestibular exercises.[32,33,34,35]

None of the studies on the use of exercises during the early postoperative stage following VS surgery reported any negative effects; however, the exercises should be used carefully. Although the exercises are performed actively and the patients are advised to make the head movements slowly so that they can see clearly, head movement increases the likelihood of exacerbating dizziness and therefore the exercises should be used only under the supervision of a trained therapist.

69.2.1 Gaze Stability Exercises

Gaze stability exercises were developed based on two concepts. The first concept is that vestibuloocular reflex (VOR) function can be improved through the process of adaptation. Adaptation refers to long-term change in the neuronal response to head movements with the goal of normalizing gaze stability and reducing symptoms. That is, the gain of the VOR can be increased by providing an error signal that the central nervous system then tries to resolve. The primary error signal for VOR adaptation is retinal slip or movement of an image across the retina.[5] To understand this process, it is important to understand that the primary function of the VOR is to keep an image on the fovea of the retina during head movements so that the person can see clearly. If, during head movements, the image moves off the fovea (retinal slip), the image will be blurry. Gaze stability exercises, based on the assumption that they promote vestibular adaptation, involve head movement while maintaining focus on a target, which may be stationary or moving. The goal is for the patient to move his or her head at a velocity that results in a very small amount of visual blurring. The exercises can be modified in numerous ways such as by changing head velocity, distance to the target, duration of maintained head movement, or the visual background against which the exercise is performed. Because the exercises involve head movement, they improve balance as well as gaze stability and symptoms.[1] The second concept underlying the gaze stabilization exercises is based on the principles of substitution. Substitution exercises were developed with the goal of promoting alternative eye movement strategies (e.g., central preprogramming of eye movements, anticipatory saccades) to substitute for lost or reduced vestibular function.[6,7,8,9] For example, in one exercise requiring active eye and head movements between two targets, an eye movement to a target is made before the head movement toward the target; when the head then moves toward the target, the goal is for the patient to keep the eyes on the target. In a healthy individual, the VOR maintains the eyes on the target. In the absence of the VOR, head movements toward the side of a vestibular loss require a different eye movement or eye movements to maintain fixation on the target. Both adaptation and substitution exercises are performed with head movements in the horizontal and vertical planes.

69.2.2 Habituation

Habituation, as a treatment approach, involves repeated exposure to the specific stimulus that provokes dizziness in order to reduce the dizziness. Cawthorne and Cooksey were the first to introduce habituation as an exercise approach in the 1940s.[10,11] Cawthorne and Cooksey based the exercises on the principle that patients who moved more did better than those who tended to be inactive. These habituation exercises were prescribed for patients with vestibular hypofunction or concussion and involved a progression of activities from eye movements only, head movements with eyes open or closed, bending, tossing a ball, to walking.[12] Patients typically did these exercises in a group. Today habituation exercises are individualized and are chosen based on specific movements (e.g., horizontal head movements) or situations (e.g., busy visual environments) that provoke symptoms.[13,14,15,16] Patients perform several repetitions of body motions, or are exposed to the visual stimulus, that cause mild to moderate symptoms several times a day. This systematic exposure to the provocative stimulus leads to a reduction in symptoms over time. As the patient's symptoms decrease, the intensity of the exercise can be increased. Other habituation approaches involve the use of optokinetic stimuli or virtual reality environments as habituation exercises.[17,18] Optokinetic stimuli involves the use of moving visual patterns while virtual reality immerses patients in realistic, visually challenging environments. Both are used to address visual motion sensitivity, also known as visual vertigo, or visually induced dizziness. In both approaches, the stimulus can be graded in intensity by altering stimulus parameters such as velocity of stimulus motion, size of stimulus, and instructions to participant. The stimulus may be provided by optokinetic drums, moving rooms or virtual reality goggles, busy screen savers on a computer, or videos of busy visual environments.

69.2.3 Balance and Gait Training

Balance and gait training under challenging sensory and dynamic conditions are typically included as part of vestibular rehabilitation. Although not unique to treatment of vestibular impairments, these exercises facilitate use of visual and/or somatosensory cues to substitute for missing vestibular function. Balance exercises include balancing under conditions of altered visual (e.g., vision removed) and/or somatosensory input (e.g., standing on compliant or moving surfaces) and may involve changes in the base of support (e.g., Romberg, tandem, single-leg stance) and the addition of head movement to increase the challenge. Weight shifting in stance is used to improve center of gravity control and balance recovery. Gait exercises include walking with head turns, walking in different environments, or performing a secondary task while walking. Equipment is available that can augment balance and gait training such as gaming technology and virtual reality systems.

69.2.4 General Conditioning

General conditioning, such as walking for endurance or aerobic exercise, is frequently an element of rehabilitation because people with peripheral vestibular dysfunction often limit physical activity to avoid symptom provocation. General conditioning exercise (e.g., stationary bicycle) by itself has not been found to improve gaze stability, reduce symptoms, or improve balance in patients with vestibular hypofunction in the more chronic period after vestibular loss.[19,20]

69.3 Evidence of Treatment Efficacy

A recently published clinical practice guideline advocates that clinicians should offer vestibular rehabilitation to patients with acute or subacute unilateral vestibular hypofunction based on the number of high-quality randomized controlled clinical trials.[21] Although there are only four studies of patients following resection of VS, these studies were all high-quality randomized, controlled trials.[1,2,3,4] The studies show improved outcomes in patients receiving vestibular rehabilitation compared to controls with either no exercise or sham exercises. These studies are supported by numerous other studies of patients with acute unilateral vestibular loss from vestibular neuritis that found the use of vestibular exercises was also beneficial when compared to patients performing sham or no exercise.[22,23,24,25,26] Furthermore, the Clinical Practice Guideline suggested that early initiation of vestibular rehabilitation resulted in higher levels of recovery of balance function, reduced symptom intensity, improved recovery of activities of daily living, reduced fall risk, and improved quality of life.[21] It is important to note, however, that individuals who have already compensated sufficiently to the vestibular loss and no longer experience symptoms or gait and balance impairments do not need formal vestibular rehabilitation.

Despite strong evidence supporting the efficacy of exercises on recovery following VS resection, there are several limitations of these studies that deserve discussion. First, these publications tend to include a relatively small number of subjects, which may limit the generalizability of the findings. Second, the investigators assume that patients developed a sudden acute unilateral vestibular hypofunction from the surgery, but this is not known. Some of the patients may have had a progressive loss of vestibular function over years as the tumor grew slowly and therefore had adapted and did not experience an acute loss of vestibular function postoperatively. This may also be the case for patients who are observed without treatment or those who receive stereotactic radiosurgery. Finally, the patients in the studies may represent a biased selection based on two factors—the surgical approach used and the occurrence of postoperative complications, both of which may exclude certain patients from inclusion in the studies.

69.3.1 Vestibular Rehabilitation (Exercises Started after Surgery)

Four randomized controlled studies have examined the effects of vestibular rehabilitation during the acute/subacute stage following resection of VS (▸ Table 69.1). All concluded that the use of exercises during the early postoperative period was beneficial. In the first study, patients scheduled for resection underwent evaluation of subjective complaints, balance and gait, and then were randomly assigned to the vestibular exercise group (vestibular; $n = 11$) or to the control group ($n = 8$).[1] Exercises were started on postoperative day 3 and continued until the patients were discharged from the hospital (mean = postoperative day 6). The vestibular group performed gaze stabilization exercises while focusing on a small stationary target for 1 minute while moving their head. The exercises were performed five times per day for a maximum of 10 to 20 minutes per day. The control group performed horizontal and vertical smooth-pursuit eye movements against a featureless background following the same schedule. The use of a featureless background decreases the likelihood of retinal slip during the eye movements. All patients walked at least once each day. Both groups were supervised while they performed the exercises. Other than age (the vestibular group was older [mean age: 59 vs. 48 years for the control group, $p < 0.04$]), both groups were similar prior to surgery and on the assessment on postoperative day 3. Both groups reported significantly more intense dizziness on postoperative day 3 than before surgery and had more postural sway on postoperative day 3 than preoperatively based on computerized posturography. By postoperative day 5 or 6, the vestibular group reported significantly less intense subjective disequilibrium compared to the control group ($p < 0.05$). Additionally, more patients in the vestibular group (50%) were able to walk with head turns without staggering than in the control group (0%).

The second study on the effectiveness of gaze stabilization exercises initiated after VS surgery examined whether or not the exercises reduced the patients' perception of dizziness based on their Dizziness Handicap Inventory score.[3] Patients were randomized into a vestibular group that performed gaze stabilization and balance exercises ($n = 30$) or control group who did not perform any exercises ($n = 27$). A sequentially randomized design (first part of study was control group; second part of the study was vestibular group) was used to assign the patients. Patients in the vestibular group performed gaze stabilization exercises starting on the third postoperative day. Each exercise was performed for 1 minute, four or five times each day. The exercises were performed initially while reclining or seated and then while standing. Patients were reassessed at 2 to 3 weeks, 6 to 7 weeks, and 10 to 12 weeks postoperatively. The main finding was that patients in the vestibular group experienced significantly less dizziness, based on the scores of the Dizziness Handicap Inventory, compared to the control group.

Table 69.1 Summary of randomized, controlled trials on acute and subacute patients following resection of vestibular schwannoma

Authors	Exercise group	Control group	Initiation of exercises	Study period	Outcome
Herdman et al[1]	Gaze stability exercises, 5 times daily (10–20 min total time daily), walking	Smooth pursuit eye movements against a featureless background 10–20 min total time daily, walking	Postoperative day 3	Until postoperative day 6	Significantly less subjective dysequilibrium, better static balance, more patients able to walk with head turns at discharge in the vestibular exercise group
Enticott et al[3]	Gaze stability exercises, 4–5 times daily (1 min each)	No exercises	Postoperative day 3	10–12 wk postoperatively	Less dizziness, based on Dizziness Handicap Inventory score, in vestibular exercise group
Mruzek et al[2,a]	Habituation exercises with and without social reinforcement	Range of motion exercises and social reinforcement	Postoperative day 5	Until 7 wk postoperative	Significantly less motion sensitivity and better scores of the physical subscale if the Dizziness Handicap Inventory in the vestibular exercise groups
Vereeck et al[4]	Gaze stabilization exercises, narrow-based walking with head turns, treadmill walking for four sessions, HEP	Walk, read, watch TV	Postoperative days 3–5		Tandem gait better in vestibular exercise group; in older subjects static and dynamic balance better and greater reduction in fall risk in exercise group compared to older control group

Abbreviation: HEP, home exercise program.
[a]Patients included both vestibular schwannoma and Meniere's disease.

In a third study, patients with either VS or Ménière's disease were randomly assigned to one of three groups—vestibular exercises only, vestibular exercises plus social reinforcement, or control exercises plus social reinforcement.[2] Vestibular exercises consisted of habituation exercises based on the results of the Motion Sensitivity Quotient Test and Cawthorne–Cooksey exercises. The control group performed range of motion exercises. Both groups started the exercises on postoperative day 5. Social reinforcement entailed periodic phone calls to praise the patients and encourage compliance. All interventions lasted 8 weeks at which time patients were reassessed. Mruzek et al found that all patients improved in the Motion Sensitivity Quotient Test and Dizziness Handicap Inventory scores and on computerized dynamic posturography.[2] However, patients who performed the vestibular exercises had significantly less motion sensitivity and better scores on the physical subscale of the Dizziness Handicap Inventory than the control group.

The final study of patients following VS surgery also started vestibular exercises 3 to 5 days postoperatively.[4] Patients were randomized to one of four groups: vestibular exercises ($n = 16$ younger, $n = 15$ older, where older was defined as > 50 years old) or to a control group ($n = 11$ younger, $n = 11$ older). All groups were reassessed after 12 weeks. Vestibular exercises included supervised gaze stabilization exercises, walking with a narrow base of support with head turning, and treadmill training for a total of four sessions as well as a home exercise program performed three times per day. The control group was told to read, watch TV, and to walk while in the hospital and then once at home, gradually to increase their activity level. Tumor size and mean caloric asymmetry did not differ between the groups preoperatively. During the acute/subacute stage, balance measures did not differ between the vestibular exercise and control group except for tandem gait, which was better in the vestibular exercise group. However, when only older patients were considered, the group who performed vestibular exercises were significantly better on measures of static balance, the Timed Up and Go test, and tandem gait than the group who watched TV, read, or simply walked. At 9 to 12 weeks, older subjects who performed vestibular exercises had better Dynamic Gait Index scores, static balance, Timed Up and Go scores, and tandem walk than did the older control group. Finally, this study found no benefit in vestibular exercises compared to general instructions in patients younger than 50 years. One reason for this age effect may be the patients' general physical activity level preoperatively. Gauchard et al suggested that the level of regular physical activity prior to surgery contributes to the rate of recovery after VS resection.[27] They reported that patients who were sedentary had a more difficult recovery during the early postoperative period than those patients who engaged in regular physical activity.

69.3.2 "PreHab": Treatment before Surgery

Several retrospective studies introduced a new concept of rehabilitation for patients scheduled for vestibular ablation, either for VS or Ménière's disease.[28,29,30] These studies suggest that treating patients with a combination of intratympanic gentamicin and vestibular exercises *before* surgery facilitates recovery. They hypothesize that by producing further loss of vestibular function through the injection of a vestibulotoxic medication and by inducing vestibular compensation with a course of vestibular exercises, better and faster recovery should occur postoperatively. They stated that patients undergoing "prehab" had faster symptom and balance recovery following surgery. However, further research is needed to determine whether there is a significant difference in recovery with prehab compared to patients performing vestibular exercises postoperatively.

69.4 Conclusion

Vestibular therapy is critical to hasten and improve the static and dynamic vestibular compensation that occurs after a unilateral loss of function. With early introduction of treatment exercises, patients experience improvements in gaze stability, balance, and dizziness handicap. With good evidence for efficacy, vestibular physical therapy should be routinely considered after VS resection.

References

[1] Herdman SJ, Clendaniel RA, Mattox DE, Holliday MJ, Niparko JK. Vestibular adaptation exercises and recovery: acute stage after acoustic neuroma resection. Otolaryngol Head Neck Surg. 1995; 113(1):77–87

[2] Mruzek M, Barin K, Nichols DS, Burnett CN, Welling DB. Effects of vestibular rehabilitation and social reinforcement on recovery following ablative vestibular surgery. Laryngoscope. 1995; 105(7, Pt 1):686–692

[3] Enticott JC, O'leary SJ, Briggs RJ. Effects of vestibulo-ocular reflex exercises on vestibular compensation after vestibular schwannoma surgery. Otol Neurotol. 2005; 26(2):265–269

[4] Vereeck L, Wuyts FL, Truijen S, De Valck C, Van de Heyning PH. The effect of early customized vestibular rehabilitation on balance after acoustic neuroma resection. Clin Rehabil. 2008; 22(8):698–713

[5] Miles FA, Eighmy BB. Long-term adaptive changes in primate vestibuloocular reflex. I. Behavioral observations. J Neurophysiol. 1980; 43(5):1406–1425

[6] Tian J, Crane BT, Demer JL. Vestibular catch-up saccades in labyrinthine deficiency. Exp Brain Res. 2000; 131(4):448–457

[7] Schubert MC, Migliaccio AA, Clendaniel RA, Allak A, Carey JP. Mechanism of dynamic visual acuity recovery with vestibular rehabilitation. Arch Phys Med Rehabil. 2008; 89(3):500–507

[8] Scherer M, Migliaccio AA, Schubert MC. Effect of vestibular rehabilitation on passive dynamic visual acuity. J Vestib Res. 2008; 18(2–3):147–157

[9] Schubert MC, Hall CD, Das V, Tusa RJ, Herdman SJ. Oculomotor strategies and their effect on reducing gaze position error. Otol Neurotol. 2010; 31(2): 228–231

[10] Cawthorne T. The physiological basis for head exercises. J Chartered Soc Physiother. 1944; 30:106

[11] Cooksey FS. Rehabilitation in vestibular injuries. Proc R Soc Med. 1946; 39(5): 273–278

[12] Hecker HC, Haug CO, Herndon JW. Treatment of the vertiginous patient using Cawthorne's vestibular exercises. Laryngoscope. 1974; 84(11):2065–2072

[13] Telian SA, Shepard NT, Smith-Wheelock M, Kemink JL. Habituation therapy for chronic vestibular dysfunction: preliminary results. Otolaryngol Head Neck Surg. 1990; 103(1):89–95

[14] Shepard NT, Telian SA, Smith-Wheelock M. Habituation and balance retraining therapy. A retrospective review. Neurol Clin. 1990; 8(2):459–475

[15] Shepard NT, Telian SA, Smith-Wheelock M, Raj A. Vestibular and balance rehabilitation therapy. Ann Otol Rhinol Laryngol. 1993; 102(3, Pt 1):198–205

[16] Shepard NT, Telian SA. Programmatic vestibular rehabilitation. Otolaryngol Head Neck Surg. 1995; 112(1):173–182

[17] Pavlou M, Kanegaonkar RG, Swapp D, Bamiou DE, Slater M, Luxon LM. The effect of virtual reality on visual vertigo symptoms in patients with peripheral vestibular dysfunction: a pilot study. J Vestib Res. 2012; 22(5–6): 273–281

[18] Pavlou M, Bronstein AM, Davies RA. Randomized trial of supervised versus unsupervised optokinetic exercise in persons with peripheral vestibular disorders. Neurorehabil Neural Repair. 2013; 27(3):208–218

[19] Horak FB, Jones-Rycewicz C, Black FO, Shumway-Cook A. Effects of vestibular rehabilitation on dizziness and imbalance. Otolaryngol Head Neck Surg. 1992; 106(2):175–180

[20] Krebs DE, Gill-Body KM, Riley PO, Parker SW. Double-blind, placebo-controlled trial of rehabilitation for bilateral vestibular hypofunction: preliminary report. Otolaryngol Head Neck Surg. 1993; 109(4):735–741

[21] Hall CD, Herdman SJ, Whitney SL, et al. Vestibular rehabilitation for peripheral vestibular hypofunction: an evidence-based clinical practice guideline: From the American Physical Therapy Association Neurology Section. J Neurol Phys Ther. 2016; 40(2):124–155

[22] Strupp M, Arbusow V, Maag KP, Gall C, Brandt T. Vestibular exercises improve central vestibulospinal compensation after vestibular neuritis. Neurology. 1998; 51(3):838–844

[23] Venosa AR, Bittar RS. Vestibular rehabilitation exercises in acute vertigo. Laryngoscope. 2007; 117(8):1482–1487

[24] Teggi R, Caldirola D, Fabiano B, Recanati P, Bussi M. Rehabilitation after acute vestibular disorders. J Laryngol Otol. 2009; 123(4):397–402

[25] Marioni G, Fermo S, Zanon D, Broi N, Staffieri A. Early rehabilitation for unilateral peripheral vestibular disorders: a prospective, randomized investigation using computerized posturography. Eur Arch Otorhinolaryngol. 2013; 270(2):425–435

[26] Sparrer I, Duong Dinh TA, Ilgner J, Westhofen M. Vestibular rehabilitation using the Nintendo® Wii Balance Board – a user-friendly alternative for central nervous compensation. Acta Otolaryngol. 2013; 133(3): 239–245

[27] Gauchard GC, Parietti-Winkler C, Lion A, Simon C, Perrin PP. Impact of pre-operative regular physical activity on balance control compensation after vestibular schwannoma surgery. Gait Posture. 2013; 37(1):82–87

[28] Magnusson M, Kahlon B, Karlberg M, Lindberg S, Siesjö P. Preoperative vestibular ablation with gentamicin and vestibular 'prehab' enhance postoperative recovery after surgery for pontine angle tumours–first report. Acta Otolaryngol. 2007; 127(12):1236–1240

[29] Tjernström F, Fransson P-A, Kahlon B, et al. Vestibular PREHAB and gentamicin before schwannoma surgery may improve long-term postural function. J Neurol Neurosurg Psychiatry. 2009; 80(11):1254–1260

[30] Magnusson M, Karlberg M, Tjernström F. 'PREHAB': Vestibular prehabilitation to ameliorate the effect of a sudden vestibular loss. NeuroRehabilitation. 2011; 29(2):153–156

[31] Zee DS. The management of patients with vestibular disorders. In Barber HO, Sharpe JA, eds. Vestibular Disorders. Chicago, IL: Year Book Medical Publisher; 1987:254

[32] Whitney SL, Wrisley DM, Marchetti GF, Furman JM. The effect of age on vestibular rehabilitation outcomes. Laryngoscope. 2002; 112(10):1785–1790

[33] Humphriss RL, Baguley DM, Moffat DA. Change in dizziness handicap after vestibular schwannoma excision. Otol Neurotol. 2003; 24(4):661–665

[34] Cohen HS, Kimball KT. Changes in a repetitive head movement task after vestibular rehabilitation. Clin Rehabil. 2004; 18(2):125–131

[35] Herdman SJ, Hall CD, Delaune W. Variables associated with outcome in patients with unilateral vestibular hypofunction. Neurorehabil Neural Repair. 2012; 26(2):151–162

70 Management of Pre- and Posttreatment Trigeminal Neuralgia in Vestibular Schwannoma

Ramsey Ashour, Siviero Agazzi, and Harry van Loveren

70.1 Introduction

Patients with vestibular schwannoma (VS) occasionally present with trigeminal neuralgia secondary to the tumor itself, or, more rarely, develop trigeminal neuralgia as a complication after radiosurgical treatment of the tumor. For the former group, the presence of "pretreatment trigeminal neuralgia" may impact the strategy for tumor management. For the latter group, the plan and resulting outcome of radiosurgical treatment can impact the management strategy for "posttreatment trigeminal neuralgia." In this chapter, we review the management of pre- and posttreatment trigeminal neuralgia in patients with VS.

70.2 Pretreatment Trigeminal Neuralgia

70.2.1 History

Early 20th century reports of trigeminal neuralgia in the setting of a posterior fossa tumor were provided by Krause,[1] Lexer,[2] Oppenheim,[3] and Weisenburg.[4] However, it was Cushing[5] who provided the clearest early description of VS case presentations in his 1917 monograph, some of whom also presented with trigeminal neuralgia. He noted that, "in true tic douloureux, unmodified by operation, there is no cutaneous hypoesthesia, whereas in the painful neuralgia from pressure of a tumor some sensory loss is demonstrable, and the conditions may thus be easily distinguished."

We once agreed with Cushing that the so-called secondary trigeminal neuralgia associated with a tumor could always be distinguished by the presence of a detectable neurologic deficit specific to the tumor (e.g., hearing loss, vestibulopathy, trigeminal numbness, and sensorimotor disturbances) that was caused by brainstem compression. We later disagreed with this premise after encountering a number of patients who had classic trigeminal neuralgia, that is, an occurrence characterized by no detectable neurologic deficit in spite of nerve distortion by tumor as the probable cause.

During his era, Cushing also documented the occasional manifestation of trigeminal neuralgia contralateral to the side of large tumors, and highlighted the high incidence of trigeminal neuropathy in VS patients. He then pointed out that, in association with cerebellopontine angle tumors, neurotrophic keratitis can develop because of trigeminal nerve compression; however, he stated that this "never occurs in true trigeminal neuralgia except as the result of the loss of sensitivity of the cornea following a neurectomy." Interestingly, Cushing emphasized that trigeminal neuralgia "is rarely if ever a significant symptom of a VS." Careful review of his classic monograph reveals a relatively high incidence (8/33 cases) of VS-related trigeminal "neuralgic" pain, perhaps reflecting the large tumor sizes at the time of diagnosis during this early era.

70.2.2 Epidemiology and Clinical Features

Trigeminal neuralgia can be attributed to the presence of tumor in 2 to 10% of cases, most often meningiomas, epidermoids, or VSs.[6,7,8,9,10,11,12] Although pretreatment trigeminal neuralgia has been reported to affect 3.5 to 7% of VS patients, its true incidence is often hindered and likely overestimated by a failure to distinguish between trigeminal neuralgia and trigeminal neuropathy.[13,14,15]

Tumor-related trigeminal neuralgia shares the same features as non–tumor-related trigeminal neuralgia. Both are characterized by paroxysmal, intense, shock-like pains in one or more ipsilateral trigeminal distributions that are often triggered by cutaneous stimulation of the affected areas, such as by touch or common oral activities. Atypical trigeminal neuralgia can also occur, characterized by concomitant background "aching" facial pain in addition to the neuralgic pains. On the other hand, compressive trigeminal neuropathy in the setting of tumor results in facial numbness and associated paresthesias and dysesthesias, and has been reported to affect almost half of large VSs.[12,13]

Even patients with non–tumor-related trigeminal neuralgia can experience subtle changes in facial sensation and/or complain of facial numbness especially when in the midst of a series of painful attacks.[14] Therefore, it is difficult to distinguish between tumor- and non–tumor-related trigeminal neuralgia on clinical grounds alone.[8] This difficulty supports obtaining an MRI whenever possible before treatment in patients with trigeminal neuralgia to elucidate any primary disorders (e.g., tumor, vascular malformation, multiple sclerosis) that might affect treatment strategy. In VS patients, vestibulocochlear nerve dysfunction (i.e., hearing loss) drives the diagnosis, but the presence of trigeminal neuralgia does not appear to result in earlier diagnosis of VS.[9]

70.2.3 Pathophysiology

Although it seems obvious that the cause of tumor-related trigeminal neuralgia is tumor contact with the nerve,[15] Cushing[5] realized that the extent of tumor compression alone could not explain the development of trigeminal neuralgia. He explained, "In the case of the trigeminus ... neuralgic pain such as one would expect is relatively uncommon. This is more remarkable when one realizes how flattened and elongated the nerve becomes as it is crowded aside by the growth."

Jannetta[16] pioneered the concept of neurovascular conflict, specifically, a blood vessel contacting the trigeminal root in either non–tumor-related or tumor-related trigeminal neuralgia. In his series of trigeminal neuralgia patients with posterior fossa tumors, vessels compressing the nerve were found in all 21 patients in whom the nerve root entry zone was examined.[8] In his hypothesis, the tumor either pushes a vessel against the nerve or the nerve against a vessel, thus reproducing a classic

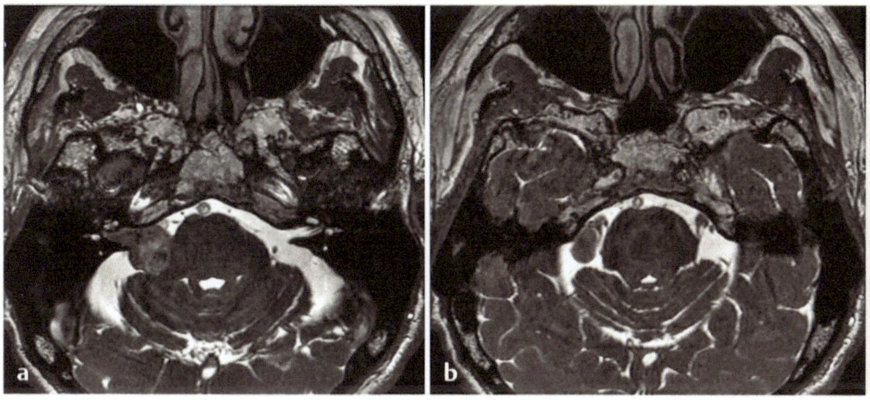

Fig. 70.1 Axial T2-weighted images of a right vestibular schwannoma in a patient with medically intractable right trigeminal neuralgia and right-sided hearing loss. (a) At the level of the internal auditory canal. (b) Above level of the internal auditory canal, demonstrating where the tumor reaches the level of the trigeminal nerve. At surgery, the trigeminal nerve was deep to the tumor and a large loop of the superior cerebellar artery was found compressing the nerve from above.

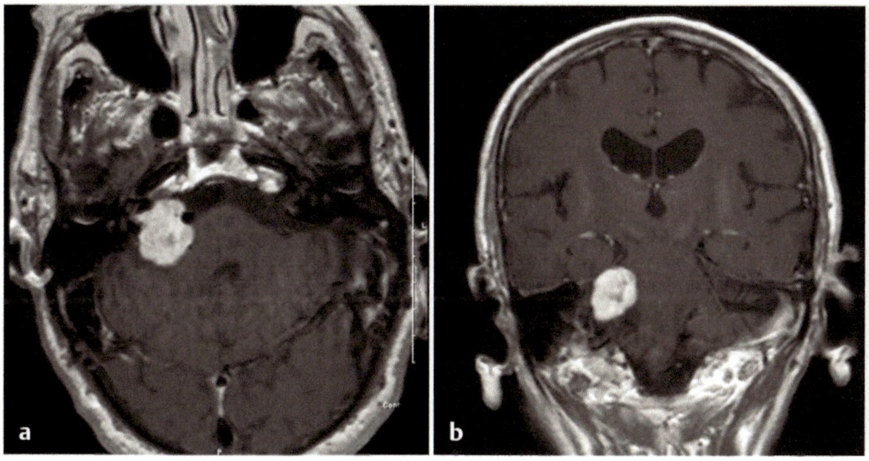

Fig. 70.2 Postcontrast T1-weighted images in a vestibular schwannoma patient with hearing loss and trigeminal neuralgia. (a) Axial view shows a prominent vertebrobasilar complex abutting the ventromedial aspect of the tumor. At surgery, multiple arterial loops were found to be compressing the trigeminal both from above and below. (b) Coronal view demonstrates tumor extending superiorly up to the petrotentorial junction in close proximity to the trigeminal nerve.

neurovascular conflict and therefore a classic trigeminal neuralgia. Some authors have also documented vascular compression of the trigeminal nerve root in cases of tumor-related trigeminal neuralgia,[17,18,19,20] whereas others searched for but did not find vascular compression in such cases.[10,21,22] Recall that even in non–tumor-related classic trigeminal neuralgia, vascular conflict is not universally present (▸ Fig. 70.1, ▸ Fig. 70.2).

70.2.4 Management

Medical Therapy

Standard pharmacotherapy for non–tumor-related trigeminal neuralgia includes carbamazepine, oxcarbazepine, lamotrigine, or baclofen.[23] Alternatives include gabapentin, pregabalin, topiramate, and older anticonvulsants. When medications prove ineffective at achieving adequate pain control or cause intolerable side effects to the patient, neurosurgical interventions (e.g., microvascular decompression, percutaneous ablative procedures, radiosurgery) are considered.[24]

Trigeminal neuralgia caused by VS is not in and of itself an absolute indication for VS treatment. This is the case when the neuralgia is well controlled by medical therapy with tolerable side effects, and the tumor is otherwise without evidence of active growth. In the majority of patients, tumor treatment whether by radiosurgery or surgery will achieve excellent relief of the associated trigeminal neuralgia so long as either treatment is specifically designed to address both disorders simultaneously. Percutaneous radiofrequency rhizotomy and glycerol rhizotomy are also part of the surgical armamentarium and should not be forgotten; however, both have been largely set aside because they address only the trigeminal neuralgia component and ignore the tumor.

Tumor Surgery

Resolution of tumor-related trigeminal neuralgia after surgical resection of the tumor is well documented.[8,10,13,25,26] In Jannetta's series of 26 patients with tumor-related trigeminal neuralgia treated surgically, there were 8 completely resected VSs. Based on Kaplan–Meier analysis, the authors estimated excellent facial pain relief in 81% at 10 years after surgery and partial relief in an additional 4%.[8] Noteworthy is that this rate and duration of "excellent relief" exceeds that of non–tumor-related trigeminal neuralgia after simple microvascular decompression. In another series of 25 patients with tumor-related trigeminal neuralgia, Nakagawa et al[10] found vascular compression at surgery in 12 patients and reported complete resolution of facial pain in all 25 patients after tumor resection, including 9 with VSs.

Resection of the tumor alone will often relieve tumor-related trigeminal neuralgia, particularly when it is large enough to compress the nerve or displace a vessel against it. However, trigeminal exploration after resection is important to identify any remaining vascular compression of the nerve, which can then be addressed in a "belt-and-suspenders" fashion. Typically, we insert one or more pieces of polyvinyl acetal sponge (Ivalon; FABCO, New London, CT) between the nerve and offending vessels to ensure that they remain separate from each other after surgery. Other widely used materials include Teflon-coated vascular pledget fibers rolled into a ball, gelatin sponge, oxidized cellulose, cotton wool pad, muscle, fascia, and others.

Microvascular decompression for trigeminal neuralgia is typically performed via a retrosigmoid approach. Given this, the question arises: "Does the presence of tumor-related trigeminal neuralgia lower the threshold to utilize a retrosigmoid approach for resection of the VS to then maximize access to the trigeminal root entry zone?" Indeed, the retrosigmoid approach gives the surgeon a familiar trajectory and more working space for microvascular decompression. In our experience, the trigeminal nerve can also be decompressed via a translabyrinthine approach for VS resection in the same setting. However, microvascular decompression of this nerve is not a realistic goal when a hearing preservation, middle fossa surgical approach, is considered for a small intracanalicular VS. In these cases, the presence of trigeminal neuralgia is not considered tumor related and should be managed independently.

Radiation Therapy

Improvement in tumor-related trigeminal neuralgia has been reported after radiosurgery that targets the tumor, the trigeminal nerve, or both. In 46 patients with tumor-related trigeminal neuralgia, including 17 VS patients, Régis et al[27] used radiosurgery for the tumor and reported complete resolution of the facial pain in 35 (79.5%) at mean follow-up of 4.5 years. Radiosurgery targeted to the trigeminal nerve itself achieved complete facial pain resolution in three-fourths of patients and radiosurgery to both the tumor and nerve was successful in two-thirds of patients treated. In 21 patients with tumor-related trigeminal neuralgia, including 9 with VS, Huang el al[28] achieved complete pain relief in 12 (57%) patients after one treatment alone; for 8 patients with persistent or recurrent pain, 7 were retreated with radiosurgery to the trigeminal nerve and 1 patient underwent reirradiation of the tumor itself. At mean follow-up of 57.8 months, 16 (76%) of the 21 patients experienced complete relief of facial pain. Although the rates and duration of complete pain relief were less than those achieved with surgery, this should be expected and is comparable with radiosurgery for non–tumor-related trigeminal neuralgia. Of note, four patients suffered new facial numbness after repeat radiosurgery.

In a 2016 study of 15 patients with tumor-related trigeminal neuralgia, including 3 VSs, Kim et al[29] targeted both the tumor and trigeminal root entry zone in a single session of radiosurgery. At mean follow-up of 38 months, complete pain relief without medication was achieved in 10 (67%) patients and persistent new-onset facial numbness occurred in 3 (20%) patients.

Decision Making

The presence of pretreatment trigeminal neuralgia may lower the threshold to offer treatment for VS. If treatment is considered, the threshold to offer surgery may also be lower because of its ability to directly decompress the trigeminal nerve with minimal risk of postoperative facial numbness. Radiosurgical options that target the tumor, nerve, or both may also be considered, particularly in patients who are high risk for surgery. Compared with surgery, this option offers less durability and an increased risk of facial numbness after treatment. Overall, the influence of pretreatment trigeminal neuralgia on VS management is incremental. By and large, we tend to decide if and how to treat the tumor based on typical factors, including tumor growth, tumor size, brainstem compression, hearing status, patient age/medical condition, and patient preference and subsequently "add on" the trigeminal component.

70.3 Posttreatment Trigeminal Neuralgia

The development of new-onset trigeminal neuralgia after VS treatment is decidedly uncommon, and when it does occur, it is almost exclusively after radiosurgery. Indeed, although VS resection can cause new trigeminal neuropathy or even anesthesia dolorosa[30] as a result of trigeminal nerve manipulation/ trauma during surgery, new-onset trigeminal neuralgia after surgery is a rare event.

70.3.1 Postradiosurgery Trigeminal Neuralgia

Epidemiology

In the early radiosurgery experience of VS by the Karolinska group[31] performed on the basis of CT, metrizamide cisternography, or pneumoencephalography, facial weakness developed in 5 (36%) and facial numbness in 2 (14%) of 14 patients after treatment. Similarly, the Pittsburgh group's[32] early radiosurgery experience for VS demonstrated high rates of facial nerve (21%) and trigeminal nerve (27%) dysfunction after treatment. Further advances in radiosurgery by the early 1990s, including the introduction of MRI, improvements in dose planning software, and reduction in the radiation dose to the margin of the tumor, led to better tumor growth control results (> 95%) and lower rates of facial (< 10%) and trigeminal (< 10%) neuropathies.[33]

The incidence of new-onset "true" trigeminal neuralgia after radiosurgery is difficult to determine because trigeminal neuralgia and neuropathy are often combined in the evaluation of trigeminal "dysfunction." For example, in a series of 123 VS patients treated with Gamma knife radiosurgery, Hempel et al[34] reported posttreatment trigeminal neuralgia in 5.8% of patients; however, their definition included facial numbness and paresthesias. In contrast, in a large retrospective review of 829 VSs treated with Gamma knife radiosurgery during a 15-year period, Lunsford et al[32] reported the complication of trigeminal neuralgia after treatment in only 0.2% of cases. In a 2005 study of 195 VS patients treated with Gamma knife radiosurgery, Chung et al[35] reported new-onset trigeminal neuralgia in 2 (1%) of the cohort. With modern imaging and dose planning, radiation-induced trigeminal neuralgia is a rare complication (< 1%).

Pathophysiology

Escalating radiation doses to the trigeminal nerve has been demonstrated in primates to cause anywhere from limited demyelination to severe derangement in nerve tissue with fragmentation, necrosis, and axonal loss.[36] On this basis, these effects have been used in a controlled fashion to treat trigeminal neuralgia. Yet, the unanswered question remains whether radiation-induced trigeminal nerve injury after VS radiosurgery can be implicated as a cause of posttreatment trigeminal neuralgia.

Notably, the radiosurgery dose used to treat trigeminal neuralgia (average maximum dose: 80 Gy)[37] is much higher than that used for VS (average margin dose: 12.5–13 Gy).[32] Compared with a normal trigeminal nerve, a nerve that is stretched or compressed by tumor may be more vulnerable to radiation injury. In one systematic review of 5,631 VS patients treated with Gamma Knife radiosurgery, the incidence of radiation-induced trigeminal neuropathy was statistically significantly higher in those patients treated with higher marginal doses: that is, 3.2% after ≥ 13 Gy versus 1.6% after < 13 Gy.[38] In another study, the incidence of delayed trigeminal neuropathy after VS radiosurgery depended more on the estimated length of nerve irradiated, as determined by the pons-petrous distance, than on tumor dose or tumor volume irradiated.[39]

Furthermore, VS radiosurgery may result in an initial period of tumor growth/swelling that is followed by size stabilization, which may also include central cystic changes within the tumor. Some have hypothesized that, in rare cases, radiation-induced tumor changes can cause further displacement of an adjacent vessel against the trigeminal nerve itself. In a study of 208 VS patients who underwent stereotactic radiosurgery, Pollock[40] observed that 30 (14%) tumors grew at least 2 mm after radiosurgery, including 1 that developed new-onset trigeminal neuralgia. In a study of radiosurgically treated VS and meningioma patients, Ganz et al[41] noted that radiation-induced clinical trigeminal and facial nerve deficits were always associated with increased T2 signal in the neighboring brainstem parenchyma. Future studies correlating the timing of trigeminal neuralgia onset after radiosurgery and associated neuroimaging changes would further contribute to our understanding of this rare complication.

Management

In VS patients treated with radiosurgery who subsequently develop trigeminal neuralgia, medical therapy remains the first option. If medical therapy fails or becomes intolerable because of medication side effects, surgical tumor resection can then be considered. In a study of four patients with radiation-induced tumor-related trigeminal neuralgia who subsequently underwent complete tumor resection, including two VS patients, Gerganov et al[42] reported complete resolution of facial pain in three patients and near-complete resolution in one patient at mean follow-up of 42.5 months. They also noted that the onset of trigeminal neuralgia after radiosurgery ranged from 12 to 60 months (mean: 39 months).

Although surgical outcomes are slightly worse after previous radiosurgery, a surgical option may be more compelling when postradiosurgery tumor growth has been demonstrated. In most cases, however, radiation-induced trigeminal neuralgia will occur without continued tumor growth after radiosurgery. In these cases after previous radiosurgery, the advantages of surgical tumor resection, with the opportunity to perform microvascular decompression of the trigeminal nerve in the same setting, must be weighed against increased surgical risks of facial nerve injury, hearing loss, trigeminal neuropathy, and persistent trigeminal neuralgia.

Radiosurgery to the trigeminal nerve itself or the previously irradiated tumor has been attempted in VS patients who present with tumor-related trigeminal neuralgia.[28] To our knowledge, the use of radiosurgery to treat radiation-induced trigeminal neuralgia has not been previously described. This is consistent with our experience and that of others that further therapeutic attempts to damage a nerve that has already exhibited a poor response to controlled "destructive" procedures (i.e., radiosurgery, percutaneous ablative procedures) are generally ineffective. In a recent systematic review of 20 studies reporting outcomes for repeat radiosurgery in cases of recurrent trigeminal neuralgia, Tuleasca et al[43] observed wide variation both in how cases are selected for retreatment and how outcomes are reported. They concluded that initial pain cessation rates after retreatment appear comparable to initial treatment, but with much higher toxicity (i.e., 33% median rate of new facial hypesthesia).

70.4 Conclusion

With earlier diagnosis and thus smaller tumor size at the time of diagnosis, pretreatment trigeminal neuralgia is rare in VS patients. Posttreatment trigeminal neuralgia is rarer still and, when it occurs, is almost exclusively after radiosurgical rather than open surgical treatment. Overall, the influence of pre- or posttreatment trigeminal neuralgia on VS management is incremental; by and large, we tend to decide if and how to treat the tumor based on the typical factors. Nevertheless, as reviewed in this chapter, in centers specializing in the management of VS, practitioners must recognize the basic features and nuances of coexistent trigeminal neuralgia in this unique patient population.

References

[1] Krause F. Operationen in der hinteren Schadelgrube. Arch f Klin Chir. 1906; lxxxi:40–60
[2] Lexer E. Zur Operation des Ganglion Gasseri nach Erfahrungen an 15 Fallen. Arch f Klin Chir. 1902; lxv:843–928
[3] Oppenheim H. Lehrbuch der Nervenkrankheiten. Fur Arzte und Studierende. Vol 1. 4th ed. Berlin: S Karger; 1905
[4] Weisenburg T. Cerebello-pontile tumor diagnosed for six years as tic douloureaux. The symptoms of irritation of the ninth and twelfth cranial nerves. JAMA. 1910; 54:1600–1604
[5] Cushing H. Tumors of the Nervus Acusticus and the Syndrome of the Cerebellopontile Angle. Philadelphia, PA: WB Saunders; 1917
[6] Gonzalez Revilla A. Tic douloureux and its relationship to tumors of the posterior fossa; analysis of twenty-four cases. J Neurosurg. 1947; 4(3):233–239
[7] Hasegawa K, Kondo A, Kinuta Y, et al. Studies concerning the pathogenesis of trigeminal neuralgia caused by cerebellopontine angle tumors. No Shinkei Geka. 1995; 23(4):315–320
[8] Barker FG, II, Jannetta PJ, Babu RP, Pomonis S, Bissonette DJ, Jho HD. Long-term outcome after operation for trigeminal neuralgia in patients with posterior fossa tumors. J Neurosurg. 1996; 84(5):818–825
[9] Samii M, Matthies C. Acoustic neurinomas associated with vascular compression syndromes. Acta Neurochir (Wien). 1995; 134(3)(/)(4):148–154
[10] Nakagawa K, Aoyagi M, Kawano Y, Ohno K. Clinical and operative findings in patients with trigeminal neuralgia caused by brain tumors. No Shinkei Geka. 2009; 37(9):863–871
[11] Khan Afridi EA, Khan SA, Qureshi WU, et al. Frequency of cerebellopontine angle tumours in patients with trigeminal neuralgia. J Ayub Med Coll Abbottabad. 2014; 26(3):331–333

[12] Matsuka Y, Fort ET, Merrill RL. Trigeminal neuralgia due to an acoustic neuroma in the cerebellopontine angle. J Orofac Pain. 2000; 14(2):147–151

[13] Karkas A, Lamblin E, Meyer M, Gay E, Ternier J, Schmerber S. Trigeminal nerve deficit in large and compressive acoustic neuromas and its correlation with MRI findings. Otolaryngol Head Neck Surg. 2014; 151(4):675–680

[14] Nurmikko TJ. Altered cutaneous sensation in trigeminal neuralgia. Arch Neurol. 1991; 48(5):523–527

[15] Dandy WE. Concerning the cause of trigeminal neuralgia. Am J Surg. 1934; 24:447–455

[16] Jannetta PJ. Treatment of trigeminal neuralgia by suboccipital and transtentorial cranial operations. Clin Neurosurg. 1977; 24:538–549

[17] Berger MS, Wilson CB. Epidermoid cysts of the posterior fossa. J Neurosurg. 1985; 62(2):214–219

[18] Bederson JB, Wilson CB. Evaluation of microvascular decompression and partial sensory rhizotomy in 252 cases of trigeminal neuralgia. J Neurosurg. 1989; 71(3):359–367

[19] Rappaport ZH. Epidermoid tumour of the cerebellopontine angle as a cause of trigeminal neuralgia. Neurochirurgia (Stuttg). 1985; 28(5):211–212

[20] Michelucci R, Tassinari CA, Plasmati R, et al. Trigeminal neuralgia associated with contralateral intracranial tumour: a false localising sign caused by vascular compression? Report of two cases. J Neurol Neurosurg Psychiatry. 1989; 52(10):1202–1203

[21] Ogleznev KYa, Grigoryan YuA, Slavin KV. Parapontine epidermoid tumours presenting as trigeminal neuralgias: anatomical findings and operative results. Acta Neurochir (Wien). 1991; 110(3–4):116–119

[22] Sabin HI, Bordi LT, Symon L. Epidermoid cysts and cholesterol granulomas centered on the posterior fossa: twenty years of diagnosis and management. Neurosurgery. 1987; 21(6):798–805

[23] Benoliel R, Zini A, Khan J, Almoznino G, Sharav Y, Haviv Y. Trigeminal neuralgia (part II): factors affecting early pharmacotherapeutic outcome. Cephalalgia. 2016; 36(8):747–759

[24] Zakrzewska JM, Akram H. Neurosurgical interventions for the treatment of classical trigeminal neuralgia. Cochrane Database Syst Rev. 2011(9): CD007312

[25] Silva J, Cerejo A, Duarte F, Silveira F, Vaz R. Surgical removal of giant acoustic neuromas. World Neurosurg. 2012; 77(5–6):731–735

[26] Schankin CJ, Gall C, Straube A. Headache syndromes after acoustic neuroma surgery and their implications for quality of life. Cephalalgia. 2009; 29(7): 760–771

[27] Régis J, Metellus P, Dufour H, et al. Long-term outcome after gamma knife surgery for secondary trigeminal neuralgia. J Neurosurg. 2001; 95(2):199–205

[28] Huang CF, Tu HT, Liu WS, Lin LY. Gamma Knife surgery for trigeminal pain caused by benign brain tumors. J Neurosurg. 2008; 109 Suppl:154–159

[29] Kim SK, Kim DG, Se YB, et al. Gamma Knife surgery for tumor-related trigeminal neuralgia: targeting both the tumor and the trigeminal root exit zone in a single session. J Neurosurg. 2016; 125(4):838–844

[30] Elahi F, Ho KW. Anesthesia dolorosa of trigeminal nerve, a rare complication of acoustic neuroma surgery. Case Rep Neurol Med. 2014; 2014:496794

[31] Norén G, Arndt J, Hindmarsh T. Stereotactic radiosurgery in cases of acoustic neurinoma: further experiences. Neurosurgery. 1983; 13(1):12–22

[32] Lunsford LD, Niranjan A, Flickinger JC, Maitz A, Kondziolka D. Radiosurgery of vestibular schwannomas: summary of experience in 829 cases. J Neurosurg. 2005; 102 Suppl:195–199

[33] Flickinger JC, Kondziolka D, Pollock BE, Lunsford LD. Evolution in technique for vestibular schwannoma radiosurgery and effect on outcome. Int J Radiat Oncol Biol Phys. 1996; 36(2):275–280

[34] Hempel JM, Hempel E, Wowra B, Schichor Ch, Muacevic A, Riederer A. Functional outcome after Gamma Knife treatment in vestibular schwannoma. Eur Arch Otorhinolaryngol. 2006; 263(8):714–718

[35] Chung WY, Liu KD, Shiau CY, et al. Gamma Knife surgery for vestibular schwannoma: 10-year experience of 195 cases. J Neurosurg. 2005; 102 Suppl:87–96

[36] Zhao ZF, Yang LZ, Jiang CL, Zheng YR, Zhang JW. Gamma Knife irradiation-induced histopathological changes in the trigeminal nerves of rhesus monkeys. J Neurosurg. 2010; 113(1):39–44

[37] Mousavi SH, Niranjan A, Huang MJ, et al. Early radiosurgery provides superior pain relief for trigeminal neuralgia patients. Neurology. 2015; 85(24):2159–2165

[38] Sughrue ME, Yang I, Han SJ, et al. Non-audiofacial morbidity after Gamma Knife surgery for vestibular schwannoma. Neurosurg Focus. 2009; 27(6):E4

[39] Linskey ME, Flickinger JC, Lunsford LD. Cranial nerve length predicts the risk of delayed facial and trigeminal neuropathies after acoustic tumor stereotactic radiosurgery. Int J Radiat Oncol Biol Phys. 1993; 25(2):227–233

[40] Pollock BE. Management of vestibular schwannomas that enlarge after stereotactic radiosurgery: treatment recommendations based on a 15 year experience. Neurosurgery. 2006; 58(2):241–248, discussion 241–248

[41] Ganz JC, Reda WA, Abdelkarim K. Adverse radiation effects after Gamma Knife Surgery in relation to dose and volume. Acta Neurochir (Wien). 2009; 151(1):9–19

[42] Gerganov VM, Giordano M, Elolf E, Osamah A, Amir S, Madjid S. Operative management of patients with radiosurgery-related trigeminal neuralgia: analysis of the surgical morbidity and pain outcome. Clin Neurol Neurosurg. 2014; 122:23–28

[43] Tuleasca C, Carron R, Resseguier N, et al. Repeat Gamma Knife surgery for recurrent trigeminal neuralgia: long-term outcomes and systematic review. J Neurosurg. 2014; 121 Suppl:210–221

71 Postoperative Headache: Clinical Evaluation and Treatment in Patients Undergoing Surgery for Vestibular Schwannoma

Narayan R. Kissoon and Kelly D. Flemming

71.1 Introduction

Headaches in patients undergoing intervention for vestibular schwannomas (VS) are a key driver of quality of life.[1,2] Headaches may reduce quality of life and have a negative impact on psychological and physical functioning.[2,3,4,5] Thus, it is important to be familiar with the pathogenesis, risk factors, and phenotypes of the different posttreatment headache syndromes. These factors help guide treatments of postoperative headache in these patients. A combination of presurgical planning, intraoperative techniques, and postoperative medication and nonmedication strategies can be employed to reduce the frequency and severity of postoperative headaches. Chapter 59 reviews the epidemiology, diagnostic criteria, and pathogenesis of headaches in patients with VS. This chapter focuses primarily on clinical evaluation and treatment.

71.2 Approach to Postoperative Headache

71.2.1 Clinical Evaluation

The temporal profile of the headache in relation to the timing of the operation can help guide evaluation and provides clues to the underlying cause of the headache. Generally, serious causes of postoperative headache would occur during the acute period, less than 3 months after the operation. The differential diagnosis of acute and chronic postoperative headaches in patients undergoing surgery for VS is listed in ▶ Table 71.1.

The history should address the location, quality, frequency, and duration of the pain in addition to aggravating and alleviating factors. Two retrospective studies reported that VS headaches were most commonly localized to the occipital[6] or neck region.[7] Headaches may also localize to the frontal region, top of the head, or entire head,[6,7,8] and have been reported to be both unilateral or bilateral.[8]

Table 71.1 Differential diagnosis of acute and chronic postoperative headaches in patients undergoing surgery for vestibular schwannoma

Acute (generally < 3 mo postoperative)	Chronic (generally > 3 mo postoperative)
Serious • Intracranial hemorrhage • CSF leak • Tension pneumocephalus • Infection (wound, meningitis) • Aseptic meningitis • Hydrocephalus • Sinus thrombosis or sacrifice Benign • Acute postcraniotomy headache • Acute migraine headache	• Chronic postcraniotomy headache • Tension headache • Occipital neuralgia • Trigeminal neuropathy • Cervicogenic headache • Migraine headache • Rebound headache (medication overuse headache) • Temporomandibular joint dysfunction or masticatory muscle injury

The examination should focus on assessing the temporomandibular joint and muscles of mastication if a temporal craniotomy was performed, examining the scar for signs of infection or neuralgic pain at the site, assessing cervical range of motion, palpation of areas of emergences of cranial or spinal nerves, funduscopic examination for papilledema, and evaluating for neurologic dysfunction. Importantly, the initial evaluation should carefully rule out serious causes of postoperative headache.

Headache severity can be assessed in the clinical and research setting. Headache severity is most commonly assessed in the clinical setting via patient questionnaire, direct questioning, or estimated using a nonstandardized rating scale, either ordinal or visual analog.[9,10,11,12,13] Several studies have retrospectively quantified headache severity by assigning a numerical value from review of medical records alone.[6,7,14,15] Standardized measures of headache severity have also been employed by a few authors. Carlson and colleagues used the Headache Disability Inventory (▶ Fig. 71.1) to assess the functional and emotional effects of headache on everyday life.[16] This 25-item standardized measure of headache severity has been shown to have good internal reliability and content validity.[17,18] Other validated instruments have been developed to assess headache and pain in the context of other quality-of-life measures. The Penn Acoustic Neuroma Quality of Life Scale is a self-report questionnaire that includes seven domains, one of which assesses head pain in the form of a single question.[19] Finally, a number of self-rated headache disability inventories exist but have not yet been employed in the VS literature, presenting an opportunity for future study. These include the Headache Impact Test (HIT),[20] Headache Disability Questionnaire (HDQ),[21] Burden of Migraine (BURMIG) questionnaire,[22] and EUROLIGHT questionnaire.[22]

71.2.2 Secondary Causes

In the acute period, serious causes should be considered and excluded. Intracranial hemorrhage (intraparenchymal or subdural) complicates VS surgery in less than 5% of patients[23] and may present with headache and change in level of awareness or consciousness with or without focal neurologic symptoms. Cerebrospinal fluid (CSF) leak is a common complication of VS surgery, but is usually associated with CSF rhinorrhea and generally not spontaneous intracranial hypotension.[24] However, spontaneous intracranial hypotension with postural headache due to a spinal source has been described in patients postoperatively after skull base tumor resection.[24] In addition, Mokri reported on a patient with postcraniotomy CSF leak that paradoxically had postural headaches worse with lying down.[25] In addition, tension pneumocephalus may concurrently develop with an active CSF leak through a "ball-valve" mechanism. The

HEADACHE DISABILITY INDEX

N AME: ____________________ D ATE: ______ A GE: ____ S CORES TOTAL: ____; E____; F____
(100) (52) (48)

INSTRUCTIONS: Please CIRCLE the correct response:

1. I have headache: [1] 1 per month [2] more than but less than 4 per month [3] more than one per week.
2. My headache is: [1] mild [2] moderate [3] severe

INSTRUCTIONS: PLEASE READ CAREFULLY: The purpose of the scale is to identify difficulties that you may be experiencing because of your headache. Please check off "YES", "SOMETIMES", or "NO" to each item. Answer each item as it pertains to your headache only.

	YES	SOMETIMES	NO
E1. Because of my headaches I feel handicapped.			
F2. Because of my headaches I feel restricted in performing my routine daily activities.			
E3. No one understands the effect my headaches have on my life.			
F4. I restrict my recreational activities (e.g. sports, hobbies) because of my headaches			
E5. My headaches make me angry.			
E6. Sometimes I feel that I am going to lose control because of my headaches			
F7. Because of my headaches I am less likely to socialize.			
E8. My spouse/significant other, or family and friends have no idea what I am going through because of my headaches.			
E9. My headaches are so bad that I feel I am going to go insane.			
E10. My outlook on the world is affected by my headaches.			
E11. I am afraid to go outside when I feel a headache is starting.			
E12. I feel desperate because of my headaches.			
F13. I am concerned that I am paying penalties at work or at home because of my headaches.			
E14. My headaches place stress on my relationships with family or friends.			
F15. I avoid being around people when I have a headache.			
F16. I believe my headaches are making it difficult for me to achieve my goals in life.			
F17. I am unable to think clearly because of my headaches.			
F18. I get tense (e.g. muscle tension) because of my headaches.			
F19. I do not enjoy social gatherings because of my headaches.			
E20. I feel irritable because of my headaches.			
F21. I avoid traveling because of my headaches.			
E22. My headaches make me feel confused.			
E23. My headaches make me feel frustrated.			
F24. I find it difficult to read because of my headaches.			
F25. I find it difficult to focus my attention away from my headaches and on other things.			

Reference: Jacobson Gary P., Ramadan NM, et al., The Henry Ford Hospital Headache Disability Inventory (HDI). Neurology 1994; 44:837-842
FORM 502

Fig. 71.1 Headache Disability Inventory.

risk of tension pneumocephalus is higher when using a lumbar drain or continuous positive air pressure (CPAP) therapy for sleep apnea. Infection (wound or meningitis) is a serious but fortunately uncommon complication of VS surgery that may result in headache.[26,27,28] Aseptic, or chemical meningitis, may develop in up to 5% of cases following cerebellopontine angle surgery and is thought to arise from the presence of residual postoperative inflammatory products, such as blood and bone dust, in the subarachnoid space. Headache from aseptic meningitis classically emerges while the patient is tapering off a perioperative steroid, and may be associated with pseudomeningocele, representing elevated intracranial pressures. In this setting, a lumbar puncture for CSF analysis, including culture, is often required to distinguish aseptic meningitis from bacterial meningitis.[29] Hydrocephalus postoperatively may result in headache, visual changes, and reduced level of consciousness. The management of perioperative hydrocephalus is discussed further in Chapter 46.

Sinus thrombosis, sinus stenosis, or sacrifice of a dural sinus could result in holocephalic, severe pain.[30] If persistent, venous hypertension could develop and result in focal neurologic deficits, vision loss, and/or seizures. Keiper and colleagues reported venous sinus thrombosis causing headache following both retrosigmoid and translabyrinthine craniotomy.[31] Patients with venous sinus thrombosis developed postoperative symptoms consistent with intracranial hypertension including headache, vision changes, and papilledema. Imaging studies in these patients revealed occlusion of their dominant transverse and/or sigmoid sinus. Another study reported that postoperative transverse sinus thrombosis was more frequent following the translabyrinthine approach.[32] In their study, all patients experience some degree of lateral sinus thrombosis following surgical resection of VSs, and it is unclear whether isolated sigmoid sinus thrombosis without concurrent transverse sinus occlusion contributes to clinically significant intracranial hypertension and postsurgical headache. The risk of dural sinus thrombosis is greatest when operating on the side with a dominant venous system, when the lateral sinus system is injured, or in patients with hypercoagulopathy. Suspected cases are optimally imaged using magnetic resonance imaging (MRI) with MR venography, or computed tomography (CT) with CT venography. Fortunately, the prevalence of clinically significant sinus thrombosis following VS surgery is very low. Chapter 45 discusses this topic further.

71.2.3 Clinical Phenotypes of Postoperative Headache in Patients with Vestibular Schwannoma

Approximately 30% of patients undergoing surgery for VS may have persistent pain lasting more than 3 to 6 months. There are several chronic headache categories that these patients may fall into. Schankin and colleagues assessed headaches in 95 patients undergoing VS surgery, all with a retrosigmoid approach.[10] Thirty-two percent of those patients had a persistent headache with a severity of at least 6 out of 10 postoperatively for more than 6 months. When using the second edition of the International Classification of Headache Disorders (ICHD2), patient's headache syndromes fell into five categories: tension type (46%), occipital nerve (16.6%), trigeminal neuropathy (16.6%), neuropathy of the intermedian nerve (10.0%), and cervicogenic headache (10.0%). This study assessed quality of headache type nearly 1 year after surgery. Some have suggested the quality of headache may change with time and therefore migrainous quality may be underrepresented.[33] Other considerations for chronic postoperative headache causes include medication overuse headaches, migraine headaches,[8] and temporomandibular joint dysfunction.[34] Each of these headache types have unique locations, quality of pain, and precipitating factors. However, they can also be encompassed into the ICHD criteria of postcraniotomy headache. When serious causes have been ruled out, it is important to assess which category a patient's headache syndrome might fit in so that treatment may be appropriately tailored (▸ Fig. 71.2 and ▸ Table 71.2).

The following section reviews general considerations and approaches to headache management followed by a section on the evaluation and treatment of more specific, common phenotypes of chronic postoperative headache.

71.3 General Headache Management

Medical management of persistent headache in postcraniotomy patients may be challenging and frequently requires a multidisciplinary approach involving the neurological, pain management, and surgical disciplines. Management strategies should be based on thorough consideration of the headache pattern including the presence of pretreatment headaches as well as their current location, quality, duration, and intensity.

71.3.1 Preoperative Considerations

There are several preoperative considerations when counseling a patient on intervention for a VS. It is important to recognize that multiple studies have shown that a major risk factor for postoperative headache is the presence of preoperative headache.[17] In this regard, it is useful to set expectations for the purpose of surgery so as to avoid unrealistic goals. In addition, one might consider determining if there is a primary headache disorder and consider preoperative proactive treatment. While no studies exist comparing the risk of postoperative headache with preemptive prophylactic treatment of the headache disorder prior to VS surgery, this could be considered. In addition, a history of anxiety and/or depression may increase the risk of postoperative headache. Identification and treatment of these comorbid conditions should be considered prior to surgery.

A careful consideration of treatment options should be discussed with the patient. For example, in a patient with severe headaches at baseline, can an approach other than retrosigmoid craniotomy be considered if surgery is pursued? Is the tumor amenable to observation, stereotactic radiosurgery, or another surgical approach?

71.3.2 Operative Considerations

Several studies have suggested that limiting nuchal muscle dissection, and the size of craniotomy[18] and avoiding craniectomy, can reduce postoperative headache.[6,13,35] This is supported by

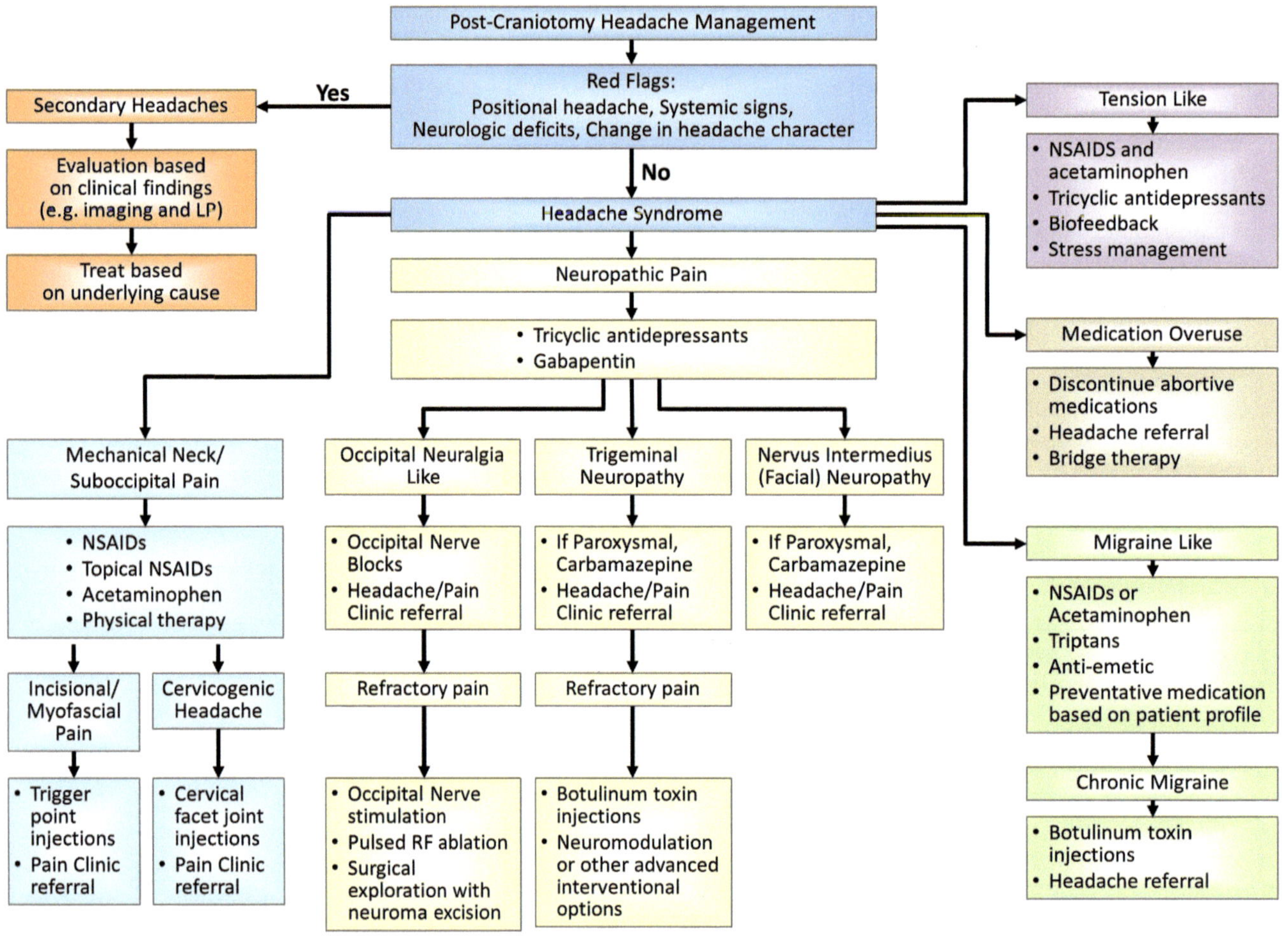

Fig. 71.2 Postcraniotomy Headache Management Algorithm. NSAIDs, nonsteroidal anti-inflammatory drugs; LP, lumbar puncture; RF, radiofrequency ablation.

Table 71.2 Common *persistent* headache types after vestibular schwannoma surgery

Craniofacial Pain Syndrome	Description of pain	Other symptoms	Abortive therapy	Prophylactic management
Tension type	Dull, aching pain Starts near incision and can spread bilaterally Often worse in morning	–	NSAIDs Acetaminophen	• Tricyclic antidepressants • SNRIs • Gabapentin • Topiramate
Occipital Neuropathy	Intermittent stabbing pain in the retromastoid region; may radiate cranially on the ipsilateral side	May have reduced sensation in distribution of occipital nerve	[a]	• Gabapentin • Tricyclic antidepressants • Occipital nerve block
Trigeminal neuropathy	Dull, drilling in distribution of trigeminal nerve (V1 or V3)	Dysesthesia of trigeminal nerve	[a]	• Gabapentin • Tricyclic antidepressants
Nervus intermedius (geniculate) neuralgia	Deep external auditory canal or preauricular	Dry eye Dysgeusia	[a]	• Gabapentin • Tricyclic antidepressants
Cervicogenic and incisional pain	Dull, drilling pain Begins in neck and radiates cranially (and can be bilateral)	Paresthesias in arms occasionally	NSAIDs Topical NSAIDs Acetaminophen	• Gabapentinoids • SNRIs • Physical therapy
Rebound (medication overuse)	Holocephalic aching pain generally worse in mornings and as the next dose of pain reliever is due Headaches more than 15 d per month	Frequent use of pain relievers, often greater than 3 mo	Limit and reduce offending agent	• Discontinue offending agent • Consider neurologic or pain consultation for establishing treatment plan
Migraine	Throbbing pulsating, bifrontal or holocephalic pain	Nausea/Vomiting Photophobia Phonophobia	NSAIDs Triptans Acetaminophen	• Tricyclic antidepressants • Anticonvulsant drugs (Topamax, Divalproex sodium, Gabapentin) • Beta-blocker • Calcium channel blocker • Botox injections

Abbreviations: NSAIDs, nonsteroidal anti-inflammatory drugs; SNRIs, serotonin-norepinephrine reuptake inhibitors.
[a]NSAIDs, acetaminophen, and narcotics can be tried but often ineffective.

the theory that postcraniotomy headache can result from attachment and scarring of nuchal musculature to exposed dura. In addition, consideration of duraplasty rather than direct dural closure has been suggested by some.[6] Minimizing intradural bone drilling, prevention of subarachnoid bone dust dissemination, and meticulous removal of bone dust after meatal drilling, is recommended as this may potentially be linked to development of aseptic meningitis and headache.[14,15] Catalano and colleagues reported a lower incidence of postoperative headache when Gelfoam was used to cover posterior fossa structures and CSF cisterns prior to commencement of drilling, in order to trap bone dust and prevent spread.[14]

Some advocate the use of local anesthesia at the scalp site as a means of reducing postoperative headache.[36,37] In a blinded study of 52 patients undergoing intracranial tumoral resection of any type, half received infiltration of the surgical site with 20 cc of ropivacaine 0.75% and half did not.[36] All received intravenous (IV) acetaminophen combined with nalbuphine. There was a trend toward reduced nalbuphine consumption during the first postoperative day. At 2 months, postoperative pain was lower in the group that received ropivacaine. While not studied in craniotomy patients, some have suggested reduction in neuropathic pain with perioperative delivery of neuropathic agents and/or ketamine.[38,39,40]

71.3.3 Postoperative Considerations

Postoperatively, it is important to assess the type of headache and if there is a secondary cause requiring intervention as discussed earlier. If craniectomy alone was performed, revision cranioplasty could be considered in the case of persistent headache, particularly if focused at the surgical site and refractory to medical therapy.

71.3.4 Lifestyle Strategies and Nonpharmacologic Alternatives

A comprehensive headache management strategy including education and counseling regarding lifestyle regulation will be critical to successful outcomes. Headaches can be exacerbated by lack of sleep. Thus, assessing a patient's sleep habits is important and also advising patients on good sleep hygiene, which may include going to bed at a regular time and removing television from the bedroom. Some headaches may be exacerbated by poor eating habits. Regular meals, cessation of caffeine use, and avoiding food triggers may limit exacerbations of headache.[41,42]

Emotional and physical stress can exacerbate headaches as well. After VS surgery, patients may be suffering from other symptoms, concerned about employment, and have fatigue. Identifying and addressing stress, depression, and anxiety is a key component of headache management. Relaxation techniques, biofeedback, and cognitive behavioral therapy may be helpful adjunctive strategies to reduce the impact of stress contributing to the patient's headaches.[41,42]

A variety of nonpharmacologic alternatives have also been utilized for the treatment of chronic postcraniotomy headaches including acupuncture, physiotherapy, biofeedback therapy, and transcutaneous electrical stimulation. Based on trial results for chronic headache, these techniques appear to be associated with low risk of serious adverse effects; however, their clinical effectiveness as a treatment for headaches after craniotomy or VS resection has not been evaluated using scientifically rigorous methods.

71.3.5 Intractable Pain

In some patients, intractable pain continues or they are limited by side effects of standard medications. In patients in whom standard treatments are not useful, a referral to a center with comprehensive headache and pain care can be considered. Physical medicine and rehabilitation, neurology, psychiatry, and pain experts may be needed to help in the treatment of these difficult cases.

71.4 Specific Craniofacial Pain Syndromes: Clinical Features and Management

71.4.1 Incisional Pain

Clinical Features

In this case, pain is generally greatest over the surgical site incision.[6,43,44] With the retrosigmoid approach, the headache often starts at the incision and extends to the midocciput and the posterior skull region.[6] The type of the pain is a dull ache with pressure. Typically, this type of pain is constant in a majority of patients.[43] During the first several months, the pain is often moderate to severe in intensity, but patients with persistent long-term headache usually describe a mild headache.[43] Patients often have tenderness to palpation at the incisional site. In a majority of patients, the pain along the incision site resolves within 4 months.[43]

Management

For patients with incisional neck pain, nonsteroidal anti-inflammatory drugs (NSAIDs) are commonly useful. In patients with persistent incisional pain, topical NSAIDs such as a diclofenac gel can be used to help minimize the use of systemic NSAIDs and the adverse events that can occur with systemic NSAID use.[45] Muscle relaxants could be considered, but are often associated with sedation. If the incisional pain persists despite the aforementioned management strategies, a serotonin-norepinephrine reuptake inhibitor (SNRI) such as duloxetine or a gabapentinoid could also be considered.[46,47]

71.4.2 Cervicogenic Headache

Clinical Features

Patients complain of a dull and drilling pain beginning in the neck and can radiate cranially, which is provoked by extension or axial rotation of the neck.[10] The most commonly treated cause of cervicogenic headache is related to cervical facet arthritis.[48,49] The distribution of headache and neck pain can be indicative of the facet joints involved (▸ Fig. 71.3).[48] Occasionally, patients may have paresthesias in the upper extremities suggestive of a cervical radiculopathy.

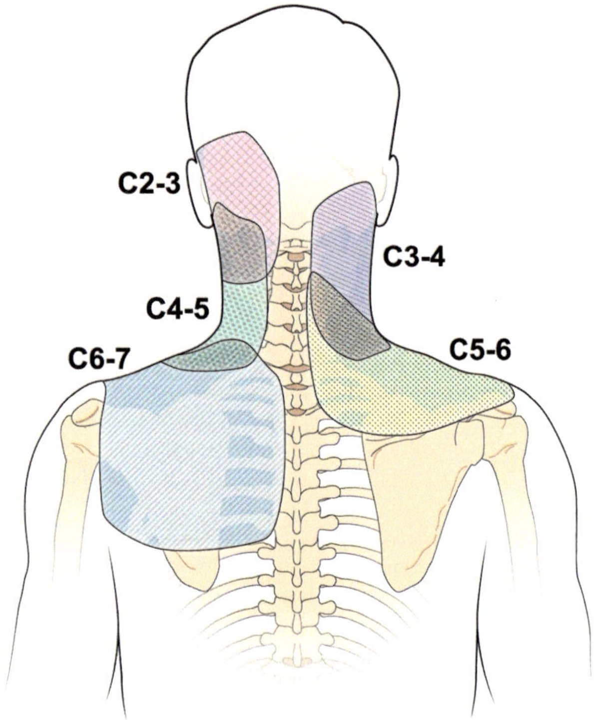

Fig. 71.3 Referral patterns of pain from cervical facet joints. (Adapted from Cooper et al.[48])

Management

Medical management is similar to that used for incisional pain as outlined earlier. However, if the pain is refractory to medications and physical therapy, then percutaneous interventions could be considered. Based on the referral pattern and findings on plain cervical spine films, cervical facet joint injections may be beneficial.[48] If there are advanced degenerative changes involving the cervical facet joints, then medial branch blocks leading to radiofrequency denervation of the respective cervical facet joints can provide long-lasting pain relief and could potentially be repeated as frequent as every 6 months if the pain recurs.[49] If there are findings of radicular pain or paresthesias in the upper extremities, then a MRI of the cervical spine and cervical epidural steroid injection could be considered as a management option.

71.4.3 Occipital Neuralgia-Like Pain

Clinical Features

An occipital neuralgia-like headache is common postoperatively and is characterized by stabbing pain in the region of the occipital nerve near the mastoid. This pain can radiate cranially (always ipsilateral) and is often triggered by wound contact and/or head movement. This pain is rarely a neuralgiform pain. More commonly, it is a constant, burning-type pain.[10] Tenderness along the occipital nerve region is a common finding on examination.

Management

If the occipital nerve is felt to be possibly the source of pain, oral analgesics are often ineffective.[50] Gabapentin and nortriptyline are often first-line medications.[51] Other medications to consider are carbamazepine, pregabalin, and baclofen.[51] A local anesthetic block with corticosteroid can be diagnostic and therapeutic.[51,52] If only short-term pain relief is obtained with occipital nerve block, then pulsed radiofrequency ablation of the nervus occipitalis is a potential therapeutic option.[52] In refractory cases, occipital nerve stimulation at an experienced center or occipital nerve excision could be considered.[50,52,53] In one study,[50] seven patients had been found where an occipital neuroma or entrapment was identified as the cause of persistent pain. In these seven patients, conservative management failed. Surgery with excision of the greater and lesser occipital nerve resulted in six of seven improving significantly.

71.4.4 Trigeminal Neuropathy

Clinical Features

With a retrosigmoid approach, some patients may develop neuropathic facial pain postoperatively. This usually occurs in the V1 or V3 region and is characterized as a dull, drilling sensation but not necessarily a lancinating or neuralgiform-type character. Unlike trigeminal neuralgia, there are no typical triggering factors. Patients may also complain of reduced sensation or dysesthesia in the same distribution of pain, altered taste, and dry mouth and eyes.[10]

Management

Patients with trigeminal neuropathic symptoms are less likely to respond well to medications. Given the pain is often not neuralgiform in nature, patients do not respond well to carbamazepine or other neuralgiform pain medications.[10] Gabapentin or tricyclic antidepressants, common neuropathic pain medications, could be considered, but no clinical trials or series have evaluated the efficacy.[54] If the pain is paroxysmal in nature, then carbamazepine and oxcarbazepine may be beneficial among other medications.[55,56] Limited data are available evaluating the efficacy of medications in postoperative trigeminal nerve distribution pain, but painful trigeminal neuropathy is often difficult to treat[57] and may require referral to a specialist in neurology and/or pain clinic. Refractory trigeminal nerve distribution pain may be responsive to intradermal botulinum toxin injections.[58,59] In experienced centers, advanced interventional techniques may be considered for refractory trigeminal nerve distribution pain.[53,55,60]

71.4.5 Nervus Intermedius Neuralgia (Geniculate Neuralgia)

Clinical Features

In rare cases, neuropathic pain centered deep in the external auditory canal can be encountered in patients undergoing VS resection. This pain can radiate to the infra- and preauricular skin. Oftentimes, patients also complain of dysgeusia.[10]

Management

Management for nervus intermedius neuralgia is similar to trigeminal neuropathic symptoms and similarly is less likely to respond well to medications.[10] The same neuropathic medications used for trigeminal nerve distribution pain may be considered for use in the management of nervus intermedius neuralgia.[54] Refractory pain may require referral to a specialist in neurology and/or pain clinic. There are no data regarding advanced interventional techniques for the management of nervus intermedius neuralgia, but neuromodulation could potentially be considered in refractory cases.[61,62] Limited reports have suggested that division of the nervus intermedius, microvascular decompression with padding of any offending vasculature, or geniculate ganglion decompression may benefit select patients.[63]

71.4.6 Tension-Type Headache

Clinical Features

In some patients, the pain extends from the occipital region to the frontal region.[8] It can be ipsilateral to the surgical site or bilateral. Most commonly, patients describe the headache as an aching or pressing pain worse with head movement, fatigue, and exercise.[6] The quality of a dull aching pain is often similar to that encountered in a tension-type headache.[6,10,43,44] In two-thirds of patients, the pain is intermittent and for others, it can be constant.[8] Headaches often last minutes to hours and can be aggravated or triggered with bending, coughing, and physical or emotional stress.[8,44] The headache may alter sleep and be present upon awakening.

Management

If a secondary cause is not determined, and the headache is felt to be acute postcraniotomy headache, a short course of NSAIDs,[8,10] opioids, or acetaminophen are commonly used. In one study, 35% of postoperative headaches ceased with NSAIDs alone.[8] However, these medications should be used sparingly due to the potential for medication overuse syndrome (rebound) or effects on other systems.

Limited data exist for prophylactic agents in the treatment of tension-type postcraniotomy headache, as few studies have stratified postcraniotomy headaches by phenotype,[8,10] but medications similar to those used for traumatic brain injury and/or chronic tension-type headaches are commonly trialed (▶ Table 71.2). The strongest evidence for treatment efficacy of chronic tension-type headaches is with tricyclic antidepressants and biofeedback.[41] There is limited evidence supporting the use of other medications such as SNRIs and anticonvulsants in chronic tension-type headache.[41,64,65] In some cases, stress management, physical therapy, and/or massage could be considered.[9] While not studied in the context of craniotomy for VS, acupuncture, TENS unit, massage, and biofeedback could be considered.[66]

71.4.7 Medication Overuse Headache

Clinical Features

Medication overuse headaches (rebound) are an uncommon type of postoperative headache.[8,10] Headaches generally occur nearly every day and are often present upon wakening. Use of a pain reliever helps the headache, but as the pain reliever wears off, the headache returns. Characteristics of the headaches are generally similar to tension or migraine types.[67] Patients may also have mild nausea, restlessness, or fatigue. Opioids are commonly offending agents, but even NSAIDs, acetaminophen, or triptans used daily can cause medication overuse headache.

Management

Medication overuse headaches can be difficult to treat. Withdrawal of the offending agent is the key to treatment, but may be difficult for the patient as the headaches can be severe. Most cases of medication overuse headaches can be treated in the outpatient setting; however, if opioids, benzodiazepines, barbiturates, or tranquilizers are the offending agent, specialized treatment programs may be needed. The treatment of medication overuse headaches is beyond the scope of this chapter. Recognition of the headache with referral to a specialist in neurology or pain medicine is important. Often a regimen of a "bridge therapy" and prophylactic agent is recommended. Bridge therapy refers to the analgesic or medication that is used to get through the acute pain while withdrawing from the offending agent.

71.4.8 Migraine-Like Headache

Clinical Features

In some patients, their preexisting migraine headache may be triggered or someone with a predisposition for migraine headache may develop new-onset migrainous headaches. It may be intermittent, or become chronic. Migraine headaches are typically characterized by a throbbing, pulsating pain that may be frontal, holocephalic, or sometimes located in the occipital region. It is often associated with photophobia, photophobia, nausea, and sometimes vomiting. Patients often report that lying down and sleeping will reduce the pain. As migraines transition to a chronic or daily headache, often the throbbing quality and associated symptoms dissipate.

Management

For patients with an exacerbation of migraine, NSAIDs, triptans, and acetaminophen can be tried for abortive therapy. In some case series and reports, sumatriptan has been found to abort headache in some patients postsurgery.[68] Often patients are knowledgeable about what works for them. If first-line agents are not helpful and the severity of the symptoms is significant, IV ketorolac, IV valproic acid, IV magnesium, subcutaneous sumatriptan, IV Dihydroergotamine (DHE), antinausea medications (prochlorperazine, chlorpromazine, metoclopramide), or IV dexamethasone can be useful. In one case of postoperative intractable migrainous headache in a patient after VS removal, IV lidocaine followed by mexiletine[69] was successful.

A number of prophylactic agent options are available. In general, this includes beta-blockers (e.g., propranolol), calcium channel blockers (e.g., verapamil), and anticonvulsant medications (topiramate, valproic acid, gabapentin). Case reports and small case series have suggested migraine prophylactic medications such as combination of divalproex sodium and verapamil,[70] divalproex sodium,[71] and tricyclic antidepressants[9] could be considered in the management of postoperative headache. Choice of medication is dependent on factors such as response of medications prior to surgery for patients on prior prophylactic medications, presence of aura, age, medication side effect profile, and medical comorbidities.[42] For women of child-bearing age, medications like topiramate and valproic acid are teratogenic; so, either contraception or use of an alternative medication would need to be considered.[42] With chronic intractable migraine, referral to a specialist in neurology and botulinum toxin injections may be considered if patient fails or is intolerant to prophylactic medications.[42] Complimentary to medications, regular meals, adequate sleep, stress reduction, and avoidance of potential triggers are a mainstay of migraine therapy.[42]

71.5 Conclusion

Patients undergoing surgical treatment for VS not uncommonly experience headache. In some, this leads to significant psychosocial dysfunction and disability. Preoperatively, careful thought as to modality of tumor management, proactive treatment of comorbid anxiety and depression, and counseling on expectations for surgery is important. Surgical technique appears to have some impact on postoperative headache and optimization of these factors intraoperatively including limiting nuchal muscle dissection, prevention of subarachnoid bone dust dissemination, use of duraplasty, and craniotomy instead of craniectomy may reduce postoperative headaches. In addition, selection of surgical approach, such as using the translabyrinthine approach instead of the retrosigmoid approach for example, may be a worthwhile consideration in patients with an existing history of problematic headache or predisposition to such. The etiology of headaches immediately postoperatively may vary from those that are chronic and careful attention to determining the correct cause is important. Chronic, persistent headaches most commonly fall into a tension-type headache, migrainous headache, cervicogenic type, or neuropathic pain type (trigeminal or occipital nerve). Identifying the category of headache can help guide abortive, prophylactic, and nonpharmacologic therapies.

References

[1] Betchen SA, Walsh J, Post KD. Self-assessed quality of life after acoustic neuroma surgery. J Neurosurg. 2003; 99(5):818–823

[2] Carlson ML, Tveiten OV, Driscoll CL, et al. What drives quality of life in patients with sporadic vestibular schwannoma? Laryngoscope. 2015; 125(7):1697–1702

[3] Ryzenman JM, Pensak ML, Tew JM, Jr. Patient perception of comorbid conditions after acoustic neuroma management: survey results from the acoustic neuroma association. Laryngoscope. 2004; 114(5):814–820

[4] Tos T, Caye-Thomasen P, Stangerup SE, Tos M, Thomsen J. Long-term socio-economic impact of vestibular schwannoma for patients under observation and after surgery. J Laryngol Otol. 2003; 117(12):955–964

[5] Tos T, Cayé-Thomasen P, Stangerup SE, Tos M, Thomsen J. Patients' fears, expectations and satisfaction in relation to management of vestibular schwannoma: a comparison of surgery and observation. Acta Otolaryngol. 2003; 123(5):600–605

[6] Schaller B, Baumann A. Headache after removal of vestibular schwannoma via the retrosigmoid approach: a long-term follow-up-study. Otolaryngol Head Neck Surg. 2003; 128:387–395

[7] Harner SG, Beatty CW, Ebersold MJ. Headache after acoustic neuroma excision. Am J Otol. 1993; 14(6):552–555

[8] Rimaaja T, Haanpää M, Blomstedt G, Färkkilä M. Headaches after acoustic neuroma surgery. Cephalalgia. 2007; 27(10):1128–1135

[9] Pedrosa CA, Ahern DK, McKenna MJ, Ojemann RG, Acquadro MA. Determinants and impact of headache after acoustic neuroma surgery. Am J Otol. 1994; 15(6):793–797

[10] Schankin CJ, Gall C, Straube A. Headache syndromes after acoustic neuroma surgery and their implications for quality of life. Cephalalgia. 2009; 29(7):760–771

[11] Schessel DA, Rowed DW, Nedzelski JM, Feghali JG. Postoperative pain following excision of acoustic neuroma by the suboccipital approach: observations on possible cause and potential amelioration. Am J Otol. 1993; 14(5):491–494

[12] Vijayan N. Postoperative headache in acoustic neuroma. Headache. 1995; 35 (2):98–100

[13] Wazen JJ, Sisti M, Lam SM. Cranioplasty in acoustic neuroma surgery. Laryngoscope. 2000; 110(8):1294–1297

[14] Catalano PJ, Jacobowitz O, Post KD. Prevention of headache after retrosigmoid removal of acoustic tumors. Am J Otol. 1996; 17(6):904–908

[15] Jackson CG, McGrew BM, Forest JA, et al. Comparison of postoperative headache after retrosigmoid approach: vestibular nerve section versus vestibular schwannoma resection. Am J Otol. 2000; 21(3):412–416

[16] Carlson ML, Tveiten OV, Driscoll CL, et al. Risk factors and analysis of long-term headache in sporadic vestibular schwannoma: a multicenter cross-sectional study. J Neurosurg. 2015; 123(5):1276–1286

[17] Jatoi A, Radecki Breitkopf C, Foster NR, et al. A mixed-methods feasibility trial of protein kinase C iota inhibition with auranofin in asymptomatic ovarian cancer patients. Oncology. 2015; 88(4):208–213

[18] Santarius T, D'Sousa AR, Zeitoun HM, Cruickshank G, Morgan DW. Audit of headache following resection of acoustic neuroma using three different techniques of suboccipital approach. Rev Laryngol Otol Rhinol (Bord). 2000; 121(2):75–78

[19] Shaffer BT, Cohen MS, Bigelow DC, Ruckenstein MJ. Validation of a disease-specific quality-of-life instrument for acoustic neuroma: the Penn Acoustic Neuroma Quality-of-Life Scale. Laryngoscope. 2010; 120(8):1646–1654

[20] Kosinski M,, Bayliss MS, Bjorner JB, et al. A six-item short-form survey for measuring headache impact: the HIT-6. Qual Life Res. 2003; 12(8):963–974

[21] Niere K, Quin A. Development of a headache-specific disability questionnaire for patients attending physiotherapy. Man Ther. 2009; 14(1):45–51

[22] Andrée C, Vaillant M, Barre J, et al. Development and validation of the EURO-LIGHT questionnaire to evaluate the burden of primary headache disorders in Europe. Cephalalgia. 2010; 30(9):1082–1100

[23] Betka J, Zverina E, Balogova Z, et al. Complications of microsurgery of vestibular schwannoma. BioMed. 2014:ID:: 315952

[24] Schievink WI, Schwartz MS, Maya MM, Moser FG, Rozen TD. Lack of causal association between spontaneous intracranial hypotension and cranial cerebrospinal fluid leaks. J Neurosurg. 2012; 116(4):749–754

[25] Mokri B. Posture-related headaches and pachymeningeal enhancement in CSF leaks from craniotomy site. Cephalalgia. 2001; 21(10):976–979

[26] Mallory GW, Wilson JW, Castner ML, Driscoll CL, Link MJ. Herpes simplex meningitis after removal of a vestibular schwannoma: case report and review of the literature. Otol Neurotol. 2012; 33(8):1422–1425

[27] Korinek AM, Golmard JL, Elcheick A, et al. Risk factors for neurosurgical site infections after craniotomy: a critical reappraisal of antibiotic prophylaxis on 4,578 patients. Br J Neurosurg. 2005; 19(2):155–162

[28] Kourbeti IS, Jacobs AV, Koslow M, Karabetsos D, Holzman RS. Risk factors associated with postcraniotomy meningitis. Neurosurgery. 2007; 60(2):317–325, discussion 325–326

[29] Sanchez GB, Kaylie DM, O'Malley MR, Labadie RF, Jackson CG, Haynes DS. Chemical meningitis following cerebellopontine angle tumor surgery. Otolaryngol Head Neck Surg. 2008; 138(3):368–373

[30] Higgins JN, Pickard JD. Intractable headache after excision of an acoustic neuroma treated by stent revascularisation of the sigmoid sinus. Br J Neurosurg. 2013; 27(6):819–821

[31] Keiper GL, Jr, Sherman JD, Tomsick TA, Tew JM, Jr. Dural sinus thrombosis and pseudotumor cerebri: unexpected complications of suboccipital craniotomy and translabyrinthine craniectomy. J Neurosurg. 1999; 91(2):192–197

[32] Moore J, Thomas P, Cousins V, Rosenfeld JV. Diagnosis and management of dural sinus thrombosis following resection of cerebellopontine angle tumors. J Neurol Surg B Skull Base. 2014; 75(6):402–408

[33] Filho PA, Schankin CJ. Post-craniotomy headache after acoustic neuroma surgery. Cephalalgia. 2010; 30(4):509–510

[34] Rocha-Filho PA, Fujarra FJ, Gherpelli JL, Rabello GD, de Siqueira JT. The long-term effect of craniotomy on temporalis muscle function. Oral Surg Oral Med Oral Pathol Oral Radiol Endod. 2007; 104(5):e17–e21

[35] Koperer H, Deinsberger W, Jödicke A, Böker DK. Postoperative headache after the lateral suboccipital approach: craniotomy versus craniectomy. Minim Invasive Neurosurg. 1999; 42(4):175–178

[36] Batoz H, Verdonck O, Pellerin C, Roux G, Maurette P. The analgesic properties of scalp infiltrations with ropivacaine after intracranial tumoral resection. Anesth Analg. 2009; 109(1):240–244

[37] de Oliveira Ribeiro MdoC, Pereira CU, Sallum AM, et al. Immediate post-craniotomy headache. Cephalalgia. 2013; 33(11):897–905

[38] Doleman B, Heinink TP, Read DJ, Faleiro RJ, Lund JN, Williams JP. A systematic review and meta-regression analysis of prophylactic gabapentin for postoperative pain. Anaesthesia. 2015; 70(10):1186–1204

[39] Humble SR, Dalton AJ, Li L. A systematic review of therapeutic interventions to reduce acute and chronic post-surgical pain after amputation, thoracotomy or mastectomy. Eur J Pain. 2015; 19(4):451–465

[40] Porter SB, McClain RL, Howe BL, et al. Perioperative ketamine for acute postoperative analgesia: the Mayo Clinic-Florida experience. J Perianesth Nurs. 2015; 30(3):189–195

[41] Bendtsen L, Evers S, Linde M, Mitsikostas DD, Sandrini G, Schoenen J, EFNS. EFNS guideline on the treatment of tension-type headache - report of an EFNS task force. Eur J Neurol. 2010; 17(11):1318–1325

[42] Silberstein SD, Goadsby PJ. Migraine: preventive treatment. Cephalalgia. 2002; 22(7):491–512

[43] Mosek AC, Dodick DW, Ebersold MJ, Swanson JW. Headache after resection of acoustic neuroma. Headache. 1999; 39(2):89–94

[44] Rocha-Filho PA. Post-craniotomy headache: a clinical view with a focus on the persistent form. Headache. 2015; 55(5):733–738

[45] Derry S, Wiffen P, Moore A. Topical nonsteroidal anti-inflammatory drugs for acute musculoskeletal pain. JAMA. 2016; 315(8):813–814

[46] Smith HS, Smith EJ, Smith BR. Duloxetine in the management of chronic musculoskeletal pain. Ther Clin Risk Manag. 2012; 8:267–277

[47] Flórez-García M, Ceberio-Balda F, Morera-Domínguez C, Masramón X, Pérez M. Effect of pregabalin in the treatment of refractory neck pain: cost and clinical evidence from medical practice in orthopedic surgery and rehabilitation clinics. Pain Pract. 2011; 11(4):369–380

[48] Cooper G, Bailey B, Bogduk N. Cervical zygapophysial joint pain maps. Pain Med. 2007; 8(4):344–353

[49] Boswell MV, Colson JD, Sehgal N, Dunbar EE, Epter R. A systematic review of therapeutic facet joint interventions in chronic spinal pain. Pain Physician. 2007; 10(1):229–253

[50] Ducic I, Felder JM, III, Endara M. Postoperative headache following acoustic neuroma resection: occipital nerve injuries are associated with a treatable occipital neuralgia. Headache. 2012; 52(7):1136–1145

[51] Dougherty C. Occipital neuralgia. Curr Pain Headache Rep. 2014; 18(5):411

[52] Vanelderen P, Lataster A, Levy R, Mekhail N, van Kleef M, Van Zundert J. 8. Occipital neuralgia. Pain Pract. 2010; 10(2):137–144

[53] Rasskazoff SY, Slavin KV. Neuromodulation for cephalgias. Surg Neurol Int. 2013; 4 Suppl 3:S136–S150

[54] Finnerup NB, Otto M, McQuay HJ, Jensen TS, Sindrup SH. Algorithm for neuropathic pain treatment: an evidence based proposal. Pain. 2005; 118(3):289–305

[55] Gronseth G, Cruccu G, Alksne J, et al. Practice parameter: the diagnostic evaluation and treatment of trigeminal neuralgia (an evidence-based review): report of the Quality Standards Subcommittee of the American Academy of Neurology and the European Federation of Neurological Societies. Neurology. 2008; 71(15):1183–1190

[56] Cheshire WP, Jr. Cranial neuralgias. Continuum (Minneap Minn). 2015; 21 4 Headache:1072–1085

[57] Haviv Y, Zadik Y, Sharav Y, Benoliel R. Painful traumatic trigeminal neuropathy: an open study on the pharmacotherapeutic response to stepped treatment. J Oral Facial Pain Headache. 2014; 28(1):52–60

[58] Wu CJ, Lian YJ, Zheng YK, et al. Botulinum toxin type A for the treatment of trigeminal neuralgia: results from a randomized, double-blind, placebo-controlled trial. Cephalalgia. 2012; 32(6):443–450

[59] Oh HM, Chung ME. Botulinum toxin for neuropathic pain: a review of the literature. Toxins (Basel). 2015; 7(8):3127–3154

[60] van Kleef M, van Genderen WE, Narouze S, et al. World Institute of Medicine. 1. Trigeminal neuralgia. Pain Pract. 2009; 9(4):252–259

[61] Arcioni R, Palmisani S, Mercieri M, et al. Cervical 10 kHz spinal cord stimulation in the management of chronic, medically refractory migraine: a prospective, open-label, exploratory study. Eur J Pain. 2016; 20(1):70–78

[62] Chivukula S, Tempel ZJ, Weiner GM, et al. Cervical and cervicomedullary spinal cord stimulation for chronic pain: efficacy and outcomes. Clin Neurol Neurosurg. 2014; 127:33–41

[63] Tang IP, Freeman SR, Kontorinis G, et al. Geniculate neuralgia: a systematic review. J Laryngol Otol. 2014; 128(5):394–399

[64] Lampl C, Marecek S, May A, Bendtsen L. A prospective, open-label, long-term study of the efficacy and tolerability of topiramate in the prophylaxis of chronic tension-type headache. Cephalalgia. 2006; 26(10): 1203–1208

[65] Spira PJ, Beran RG, Australian Gabapentin Chronic Daily Headache Group. Gabapentin in the prophylaxis of chronic daily headache: a randomized, placebo-controlled study. Neurology. 2003; 61(12):1753–1759

[66] Acoustic Neuroma Association. Headache associated with acoustic neuroma treatment. 2015

[67] Limmroth V, Katsarava Z, Fritsche G, Przywara S, Diener HC. Features of medication overuse headache following overuse of different acute headache drugs. Neurology. 2002; 59(7):1011–1014

[68] Levo H, Blomstedt G, Hirvonen T, Pyykkö I. Causes of persistent postoperative headache after surgery for vestibular schwannoma. Clin Otolaryngol Allied Sci. 2001; 26(5):401–406

[69] Schere D, Silberstein SD. Intravenous lidocaine infusion for the treatment of post-acoustic neuroma resection headache: a case report. Headache. 2009; 49(2):302–303

[70] Hanson MB, Glasscock ME, III, Brandes JL, Jackson CG. Medical treatment of headache after suboccipital acoustic tumor removal. Laryngoscope. 1998; 108(8, Pt 1):1111–1114

[71] Hendler N, Cashen A, Morrison C, Long D, Holliday M. Divalproex sodium and other medications for headache following craniotomy for acoustic neuroma. Headache. 1995; 35(8):490–493

72 The Acoustic Neuroma Association and Social Aspects of Support Group Care for Patients with Vestibular Schwannoma

Judy B. Vitucci

72.1 Introduction

You have just been told you have a brain tumor. It is called a vestibular schwannoma (VS), also known as an acoustic neuroma. The diagnosis leaves you and your family numb with fear and disbelief. Your mind is flooded with questions. Why me? How did this happen? Sure, your hearing has been gradually declining and it's been a little harder to hear over the phone lately. But a *brain tumor*? You are informed that there is no known cause and, though benign, the tumor may grow. You'll feel an urge to take action, but where do you even begin?

The physician who frequently deals with cranial tumors may be relieved that the etiology of the patient's symptoms is discovered and that the cause is a benign brain tumor. The patient, on the other hand, has never heard of a VS and may be devastated by the words "brain tumor" and all the new and uncertain information, fearing the worst. Never knowing anyone who has been diagnosed and treated for a VS makes the future feel very uncertain.

Diagnosis and treatment of a VS is a pivotal event in the patient's life. Much of the rest of his or her life is defined in terms of "before or after my VS." Whether pre- or posttreatment, many patients and their caregivers live a life where the impact of their tumor is felt every day as they adjust to their new normal situation (▶ Fig. 72.1). After treatment, the physician's appraisal of the patient's results may be quite positive with the tasks completed—the brain tumor treated—while the patient's assessment of the same results can differ. Treatment may lead to hearing loss, tinnitus, balance issues, or perhaps some loss of facial function. These issues among others are often a source of ongoing distress to the VS patient.

72.2 Acoustic Neuroma Association—www.ANAUSA.org

The Acoustic Neuroma Association (ANA) was established to provide educational information and support in an effort to improve the patient experience—both pre- and posttreatment. Early patient education can provide realistic and accurate expectations regarding potential treatment options and long-term outlook. In addition, networking and social support offers opportunities for positive interaction with other VS patients who can offer valuable insight and reassurance to the newly diagnosed patient. Finally, finding a medical provider with substantial experience in VS treatment is critical to the patient's long-term health and well-being. The ANA was established to improve patients' overall experience with VS, and remains an important medium for connecting patients to other patients and to medical professionals.

The ANA was founded in 1981 by a VS patient, Virginia (Ginny) Fickel Ehr in Carlisle, PA. She found no patient information or patient support available when she had surgery for a VS in 1977. Ginny experienced significant neurological deficits before and after surgery and sought information about VS that could be understood by a layperson; however, none was available at that time. From this experience, she resolved that future patients diagnosed with VS would not face the same difficulties. With the support of her surgeon, she assembled eight patients who made up ANA's first volunteer Board of Directors. The association was incorporated in 1981 and received tax-exempt status 501(c)(3). The ANA was thus founded to provide ongoing support and services to VS patients, family members, and caregivers through their VS journey. A mission statement was subsequently adopted by the Board in April 2006: *The mission of Acoustic Neuroma Association is to inform, educate, and provide national and local support networks for those affected by acoustic neuromas, and to be an essential resource for health care professionals who treat acoustic neuroma patients.*

Since its inception, the ANA has worked with tens of thousands of patients worldwide. Today, the ANA is the premier organization for VS patients and actively serves a membership of nearly 5,000 and communicates directly with nearly 10,000 VS patients, friends, family, and medical professionals. The ANA website receives 60,000 visits monthly, and ANA coordinates nearly 60 registered support groups. Patients involved in the ANA consistently report that they:

- Find encouragement through the ANA support groups.
- Appreciate the realistic and practical patient information the ANA provides.
- Are grateful for the connection ANA provides to medical professionals who excel in VS treatment and posttreatment care, resulting in improved outcomes.
- Are motivated by helping others and learning more, as they were helped, thus perpetuating the existence and need for the ANA.

72.3 Support Groups

Very early on the ANA recognized the need for support groups, a concept that patients across the United States quickly embraced. Support groups provide a unique and critical service: acceptance. Today the annual attendance includes more than 2,000 participants who are served by nearly 60 support groups nationwide. Individual support groups are led by ANA volunteer patients and caregivers, and regularly convene two to five times per year. In 2016 alone, there were 124 ANA support group meetings in 32 states (▶ Table 72.1). All support groups are unique, yet ultimately share many similarities. The structure of individual support group meetings varies to some extent, but usually the meeting includes a general "Caring and Sharing" time and, in many instances, a presentation by medical professionals on topics of interest to VS patients.

A PATIENT'S GUIDE TO DISCOVERY, DIAGNOSIS, AND TREATMENT

Begin to experience symptoms - loss of hearing on one side only, tinnitus (a noise produced in the inner ear, such as ringing, buzzing, roaring, clicking, etc.), problems with balance and vertigo (dizziness, a symptom sometimes caused by a vestibular schwannoma), feeling of fullness in the ear.

↓

See physician, typically an ENT and then a neurotologist (a physician specializing in the neurological aspects of the auditory and vestibular apparatus) if possible. Consider a physician who has substantial experience in treating vestibular schwannoma, even if not in your hometown.

↓

A **hearing test** (audiogram, a chart of hearing acuity recorded during hearing test) and **MRI** with contrast should be performed to determine a diagnosis.

↓

Vestibular schwannoma diagnosis

↓

Next Steps for Patient

1. Learn as much as possible about vestibular schwannoma at www.ANAUSA.org.
2. Order free ANA information packet, which includes Local Support Group leader information and the ANetwork list, Nationwide Peer Support Program.
3. Contact the Support Group leader in your area and others who have a vestibular schwannoma.
4. Proceed with getting an MRI with contrast and review with your physician.
5. Review all treatment options available based on the size of the tumor, its location, your age, symptoms, status of hearing and overall health.
6. After MRI, get copy on disk to share with other physicians when seeking additional opinions.
7. Consulting with a minimum of two to four physicians is perfectly acceptable, including a neurosurgeon (a physician with a surgical specialty concerned with the treatment of diseases and disorders of the brain, spinal cord and peripheral and sympathetic nervous system), neurotologist (physician specializing in the neurological aspects of the auditory and vestibular apparatus) and radiation oncologist.
8. Investigate health insurance coverage and ask the physician's office about whether or not they are in network to determine if they will take your insurance. They can also assist you to address insurance questions and getting pre-approved. Refer to the ANA website for additional insurance information.

↓

Patient works with medical team to **choose best course of action**:
Watch and Wait
Microsurgery
Radiosurgery

Fig. 72.1 A patient's guide to discovery, diagnosis, and treatment.

Table 72.1 ANA Local Support Group Meeting attendance

Year	Attendance
2005	807
2006	928
2007	853
2008	1,243
2009	1,255
2010	1,624
2011	1,592
2012	1,713
2013	1,949
2014	2,007
2015	2,011

72.4 Support Group Benefits

72.4.1 Communication

At support group meetings, VS patients and family members are able to communicate in a nurturing, nonjudgmental, and confidential environment with others who have shared a common VS experience. The open format allows participants to feel some degree of anonymity and to participate as they are comfortable. For some, simply attending meetings and listening to the experiences of others can be helpful.

In addition, the support groups provide an opportunity for networking on all issues relevant to VS patients. As VSs are relatively rare, most newly diagnosed patients find that the education and support provided by other patients is invaluable. Interactions with other patients and family members provide an opportunity to learn new ways to handle challenges and cope with changes.

Likely, the largest benefit of support group attendance is helping a patient realize that he or she is not alone—that there are other people who have the same problems. Support group participants learn to develop effective coping skills and ways to come to terms with difficult emotions and stresses inherent to the situation. By sharing information and resources, participants learn how others have coped with similar problems.

A major component of most support group meetings is the "Caring and Sharing" session, in which each person briefly reviews their personal journey and current challenges. Support group members often realize how their experiences in the group have created a special bond and identity between members. After all, no one understands the experience of someone affected by a VS more than somebody else in the same situation. For the newly diagnosed patient, merely hearing about a positive surgical or radiation treatment outcome often brings enormous comfort.

72.4.2 Sharing Information

For those who have been recently diagnosed, receiving tips about hearing devices, how to cope with balance and tinnitus issues, and living with facial paresis, eye problems, and headache from those with more experience is invaluable. This sharing of information includes how to deal with specific challenges, overcoming handicaps, and transitioning to the "new normal." The exchange of information at support group sessions is not unidirectional, but rather the collaboration between members often leads to creative problem solving and attendees frequently leave invigorated.

72.4.3 Education

Guest speakers from the health care profession often contribute to support group meetings. These medical professionals who have experience treating VS patients are able to present detailed information about various aspects of VS treatment and address questions and issues in a personal environment. Guest speakers may cover a range of topics such as treatment, dizziness and imbalance, facial nerve issues, tinnitus, hearing loss, hearing rehabilitation, and headache. At times, the support group will include presentations and demonstrations from industry. For example, a hearing device company may present different products and allow members to briefly trial various technologies. When a physical therapist discusses balance issues at the support group meeting, there are usually opportunities to learn new exercises to help with balance rehabilitation.

72.4.4 Emotional Support

Since the members who attend support group meetings have direct personal experience with VS, they can provide important emotional support that others cannot offer. Family members and friends often do not fully understand the burden that VS patients face and the daily challenges that commonly exist. For example, participants at meetings often share instances where they inadvertently offended someone they could not hear due to hearing loss. Others may share about a time when they lost their balance and bumped into someone accidentally. The constant attentiveness required to compensate for hearing loss and balance issues can oftentimes lead to progressive fatigue throughout the day. For others it may be facial paralysis or constant tinnitus.

72.5 ANA Website Discussion Forum and Social Media

For some patients who live in smaller cities, there may not be a local support group immediately available. Others might prefer to remain anonymous and not attend face-to-face meetings with other members. In these cases, there are several online options available that can provide many of the benefits that an in-person support group can provide—in essence a virtual support group. Just like the in-person meeting, online avenues provide VS patients the opportunity to offer mutual support and information to other members. In many ways, online interactions can provide certain advantages over in-person meetings. Most notably, responses to questions and concerns can be provided around the clock in real time, with no need to wait for a scheduled meeting.

72.6 ANA Discussion Forum

The ANA Discussion Forum on the ANA website was established in 2005 and provides an important online tool for VS patients. There is a key group of regular members who provide a wealth of information and support to new patients who have been just diagnosed or who have just found this important resource. The forum is organized by categories; so, one can choose the area of interest to post questions or comments. Seasoned VS patients volunteer as moderators on the forum and keep the site on track, both structurally and attitudinally.

72.7 Social Media

The ANA has had a strong presence in the social media arena since 2011, and this is another channel for communication for those who either do not want to or do not have an option to attend an in-person support group meeting. Members can post questions and comments of interest to them. This option also provides the benefit of getting real-time responses to questions. ANA is represented on Facebook, Twitter, YouTube, and LinkedIn.

72.8 ANetwork

Another networking tool available to VS patients is the ANetwork, a nationwide peer-support program. This program, formerly known as the "Willing to Talk" list, consists of VS patients who have undergone all types of treatment, with various tumor sizes, and representative demographics from across the United States. This list is sent to all who request a complimentary packet of ANA information and includes contact information along with tumor size, treatment dates, and types of treatment, to assist the patient in locating someone with similar experiences.

72.9 Testimonials

This chapter concludes with the testimonials of several ANA members describing the positive impact of support group participation:

"We have faced a common trauma – coping with an acoustic neuroma. Face-to-face group meetings give the opportunity to be with others who truly understand. By sharing how we have coped and been helped by receiving medical information from professionals who may be new to us, we can restore ourselves by the strength furnished by a caring community." Ginny Fickel Ehr, ANA Founder.

"I remember how desperately I wanted to be able to talk with someone. I feel one of the many benefits provided by our group is its ability to provide encouragement and compassion for the newly diagnosed." Greg from DC.

"My greatest reward from attending this group is watching newly diagnosed patients attend a meeting and having the opportunity to meet a variety of people with many treatment types as they weigh all their options. I see the hope in their eyes appear as they learn we have all survived, and life after an AN is possible." Joan from Florida.

"I had great support from my family and friends, but they could not understand my concerns, thoughts and feelings. I never knew anyone who had any type of brain tumor, so it seemed, at times, that I was going through this alone. Coming to the support group allowed me to meet people who also had a vestibular schwannoma. Even though our conditions may differ, it is a great feeling to relate to others." Jennifer from Illinois.

"The group gave me hope and made me realize that I wasn´t alone. There were many others out there who shared similar problems to mine, and we were bonded on that basis. Together, we can make a difference for others who are newly diagnosed and those who have difficulty dealing with their present reality." Carol from California.

Part IX

Controversial or Challenging Aspects of Care

IX

73 Management of Small Vestibular Schwannoma in Patients with Minimal Symptoms

Erling Myrseth, Morten Lund-Johansen, and Øystein V. Tveiten

73.1 Introduction

Treatment of small, slow-growing, benign tumors may be challenging as the treatment should not increase the patient's symptoms or complaints. Treatment of small vestibular schwannomas (VSs) is no exception. More recently, in the past one to two decades, there has been an increase in the detection of small VS, especially in the elderly population and those with minimal symptoms. The most plausible explanation for the observed increase in incidence is greater access to magnetic resonance imaging (MRI).[1] A thorough knowledge of the natural course of growth and symptomatology is mandatory so that the best treatment option can be chosen, and the patient can be convinced and reconciled that the right decision has been made.

The management of small VSs in patients with minimal complaints is a matter of debate, and currently there is no consensus on initial treatment strategy. The chosen treatment is strongly influenced by the physicians' and patients' preference. The goal of this chapter is to review the latest evidence regarding treatment outcomes for patients with small, asymptomatic, incidentally discovered, or minimally symptomatic VS.

73.2 Definition of Small Vestibular Schwannoma

In this context, small VSs are defined as tumors according to Koos grades I and IIA: grade I tumors are purely intracanalicular, and grade IIA tumors are protruding not more than 10 mm into the cerebellopontine angle (CPA) measured from the lip of the porus acusticus, and not in contact with the brain stem (▶ Fig. 73.1).[2]

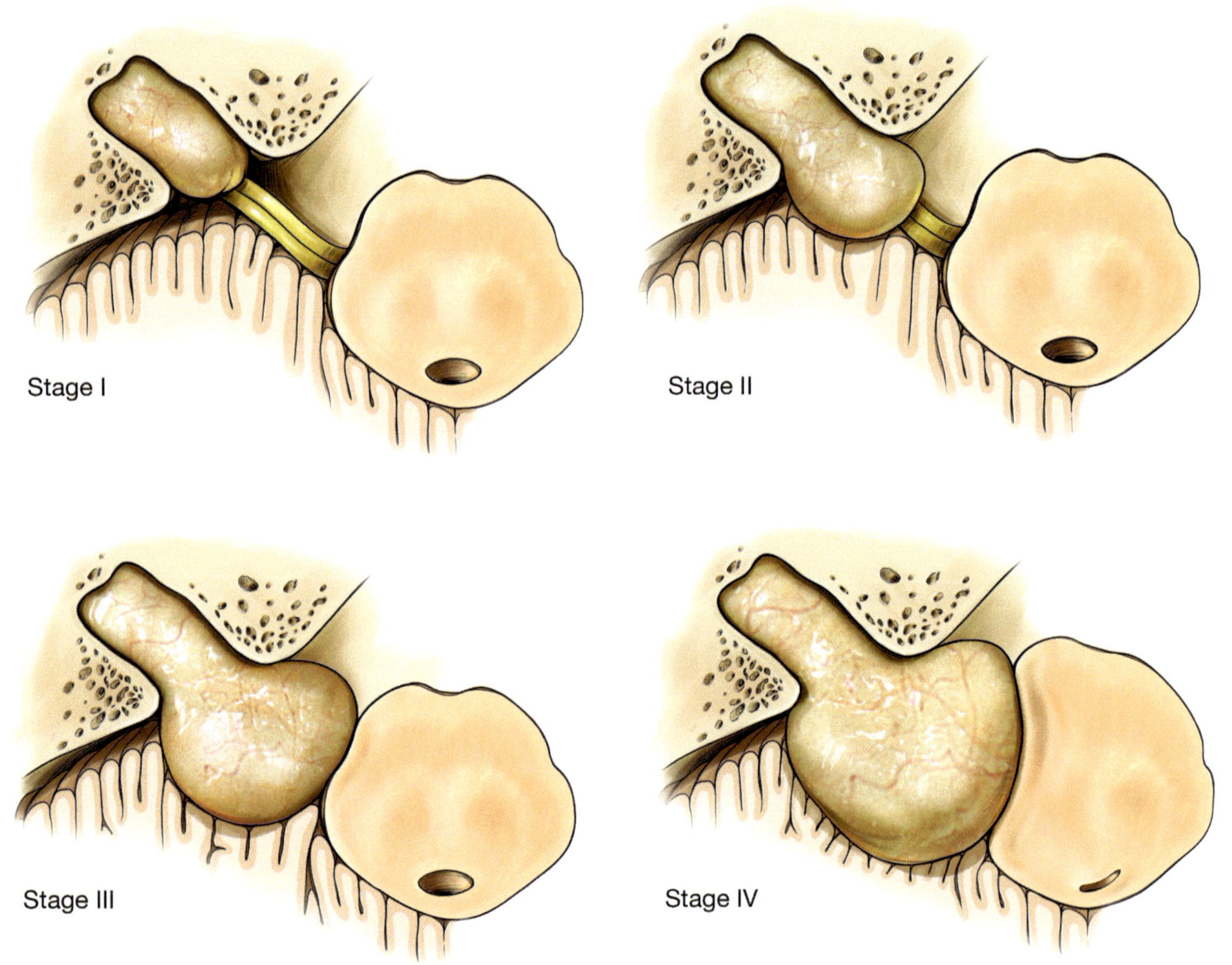

Fig. 73.1 Koos stages 1 to 4 tumor staging system for vestibular schwannoma.

73.3 The Natural History of Vestibular Schwannoma

Vestibular schwannoma usually grows slowly, but the growth pattern is heterogeneous. The typical growth rate for a growing tumor is 1 to 2 mm/year. However, some may enlarge much more rapidly, and yet others may actually involute. Growth patterns may be characterized by saltatory growth, linear growth, exponential growth, stable size, and decreasing size. There is a common belief that after growth is witnessed, most tumors will continue to grow indefinitely. However, this notion is easily discredited by the simple observation that many tumors do not grow for extended periods following diagnosis, but of course, the tumor must have grown at some point to reach its current size. Especially intrameatal tumors often do not grow for years.[1] Risk of growth and growth rates are shown in ▶ Table 73.1 and further summarized in Chapter 14. Not surprisingly, the proportion of growing tumors seems to increase with longer follow-up.[3] No strong predictor of tumor growth has been detected, except for cystic tumors which tend to have a higher growth rate than completely solid tumors.[4]

Gradual hearing deterioration is common in untreated VS patients, even in the absence of tumor growth. Overall, a hearing preservation rate of approximately 50% during a mean follow-up period ranging from 2 to 5 years is to be expected.[5,6,7,8] In one series, 100% speech discrimination at diagnosis was a positive prognostic factor for maintaining long-term useful hearing with conservative treatment.[9] Sudden sensorineural hearing loss (SSNHL), defined as 30 dB or greater hearing loss over less than 72 hours, in VS patients occurs in approximately 10 to 20% of cases.[10,11] Contrary to what might be expected, tumor size was significantly smaller in VS with SSNHL compared to other VSs.[11]

In small- and medium-sized VS, the difference in long-term quality of life (QoL) between treatment strategies when evaluated by disease-specific questionnaires is small and not necessarily clinically significant.[12,13]

73.4 Treatment Options

There are three main treatment options for VS: (1) conservative management with observation/serial radiological follow-up, (2) radiation, and (3) surgery. This results in five possible treatment strategies: (1) observation, (2) observation followed by radiosurgery if tumor growth, (3) observation followed by microsurgery if tumor growth, (4) immediate radiosurgery, and (5) immediate microsurgery. Each modality has pros and cons, and several factors have to be taken into account when advising patients about treatment options. Usually, the tumor size is the most important determining factor, but age, medical condition, hearing level as well as other complaints, and patients' preferences also have to be considered.

For patients with small tumors and mild or no symptoms, the controversy is especially pointed. According to the Hippocratic Oath, treatment should not cause more morbidity to the patient than the natural course of the disease, neither in the short or long term. Therefore, it is most important to have a thorough knowledge about the natural course of the disease, both regarding tumor growth, QoL, and symptom development. Unnecessary treatment should be avoided. The dilemma in patients with small tumors and good ipsilateral hearing is to evaluate the treatment choice regarding chance of hearing preservation and tumor control, both immediately and in the long term.

Table 73.1 Natural growth rate in vestibular schwannoma

Author (year)	Follow-up period	Percentage of growth (range)	Growth rate (mean)
Nikolopoulos et al (2010)	NR	NR (7-73)	1–2 mm/y
Yoshimoto (2005)	38 mo	46 (15–85)	1.2 mm/y
Thakur et al (2012)	3 y	44 (29–54)	NR
Whitehouse et al (2010)	3.65 y	51.1	1.24 mm/y
Hajioff et al (2008)	10 y	78	1.0 mm/y

Abbreviations: NR=not reported

73.4.1 Conservative Treatment

Conservative treatment, also called "wait-and-see" or "wait-and-scan," implies clinical and MRI follow-up at regular intervals. There are different follow-up algorithms regarding imaging intervals and duration of follow-up needed. Most authors recommend the first scan 6 months after the initial scan to identify rapid growing tumors. In case of no growth, further MRI scans should be taken annually for at least 5 years. Stangerup et al suggested further MRI scans at 7, 9, and 14 years after the initial MRI scan.[14] Martin et al recommended follow-up scans every 5 years for the rest of the patient's life.[15] Smouha et al recommended continuation of annual MRI scans.[16]

For small tumors with minimal symptoms, the "wait-and-scan" treatment strategy hopes to prolong the period of minimal complaints, avoiding the risk of new symptoms or complications related to the treatment. Several authors recommended conservative treatment, or no treatment, for most small tumors with minor or no complaints.[3,6,12,13,17,18,19,20,21,22,23,24] One objection against this strategy is the risk of early progressive or SSNHL. This risk needs to be compared with the likelihood of preserving hearing if the tumor is treated by surgery or radiosurgery.

Tveiten et al analyzed the hearing status in small- and medium-sized VS at a mean time of almost 8 years after initial treatment, and found that treatment modality was an independent risk factor for hearing deterioration; patients treated by observation had the best prognosis.[25] Among ears with serviceable hearing at baseline, functional hearing was maintained in 68% of observed patients, 40% of those receiving Gamma Knife radiosurgery (GKRS; Elekta AB, Stockholm, Sweden), and 14% treated with surgery ($p < 0.005$). These results may be biased by the fact that observed tumors were not growing and that larger tumors tended to receive microsurgical resection.

Jeyakumar et al suggested that small incidentally discovered VSs tend to follow a more benign course requiring intervention less frequently than symptomatic larger lesions (47 vs. 76%, respectively).[26] However, other studies have found that the biological behavior and eventual need for treatment of an asymptomatic tumor is no different than one causing hearing loss or other symptoms when comparing VS of equal size.[27]

Failure of conservative management is most often due to tumor growth and rarely due to symptom progression. Tumor growth is usually defined as linear increase or tumor volume doubling time, but growth of intrameatal tumors to extrameatal extension is also used.[1] This variation, as well as length of follow-up period, might obviously influence the reported growth rate results and treatment failure rates.

The efficacy of conservative treatment, as defined as freedom from active treatment, is reported in several studies. Breivik et al studied a cohort of 193 consecutive VS patients prospectively for a minimum of 24 months (median: 43 months), and found that 74 patients (38%) underwent active treatment (microsurgery or radiosurgery) during the period of observation, 37 patients (19%) before 3 years.[28] This result is comparable with other series.[3,23] However, the need for active treatment is reported in the range of 18 to 49%.[26,29,30]

73.4.2 Gamma Knife Radiosurgery

The tumor control rate after GKRS is reported to be 93 to 98%, comparable to tumors treated by microsurgery, and the reported side effects are minimal.[24,31,32,33,34,35] A meta-analysis comparing stereotactic radiosurgery (SRS) and conservative management showed that hearing preservation was not significantly different between the groups, although there was a trend toward better useful hearing preservation in the SRS group.[35] Régis et al compared conservative treatment with GKRS in two cohorts of patients with intracanalicular tumors and useful hearing, and reported that hearing preservation was significantly better in the GKRS group at 3, 4, and 5 years.[29] However, this study was not randomized, and the patient population was small. With a tumor margin dose of ≤ 13 Gy, 60 to 75% serviceable hearing preservation is reported with a mean follow-up period of 3 to 5 years.[31,32,36]

Kondziolka et al found that an average cochlea dose of less than 4.2 Gy was associated with better hearing preservation.[24] In a recent study, favorable hearing outcomes were found if GKRS was performed before the onset of subjective hearing loss.[37]

In a meta-analysis of 381 VS patients receiving GKRS for tumors less than 2 cm, hearing preservation was 68.8% after a mean follow-up period of 7 years.[35] Another meta-analysis reported 51% serviceable hearing preservation after a mean follow-up of 35 months, reaching 60.5% if tumor margin dose was ≤ 13 Gy.[36] Tveiten et al found a lower figure in a large, dual-center study on long-term hearing status following treatment: 40% of patients with serviceable hearing at treatment maintained good hearing status almost 8 years following GKRS.[25] GKRS is a good treatment option for small VS. However, it has not been shown in randomized controlled studies if GKRS prevents or accelerates hearing loss in the long run.

73.4.3 Microsurgical Treatment

For VS patients with small tumors and minimal symptoms, any surgery should aim at preserving facial nerve function and hearing, which can be achieved through the middle fossa (MF) or retrosigmoid (RS) approach. These two approaches yield quite similar hearing preservation rates when performed at experienced centers.[35,38,39] Some studies report more facial weakness, at least in the early postoperative period, if surgery is carried out through the MF approach. Hearing preservation is reportedly achieved in about 50 to 70% of selected cases, with extreme good results (100%) in one series.[2,35,40] However, in subsequent follow-up, some patients may experience a gradual deterioration to nonserviceable levels.[41,42,43,44]

Prognostic factors for hearing preservation are good preoperative hearing level, space between the fundus and lateral tumor margin, the presence of a wave V in auditory brainstem response at the end of the procedure, and, of course, smaller tumor size.[39,40,45,46,47]

The large variability of hearing preservation results after microsurgery is obviously influenced by patient selection and surgeon's skill. The literature on this topic is largely characterized by single institution, even single-surgeon series—and there are likely tremendous inclusion and treatment biases.

73.5 Discussion

Hearing loss in VS patients is a part of the natural course of the disease; the overall prognosis regardless of treatment is poor.[25] The hearing loss is typically gradual over years, but in some cases SSNHL may occur. The risk of SSNHL is greater with intracanalicular and small tumors, and it has to be considered as a risk factor during conservative management.

So far, we do not know for certain if radiosurgery protects or aggravates hearing loss. Two nonrandomized studies have shown better hearing preservation in GKRS-treated patients than in observed patients, but according to Quesnel and McKenna, hearing preservation rates for either radiation or surgical treatment have not been consistently better than that observed in tumors managed conservatively.[17,29,37] Again, Tveiten et al compared the three management options and found favorable outcomes in the observed group of patients; the greatest long-term hearing loss was seen in the microsurgical cohort. In a meta-analysis of VS patients with tumors less than 2 cm and a pretreatment hearing level according to Gardner–Robertson grades I to II, the overall useful hearing preservation outcome was 70.2% for the stereotactic radiation group, compared to 50.3% for the microsurgery group.[35] This difference was highly significant ($p < 0.001$).

Even if hearing preservation surgery can be successfully performed in a substantial number of small VSs using either the MF or the RS approach, the procedure carries a risk of profound hearing loss in about 25 to 50% of cases.[48,49,50] Sudden loss of all ipsilateral hearing might be more incapacitating than a gradual hearing loss over years.

Interestingly, Morrison evaluated the management of small VS (< 1.5 cm) using a Markov decision model by constructing cohorts of patients entering one of four management strategies: (1) initial observation followed by GKRS if tumor grows, (2) initial observation followed by microsurgery if tumor grows, (3) primary GKRS, and (4) primary microsurgery.[22] Key parameters for each management strategy were identified from the best available evidence in the literature. The outcome measure was quality-adjusted life years (QALYs). He found that the management strategy with the highest QALY was observation followed by radiosurgery, and observation followed by microsurgery as the second highest QALY. Sensitivity tests and threshold analyses showed that observation followed by radiosurgery gave the best QoL value until a hearing loss exceeds 12.4%. Primary radiosurgery was best if the hearing loss is more pronounced. The microsurgical group sensitivity analyses failed to reach significant thresholds. Even with a hearing preservation rate of 100%, observation followed by radiosurgery strategy had the best QALY. Morrison concluded that a period of observation for all patients with small VS, regardless of age and sex, is beneficial. If careful monitoring of tumor size and hearing level show changes, definitive treatment should be considered. Similarly, Carlson et al demonstrated that patients who underwent radiosurgery or observation reported a better total QoL score on a VS-specific questionnaire than the microsurgical cohort ($p < 0.02$).[12] However, the difference was very small and the overall conclusion from this study was that choice of treatment strategy of VS has little impact on QoL.

The best way of preserving serviceable hearing as long as possible might therefore be observation, eventually followed by radiosurgery.[12,13,51] Nevertheless, both the Pittsburgh group and the Marseille group advocated GKRS as the best hearing preservation modality for patients with small VS and good hearing.[29,31,32,37] However, prospective randomized trials are necessary to prove the superiority of radiosurgery compared to "wait-and-scan" and microsurgery for long-term hearing preservation.

73.6 Conclusion

Provided a patient is compliant with follow-up, conservative treatment with serial MRI scans seems to be the best for patients with small VS and minimal symptoms, especially if the patient has 100% speech discrimination.[9,17] In some studies, however, GKRS has shown better hearing preservation rates than conservative management.[29,31,32,37] If a small tumor demonstrates growth, treatment should be strongly considered—as both radiosurgery and microsurgery are safe and effective when the tumor is small. Unfortunately, high-level scientific evidence comparing treatment modalities with respect to hearing outcome is lacking.

References

[1] Stangerup SE, Caye-Thomasen P. Epidemiology and natural history of vestibular schwannomas. Otolaryngol Clin North Am. 2012; 45(2):257–268, vii

[2] Koos WT, Day JD, Matula C, Levy DI. Neurotopographic considerations in the microsurgical treatment of small acoustic neurinomas. J Neurosurg. 1998; 88 (3):506–512

[3] Hajioff D, Raut VV, Walsh RM, et al. Conservative management of vestibular schwannomas: third review of a 10-year prospective study. Clin Otolaryngol. 2008; 33(3):255–259

[4] Nikolopoulos TP, Fortnum H, O'Donoghue G, Baguley D. Acoustic neuroma growth: a systematic review of the evidence. Otol Neurotol. 2010; 31(3):478–485

[5] Stangerup SE, Caye-Thomasen P, Tos M, Thomsen J. Change in hearing during 'wait and scan' management of patients with vestibular schwannoma. J Laryngol Otol. 2008; 122(7):673–681

[6] Breivik CN, Nilsen RM, Myrseth E, et al. Conservative management or gamma knife radiosurgery for vestibular schwannoma: tumor growth, symptoms, and quality of life. Neurosurgery. 2013; 73(1):48–56, discussion 56–57

[7] Caye-Thomasen P, Dethloff T, Hansen S, Stangerup SE, Thomsen J. Hearing in patients with intracanalicular vestibular schwannomas. Audiol Neurootol. 2007; 12(1):1–12

[8] Sughrue ME, Yang I, Aranda D, et al. The natural history of untreated sporadic vestibular schwannomas: a comprehensive review of hearing outcomes. J Neurosurg. 2010; 112(1):163–167

[9] Stangerup SE, Thomsen J, Tos M, Caye-Thomasen P. Long-term hearing preservation in vestibular schwannoma. Otol Neurotol. 2010; 31(2):271–275

[10] Moffat DA, Baguley DM, von Blumenthal H, Irving RM, Hardy DG. Sudden deafness in vestibular schwannoma. J Laryngol Otol. 1994; 108(2):116–119

[11] Sauvaget E, Kici S, Kania R, Herman P, Tran Ba Huy P. Sudden sensorineural hearing loss as a revealing symptom of vestibular schwannoma. Acta Otolaryngol. 2005; 125(6):592–595

[12] Carlson ML, Tveiten OV, Driscoll CL, et al. Long-term quality of life in patients with vestibular schwannoma: an international multicenter cross-sectional study comparing microsurgery, stereotactic radiosurgery, observation, and nontumor controls. J Neurosurg. 2015; 122(4):833–842

[13] Carlson ML, Link MJ, Wanna GB, Driscoll CL. Management of sporadic vestibular schwannoma. Otolaryngol Clin North Am. 2015; 48(3):407–422

[14] Stangerup SE, Caye-Thomasen P, Tos M, Thomsen J. The natural history of vestibular schwannoma. Otol Neurotol. 2006; 27(4):547–552

[15] Martin TP, Senthil L, Chavda SV, Walsh R, Irving RM. A protocol for the conservative management of vestibular schwannomas. Otol Neurotol. 2009; 30(3):381–385

[16] Smouha EE, Yoo M, Mohr K, Davis RP. Conservative management of acoustic neuroma: a meta-analysis and proposed treatment algorithm. Laryngoscope. 2005; 115(3):450–454

[17] Quesnel AM, McKenna MJ. Current strategies in management of intracanalicular vestibular schwannoma. Curr Opin Otolaryngol Head Neck Surg. 2011; 19(5):335–340

[18] Myrseth E, Pedersen PH, Møller P, Lund-Johansen M. Treatment of vestibular schwannomas. Why, when and how? Acta Neurochir (Wien). 2007; 149(7): 647–660, discussion 660

[19] Whitehouse K, Foroughi M, Shone G, Hatfield R. Vestibular schwannomas - when should conservative management be reconsidered? Br J Neurosurg. 2010; 24(2):185–190

[20] Bakkouri WE, Kania RE, Guichard JP, Lot G, Herman P, Huy PT. Conservative management of 386 cases of unilateral vestibular schwannoma: tumor growth and consequences for treatment. J Neurosurg. 2009; 110(4):662–669

[21] Maniakas A, Saliba I. Conservative management versus stereotactic radiation for vestibular schwannomas: a meta-analysis of patients with more than 5 years' follow-up. Otol Neurotol. 2012; 33(2):230–238

[22] Morrison D. Management of patients with acoustic neuromas: a Markov decision analysis. Laryngoscope. 2010; 120(4):783–790

[23] Godefroy WP, Kaptein AA, Vogel JJ, van der Mey AG. Conservative treatment of vestibular schwannoma: a follow-up study on clinical and quality-of-life outcome. Otol Neurotol. 2009; 30(7):968–974

[24] Kondziolka D, Mousavi SH, Kano H, Flickinger JC, Lunsford LD. The newly diagnosed vestibular schwannoma: radiosurgery, resection, or observation? Neurosurg Focus. 2012; 33(3):E8

[25] Tveiten OV, Carlson ML, Goplen F, Vassbotn F, Link MJ, Lund-Johansen M. Long-term auditory symptoms in patients with sporadic vestibular schwannoma: an international cross-sectional study. Neurosurgery. 2015; 77(2): 218–227, discussion 227

[26] Jeyakumar A, Seth R, Brickman TM, Dutcher P. The prevalence and clinical course of patients with 'incidental' acoustic neuromas. Acta Otolaryngol. 2007; 127(10):1051–1057

[27] Carlson ML, Lees KA, Patel NS, et al. The clinical behavior of asymptomatic incidental vestibular schwannomas is similar to that of symptomatic tumors. Otol Neurotol. 2016; 37(9):1435–1441

[28] Breivik CN, Varughese JK, Wentzel-Larsen T, Vassbotn F, Lund-Johansen M. Conservative management of vestibular schwannoma–a prospective cohort study: treatment, symptoms, and quality of life. Neurosurgery. 2012; 70(5): 1072–1080, discussion 1080

[29] Régis J, Carron R, Park MC, et al. Wait-and-see strategy compared with proactive Gamma Knife surgery in patients with intracanalicular vestibular schwannomas. J Neurosurg. 2010; 113 Suppl:105–111

[30] Yoshimoto Y. Systematic review of the natural history of vestibular schwannoma. J Neurosurg. 2005; 103(1):59–63

[31] Flickinger JC, Kondziolka D, Niranjan A, Lunsford LD. Results of acoustic neuroma radiosurgery: an analysis of 5 years' experience using current methods. J Neurosurg. 2001; 94(1):1–6

[32] Kondziolka D, Lunsford LD, McLaughlin MR, Flickinger JC. Long-term outcomes after radiosurgery for acoustic neuromas. N Engl J Med. 1998; 339 (20):1426–1433

[33] Myrseth E, Møller P, Pedersen PH, Vassbotn FS, Wentzel-Larsen T, Lund-Johansen M. Vestibular schwannomas: clinical results and quality of life after microsurgery or gamma knife radiosurgery. Neurosurgery. 2005; 56(5):927–935, discussion 927–935
[34] Liu W, Ni M, Jia W, et al. How to address small- and medium-sized acoustic neuromas with hearing: a systematic review and decision analysis. World Neurosurg. 2015; 84(2):283–291.e1
[35] Maniakas A, Saliba I. Microsurgery versus stereotactic radiation for small vestibular schwannomas: a meta-analysis of patients with more than 5 years' follow-up. Otol Neurotol. 2012; 33(9):1611–1620
[36] Yang I, Sughrue ME, Han SJ, et al. A comprehensive analysis of hearing preservation after radiosurgery for vestibular schwannoma. J Neurosurg. 2010; 112(4):851–859
[37] Mousavi SH, Niranjan A, Akpinar B, et al. Hearing subclassification may predict long-term auditory outcomes after radiosurgery for vestibular schwannoma patients with good hearing. J Neurosurg. 2016; 125(4): 845–852
[38] Sameshima T, Fukushima T, McElveen JT, Jr, Friedman AH. Critical assessment of operative approaches for hearing preservation in small acoustic neuroma surgery: retrosigmoid vs middle fossa approach. Neurosurgery. 2010; 67(3): 640–644, discussion 644–645
[39] Phillips DJ, Kobylarz EJ, De Peralta ET, Stieg PE, Selesnick SH. Predictive factors of hearing preservation after surgical resection of small vestibular schwannomas. Otol Neurotol. 2010; 31(9):1463–1468
[40] Sughrue ME, Yang I, Aranda D, Kane AJ, Parsa AT. Hearing preservation rates after microsurgical resection of vestibular schwannoma. J Clin Neurosci. 2010; 17(9):1126–1129
[41] Woodson EA, Dempewolf RD, Gubbels SP, et al. Long-term hearing preservation after microsurgical excision of vestibular schwannoma. Otol Neurotol. 2010; 31(7):1144–1152
[42] McKenna MJ, Halpin C, Ojemann RG, et al. Long-term hearing results in patients after surgical removal of acoustic tumors with hearing preservation. Am J Otol. 1992; 13(2):134–136
[43] Friedman RA, Kesser B, Brackmann DE, Fisher LM, Slattery WH, Hitselberger WE. Long-term hearing preservation after middle fossa removal of vestibular schwannoma. Otolaryngol Head Neck Surg. 2003; 129(6):660–665
[44] Hilton CW, Haines SJ, Agrawal A, Levine SC. Late failure rate of hearing preservation after middle fossa approach for resection of vestibular schwannoma. Otol Neurotol. 2011; 32(1):132–135
[45] Nadol JB, Jr, Chiong CM, Ojemann RG, et al. Preservation of hearing and facial nerve function in resection of acoustic neuroma. Laryngoscope. 1992; 102 (10):1153–1158
[46] Tringali S, Ferber-Viart C, Fuchsmann C, Buiret G, Zaouche S, Dubreuil C. Hearing preservation in retrosigmoid approach of small vestibular schwannomas: prognostic value of the degree of internal auditory canal filling. Otol Neurotol. 2010; 31(9):1469–1472
[47] Goddard JC, Schwartz MS, Friedman RA. Fundal fluid as a predictor of hearing preservation in the middle cranial fossa approach for vestibular schwannoma. Otol Neurotol. 2010; 31(7):1128–1134
[48] Kutz JW, Jr, Scoresby T, Isaacson B, et al. Hearing preservation using the middle fossa approach for the treatment of vestibular schwannoma. Neurosurgery. 2012; 70(2):334–340, discussion 340–341
[49] Ginzkey C, Scheich M, Harnisch W, et al. Outcome on hearing and facial nerve function in microsurgical treatment of small vestibular schwannoma via the middle cranial fossa approach. Eur Arch Otorhinolaryngol. 2013; 270(4):1209–1216
[50] Samii M, Gerganov V, Samii A. Improved preservation of hearing and facial nerve function in vestibular schwannoma surgery via the retrosigmoid approach in a series of 200 patients. J Neurosurg. 2006; 105(4):527–535
[51] Thakur JD, Banerjee AD, Khan IS, et al. An update on unilateral sporadic small vestibular schwannoma. Neurosurg Focus. 2012; 33(3):E1

74 What Is the Best Treatment for Small- to Medium-Sized Vestibular Schwannoma?

Michael J. Link and Colin L. W. Driscoll

74.1 Introduction

There is probably not a more controversial topic in all of neurosurgery or neurotology than the question of optimal treatment for a small- to medium-sized vestibular schwannoma (VS). Even before there was much of an opportunity to diagnose and treat smaller VSs, controversy surrounded the diagnosis of any VS (typically quite large and life-threatening in the early 1900s). At the beginning of the last century, the surgical mortality from the treatment of a VS was as high as 70 to 80%. It was quite questionable at that time whether surgery of the cerebellopontine angle (CPA) should be undertaken at all. Harvey Cushing, the father of American neurosurgery, advocated a wide bilateral suboccipital craniectomy to decompress the posterior fossa, facilitating safe dural opening, and intracapsular subtotal resection of VS, which reduced operative mortality significantly. This paradigm was relatively quickly challenged by one of Cushing's most accomplished pupils, Walter Dandy, who alternatively, strongly advocated for a complete resection via a unilateral exposure of the CPA and partial resection of the lateral cerebellar hemisphere to aid safe exposure. A fascinating discussion of this history can be found in Chapter 1, authored by Richard T. Ramsden. Additionally, the article by Akard et al likewise reviews the early evolution of surgical treatment of VS.[1] Once again, one of the main difficulties of that time was that there were no small- or medium-sized VS being diagnosed. They were all large and life-threatening at the time of diagnosis. In fact, in 1921, Cushing opined, "It is possible that someone may someday be able to completely enucleate one of these lesions, but it is not likely until earlier diagnoses are made and tumors of smaller size are exposed."

Following this contentious debate came the question of which surgical approach should be used; in the 1960s, primarily retrosigmoid versus translabyrinthine. In the 1980s, the role of stereotactic radiosurgery (SRS) versus microsurgery became the primary debate for the next few decades. Most recently, with a better understanding of the benign natural history of many small VSs, the original debate of more than 100 years ago regarding whether treatment is even indicated has emerged again as perhaps the most prominent controversy, especially as it relates to small- and medium-sized VS.

For the past almost two decades, we have had the opportunity to be on various panels, discussion groups, and guideline writing committees and attended national and international meetings during which this important and contentious issue has been debated. Perhaps, most importantly, we have worked together on an essentially daily basis counseling thousands of patients with small- to medium-sized VS. We evaluate approximately 150 brand new VS patients per year. The purpose of this chapter is to relate to the reader our approach in advising patients regarding their options, and try and provide a rationale for how we determine the best treatment for a small- to medium-sized VS in any individual patient.

74.2 Case Example

We recently evaluated a 49-year-old Caucasian woman with no significant past medical history. She reported a several-month history of right-sided tinnitus that sounded "like water running." It was not particularly intrusive, was not interfering with sleep or concentration, but was present most of the time and in retrospective she noted "fullness" in that ear as well. She also admitted to several episodes of imbalance without true vertigo. She had no history or facial numbness, weakness, or hemifacial spasm. She had no history of prior ear or cranial surgery, radiation exposure to the head or neck, and there was no family history of brain or peripheral nerve tumors. An audiogram confirmed mild high-frequency right-sided sensorineural hearing loss with a pure-tone average of 4 dB on the right and 1 dB on the left. Word recognition scores (WRSs) were 100% bilaterally (▶ Fig. 74.1). An MRI scan of the head with and without gadolinium was performed to investigate her mild asymmetric hearing loss and unilateral tinnitus. The scan revealed an intracanalicular enhancing tumor consistent with a VS (▶ Fig. 74.2a–c). It was not readily apparent, even on very thin cut coronal images (▶ Fig. 74.2b) whether the tumor was arising from the superior or inferior vestibular nerve. There was a small fundal cap of CSF (▶ Fig. 74.2c) indicating the tumor did not extend lateral to the transverse crest. What is the best treatment going forward for this patient?

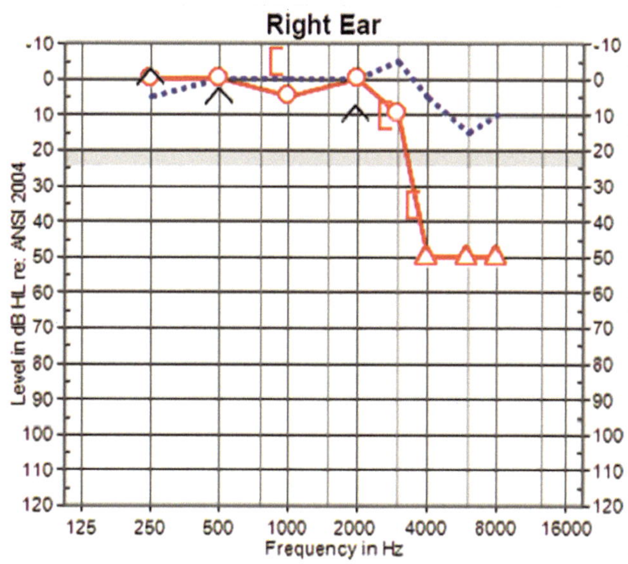

Fig. 74.1 Presenting audiogram shows high-frequency, right-sided (*red*) sensorineural hearing loss above 4,000 Hz compared to the left (*blue*). Word recognition scores were 100% bilaterally.

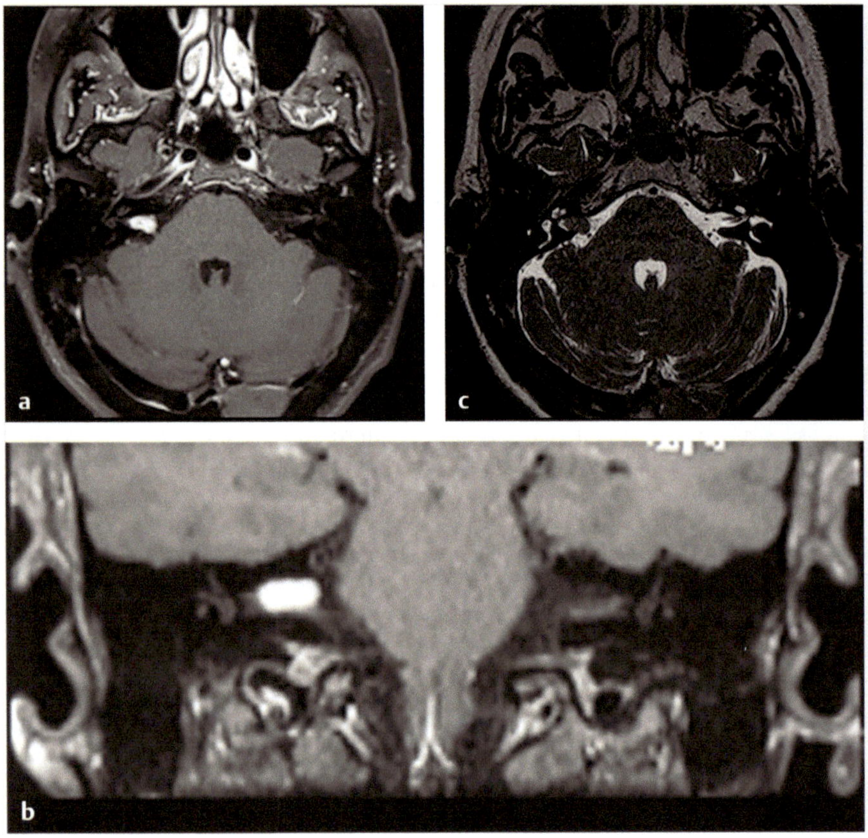

Fig. 74.2 **(a)** Axial 1-mm thickness postgadolinium T1-weighted MRI scan reveals a right-sided intracanalicular tumor consistent with a VS. **(b)** Coronal 1-mm thickness postgadolinium T1-weighted MRI scan does not show preferential extension along either the superior or inferior internal auditory canal that is sometimes helpful in distinguishing a superior vestibular nerve tumor from an inferior vestibular nerve tumor. **(c)** Axial 0.5-mm thickness heavily T2-weighted in steady-state MRI scan shows a small cap of cerebrospinal fluid in the distal fundus of the internal auditory canal (*arrow*).

74.3 What We Think We Know...

74.3.1 Microsurgery

As outlined in Chapter 31, in select patients, microsurgery has an excellent chance of complete tumor removal and preservation of useful hearing and normal facial nerve function. The likelihood of this positive scenario depends on tumor size, extent of tumor involvement of the fundus of the internal auditory canal (IAC), baseline hearing prior to surgery, and experience of the operative team. As has been reviewed elsewhere, smaller tumors centered near the porous (▶ Fig. 74.3a), rather than the fundus of the IAC (▶ Fig. 74.3b), with 100% WRS are optimal for surgical removal.

For the case example presented, we would offer the patient resection through either a middle fossa or retrosigmoid approach. It is not readily apparent on coronal imaging whether the tumor is more likely from superior or inferior vestibular nerve origin. Typically, tumors that arise from the superior vestibular nerve are better candidates for middle fossa surgery, whereas tumors that extend below the transverse crest are much more challenging (▶ Fig. 74.3b). We would estimate a 99% chance that we would remove the tumor in the case example (▶ Fig. 74.2a–c) completely and there would be no recurrence in her remaining lifetime. There would be a 95% chance of normal or near-normal facial nerve function (House–Brackmann grades 1–2) 1 year following surgery with an approximately 10 to 15% risk of temporary facial weakness immediately following removal. The chance of maintaining American Academy of Otolaryngology – Head and Neck Surgery (AAO–HNS) class A hearing (> 70% WRS and < 30 dB pure-tone average) we would estimate to be approximately 50 to 60%. We always include small (1–2%) risks of bleeding, infection, and a 5% risk of cerebrospinal fluid leak. This is based on our experience operating on approximately 650 VSs as the primary surgeons over the past 17 years. We emphasize that most patients are vertiginous or at least have a great deal of disequilibrium for the first 48 hours, postoperatively. The majority of patients spend the first 24 hours at bed rest for this reason and the typical hospital stay is 3 to 4 days. We ask patients to limit exertional activities for 3 months after surgery and feel the same amount of time off work is reasonable, but if the patient has a more or less sedentary occupation, they can return to work 4 to 6 weeks following surgery if they feel ready; however, in our experience, few patients do, usually related to a general feeling of fatigue. We obtain a follow-up MRI and audiogram and see the patient back in 3 months at which time they are released to all activities without restriction. If the 3-month MRI confirms gross total resection, we obtain another MRI at 2 years to look for early recurrence and one 5 years after that (7 years postoperatively) to investigate for later recurrence, which we think is very important in hearing preservation cases. If the 7-year scan is negative for tumor recurrence, we try and get another MRI in 7 to 10 years to look for extremely late recurrence. There remains a gap in the literature, in our opinion, regarding the durability of retained hearing following microsurgery. Most studies addressing this issue have approximately only 5 years of audiometric data and there are a large number of patients in the cohorts that are lost to follow-up.[2,3,4,5,6] We have seen rare patients who have late deterioration in their functional hearing

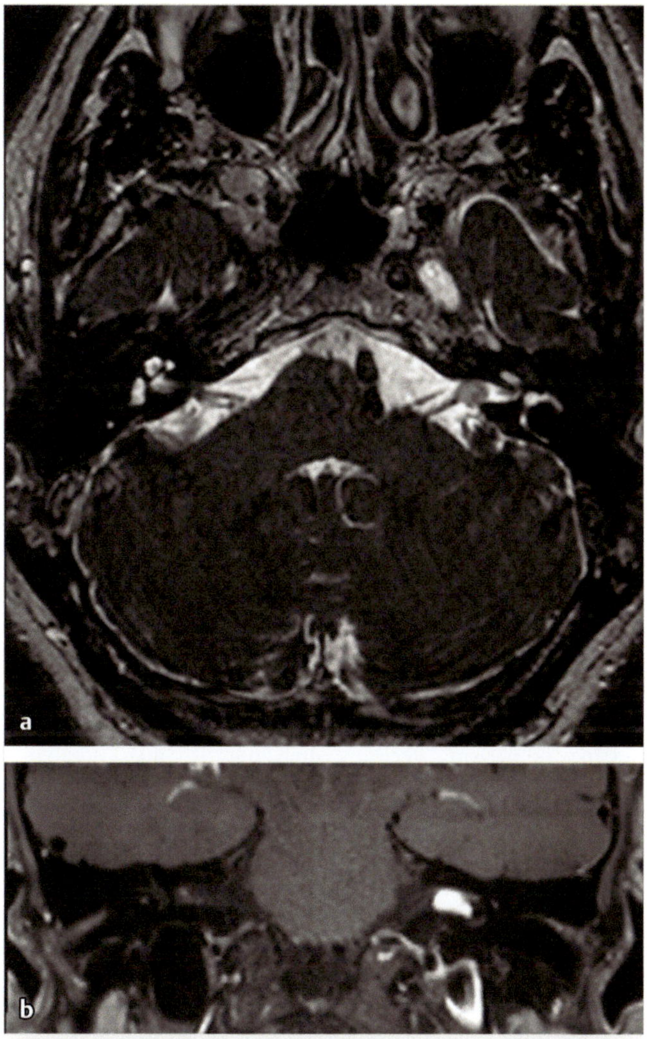

Fig. 74.3 (a) A second case example. Axial 0.5-mm thickness heavily T2-weighted in steady-state MRI shows a small left-sided VS at the porus of the internal auditory canal (*arrow*) that would be ideal for removal via a retrosigmoid or middle fossa approach, or treatable with SRS with very low dose to the cochlea. (b) A third case example. Coronal 1-mm thickness postgadolinium T1-weighted MRI scan reveals a left-sided intracanalicular VS that extends below the transverse crest to the fundus of the internal auditory canal (*arrow*). Middle fossa surgery to achieve a gross total resection and preserve hearing would be very challenging in this case. Likewise, the cochlea would likely receive greater than 6 Gy during single-fraction SRS.

with no tumor recurrence. However, we typically counsel patients if they maintain useful hearing following surgery they are likely to keep it long term.

74.3.2 Stereotactic Radiosurgery

The results of SRS to treat VS are well reviewed in Chapters 16 through 19. We have treated more than 800 VSs at the Mayo Clinic over the past 26 years using the Leksell Gamma Unit (Elekta AB, Stockholm, Sweden). For the tumor presented here, we would estimate a 93% chance of long-term tumor control.[7] There is a less than 1% chance of any adverse facial nerve effects (hemifacial spasm or weakness), and an at least 50% chance of retained AAO–HNS class A or B hearing at 5 years which likely drops to only a 25% chance of maintaining useful hearing by 10 years post-SRS.[8] Similar to the expected outcomes from microsurgery, a smaller tumor, not impacted in the fundus of the IAC and occurring in a patient with excellent baseline hearing, is the optimal candidate for SRS. We emphasize to patients, SRS is a 1-day outpatient procedure. Most patients experience mild postprocedure discomfort and swelling at the pin sites for a few days afterward but can resume a completely normal lifestyle with no restrictions usually within 48 hours of treatment, including return to full-time occupation. We obtain follow-up MRI scans and audiograms at 6-month intervals for the first year, then yearly for 2 more years, then every other year for the next 4 years, then every third year for the next 6 years, then every fourth year for the next 8 years and so on. Based on our recent analysis of growing tumors prior to SRS, we strongly prefer to determine if or at what rate the tumor is growing prior to SRS. We found extracanalicular tumors growing more than 2.5 mm/year were less likely to be controlled (69% tumor control rate) with radiation compared to tumors growing less than 2.5 mm/year (97% tumor control rate).[9] We do counsel patients that if the tumor fails SRS, we almost always recommend surgical resection. Surgery after failed SRS is generally more difficult, in particular obtaining gross total resection, but for an intracanalicular tumor, this is much less of a concern compared, for instance, to a tumor 2.5 cm in posterior fossa diameter that fails SRS.[10,11,12,13,14] We have recommended repeat SRS four times in almost 20 years in patients who we thought were too ill to safely undergo a general anesthetic for surgery to treat their enlarging VS following prior SRS. Similar to other limited reports in the literature, this has proven safe and, with very limited follow-up, effective to date.[15,16,17,18,19] Based on best evidence, the risk of a secondary radiation-associated malignancy or malignant degeneration of a benign VS is extremely low—probably, less than or equal to the risk of dying from an intraoperative or postoperative complication if microsurgery is chosen.[20] The topic of secondary malignancy following radiosurgery for VS is reviewed in Chapter 24.

74.3.3 Observation

Observation is the most common "treatment" option selected by most of the new VS patients seen in our practice, especially for patients with intracanalicular tumors, as in this patient example. This mirrors the trend across the United States, essentially, with a shift toward conservatism as opposed to active treatment at the time of diagnosis.[21] There are a variety of reasons for this: The majority of tumors will not show any growth in the first approximately 3 to 10 years of follow-up based on studies from Denmark, Italy, and the United States.[22,23,24,25] Second, almost 4% of tumors in some large series will actually display spontaneous tumor regression with no treatment.[26] For patients who start with 100% WRS, as in this example, up to 70% of patients will still have good hearing up to 10 years after diagnosis.[27,28] Third, following the tumor will potentially provide an opportunity to determine if it is actually growing and at what rate. As discussed earlier, we are less eager to radiate faster growing tumors as the risk of failure is higher compared to tumors growing less than 2.5 mm/year. We also believe that the patient will be more accepting of a treatment-related deficit, such as hearing loss, if there is evidence to support the need for active treatment. Finally, and perhaps most importantly, a period of initial observation allows the patient time to reflect upon the potential treatment options and get to know us before any future potential intervention. We obtain a follow-up MRI 6 months after the original diagnostic study along with a new audiogram and then annually thereafter. In all cases, we emphasize to the patient the importance of consistent follow-up. We almost always recommend treatment if tumor growth is documented. Rarely, we will continue to follow a very slowly growing small tumor (e.g., intracanalicular tumor or a tumor in an only hearing ear) when there is no decrement in very good hearing in the ipsilateral ear—especially if we judge the risk to hearing with active treatment to be greater than 50% based on criteria such as nerve of origin, fundal extension, and other patient- and tumor-related variables. Chapters 14 and 51 provide an excellent review of the natural history of sporadic VS.

74.3.4 Symptom-Specific Outcomes

Early in our practice we were keen to know if one treatment strategy would benefit certain patients with specific symptom complaints. This way, we might best advise patients with small- to medium-sized VS, optimally. For instance, if a patient presented with the primary complaint of "dizziness," we thought perhaps if we eliminated the hypofunctioning (or inconsistently functioning) vestibular system by surgically removing the tumor, the patient would do better in the long run. However, our analysis of long-term quality of life (QoL), along with our colleagues from Bergen, Norway, convincingly shows that treatment strategy has little effect on individual symptoms such as tinnitus, dizziness, or headache, for example, and long-term QoL.[29,30,31,32] Unfortunately, then, we almost always counsel patients that the treatment of their presenting symptoms has to often be separated from the treatment of their tumor. That is, if disequilibrium is a significant problem, then vestibular rehabilitation is the best treatment going forward; if tinnitus is the primary problem, tinnitus retraining therapy may be helpful; if intractable headache led to the diagnosis of a small VS, consultation with a neurologist with interest and expertise in headache management will almost certainly result in improved QoL for the patient. Surprisingly, we have also shown that it is dizziness and headache that actually impact patients' QoL more than, for instance, unilateral hearing loss or even facial weakness.[33]

74.3.5 Face-to-Face Consultation

We cannot emphasize enough, trying to decide the best treatment of a small- or medium-sized VS based on MRI and audiology data alone, is a perilous undertaking. We have often looked at a case as the one presented here, and walked into the room feeling like we knew what we would recommend and, after spending as little as 30 minutes with the patient, realized a different course of action would be preferable. For example, some patients with the tumor demonstrated here would want it removed to have finality to the treatment—people who want to take all the risk upfront and hope for a "homerun." Other patients may want treatment, but not be able to take much time off work and would prefer to avoid an invasive intracranial operation and choose SRS. Additionally, some people, in learning that treatment is unlikely to make them "better" in any way, would be content with just following a small, minimally symptomatic benign lesion. In summary, it is the face-to-face consultation that is critically important to helping the patient make the right decision.

We would provide this patient with all the information detailed here in a hopefully, nonbiased fashion. We then give the patient ample time to ask questions to clarify what we have told them and try to reconcile it with the information they bring with them from other consultations or the internet. We are certainly keenly aware that treatment biases exist with different providers, treatment centers, and even regions of the country.[34] We emphasize that we do not want patients to tell us upfront what has been recommended elsewhere, as many patients often do get second, third, or even fourth opinions about their VS, and we do not want to be biased by what experts elsewhere may have advised. In a case like we present here, we feel it is our primary responsibility to make sure the patient has accurate information and importantly is not making a decision based on strongly erroneous facts (e.g., "I don't want radiation because it will make the tumor cancerous," "I'll be left with crippling headaches if I have surgery," etc.). It is usually during this process that we can get a fairly good idea, which way the patient is leaning in terms of preference of treatment. We try and reinforce their decision and feel confident in supporting the patient's decision when there is clinical equipoise, which is often the case.

We often advise patients *not* to make a decision during the initial consultation but take some time to consider all the options. While as health care providers we often think of three main options for small- to medium-sized VS as microsurgery, radiation, or observation, from patients' standpoint the decision making may be much more complex. Even if they decide to have surgery, they may be confused about which of the three primary surgical approaches is optimal for them. Similarly, if radiation is selected, there is single fraction treatment with either the Gamma Knife (Elekta AB, Stockholm, Sweden) or a linear accelerator system, hypofractionated treatment with Cyberknife (Accuray, Sunnyvale, CA) or other linear accelerator systems, or hyperfractionated treatment as reviewed in Chapter 18. Even if a "wait-and-scan" strategy is chosen, the patient needs to decide if they are going to follow up near their home or travel back to a tertiary referral center. There is now even mild controversy about whether gadolinium should be administered for every MRI follow-up imaging interval.[35] Without any question, the decision-making process can be overwhelming for some patients. We encourage the interested reader to also review Chapter 13 for a thoughtful discussion regarding the nuances of patients counseling.

We have been gratified that the great majority of patients, when surveyed many years after their diagnosis, report they are happy with the decision they made, would make the same decision again, and would recommend the treatment choice they chose to a friend or family member with the diagnosis of a small- or medium-sized VS.[36]

74.4 Conclusion

There is rarely a single "best" treatment for a small- to medium-sized VS. We debated extensively if it was even appropriate to have such a chapter title in this book. Each option, microsurgery, radiation, or observation, has distinct advantages and drawbacks, and we have tried to review our analysis of these pros and cons and how we approach counseling patients. Most patients with VS will eventually lose hearing in the ipsilateral ear regardless of treatment choice, and our analysis of what effect QoL indicates unilateral deafness is a minor contributor in the decline of overall QoL that most VS patients experience. We try to get patients to articulate their one or two main priorities in dealing with their VS: Do they voice a strong desire to be "cured" and "have the tumor out of their head"? Then, surgery may be optimal. Do they desire treatment but do not want to take any time off work? Then, SRS may be the best option. Was the tumor discovered incidentally and they are content with the information this is a benign, often slow-growing tumor? Then observation offers the least short-term risk. Are they mostly bothered by ipsilateral tinnitus? Treatment modality is not going to strongly influence that symptom, and they need to understand that before they undertake a treatment for which they may be severely disappointed with the outcome.

Almost always, when this debate is raised, there is question made of conducting a prospective, randomized trial to try and answer this perplexing dilemma. Admittedly, we have considered it from time to time, but unofficially polling patients as to whether they would be willing to let random chance decide if they will simply watch their tumor, have radiation, or undergo a major intracranial operation under general anesthesia, most patients have indicated they would likely not be comfortable with that. However, on a very positive note, our colleagues in Bergen, Norway, are successfully enrolling patients in a prospective outcomes study comparing observation with SRS (Vestibular Schwannoma – Radiosurgery or Expectation, V-REX; NCT02249572). At the time of this writing, enrollment is going very well and undoubtedly the results will be extremely insightful in the years ahead.

We resist offering advice to patients or physicians who only send an MRI scan and audiogram. The decision making is highly nuanced but we feel moderately confident that after a thoughtful discussion with the patient and their family, we can help them make the right decision for their individual circumstances.

References

[1] Akard W, Tubbs RS, Seymour ZA, Hitselberger WE, Cohen-Gadol AA. Evolution of techniques for the resection of vestibular schwannomas: from saving life to saving function. J Neurosurg. 2009; 110(4):642–647

[2] Friedman RA, Kesser B, Brackmann DE, Fisher LM, Slattery WH, Hitselberger WE. Long-term hearing preservation after middle fossa removal of vestibular schwannoma. Otolaryngol Head Neck Surg. 2003; 129(6):660–665

[3] Woodson EA, Dempewolf RD, Gubbels SP, et al. Long-term hearing preservation after microsurgical excision of vestibular schwannoma. Otol Neurotol. 2010; 31(7):1144–1152

[4] Wang AC, Chinn SB, Than KD, et al. Durability of hearing preservation after microsurgical treatment of vestibular schwannoma using the middle cranial fossa approach. J Neurosurg. 2013; 119(1):131–138

[5] Nakamizo A, Mori M, Inoue D, et al. Long-term hearing outcome after retrosigmoid removal of vestibular schwannoma. Neurol Med Chir (Tokyo). 2013; 53(10):688–694

[6] Quist TS, Givens DJ, Gurgel RK, Chamoun R, Shelton C. Hearing preservation after middle fossa vestibular schwannoma removal: are the results durable? Otolaryngol Head Neck Surg. 2015; 152(4):706–711

[7] Pollock BE, Link MJ, Foote RL. Failure rate of contemporary low-dose radiosurgical technique for vestibular schwannoma. J Neurosurg. 2009; 111(4): 840–844

[8] Carlson ML, Jacob JT, Pollock BE, et al. Long-term hearing outcomes following stereotactic radiosurgery for vestibular schwannoma: patterns of hearing loss and variables influencing audiometric decline. J Neurosurg. 2013; 118 (3):579–587

[9] Marston AP, Jacob JT, Carlson ML, Pollock BE, Driscoll CLW, Link MJ. Pretreatment growth rate as a predictor of tumor control following Gamma Knife radiosurgery for sporadic vestibular schwannoma. J Neurosurg. 2017; 127(2): 380–387

[10] Friedman RA, Brackmann DE, Hitselberger WE, Schwartz MS, Iqbal Z, Berliner KI. Surgical salvage after failed irradiation for vestibular schwannoma. Laryngoscope. 2005; 115(10):1827–1832

[11] Friedman RA, Berliner KI, Bassim M, et al. A paradigm shift in salvage surgery for radiated vestibular schwannoma. Otol Neurotol. 2011; 32(8):1322–1328

[12] Gerganov VM, Giordano M, Samii A, Samii M. Surgical treatment of patients with vestibular schwannomas after failed previous radiosurgery. J Neurosurg. 2012; 116(4):713–720

[13] Husseini ST, Piccirillo E, Taibah A, Almutair T, Sequino G, Sanna M. Salvage surgery of vestibular schwannoma after failed radiotherapy: the Gruppo Otologico experience and review of the literature. Am J Otolaryngol. 2013; 34 (2):107–114

[14] Wise SC, Carlson ML, Tveiten OV, et al. Surgical salvage of recurrent vestibular schwannoma following prior stereotactic radiosurgery. Laryngoscope. 2016; 126(11):2580–2586

[15] Yomo S, Arkha Y, Delsanti C, Roche PH, Thomassin JM, Régis J. Repeat gamma knife surgery for regrowth of vestibular schwannomas. Neurosurgery. 2009; 64(1):48–54, discussion 54–55

[16] Liscak R, Vladyka V, Urgosik D, Simonova G, Vymazal J. Repeated treatment of vestibular schwannomas after gamma knife radiosurgery. Acta Neurochir (Wien). 2009; 151(4):317–324, discussion 324

[17] Kano H, Kondziolka D, Niranjan A, Flannery TJ, Flickinger JC, Lunsford LD. Repeat stereotactic radiosurgery for acoustic neuromas. Int J Radiat Oncol Biol Phys. 2010; 76(2):520–527

[18] Lonneville S, Delbrouck C, Renier C, Devriendt D, Massager N. Repeat Gamma Knife surgery for vestibular schwannomas. Surg Neurol Int. 2015; 6:153

[19] Fu VX, Verheul JB, Beute GN, et al. Retreatment of vestibular schwannoma with Gamma Knife radiosurgery: clinical outcome, tumor control, and review of literature. J Neurosurg. 2017; 6:1–9

[20] Pollock BE, Link MJ, Stafford SL, Parney IF, Garces YI, Foote RL. The risk of radiation-induced tumors or malignant transformation after single-fraction intracranial radiosurgery: results based on a 25-year experience. Int J Radiat Oncol Biol Phys. 2017; 97(5):919–923

[21] Carlson ML, Habermann EB, Wagie AE, et al. The changing landscape of vestibular schwannoma management in the United States – a shift toward conservatism. Otolaryngol Head Neck Surg. 2015; 153(3):440–446

[22] Stangerup SE, Caye-Thomasen P, Tos M, Thomsen J. The natural history of vestibular schwannoma. Otol Neurotol. 2006; 27(4):547–552

[23] Patnaik U, Prasad SC, Tutar H, Giannuzzi AL, Russo A, Sanna M. The long-term outcomes of wait-and-scan and the role of radiotherapy in the management of vestibular schwannomas. Otol Neurotol. 2015; 36(4):638–646

[24] Hunter JB, Francis DO, O'Connell BP, et al. Single institutional experience with observing 564 vestibular schwannomas: factors associated with tumor growth. Otol Neurotol. 2016; 37(10):1630–1636

[25] Kirchmann M, Karnov K, Hansen S, Dethloff T, Stangerup SE, Caye-Thomasen P. Ten-year follow-up on tumor growth and hearing in patients observed with an intracanalicular vestibular schwannoma. Neurosurgery. 2017; 80(1): 49–56

[26] Huang X, Caye-Thomasen P, Stangerup SE. Spontaneous tumour shrinkage in 1261 observed patients with sporadic vestibular schwannoma. J Laryngol Otol. 2013; 127(8):739–743

[27] Stangerup SE, Caye-Thomasen P, Tos M, Thomsen J. Change in hearing during 'wait and scan' management of patients with vestibular schwannoma. J Laryngol Otol. 2008; 122(7):673–681

[28] Stangerup SE, Tos M, Thomsen J, Caye-Thomasen P. Hearing outcomes of vestibular schwannoma patients managed with 'wait and scan': predictive value of hearing level at diagnosis. J Laryngol Otol. 2010; 124(5):490–494

[29] Carlson ML, Tveiten OV, Driscoll CL, et al. Long-term dizziness handicap in patients with vestibular schwannoma: a multicenter cross-sectional study. Otolaryngol Head Neck Surg. 2014; 151(6):1028–1037

[30] Carlson ML, Tveiten OV, Driscoll CL, et al. Long-term quality of life in patients with vestibular schwannoma: an international multicenter cross-sectional

study comparing microsurgery, stereotactic radiosurgery, observation, and nontumor controls. J Neurosurg. 2015; 122(4):833–842
[31] Tveiten OV, Carlson ML, Goplen F, Vassbotn F, Link MJ, Lund-Johansen M. Long-term auditory symptoms in patients with sporadic vestibular schwannoma: an international cross-sectional study. Neurosurgery. 2015; 77(2): 218–227, discussion 227
[32] Carlson ML, Tveiten OV, Driscoll CL, et al. Risk factors and analysis of long-term headache in sporadic vestibular schwannoma: a multicenter cross-sectional study. J Neurosurg. 2015; 123(5):1276–1286
[33] Carlson ML, Tveiten OV, Driscoll CL, et al. What drives quality of life in patients with sporadic vestibular schwannoma? Laryngoscope. 2015; 125(7): 1697–1702
[34] Carlson ML, Glasgow AE, Grossardt BR, Habermann EB, Link MJ. Does where you live influence how your vestibular schwannoma is managed? Examining geographical differences in vestibular schwannoma treatment across the United States. J Neurooncol. 2016; 129(2):269–279
[35] Gulani V, Calamante F, Shellock FG, Kanal E, Reeder SB, International Society for Magnetic Resonance in Medicine. Gadolinium deposition in the brain: summary of evidence and recommendations. Lancet Neurol. 2017; 16(7): 564–570
[36] Carlson ML, Tvieten OV, Lund-Johansen M, Tombers NM, Lohse CM, Link MJ. Patient motivation and long-term satisfaction with treatment choice in vestibular schwannoma. J Neurosurg. 2017

75 Management of Sporadic Vestibular Schwannoma in the Only Hearing Ear

Neil S. Patel and Colin L. W. Driscoll

75.1 Introduction

When determining optimal management of vestibular schwannoma (VS), the hearing status of both ears must be considered. While unilateral deafness impairs sound localization and speech understanding in noise, many patients with good hearing in the contralateral ear eventually accommodate to these changes and do not seek aural rehabilitation. This is in sharp contrast to patients with acquired severe-to-profound *bilateral* sensorineural hearing loss, where the disability of deafness is usually devastating.

Fortunately, the vast majority of sporadic VSs are diagnosed in patients with normal or serviceable hearing in the contralateral ear. The clinical scenario of VS in an only hearing ear is distressing for patients and surgeons alike. In these cases, the standard treatment paradigm for VS is disrupted and the goals of hearing preservation and aural rehabilitation come to the forefront of the discussion. A standard algorithm cannot be applied and the path forward is influenced by auditory and vestibular function of the ipsilateral and contralateral ear, tumor size, growth rate, patient health, and preferences. All patients need support and guidance as they adapt and accept the diagnosis and implications. A successful treatment plan addresses their fears and anxiety, engages them in decision making, and sets realistic expectations.

The primary objectives of the current chapter are to (1) identify the key steps in assessing the contralateral (deaf) ear for hearing restoration potential; (2) discuss management of tumors of varying sizes and pretreatment hearing status; (3) comment on hearing rehabilitation options in the ipsilateral tumor ear; (4) evaluate the modern experience with cochlear implantation (CI) following stereotactic radiosurgery (SRS) and microsurgery; and (5) highlight important patient factors that drive decision making in this challenging situation.

75.2 Auditory Rehabilitation of the Contralateral Ear

The first practical step is to sort out rehabilitative options for the contralateral ear. What was long thought to be a "useless" ear may now become valuable. If there is residual hearing, a hearing aid trial can be initiated. If the ear has not been used for many years, it may take some time before the patient maximizes performance with the aid. Even poor hearing in the contralateral ear may be reassuring for the patient, as they consider treatment options for their tumor, as well as for the surgeon, as this assures an intact auditory pathway for potential treatment options such as CI.

The modern CI has revolutionized management of sensorineural hearing loss. If the patient performs very poorly with a conventional hearing aid or lacks any hearing, a standard CI evaluation is initiated. If hearing in the tumor ear is significantly compromised already or if the tumor is large and hearing preservation with treatment is unlikely, this evaluation may be started early. In the case of a small tumor and good hearing, a CI evaluation for the contralateral ear may be either postponed or pursued upfront. With the latter option, the benefits of implantation will gradually increase, as hearing loss in the tumor ear inevitably declines either from treatment or the natural history of disease.

In addition to audiometric testing, CI candidacy workup should include magnetic resonance (MR) imaging with appropriate T2-weighted sequences to evaluate cochlear patency plus parasagittal reconstructions of the internal auditory canal establish presence of the cochlear nerve in cases of congenital deafness. If there is concern for ossification of the cochlea, a CT will be beneficial for surgical planning. The role of electrical promontory stimulation testing (EPST) in determining CI candidacy remains controversial and will be discussed later in this chapter.

Unfortunately, it is common that the diagnosis of VS in an only hearing ear occurs in patients with long-standing and even congenital contralateral hearing loss.[1] We would normally consider these patients to be poor candidates for CI, as the results are often suboptimal by standard outcome criteria; however, in this setting, there is little to lose. It is possible the patient will still gain open-set speech understanding; however, even access to environmental sound, enhanced lip-reading, and voice modulation may be valuable to the patient over time.

If a patient is a CI candidate, the sequence of tumor treatment and implantation must be considered. If the patient is considering radiation therapy for a growing tumor, it is preferable to perform radiosurgery first as MRI-based lesion targeting becomes increasingly complex in the presence of device or magnet artifact and hearing loss from radiosurgery generally occurs in a protracted manner. If surgery or observation is being contemplated, it is preferable in most cases to proceed with implantation first as the outcome of the CI in this context has a direct influence on the approach to the tumor. Hearing preservation may not be prioritized as highly as in the tumor ear if the patient has enjoyed a good result with their CI. In contrast, a patient with a poor result may favor a more conservative approach or cochlear nerve-sparing surgery that may permit a CI in the ear affected should serviceable hearing be lost.

75.3 Tumor Management

While hearing preservation and rehabilitation are tenable goals when evaluating any patient with a VS, the order of priorities shifts dramatically when a tumor is diagnosed in an only hearing ear. Given the remarkable variability in treatment approaches for small- and medium-sized tumors in the setting of normal hearing in the contralateral ear, the present discussion focuses on situations where a change in approach can be attributed to deafness in the contralateral ear, rather than attempting to reestablish treatment paradigms for all scenarios.

75.3.1 The Small Tumor

In patients with unilateral functional hearing, even minor auditory symptoms are typically noticed and reported promptly. Thus, most tumors in this population are identified at a small size when hearing is often still serviceable. Following diagnosis, a period of radiologic surveillance is almost always the initial course of action. Intuitively, the best scenario for the patient is for the tumor to remain stable. Recent epidemiologic studies have substantially increased our understanding of growth and preservation of long-term serviceable hearing among small tumors. In line with the authors' experience, less than 30% of purely intracanalicular tumors exhibit growth into the cerebellopontine angle (CPA) over long-term follow-up.[2] Tumors that extend into the CPA may exhibit slightly higher growth rates. The interested reader may refer to Chapters 14 and 51 for an in-depth review of the natural history of VS growth and hearing decline. Unfortunately, hearing can progressively deteriorate even when a tumor remains radiographically stable. Sudden changes or fluctuating hearing loss may respond favorably to a course of steroids. If the tumor remains stable but the patient no longer benefits from a conventional hearing aid, then CI should be pursued with or without treating the tumor. This strategy is discussed in greater depth later in the chapter.

Surgical intervention is generally considered only after there has been definite radiological evidence of tumor growth. The couple of exceptions to this rule may be in the setting of a very small tumor that is favorably located from a hearing preservation standpoint or a nongrowing (or slowly growing) tumor with progressive audiometric decline. A small tumor originating from the superior vestibular nerve medially in the internal auditory canal can be removed with a low risk of hearing loss by an experienced surgeon (▶ Fig. 75.1). In the case of a stable tumor with progressive hearing loss, internal auditory canal decompression via middle cranial fossa may prolong serviceable hearing in select cases.[3] However, even in this setting, it is our general practice to advocate observation. If a small tumor follows a typical slow-growing course, the decision to undertake surgery requires thoughtful and honest assessment of hearing preservation outcome. In the setting of an only hearing ear, one must take into account tumor and patient characteristics and select for surgery-only tumors with the highest likelihood of successful hearing preservation. Patients with good preoperative word recognition score, superior vestibular nerve tumors,[4,5] and those with evidence of fundal fluid on T2-weighted MRI sequences[6] may enjoy an increased likelihood of hearing preservation. Consistent with our experience, the realistic likelihood of hearing preservation for a small favorably located tumor based on early postoperative audiometry is in the range of 50 to 80% range, with estimates varying substantially in the literature.[7] A small tumor that extends to the fundus, under the transverse crest and into the base of the modiolus, is much more difficult to remove successfully. If the surgeon is not highly confident that a complete removal can be obtained with hearing preservation, strong consideration needs to be given to continued observation or SRS. Patient preference also has a large role in this decision. When hearing is successfully preserved with surgery, it is felt to be durable in most cases. Estimates of long-term serviceable hearing following microsurgical resection demonstrate hearing preservation rates from 65 to 89%; however, a large subset of patients in these studies were lost to follow-up.[8,9,10,11,12,13]

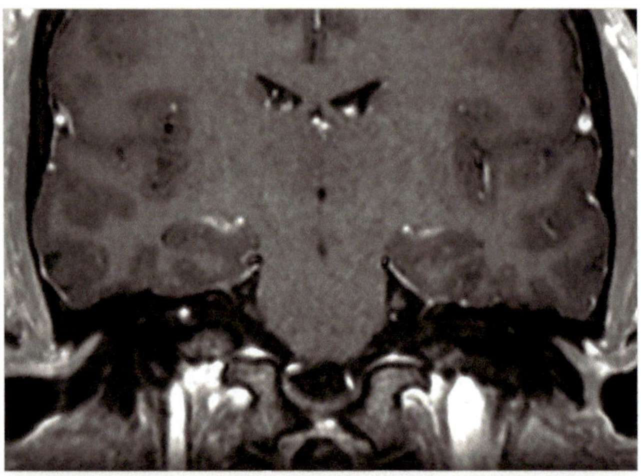

Fig. 75.1 Example of small right-sided vestibular schwannoma of superior vestibular nerve origin, located in the midportion of the internal auditory canal.

If the tumor is not favorable for microsurgical removal or the patient declines surgery, then SRS is a viable alternative. Even in the presence of slow growth, it may be beneficial to delay treatment, as radiosurgery will most likely accelerate hearing loss. Treating upfront or the so-called proactive treatment to protect hearing is controversial and not our practice. An in-depth understanding of the factors that determine hearing preservation following SRS is needed to decide when to intervene (see Chapter 52).

75.3.2 The Growing Medium- or Large-Size Tumor

Even in the setting of medium- or large-size tumors in an only hearing ear, we often prefer an initial period of observation whenever feasible. The obvious caveat is the situation of a very large tumor with hydrocephalus, where priorities shift from maintenance of hearing to prevention of significant neurological sequelae. Not only may the tumor not grow, but if it does, the rate of growth can guide decision making. If a tumor grows rapidly, the authors favor surgical intervention rather than SRS, as in our experience, tumors that grow more rapidly than 2.5 mm/year have a higher rate of radiation failure.[14]

Generally, treatment of a growing medium- or large-size tumor in an only hearing ear centers on the ability to preserve a functional cochlear nerve in order to maintain serviceable hearing or support a CI, all while maintaining tumor control. While a slow-growing tumor may still be observed for a period of time, ultimately, treatment with microsurgery or SRS will be required in most cases.

With regard to surgical intervention, we often consider as a first choice aggressive subtotal tumor removal, as it is very rare that functional hearing or an anatomically intact cochlear nerve can be preserved in tumors larger than 2 cm with gross total resection.[15] If functional hearing is preserved, the residual tumor remnant can be observed and treated with SRS only after definitive evidence of progressive radiologic growth is seen. If functional hearing is lost after subtotal removal, the residual tumor volume can be treated with SRS and a CI can be placed in order to maximize both tumor control and auditory rehabilitation. Because hearing can be preserved on occasion with large tumors, we approach all these cases with a retrosigmoid craniotomy rather than the translabyrinthine approach. In cases where the cochlear nerve is lost, auditory brainstem implant (ABI) placement should be considered.

In general, radiosurgery is rarely used in VS larger than 2.5 cm in maximum posterior fossa diameter given greater risks of tumor swell, hydrocephalus, and other adverse events. However, several studies have demonstrated that SRS can be considered for select situations including cases of a large tumor in an only hearing ear[16,17] (Chapter 22). The advantages of SRS over microsurgery include greater potential for hearing preservation, less risk of cochlear nerve injury to support future CI, and avoidance of other surgical complications. Failure to control tumor growth, acceleration of hearing loss beyond the expected rate from tumor effect alone, hydrocephalus, and the development of new neurologic symptoms due to radiation effect on the cerebellum or brainstem are all disadvantages.[18,19,20] If SRS fails and the tumor continues to grow, it is very unlikely it can be removed with preservation of a viable cochlear nerve; so, an ABI may be the only viable option for hearing rehabilitation.

For growing medium-sized tumors (~1–2.5 cm), the majority of patients choose to undergo SRS. The rationale for this approach centers on the fact that tumor control rates are similar to those obtained with surgery when the percentage of subtotal removals is considered, the chance of short- and intermediate-term hearing preservation greater, and ultimately performance with a CI may be better if required.[20,21,22] While factors such as young patient age, low dose to the cochlea, and small tumor size have been associated with good hearing outcomes after SRS, pretreatment hearing remains the most significant predictor of hearing preservation after SRS.[21]

Ultimately, management of a medium- or large-sized VS in an only hearing ear is challenging, and each case must be carefully evaluated in order to maintain serviceable hearing for as long as possible, while balancing other priorities including tumor control and facial nerve function. Unfortunately, in most cases, serviceable hearing will ultimately be lost and there is no way to adequately prepare for the consequences of bilateral deafness and the immediate and dramatic effect on patient function and quality of life.

75.4 Hearing Rehabilitation in the Ipsilateral Ear after Treatment

The ability to restore useful hearing following treatment of a VS in an only hearing ear depends on the viability of remaining structures in the peripheral auditory pathway. Candidates for CI must have a patent cochlea and an intact cochlear nerve capable of transmitting an electrical signal—if absent, ABI is the only widely available remaining option for hearing rehabilitation. This section will address the feasibility, timing, and outcomes of CI after microsurgery or radiosurgery.

75.4.1 Cochlear Implantation after Microsurgical Resection

If an anatomically intact cochlear nerve is maintained at the time that a tumor is removed from an only hearing ear, but functional hearing is lost, CI should be considered. The decision to pursue CI can only be determined after a postoperative audiogram can be reviewed. Even in the case where the intraoperative ABR or cochlear nerve action potential (CNAP) is lost, simultaneous implantation should not be considered as unfavorable results of intraoperative testing do not guarantee that functional hearing is lost. That is, some patients will maintain serviceable hearing after surgery even when intraoperative testing indicates otherwise (Chapter 28). If useful hearing is lost, CI is usually pursued soon after the patient has recovered from surgery. This will minimize the time the patient is left without hearing and also reduces the risk of difficult electrode insertion, as fibrosis and cochlear ossification can even occur in cases of middle fossa and retrosigmoid tumor resection.[22] If for some reason a translabyrinthine approach was chosen, simultaneous CI placement should be considered, as this avoids a second surgery and there is a potential to develop fibrosis or ossification of the cochlea complicating CI placement.[23,24]

Of course, any patient who maintains detectable pure-tone thresholds after surgery but has lost serviceable hearing indeed has an intact cochlear nerve and is a candidate for CI. However, CI candidacy assessment in patients who have complete hearing loss immediately after surgery remains somewhat controversial. Many have debated the timing and overall value of EPST in the context of CI candidacy assessment after tumor removal with complete hearing loss. Should testing be pursued, it should not be performed immediately after tumor removal to avoid false-negative results related to neurapraxia.[25] Several published cases of negative testing 1 month after surgery with positive testing 6 to 8 weeks later exist in the neurofibromatosis type 2 (NF2) literature.[24] The question of whether CI should be pursued with negative testing results is more challenging. The *a priori* assumption that poor EPST results would preclude benefit from CI has been disproven in multiple reports in the NF2 literature.[26,27,28] The actual false-negative rate of EPST is unknown, given that the present literature on EPST after VS surgery is limited to small case series without uniform testing protocols. Given that an absent response to EPST does exclude the chance that the patient will still benefit from implantation, we do not routinely employ EPST in candidacy assessment. Rather, the primary consideration to pursue implantation should be based on evidence (e.g., operative report) regarding the anatomical continuity of the cochlear nerve. CI provides patients with the best chance of attaining useful hearing and therefore it is worthwhile to attempt CI in this situation. Even in poor performers, patients often continue to use their devices for voice modulation, sound awareness, and lip reading—outcomes that might be expected with ABI. These patients may still undergo CI explantation and ABI placement as a salvage option.

75.4.2 Cochlear Implantation after Stereotactic Radiosurgery

In many ways, assessing a patient for CI following SRS of a VS in an only hearing ear is more straightforward. In these cases, an anatomically intact cochlear nerve is virtually guaranteed and the only obstacle to successful stimulation comes from cochlear nerve compression or radiation-associated injury of the cochlea, cochlear nerve, or cochlear nucleus. To date, most of the data regarding CI outcomes in VS come from the NF2 literature. While not perfect, it is reasonable to assume that outcomes in patients with sporadic VS will be at least on par, or better than NF2-associated VS, given a greater propensity for multicentric tumors and cochlear nerve invasion with NF2. In a recent literature review of NF2 patients who underwent CI after SRS, the majority of patients use their devices on a daily basis, with six of eight achieving open-set performance scores comparable to conventional CI users.[27] In this population, perhaps the most difficult decision is when to proceed to a CI when any degree of native residual hearing is present. Paralleling conventional CI candidates, implantation is usually pursued when the patient no longer gains significant benefit from conventional amplification.

Provided that SRS has only been in widespread use since the 1990s, long-term audiometric results in the subset that has received a CI is not available. Given the progressive decline in hearing that results from SRS,[29] it remains unclear whether CI performance will be durable in spite of delayed radiation effect, excluding situations with tumor recurrence. There has even been a case of deteriorating CI performance that improved after internal auditory canal decompression.[30] Nevertheless, eventual ABI placement remains an option if a CI is no longer beneficial or salvage surgery is required. Further studies of long-term CI use in NF2 and sporadic VS patients after radiosurgery will be helpful in counseling patients (Chapters 61 and 84).

75.5 Case

In order to highlight several of the nuances of VS management in patients with an only hearing ear, we present an illustrative case. A 56-year-old woman was referred to our clinic in 2006 for a right-sided VS in her only hearing ear. The etiology of her profound left-sided deafness was unknown but thought to be related to mastoiditis at age 3 or 4. She never used amplification. Initial audiometry revealed a sloping normal to severe sensorineural hearing loss in her right (tumor) ear with 90% word recognition and profound deafness in the left ear. She underwent MRI to evaluate the status of the left cochlear nerve and the previously diagnosed right-sided VS. Imaging revealed a 1.4-cm VS contacting the brainstem. The tumor extended laterally to the fundus but did not completely fill the internal auditory canal. The left cochlear nerve was anatomically intact and there were no inner ear malformations or ossification present.

Pure-tone audiometry demonstrated a gradual decline in her right ear over several years with fluctuations in word recognition scores between 40 and 85% (▶ Fig. 75.2). At her functional nadir, she underwent CI testing and was found to be a candidate based on sentence testing in noise. She then underwent left-side implantation and has received benefit in sound perception but has not yet achieved open-set speech recognition with the implant alone 1 year after surgery. Nevertheless, she uses her device full time.

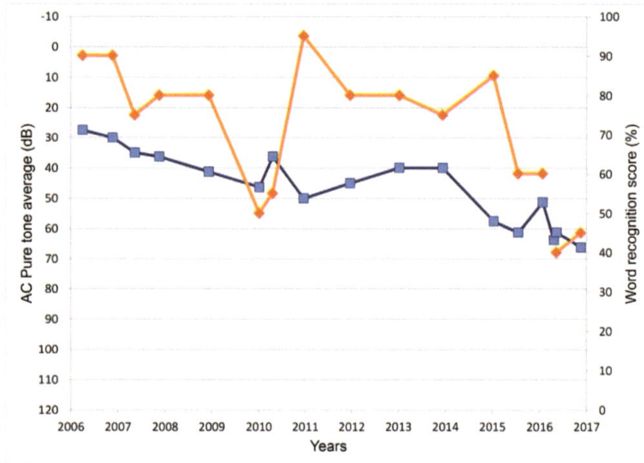

Fig. 75.2 Progression of hearing loss during a period of tumor observation. Significant fluctuations became more frequent over time and were periodically treated with courses of oral steroid. Orange line depicts word recognition score change over time and blue line indicates pure tone average change over time.

The tumor was observed for a total of 10 years during which her hearing remained functional and the tumor demonstrated limited but definite growth (▶ Fig. 75.3). Of note, the implant presented no difficulty in tumor surveillance. As her hearing has reached more marginal functional levels and the tumor growth continued, we elected to proceed with SRS. She underwent Gamma Knife radiosurgery with a marginal tumor dose of 13 Gy (maximum dose: 26 Gy) in September 2016 without incident. Given the expected decline in her hearing after SRS, she is prepared to undergo right-sided CI when she feels ready.

75.6 Conclusion

The delicate balance between tumor control and hearing preservation forms the crux of the complex care of a patient affected by a VS in an only hearing ear. The surgeon must recognize that hearing impairment caused by the tumor or its treatment exerts a strongly negative effect on daily function and overall quality of life. In most cases, the first step that should be attempted is auditory rehabilitation in the contralateral ear, as the outcome will often greatly influence subsequent tumor management. Almost all tumors in an only hearing ear should undergo an initial period of radiographic observation. Small tumors with excellent pretreatment hearing and very favorable anatomic characteristics are the best candidates for hearing preservation microsurgical approaches. In contrast, for larger, growing, and less favorable tumors, SRS or subtotal resection with cochlear nerve preservation may offer the longest duration of serviceable hearing or best CI functionality. With the exception of anatomic disruption of the cochlear nerve, CI should be the first hearing rehabilitation option pursued in the tumor ear, before ABI.

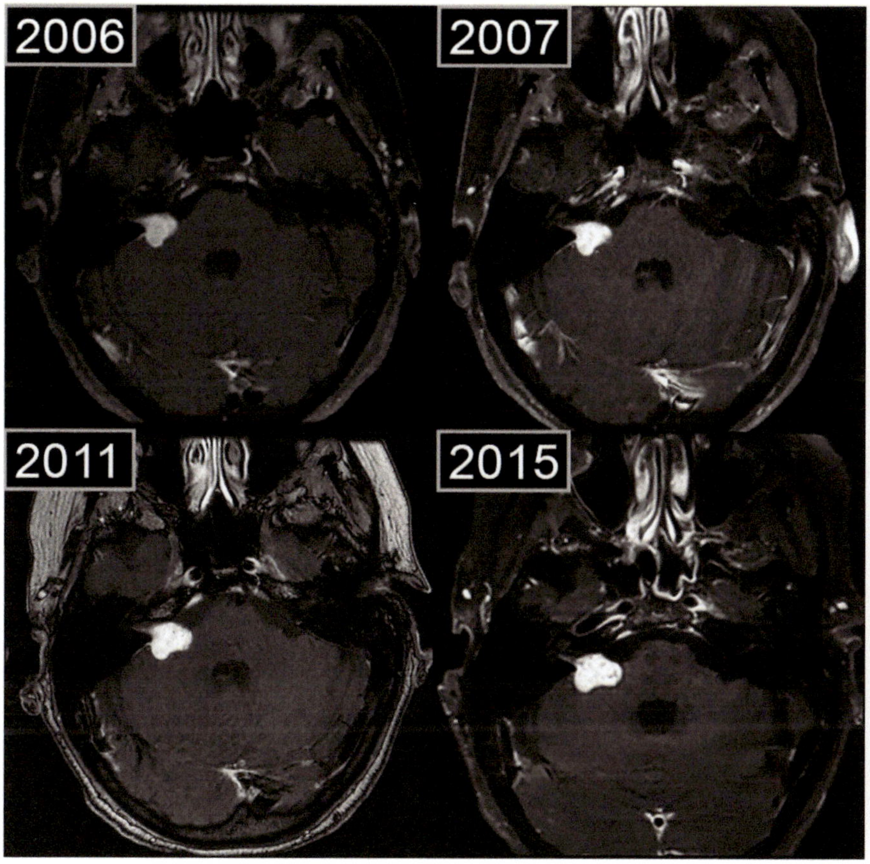

Fig. 75.3 Axial contrast-enhanced T1-weighted MR images demonstrating slow tumor growth over 9 years.

References

[1] Di Lella F, Merkus P, Di Trapani G, Taibah A, Guida M, Sanna M. Vestibular schwannoma in the only hearing ear: role of cochlear implants. Ann Otol Rhinol Laryngol. 2013; 122(2):91–99

[2] Kirchmann M, Karnov K, Hansen S, Dethloff T, Stangerup SE, Caye-Thomasen P. Ten-year follow-up on tumor growth and hearing in patients observed with an intracanalicular vestibular schwannoma. Neurosurgery. 2017; 80(1): 49–56

[3] Slattery WH, Hoa M, Bonne N, et al. Middle fossa decompression for hearing preservation: a review of institutional results and indications. Otol Neurotol. 2011; 32(6):1017–1024

[4] Jacob A, Robinson LL, Jr, Bortman JS, Yu L, Dodson EE, Welling DB. Nerve of origin, tumor size, hearing preservation, and facial nerve outcomes in 359 vestibular schwannoma resections at a tertiary care academic center. Laryngoscope. 2007; 117(12):2087–2092

[5] Rachinger J, Rampp S, Prell J, Scheller C, Alfieri A, Strauss C. Tumor origin and hearing preservation in vestibular schwannoma surgery. J Neurosurg. 2011; 115(5):900–905

[6] Goddard JC, Schwartz MS, Friedman RA. Fundal fluid as a predictor of hearing preservation in the middle cranial fossa approach for vestibular schwannoma. Otol Neurotol. 2010; 31(7):1128–1134

[7] Ansari SF, Terry C, Cohen-Gadol AA. Surgery for vestibular schwannomas: a systematic review of complications by approach. Neurosurg Focus. 2012; 33 (3):E14

[8] Friedman RA, Kesser B, Brackmann DE, Fisher LM, Slattery WH, Hitselberger WE. Long-term hearing preservation after middle fossa removal of vestibular schwannoma. Otolaryngol Head Neck Surg. 2003; 129(6):660–665

[9] Hilton CW, Haines SJ, Agrawal A, Levine SC. Late failure rate of hearing preservation after middle fossa approach for resection of vestibular schwannoma. Otol Neurotol. 2011; 32(1):132–135

[10] Quist TS, Givens DJ, Gurgel RK, Chamoun R, Shelton C. Hearing preservation after middle fossa vestibular schwannoma removal: are the results durable? Otolaryngol Head Neck Surg. 2015; 152(4):706–711

[11] Wang AC, Chinn SB, Than KD, et al. Durability of hearing preservation after microsurgical treatment of vestibular schwannoma using the middle cranial fossa approach. J Neurosurg. 2013; 119(1):131–138

[12] Woodson EA, Dempewolf RD, Gubbels SP, et al. Long-term hearing preservation after microsurgical excision of vestibular schwannoma. Otol Neurotol. 2010; 31(7):1144–1152

[13] Shelton C, Hitselberger WE, House WF, Brackmann DE. Hearing preservation after acoustic tumor removal: long-term results. Laryngoscope. 1990; 100(2, Pt 1):115–119

[14] Marston AP, Jacob JT, Carlson ML, Pollock BE, Driscoll CLW, Link MJ. Pretreatment growth rate as a predictor of tumor control following Gamma Knife radiosurgery for sporadic vestibular schwannoma. J Neurosurg. 2017; 127(2):380–387

[15] Pan HC, Sheehan J, Sheu ML, Chiu WT, Yang DY. Intracapsular decompression or radical resection followed by Gamma Knife surgery for patients harboring a large vestibular schwannoma. J Neurosurg. 2012; 117 Suppl:69–77

[16] Williams BJ, Xu Z, Salvetti DJ, McNeill IT, Larner J, Sheehan JP. Gamma Knife surgery for large vestibular schwannomas: a single-center retrospective case-matched comparison assessing the effect of lesion size. J Neurosurg. 2013; 119(2):463–471

[17] Milligan BD, Pollock BE, Foote RL, Link MJ. Long-term tumor control and cranial nerve outcomes following γ knife surgery for larger-volume vestibular schwannomas. J Neurosurg. 2012; 116(3):598–604

[18] van de Langenberg R, Hanssens PE, Verheul JB, et al. Management of large vestibular schwannoma. Part II. Primary Gamma Knife surgery: radiological and clinical aspects. J Neurosurg. 2011; 115(5):885–893

[19] Link MJ, Driscoll CL, Foote RL, Pollock BE. Radiation therapy and radiosurgery for vestibular schwannomas: indications, techniques, and results. Otolaryngol Clin North Am. 2012; 45(2):353–366, viii–ix

[20] Klijn S, Verheul JB, Beute GN, et al. Gamma Knife radiosurgery for vestibular schwannomas: evaluation of tumor control and its predictors in a large patient cohort in The Netherlands. J Neurosurg. 2016; 124(6):1619–1626

[21] Jacob JT, Pollock BE, Carlson ML, Driscoll CL, Link MJ. Stereotactic radiosurgery in the management of vestibular schwannoma and glomus jugulare: indications, techniques, and results. Otolaryngol Clin North Am. 2015; 48(3): 515–526

[22] Roehm PC, Mallen-St Clair J, Jethanamest D, et al. Auditory rehabilitation of patients with neurofibromatosis Type 2 by using cochlear implants. J Neurosurg. 2011; 115(4):827–834
[23] Chen DA, Linthicum FH, Jr, Rizer FM. Cochlear histopathology in the labyrinthectomized ear: implications for cochlear implantation. Laryngoscope. 1988; 98(11):1170–1172
[24] Neff BA, Wiet RM, Lasak JM, et al. Cochlear implantation in the neurofibromatosis type 2 patient: long-term follow-up. Laryngoscope. 2007; 117(6):1069–1072
[25] Vrabec JT, Lambert PR, Arts HA, Ruth RA. Promontory stimulation following translabyrinthine excision of acoustic neuroma with preservation of the cochlear nerve. Am J Otol. 1995; 16(5):643–647
[26] Vincenti V, Pasanisi E, Guida M, Di Trapani G, Sanna M. Hearing rehabilitation in neurofibromatosis type 2 patients: cochlear versus auditory brainstem implantation. Audiol Neurootol. 2008; 13(4):273–280
[27] Carlson ML, Breen JT, Driscoll CL, et al. Cochlear implantation in patients with neurofibromatosis type 2: variables affecting auditory performance. Otol Neurotol. 2012; 33(5):853–862
[28] Celis-Aguilar E, Lassaletta L, Gavilán J. Cochlear implantation in patients with neurofibromatosis type 2 and patients with vestibular schwannoma in the only hearing ear. Int J Otolaryngol. 2012; 2012:157497
[29] Carlson ML, Jacob JT, Pollock BE, et al. Long-term hearing outcomes following stereotactic radiosurgery for vestibular schwannoma: patterns of hearing loss and variables influencing audiometric decline. J Neurosurg. 2013; 118 (3):579–587
[30] Bernardeschi D, Peyre M, Collin M, Smail M, Sterkers O, Kalamarides M. Internal auditory canal decompression for hearing maintenance in neurofibromatosis type 2 patients. Neurosurgery. 2016; 79(3):370–377

76 Treatment of Cystic Vestibular Schwannoma

Brian A. Neff

76.1 Introduction

Cystic vestibular schwannomas (CVSs) are a subtype of vestibular schwannoma (VS) that contain solid portions of tumor mixed with single or multiple, xanthochromic, fluid-filled cysts making up the other part of the tumor. CVSs represent anywhere from 5.7 to 48% of all VSs, with most recent study estimates reporting approximately 10 to 20%. The true incidence varies because there is not a universally accepted definition of what constitutes a CVS.[1,2,3,4]

CVS patients are often characterized as presenting with larger tumors, having faster tumor growth rates, shorter symptomatic periods before presentation, worse outcomes from surgical intervention, and poorer stereotactic radiosurgery (SRS) results. However, all of these generalizations are disputable, and the literature covering CVS outcomes is limited to retrospective case series and retrospective analysis of prospectively collected databases. This chapter will cover patient presentation, radiologic differential classification, pathophysiology, and treatment results for CVS.

76.2 Patient Presentation

Many authors have reported that CVSs have a more aggressive growth rate and present as larger tumors than their solid vestibular schwannoma (SVS) counterparts.[1,4,5,6,7] Recent retrospective series disagree on the percentage of CVSs that present at a large size with 17 to 77.6% of tumors presenting greater than 4.0 cm at diagnosis.[2,4] In the presence of a cyst, there can be rapid expansion of the lesion, intratumoral hemorrhage, brainstem compression, and hydrocephalus associated with elevated intracranial pressure, papilledema, cranial nerve paresis, and facial paresthesias.[3,8] Up to 17 to 27% of CVS patients can present with acute worsening of symptoms due to rapid cyst enlargement.[1,9] In VS greater than 3 cm in diameter, hydrocephalus was seen in 21 of the 22 cystic tumors (95.5%) compared to 33 of the 40 solid tumors (82.5%).[9]

In contrast to the aforementioned points, a literature review of nine studies containing 428 CVS and 1,287 SVS showed no difference in age or sex distribution. The average size at presentation was not significantly different between CVS at 3.9 ± 0.84 cm and SVS at 3.7 ± 1.2 cm ($p = 0.7$).[10] In compiling data from three studies, the difference in symptom duration was not statistically significant (18.7 vs. 23.3 months, respectively, $p = 0.3$).[10]

76.3 Radiology and Differential Diagnosis

CVSs are best characterized by magnetic resonance imaging (MRI) studies. The solid portions of CVS appear identical to SVS and are isointense or hypointense with the brain on T1-weighted imaging.[8] Additionally, the solid tumor component and the cystic wall enhance with the addition of gadolinium contrast, and thus, this imaging characteristic can be used to differentiate CVS from arachnoid cysts and epidermoids.[3] Conversely, the cystic portions of CVS appear as fluid-filled compartments that are hypointense on T1-weighted and hyperintense on T2-weighted images[8] (▶ Fig. 76.1). The radiographic differential diagnosis of cystic lesions of the cerebellopontine angle (CPA) is summarized in ▶ Table 76.1.

Table 76.1 Radiologic differential for a cystic vestibular schwannoma, cystic CPA tumor, or cystic posterior fossa lesion

Cystic extra-axial lesions in the posterior fossa	Cystic intraxial tumors with CPA extension
Arachnoid cyst (adjacent to non-cystic meningioma or solid vestibular schwannoma)	Hemangioblastoma
Epidermoid	Dysembryoplastic Neuroepithelial tumor (DNET)
Endolymphatic sac tumor	Ganglioglioma
Neurenteric cyst (usually midline, pre-pontine)	Pilocytic Astrocytoma
Thrombosed aneurysm	
Cholesterol granuloma (extending to involve CPA)	
CPA cysticercosis	
Cavernous angioma	

Abbreviations: DNET, dysembryoplastic neuroepithelial tumor; CPA, cerebellopontine angle.

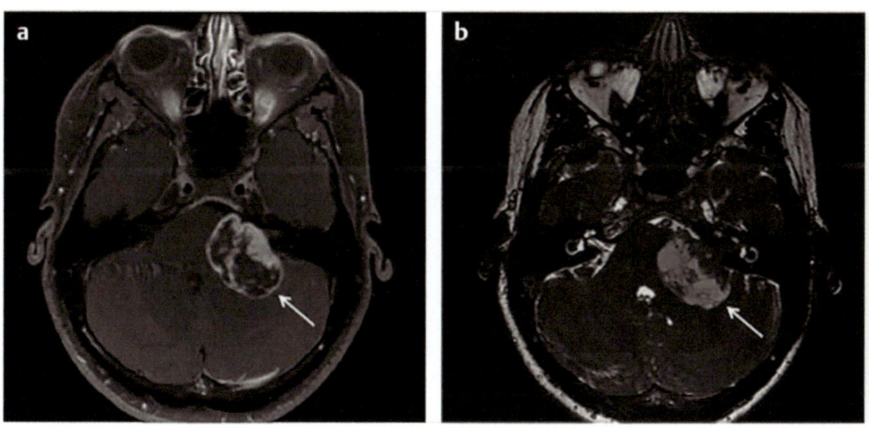

Fig. 76.1 MRI of the brain and IACs with gadolinium contrast of patient with a large left CPA cystic vestibular schwannoma. **(a)** Axial, T1-weighted scan with gadolinium; *white arrow* pointing at cystic tumor; **(b)** axial, T2-weighted FIESTA image; *white arrow* is highlighting the largely hyperintense cyst fluid that makes up the majority of the CPA portion of the tumor.

76.4 Definition and Classification

There is wide variability in the reported prevalence of CVS that is in large part due to a lack of consensus regarding the definition of what constitutes a cystic tumor. Several classification schemes have been proposed over the last few decades; however, a single classification system has yet to be universally adopted. The simplest and earliest definitions relied on radiographic demonstration of cyst formation and the presence of "significant" cysts at the time of surgery.[2,3] However, it was suggested that there were a lot of radiologic false positives; so, definitions were revised to include cystic radiologic appearance, perioperative identification of cystic elements, and histological verification of S100 positive membranes.[11] The definition of CVS has since evolved to attempt to quantify the amount of tumor that is cystic and to classify the tumors by cyst location: central versus peripheral. For example, "cystic VS" has been defined as all VSs for which the MRI exhibits evidence of cyst formation and for which the pathologic specimens are larger than 3 mm.[12] Other retrospective case series have defined "cystic VS" as tumors with cysts making up anywhere from one-third to two-thirds of the mean CPA tumor diameter or the estimated whole tumor volume.[9,10,13,14] Most of these definitions include both intramural and extramural/arachnoid cysts.

Other classification systems emphasized the importance of multicystic tumors and the cyst location. Tumors were first classified based on overall cyst location and cyst wall thickness: central and thick-walled (type A) or peripheral and thin-walled (type B). Type A lesions were then subdivided by cyst characteristics (polycystic or monocystic) and cyst size or volume (small/medium/large). Type B lesions were classified according to cyst orientation with respect to the internal auditory canal (anterior, medial, posterior, or a combination of these).[3] However, determination of the gross total volume (GTV) of cystic tumors is sometimes difficult when the cyst is extramural. If the extramural cyst is a pathologically pure arachnoid cyst, some authors argue that they should not be factored into the tumor volume if they are broadly based against the dura without any enhancement of the cyst wall.[14] As a final thought on the classification of CVS, a VS consensus group defined CVS to only include tumors with extramural cysts, and central cystic tumors should not be labeled CVS.[15] This definition has largely not been adhered to in most subsequent reports on CVS which often include intratumoral cystic tumors.

76.5 Pathophysiology

A precise understanding of cyst formation and growth in CVS remains elusive; nonetheless, various hypotheses have been created. Originally, it was thought that cyst formation was due to an increased cell growth rate that outpaced the tumor's blood supply, thus leading to tumor degeneration and cyst formation.[16,17] However, later studies did not find any difference in the Ki-67 proliferative index of CVS compared with SVS.[18] Now it is believed that the unpredictable and rapid growth in CVS is due to the expansion of the cysts themselves.[5,9]

CVS may expand due to the production of a myxomatous material in small cystic areas within Antoni type B tissue in which the smaller cysts coalesce into larger cysts and compress the surrounding Antoni type A cells. This is consistent with the reported finding that the cyst portions of the CVS were predominantly observed in the Antoni B areas.[18,19] More recent studies have shown that the cyst wall is histologically more complex consisting of an outer capsular portion, showing S100 and vimentin-positive fibrils, and an inner luminal portion, which has an epithelium-lined appearance. Therefore, the cyst wall consists of a compressed outer type A tissue and an inner layer with type B tissue.[6] In contrast to this view, other studies have not found any relationship between the distribution of cysts and the Antoni A and B tissues.[5,9]

Microhemorrhages within the tumor have been hypothesized to cause the initial presence of microcysts that may coalesce to form larger cysts.[13,20] Park et al documented the presence of significantly increased histological evidence of microhemorrhage, such as hemosiderin-laden macrophages, hemosiderin deposits, thrombotic vessels, and abnormal vessel proliferation in CVS compared with SVS.[5,21] However, the factor that triggers this hemorrhagic tendency in CVS still needs to be elucidated. Once formed, an increase in cyst size is promoted by fluid accumulation due to a direct osmotic effect or extravasation of serum proteins from an impaired blood–tumor barrier.[10,22,23]

A final hypothesis on cyst formation explains that extramural tumor cysts associated with CVS have a higher protein and/or colloid content than that observed in usual arachnoid cysts as a result of secretions from the tumors. Most extramural cysts have epicenters between the tumor and brain, suggesting that the most likely mechanism of formation is peritumoral adhesions. These adhesions lead to the development of pseudoduplication due to the trapping of fluid between the leptomeninges and the mass, resulting in an acquired type of arachnoid cyst that differs slightly from a primary arachnoid cyst not associated with VS.[3,14]

76.6 Molecular Biology of Cystic Schwannomas

In a study of differential gene expression between 11 cystic and 6 solid VSs, 46 total genes showed differential expression between CVS and SVS. Of these 46 genes, 5 genes were found to have a 10-fold expression differential on cDNA microarray confirmed by quantitative real-time polymerase chain reaction experiments. The following genes were downregulated in CVS: CLORF130 (chromosome 1 open reading frame 130 gene) whose function is unknown, CNTF gene (ciliary neurotrophic factor gene), FGFBP2 (fibroblast growth binding protein 2 gene), COL4A3 gene (collagen type IV α3 gene), and the COL4A4 gene (collagen type IV α4 gene).[24] In contrast to this aforementioned publication, another gene expression study in CVS did not find any genes that were differentially expressed between 7 CVS and 18 SVS.[25] The implications of these findings and proposed molecular mechanism for VS cyst formation are still unclear.

Matrix metalloproteinases, which are proteolytic enzymes found naturally during embryogenesis and tissue remodeling, were identified via immunohistochemistry within the cyst fluid and intraluminal cyst walls of CVS. Hence, the authors put forth an unproven hypothesis that matrix metalloproteinase-2 (MMP-2) may contribute to cyst formation as well as tumor adhesion to the facial nerve by promoting tumor expansion and growth or by stimulating proteolytic degradation at the tumor–nerve interface.[6] The utility of this finding is currently questionable as a different study showed MMP-2 expression in interstitial and extracellular matrix labeling within solid VS and normal human brain.[26] Much future work analyzing the molecular mechanism of VS cyst formation is still needed.

76.7 Surgery

Surgical excision has long been considered the primary treatment modality for CVS. However, support for this viewpoint is primarily expert opinion, and there is a great heterogeneity in reported outcomes. In no place is this seen more clearly than in postsurgical facial nerve results. Many studies, especially earlier reports, found facial nerve outcomes after CVS resection to be less favorable in comparison to SVS (▶ Table 76.2).[1,2,5,6,11,27] Both a lower rate of facial nerve anatomic preservation and worse functional outcomes with intact nerves were usually demonstrated. Conversely, a few reports showed a trend toward worse facial nerve outcomes after CVS that did not reach statistical significance (▶ Table 76.2).[8,28] Moreover, a few additional studies have found no significant difference in facial nerve outcomes when comparing CVS and SVS (▶ Table 76.2).[3,4,7,29] Because of these inconsistencies, a recent literature review of seven CVS studies evaluating facial nerve function was published. A good facial functional outcome was defined as House–Brackmann (HB) grade I or II at the latest follow-up. A total of 302 patients with CVS and 959 patients with SVS were analyzed. HB grade I to II facial nerve outcomes at the last follow-up were significantly better in the cohort of patients with SVS than in those with CVS (52.1 and 39%, respectively; $p = 0.0001$).[10] Unfortunately, this study cannot be interpreted as conclusive, as the included studies were mostly retrospective and not individually controlled for tumor size or completeness of resection. There are many probable reasons for the differing facial nerve results between studies including early nonuniform use of intraoperative facial nerve monitoring, differing degrees of tumor removal (gross total resection [GTR] vs. subtotal resection), a lack of consensus as to what defines a cystic schwannoma, failure to control for tumor size, and no agreement on what defines an acceptable facial nerve outcome. For the authors who espoused a less favorable CVS facial functional result, several reasons have been offered. Surgery on CVS can be more difficult because of the cyst's engulfment and adherence to neurovascular structures, the removal of large cystic components can cause deformation of the tumor altering the relationship to the facial nerve, hypervascular solid portions of the tumor, unpredictable cyst displacement of the facial nerve,

Table 76.2 Review of published CVS studies

Author (date)	Type	Control	No. of CVS	Summary
Wallace et al (1993)[30]	Retro	None	7	Descriptive radiology study; no SVS comparison
Tali et al (1993)[12]	Retro	None	16	Descriptive radiology study; CVS incidence of 11.3%
Charabi et al (1994)[1]	Retro	SM	23	Symptom duration shorter for CVS; surgical FN outcomes worse in CVS
Jeng et al (1995)[31]	Retro	None	15	Descriptive MRI study mentioning CVS
Pendl et al (1996)[13]	Retro	None	6	Descriptive CVS SRS paper; 3 cases with rapid, post-SRS cyst enlargement requiring surgery
Fundová et al (2000)[11]	Retro	None	44	Surgical FN outcomes worse in CVS, shorter symptom duration in CVS
Shirato et al (2000)[14]	Retro	None	20	No difference in 2-y SRS tumor control for CVS
Delsanti and Régis (2004)[32]	Retro	None	54	No difference in tumor control rate with SRS[a]
Benech et al (2005)[28]	Retro	None	26	No difference in surgical FN outcomes; shorter symptom duration in CVS[a]
Wandong et al (2005)[27]	Retro	None	22	No SVS comparison; FN outcome HB I–II in 5/22 (23%)
Jones et al (2007)[29]	Retro	SM	70	No difference in surgical FN outcomes
Moon et al (2007)[6]	Retro	None	24	Surgical facial nerve outcomes worse in CVS; shorter symptom duration in CVS; CVS tumors larger at presentation
Mehrotra et al (2008)[9]	Retro	None	22	No difference in surgical FN outcomes in giant tumors (>4 cm); higher incidence of hydrocephalus with CVS
Sinha and Sharma (2008)[2]	Retro	None	58	Surgical FN outcomes worse in CVS; lower GTR rates with CVS
Piccirillo et al (2009)[3]	Retro	SM, GTRM	96	No difference in surgical FN outcomes
Jian et al (2011)[7]	Retro (prospective database)	None	58	CVS tumors larger at presentation; no difference in surgical FN outcomes; lower GTR rates with CVS
Yashar et al (2012)[8]	Retro	GTRM	23	No difference in surgical FN outcomes[a]
Thakur et al (2012)[10]	Literature review	None	341	No difference in size, age, surgical FN outcomes, or symptom duration
Tang et al (2014)[4]	Retro	None	131	No difference in surgical FN outcome; no difference in GTR rate

Abbreviations: CVS, cystic vestibular schwannoma; FN, facial nerve; GTR, gross total resection; GTRM, groups evenly matched for gross total resection; HB, House–Brackmann score; Retro, retrospective; SM, size-matched tumors; SRS, stereotactic radiosurgery; SVS, solid vestibular schwannoma.
[a]Outcomes may have shown a trend, but were not statistically significant. The authors incorrectly concluded that this was a significant difference.

and the absence of an adequate subarachnoid dissection plane especially when the cysts are located anteromedially to the IAC.[1,3,4,10]

Authors also cannot agree on other surgical issues with CVS. For example, studies have reported significantly increased adherence of cystic tumors to neural structures with increased complications related to dissection of adhesions from the brainstem.[6] In contrast, CVSs have been subjectively evaluated to be less adherent to intracranial structures (brainstem, cranial nerves) than SVS.[3,28] In a small literature review of the comparative frequencies of tumor-brainstem adherence, it was concluded that patients with SVS had a significantly higher rate of brainstem adherence than those with CVSs (86.8 and 77.6%, respectively; $p = 0.03$).[10] These differences of opinion probably lead to differing descriptions on the possibility of complete CVS tumor resection. It has been reported that complete GTR was not as commonly possible with CVS (9–76%) compared with SVS (70–91%).[1,2,7] Conversely, another study showed no difference in the rate of subtotal removal between CVS and SVS (39/131 [29.8%] vs. 29/131 [22.1%], respectively; $p = 0.15$).[4] A literature review of 341 CVSs and 1,210 SVSs that were not matched for tumor size concluded there was no significant difference in the extent of GTR for CVS and SVS (81.2 and 80.7%, respectively; $p = 0.87$).[10] Most of these differences are likely related to retrospective patient selection bias and nonuniformity of tumor size, but discrepancies could depend on whether the surgical series had differing percentages of tumors with intratumoral or peripheral located cysts. CVS with intratumoral, centrally located cysts, and thick cyst walls tend to be less difficult to remove. Thin-walled, extratumoral cysts can be more challenging, and subtotal resection, leaving cyst wall on critical structures, is frequently warranted.[3]

The incidence of tumor regrowth after incomplete CVS removal is reported to be 25 to 46%.[14,33,34] Early reports demonstrated that residual CVS had more rapid regrowth and required repeat surgery more frequently than SVS.[17,35] Some of these rapid recurrences were due to rapid expansion of recurrent cysts. As a counterpoint, in a study that found 10 patients with residual CVS, 6 patients (60%) required repeat surgery or radiosurgery which was similar to 5 out of 8 (62.5%) tumors requiring retreatment in the SVS group.[4]

Very little data are available evaluating hearing preservation results after microsurgery for CVS. Only one study found that the hearing preservation rates were not significantly different for CVS patients compared with SVS ($p = 0.339$). Although not controlled for tumor size or extent of resection, 10 CVS patients (62%) had hearing preservation of American Academy of Otolaryngology – Head and Neck Surgery (AAO-HNS) class A or B compared to 122 patients (73%) with SVS.[7]

76.8 Stereotactic Radiosurgery

To date, there is a relative paucity of data evaluating outcomes following SRS for CVS. What is available is limited to case reports and small case series. Several early reports highlighted cases of rapid and significant cystic expansion or rupture after SRS requiring urgent surgery for neurologic compromise.[13,36] Hirato et al revealed evidence suggesting that high-dose single-fraction SRS results in subacute enlargement of many tumors especially in cases of CVS.[37] Similarly, Shirato et al reported transient enlargement of CVS after fractionated stereotactic radiotherapy, although the long-term tumor reduction rates were higher in CVS than in SVS.[14] There are probably varying thresholds of concern between these physicians when differentiating temporary CVS enlargement or "swell" from disturbing, progressive post-SRS cyst growth.

More recent, larger, retrospective SRS series have shown efficacy in CVS treatment in tumors less than 3.0 cm in greatest CPA dimension. Delsanti and Régis reported SRS results for 54 patients with CVS with a mean follow-up of 33 months. Tumor control rates were statistically equivalent between CVS (93.6%) and SVS (98%).[32] A second study evaluated 20 CVS patients receiving linear accelerator (LINAC) fractionated stereotactic radiotherapy to a total dose of 36 to 50 Gy in 20 to 25 fractions being administered to the isocenter and 80% to the tumor periphery. Overall tumor control was defined as no tumor growth greater than 2.0 mm after 2 years or no requirement of salvage surgery. Tumor enlargement was defined as an enlargement in tumor diameter of 2 mm or more compared to the size before irradiation. Corticosteroids were used to treat the subacute, transient tumor enlargement. The actuarial 3-year rates of no episode of enlargement were 75% in SVS and 55% in CVS, with the difference being statistically significant ($p = 0.023$). The 3-year tumor reduction rates were 31% for solid tumors and 93% for cystic tumors, with the difference being significant ($p = 0.0006$). The 3-year class hearing preservation rates for cystic and solid tumors were 76 and 50%, respectively. This difference did not reach a statistically significant level ($p = 0.07$).[14] Neither of these studies reported any rapid neurological decline from massive, rapid cyst enlargement. To date, there has not been a large series reported on CVS treated with modern single-fraction, low-dose SRS or current low-dose fractionated schedules.

76.9 Observation

It has been recommended that wait and scan should not be employed in CVS due to a small number of tumors 4/23 (20%) that rapidly and spontaneously increase in size due to rapid cyst enlargement which can cause displacement of the brainstem and compression of the fourth ventricle, resulting in hydrocephalus.[1,6,14,38] Although most centers do not employ wait and scan for CVS, especially those larger than 3 cm, this expert opinion has really not been evaluated in any of the current large wait-and-scan studies which did not subcategorize or comment on the natural history of CVS.[39]

76.10 Conclusion

Cystic vestibular schwannomas are a relatively rare subgroup of VS that are defined by their intratumoral or extratumoral fluid-filled cysts. To date, microsurgical resection has been the favored treatment especially for tumors larger than 3 cm or with mass effect; however, cranial nerve outcomes compared to surgery for SVS are highly discordant. In the future, an MRI cyst volume-based definition needs to be agreed upon as well as better experimental design with matching tumor sizes with SVS to better report surgical outcomes. The role of SRS when employing conventional 12-13 Gy marginal doses and wait-

and-scan treatment paradigms also need to be assessed to better define their roles in the treatment of small- and medium-sized CVS.

References

[1] Charabi S, Tos M, Børgesen SE, Thomsen J. Cystic acoustic neuromas. Results of translabyrinthine surgery. Arch Otolaryngol Head Neck Surg. 1994; 120 (12):1333–1338

[2] Sinha S, Sharma BS. Cystic acoustic neuromas: surgical outcome in a series of 58 patients. J Clin Neurosci. 2008; 15(5):511–515

[3] Piccirillo E, Wiet MR, Flanagan S, et al. Cystic vestibular schwannoma: classification, management, and facial nerve outcomes. Otol Neurotol. 2009; 30(6): 826–834

[4] Tang IP, Freeman SR, Rutherford SA, King AT, Ramsden RT, Lloyd SK. Surgical outcomes in cystic vestibular schwannoma versus solid vestibular schwannoma. Otol Neurotol. 2014; 35(7):1266–1270

[5] Park CK, Kim DC, Park SH, et al. Microhemorrhage, a possible mechanism for cyst formation in vestibular schwannomas. J Neurosurg. 2006; 105(4):576–580

[6] Moon KS, Jung S, Seo SK, et al. Cystic vestibular schwannomas: a possible role of matrix metalloproteinase-2 in cyst development and unfavorable surgical outcome. J Neurosurg. 2007; 106(5):866–871

[7] Jian BJ, Sughrue ME, Kaur R, et al. Implications of cystic features in vestibular schwannomas of patients undergoing microsurgical resection. Neurosurgery. 2011; 68(4):874–880, discussion 879–880

[8] Yashar P, Zada G, Harris B, Giannotta SL. Extent of resection and early postoperative outcomes following removal of cystic vestibular schwannomas: surgical experience over a decade and review of the literature. Neurosurg Focus. 2012; 33(3):E13

[9] Mehrotra N, Behari S, Pal L, Banerji D, Sahu RN, Jain VK. Giant vestibular schwannomas: focusing on the differences between the solid and the cystic variants. Br J Neurosurg. 2008; 22(4):550–556

[10] Thakur JD, Khan IS, Shorter CD, et al. Do cystic vestibular schwannomas have worse surgical outcomes? Systematic analysis of the literature. Neurosurg Focus. 2012; 33(3):E12

[11] Fundová P, Charabi S, Tos M, Thomsen J. Cystic vestibular schwannoma: surgical outcome. J Laryngol Otol. 2000; 114(12):935–939

[12] Tali ET, Yuh WT, Nguyen HD, et al. Cystic acoustic schwannomas: MR characteristics. AJNR Am J Neuroradiol. 1993; 14(5):1241–1247

[13] Pendl G, Ganz JC, Kitz K, Eustacchio S. Acoustic neurinomas with macrocysts treated with Gamma Knife radiosurgery. Stereotact Funct Neurosurg. 1996; 66 Suppl 1:103–111

[14] Shirato H, Sakamoto T, Takeichi N, et al. Fractionated stereotactic radiotherapy for vestibular schwannoma (VS): comparison between cystic-type and solid-type VS. Int J Radiat Oncol Biol Phys. 2000; 48(5):1395–1401

[15] Kanzaki J, Tos M, Sanna M, Moffat DA, Monsell EM, Berliner KI. New and modified reporting systems from the consensus meeting on systems for reporting results in vestibular schwannoma. Otol Neurotol. 2003; 24(4):642–648, discussion 648–649

[16] Lunardi P, Missori P, Mastronardi L, Fortuna A. Cystic acoustic schwannomas. Acta Neurochir (Wien). 1991; 110(3–4):120–123

[17] Kameyama S, Tanaka R, Honda Y, Hasegawa A, Yamazaki H, Kawaguchi T. The long-term growth rate of residual acoustic neurinomas. Acta Neurochir (Wien). 1994; 129(3–4):127–130

[18] Charabi S, Klinken L, Tos M, Thomsen J. Histopathology and growth pattern of cystic acoustic neuromas. Laryngoscope. 1994; 104(11, Pt 1):1348–1352

[19] Charabi S, Mantoni M, Tos M, Thomsen J. Cystic vestibular schwannomas: neuroimaging and growth rate. J Laryngol Otol. 1994; 108(5):375–379

[20] Muzumdar DP, Goel A, Pakhmode CK. Multicystic acoustic neurinoma: report of two cases. J Clin Neurosci. 2002; 9(4):453–455

[21] Lohle PN, Wurzer HA, Seelen PJ, Kingma LM, Go KG. Cystic lesions accompanying extra-axial tumours. Neuroradiology. 1999; 41(1):13–17

[22] Kingsley DP, Thornton A, Furneaux C, King TT. Transmural passage of subarachnoid metrizamide into a cystic acoustic schwannoma of the cerebellopontine angle: a diagnostic dilemma. Neuroradiology. 1984; 26(4):319–321

[23] Schober R, Vogeley KT, Urich H, Hölzle E, Wechsler W. Vascular permeability changes in tumours of the peripheral nervous system. Virchows Arch A Pathol Anat Histopathol. 1992; 420(1):59–64

[24] Zhang Z, Wang Z, Sun L, et al. Mutation spectrum and differential gene expression in cystic and solid vestibular schwannoma. Genet Med. 2014; 16 (3):264–270

[25] Aarhus M, Bruland O, Sætran HA, Mork SJ, Lund-Johansen M, Knappskog PM. Global gene expression profiling and tissue microarray reveal novel candidate genes and down-regulation of the tumor suppressor gene CAV1 in sporadic vestibular schwannomas. Neurosurgery. 2010; 67(4):998–1019, discussion 1019

[26] Møller MN, Werther K, Nalla A, et al. Angiogenesis in vestibular schwannomas: expression of extracellular matrix factors MMP-2, MMP-9, and TIMP-1. Laryngoscope. 2010; 120(4):657–662

[27] Wandong S, Meng L, Xingang L, et al. Cystic acoustic neuroma. J Clin Neurosci. 2005; 12(3):253–255

[28] Benech F, Perez R, Fontanella MM, Morra B, Albera R, Ducati A. Cystic versus solid vestibular schwannomas: a series of 80 grade III-IV patients. Neurosurg Rev. 2005; 28(3):209–213

[29] Jones SE, Baguley DM, Moffat DA. Are facial nerve outcomes worse following surgery for cystic vestibular schwannoma? Skull Base. 2007; 17(5):281–284

[30] Wallace CJ, Fong TC, Auer RN. Cystic intracranial schwannoma. Can Assoc Radiol J. 1993; 44(6):453–459

[31] Jeng CM, Huang JS, Lee WY, Wang YC, Kung CH, Lau MK. Magnetic resonance imaging of acoustic schwannomas. J Formos Med Assoc. 1995; 94(8):487–493

[32] Delsanti C, Régis J. Cystic vestibular schwannomas. [in French]. Neurochirurgie. 2004; 50(2–3, Pt 2):401–406

[33] Sakaki S, Nakagawa K, Hatakeyama T, Murakami Y, Ohue S, Matsuoka K. Recurrence after incompletely resected acousticus neurinomas. Med J Osaka Univ. 1991; 40(1–4):59–66

[34] Schessel DA, Nedzelski JM, Kassel EE, Rowed DW. Recurrence rates of acoustic neuroma in hearing preservation surgery. Am J Otol. 1992; 13(3):233–235

[35] Kameyama S, Tanaka R, Kawaguchi T, Fukuda M, Oyanagi K. Cystic acoustic neurinomas: studies of 14 cases. Acta Neurochir (Wien). 1996; 138(6):695–699

[36] de Ipolyi AR, Yang I, Buckley A, Barbaro NM, Cheung SW, Parsa AT. Fluctuating response of a cystic vestibular schwannoma to radiosurgery: case report. Neurosurgery. 2008; 62(5):E1164–E1165, discussion E1165

[37] Hirato M, Inoue H, Zama A, Ohye C, Shibazaki T, Andou Y. Gamma Knife radiosurgery for acoustic schwannoma: effects of low radiation dose and functional prognosis. Stereotact Funct Neurosurg. 1996; 66 Suppl 1:134–141

[38] Charabi S, Thomsen J, Mantoni M, et al. Acoustic neuroma (vestibular schwannoma): growth and surgical and nonsurgical consequences of the wait-and-see policy. Otolaryngol Head Neck Surg. 1995; 113(1):5–14

[39] Stangerup SE, Caye-Thomasen P. Epidemiology and natural history of vestibular schwannomas. Otolaryngol Clin North Am. 2012; 45(2):257–268, vii

77 Primary Inner Ear (Intralabyrinthine) Schwannomas

Brian A. Neff

77.1 Introduction

Although there is ongoing debate over the specifics of tumor origin, most agree that vestibular schwannomas (VSs) arise from Schwann cells within the internal auditory canal (IAC). As will be discussed, these progenitor Schwann cells are also found beyond the confines of the IAC in the more distal inner ear labyrinth.[1] Tumors arising in this area are termed "primary inner ear schwannomas" or "intralabyrinthine schwannomas (ILSs)" and are far less common than the typical schwannoma involving the IAC. This chapter reviews primary ILS (i.e., schwannomas that develop from within the labyrinth), which are a separate clinical entity from VS that secondarily invade the inner ear via extension from the IAC through the fundus (▶ Fig. 77.1 and ▶ Fig. 77.2). First described by Mayer in 1917, the most recent systematic review of the literature revealed 234 ILSs which have now been described.[2,3]

Prior to the advent of magnetic resonance imaging (MRI), ILS tumors were found exclusively at the time of autopsy, or as an unexpected discovery during neurotologic surgery for another reason, such as labyrinthectomy for Ménière's disease.[4] Due to their rarity and presentation overlap with Ménière's disease, diagnosis can be delayed. Visualizing these tumors is also a challenge because the MRI quality and sequences utilized are critical in avoiding a missed diagnosis.

77.2 Anatomy

Within the modiolus are numerous bony channels called Rosenthal's canals, which are adjacent to the scala tympani and contain the spiral ganglia. The afferent branches of the cochlear nerve originate between the hair cells and the spiral ganglia. These nerve endings pierce the organ of Corti through multiple small openings called the habenula perforata. It is at this most distal location where Schwann cell myelination terminates. The afferent branches then run from the spiral ganglia through multiple small openings at the distal IAC called "the cribriform plate." Just proximal to Scarpa's ganglia and just distal to the cribriform plate is the Schwann-glial cell junction of the cochlear division of the eighth cranial nerve.[5]

The bony vestibule, located between the cochlea and three semicircular canals, contains the utricle and saccule. The ampulated ends of the semicircular canals open into the utricle. The saccule communicates with the scala media of the cochlea via the ductus reuniens. Two small ducts, one each from the saccule and utricle, unite to form the endolymphatic duct. As its name implies, this endolymph-containing duct is also part of the membranous labyrinth, and is housed within the bony vestibular aqueduct. The afferent nerve fibers traveling from the vestibular hair cells of the semicircular canals, utricle, and saccule pierce the cribriform plate of the distal IAC en route to the

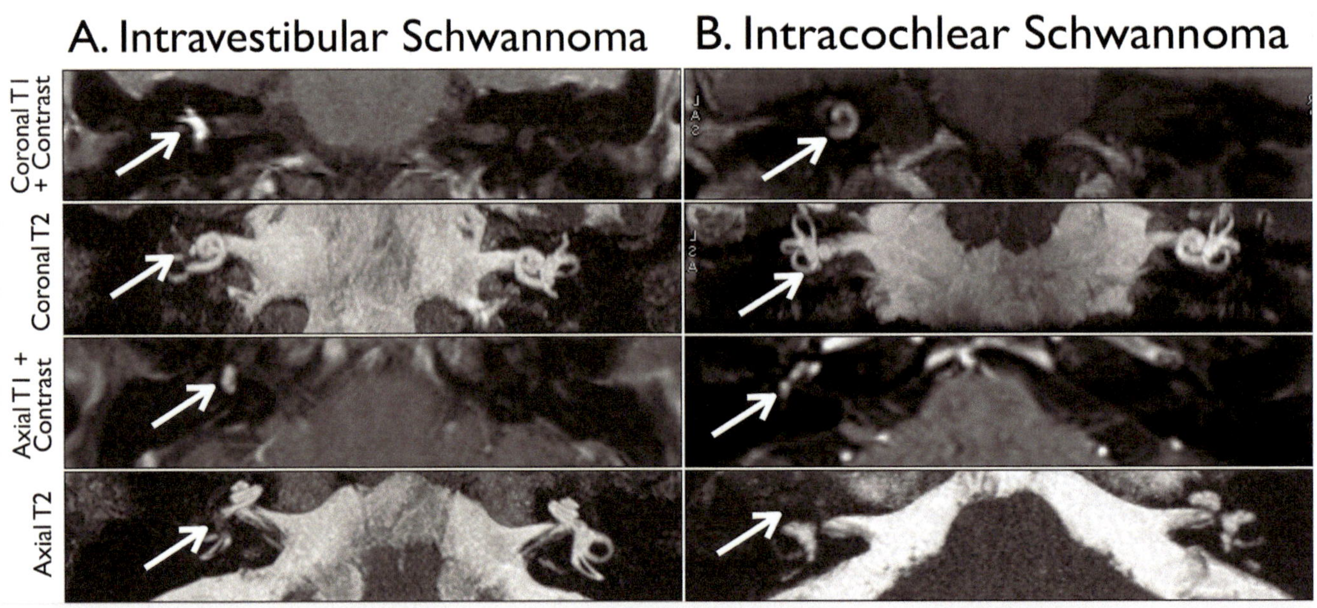

Fig. 77.1 (a) Intravestibular schwannoma and (b) intracochlear schwannoma on axial and coronal postcontrast T1-weighted images and 3D T2-SPACE images demonstrating tumoral enhancement and filling defects (hypointensity) within the bright inner ear fluid signal.

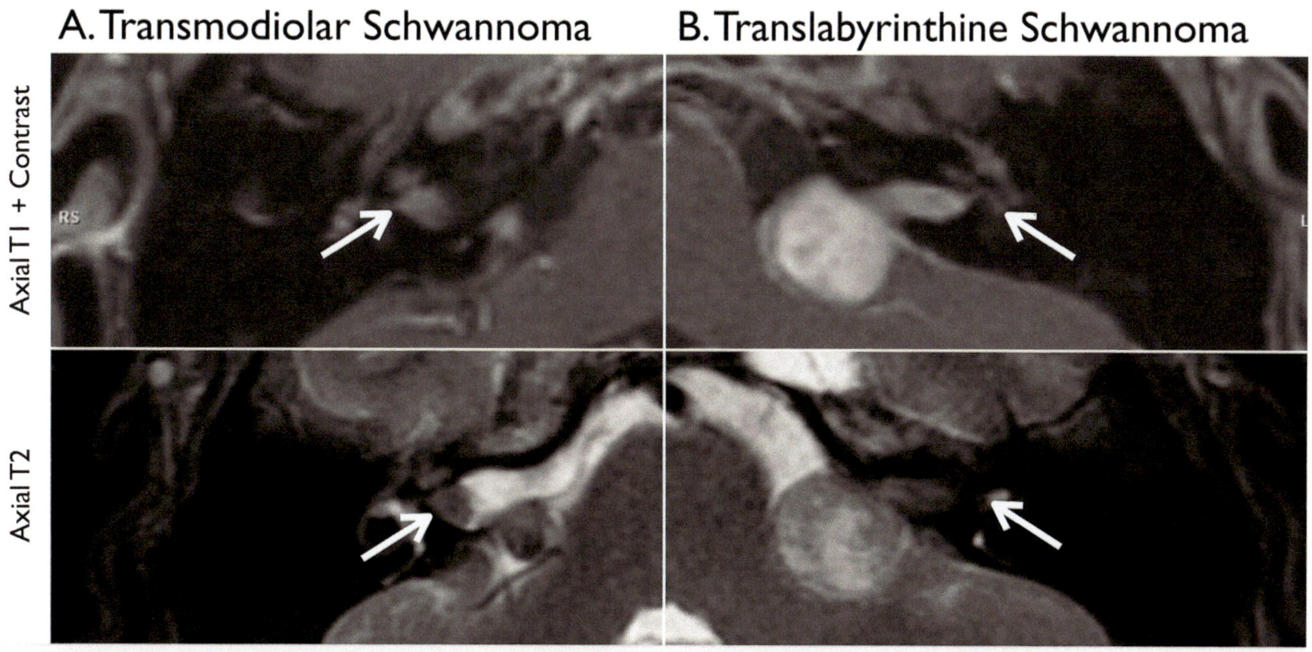

Fig. 77.2 (**a**) Transmodiolar and (**b**) translabyrinthine growth of vestibular schwannomas demonstrated on axial postcontrast T1- and T2-weighted images in a patient with neurofibromatosis type 2.

Scarpa ganglia within the IAC. Unlike the cochlear division, the Schwann-glial cell junction of the vestibular divisions is at the Scarpa ganglia.[6] With this anatomy in mind, it is helpful to refer to the revised Kennedy classification system in order to describe tumor locations (▶ Fig. 77.3).

77.3 Pathogenesis

Schwann cells occur in higher density within the IAC near the Schwann-glial junction, and controversially, this is felt by some to be the site of origin of the more common VS of the IAC and CPA.[7,8] Similarly, it has been hypothesized that cochlear ILS might originate in the more distal cochlear nerve Schwann-glial junction in the modiolus, where Schwann cell concentration is also high.[3]

As will be discussed further in section "Clinical Presentation," these tumors can cause variable symptoms depending on location of origin, as well as pathway of growth. As postulated earlier, it is possible that a majority of these tumors originate in the terminal Schwann cells of the modiolus, and then easily grow directly into the cochlea. This could explain why the cochlea, specifically the basal turn, is the most common location for ILS, with many reports of tumors isolated to the modiolus or basal turn of the cochlea.[3,9,10,11,12] Lastly, the anatomy is relevant in terms of adjacent spaces into which these tumors may spread, thus influencing their presentation. Tumor spread is likely to occur along the path of least resistance and, therefore, is unlikely to spread beyond the highly dense otic capsule. Reports of tumor spreading to the middle ear by passing through the round window or displacing the stapes footplate are relatively rare, termed "tympanolabyrinthine or transotic growth."[13,14] However, tumor can easily spread throughout the labyrinth from cochlea to vestibule to semicircular canal and vice versa. Though not occurring frequently, tumor may break through the cribriform plate located at the distal end of the IAC and then grow more proximally toward the CPA.

77.4 Clinical Presentation

The average age for ILS diagnosis is 49 years (range: 14–89), with no male–female predilection. Due to relative rarity, overlap with other diagnoses, and difficult radiologic detection, the current average delay until diagnosis is approximately 7 years.[3] As mentioned previously, the overlap in ILS symptoms with other more common neurotologic diseases such as Ménière's disease, vestibular migraine, and VS of the IAC and CPA makes diagnosis challenging. As the most common symptoms are hearing loss and vertigo, we will examine these in greatest detail in the following section.

77.4.1 Hearing Loss

Early reports of ILS series demonstrated that nearly all patients initially presented with hearing loss.[4,15,16] In 2013, a large literature review examined 234 cases and reported a 99% rate of hearing loss, with the vast majority (87%) presenting with American Academy of Otolaryngology – Head and Neck Surgery (AAO–HNS) class D hearing.[3,17] The pattern of hearing loss is

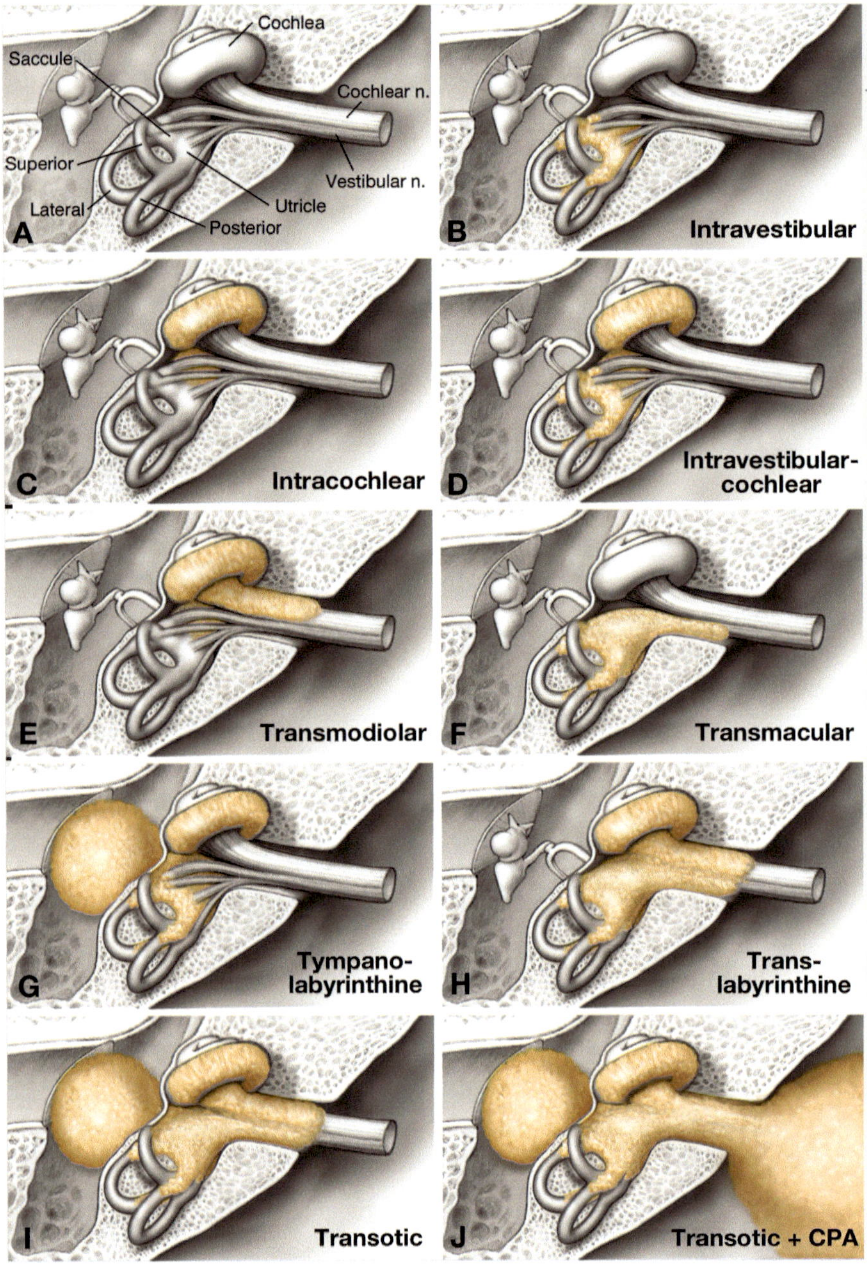

Fig. 77.3 Modified Kennedy classification (reproduced with permission from Van Abel et al[1]).

variable, and may not provide a means of discriminating these tumors from patients with Ménière's disease. ILSs have presented with progressive, sudden, and fluctuating patterns of hearing loss. One case series found rates of 61% progressive loss, 32% sudden loss, and 7% fluctuating hearing loss.[15] Another literature review showed that fluctuating hearing loss occurred only 3% of the time for ILS, while many ILS patients (39%) were misdiagnosed with Ménière's disease.[3]

Although there have been histologic reports of isolated neural damage at only the tumor site, potentially causing isolated frequencies of hearing loss, this presentation is not seen in many ILSs. The fact that many ILSs do not involve the cochlea (30%), yet 99% of patients report hearing loss, means that other pathophysiologic mechanisms of hearing loss, other than direct cochlear invasion, must exist. One hypothesis is that isolated tumors of the vestibule and semicircular canals still may cause hearing loss by either direct compression of the ductus reuniens or any other site along the pathway of endolymph flow toward the endolymphatic sac, thus leading to endolymphatic hydrops.[15] Others feel that the presence of abnormal metabolites or interruption of potassium cycling within the tumor-containing labyrinth may directly damage or alter function of the organ of Corti.[18,19]

Lastly, the clinician should be aware of the possibility of a mixed hearing loss occurring in a small subset of patients with ILS. Stapes footplate fixation or displacement into the middle ear from extension of intracochlear tumors can occur.[14,20] Hamed and Linthicum captured an example of this in a temporal bone histology section of the cochlea and stapes footplate.[21] In this patient, tumor was discovered filling the vestibule, primarily, but had extended into the proximal scala vestibuli. The tumor extended along the superior vestibular nerve as far as its entry point into the IAC, but abruptly stopped at that point. Instead of growing into the IAC, stapes footplate dislocation into the middle ear had occurred. These examples of "inner ear" conductive hearing loss would appear as a mixed pattern on audiologic testing.

77.4.2 Vertigo and Dysequilibrium

Patients with ILS may describe variable vestibular symptoms including vertigo, motion-induced dizziness, and disequilibrium. Abnormal balance and unsteadiness were found to be more common than vertigo.[3] Vertigo has been reported in 59% of patients, and the vertigo was episodic in all but one patient, who described constant vertigo. The relatively high rate of episodic vertigo described by these patients, in addition to the near-uniform presence of sensorineural hearing loss (SNHL) and tinnitus, makes differentiating these lesions from Ménière's disease challenging.

The pathophysiologic mechanism to explain episodic vertigo is not definitively established. A greater rate of vestibular subsite involvement has been reported in patients presenting with vestibular symptoms, but vertigo can also occur with isolated cochlear lesions.[3] One report found that 26% (7/27) of patients with vertigo had isolated cochlear ILS. One possible explanation for this occurrence was hypothesized from temporal bone examinations. Three of seven cochlear ILS patients had histologic evidence of endolymphatic hydrops, and perhaps, this is the reason for vestibular symptoms in patients having isolated cochlear involvement.[4]

Lastly, it should be noted that the percentage of patients with ILS having vertiginous symptoms seems to be higher than that of patients with the more common VS of the IAC in whom the presentation is often disequilibrium without vertigo.[4] This might be because ILSs arise from a more distal site within the vestibular system. Distal vestibular damage might create abnormal or fluctuating neural input to the more proximal vestibular system, whereas IAC schwannoma originating near the Scarpa ganglion might lead to a more stable, yet reduced, vestibular input to the brainstem.

77.5 Imaging

The diagnosis of an ILS is ultimately made with MRI in the context of the clinical presentation. Unfortunately, there are no pathognomonic clinical symptoms, physical exam findings, or audiologic criteria that will definitively suggest ILS pathology. MRI is an integral test for preoperative localization and surgical planning, or as a method of following stable tumors. Early MRI reports describe a lack of normal fluid density on T2-weighted imaging, with corresponding enhancement seen on gadolinium-enhanced T1-weighted scans.[6] However, other specific MRI sequences are also important for accurate diagnosis. The standard two-dimensional fast-spin T2 sequence, typically acquired at a slice thickness of 3 mm, may miss smaller tumors.[3] Three-dimensional (3D) imaging techniques to include constructive interference in a steady state (CISS) and variable flip angle 3D fast-spin echo T2-weighted sequences (T2 SPACE), acquired at a 1-mm slice thickness or less, have become critical for the evaluation of pathology involving the membranous labyrinth and inner ear.[22] At the authors' institution, we also employ variable flip angle 3D FSE T1-weighted sequences (T1 SPACE) which can be acquired at 0.6 mm sections through the labyrinth. Utilizing both the 3D T2-weighted sequences and fat-saturated postgadolinium 3D T1-weighted images allows for precise localization of tumor margins (▶ Fig. 77.1).[23] Physicians evaluating for ILS must make sure these sequences are performed because many routine MRI protocols may not include these sequences unless they are specifically requested.

77.5.1 Differential Diagnosis: Clinical and Radiographic

The clinical differential diagnosis of ILS depends on whether the patient is presenting with complaints of hearing loss, disequilibrium, vertigo, or a combination of these symptoms. Ménière's disease, vestibular migraine, labyrinthitis, vestibular neuritis, autoimmune hearing loss, otosyphilis, and classic VSs of the IAC or CPA are all considered. Typically, the clinician has to decide between possible diagnoses based on the appearance of an enhancing inner ear lesion seen on a MRI. This list can generally be divided into primary enhancing lesions confined to the inner ear or enhancing lesions that extend to and include the inner ear. Labyrinthine hemorrhage is a relatively rare diagnosis, which presents similar to acute viral labyrinthitis in patients with concussive head trauma or spontaneously in patients on anticoagulant therapy (▶ Fig. 77.4). Chronic labyrinthitis with or without ossification is a cause of SNHL secondary to bacterial meningitis in children and adults. All of these MRI abnormalities show a more diffuse inner ear enhancement without discrete borders. Alternatively, ILS presents as a discrete enhancement with sharply marginated borders on both contrast-enhanced T1-weighted and T2-SPACE sequences (▶ Fig. 77.1).

There are several very rare case reports of other primary tumors arising within the labyrinth. A few intralabyrinthine lipomas have been reported, and these were diagnosed by suppression of tumor hyperintensity on fat suppression T1-weighted MRI sequences.[24] Another case report highlighted a traumatic neuroma following labyrinthectomy.[25] This patient had a remote history of Ménière's disease treated with labyrinthectomy and then later developed a more chronic dysequilibrium.[1] However, it is not entirely certain if the traumatic neuroma was truly causative of the imbalance. Lastly, the author of this chapter has treated a patient who presented with unilateral deafness and a MRI showing a discrete inner ear lesion similar to an ILS. However, the tumor showed atypical T1 hyperintensity without contrast and an extremely rapid growth rate to involve the CPA. Surgical pathology confirmed the diagnosis of melanocytic schwannoma arising from the vestibule.

There are also rare instances where tumors or inflammatory lesions arise outside the inner ear but extend to involve the cochlea or vestibule. Meningiomas of the IAC, lymphoma, post-transplant lymphoproliferative disease (PTLD), and paraganglioma all can present with unilateral SNHL and vestibular complaints. The MRI appearance can be similar to an ILS that has extended to involve the IAC or middle ear.

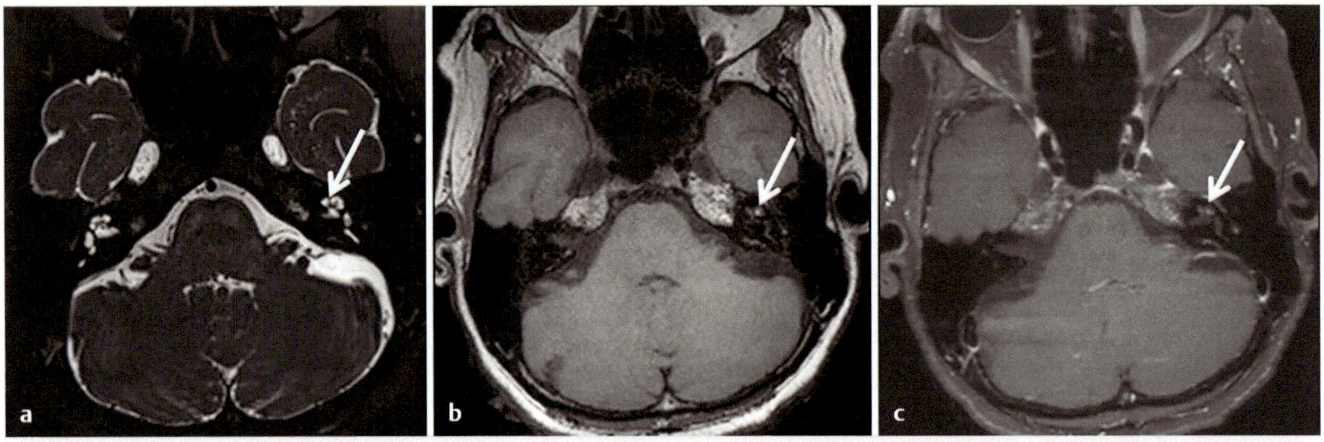

Fig. 77.4 Acute labyrinthitis with hemorrhage, left ear. (**a**) Axial 3D fast-spin echo T2-weighted image shows normal fluid signal within the inner ear and cochlea (*arrow*); (**b**) axial precontrast 3D fast-spin echo T1-weighted image shows signal hyperintensity of the cochlea (*arrow*); (**c**) axial fat-saturated postcontrast 3D fast-spin echo T1-weighted image demonstrates no substantial enhancement (*arrow*).

77.6 Management and Outcomes

77.6.1 Management

The treatment approach for ILS is dictated by patient symptoms, tumor size, and tumor location. Surgical indications for ILS removal are intractable vertigo, growth into the IAC or middle ear, and uncertainty regarding diagnosis.[1,3,4,14,15] Management options primarily include observation with serial MRI imaging versus surgical removal, with approach dictated by tumor size and location. To our knowledge, only two patients have been reported who received stereotactic radiosurgery (SRS) for their ILS.[3,15] There has also been a single report utilizing transtympanic steroid injections for an ILS patient with sudden SNHL.[26] This patient experienced short-term hearing improvement until the inevitable, permanent, tumor-induced SNHL.

In a 2013 ILS review, 53% of patients (109/189) were observed with serial MRI scans. Only 3% of observed patients went on to need surgical removal due to vestibular symptoms or significant tumor growth. This was despite MRI evidence of slow tumor growth in 52% of these patients. Interestingly, they found that in the observation group, 93% (55/59) had stable or improved vertigo, tinnitus, or unsteadiness.[3] These findings provide support for a more conservative approach to the management of these tumors.

When patients experience severe vertigo or tumor growth into the IAC, CPA, or middle ear, treatment is required. Earlier removal of these tumors prior to extensive IAC involvement is likely to have less risk of postoperative facial paralysis.[27] Middle ear ILS extension has also historically been an indication for tumor removal. The provided reasoning for this is that the tumor lacks a barrier to spread once it has reached the middle ear. This decision is probably sound in more quickly growing tumors, but it can be questioned in the majority of slow-growing tumors. The middle ear may provide slow-growing tumors an increased area to asymptomatically expand without consequence. In general, the author of this chapter prefers to resect tumors when there is extension through the oval window due to the proximity of the tympanic facial nerve. This allows tumor removal when facial nerve contact is at a minimum and may provide easier dissection and facial nerve preservation. Additionally, middle ear ILSs are also removed prior to significant eustachian tube involvement as this can add a degree of difficulty to complete tumor resection. Slow-growing tumors extending through the round window into the hypotympanum might be observed if they have not radiographically encroached upon the facial nerve.

Clinicians may rarely be faced with an ILS patient experiencing severe vertigo without tumor growth or hearing loss. Transtympanic gentamicin injection could be done in these instances especially if that patient did not wish to have surgery or was medically unfit for surgery. Patients should be counseled that this treatment does not prevent tumor growth and any remaining hearing could be lost due to the injection.

Ultimately, the vast majority of patients requiring treatment will undergo surgical removal. It is helpful to have ILS classification schemes in order to choose an appropriate surgical approach for the tumor location. It is important that patients understand that they will no longer have any hearing regardless of the surgical approach selected, although most patients with these ILSs present with nonserviceable hearing.[3] Patients with tumors isolated to the vestibular system (vestibule or semicircular canals) can effectively undergo tumor removal via a transmastoid labyrinthectomy. For a transmacular ILS, the translabyrinthine approach provides adequate exposure for tumor resection. Patients with cochlear involvement are likely to require a transotic approach for ILS removal, regardless of whether there is tumor extension into the IAC. This would also provide adequate exposure for cochlear tumors involving the middle ear. The transotic approach requires over-closure of the external auditory meatus, packing of the middle ear, and eustachian tube obliteration to prevent cerebrospinal fluid (CSF) leak from the IAC through the basal cochlear modiolus. Tumors with only minimal cochlear involvement could potentially be removed without a transotic approach. Case reports of transmastoid removal of small cochlear, basal turn ILSs have been published. The authors describe a standard facial recess approach and enlarged cochleostomy for tumor removal.[28] Finally, an endoscopic transcanal transpromontory approach could be employed depending on the experience and preference of the surgeon. This approach is described further in Chapter 39. Older reports exist of microscopic transcanal removal of ILS found unexpectedly in patients undergoing transcanal labyrinthectomy.[1] However, this is probably not advisable as a planned procedure unless the tumor is isolated to the cochlea as tumor exposure and removal might be incomplete if the lesion extends beyond the confines of the cochlea.

77.6.2 Outcomes

To date, no operated patient has developed tumor recurrence after gross total ILS excision, but long-term imaging follow-up was not available for many case series. One patient, who underwent subtotal tumor removal, required a second surgery due to residual tumor growth in the cochlea after an initial transotic approach.[29] Surgical excision of ILS has resulted in vertigo resolution in many patients, although patient selection for surgery was not uniformly applied.[4,15] Additionally, utilization of standardized vestibular symptom definitions was also not performed. It is unlikely that spontaneous-onset vertigo was systematically distinguished from head-motion–induced vertigo, dysequilibrium while walking, or constant dizziness present in all positions and activities. Spontaneous vertigo from tumor irritation would likely respond well to surgical vestibular ablation, whereas the latter chronic symptoms, which are indicative of poor central vestibular compensation, are unlikely to improve after surgery.

Complications after ILS surgery are seemingly rare. Unfortunately, facial nerve outcomes are difficult to assess due to sporadic reporting practices in the literature. Postoperative facial nerve paresis or paralysis was an unusual complication seen in 4% (2/55) of surgical patients. One patient initially had House–Brackmann (HB) grade III/VI facial paresis that completely resolved by 1 year, and another patient had HB grade IV function 12 months postoperatively.[4,15] There have been three cases of patients experiencing postsurgical CSF leak.[30,31] One of these was managed conservatively, one had an unknown clinical course, and one underwent an operation upon the development of meningitis.

There are a few controversies regarding the management of ILS. The first is regarding whether young patients (≤ 50 years old) with a slowly growing ILS should undergo prolonged observation, even if they lack vestibular symptoms. As previously highlighted, many surgeons promote a wait-and-scan policy in all nonvertiginous ILS patients, irrespective of age, because surgery will not offer any hearing or tinnitus improvement. On the other hand, even if growth is limited to 1 mm every 2 to 3 years, the tumor will likely run out of room within the inner ear and extend to the IAC at some point over the next 30 to 40 years. This would then need treatment in a more elderly patient group. Of course, treatment could be accomplished with SRS with a subsequent unclear prognosis, but because of this probable need to treat within the patient's lifetime, surgery should probably be a treatment option discussed with the younger (≤ 50 years old), asymptomatic patient with a slowly growing ILS. Moreover, even with conservative MRI follow-up schedules every 2 to 5 years, this is a large commitment of patient's time and medical resources over the younger patient's lifetime.

The second controversy surrounding ILS management is whether SRS should be considered a valid, first-line treatment option. There have been two reports of SRS treatment for ILS. One of these patients who underwent SRS had no clinical or radiographic follow-up.[15] The second patient underwent successful SRS following tumor growth on serial MRI scans.[3] Hearing preservation is probably not possible in the rare patient with serviceable hearing due to the high cochlear radiation dose, and SRS treatment should not be considered until AAO–HNS class D hearing levels are reached. The indications for SRS could potentially be similar for ILS and IAC schwannomas, and this would include tumor growth on serial MRI scans, growth of the tumor to involve the IAC, and intractable spontaneous vertigo. Imbalance, constant dizziness, and motion-provoked vertigo are not good SRS (or surgical) indications as these are more likely resultant from poor central compensation rather than an irritative tumor phenomena. There is some hesitancy to recommend SRS to treat ILS tumors causing spontaneous vertigo, as theoretically, the tumor that is causing abnormal vestibular input has not been removed. Surgical removal of ILS tumors also accomplishes total vestibular ablation which may allow patients better spontaneous vertigo control. These hypotheses have not really been well studied in the treatment of ILS or standard VSs. Lastly, the risk–benefit analysis for ILS tumors is different from that of standard IAC or CPA tumors. Complete microsurgical removal of ILS tumors without IAC involvement is generally easily accomplished, and the risk of facial nerve morbidity is limited compared to standard VSs. Currently, SRS for the treatment of ILS has been reserved for the medically infirm patient who cannot undergo surgical anesthesia. With the relative infrequency of these tumors, the slow growth, and the difficulty in measuring growth on serial scans, it is unlikely that a randomized, prospective trial comparing SRS, microsurgery, and observation will ever occur. Future systematic reviews will be needed to assist in defining best treatment practices.

77.7 Hearing Rehabilitation

Increasingly, patients with unilateral, profound SNHL are finding significant benefit from cochlear implantation (CI). CI restores a degree of bilateral hearing that may help with sound localization and hearing in noise that cannot be provided by contralateral routing of sound strategies.[32] Currently, in the United States, insurance companies do not routinely provide reimbursement for CI when the contralateral ear has normal or near-normal hearing. Although speculative, the authors postulate that eventually CI for unilateral hearing loss will become more mainstream with consistent outcome studies to demonstrate benefit. This is significant for patients with ILS as most of these patients will have unilateral, profound SNHL in need of rehabilitation. CI rehabilitation might also shift the current ILS treatment paradigm away from observation to early SRS or surgical removal at a time when the tumor is at its smallest. Obviously, there are many unanswered questions as to whether this will be possible for ILS patients. Most likely, patients with tumors limited to the vestibule and semicircular canals will be able to undergo simultaneous tumor removal and successful CI with resultant hearing benefit. Alternatively, cochlear ILS may be difficult to remove while still maintaining enough cochlear spiral ganglion cells and distal cochlear nerve branches to ensure significant CI benefit. Two cases of resection of limited cochlear schwannomas involving only the basal turn have been reported with simultaneous CI placement.[28,33] Initial hearing results were good in one patient, although long-term follow-up and standardized sentence testing comparison to typical CI patients were not performed. Additionally, there are emerging reports of CI in patients with stable, nongrowing ILS (SRS treated or observed) who have had a CI placed through the soft intracochlear tumor to maximize surviving spiral ganglion cells. Preliminary outcomes over a relatively short follow-up period have shown benefit in seven out of nine patients with a median CNC word score of 57% (range: 28–88%).[34]

It is also not clear if CI would need to be performed at primary tumor extirpation or whether it could be done in a delayed fashion. If CI placement was staged over concerns of CSF leakage, the window of time for successful CI insertion is also not established. Worry over delayed labyrinthitis ossificans development, and subsequent implantation failure, has been highlighted in case studies of patients who previously underwent labyrinthectomy.[35] However, how quickly this develops and in what percentage of patients is currently not clear.

77.8 Conclusion

Intralabyrinthine schwannomas are uncommon tumors that were historically found either at the time of autopsy or unexpectedly during surgery for control of vertigo in patients thought to have Ménière's disease. Numerous retrospective case reports, case series, and literature reviews have increased our knowledge of these tumors. The routine use of high-resolution MRI has increased the likelihood of discovering these tumors, and has subsequently increased their incidence. Armed with the knowledge of their clinical presentation and overlap with other neurotologic pathology, as well as the imaging specifics required to visualize these tumors, clinicians will certainly decrease delays in diagnosis. Though a conservative "wait-and-scan approach" can be used for most patients, operative management is sometimes indicated and results in rare morbidity. Future reports may help in both better defining surgical indications and further clarifying if there is a role for primary SRS.

References

[1] Green J. Intralabyrinthine schwannoma. In: Jackler RK, Driscoll CLW, eds. Tumors of the Ear and Temporal Bone. Philadelphia, PA: Lippincott Williams & Wilkins; 2000:146–155

[2] Mayer O. Ein Fall von multiplen Tumoren in den Endansbreitungen des Akustikus. Z Ohrenheilk. 1917; 75:95–113

[3] Van Abel KM, Carlson ML, Link MJ, et al. Primary inner ear schwannomas: a case series and systematic review of the literature. Laryngoscope. 2013; 123 (8):1957–1966

[4] Neff BA, Willcox TO, Jr, Sataloff RT. Intralabyrinthine schwannomas. Otol Neurotol. 2003; 24(2):299–307

[5] Anson BJ, Donaldson JA. Surgical Anatomy of the Temporal Bone. Philadelphia, PA: WB Saunders; 1981:475–481

[6] Donnelly MJ, Daly CA, Briggs RJ. MR imaging features of an intracochlear acoustic schwannoma. J Laryngol Otol. 1994; 108(12):1111–1114

[7] Sterkers JM, Perre J, Viala P, Foncin JF. The origin of acoustic neuromas. Acta Otolaryngol. 1987; 103(5–6):427–431

[8] Xenellis JE, Linthicum FH, Jr. On the myth of the glial/Schwann junction (Obersteiner-Redlich zone): origin of vestibular nerve schwannomas. Otol Neurotol. 2003; 24(1):1

[9] Gussen R. Intramodiolar acoustic neurinoma. Laryngoscope. 1971; 81(12): 1979–1984

[10] Babin RW, Harker LA. Intralabyrinthine acoustic neurinomas. Otolaryngol Head Neck Surg. 1980; 88(4):455–461

[11] Jorgensen MB. Intracochlear neurinoma. Acta Otolaryngol. 1962; 54:227–232

[12] Johnsson LG, Kingsley TC. Asymptomatic intracochlear neurinoma. A temporal bone report. Arch Otolaryngol. 1981; 107(6):377–381

[13] Amoils CP, Lanser MJ, Jackler RK. Acoustic neuroma presenting as a middle ear mass. Otolaryngol Head Neck Surg. 1992; 107(3):478–482

[14] Stoney PJ, Rutka J, Dolan E, Hawke M. Acoustic neuroma presenting as a middle ear mass. J Otolaryngol. 1991; 20(2):141–143

[15] Kennedy RJ, Shelton C, Salzman KL, Davidson HC, Harnsberger HR. Intralabyrinthine schwannomas: diagnosis, management, and a new classification system. Otol Neurotol. 2004; 25(2):160–167

[16] Doyle KJ, Brackmann DE. Intralabyrinthine schwannomas. Otolaryngol Head Neck Surg. 1994; 110(6):517–523

[17] Committee on Hearing and Equilibrium guidelines for the evaluation of hearing preservation in acoustic neuroma (vestibular schwannoma). American Academy of Otolaryngology-Head and Neck Surgery Foundation, INC. Otolaryngol Head Neck Surg. 1995; 113(3):179–180

[18] DeLozier HL, Gacek RR, Dana ST. Intralabyrinthine schwannoma. Ann Otol Rhinol Laryngol. 1979; 88(2, Pt 1):187–191

[19] Miyamoto RT, Isenberg SF, Culp WM, Tubergen LB. Isolated intralabyrinthine schwannoma. Am J Otol. 1980; 1(4):215–217

[20] Hallpike CS. Stapes fixation by an intra-labyrinthine "seedling" neurofibroma as a cause of conductive deafness in a case of von Recklinghausen's disease. Acta Otolaryngol Suppl. 1963; 183:62–65

[21] Hamed A, Linthicum FH, Jr. Intralabyrinthine schwannoma. Otol Neurotol. 2005; 26(5):1085–1086

[22] Lane JI, Witte RJ, Bolster B, Bernstein MA, Johnson K, Morris J. State of the art: 3T imaging of the membranous labyrinth. AJNR Am J Neuroradiol. 2008; 29 (8):1436–1440

[23] Casselman JW, Kuhweide R, Deimling M, Ampe W, Dehaene I, Meeus L. Constructive interference in steady state-3DFT MR imaging of the inner ear and cerebellopontine angle. AJNR Am J Neuroradiol. 1993; 14(1):47–57

[24] Dahlen RT, Johnson CE, Harnsberger HR, et al. CT and MR imaging characteristics of intravestibular lipoma. AJNR Am J Neuroradiol. 2002; 23(8):1413–1417

[25] Linthicum FH, Jr, Alonso A, Denia A. Traumatic neuroma: a complication of transcanal labyrinthectomy. Arch Otolaryngol. 1979; 105(11):654–655

[26] Iseri M, Ulubil SA, Topdag M, Oran A. Hearing loss owing to intralabyrinthine schwannoma responsive to intratympanic steroid treatment. J Otolaryngol Head Neck Surg. 2009; 38(3):E95–E97

[27] Moffat DA, Parker RA, Hardy DG, Macfarlane R. Factors affecting final facial nerve outcome following vestibular schwannoma surgery. J Laryngol Otol. 2014; 128(5):406–415

[28] Schutt CA, Kveton JF. Cochlear implantation after resection of an intralabyrinthine schwannoma. Am J Otolaryngol. 2014; 35(2):257–260

[29] Falcioni M, Taibah A, Di Trapani G, Khrais T, Sanna M. Inner ear extension of vestibular schwannomas. Laryngoscope. 2003; 113(9):1605–1608

[30] Storrs LA. Acoustic neurinomas presenting as middle ear tumors. Laryngoscope. 1974; 84(7):1175–1180

[31] Tran Ba Huy P, Hassan JM, Wassef M, Mikol J, Thurel C. Acoustic schwannoma presenting as a tumor of the external auditory canal. Case report. Ann Otol Rhinol Laryngol. 1987; 96(4):415–418

[32] Blasco MA, Redleaf MI. Cochlear implantation in unilateral sudden deafness improves tinnitus and speech comprehension: meta-analysis and systematic review. Otol Neurotol. 2014; 35(8):1426–1432

[33] Kronenberg J, Horowitz Z, Hildesheimer M. Intracochlear schwannoma and cochlear implantation. Ann Otol Rhinol Laryngol. 1999; 108(7, Pt 1): 659–660

[34] Carlson ML, Neff BA, Sladen DP, et al. Cochlear Implantation in Patients with Intracochlear and Intralabyrinthine Schwannomas. Otol Neurotol. 2016; 37 (6): 647–53

[35] Chen DA, Linthicum FH, Jr, Rizer FM. Cochlear histopathology in the labyrinthectomized ear: implications for cochlear implantation. Laryngoscope. 1988; 98(11):1170–1172

Part X

Neurofibromatosis Type 2

X

78 Genetics of Neurofibromatosis Type 2

Simon K. W. Lloyd and D. Gareth R. Evans

78.1 Introduction

Neurofibromatosis type 2 (NF2) is an autosomal dominant disorder characterized by the development of multiple tumors of the nervous system, most typically bilateral vestibular schwannomas.[1,2] Other tumors may also occur including schwannomas of other cranial, spinal, peripheral, and intracutaneous nerves; cranial and spinal meningiomas; and ependymomas. NF2 is also associated with ocular changes including cataract formation, epiretinal membranes, and retinal hamartomas, as well as cutaneous changes such as skin plaques. The symptomatic prevalence of NF2 is approximately 1 per 60,000 people.[3] The Manchester criteria has been used for the clinical diagnosis of NF2 (▸ Table 78.1).[4]

78.2 Inheritance of Neurofibromatosis Type 2

The genetic nature of NF2 was first described by Feiling and Ward in 1920[5] and its autosomal dominant inheritance was described by Gardner and Frazier in 1930.[6] While many patients inherit the disease from their parents, more than half of patients with NF2 have *de novo* mutations.[1] Of these, approximately 35% display mosaicism. First described in 1995 by Bourn et al,[7] mosaicism is a phenomenon in which only some cells within the affected individual carry the *NF2* gene mutation.[8,9,10] It results from postzygotic mutation of the *NF2* gene such that two distinct cell lines develop—one normal and the other carrying the *NF2* gene mutation. Mosaicism is more common in NF2 than in almost any other condition. In NF2 patients with unilateral vestibular schwannomas, the rate of mosaicism is as high as 60%.[11] The remaining 65% of *de novo* cases have the *NF2* gene mutation throughout their body.

In order to develop NF2-related tumors, both alleles of the *NF2* gene must become mutated/deleted. NF2 patients carry a germline mutation that constitutes the first hit. The second hit is not, however, present as a germline mutation but is acquired at a later stage. This second hit is especially likely in Schwann cells where Merlin expression is particularly high, hence the propensity of NF2 patients to develop vestibular schwannomas.

Table 78.1 Manchester criteria for the clinical diagnosis of NF2

Primary criteria	Additional criteria required
Bilateral vestibular schwannomas	None
First-degree relative	Unilateral vestibular schwannoma *or* two NF2-associated lesions (meningioma, schwannoma, glioma, neurofibroma, cataract)
Unilateral vestibular schwannoma	Two NF2-associated lesions (meningioma, schwannoma, glioma, neurofibroma, cataract)
Multiple meningiomas	Unilateral vestibular schwannoma *or* two NF2-associated lesions (schwannoma, glioma, neurofibroma, cataract)

Abbreviation: NF2, neurofibromatosis type 2.

78.3 The *NF2* Gene

NF2 results from inactivation of the *NF2* gene. There is no current evidence that a mutation of any other gene is implicated in classical NF2. However, cases with unilateral vestibular schwannomas and other schwannomas may have an underlying *LZTR1* mutation.[12] The NF2 gene was identified by two separate groups in 1993[13,14] and is located on chromosome 22, band 22q12.2. Its promoter and major transcription ignition sites have also been described.[15] Its protein product is called Merlin, also known as Schwannomin. Merlin is a 69-kDa protein with 595 amino acids and is part of the band 4.1 family of cytoskeletal proteins known as ERM proteins, ERM being an abbreviation of ezrin–radixin–moesin-like protein.[13,14] It has three functional domains: a conserved FERM (4.1 ERM) amino terminal domain (exons 1–9), an alpha-helical domain (exons 10–13), and a carboxy terminal domain (exons 14–17).[16] Most truncating mutations map to the FERM domain suggesting that this has a particularly important tumor suppression role.

Merlin is found ubiquitously throughout the body, but it is particularly well expressed in the cell membranes of Schwann cell, in nerve tissue, in lens tissue, and in meningeal tissues.[17] It has two isoforms, Merlin-1 and Merlin-2, resulting from alternative splicing of exons 16 and 17. Its activity is regulated by phosphorylation of serine 518.[18] Phosphorylation results in conformational change such that Merlin becomes open and inactive. Dephosphorylation results in a closed confirmation and activation of the molecule. This is controlled by a family of ras-related kinases including protein kinase A and p21 activated kinases. The unphosphorylated active form may have a number of roles, all of which act to inhibit cell growth[19]:

1. Linkage of cell surface glycoproteins such as CD44, β1integrin, and β catenin to intracellular adhesion molecules and cytoskeletal actin regulating cell:cell adhesion and contact inhibition.[20]
2. An upstream regulator of the Hippo pathway, a regulator of cell growth by contact inhibition.[21] This may be mediated through translocation of Merlin to the nucleus where it inhibits E3 ubiquitin ligase $CRL4^{DCAF1}$.[22]
3. Promotion of inactivation of membrane growth factor receptors, e.g., EGFR, PDGFR.[23]

Loss of this tumor suppressor function is the underlying reason for the propensity for tumor development in individuals carrying a mutated form of the gene.

78.4 Types of Mutation and the Association with Phenotype

Traditionally, NF2 patients have been divided into two broad phenotypic groups: those with milder disease, termed "Gardner type," and those with more severe disease, termed "Wishart type." These terms have now become outdated in the knowledge that there is a spectrum of disease severity with enormous variability in disease location and severity between and within individuals.

Members of the same family tend to have similar disease severity, but there is significant variability in the phenotype of unrelated patients with NF2.[3,24] This partly relates to the presence of mosaicism but is also dependent on the type of mutation.

Patients with mosaicism often have less severe disease and the severity of disease is related to the proportion of cells affected.[11] This is, in turn, related to the point during development at which the mutation takes place. The earlier the mutation takes place, the more affected cells are present and the more severe the disease. Mosaic patients may also have segmental involvement resulting from proliferation of cells with the mutated form of the *NF2* gene in isolated areas of the body.[25]

There are a number of different types of mutations of the *NF2* gene that have been described and the frequencies of the recorded mutations from the Manchester cohort are shown in ▶ Table 78.2.

While it is not an invariable correlation, the type of mutation often determines disease severity. Truncating mutations, including non-sense and frameshift mutations, are associated with a younger age of disease presentation and more severe phenotype[24,26,27,28] and poorer survival[29] than that seen with missense mutations, in-frame mutations, or large deletions. Splice-site mutations, in contrast, can result in a range of disease severity depending on the site of the mutation. For example, mutations in the first five exons are associated with more severe disease than those occurring in exons 11 to 15.[30] The reason why truncating mutations are associated with more severe phenotypes is unclear. It has been hypothesized that the mutant protein dimerizes with the normal product resulting in less normal product to suppress tumor development. Ring 22 is another genetic defect that can lead to NF2 and is associated with mental retardation.[31]

Paradoxically, truncating mutations are more common in mosaic cases than in inherited cases, presumably because of reduced "genetic fitness." Conversely, missense mutations are much less frequent in mosaic cases compared to inherited cases. Truncating mutations have a higher prevalence of meningioma compared to missense or splice-site mutations.[32] Truncating and nonsense mutations are associated with a higher risk of developing spinal tumors.[33] Nonsense and frameshift mutations are also associated with greater mortality.[29]

The site of mutation may also influence disease severity. For example, splice-site mutations in exons 11 to 15 are associated with less severe disease than splice-site mutations in exons 1 to 5[30] and risk of meningioma development is higher if a mutation is in exons 1 to 3 compared to exons 14 to 15.[34] Recently, a positional effect has also been shown for truncating mutations with those in exons 1 and 14 to 15 being associated with milder disease, less meningiomas, and improved survival.[35]

There may also be epigenetic factors that influence *NF2* gene inactivation as well as gene mutation. For example, it has been suggested that methylation of the NF2 gene may be responsible for inactivation in some cases.[36]

Although disease severity is often determined by the type of mutation, it is not unusual to see differences in phenotype between individuals in the same family and even between monozygotic twins.[37] There is also variability in the behavior of tumors within individuals.[38] This suggests that there are certainly other factors involved in determining severity other than mutation type and mosaicism. This may relate to expression of cytokine or hormone receptors such as vascular endothelial growth factor (VEGF) receptor[39] or androgen receptor. The interested reader may also review Chapter 5, further detailing the molecular biology of sporadic and NF2-associated vestibular schwannomas.

Table 78.2 Frequencies of germline (first hit) and tumor (second hit) mutations in the Manchester NF2 cohort (unpublished data)

	NF2 VS first hit (*n* = 531)	NF2 VS second hit (*n* = 146)
Nonsense	155 (29%)	3 (2.0%)
Frameshift insertions/ deletions	125 (25%)	9 (6.0%)
Missense	24 (4.5%)	0
In-frame deletions	5 (1.0%)	0
Splice site	115 (22%)	5 (3.5%)
Ring 22	3 (0.5%)	*NA*
Chromosome translocation	2 (0.5%)	*NA*
MLPA exon deletions/ duplications	102 (19%)	3 (2.0%)
Loss of most/all of chromosome 22q	0	80 (55%)
Mitotic recombination	0	20 (14%)
Methylation	0	0

Abbreviations: NF2, neurofibromatosis type 2; NA*, not assessed; VS, vestibular schwannoma.

78.5 Genetic Testing

Patients with NF2 can be screened for an *NF2* gene mutation in blood or in affected tissue. The latter is obtained from biopsy of NF2-related tumors. This does not need to be the index tumor and may be a more accessible tumor such as a cutaneous tumor. Screening is helpful for a number of reasons. First, it may confirm the diagnosis of NF2 in patients who do not have a definite NF2 phenotype at presentation. Second, it provides some measure of likely severity of disease depending on the type of mutation identified. Third, it can aid in differentiating NF2 from schwannomatosis. Fourth, if a mutation is identified, it facilitates screening of currently unaffected family members for the mutation.

The rate of identification of a *NF2* gene mutation in blood is 37 to 60% in patients with typical NF2.[40,41] This figure is, however, affected by the high proportion of mosaicism, as it is harder to identify a mutation in mosaic individuals because the mutant alleles may only be present in blood at very low levels (as low as 2.6%).[42] If second-generation patients, who will not display mosaicism, are separated out, this group has a 93% chance of having the mutation identified in blood.[41] Techniques such as deep sequencing and next-generation sequencing are likely to significantly improve the rate of identification of mutations.[42]

The optimal means for testing for NF2 mutations is by sequencing ideally with next-generation sequencing with testing for large single or multiple exon deletions or duplications with multiple ligation-dependent probe amplification (MLPA).

78.6 At-Risk Patients

Individuals who meet the Manchester criteria for NF2 or who have genetic testing confirming mutation of the *NF2* gene should be considered as having NF2. Those who meet the Manchester criteria should be considered as having NF2 even if blood or tumor genetic analysis is negative. There are, however, two main groups of patients who do not have proven NF2 but are at risk of having it: those who have one or more potential NF2 tumors but fall short of the Manchester criteria and those whose parents have NF2. It is important to screen these patients. Evans et al have defined "at risk" as a greater than 1% chance of having NF2.[41]

Patients who do not meet the Manchester criteria but are at high risk (> 20% chance) of having NF2 include[41]:

- Isolated unilateral vestibular schwannoma < 20 years.
- Isolated cranial meningioma < 20 years.
- Childhood isolated schwannoma at another site.
- Childhood typical retinal hamartoma.
- Individuals fulfilling two criteria of the Manchester criteria < 50 years of age but including childhood mononeuropathy as a criterion.

Other patients with lower risk (but still at risk) include those with unilateral vestibular schwannomas aged between 20 and 30 years and those fulfilling two Manchester criteria over 50 years of age.

The most common situation in which counseling regarding risk of NF2 is required is the young patient presenting with an isolated unilateral vestibular schwannoma. The age-related risk of having NF2 in the presence of an isolated vestibular schwannoma is shown in ▶ Table 78.3.[43] In an individual presenting below the age of 20 years, the risk of NF2 is 20%. In an individual over the age of 60 years, this risk reduces to 0.1%. It should also be noted that it is possible for bilateral vestibular schwannomas to be two sporadic tumors rather than related to NF2. The incidence of this is approximately 1 in 2 million. We have recently confirmed that both vestibular schwannomas in an older patient presenting with bilateral tumors had occurred independently and that those with bilateral vestibular schwannomas and no other NF2 features after 70 years of age have close to a 50% likelihood that these occurred by chance.

Table 78.3 Age-related risk of having NF2 for patients presenting with VSs

Age at diagnosis of VS (y)	Proportion of VS having NF2 (%)	Proportion of VS in NF2 presenting unilaterally (%)	Proportion of NF2 presenting as a unilateral sporadic VS (%)	Proportion of sporadic VS having NF2
< 20	83	18	5	20
20–29	43	24	8	5.7
30–39	7	23	8	0.6
40–49	3	29	9	0.3
50–59	3.5	33	9.5	0.3
60 +	2	26	7	0.1
Total	7.7	24	7.5	–

Abbreviations: NF2, neurofibromatosis type 2; NA, not available; VS, vestibular schwannoma.

For children of affected individuals, screening may begin at birth with an examination of the eyes to identify cataracts. Screening with serial magnetic resonance imaging (MRI) should then begin at age 10 years with scans undertaken every other year up until the age of 20 years. The practicalities of scanning at younger ages are difficult and development of symptomatic tumors before 10 years of age is very rare. Above the age of 20 years, the scanning interval can be increased to 3 to 5 years as tumors tend to grow less aggressively with increasing age. If an individual has a proven mutation, then cranial imaging should be undertaken annually and spinal imaging undertaken every 3 years. If no tumor has been identified by the age of 40 years, then scanning can be discontinued. If there is a known mutation within a family, targeted testing for that mutation can be undertaken. This should ideally be undertaken from tumor, but testing in blood is also likely to be helpful.

For second-generation patients with NF2, the risk of transmission to their offspring is 50%. For de novo patients, the risk of transmission is significantly less because of mosaicism. ▶ Table 78.4 shows the risk of transmission of NF2 in a large cohort of patients from the Manchester program broken down according to age.[41] Young individuals with bilateral disease at presentation have a high risk of transmission because they are less likely to have mosaic disease. For example, there is a 29% risk of transmission of NF2 in individuals presenting with bilateral vestibular schwannoma under the age of 20 years. In contrast, patients who are older and have unilateral disease are very much less likely to pass on the disease as most of these individuals will have milder forms of mosaic NF2.[43,44] For example, over the age of 40 years, the risk of transmitting NF2 drops to 9% in individuals with bilateral disease. Offspring who do inherit the NF2 mutation will develop full NF2 and are therefore likely to have more severe disease than their mosaic parent.[41,45]

At-risk patients should undergo germline mutation testing in blood and in fresh frozen tumor, where possible. They should also have a full evaluation for other NF2-related conditions including MRI of the head and spine, audiological and ophthalmic assessments, and a cutaneous examination at baseline and at 18 to 20 years of age.

Follow-up cranial imaging should take place at 5, 10, and 20 years after initial assessment for all at-risk patients. If there is no evidence of NF2 after 20 years, then the risk of having NF2 is less than 1% and the patient can be reasonably discharged.

78.7 Schwannomatosis

Schwannomatosis is an autosomal dominant condition, separate from NF2, in which the affected individual is prone to developing multiple schwannomas, but vestibular schwannomas are not usually seen.[46] It may be mistaken for mosaic NF2. Ninety percent of cases are sporadic with 10% being familial. About 50% of familial cases have a mutation in the *SMARCB1*

Table 78.4 Chances of mosaicism and risk to offspring based on testing 402 de novo NF2 patients fulfilling Manchester criteria

Age at VS diagnosis	Number of patients	Mutation nonmosaic	Mosaic found blood	Mosaic found tumor	Mosaic inferred pre-blood genetic test (%)	Transmission risk pre-blood genetic test (%)	Likelihood of missed full mutation after negative blood testing	Mosaic inferred post-negative blood test (%)	Transmission risk post-negative blood test
<20 BVS	99	81 (81%)	5 (5%)	1 (1%)	12	45	7/13 (54%)	46	29%, 1 in 3
<20 UVS	21	13 (62%)	3 (14%)	3 (14%)	33	33	1.1/5 (22%)	78	15%, 1 in 7
20–29 BVS	77	49 (64%)	7 (9%)	2 (3%)	30	36	4.3/21 (20%)	80	15%, 1 in 7
20–29 UVS	28	5 (18%)	4 (14%)	6 (21%)	78	19	0.44/19 (2%)	98	6%, 1 in 16
30–39 BVS	54	25 (45%)	9 (17%)	7 (13%)	50	28	2.2/20 (11%)	89	11%, 1 in 9
30–39 UVS	20	3 (15%0	1 (5%)	6 (30%)	83	12	0.26/16 (2%)	98	6%, 1 in 16
40 + BVS	59	18 (31%)	5 (8%)	7 (12%)	66	22	1.56/26 (6%)	94	9%, 1 in 11
40 + UVS	44	4 (9%)	2 (5%)	8 (18%)	90	10	0.35/36 (1%)	99	5.5%, 1 in 20
Total	402	198 (49%)	36 (9%)	40 (10%)					

Abbreviations: BVS, bilateral vestibular schwannoma; NF2, neurofibromatosis type 2; UVS, unilateral vestibular schwannoma; VS, vestibular schwannoma.

gene with a further 30% due to *LZTR1*.[12] Although vestibular schwannomas have not been reported with *SMARCB1*, *LZTR1* does appear to confer a risk.[12] Sporadic cases are only positive for *SMARCB1* in 10% of cases[47,48,49,50] with a similar proportion being due to *LZTR1*. In those who do not carry a *SMARCB1* mutation, 80% of schwannomatosis patients who had typical NF2 inactivation with an NF2 mutation and loss of chromosome 22q were reported as having a mutation of the *LZTR1* gene.[51] However, this is likely to be an overestimate.[12] Patients with schwannomatosis demonstrate a four-hit, three-step model rather than the two-hit model demonstrated by patients with NF2. Patients with two or more nonvestibular schwannomas should be assessed for this condition by tumor and blood analysis.

78.8 Conclusion

NF2 is an autosomal dominant condition with a high incidence of mosaicism. It results from mutation of the *NF2* gene, residing on chromosome 22, that encodes Merlin, a tumor suppressor protein that is expressed particularly avidly in the cell membrane of Schwann cells. Various types of mutations of the gene have been identified with truncating mutations being the most common. Severity of disease is associated with the type of mutation, with truncating mutations being associated with more severe disease than deletions. Mosaic cases are also associated with milder and often segmental disease. Identification of the mutation in blood is possible in 93% of cases in nonmosaic individuals but is significantly lower in mosaic patients. At-risk patients should undergo screening in order to identify disease early. This includes ophthalmological, audiological, and cutaneous assessments, as well as MRI imaging of the head and spine.

References

[1] Evans DG, Huson SM, Donnai D, et al. A clinical study of type 2 neurofibromatosis. Q J Med. 1992; 84(304):603–618

[2] Lloyd SK, Evans DG. Neurofibromatosis type 2 (NF2): diagnosis and management. Handb Clin Neurol. 2013; 115:957–967

[3] Evans DG, Huson SM, Donnai D, et al. A genetic study of type 2 neurofibromatosis in the United Kingdom. I. Prevalence, mutation rate, fitness, and confirmation of maternal transmission effect on severity. J Med Genet. 1992; 29 (12):841–846

[4] Evans DG, Baser ME, O'Reilly B, et al. Management of the patient and family with neurofibromatosis 2: a consensus conference statement. Br J Neurosurg. 2005; 19(1):5–12

[5] Feiling A, Ward E. A familial form of acoustic neuroma. BMJ. 1920; 1(3093): 496–497

[6] Gardner WJ, Fraszier CH. Bilateral acoustic neurofibromas: a clinical study and field survey of a family of five generations with bilateral deafness in thirty eight members. Arch Neurol Psychiatry. 1930; 23:266–302

[7] Bourn D, Carter SA, Evans DG, Goodship J, Coakham H, Strachan T. A mutation in the neurofibromatosis type 2 tumor-suppressor gene, giving rise to widely different clinical phenotypes in two unrelated individuals. Am J Hum Genet. 1994; 55(1):69–73

[8] Evans DG, Wallace AJ, Wu CL, Trueman L, Ramsden RT, Strachan T. Somatic mosaicism: a common cause of classic disease in tumor-prone syndromes? Lessons from type 2 neurofibromatosis. Am J Hum Genet. 1998; 63(3):727–736

[9] Moyhuddin A, Baser ME, Watson C, et al. Somatic mosaicism in neurofibromatosis 2: prevalence and risk of disease transmission to offspring. J Med Genet. 2003; 40(6):459–463

[10] Kluwe L, Mautner V, Heinrich B, et al. Molecular study of frequency of mosaicism in neurofibromatosis 2 patients with bilateral vestibular schwannomas. J Med Genet. 2003; 40(2):109–114

[11] Kluwe L, Mautner VF. Mosaicism in sporadic neurofibromatosis 2 patients. Hum Mol Genet. 1998; 7(13):2051–2055

[12] Smith MJ, Isidor B, Beetz C, et al. Mutations in LZTR1 add to the complex heterogeneity of schwannomatosis. Neurology. 2015; 84(2):141–147

[13] Trofatter JA, MacCollin MM, Rutter JL, et al. A novel moesin-, ezrin-, radixin-like gene is a candidate for the neurofibromatosis 2 tumor suppressor. Cell. 1993; 72(5):791–800

[14] Rouleau GA, Merel P, Lutchman M, et al. Alteration in a new gene encoding a putative membrane-organizing protein causes neuro-fibromatosis type 2. Nature. 1993; 363(6429):515–521

[15] Kino T, Takeshima H, Nakao M, et al. Identification of the cis-acting region in the NF2 gene promoter as a potential target for mutation and methylation-dependent silencing in schwannoma. Genes Cells. 2001; 6(5):441–454

[16] Pećina-Šlaus N. Merlin, the NF2 gene product. Pathol Oncol Res. 2013; 19(3): 365–373

[17] Hanemann CO. Magic but treatable? Tumours due to loss of merlin. Brain. 2008; 131(Pt 3):606–615

[18] Neff BA, Welling DB, Akhmametyeva E, Chang LS. The molecular biology of vestibular schwannomas: dissecting the pathogenic process at the molecular level. Otol Neurotol. 2006; 27(2):197–208

[19] Petrilli AM, Fernández-Valle C. Role of Merlin/NF2 inactivation in tumor biology. Oncogene. 2016; 35(5):537–548

[20] Pelton PD, Sherman LS, Rizvi TA, et al. Ruffling membrane, stress fiber, cell spreading and proliferation abnormalities in human Schwannoma cells. Oncogene. 1998; 17(17):2195–2209

[21] Hamaratoglu F, Willecke M, Kango-Singh M, et al. The tumour-suppressor genes NF2/Merlin and expanded act through Hippo signalling to regulate cell proliferation and apoptosis. Nat Cell Biol. 2006; 8(1):27–36

[22] Li W, Cooper J, Zhou L, et al. Merlin/NF2 loss-driven tumorigenesis linked to CRL4(DCAF1)-mediated inhibition of the hippo pathway kinases Lats1 and 2 in the nucleus. Cancer Cell. 2014; 26(1):48–60

[23] Chiasson-MacKenzie C, Morris ZS, Baca Q, et al. NF2/Merlin mediates contact-dependent inhibition of EGFR mobility and internalization via cortical actomyosin. J Cell Biol. 2015; 211(2):391–405

[24] Parry DM, MacCollin MM, Kaiser-Kupfer MI, et al. Germ-line mutations in the neurofibromatosis 2 gene: correlations with disease severity and retinal abnormalities. Am J Hum Genet. 1996; 59(3):529–539

[25] Castellanos E, Bielsa I, Carrato C, et al. NF2 Multidisciplinary Clinics HUGTiP-ICO-IMPPC. Segmental neurofibromatosis type 2: discriminating two hit from four hit in a patient presenting multiple schwannomas confined to one limb. BMC Med Genomics. 2015; 8:2

[26] Evans DG, Trueman L, Wallace A, Collins S, Strachan T. Genotype/phenotype correlations in type 2 neurofibromatosis (NF2): evidence for more severe disease associated with truncating mutations. J Med Genet. 1998; 35(6):450–455

[27] Ruttledge MH, Andermann AA, Phelan CM, et al. Type of mutation in the neurofibromatosis type 2 gene (NF2) frequently determines severity of disease. Am J Hum Genet. 1996; 59(2):331–342

[28] Kluwe L, MacCollin M, Tatagiba M, et al. Phenotypic variability associated with 14 splice-site mutations in the NF2 gene. Am J Med Genet. 1998; 77(3): 228–233

[29] Baser ME, Friedman JM, Aeschliman D, et al. Predictors of the risk of mortality in neurofibromatosis 2. Am J Hum Genet. 2002; 71(4):715–723

[30] Baser ME, Kuramoto L, Woods R, et al. The location of constitutional neurofibromatosis 2 (NF2) splice site mutations is associated with the severity of NF2. J Med Genet. 2005; 42(7):540–546

[31] Tsilchorozidou T, Menko FH, Lalloo F, et al. Constitutional rearrangements of chromosome 22 as a cause of neurofibromatosis 2. J Med Genet. 2004; 41(7): 529–534

[32] Selvanathan SK, Shenton A, Ferner R, et al. Further genotype–phenotype correlations in neurofibromatosis 2. Clin Genet. 2010; 77(2):163–170

[33] Patronas NJ, Courcoutsakis N, Bromley CM, Katzman GL, MacCollin M, Parry DM. Intramedullary and spinal canal tumors in patients with neurofibromatosis 2: MR imaging findings and correlation with genotype. Radiology. 2001; 218(2):434–442

[34] Smith MJ, Higgs JE, Bowers NL, et al. Cranial meningiomas in 411 neurofibromatosis type 2 (NF2) patients with proven gene mutations: clear positional effect of mutations, but absence of female severity effect on age at onset. J Med Genet. 2011; 48(4):261–265

[35] Hexter A, Jones A, Joe H, et al. English Specialist NF2 Research Group. Clinical and molecular predictors of mortality in neurofibromatosis 2: a UK national analysis of 1192 patients. J Med Genet. 2015; 52(10):699–705

[36] Gonzalez-Gomez P, Bello MJ, Alonso ME, et al. CpG island methylation in sporadic and neurofibromatis type 2-associated schwannomas. Clin Cancer Res. 2003; 9(15):5601–5606

[37] Baser ME, Ragge NK, Riccardi VM, Janus T, Gantz B, Pulst SM. Phenotypic variability in monozygotic twins with neurofibromatosis 2. Am J Med Genet. 1996; 64(4):563–567

[38] Fisher LM, Doherty JK, Lev MH, Slattery WH. Concordance of bilateral vestibular schwannoma growth and hearing changes in neurofibromatosis 2: neurofibromatosis 2 natural history consortium. Otol Neurotol. 2009; 30(6): 835–841

[39] Cayé-Thomasen P, Baandrup L, Jacobsen GK, Thomsen J, Stangerup SE. Immunohistochemical demonstration of vascular endothelial growth factor in vestibular schwannomas correlates to tumor growth rate. Laryngoscope. 2003; 113(12):2129–2134

[40] Pasmant E, Louvrier C, Luscan A, et al. Neurofibromatosis type 2 French cohort analysis using a comprehensive NF2 molecular diagnostic strategy. Neurochirurgie. 2015:[Epub ahead of print]

[41] Evans DG, Raymond FL, Barwell JG, Halliday D. Genetic testing and screening of individuals at risk of NF2. Clin Genet. 2012; 82(5):416–424

[42] Spyra M, Otto B, Schön G, Kehrer-Sawatzki H, Mautner VF. Determination of the mutant allele frequency in patients with neurofibromatosis type 2 and somatic mosaicism by means of deep sequencing. Genes Chromosomes Cancer. 2015; 54(8):482–488

[43] Evans DG, Ramsden RT, Shenton A, et al. Mosaicism in neurofibromatosis type 2: an update of risk based on uni/bilaterality of vestibular schwannoma at presentation and sensitive mutation analysis including multiple ligation-dependent probe amplification. J Med Genet. 2007; 44(7):424–428

[44] Evans DG, Wallace A. An update on age related mosaic and offspring risk in neurofibromatosis 2 (NF2). J Med Genet. 2009; 46(11):792

[45] Mohyuddin A, Neary WJ, Wallace A, et al. Molecular genetic analysis of the NF2 gene in young patients with unilateral vestibular schwannomas. J Med Genet. 2002; 39(5):315–322

[46] Plotkin SR, Blakeley JO, Evans DG, et al. Update from the 2011 International Schwannomatosis Workshop: from genetics to diagnostic criteria. Am J Med Genet A. 2013; 161A(3):405–416

[47] Boyd C, Smith MJ, Kluwe L, Balogh A, Maccollin M, Plotkin SR. Alterations in the SMARCB1 (INI1) tumor suppressor gene in familial schwannomatosis. Clin Genet. 2008; 74(4):358–366

[48] Hadfield KD, Newman WG, Bowers NL, et al. Molecular characterisation of SMARCB1 and NF2 in familial and sporadic schwannomatosis. J Med Genet. 2008; 45(6):332–339

[49] Rousseau G, Noguchi T, Bourdon V, Sobol H, Olschwang S. SMARCB1/INI1 germline mutations contribute to 10% of sporadic schwannomatosis. BMC Neurol. 2011; 11:9

[50] Smith MJ, Wallace AJ, Bowers NL, et al. Frequency of SMARCB1 mutations in familial and sporadic schwannomatosis. Neurogenetics. 2012; 13(2):141–145

[51] Piotrowski A, Xie J, Liu YF, et al. Germline loss-of-function mutations in LZTR1 predispose to an inherited disorder of multiple schwannomas. Nat Genet. 2014; 46(2):182–187

79 Diagnosis and Evaluation of Neurofibromatosis Type 2

Bryan K. Ward, Shannon Langmead, and Jaishri O. Blakeley

79.1 Introduction

Neurofibromatosis type 2 (NF2) is a rare neurogenetic syndrome inherited in an autosomal dominant pattern, with an estimated incidence of roughly 1:30,000.[1] Although heritable, approximately 50% of people with NF2 have a *de novo* mutation. The causative mutation on chromosome 22q11.2 leads to inactivation of the tumor suppressor protein Merlin. The lack of functional Merlin has been shown to decrease apoptosis and increase proliferation indexes in Schwann cells. Loss of both copies of normal *NF2* results in tumor formation in multiple different cell types (Schwann, arachnoidal, and ependymal cells) leading to nervous system tumors including schwannomas of the cranial and peripheral nerves, meningiomas, and ependymomas (▶ Fig. 79.1). A more detailed discussion regarding the molecular biology and genetics of NF2 can be found in Chapters 5 and 78.

Neurofibromatosis was first described by the German pathologist Friedrich Daniel von Recklinghausen in 1882, and was subsequently stratified into types 1 and 2 when the associated genes for the two conditions were identified on separate chromosomes. Neurofibromatosis type 1 (NF1) and NF2 are now known to be distinct clinical entities. NF1 is far more common (estimated 1:3,000) and often diagnosed at an earlier age based on the high frequency of dermatologic findings such as café au lait spots and cutaneous neurofibromas. In contrast, NF2 is often diagnosed in the teenage years or later when the initial signs and symptoms related to intracranial or spinal tumors begin to manifest. The most common presenting symptoms of NF2 include hearing loss, tinnitus, balance dysfunction, cranial neuropathy, and/or focal weakness suggestive of expanding intracranial or spinal lesions.[2,3]

The diagnosis of NF2 can be made on the basis of either clinical or molecular evidence. Patients with an established family history of NF2 are often identified early in the course of disease from screening protocols or heightened suspicion. This is particularly true in cases where a causative mutation for a specific individual is known, as family members can be screened for the same mutation in order to confirm the diagnosis, even before clinical symptoms develop. In contrast, an early clinical diagnosis of NF2 in patients without a family history of the disease can be challenging, as the presenting signs and symptoms are frequently nonspecific.[4,5] Furthermore, even with radiographic evidence of a tumor, the diagnosis of NF2 can be initially missed

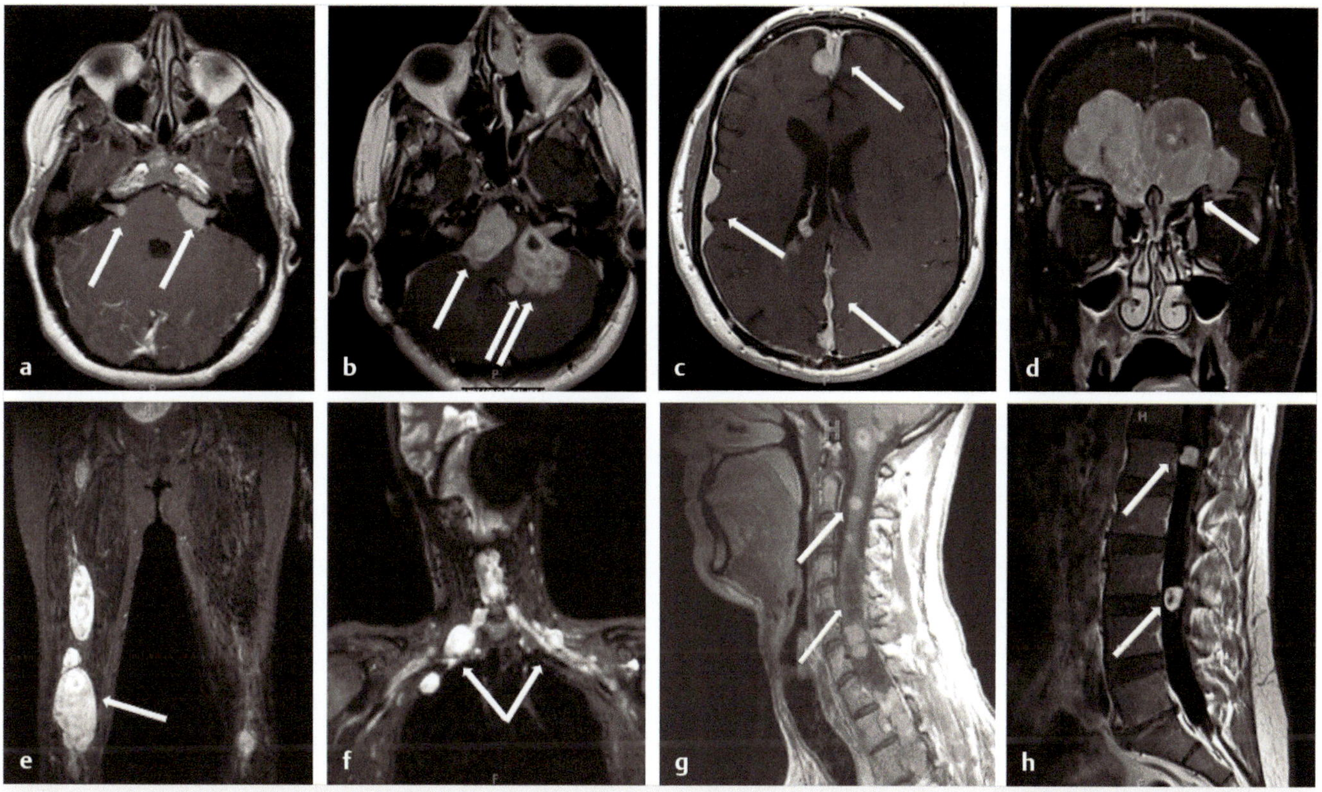

Fig. 79.1 Representative images from patients with NF2 of various ages from childhood to late adulthood. (**a**) Bilateral vestibular schwannomas in a 20-year-old with no hearing loss to date; (**b**) bilateral vestibular schwannomas complicated by "collision tumors" likely composed of multiple schwannomas (*two arrows*) and meningioma (*one arrow*); (**c**) multiple meningiomas suggestive of meningiomatosis; (**d**) complex, "giant" meningioma encasing the cavernous sinus resulting in multiple cranial neuropathies; (**e**) peripheral schwannomas in a 20-year-old; (**f**) multiple spinal tumors consistent with schwannomas; (**g**) multiple intramedullary tumors suggestive of ependymoma including a cystic ependymoma C4–T1(*lower arrow*); (H) intradural, extramedullary paraspinal lesions consistent with spinal schwannomas.

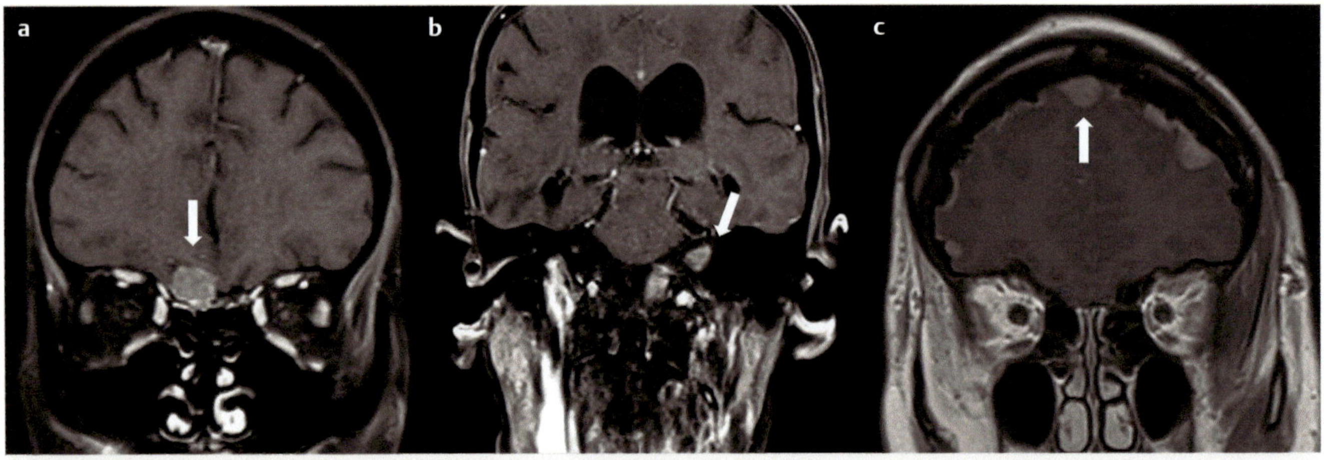

Fig. 79.2 **(a, b)** Leptomeningeal deposits from choroid plexus papillomas that mimic meningioma in **(a)** and vestibular schwannoma in **(b)**. **(c)** Image demonstrates meningiomatosis in the setting of NF2. The same involvement can be seen in people confirmed not to have NF2.

or overlooked, as tumors occurring in NF2 are common tumors in the general population and can occur metachronously or in a nonconventional pattern. Although the constellation of multiple schwannomas and meningiomas is a hallmark of NF2, some patients may initially present with only one or two tumors—findings that may not directly suggest NF2 or reach diagnostic criteria at initial presentation.[6,7,8,9,10] Furthermore, nodular enhancement of cranial nerves from leptomeningeal disease related to malignant or inflammatory conditions, or multiple meningiomas as seen in meningiomatosis not associated with NF2, can mimic NF2 (▶ Fig. 79.2). Importantly, it is now known that intracranial schwannomas and meningiomas can occur in some patients with schwannomatosis, a distinct syndrome that has many overlapping features with NF2, making the accurate diagnosis of NF2 even more challenging.[8,10,11] Given that NF2 is rare and that the presenting symptoms and imaging findings can occur coincidentally or in the setting of other disease processes, clinicians need to be knowledgeable about the spectrum of NF2 and have a high index of suspicion to make the correct diagnosis in a timely manner.

79.2 Diagnostic Criteria for Neurofibromatosis Type 2

Clinical diagnostic criteria for NF2 were originally proposed by the National Institutes of Health (NIH) in 1987 to distinguish NF2 from NF1, and were subsequently revised in 1991.[4] Additional groups such as the Manchester group in 1992[12] and a panel of experts convened by the National Neurofibromatosis Foundation (NNFF) in 1997 developed independent guidelines.[13] In all proposed criteria, the presence of bilateral vestibular schwannomas (VSs) is pathognomonic for NF2 because of the rarity of such an event occurring spontaneously. Since NF2 is autosomal dominant, all guidelines also allow a first-degree relative with NF2 paired with either a unilateral VS or the presence of two other features that are part of the NF2 spectrum (i.e., meningioma, schwannoma, ependymoma, or juvenile cataract) as diagnostic criteria. While the presence of bilateral VS is a clear criterion for the diagnosis of NF2, some clinicians were concerned that the initial diagnostic criteria were overly restrictive, missing younger patients who would later develop full features of NF2. To address this, the NNFF recommended differentiating between "confirmed NF2" and "presumed NF2" in order to encourage regular clinical evaluation in those suspected of having NF2.[13] The finding of a VS or meningioma in a young person less than 30 years of age, for instance, raises suspicion for NF2[14] and although not all cases of VS in a young patient lead to later development of NF2,[15] several patients will eventually develop NF2 based on clinical criteria.[7]

In 2002, Baser et al reviewed the sensitivity and specificity of the four previously proposed clinical diagnostic criteria against a large series of patients in the United Kingdom NF2 registry that presented without bilateral VSs, but later met criteria for NF2. While the specificity was 100% with each of the existing criteria, the sensitivity of any one of the criteria was ≤ 70%.[16] Baser et al then offered revised criteria to increase the diagnostic sensitivity by developing a scoring system that ascribed points to family history, presence of unilateral or bilateral schwannoma, one or more meningiomas, cutaneous schwannoma, other cranial nerve tumors, mononeuropathy, or cataract with more points ascribed when any of the aforementioned occurred in people younger than 30 years. With these criteria, the sensitivity increased to 80% while maintaining 100% specificity. The Baser revised system also allows for additional genetic testing for indeterminate cases.[7] As mentioned earlier, there are recent calls to further revise the criteria to clarify between NF2 and schwannomatosis based on LZTR1 testing.[10] The clinical diagnostic criteria currently in use are shown in ▶ Table 79.1.

79.3 Other Conditions with Overlapping Clinical Features

The complexity of appropriately applying even the most exacting diagnostic criteria still leaves uncertainty in diagnosis and difficulty in discerning NF2 from overlapping conditions. For example, another neurogenetic condition, schwannomatosis, is clinically and genetically distinct from NF2, but the syndromes share several clinical and molecular features. Like NF2,

Table 79.1 Existing Clinical Diagnostic Criteria for Neurofibromatosis 2

NIH criteria (NIH Consensus Statement)	Manchester criteria (D. G. Evans et al. 1992)	National Neurofibromatosis Foundation (NNFF) criteria (Gutmann et al. 1997)	Baser criteria (Michael E Baser et al. 2011)	< 30 yrs	≥ 30 yrs
				Points assigned (>6 points = definite NF2)	
Bilateral VS *or*	A. Bilateral VS *or*	*Confirmed or definite NF2:*	First-degree family relative with NF2	2	2
First-degree relative with NF2 and either unilateral VS *or* any *one* of the following:	B. Family history of NF2 plus:	Bilateral VS *or*			
	(1) Unilateral acoustic *or*	First-degree family relative with NF2 and unilateral VS, 30 y or any two of meningioma, glioma, schwannoma, juvenile lens opacity (posterior subcapsular cataract or cortical cataract)	Unilateral VS	2	1 *(if < 70 y)*
Neurofibroma	(2) Any *two* of: meningioma, glioma, neurofibroma, schwannoma, posterior subcapsular lenticular opacities.		Second VS	4	3 *(if < 70 y)*
Meningioma					
Glioma					
Schwannoma					
			One meningioma	2	1
Juvenile posterior subcapsular lens opacity	C. Unilateral VS *and* any *two* of neurofibroma, meningioma, glioma, schwannoma, or posterior subcapsular lenticular opacities.	*Presumptive or probable NF2:*			
		Unilateral VS < 30 y and at least one of meningioma, glioma, schwannoma, juvenile lens opacity	Second meningioma	2	1
	D. Multiple meningiomas (two or more) *and* unilateral VS *or* any *two* of neurofibroma, glioma, schwannoma, or cataract		Cutaneous schwannoma	2	1
		Multiple meningiomas (two or more) and unilateral VS < 30 y or at least one of meningioma, glioma, schwannoma, juvenile lens opacity	Cranial nerve tumor; one or more; excluding VS	2	1
			Mononeuropathy	2	1
			Cataract (one or more)	2	0

Abbreviations: NNFF, National Neurofibromatosis Foundation; VS, vestibular schwannoma.
("National Institutes of Health Consensus Development Conference Statement on Acoustic Neuroma, December 11–13, 1991. The Consensus Development Panel." 1994)

schwannomatosis is characterized by multiple schwannomas of the spine and peripheral nerves but without bilateral VS (▶ Table 79.2).[17] As mentioned earlier, it is now recognized that patients with schwannomatosis may have unilateral VS or meningioma.[8,11] Some families have been described with multiple meningiomas without VS or with unilateral VS.

There is also mosaicism of *NF2* that complicates the ability to clinically diagnose NF2. In these cases, the mutation affects only a portion of the individual's cells and therefore only a segment of the body develops tumors. This localized effect makes the distinction between sporadic tumors, segmental NF2, and schwannomatosis challenging. Genetic mosaicism can also lead to difficulties in acquiring a molecular diagnosis, as lymphocyte blood testing is often negative. In such cases, the diagnosis can only be confirmed via molecular testing of several individual tumors and serum. However, access to multiple tissue samples is rarely feasible and tumor biopsy is not advised if performed only for the purpose of establishing a genetic diagnosis.[18]

Finally, when assessing a patient with apparent bilateral VS, with or without additional cranial nerve schwannomas or meningiomas, it is important to take a detailed history to ensure that there has not been prior radiation involving the affected area resulting in radiation-induced neoplasia rather than NF2-driven neoplasms. It is also important to ensure that there are no other signs of a systemic process that can lead to leptomeningeal thickening, or multiple cranial neuropathies such as Lyme's disease, neurosarcoidosis, or cancer with leptomeningeal involvement.

79.4 Vestibular Schwannomas

In NF2, schwannomas can occur along any cranial nerve, either in isolation or with multiple contiguous or clusters of tumors. Compared to other cranial nerves, schwannomas develop on the vestibular nerves with much greater frequency—approximately 60% of patients with NF2 have bilateral VS on their initial assessment, and over 95% will have bilateral VS by the age of 30 years.[18,19] As discussed elsewhere in this text, the consequences of VS growth are numerous but can include hearing and vestibular loss, trigeminal neuropathy or neuralgia, facial nerve paralysis, and eventually brainstem compression, hydrocephalus, and death.

The behavior of VS in people with NF2 is highly variable with individual tumors following linear, sigmoid, logarithmic, and

Table 79.2 The diagnostic criteria for schwannomatosis

Schwannomatosis	
Definite schwannomatosis	**Possible schwannomatosis**
Age > 30 y *and* 2 or more non-intradermal schwannomas, at least 1 with histologic confirmation *and* no evidence of vestibular tumor on high-resolution MRI *and* no known constitutional NF2 mutation *or* One pathologically confirmed nonvestibular schwannoma plus a first-degree relative who meets above criteria	Age < 30 y *and* 2 or more non-intradermal schwannomas, at least 1 with histologic confirmation *and* no evidence of vestibular tumor on high-resolution MRI *and* no known constitutional NF2 mutation *or* Age > 45 y *and* 2 or more non-intradermal schwannomas, at least 1 with histologic confirmation *and* no symptoms of 8th nerve dysfunction *and* no known constitutional NF2 mutation *or* Radiographic evidence of nonvestibular schwannoma and first-degree relative meeting criteria for definite schwannomatosis

Abbreviation: NF2, neurofibromatosis type 2.
Source: Used with permission from MacCollin M, Chiocca EA, Evans DG, et al. Diagnostic criteria for schwannomatosis. Neurology. 2005; 64 (11):1838–1845.

overall irregular growth curves based on traditional linear measurements on MRI.[20] Despite this variability, there is consensus that these tumors grow over time with the majority of NF2-associated VS doubling their volume within 5 years.[21] Further, left and right VSs often grow at similar rates in people with NF2, but the onset of growth is variable resulting in different tumor volumes on either side.[22] Overall, VSs tend to slow in growth as patients age, with being more rapid growth in children and young adults, but growth can occur life-long.[20,22,23] A recent natural history study assessing volumetric growth of 39 VSs in 52 patients with NF2 over a median of 36 months showed that with volumetric measures, growth patterns are most commonly saltatory, followed with equal frequency by exponential or linear growth but intermixed with long periods of stability.[21] Given this variability, patients with NF2 are recommended to undergo MRI brain with thin cuts through the internal auditory canals at least annually and more frequently if there is evidence of active growth or if receiving treatment.[24]

Several studies have demonstrated that there is not a strong association between absolute tumor size (as assessed with MRI volumetrics) and hearing function based on both retrospective and prospective evaluations.[25,26,27,28,29,30] Given the weak association between these two parameters, it is important to pair MRI and audiometric testing together during clinical surveillance. Hearing loss in the absence of tumor growth commonly occurs, suggesting that other tumor, paracrine, or systemic factors play a role in hearing deterioration. The converse is also true, which a tumor may increase in size without clear progression of sensorineural hearing loss. Hence, both evaluations are needed and audiometry should be performed at least annually, but for young patients, people with recent changes in hearing, or those in active treatment, audiometry should be done more frequently as clinically indicated.

79.5 Nonvestibular Cranial Nerve Schwannomas

Patients with NF2 may also have schwannomas of the trigeminal, vagus, glossopharyngeal, and hypoglossal nerves.[31] In fact, approximately half of patients with NF2 will present with at least one non-VS. Of those patients with non-VS, the most common is the trigeminal nerve (72%), followed by oculomotor (15%), and vagus nerves (5%).[31] In adults, these tumors are often silent and do not require intervention. The exception to this is schwannomas of the lower cranial nerves that can affect swallow and speech. Hence, patients with NF2 should be screened for swallow dysfunction and hypophonia in routine clinical evaluations and referred for formal swallow evaluation prior to surgeries that could impact the lower cranial nerves or if there are signs or symptoms of swallow difficulty.

In contrast to adults, children with NF2 are more likely to present with third nerve palsy or other mononeuropathies such as a facial paralysis or foot drop. These deficits are often due to meningiomas rather than schwannomas. The fact that there are multiple tumor types that can be active in people with NF2 highlights the importance of confirming that a particular tumor is causing the symptom of concern before proceeding with intervention.

Since neighboring cranial nerves are affected by VS and other cranial nerves also can develop schwannomas in NF2, there is an effort to develop specific measures for facial nerve, swallowing, and peripheral nerve function.[32] Specifically, the scaled measurement of improvement in lip excursion (SMILE) system has been recommended for assessing facial nerve function[32] and studies are ongoing to develop measures for swallow function in people with NF2.

79.6 Meningioma

Meningiomas are the second most common tumor type in patients with NF2, present in over half of patients. Although sporadic meningiomas in the general population are more common in women, in NF2 there is no apparent gender preference,[33] suggesting the presence of meningiomas in NF2 is more dependent on an underlying mutation rather than hormonal influence. In patients with NF2, the presence of meningiomas is also a poor prognostic factor in that they are associated with a more severe overall disease course.[3] Meningiomas are often multiple, with NF2 patients having on average three to five meningiomas.[33,34] They can develop on any portion of the meninges, but appear to occur more frequently around the falx cerebri.[34] Some patients with NF2 develop a condition known as meningiomatosis, in which diffuse plaque-like or nodular thickening of the meninges occurs. When growing, meningiomas can result in focal neurological deficits, hydrocephalus, or seizures. However, in many NF2 patients, meningiomas are clinically silent. In a long-term follow-up study of patients with NF2-associated meningiomas, the mean annual growth rate was 1.5 mm, but two-thirds of tumors showed no growth during a mean follow-up of approximately 9 years.[33] *De novo* tumors, those tumors arising during observation, are rare. However, when they occur, they have more rapid growth rates and are more likely to cause local edema. As such, these *de novo* tumors may be more likely to require surgery. Approximately 45% of patients with NF2 require surgery for their meningiomas in the course of their disease. For the patients who do require intervention for their meningiomas, the course can be very complicated, as there are often multiple tumors that are impacting one another and there can be unpredictable changes in intracranial pressure due to abnormal cerebrospinal fluid reabsorption or venous hypertension in patients with meningiomatosis. Given the limitation of surgery and radiation in patients with multiple meningiomas, efforts are underway to develop drug therapies for NF2-driven meningiomas (NCT02831257, NCT02523014).[30]

79.7 Ependymoma

Spinal tumors in NF2 include extradural nerve sheath schwannomas, meningiomas, or intradural ependymomas.[35] At diagnosis, the prevalence of spinal tumors (intra- or extramedullary) has been reported as high as 90%, with approximately 30% of these tumors being intramedullary.[36] The intramedullary tumors were initially called by the global term "glioma." Later detailed pathologic studies showed the vast majority of these tumors to specifically be low-grade ependymomas.[37] Ependymomas are often viewed as a marker of aggressive NF2 phenotype, being associated with more intracranial tumors, a younger age at presentation, and harboring genetic mutations associated with poorer prognosis.[37] Ependymomas are often multiple and occur more commonly in the cervical spinal cord or cervicomedullary junction, with rare involvement of the lumbar cord and no involvement of the brain.[38] This is in stark contrast to sporadic ependymomas, which are commonly intracranial. In NF2, ependymomas are often asymptomatic, particularly at the time of diagnosis, and incidentally discovered on surveillance imaging.[38] Fortunately, many of these tumors do not require intervention ever or for many years, even when cystic components are present. Eventually, however, approximately 20 to 40% of patients are referred for treatment due to pain, motor weakness, or sensory deficits (▸ Fig. 79.3).[34,38,39] Again, given the multiplicity of tumors in a person with NF2, it is imperative to show that the ependymoma is the source of the symptoms prior to intervention.

79.8 Peripheral Schwannoma and Skin Manifestations

Tumors of the skin and subcutaneous tissue are common in NF2 occurring in approximately 56% of cases, especially in patients with the more severe presentation of disease (▸ Fig. 79.4).[13] Tumors of the skin often present as flat lesions involving the dermis or spherical subcutaneous nodules involving peripheral nerves. The histology of peripheral tumors in NF2 is typically consistent with a schwannoma rather than a neurofibroma, in contrast to NF1 in which neurofibromas predominate. The pathologic distinction between a schwannoma and a neurofibroma can be challenging, even for an experienced pathologist. While the occurrence of a neurofibroma in a person with NF2 is possible, this finding creates nosological challenges. To further complicate matters, café au lait spots are present in some patients with NF2, albeit fewer and much less commonly than in people with NF1 such that patients with NF2 will not meet the clinical criteria for NF1.

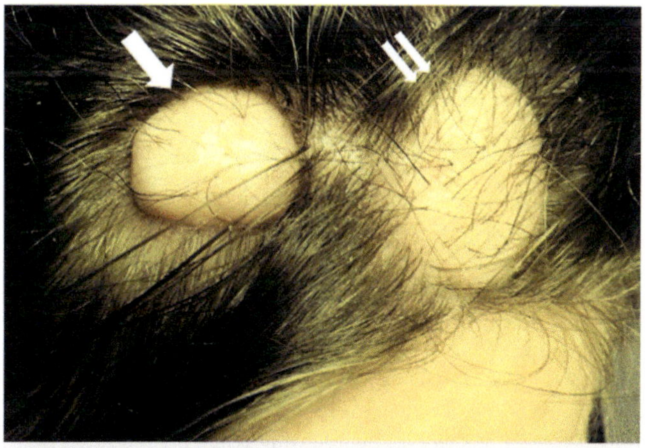

Fig. 79.4 Subcutaneous schwannomas of the scalp: the *large white arrow* showing a nodular lesion and the *small white arrows* showing a flat lesion. Both were pathologically schwannomas.

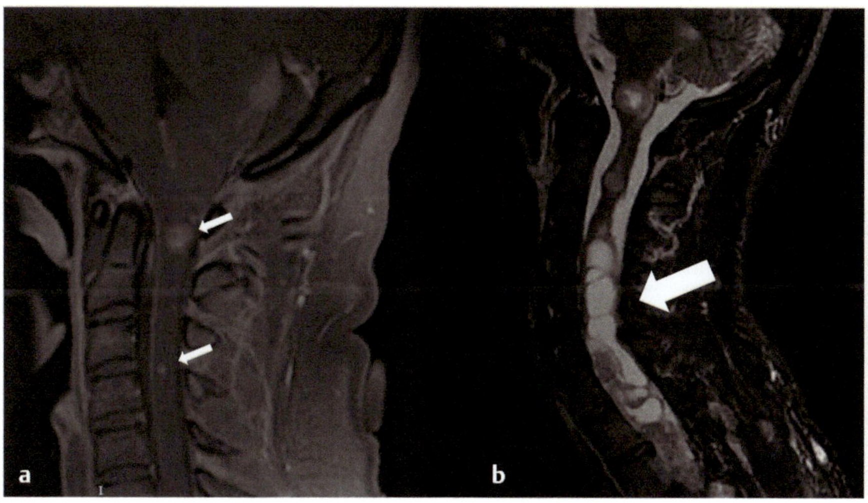

Fig. 79.3 Panel **a** demonstrates two foci of asymptomatic ependymoma (*small white arrows*) and panel **b** demonstrates a high burden of tumor with associated cystic changes in a person with NF2 (*large white arrow*).

79.9 Ophthalmologic Manifestations

Abnormalities affecting the eye are common in NF2, and include epiretinal membranes, retinal hamartomas, cataracts at a young age, and meningiomas of the optic nerve sheath. These conditions are different from ophthalmologic abnormalities commonly seen in NF1 in which optic nerve gliomas and Lisch nodules (hamartomas of the iris) predominate. These diagnostic distinctions highlight the importance of early involvement of an ophthalmologist or neuro-ophthalmologist in the diagnosis and management of patients with NF2.

In particular, posterior subcapsular–capsular cataracts have been found in 80% of individuals with NF2. Peripheral cortical cataracts are also prevalent in NF2.[40] These cataracts rarely result in significant visual impairment and if they do cause any visual symptoms, they occur later in life.[41] The ophthalmologic manifestations in NF2 result from alterations in the surface ectoderm and neuroectoderm of the eye, as during development neural crest cells are located at the interface of these structures.[42] Meyers et al have speculated that the factors that lead to proliferation of neural crest cells elsewhere in the body in NF2 patients may also lead to the epiretinal membranes, retinal hamartomas, and presenile cataracts.[42]

79.10 Diagnostic Imaging

Imaging is central to NF2 evaluation as outlined by established clinical diagnostic criteria (▶ Table 79.1). If NF2 is suspected, MRI of the brain with thin submillimeter cuts through the internal auditory canals, with and without gadolinium, is required as they are able to detect even very small tumors (< 2 mm) with good reliability.[43,44] Specific imaging guidelines for NF2-associated VS were outlined in a 2013 consensus statement and are detailed in consensus imaging recommendations.[43] Recommendations allow identification of both bilateral VS and schwannomas involving other lower cranial nerves, as seen in up to 38% of patients presenting with NF2.[36] Initial radiological workup should include MRI of the head as detailed earlier, in addition to imaging of the entire spine with and without gadolinium to evaluate tumor burden. Standard tumor-based imaging (at 1.5 or 3 T, including short tau inversion recovery and gadolinium sequences) is sufficient for initial screening for spine involvement[43] (▶ Table 79.3).

After completing an initial evaluation, patients with NF2 should undergo surveillance brain MRI every 6 to 12 months to establish the rate of progression of any tumors identified at initial diagnosis. If the rate of growth is slow, or there is no change after several scans, the time interval between imaging may be prolonged to annually or in rare cases with prolonged stability up to every 2 years. In patients with changing lesions or on active treatment, MRI is indicated as often as every 3 months. It is important that the images consistently be obtained with thin cuts through the brainstem using similar imaging characteristics (magnet strength, views, contrast, and cuts), such that comparisons can readily be made to assess for any growth or change in tumor characteristics.

The radiological evaluation of NF2 can be particularly challenging, even for specialized neuroradiologists. Patients with severe phenotypic disease often have multiple overlapping or "collision tumors" (▶ Fig. 79.1). Postoperative changes, such as after obliteration of a tumor resection cavity with fat, can also distort the normal anatomy, requiring fat-saturation image acquisition procedures that are not otherwise routinely performed. Additionally, patients with NF2 may have ventricular shunts, auditory brainstem implants, or cochlear implants, all of which add additional safety concerns with MRI scanning and introduce the potential for significant image artifact. Given these considerations, it is generally optimal for patients with NF2 to consistently undergo imaging at the same center for all evaluations in order to minimize factors that may make comparisons difficult and to ensure the images are interpreted at a center that specializes in NF2.

Table 79.3 Consensus imaging recommendations for NF2-associated intracranial tumors

Volumetric sequence for vestibular schwannoma and meningiomas			
Axial T1 post-contrast	**Recommended range**	**Internal auditory canal**	**Whole brain**
Echo train length	1–3	1–3	1–3
TR	5–800	5–800	5–800
TE	2–20	2–20	2–20
Slice thickness	1–5 mm	1 mm	1–5 mm
Skip	0	0	0
Matrix	216 × 216 – 512 × 512	216 × 216 – 512 × 512	320 × 256 – 512 × 512
FOV	15–25 cm	15–18 cm	15–25 cm

Abbreviations: FOV, field of view; NF2, neurofibromatosis type 2; TE, echo time; TR, repetition time.
Source: Used with permission from Dombi E, Ardern-Holmes SL, Babovic-Vuksanovic D, et al. REiNS International Collaboration. Recommendations for imaging tumor response in neurofibromatosis clinical trials. Neurology. 2013; 81(21) Suppl 1:S33–S40.

Detecting tumor progression can be challenging, as there is variability in the approaches to assessment of tumor size. The recommended standard based on test–retest and intraobserver reliability and improved sensitivity for detection of change is volumetric analysis.[43] Currently, the process required for volumetric assessment is not uniformly supported by third-party payers and therefore is not yet widely available despite the evidence that supports its use. Furthermore, volumetric analysis of multiple tumors on serial MRI studies may be time consuming and not practical during the time allotted for a patient's clinical consult, although this is the most accurate assessment for VS change over time. As discussed earlier, growth rates for tumors in NF2 are highly variable with periods of growth and plateau that cannot be predicted. It is this variability in tumor growth behavior in NF2 that makes regular follow-up with specialized and consistent brain imaging as well as detailed assessment for both long- and short-term changes an important recommendation.

79.11 Audiometric Parameters

Audiometric findings in NF2 are often nonspecific and variable. Patients with asymmetrical or sudden sensorineural hearing loss (SNHL) are likely to be referred early for MRI screening; however, those with more symmetrical patterns of SNHL or indolent progression are at greater risk of experiencing diagnostic delay. Patients will commonly have a decrease in word recognition score (WRS) out of proportion to pure-tone thresholds—a characteristic finding of retrocochlear lesions. While other screening methods such as acoustic immittance testing or auditory brain responses are commonly discussed when reviewing diagnostic evaluation for NF2, these measures are now primarily of historical interest.

Following diagnosis, patients with NF2 are commonly followed with serial audiometry to assist in optimal aural rehabilitation and guide clinical decision making. Given that hearing loss affects almost all patients with NF2 by their third decade, hearing function is a critical endpoint in clinical trials for patients with NF2. A consensus statement was issued in 2013, endorsing clinically meaningful improvement in WRS, defined as exceeding the 95% confidence interval for the WRS change, as a primary hearing endpoint in an effort to provide a uniform reporting method for clinical trials.[32] This statement may be applicable to other studies involving VS in the non-NF2 population and is commonly used as a prime consideration for initiating therapy, as the WRS is the measure that most closely reflects a person's ability to communicate socially and therefore has a major impact on meaningful function.

79.11.1 Vestibular Function

In addition to bilateral hearing loss, patients inevitably experience bilateral loss of vestibular function, leading to oscillopsia (the movement of the visual scene with head movements) and risk of falling or even drowning. With absence of visual cues (e.g., in a dark room or at night) and proprioception (walking on thick carpet or sand, or while swimming), humans are dependent on their vestibular system to maintain upright posture and to keep their gaze fixed on a target. Patients with advanced NF2 are at risk for falls related to loss of vestibular function or drowning due to an inability to orient underwater without the benefit of inner ear gravity receptors. Training with a physical therapist who specialized in vestibular physical therapy may benefit patients, and educating patients and their families about these risks is required.

79.11.2 Genetic Testing

Molecular diagnosis includes testing for mutations involving chromosome 22. The specifics of the types of mutations in chromosome 22 that lead to symptomatic expression of NF2 are addressed in detail in Chapters 5 and 78. However, it is important to bear in mind a few specific points about molecular testing in NF2 as they pertain to clinical presentation and manifestations. Patients with protein-truncating mutations (frameshift or nonsense mutations) tend to present at an early age (< 20 years), have multiple intracranial and spinal tumors, and consequently have a poorer overall prognosis. Missense mutations generally lead to a milder presentation of the disease.[3,16] In the approximately 50% of cases that are familial, there tends to be less phenotypic variability among the family members compared to between families. About half of cases of NF2 are *de novo* mutations, and 20 to 30% of these patients are mosaic for an *NF2* mutation.[45] Approximately 60% of patients who meet the Manchester diagnostic criteria for NF2 without a family history of NF2 will have an identifiable mutation in blood.[46] This sensitivity is higher in patients with a family history of NF2 (93%) and in younger patients (80% in patients < 20 years).[46] The false-negative rate is likely the result of mosaicism or patients with schwannomatosis and overlapping findings.[10]

79.11.3 Counseling Families at the Time of Diagnosis

After the initial diagnosis of NF2 is established, ongoing clinical management from a multidisciplinary team with expertise in NF2 is important. It is critical to emphasize to patients and their families at the time of diagnosis that NF2 requires long-term, regular follow-up with a team of experts including otolaryngologists, neurologists, neurosurgeons, ophthalmologists, geneticists, and physiatrists in coordination with the primary care team due to the likelihood of acquiring additional lesions or disease progression requiring serial interventions that all need to balance short- and long-term cumulative risks and benefits.[30] In fact, there is evidence to suggest that care at an NF2 specialty clinic with multidisciplinary decision making is associated with improved long-term outcomes.[22,47]

References

[1] Evans DG, Howard E, Giblin C, et al. Birth incidence and prevalence of tumor-prone syndromes: estimates from a UK family genetic register service. Am J Med Genet A. 2010; 152A(2):327–332

[2] Evans DG, Huson SM, Donnai D, et al. A clinical study of type 2 neurofibromatosis. Q J Med. 1992; 84(304):603–618

[3] Hexter A, Jones A, Joe H, et al. English Specialist NF2 Research Group. Clinical and molecular predictors of mortality in neurofibromatosis 2: a UK national analysis of 1192 patients. J Med Genet. 2015; 52(10):699–705

[4] The Consensus Development Panel. National Institutes of Health Consensus Development Conference Statement on Acoustic Neuroma, December 11–13, 1991. Arch Neurol. 1994; 51(2):201–207

[5] Evans DGR. Neurofibromatosis type 2 (NF2): a clinical and molecular review. Orphanet J Rare Dis. 2009; 4(1):16

[6] Hadfield KD, Smith MJ, Urquhart JE, et al. Rates of loss of heterozygosity and mitotic recombination in NF2 schwannomas, sporadic vestibular schwannomas and schwannomatosis schwannomas. Oncogene. 2010; 29(47):6216–6221

[7] Baser ME, Friedman JM, Joe H, et al. Empirical development of improved diagnostic criteria for neurofibromatosis 2. Genet Med. 2011; 13(6):576–581

[8] van den Munckhof P, Christiaans I, Kenter SB, Baas F, Hulsebos TJM. Germline SMARCB1 mutation predisposes to multiple meningiomas and schwannomas with preferential location of cranial meningiomas at the falx cerebri. Neurogenetics. 2012; 13(1):1–7

[9] Evans DG, Freeman S, Gokhale C, et al. Manchester NF2 service. Bilateral vestibular schwannomas in older patients: NF2 or chance? J Med Genet. 2015; 52(6):422–424

[10] Smith MJ, Bowers NL, Bulman M, et al. Revisiting neurofibromatosis type 2 diagnostic criteria to exclude LZTR1-related schwannomatosis. Neurology. 2017; 88(1):87–92

[11] Melean G, Velasco A, Hernández-Imaz E, et al. RNA-based analysis of two SMARCB1 mutations associated with familial schwannomatosis with meningiomas. Neurogenetics. 2012; 13(3):267–274

[12] Evans DG, Huson SM, Donnai D, et al. A genetic study of type 2 neurofibromatosis in the United Kingdom. II. Guidelines for genetic counselling. J Med Genet. 1992; 29(12):847–852

[13] Gutmann DH, Aylsworth A, Carey JC, et al. The diagnostic evaluation and multidisciplinary management of neurofibromatosis 1 and neurofibromatosis 2. JAMA. 1997; 278(1):51–57

[14] Holman MA, Schmitt WR, Carlson ML, Driscoll CLW, Beatty CW, Link MJ. Pediatric cerebellopontine angle and internal auditory canal tumors: clinical article. J Neurosurg Pediatr. 2013; 12(4):317–324

[15] Walcott BP, Sivarajan G, Bashinskaya B, Anderson DE, Leonetti JP, Origitano TC. Sporadic unilateral vestibular schwannoma in the pediatric population. Clinical article. J Neurosurg Pediatr. 2009; 4(2):125–129

[16] Baser ME, Friedman JM, Wallace AJ, Ramsden RT, Joe H, Evans DGR. Evaluation of clinical diagnostic criteria for neurofibromatosis 2. Neurology. 2002; 59(11):1759–1765

[17] MacCollin M, Chiocca EA, Evans DG, et al. Diagnostic criteria for schwannomatosis. Neurology. 2005; 64(11):1838–1845

[18] Plotkin SR, Albers AC, Babovic-Vuksanovic D, et al. Update from the 2013 international neurofibromatosis conference. Am J Med Genet A. 2014; 164A (12):2969–2978

[19] Asthagiri AR, Parry DM, Butman JA, et al. Neurofibromatosis type 2. Lancet. 2009; 373(9679):1974–1986

[20] Mautner V-F, Baser ME, Thakkar SD, Feigen UM, Friedman JM, Kluwe L. Vestibular schwannoma growth in patients with neurofibromatosis Type 2: a longitudinal study. J Neurosurg. 2002; 96(2):223–228

[21] Lawson McLean AC, Rosahl SK. Growth dynamics of intracranial tumors in patients with neurofibromatosis type 2. World Neurosurg. 2017; 98: 152–161

[22] Baser ME, Makariou EV, Parry DM. Predictors of vestibular schwannoma growth in patients with neurofibromatosis type 2. J Neurosurg. 2002; 96(2): 217–222

[23] Choi JW, Lee JY, Phi JH, et al. Clinical course of vestibular schwannoma in pediatric neurofibromatosis type 2. J Neurosurg Pediatr. 2014; 13(6):650–657

[24] Blakeley JO, Evans DG, Adler J, et al. Consensus recommendations for current treatments and accelerating clinical trials for patients with neurofibromatosis type 2. Am J Med Genet A. 2012; 158A(1):24–41

[25] Lalwani AK, Abaza MM, Makariou EV, Armstrong M. Audiologic presentation of vestibular schwannomas in neurofibromatosis type 2. Am J Otol. 1998; 19 (3):352–357

[26] Slattery WH, III, Fisher LM, Iqbal Z, Oppenhiemer M. Vestibular schwannoma growth rates in neurofibromatosis type 2 natural history consortium subjects. Otol Neurotol. 2004; 25(5):811–817

[27] Masuda A, Fisher LM, Oppenheimer ML, Iqbal Z, Slattery WH, Natural History Consortium. Hearing changes after diagnosis in neurofibromatosis type 2. Otol Neurotol. 2004; 25(2):150–154

[28] Fisher LM, Doherty JK, Lev MH, Slattery WH. Concordance of bilateral vestibular schwannoma growth and hearing changes in neurofibromatosis 2: neurofibromatosis 2 natural history consortium. Otol Neurotol. 2009; 30(6):835–841

[29] Plotkin SR, Merker VL, Muzikansky A, Barker FG, II, Slattery W, III. Natural history of vestibular schwannoma growth and hearing decline in newly diagnosed neurofibromatosis type 2 patients. Otol Neurotol. 2014; 35(1):e50–e56

[30] Blakeley JO, Plotkin SR. Therapeutic advances for the tumors associated with neurofibromatosis type 1, type 2, and schwannomatosis. Neuro-oncol. 2016; 18(5):624–638

[31] Fisher LM, Doherty JK, Lev MH, Slattery WH, III. Distribution of nonvestibular cranial nerve schwannomas in neurofibromatosis 2. Otol Neurotol. 2007; 28 (8):1083–1090

[32] Plotkin SR, Ardern-Holmes SL, Barker FG, II, et al. REiNS International Collaboration. Hearing and facial function outcomes for neurofibromatosis 2 clinical trials. Neurology. 2013; 81(21) Suppl 1:S25–S32

[33] Goutagny S, Bah AB, Henin D, et al. Long-term follow-up of 287 meningiomas in neurofibromatosis type 2 patients: clinical, radiological, and molecular features. Neuro-oncol. 2012; 14(8):1090–1096

[34] Aboukais R, Zairi F, Baroncini M, et al. Intracranial meningiomas and neurofibromatosis type 2. Acta Neurochir (Wien). 2013; 155(6):997–1001, discussion 1001

[35] Halliday AL, Sobel RA, Martuza RL. Benign spinal nerve sheath tumors: their occurrence sporadically and in neurofibromatosis types 1 and 2. J Neurosurg. 1991; 74(2):248–253

[36] Mautner VF, Lindenau M, Baser ME, et al. The neuroimaging and clinical spectrum of neurofibromatosis 2. Neurosurgery. 1996; 38(5):880–885, discussion 885–886

[37] Hagel C, Stemmer-Rachamimov AO, Bornemann A, et al. Clinical presentation, immunohistochemistry and electron microscopy indicate neurofibromatosis type 2-associated gliomas to be spinal ependymomas. Neuropathology. 2012; 32(6):611–616

[38] Plotkin SR, O'Donnell CC, Curry WT, Bove CM, MacCollin M, Nunes FP. Spinal ependymomas in neurofibromatosis Type 2: a retrospective analysis of 55 patients. J Neurosurg Spine. 2011; 14(4):543–547

[39] Morris KA, Afridi SK, Evans DG, et al. on behalf of the UK NF2 Research Group. The response of spinal cord ependymomas to bevacizumab in patients with neurofibromatosis Type 2. J Neurosurg Spine. 2017; 26(4):474–482

[40] Bouzas EA, Freidlin V, Parry DM, Eldridge R, Kaiser-Kupfer MI. Lens opacities in neurofibromatosis 2: further significant correlations. Br J Ophthalmol. 1993; 77(6):354–357

[41] Evans DG. Neurofibromatosis 2. In: Pagon RA, Adam MP, Ardinger HH, eds. GeneReviews. Seattle: University of Washington; 1993

[42] Meyers SM, Gutman FA, Kaye LD, Rothner AD. Retinal changes associated with neurofibromatosis 2. Trans Am Ophthalmol Soc. 1995; 93:245–252, discussion 252–257

[43] Dombi E, Ardern-Holmes SL, Babovic-Vuksanovic D, et al. REiNS International Collaboration. Recommendations for imaging tumor response in neurofibromatosis clinical trials. Neurology. 2013; 81(21) Suppl 1:S33–S40

[44] Harris GJ, Plotkin SR, Maccollin M, et al. Three-dimensional volumetrics for tracking vestibular schwannoma growth in neurofibromatosis type II. Neurosurgery. 2008; 62(6):1314–1319, discussion 1319–1320

[45] Kluwe L, Mautner V, Heinrich B, et al. Molecular study of frequency of mosaicism in neurofibromatosis 2 patients with bilateral vestibular schwannomas. J Med Genet. 2003; 40(2):109–114

[46] Evans DG, Raymond FL, Barwell JG, Halliday D. Genetic testing and screening of individuals at risk of NF2. Clin Genet. 2012; 82(5):416–424

[47] Evans DGR, Baser ME, O'Reilly B, et al. Management of the patient and family with neurofibromatosis 2: a consensus conference statement. Br J Neurosurg. 2005; 19(1):5–12

80 Natural History of Vestibular Schwannoma Growth and Hearing in Neurofibromatosis Type 2

Michel Kalamarides, Matthieu Peyre, Daniele Bernardeschi, and Olivier Sterkers

80.1 Introduction

Bilateral vestibular schwannomas (VSs) are the hallmark of neurofibromatosis type 2 (NF2) and are present in 90 to 95% of patients with NF2.[1] VSs are slow-growing benign tumors and inescapably cause bilateral deafness in most patients. To critically evaluate the results of the available treatments, the authors have reviewed the published natural history of VS in NF2, focusing on the patterns and factors influencing tumor growth and the patterns and mechanisms of hearing loss.

80.2 Growth Rate and Growth Patterns

During the last decade, the evolution of imaging techniques has led to the consensus that three-dimensional volumetric measurements are significantly more sensitive to change than single linear diameter measurements.[2] Linear measures underestimate the volumetric growth of VS. This finding was seen for overall growth rates, annual growth rates, and determination of tumor progression. While linear measurements are performed for ease of use and are suitable for most malignant lesions that rapidly change in size, they are inappropriate for benign slow-growing tumors such as VSs, for which volumetric analysis of MRIs has been recommended.[3]

The natural history of bilateral VS in NF2 has been thoroughly described in several studies, emphasizing their highly variable growth rates[4,5,6,7,8,9,10,11] (▶ Table 80.1). In publications focusing on patients treated with conservative management, the mean VS growth rates ranged from 0.4 mm/year[12] to 1.8 mm/year.[13] In other cohorts, the mean annual growth rates of NF2-related VS were higher (Harris et al[2]: 8.9 mm/year, Dirks et al[8]: 8.4 mm/year). The first two cohorts suffer from selection bias, as fast-growing tumors ineligible for conservative treatment were excluded from their studies. The last two cohorts suffer from a small cohort size—15 and 18 tumors, respectively. When attempting to classify enlarging VSs according to growth rate, 31% may be defined as slow-growing (growth rate: < 1 mm/year) and 25% as fast-growing (growth rate: > 3 mm/year), while 44% have intermediate growth rates.

Several studies have reported that linear diameter growth rates, but not volumes, of left- and right-sided VS in the same patient are strongly correlated.[4,6,7,13] Conversely, in their cohort of 29 patients harboring 58 VSs, Slattery and colleagues[9] found a significant relationship between the sizes of left and right VS at a precise time point (baseline and end of follow-up) but not between the growth rates of the tumors. In a 2013 publication from our center, we showed that before the first surgery, bilateral VSs tend to have similar growth rates. We postulated that despite their intrinsic similar growth rates, bilateral VSs often present at different sizes at diagnosis, depending on the timing of the second hit leading to biallelic inactivation of the *NF2* gene (the first hit being the germline or mosaic mutation).[14] However, we believe that this small correlation does not validate the use of a contralateral VS as an internal control for studies evaluating unilateral radiosurgery effects on tumor growth, as previously reported.

In a recent study by Dirks et al with long-term follow-up of VS in NF2 patients, the authors suggested that all VSs eventually grow over time.[8] Despite long follow-up (mean: 9.5 years), this study suffers from a small cohort size (17 patients) and from selection bias with most patients presenting with more severe phenotypes and high tumor burden.

Spontaneous shrinkage can also occur during radiological follow-up, which must be taken into consideration when examining the efficacy of radiosurgery and medical therapy. In our study, we found that 14% (13/92) displayed shrinkage or no growth but with a shorter radiological follow-up (mean: 4.2 years).[13] Similarly, others have shown that VS may spontaneously decrease in size over time.[9] In a series of 56 patients with 84 VSs, Slattery et al found some degree of size regression in 19% of tumors (16 of 84): 7 of 16 decreased less than 1 mm in size and 13 tumors less than 2 mm. Most interestingly, one tumor regressed almost 7 mm in short-term follow-up. In the most recent and largest study to date on 102 patients, Plotkin et al[15] reported a 25% rate of spontaneous tumor shrinkage, defined as a decrease in tumor volume of 20% or greater. However, about one-third of tumors failed to maintain tumor shrinkage during follow-up and 25% of concerned patients demonstrated tumor shrinkage only at their last study visit, questioning the durability of such a phenomenon. Dirks et al demonstrated the existence of saltatory growth patterns for 47% of VSs and suggested that previous studies may have incorrectly classified tumors as nongrowing while they were actually quiescent over the course of the study.[8] However, this observation relies on a small number of tumors (18 tumors in 12 patients) and nonvolumetric analysis of growth.

80.3 Factors Influencing Vestibular Schwannoma Growth

Patients with NF2 may present with disease phenotypes of varying severity—mild NF2 with bilateral VSs presenting in adulthood (mean age: 22–27 years) often as the only feature and severe NF2 with multiple rapidly progressing CNS tumors other than VS, which may present first usually in childhood. As young age is classically a characteristic of the most severe disease form, there is a preconception that VS will grow more rapidly in younger patients. Most natural history studies confirm that VS growth rates tend to decrease with increasing age. Ito and colleagues[7] have also suggested that in NF2 patients, age at onset represents a more important factor than multiplicity of tumors for predicting clinical course. One may therefore speculate that the younger the age at onset, the faster the tumor will grow. Case reports of NF2 with onset before the age of 1 year have demonstrated that VS growth was not progressive over

Table 80.1 Natural history of vestibular schwannomas in NF2 patients

	Number of patients	Number of vestibular schwannomas	Mean age at onset of signs (y)	Mean clinical follow-up (y)	Mean radiological follow-up (y)	Mean tumor size at baseline (mm)	Mean growth rate (mm or mm^3/y)	Growth patterns[a]	Factors influencing tumor growth
Mautner et al (2002)	37	64	12	–	3.9	–	–	Linear, logarithmic, **sigmoid**, irregular	Age at diagnosis
Baser et al (2002)	25	38	17.6	–	4	–	–	–	Age at diagnosis
Slattery et al (2004)	56	84	–	1.1	1	10	1.3	–	Age at diagnosis
Harris et al (2008)	10	15	29.4	–	2.6	–	8.9	–	–
Dirks et al (2012)	17	18	33.2	9.5	–	–	8.4	Linear, exponential, **saltatory**	None
Peyre et al (2013)	46	92	25.5	6.0	4.2	17	1.8	–	Age at diagnosis
Kontorinis et al (2014)	56	89	28.9	7	–	13	0.4	–	–
Li et al (2015)	66	74	29.1	–	4.9	*642 mm^3*	*257 mm^3*	–	Age at diagnosis
Picry et al (2016)	18	26	26.1	–	5.6	*731 mm^3*	*218 cm^3* (0.9 mm)	–	*NF2* mutation

Abbreviation: NF2, neurofibromatosis type 2.
[a]Dominant growth patterns are indicated in bold.

the years but was rather found to be slow with bursts of acceleration during pubertal period.[16]

Another factor influencing VS growth is surgical resection of the contralateral tumor. In a recent study on 11 NF2 patients,[17] an increase of VS growth in the remaining VS was observed after the removal of the first tumor when both tumors threaten the brainstem. Before the first surgery, growth patterns were similar in 9 of 11 cases. After the first surgery, the growth rate of the remaining VS was significantly accelerated compared with the preoperative period (2.5 ± 2.2 vs. 4.4 ± 3.4 mm/year; p = 0.01, Wilcoxon's test). This result has been recently confirmed in a larger series of VS.[10] One can speculate on two main mechanisms accounting for this result. On the one hand, a pure mechanic effect could be suggested. Because both tumors compress the brainstem, the importance of the global tumor burden in the posterior fossa could slow down tumor growth. Therefore, surgery of one of the VS might accelerate the growth rate of the remaining tumor as a result of the absence of counterpressure. On the other hand, the presence of paracrine factors in the cerebrospinal fluid could explain this observation. The increase of VS growth was statistically more important in young NF2 patients. In addition, von Eckardstein et al[18] published two astonishing cases of spontaneous VS regression occurring after resection of the contralateral tumor. In the first case, the maximum posterior fossa diameters of the tumors were 39 and 27 mm, but in the other patient, tumors were smaller and one of them was a recurrence. In our study, the most striking increases in postoperative velocity of diametric expansion were seen in the youngest patients, and one may therefore postulate that similar to basal tumor growth, postoperative tumor growth may be highly dependent on patient age.[17] Circulating growth factors might also influence VS growth. In our study, we were able to show that in two patients who had similar VS sizes at diagnosis, the discrepancy of growth over time was potentially due to the contact of an NF2-related tumor. Pallini et al[19] have also reported the case of an NF2 patient in whom the contact established by a VS and a meningioma at the tentorial incisura may have increased the growth rate of both VS. In this study, the authors demonstrated the presence of growth factor with EGF-like properties in the CSF of the corresponding patient. Together, these two cases raise the question of a possible autocrine/paracrine mechanism responsible for tumor growth in adjacent tumors of NF2 patients. Further analysis of growth factors in the CSF of NF2 patients is mandatory to explore this interesting hypothesis.

80.4 Hearing Evaluation, Natural History of Hearing, and Mechanisms of Hearing Loss

As hearing preservation is one of the main goals in NF2 management, a thorough evaluation of hearing in all patients with NF2 is mandatory in order to detect early audiometric decline. Following recent recommendations for hearing endpoints in NF2-related VS trials,[20] maximum speech discrimination score (SDS) was defined as the primary endpoint and hearing decline was defined as a statistically significant decrease in speech discrimination.

Table 80.2 Hearing outcome of NF2 patients with vestibular schwannoma

	Number of patients	Number of ears	Mean age at onset of signs (y)	Mean clinical follow-up (y)	Serviceable hearing at presentation	Serviceable hearing at the end of follow-up	Time to loss of serviceability (y)	Factors influencing hearing loss
Asthagiri et al (2012)	56	84	21.7	–	50 (62%)	–	–	Tumor size
Peyre et al (2013)	46	92	25.5	6.0	39 (85%)	34 (74%)	5	No correlation with tumor size and growth rate
Kontorinis et al (2014)	56	89	28.9	7	70 (78.6%)	59 (66.3%)	7.6	No correlation with tumor size and growth rate

Abbreviation: NF2, neurofibromatosis type 2.

Patterns of hearing loss in NF2 have been investigated (▶ Table 80.2). In the publication by Asthagiri et al[21] focusing on 89 ears in 56 patients, the authors reported that hearing loss occurred gradually over months to years in 35% of ears, in a stepwise manner characterized by periodic decrements of hearing associated with intervening periods of stable hearing in 29% of patients, in a relapsing-remitting pattern defined by periodic decrements in hearing coupled with periods of partial recovery in 12% of patients, or in a sudden and complete fashion in 15% of patients.

The mechanisms of hearing loss in NF2 patients are not well understood. Direct compression and stretching of the cochlear nerve by the enlarging tumor has been implicated, directly linking tumor enlargement and hearing loss. However, this somewhat intuitive relationship has never been adequately confirmed. Fisher et al[22] focused on 1-year evaluations and used only pure-tone average (PTA) for the evaluation of hearing. The authors concluded that a significant worsening in hearing occurred over a 1-year period without a significant statistical association with concomitant tumor growth. In our study of bilateral VS in NF2 patients managed with conservative observation,[13] we identified a high rate of serviceable hearing preservation at the end of a 6-year follow-up (74%) but with only 66% of patients (22/33) conserving binaural serviceable hearing. We confirmed that hearing progression in NF2 patients with bilateral VS was not statistically correlated with tumor growth rate. In the series of 56 NF2 patients published by Kontorinis et al,[12] the authors demonstrated that patients with NF2 and indolently behaving tumors had a slow deterioration in hearing, with approximately 65% of patients with serviceable hearing at presentation preserving serviceable hearing over a 7-year period. There was no correlation between tumor size and change in PTA. Despite the absence of a statistical correlation, Bernardeschi et al[23] demonstrated in a series of 21 NF2 patients that middle fossa decompression, consisting of a drilling and enlargement of the roof of the internal auditory canal, could prolong hearing in patients with hearing changes in an only hearing ear. Moreover, the presence of hearing loss was statistically correlated with larger tumor volume at presentation in our series and the study by Asthagiri et al.[21] This correlation was not supported by Plotkin et al,[15] while they found an association between large tumor volume at presentation and increased risk of hearing decline during the study period. In their series of 54 NF2 patients harboring 76 VSs, they demonstrated that the median time to hearing decline was 62 months after a mean follow-up of 31.3 months. However, the serviceability of hearing was not specifically analyzed. In the same study, the median time to tumor growth (14 months) was significantly shorter than the time to hearing decline, making it unlikely to be captured in short-term study.

As most natural history studies do not find any correlation between tumor growth rate and hearing loss, Asthagiri et al studied the role of elevated intralabyrinthine protein, demonstrated on T2-FLAIR MRI sequences, and cochlear aperture obstruction, as defined by the absence of a patent cerebrospinal fluid pathway between the posterior fossa and the cochlear aperture.[21] In a series of 89 ears in 56 consecutive patients, there was a strong correlation between normal intralabyrinthine protein and normal hearing (20/22 ears, 91%), while ears with hearing loss had frequent elevated intralabyrinthine protein (35/37 ears, 91%). In another series of 49 ears in 32 NF2 patients reported by the same authors,[24] they found a significant association between elevated intralabyrinthine protein and hearing loss; yet, 36.7% of ears had elevated protein with normal hearing. Cochlear aperture obstruction was not correlated to hearing loss. The presence of intralabyrinthine tumor may also explain elevation of intralabyrinthine protein. In a cadaveric study of 26 temporal bones in 16 patients harboring NF2, Nam et al[25] reported multicentric tumors in 81% of patients and 73% of ears. Intralabyrinthine schwannomas were discovered in 88% of ears (developed in the cochlea, vestibule, and/or semicircular canals) that were, most of the time, anatomically separated from the tumor within the internal auditory canal.

Other mechanisms of hearing loss have been hypothesized in NF2 such as intralabyrinthine hemorrhage and endolymphatic hydrops. In the study of Asthagiri et al,[21] intralabyrinthine hemorrhage was never encountered and endolymphatic hydrops was found in 8% of ears but was equally distributed between normal hearing ears and ears with hearing loss. The interested reader is encouraged to review Chapters 14 and 51 for additional discussion pertaining to the topic of this chapter.

80.5 Conclusion

In order to accurately monitor VS natural history in NF2 patients, tumor growth should be assessed using three-dimensional volumetric analysis every 6 months in the case of growing tumors or annually in stable tumors. Hearing should be evaluated using PTA and SDS with monosyllabic words. Monitoring of tumor growth could be reported using time to tumor progression and monitoring of hearing loss using time to hearing decline.

References

[1] Evans DG. Neurofibromatosis type 2 (NF2): a clinical and molecular review. Orphanet J Rare Dis. 2009; 4:16

[2] Harris GJ, Plotkin SR, Maccollin M, et al. Three-dimensional volumetrics for tracking vestibular schwannoma growth in neurofibromatosis type II. Neurosurgery. 2008; 62(6):1314–1319, discussion 1319–1320

[3] Dombi E, Ardern-Holmes SL, Babovic-Vuksanovic D, et al. REiNS International Collaboration. Recommendations for imaging tumor response in neurofibromatosis clinical trials. Neurology. 2013; 81(21) Suppl 1:S33–S40

[4] Baser ME, Makariou EV, Parry DM. Predictors of vestibular schwannoma growth in patients with neurofibromatosis Type 2. J Neurosurg. 2002; 96(2): 217–222

[5] Baser ME, Mautner VF, Parry DM, Evans DG. Methodological issues in longitudinal studies: vestibular schwannoma growth rates in neurofibromatosis 2. J Med Genet. 2005; 42(12):903–906

[6] Mautner VF, Baser ME, Thakkar SD, Feigen UM, Friedman JM, Kluwe L. Vestibular schwannoma growth in patients with neurofibromatosis Type 2: a longitudinal study. J Neurosurg. 2002; 96(2):223–228

[7] Ito E, Saito K, Yatsuya H, Nagatani T, Otsuka G. Factors predicting growth of vestibular schwannoma in neurofibromatosis type 2. Neurosurg Rev. 2009; 32(4):425–433

[8] Dirks MS, Butman JA, Kim HJ, et al. Long-term natural history of neurofibromatosis Type 2-associated intracranial tumors. J Neurosurg. 2012; 117(1): 109–117

[9] Slattery WH, III, Fisher LM, Iqbal Z, Oppenhiemer M. Vestibular schwannoma growth rates in neurofibromatosis type 2 natural history consortium subjects. Otol Neurotol. 2004; 25(5):811–817

[10] Li H, Hao SY, Wang L, et al. Factors influencing the growth rate of vestibular schwannoma in patients with neurofibromatosis type 2. Acta Neurochir (Wien). 2015; 157(11):1983–1990

[11] Picry A, Bonne NX, Ding J, et al. Long-term growth rate of vestibular schwannoma in neurofibromatosis 2: a volumetric consideration. Laryngoscope. 2016; 126(10):2358–2362

[12] Kontorinis G, Nichani J, Freeman SR, et al. Progress of hearing loss in neurofibromatosis type 2: implications for future management. Eur Arch Otorhinolaryngol. 2015; 272(11):3143–3150

[13] Peyre M, Goutagny S, Bah A, et al. Conservative management of bilateral vestibular schwannomas in neurofibromatosis type 2 patients: hearing and tumor growth results. Neurosurgery. 2013; 72(6):907–913, discussion 914, quiz 914

[14] Hadfield KD, Smith MJ, Urquhart JE, et al. Rates of loss of heterozygosity and mitotic recombination in NF2 schwannomas, sporadic vestibular schwannomas and schwannomatosis schwannomas. Oncogene. 2010; 29 (47):6216–6221

[15] Plotkin SR, Merker VL, Muzikansky A, Barker FG, II, Slattery W, III. Natural history of vestibular schwannoma growth and hearing decline in newly diagnosed neurofibromatosis type 2 patients. Otol Neurotol. 2014; 35(1):e50–e56

[16] Ruggieri M, Gabriele AL, Polizzi A, et al. Natural history of neurofibromatosis type 2 with onset before the age of 1 year. Neurogenetics. 2013; 14(2):89–98

[17] Peyre M, Goutagny S, Imbeaud S, et al. Increased growth rate of vestibular schwannoma after resection of contralateral tumor in neurofibromatosis type 2. Neuro-oncol. 2011; 13(10):1125–1132

[18] von Eckardstein KL, Beatty CW, Driscoll CL, Link MJ. Spontaneous regression of vestibular schwannomas after resection of contralateral tumor in neurofibromatosis Type 2. J Neurosurg. 2010; 112(1):158–162

[19] Pallini R, Tancredi A, Casalbore P, et al. Neurofibromatosis type 2: growth stimulation of mixed acoustic schwannoma by concurrent adjacent meningioma: possible role of growth factors. Case report. J Neurosurg. 1998; 89(1): 149–154

[20] Plotkin SR, Ardern-Holmes SL, Barker FG, II, et al. REiNS International Collaboration. Hearing and facial function outcomes for neurofibromatosis 2 clinical trials. Neurology. 2013; 81(21) Suppl 1:S25–S32

[21] Asthagiri AR, Vasquez RA, Butman JA, et al. Mechanisms of hearing loss in neurofibromatosis type 2. PLoS One. 2012; 7(9):e46132

[22] Fisher LM, Doherty JK, Lev MH, Slattery WH. Concordance of bilateral vestibular schwannoma growth and hearing changes in neurofibromatosis 2: neurofibromatosis 2 natural history consortium. Otol Neurotol. 2009; 30(6): 835–841

[23] Bernardeschi D, Peyre M, Collin M, Smail M, Sterkers O, Kalamarides M. Internal auditory canal decompression for hearing maintenance in neurofibromatosis type 2 patients. Neurosurgery. 2015

[24] Holliday MA, Kim HJ, Zalewski CK, et al. Audiovestibular characteristics of small cochleovestibular schwannomas in neurofibromatosis type 2. Otolaryngol Head Neck Surg. 2014; 151(1):117–124

[25] Nam S-I, Linthicum FH, Jr, Merchant SN. Temporal bone histopathology in neurofibromatosis type 2. Laryngoscope. 2011; 121(7):1548–1554

81 Microsurgery for Neurofibromatosis Type 2 Focusing on Vestibular Schwannoma

Marc S. Schwartz and Gregory P. Lekovic

81.1 Introduction

The hallmark of neurofibromatosis type 2 (NF2) is the development of bilateral vestibular schwannomas (VSs). NF2 is caused by mutation of the *NF2* gene on the 22nd chromosome, which is inherited in an autosomal dominant fashion. About half of all NF2 patients are originators, presenting with a new mutation. The incidence of NF2 is approximately 1/33,000, with no ethnic or racial predilections.[1]

In addition to VSs, patients with NF2 develop other tumors, including schwannomas, meningiomas, and ependymomas, in other locations in the neuroaxis. The phenotypic expression of NF2 is highly variable. Patients with more severe disease may present in adolescence with numerous large, rapidly growing tumors, while more mildly affected individuals present in middle age with only small VSs. Traditionally, NF2 has been subcategorized into either the more severe Wishart type or the more mild Gardner type.[2] More recently, mosaic forms of NF2 have also been recognized.[3] It is probably best, however, to view NF2 as occurring along a continuum of severity.

Since NF2 is not uniform in its presentation, it is impossible to make firm recommendations as to the best surgical treatment in all cases. Indeed, it is critical to understand that treatment must be individualized. Over-riding pronouncements about "the best" or "the worst" treatment must be taken with due skepticism.

81.2 General Considerations

In considering microsurgical resection of NF2-associated VSs, there are three issues that differentiate these tumors from those seen in sporadic cases.

First and most obvious is the fact that patients with bilateral VSs are at risk for total deafness. Indeed the natural history of NF2 is one that eventually leads to profound hearing loss in most cases. Thus, preservation and rehabilitation of hearing becomes much more critical in NF2 patients than in those with sporadic tumors, who are generally at risk only for unilateral hearing loss. The goal of hearing preservation may lead in a limited number of cases to a more proactive approach to small tumors; however, in most other cases, it may lead to a less aggressive strategy of continued observation.

In addition, the risk of bilateral profound hearing loss in NF2 mandates consideration of other methods of auditory rehabilitation. Auditory brainstem implants (ABIs) have been used to restore auditory perception to patients with NF2.[4] These are generally placed at the same time as tumor resection because, in general, it is usually not feasible to preserve the cochlear nerve either anatomically or functionally. More recently, cochlear implantation has been utilized in patients with NF2 in whom cochlear nerve integrity can be maintained.[5] It is critical to understand that no current method of auditory rehabilitation can be expected to restore normal hearing. A detailed discussion regarding auditory rehabilitation for NF2 can be found in Chapter 84.

The second consideration is that NF2-associated VSs are frequently seen in combination with other tumors, either meningiomas or schwannomas of other nerves. These must be considered in the plan of resection. Most notably, tumors of the facial nerve are often encountered, making differentiation and preservation of this structure more problematic. In addition, VSs are frequently seen in collision with schwannomas of either the trigeminal nerve or of the jugular foramen. Resection of either of these types of tumor together with a VS may lead to additional morbidity. In the case of trigeminal involvement, any combination of facial and trigeminal dysfunction is likely to result in significant corneal pathology and possible vision loss. In the case of lower cranial nerve involvement, swallowing difficulties are likely to ensue.

The third consideration is the often polyclonal nature of NF2-associated VSs.[6] Although in sporadic tumors the cochlear nerve can reliably be found on the surface of the tumor mass, in NF2 all eight nerve components may run between tumor lobes. That is, it is often more useful to think of an NF2-associated tumor as a "bunch of grapes" rather than as an "orange or apple." This fact makes consideration of hearing preservation much more daunting. Indeed, the results of hearing preservation surgery in NF2, at least for larger tumors, are generally considered to be poor. Similarly, results of hearing preservation with radiosurgery are considered to be poorer than for sporadic tumors as well.[7]

81.3 Decision Making: When to Proceed with Surgery

In the setting of NF2, the decision to proceed with microsurgery, or indeed with any treatment, may be considerably more complicated than with sporadic tumors. Of course, this is not always the case. For instance, one patient may present with a large and growing tumor on a side with poor hearing, while having a small tumor and good hearing on the contralateral side. In this case, the decision to proceed with resection of the larger tumor is straightforward. Another patient may present with a large and growing tumor in his or her only hearing ear—a much more difficult problem (see Chapter 75; ▶ Fig. 81.1).

The goal of hearing preservation can be expected to hinder the achievement of other objectives in many instances. Not infrequently, a patient will present with a giant tumor on the side of an only hearing ear at the point that the goal of facial nerve preservation has already been made difficult and the goal of safe tumor resection has even been called into question. Furthermore, patients and their caregivers often deliberately watch and wait until this point is reached. It has been postulated that large NF2 tumors are apt to maintain good hearing due to the fact that cochlear fibers may traverse them rather than being stretched around them as with sporadic tumors.[8] Thus with

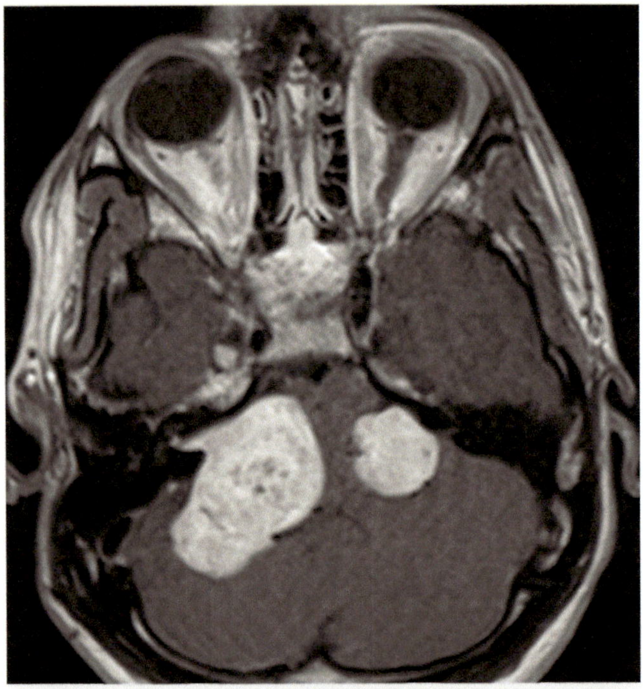

Fig. 81.1 Contrast-enhanced axial T1 MRI in a patient who presented with total hearing loss on the left and near-normal hearing on the right. The decision to remove the giant right vestibular schwannoma resulted in total deafness.

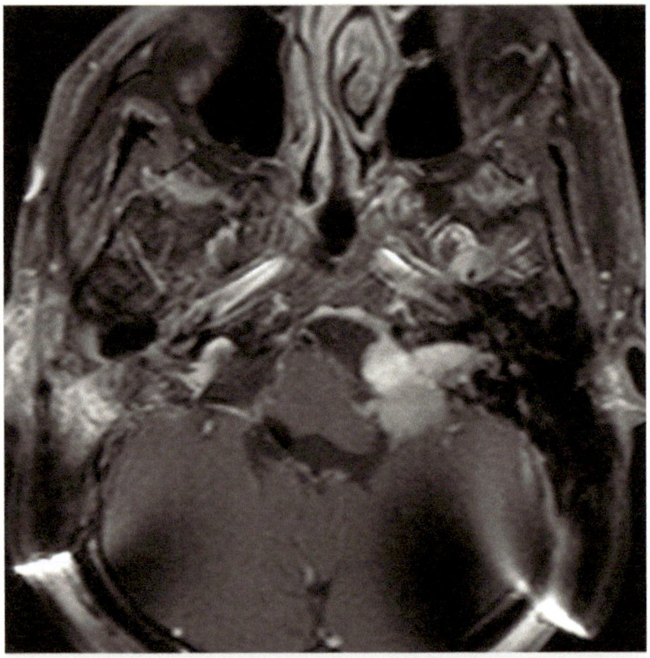

Fig. 81.2 This contrast-enhanced axial T1 MRI shows collision between a vestibular schwannoma filling the left internal auditory canal and extending into the cerebellopontine angle and a slightly less avidly enhancing meningioma based on the dura posteroinferior to the canal. The patient had previously undergone cochlear implantation on the ipsilateral side.

NF2 patients, surgeons may be placed in a position of advocating tumor resection in cases in which bilateral profound hearing loss will be the known result. Of course, this should be done only after other options, such as the use of bevacizumab, and other potential medical therapies have been exhausted (see Chapter 83).

81.4 Preoperative Evaluation

In addition to the usual considerations with VSs, potential impairment of other functions in NF2 makes further evaluation critical. Magnetic resonance imaging (MRI) of the entire brain and spine should be carried out prior to surgery. Other, larger tumors may take precedence over VSs. This depends on both tumor appearance and symptomatology. Furthermore, pathology in the cervical spine may limit operative positioning, and in cases with spinal disease somatosensory evoked potential monitoring is mandatory.

Thorough preoperative vision assessment is also necessary prior to proceeding with VS surgery in NF2 patients. Unilateral vision loss in NF2 patients is frequent and may be unrecognized.[9] Vision loss on the side contralateral to the side of planned VS surgery is of particular concern as even transient facial nerve weakness may result in significant disability in patients with good vision only ipsilaterally.

Even more critical is evaluation of vocal cord and swallowing function. Again, the particular concern is possibility of preexisting contralateral lower cranial neuropathy. Rather than being directly related to VSs, the most common cause of mortality in NF2 is lower cranial nerve dysfunction.[10] These nerves may be put at risk with VS tumor resection, and the creation of bilateral difficulties could be expected to lead to severe morbidity. Especially when resection of larger tumors is being considered, in-office flexible laryngoscopy should be part of the routine preoperative evaluation.

81.5 Tumor Resection: General Considerations

Except in cases of surgical misadventure, VSs are rarely the cause of death in patients with NF2. Medium- to giant-sized VSs may be approached via either the translabyrinthine or the retrosigmoid route, the most important consideration being surgeons' comfort.

As with sporadic tumors, there is considerable variability in tumor consistency, adherence, and vascularity. NF2-associated VSs have been shown to express more vascularity-associated growth factors than sporadic tumors, a finding which served as the basis for the initial trials with bevacizumab.[11] While the vascularity of these tumors may provide significant challenges in resection, it is the authors' experience that excessive bleeding occurs primarily from discrete vascular channels between areas of tumors of likely distinct clonal origins.

NF2-associated VSs may also be found in collision with other tumors, including meningiomas, trigeminal schwannomas, and jugular foramen schwannomas (▸ Fig. 81.2). Meningioma tissue may be found interspersed with schwannoma.[12] Resection of trigeminal schwannomas should only be considered for large trigeminal tumors with significant brainstem compression.

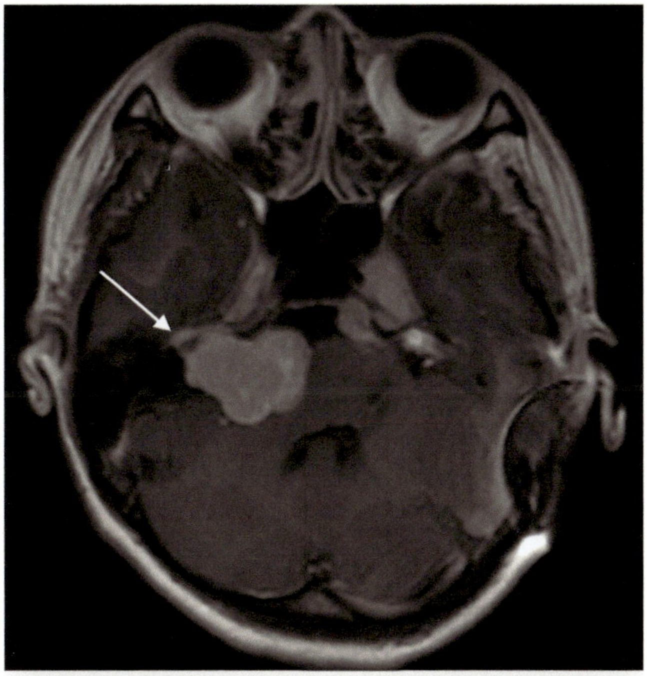

Fig. 81.3 Contrast-enhanced axial T1 MRI of an NF2 patient who had previously undergone resection of a left vestibular schwannoma with placement of an auditory brainstem implant. On the right, there is a large vestibular schwannoma, and evidence of an enhancing mass at the geniculate ganglion (*arrow*) demonstrating presence of a facial nerve schwannoma as well.

Indeed, the trigeminal nerve should be handled with great care. Surgery resulting in both motor and sensory deficits involving the eye is likely to lead to considerable disability.

Failure of airway protection is the most common cause of mortality in patients with NF2.[10] Because of this, preservation of lower cranial nerve function must be of utmost importance. It is our practice to never resect tumors arising from the lower cranial nerves unless absolutely necessary, which typically grow slowly. Indeed, even patients with preexisting ipsilateral dysfunction are likely to suffer further decline after disruption of these nerves in the posterior fossa. In the absence of ipsilateral vocal cord movement, for example, the vagal nerve may still provide laryngopharyngeal tone and sensation that may worsen considerably after lower cranial nerve schwannoma resection.

81.6 Tumor Resection: Facial Nerve

Especially in cases of more severe phenotypic expression, direct involvement of the facial nerve with tumor is common in NF2.[13] In many cases, the presence of facial nerve schwannoma can be demonstrated preoperatively on MRI (▶ Fig. 81.3). Lack of abnormal enhancement along the course of the facial nerve in the temporal bone does not, however, preclude the possibility of encountering a facial nerve tumor intraoperatively.

Of course, one of the major goals of VS resection is preservation of facial nerve function, which may be a more difficult task than in sporadic tumors. Facial nerve results have been shown to be poorer after resection of NF2-associated VSs.[13] In the interests of facial nerve preservation, surgeons should be focused on early identification of the facial nerve, which may be expanded or otherwise abnormal in appearance. Especially since schwannoma growing from the facial nerve typically grows more slowly than tumors of vestibulocochlear origin, preservation of function takes precedence over resection of facial nerve tumor.

It should also be understood that all options for facial nerve rehabilitation may not be available in NF2 patients. If continuity of the facial nerve is lost, direct grafting can be attempted. However, the peripheral sources of nerve graft may also be involved with tumor. Nerve substitution techniques, such as hypoglossal-facial anastomosis or cross-facial grafting, may not be possible due to dysfunction of donor nerves. A review of published facial nerve outcomes following microsurgical resection of NF2-associated VS is presented in ▶ Table 81.1.

81.7 Tumor Resection: Hearing

In most cases, hearing results with microsurgical resection of NF2-associated VSs are poor. While there are reports of hearing preservation with either total or partial tumor resection via the retrosigmoid route, it is our experience that this goal is rarely, if ever, accomplished, at least with larger tumors or in cases of more severe disease.[14] Unfortunately, patients with a large tumor in an only hearing ear often find themselves facing the prospect of tumor resection with certain knowledge of resulting deafness. Promises of "tumor debulking with hearing preservation" should be viewed with suspicion.

Primarily with smaller tumors and in patients with less severe forms of NF2, resection of tumor with attempted anatomic preservation of the cochlear nerve in the interest of later cochlear implantation has been reported.[15] Results of this approach are variable, with successful auditory benefit seen in only a portion of patients. With larger tumors and in more severe NF2, it is probably not reasonable to expect similar results due to the difficulty of preserving cochlear nerves likely to be traversing tumor.

81.7.1 Proactive Middle Fossa Tumor Resection

The role of early resection of small NF2-associated VSs for the purpose of hearing preservation remains controversial. Similar to patients with sporadic tumors, maintenance of useful hearing can be achieved in a significant portion of patients with an otherwise low complication rate.[16] Of course, as with any operative attempt at hearing preservation, the risk of total hearing loss remains significant. In most cases, this limits the option of early surgical intervention to "first side" treatment in those who retain good hearing bilaterally.

The choice of early surgical intervention should be offered only to patients with proven growing tumors with favorable imaging characteristics. Fundal tumor impaction, as well as involvement of the cochlea or vestibule, precludes successful hearing preservation in most cases.[8] Despite the significant chance of poor hearing outcome even in favorable cases, a

Table 81.1 Summary of published outcomes following microsurgery of NF2-associated vestibular schwannoma

Study	Center	Years	Case no.	Follow-up	Tumor size	Surgical approach	Degree of resection	Recurrence	FN outcome	HP outcome	Other complications
Glasscock et al (1989)	Vanderbilt University, Nashville, TN	1970–1988	34 pts, 44 VS	Mean: 8.2 y (1–13 y)	Mean: 2.5 cm	16 TL 16 RS 12 MCF	NR	5%	HB I: 15 HB II: 8 HB III: 4 HB IV: 2 HB V: 1	67% (4 of 6) retained SH	Hydrocephalus: 5% CSF leak: 11%
Slattery et al (2011)	House Ear Institute, Los Angeles, CA	1992–2004	35 pts, 47 VS	Mean: 2.8 y	Mean: 1.1 cm (0.4–3.2 cm)	100% MCF	NR	NR	HB I: 76% HB II: 7% HB III: 7% HB IV: 2% HB V: 5% HB VI: 2%	58% (23 of 40) retained SH	NR
Samii et al (2008)	International Neuroscience Institute, Hannover, Germany	More than 35 y	145 pts, 195 VS	NR	NR	NR	GTR: 85% STR: 15%	NR	"Anatomic integrity" preserved in 89%	65% retained "useful hearing"	NR
Friedman et al (2011)	House Clinic, Los Angeles, CA	2000–2010	37 pts, 55 VS	Mean: 60.7 mo	Mean: 1.0 cm (0.3–2.1)	100% MF	GTR: 96% Less than GTR: 4%	60% with tumor present in surgical field; 9% underwent salvage microsurgery	HB I: 75% HB II: 19% HB III: 4% HB IV: 0% HB V: 2% HB VI: 0%	50% retained SH	NR
Odat et al (2011)	Gruppo Otologico, Paicenza, Italy	1988–2008	38 pts, 48 VS	Mean: 3.7 y (1 mo–20 y)	Mean: 3.1 cm (0.6–6 cm)	ETLA-TA: 75% Transotic: 8% Transcochlear: 2% RS: 12% MCF: 2%	GTR: 92% STR: 8%	2%	HB I: 35% HB II: 17% HB III: 23% HB IV: 2% HB V: 2% HB VI: 21%	43% (3 of 7) retained SH	Perioperative mortality: 0% CSF leak: 0% Lower CN paralysis: 6%
Tysome et al (2012)	Cambridge University Hospitals NHS Trust, Cambridge, UK	1981–2011	44 pts, 50 VS	Median: 8 y (1–28 y)	Median: 2.8 cm	90% TL 10% RS	GTR: 78% NTR: 21%	None with regrowth or recurrence	HB I: 33% HB II: 21% HB III: 30% HB IV: 2% HB V: 9% HB VI: 5%	20% (1 of 5) retained SH	1 perioperative death from PE
Moffat et al (2013)	Cambridge University Teaching Hospitals NHS Trust, UK; Manchester Royal Infirmary, UK	NR	128 pts, 148 VS	Mean: 12.4 y (1–30 y)	Mean: 3.1 cm (1.1–5.5 cm)	100% TL	GTR: 66% NTR: 24% STR: 5% Partial: 5%	13.9% (0% after GTR)	HB I: 53% HB II: 8%% HB III: 22% HB IV–VI: 17%	NA (TL approach)	Perioperative mortality: 1.6% CSF leak: 2.5%
Nowak et al (2015)	Warszawski Uniwersytet Medyczny, Poland	1998–2014	30 pts, 51 VS	Mean: 5.3 y (1.5–15 y)	Mean: 2.8 cm (0.8–5 cm)	90% RS 4% TL 6% MCF	100% GTR and NTR (not separated)	10%	HB I: 14% HB II: 35% HB III: 35% HB IV: 8% HB V: 0% HB VI: 8%	14% (3 of 22) retained SH	Lower CN paralysis: 12% CN VI paralysis: 4% Hydrocephalus: 2% CSF leak: 4%

Abbreviations: CN, cranial nerve; CSF, cerebrospinal fluid; ETLA-TA, Enlarged translabyrinthine with transapical extension; GTR, gross total resection; HB, House–Brackmann; MCF, Middle cranial fossa; NR, not reported; NTR, near total resection; pts, patients; RS, retrosigmoid; SH, serviceable hearing; STR, subtotal resection; TL, translabyrinthine; VS, vestibular schwannomas; PE, pulmonary embolism.

number of patients will choose this option rather than continuing to wait until tumors grow too large to consider any attempt at hearing preservation surgery.

While long-term hearing prognosis is thought to be improved in patients who have had hearing preserved after proactive surgery, follow-up studies have shown that new or recurrent tumors develop in a significant percentage of cases.[16] Thus, a lifetime of good hearing cannot be promised even if all operative goals are met. A review of published hearing preservation outcomes following microsurgical resection of NF2-associated VS is presented in ▶ Table 81.1.

81.7.2 Middle Fossa Decompression

Decompression of the internal auditory canal via the middle fossa approach has been proposed as a means of maintaining auditory function in NF2 patients with actively deteriorating hearing.[17] Using this technique, the majority of patients may maintain useful hearing for several years with little risk of operative complications including facial nerve injury or acute hearing loss.

Of course, middle fossa decompression is a palliative measure that does not affect tumor growth and may indeed make further interventions more complicated. The combination of middle fossa decompression and bevacizumab or other novel therapies may hold promise in preserving function.

81.8 Tumor Resection and Auditory Brainstem Implantation

Auditory brainstem implants have been utilized to restore auditory sensation in patients with NF2 deafened due to destruction of the cochlear nerves. Typically, ABIs are placed at the same time as tumor resection, via either the translabyrinthine or the retrosigmoid route. In this way, the risk of ABI implantation can be assumed primarily by the need for tumor resection. Attempts at ABI placement via reoperation following tumor resection are typically made more difficult due to scarring and other postoperative changes.

Historically, auditory results from ABI implantation have been shown to vary considerably from patient to patient with generally modest outcomes.[18] While most patients utilize their ABIs on a daily basis and report a high degree of satisfaction, measurable auditory perception usually consists only of the ability to hear environmental sounds and to understand speech on only a limited basis. In the initial series, only about 5% of patients were capable of significant open-set speech discrimination.

More recent studies have shown the potential for improved audiological outcomes from ABI.[19] Most of these patients were implanted via the retrosigmoid approach in the sitting position. Possible factors for improved performance include choice of approach, positioning, choice of device, and nuances of surgical technique. A consensus of ABI surgeons concluded that meticulous handling of tissues, along the brainstem and including its vasculature, akin to hearing preservation surgery, is necessary to achieve optimal ABI results.[20] Chapter 84 discusses the topic of hearing rehabilitation in NF2 using ABI and CI in further detail.

81.9 Conclusion

Since NF2 is a disorder with variable presentation, blanket statements regarding the best care of NF2-associated VSs cannot be made. Treatment must be individualized. Surgical treatment of NF2-associated VSs carries with it additional challenges compared to the treatment of sporadic tumors, including a greater risk of cranial nerve injury, greater implications of cranial nerve injury, and patients facing the prospect of profound bilateral hearing loss.

References

[1] Evans DG, Howard E, Giblin C, et al. Birth incidence and prevalence of tumor-prone syndromes: estimates from a UK family genetic register service. Am J Med Genet A. 2010; 152A(2):327–332

[2] Parry DM, Eldridge R, Kaiser-Kupfer MI, Bouzas EA, Pikus A, Patronas N. Neurofibromatosis 2 (NF2): clinical characteristics of 63 affected individuals and clinical evidence for heterogeneity. Am J Med Genet. 1994; 52(4):450–461

[3] Evans DG, Ramsden RT, Shenton A, et al. Mosaicism in neurofibromatosis type 2: an update of risk based on uni/bilaterality of vestibular schwannoma at presentation and sensitive mutation analysis including multiple ligation-dependent probe amplification. J Med Genet. 2007; 44(7):424–428

[4] Schwartz MS, Otto SR, Shannon RV, Hitselberger WE, Brackmann DE. Auditory brainstem implants. Neurotherapeutics. 2008; 5(1):128–136

[5] Mukherjee P, Ramsden JD, Donnelly N, et al. Cochlear implants to treat deafness caused by vestibular schwannomas. Otol Neurotol. 2013; 34(7): 1291–1298

[6] Dewan R, Pemov A, Kim HJ, et al. Evidence of polyclonality in neurofibromatosis type 2-associated multilobulated vestibular schwannomas. Neuro-oncol. 2015; 17(4):566–573

[7] Mallory GW, Pollock BE, Foote RL, Carlson ML, Driscoll CL, Link MJ. Stereotactic radiosurgery for neurofibromatosis 2-associated vestibular schwannomas: toward dose optimization for tumor control and functional outcomes. Neurosurgery. 2014; 74(3):292–300, discussion 300–301

[8] Nam SI, Linthicum FH, Jr, Merchant SN. Temporal bone histopathology in neurofibromatosis type 2. Laryngoscope. 2011; 121(7):1548–1554

[9] Feucht M, Griffiths B, Niemüller I, Haase W, Richard G, Mautner VF. Neurofibromatosis 2 leads to higher incidence of strabismological and neuro-ophthalmological disorders. Acta Ophthalmol. 2008; 86(8):882–886

[10] Aboukais R, Zairi F, Bonne NX, et al. Causes of mortality in neurofibromatosis type 2. Br J Neurosurg. 2014; 25:1–4

[11] Plotkin SR, Stemmer-Rachamimov AO, Barker FG, II, et al. Hearing improvement after bevacizumab in patients with neurofibromatosis type 2. N Engl J Med. 2009; 361(4):358–367

[12] Matyja E, Kunert P, Grajkowska W, Marchel A. Coexistence of meningioma and schwannoma in the same cerebellopontine angle in a patients with NF2. Folia Neuropathol. 2012; 50(2):166–172

[13] Tysome JR, Macfarlane R, Durie-Gair J, et al. Surgical management of vestibular schwannomas and hearing rehabilitation in neurofibromatosis type 2. Otol Neurotol. 2012; 33(3):466–472

[14] Samii M, Gerganov V, Samii A. Microsurgery management of vestibular schwannomas in neurofibromatosis type 2: indications and results. Prog Neurol Surg. 2008; 21:169–175

[15] Lloyd SK, Glynn FJ, Rutherford SA, et al. Ipsilateral cochlear implantation after cochlear nerve preserving vestibular schwannoma surgery in patients with neurofibromatosis type 2. Otol Neurotol. 2014; 35(1):43–51

[16] Friedman RA, Goddard JC, Wilkinson EP, et al. Hearing preservation with the middle cranial fossa approach for neurofibromatosis type 2. Otol Neurotol. 2011; 32(9):1530–1537

[17] Slattery WH, Hoa M, Bonne N, et al. Middle fossa decompression for hearing preservation: a review of institutional results and indications. Otol Neurotol. 2011; 32(6):1017–1024

[18] Otto SR, Brackmann DE, Hitselberger WE, Shannon RV, Kuchta J. Multichannel auditory brainstem implant: update on performance in 61 patients. J Neurosurg. 2002; 96(6):1063–1071

[19] Matthies C, Brill S, Varallyay C, et al. Auditory brainstem implants in neurofibromatosis Type 2: is open speech perception feasible? J Neurosurg. 2014; 120(2):546–558

[20] Behr R, Colletti V, Matthies C, et al. New outcomes with auditory brainstem implants in NF2 patients. Otol Neurotol. 2014; 35(10):1844–1851

[21] Glasscock ME 3rd, Woods CI, Jackson CG, Welling DB. Management of bilateral acoustic tumors. Laryngoscope. 1989 May;99(5):475-84. PubMed PMID: 2709934

[22] Odat HA, Piccirillo E, Sequino G, Taibah A, Sanna M. Management strategy of vestibular schwannoma in neurofibromatosis type 2. Otol Neurotol. 2011 Sep;32(7):1163-70. doi: 10.1097/MAO.0b013e3182267f17. PubMed PMID: 21817944

[23] Moffat DA, Lloyd SK, Macfarlane R, Mannion R, King A, Rutherford S, Axon PR, Donnelly N, Freeman S, Tysome JR, Evans DG, Ramsden RT. Outcome of translabyrinthine surgery for vestibular schwannoma in neurofibromatosis type 2. Br J Neurosurg. 2013 Aug;27(4):446-53. doi: 10.3109/02688697.2013.771143. Epub 2013 Mar 8. PubMed PMID: 23472624

[24] Nowak A, Dziedzic T, Czernicki T, Kunert P, Morawski K, Niemczyk K, Marchel A. Strategy for the surgical treatment of vestibular schwannomas in patients with neurofibromatosis type 2. Neurol Neurochir Pol. 2015;49(5):295-301. doi: 10.1016/j.pjnns.2015.06.008. Epub 2015 Jul 3. PubMed PMID: 26377980

82 Radiosurgery and Radiotherapy for Neurofibromatosis Type 2 Focusing on Vestibular Schwannoma

Amparo Wolf and Douglas Kondziolka

82.1 Introduction

Neurofibromatosis type 2 (NF2) is an autosomal dominant disease with an incidence of approximately 1 in 25,000 to 1 in 60,000.[1] A hallmark feature of NF2 is the presence of bilateral vestibular schwannomas (VSs). Additional nervous system tumors in NF2 include schwannomas of other cranial and spinal nerves, meningiomas, ependymomas, and gliomas. Approximately 90 to 95% of patients with NF2 will develop bilateral VSs.[2] NF2-associated tumors develop from the inactivation of both alleles of the *NF2* tumor-suppressor gene, located on chromosome 22q12. NF2-associated VSs tend to infiltrate and involve the cochlear nerve,[3] resulting in gradual sensorineural hearing loss (SNHL) and high-pitched tinnitus as the presenting symptoms in 60% of adults and up to 30% of children.[2,4] Furthermore, NF2-related VSs tend to behave more aggressively than sporadic tumors in terms of recurrence and result in a greater incidence of cranial nerve deficits.[2,5]

Treatment options for NF2-associated VS include observation, medical therapies, microsurgery, and stereotactic radiosurgery (SRS). As in sporadic tumors, surgery is indicated in patients with large VS resulting in significant brainstem compression or hydrocephalus. In some NF2 patients, there is an important role for SRS. The purpose of this chapter is to review the current evidence on single-session SRS and multisession stereotactic hypofractionated or conventionally fractionated radiotherapy in NF2-associated VS, as it relates to tumor control rates, hearing, and facial nerve outcomes.

82.2 The Natural History of NF2-Associated Vestibular Schwannomas

The natural history of VS in NF2 is characterized by highly variable growth rates that decrease inversely with age.[6,7] From a recent natural history study of a select group of 46 NF2 patients with 74 tumors followed up for a mean of 6 years, in which patients with more severe forms of the disease were excluded, the median growth rate was 1.4 mm per year (0–8 mm/year).[6] However, growth rates as high as 10 mm/year have been reported.[8,9] Rare studies have shown that VS may spontaneously decrease in size over time, particularly after the resection of contralateral tumors in NF2 patients.[10] The heterogeneity in growth rates may be partly attributable to the type of NF2 gene mutation (e.g., nonsense or frame shift mutations producing a truncated protein vs. missense mutations) and phenotype (Wishart vs. Gardner).[11]

The natural history of SNHL in untreated VS is also unpredictable. In a study investigating hearing outcomes in relation to tumor growth following conservative management of bilateral VS in NF2 patients, a serviceable hearing preservation rate of 74% was reported at a mean follow-up of 6 years, but with only 66% of patients conserving binaural serviceable hearing.[6] Initial tumor size and growth rate are not predictive of hearing status in NF2 patients.[12,13] Chapter 80 further reviews the natural history of VS in patients with NF2.

82.2.1 Stereotactic Radiosurgery in NF2-Associated Vestibular Schwannomas: Control Rates

▶ Table 82.1 summarizes the published studies to date that evaluated tumor control rates in patients with NF2-associated VS after SRS. SRS provides tumor control in reportedly 70 to 100% of cases with reported long-term local control rates of 80% at 15 years in NF2 patients.[14] Overall, the results for VS in NF2 patients after SRS support good local control, although comparatively less favorable than sporadic VS patients in the long term, where up to 98% control is seen at 10 years.[15] ▶ Fig. 82.1 demonstrates a 50-year-old NF2 patient with bilateral hearing loss and a growing right-sided VS. The left-sided VS has been stable over serial MRIs. The patient underwent SRS at a margin dose of 12 Gy. At 4-year follow-up, the right-sided VS has reduced in size.

Predictors of local control include age, tumor volume, margin dose, and NF2 phenotype.[23,24] Higher margin doses in NF2 tumors may result in improved tumor control; however, no study has directly investigated this prospectively and in a randomized fashion. One retrospective report from the Mayo Clinic examined the effect of dose on tumor response, taking into account that their institution continued to use a margin dose of 14 Gy until 1996. They reported that the median margin dose for tumors that decreased in size after SRS was 15.5 Gy compared with 13 Gy for tumors with continued growth after treatment.[23] In the study of Mathieu et al,[14] higher radiation dose did not have an impact on tumor control, but it did impact hearing preservation and complication rates. Progression-free survival rates after SRS for patients with the more aggressive phenotype NF2 are reportedly reduced compared to patients with less severe phenotype NF2.[24]

82.2.2 Stereotactic Radiosurgery in NF2-Associated Vestibular Schwannomas: Functional Outcomes

Patients with NF2 frequently develop bilateral VS and are at risk of complete hearing loss over time. In order to maximize hearing longevity, typically a conservative treatment approach is recommended in NF2 patients who have small VS, with SRS or microsurgery employed only after progressive tumor growth has been documented. Overall, the studies reviewed in ▶ Table 82.1 suggest a serviceable hearing preservation rate of 25 to 78% after SRS.

Hearing outcomes after SRS for VS are partly related to the radiation dose employed.[14,20] Even at a reduced margin dose

Table 82.1 Summary of studies of stereotactic radiosurgery in NF2-associated vestibular schwannomas

Study	#patients/ #tumors	Dose (Gy)	Tumor volume (cm^3)	Local tumor control	Median follow-up time (mo)	Hearing preservation (%)	CN VII weakness	CN V dysfunction	MT
Subach et al (1999)[16]	40/45	15	4.8 (mean)	98%	36 (median)	43% (pre 1992); 67% (post 1992)	19%	6%	NR
Kida et al (2000)[17]	20/20	13	2.4 (mean)	100%	33.6 (mean)	33.3%	0	0	NR
Rowe et al (2003)[18]	96/122	15.2	4.6 (mean)	52% at 8 y	51 (median)	38% at 3 y	5%	2%	NR
Roche et al (2004)[19]	37/50	12.3	3.5 (mean)	85% at 10 y	62 (median)	36% at 5 y	2%	NA	NA
Mathieu et al (2007)[14]	62/74	14	5.7 (mean)	81% at 15 y	53 (median)	48% at 5 y	8%	4%	0
Phi et al (2009)[20]	30/36	12.1	3.2 (median)	66% at 5 y	36.5	33% at 5 y	3.3%	3.3%	0
Sharma et al (2010)[21]	30/54	12	3.7 (mean)	67.3% at 5 y	26.6	66.7%	3.1%	0	0
Massager et al (2013)[22]	18/25	12	2.04 (median)	80.2% at 5 y	52.8	78%	0	0	0
Mallory et al (2014)[23]	26/32	14	2.7 (median)	85% at 5 y	91.2 (median)	25%	50%	NR	NR
Sun et al (2014)[24]	46/73	12.9	5.1 (mean)	87% at 5 y 41% at 10 y	109 (median)	31.9%	5%	8%	NR

Abbreviations: MT, malignant transformation; NA, not available; NR, not reported.

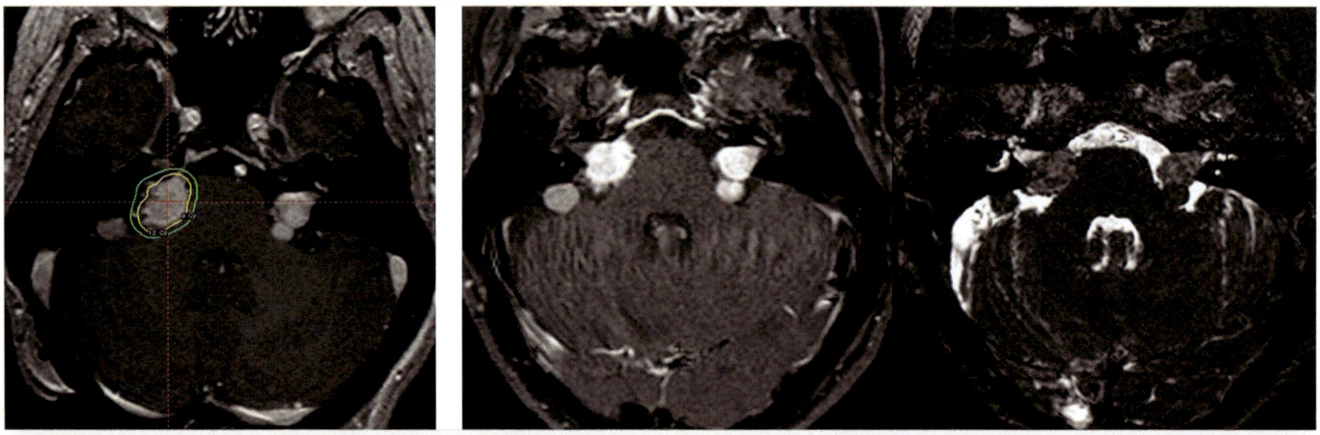

Fig. 82.1 MR images of a 50-year-old NF2 patient who underwent SRS for a right-sided vestibular schwannoma. **(a)** SRS treatment plan at a margin dose of 12 Gy at the 50% isodose volume. **(b)** Axial T1-gadolinium and T2-weighted MRI 4 years after SRS showing reduction in size of the right vestibular schwannoma and stable left vestibular schwannoma.

(< 13 Gy), NF2 patients may experience hearing loss after SRS and at the potential expense of tumor control.[6,20] Preoperative hearing status is an important determinant of retained serviceable hearing after SRS.[14] Earlier intervention at first signs of tumor growth followed by cochlear or auditory brainstem implantation has been advocated by some, although with varying success.[23,25,26] Some groups have used SRS to treat bilateral VS, either in staged or at one procedure, and have found similar hearing outcomes to unilateral treatment.[19,22]

With respect to facial nerve outcomes, as with hearing, it can be difficult to differentiate between the natural history of NF2 VS and delayed complications arising from SRS. Overall, the studies reviewed in ▶ Table 82.1 suggest facial nerve function preservation in 92 to 100% of patients, lower than reported outcomes for sporadic tumors (> 99%).[27] From these studies, we can also extrapolate that there is a trend toward poorer facial nerve function with higher margin doses.[28] Maximum doses greater than 28 Gy predicted development of complications such as facial weakness, trigeminal neuropathy, or vestibular dysfunction.[14] Furthermore, facial nerve outcomes in NF2 may be confounded by prior surgery and possibly the existence of facial schwannomas. Of note, some of the studies in Table 1 reported on patients treated prior to 1992 and, as such, did not use current radiosurgery techniques including MRI for targeting and more sophisticated treatment planning. Current functional outcomes should be superior with advanced radiosurgery techniques,[23] as with other tumor types.

82.3 Fractionated Radiotherapy in NF2-Associated Vestibular Schwannomas

There are few studies using linear accelerator (LINAC)-based single-session radiosurgery or multisession hypofractionated or conventionally fractionated radiotherapy for bilateral VS in NF2 patients.[29,30,31] Fuss et al[29] reported on 10 patients with NF2 who had bilateral VS treated with conventionally fractionated LINAC-based stereotactic radiotherapy and found no ipsilateral progression after a mean follow-up of 42 months. Meijer et al[30] looked at 25 NF2 patients who underwent either LINAC single-session radiosurgery or multisession fractionated radiotherapy and also reported no progression of tumors by 109 months. In another study comparing 200 VS patients undergoing either LINAC-based single-session radiosurgery or multisession fractionated radiotherapy, tumor control rates and hearing preservation rates were similar in both groups when the margin dose of SRS was less than 13 Gy,[31] which included 16 patients with NF2. In NF2 patients with serviceable hearing, the actuarial hearing preservation rate was 85% at 1 year, 83% at 2 years, and 78% at 5 years.[31]

82.4 Stereotactic Radiosurgery in Other NF2-Associated Tumors

Meningiomas occur in 45 to 58% of patients with NF2.[2] In a small-sample, single-institution study looking at the effectiveness of SRS in NF2-associated meningiomas, which were not verified histologically, Liu et al[32] reported a 5-year local tumor control rate of 92% and the development of new distant tumors at a rate of 77%. The mean time to repeat treatment, either radiosurgery or surgery, was 38 months. In a study of 46 patients with 122 non-VS NF2 tumors (other schwannomas, meningiomas) with longer-term follow-up, a local tumor control rate of 85% was reported with a median duration of follow-up of 109 months. Although there are limited studies to date, SRS may provide good local tumor control in NF2-associated meningiomas and other schwannomas.

82.5 Malignant Transformation in NF2

There is a potential for malignant transformation or the formation of new malignancies after SRS particularly given the genetic predisposition of NF2 patients. In a recent published literature review, there have been 29 reports of malignant transformation of VS after irradiation (SRS, fractionated radiotherapy), approximately 40% of who had NF2.[33] However, current data suggest that this risk is very low. Of the studies that reported on malignant transformation in Table 1, none were observed. In a population study of nearly 5,000 cases from Sheffield, England, there was no increased rate of malignancy of any kind after radiosurgery.[34] In a retrospective analysis of 118 NF2 patients with greater than 900 patient-years of follow-up, 1 patient may have developed malignant transformation of VS, although the tumor behaved aggressively with rapid growth prior to radiosurgery.[28] Another patient developed a new glioblastoma 3 years after SRS, with no details reported as to where it arose in relation to the VS.[28] Furthermore, up to 4% of NF2 patients can develop gliomas. Based on the analysis of Seferis et al,[33] the reported overall risk of malignant transformation after radiation treatment over 20 years is 25.1 per 100,000, decreasing to 15.6 per 100,000 if cases of NF2 are excluded,[33] compared to 1.32 to 2.08 per 100,000 in patients who did not receive radiation treatment. A limitation with many of these studies is that there lacks histology to confirm a previously benign lesion. Thus, at this time, patients with NF2 may be more prone to malignant transformation than patients with sporadic VS, although the overall risk remains quite low. Chapter 24 reviews the subject of malignant transformation in VS further.

82.6 Conclusion

Stereotactic radiosurgery provides high rates of long-term tumor control in NF2 patients with VS, with a low risk of facial nerve injury and the possibility of maintaining serviceable hearing. The management of NF2 is evolving with ongoing studies looking at newer treatment strategies including the combination of radiosurgery with pharmacological agents (bevacizumab, tyrosine kinase inhibitors), with the hope of improving bilateral tumor control and maintaining long-term hearing and facial nerve function.

References

[1] Evans DG, Howard E, Giblin C, et al. Birth incidence and prevalence of tumor-prone syndromes: estimates from a UK family genetic register service. Am J Med Genet A. 2010; 152A(2):327–332

[2] Asthagiri AR, Parry DM, Butman JA, et al. Neurofibromatosis type 2. Lancet. 2009; 373(9679):1974–1986

[3] Jääskeläinen J, Paetau A, Pyykkö I, Blomstedt G, Palva T, Troupp H. Interface between the facial nerve and large acoustic neurinomas. Immunohistochemical study of the cleavage plane in NF2 and non-NF2 cases. J Neurosurg. 1994; 80(3):541–547

[4] Ruggieri M, Praticò AD, Evans DG. Diagnosis, management, and new therapeutic options in childhood neurofibromatosis type 2 and related forms. Semin Pediatr Neurol. 2015; 22(4):240–258

[5] Samii M, Matthies C, Tatagiba M. Management of vestibular schwannomas (acoustic neuromas): auditory and facial nerve function after resection of 120 vestibular schwannomas in patients with neurofibromatosis 2. Neurosurgery. 1997; 40(4):696–705

[6] Peyre M, Goutagny S, Bah A, et al. Conservative management of bilateral vestibular schwannomas in neurofibromatosis type 2 patients: hearing and tumor growth results. Neurosurgery. 2013; 72(6):907–913, discussion 914, quiz 914

[7] Baser ME, Mautner VF, Parry DM, Evans DG. Methodological issues in longitudinal studies: vestibular schwannoma growth rates in neurofibromatosis 2. J Med Genet. 2005; 42(12):903–906

[8] Dirks MS, Butman JA, Kim HJ, et al. Long-term natural history of neurofibromatosis Type 2-associated intracranial tumors. J Neurosurg. 2012; 117(1):109–117

[9] Harris GJ, Plotkin SR, Maccollin M, et al. Three-dimensional volumetrics for tracking vestibular schwannoma growth in neurofibromatosis type II. Neurosurgery. 2008; 62(6):1314–1319, discussion 1319–1320

[10] von Eckardstein KL, Beatty CW, Driscoll CLW, Link MJ. Spontaneous regression of vestibular schwannomas after resection of contralateral tumor in neurofibromatosis Type 2. J Neurosurg. 2010; 112(1):158–162

[11] Evans DG, Trueman L, Wallace A, Collins S, Strachan T. Genotype/phenotype correlations in type 2 neurofibromatosis (NF2): evidence for more severe disease associated with truncating mutations. J Med Genet. 1998; 35(6):450–455

[12] Fisher LM, Doherty JK, Lev MH, Slattery WH. Concordance of bilateral vestibular schwannoma growth and hearing changes in neurofibromatosis 2:

neurofibromatosis 2 natural history consortium. Otol Neurotol. 2009; 30(6): 835–841
[13] Masuda A, Fisher LM, Oppenheimer ML, Iqbal Z, Slattery WH, Natural History Consortium. Hearing changes after diagnosis in neurofibromatosis type 2. Otol Neurotol. 2004; 25(2):150–154
[14] Mathieu D, Kondziolka D, Flickinger JC, et al. Stereotactic radiosurgery for vestibular schwannomas in patients with neurofibromatosis type 2: an analysis of tumor control, complications, and hearing preservation rates. Neurosurgery. 2007; 60(3):460–468, discussion 468–470
[15] Chopra R, Kondziolka D, Niranjan A, Lunsford LD, Flickinger JC. Long-term follow-up of acoustic schwannoma radiosurgery with marginal tumor doses of 12 to 13 Gy. Int J Radiat Oncol Biol Phys. 2007; 68(3):845–851
[16] Subach BR, Kondziolka D, Lunsford LD, Bissonette DJ, Flickinger JC, Maitz AH. Stereotactic radiosurgery in the management of acoustic neuromas associated with neurofibromatosis Type 2. J Neurosurg. 1999; 90(5):815–822
[17] Kida Y, Kobayashi T, Tanaka T, Mori Y. Radiosurgery for bilateral neurinomas associated with neurofibromatosis type 2. Surg Neurol. 2000; 53(4):383–389, discussion 389–390
[18] Rowe JG, Radatz MWR, Walton L, Soanes T, Rodgers J, Kemeny AA. Clinical experience with gamma knife stereotactic radiosurgery in the management of vestibular schwannomas secondary to type 2 neurofibromatosis. J Neurol Neurosurg Psychiatry. 2003; 74(9):1288–1293
[19] Roche P-H, Robitail S, Thomassin J-M, Pellet W, Régis J. [Surgical management of vestibular schwannomas secondary to type 2 neurofibromatosis]. Neurochirurgie. 2004; 50(2–3, Pt 2):367–376
[20] Phi JH, Kim DG, Chung H-T, Lee J, Paek SH, Jung H-W. Radiosurgical treatment of vestibular schwannomas in patients with neurofibromatosis type 2: tumor control and hearing preservation. Cancer. 2009; 115(2):390–398
[21] Sharma MS, Singh R, Kale SS, Agrawal D, Sharma BS, Mahapatra AK. Tumor control and hearing preservation after Gamma Knife radiosurgery for vestibular schwannomas in neurofibromatosis type 2. J Neurooncol. 2010; 98(2): 265–270
[22] Massager N, Delbrouck C, Masudi J, De Smedt F, Devriendt D. Hearing preservation and tumour control after radiosurgery for NF2-related vestibular schwannomas. B-ENT. 2013; 9(1):29–36
[23] Mallory GW, Pollock BE, Foote RL, Carlson ML, Driscoll CL, Link MJ. Stereotactic radiosurgery for neurofibromatosis 2-associated vestibular schwannomas: toward dose optimization for tumor control and functional outcomes. Neurosurgery. 2014; 74(3):292–300, discussion 300–301
[24] Sun S, Liu A. Long-term follow-up studies of Gamma Knife surgery for patients with neurofibromatosis Type 2. J Neurosurg. 2014; 121(December) Suppl:143–149
[25] Carlson ML, Breen JT, Driscoll CL, et al. Cochlear implantation in patients with neurofibromatosis type 2: variables affecting auditory performance. Otol Neurotol. 2012; 33(5):853–862
[26] Matthies C, Brill S, Kaga K, et al. Auditory brainstem implantation improves speech recognition in neurofibromatosis type II patients. ORL J Otorhinolaryngol Relat Spec. 2013; 75(5):282–295
[27] Flickinger JC, Kondziolka D, Niranjan A, Maitz A, Voynov G, Lunsford LD. Acoustic neuroma radiosurgery with marginal tumor doses of 12 to 13 Gy. Int J Radiat Oncol Biol Phys. 2004; 60(1):225–230
[28] Rowe J, Grainger A, Walton L, Radatz M, Kemeny A. Safety of radiosurgery applied to conditions with abnormal tumor suppressor genes. Neurosurgery. 2007; 60(5):860–864, discussion 860–864
[29] Fuss M, Debus J, Lohr F, et al. Conventionally fractionated stereotactic radiotherapy (FSRT) for acoustic neuromas. Int J Radiat Oncol Biol Phys. 2000; 48 (5):1381–1387
[30] Meijer OWM, Vandertop WP, Lagerwaard FJ, Slotman BJ. Linear accelerator-based stereotactic radiosurgery for bilateral vestibular schwannomas in patients with neurofibromatosis type 2. Neurosurgery. 2008; 62(5) Suppl: A37–A42, discussion A42–A43
[31] Combs SE, Welzel T, Schulz-Ertner D, Huber PE, Debus J. Differences in clinical results after LINAC-based single-dose radiosurgery versus fractionated stereotactic radiotherapy for patients with vestibular schwannomas. Int J Radiat Oncol Biol Phys. 2010; 76(1):193–200
[32] Liu A, Kuhn EN, Lucas JT, Jr, Laxton AW, Tatter SB, Chan MD. Gamma Knife radiosurgery for meningiomas in patients with neurofibromatosis Type 2. J Neurosurg. 2015; 122(3):536–542
[33] Seferis C, Torrens M, Paraskevopoulou C, Psichidis G. Malignant transformation in vestibular schwannoma: report of a single case, literature search, and debate. J Neurosurg. 2014; 121(December) Suppl:160–166
[34] Rowe J, Grainger A, Walton L, Silcocks P, Radatz M, Kemeny A. Risk of malignancy after gamma knife stereotactic radiosurgery. Neurosurgery. 2007; 60 (1):60–65, discussion 65–66

83 Medical Therapy for Neurofibromatosis Type 2 Focusing on Vestibular Schwannoma

Nicholas L. Deep, Matthew L. Carlson, and Scott R. Plotkin

83.1 Introduction

The hallmark of neurofibromatosis type 2 (NF2) is the development of bilateral vestibular schwannomas (VSs).[1] While histologically benign, VSs are a source of significant morbidity in NF2 patients, given their bilateral presentation, earlier age of onset, proximity to other critical neurovascular structures, and greater tendency to recur after treatment.[1,2] The coexistence of lower cranial nerve schwannomas, meningiomas, and spinal cord ependymomas further complicate clinical decision making.[1] The conventional treatment options for VS include surgical excision, stereotactic radiation, and observation. Currently, there is no approved medical therapy for VS in the United States. Due to the potential high morbidity of treating VS, particularly in the NF2 population, developing novel medical therapies as an alternative has become a high priority. Fortunately, in recent years, there have been breakthroughs in the understanding of NF2 tumor biology which has led to the discovery of several important surface receptors and intracellular signaling pathways that are responsible for the growth and survival of NF2-related tumors (reviewed further in Chapter 5).[3] As a result, rationally designed drugs targeting various components of this molecular pathway have been developed and tested in preclinical and clinical trials (▶ Fig. 83.1, ▶ Fig. 83.2).[3] In this

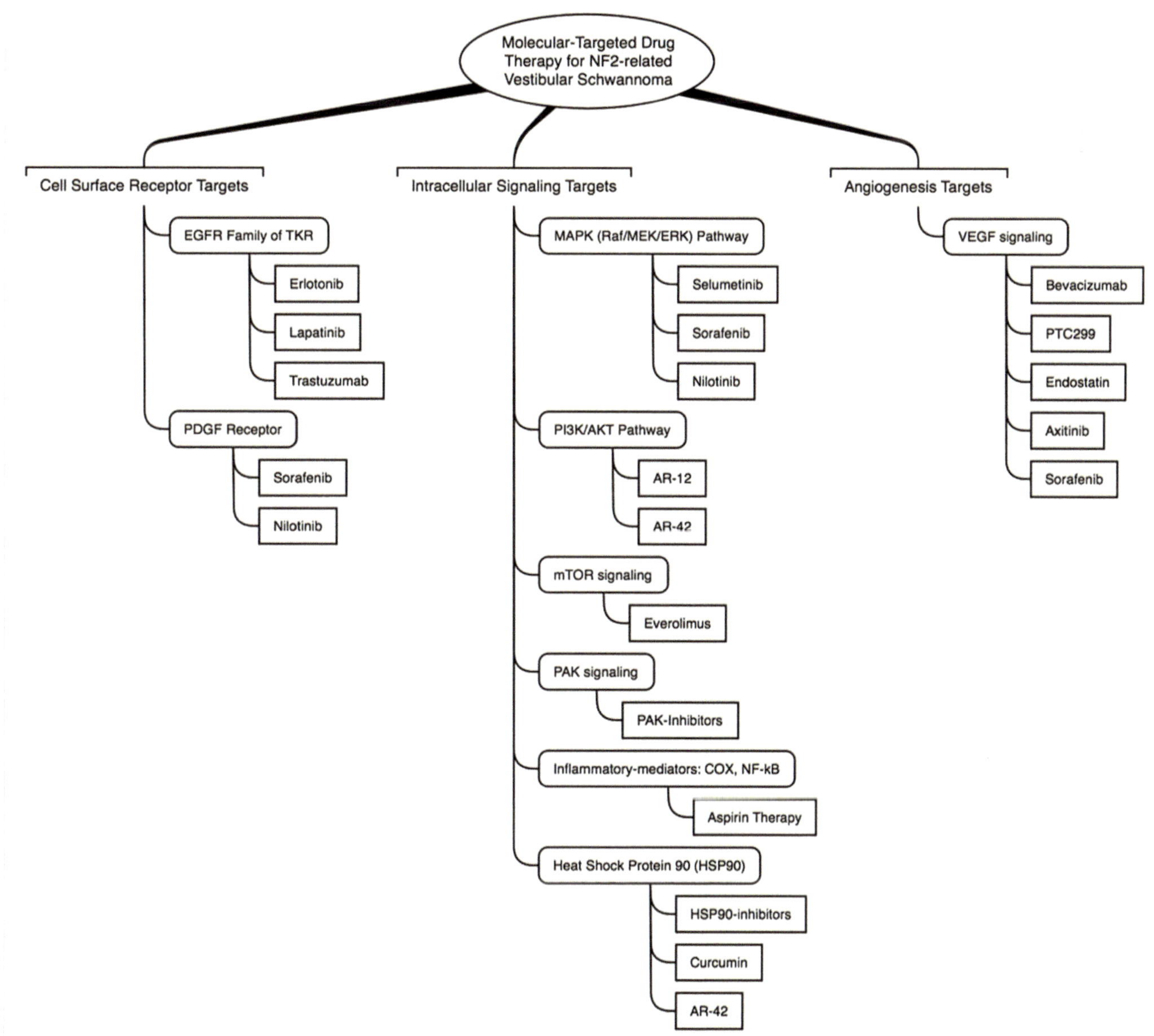

Fig. 83.1 Overview of molecular-targeted drug therapies.

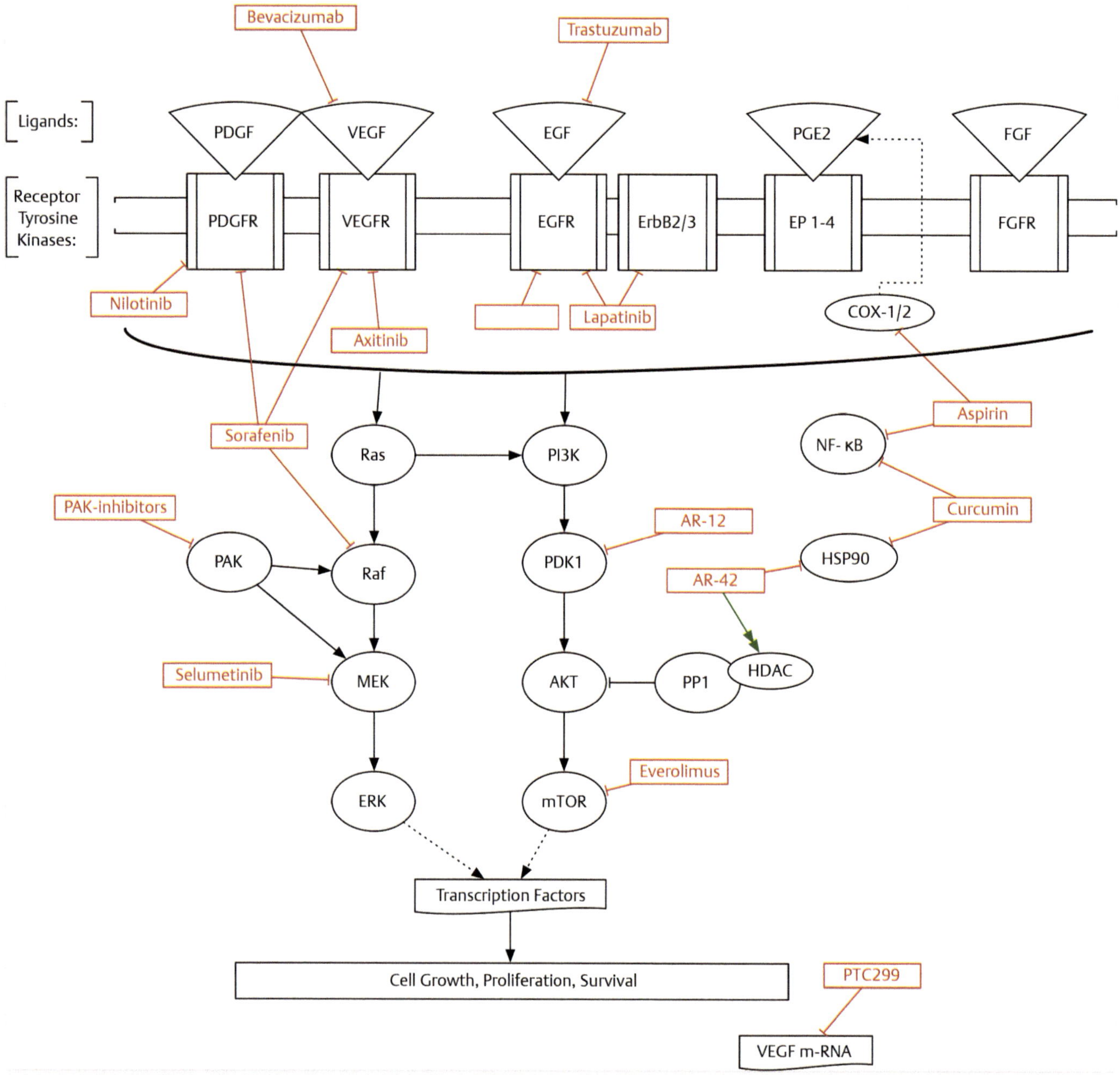

Fig. 83.2 Targets of therapeutic drugs for vestibular schwannoma. Current strategies target the abnormal merlin-controlled growth regulator pathways through blockade of surface receptors or intracellular signaling pathways, and/or target the tumors microenvironment (endothelial cells) by inhibiting neoangiogenesis. Receptor tyrosine kinases (VEGFR, PDGFR, EGFR, and ErbB2/3) are overly expressed in *NF2*-deficient cells leading to tumorigenesis. Inhibiting their ligands (e.g., VEGF, EGF, PGE2) or the receptors themselves have been shown to suppress downstream signaling, thereby preventing tumor growth. Multiple proneoplastic pathways are activated in merlin-deficient cells and significant "cross-talk" exists, leading to treatment failure or development of drug resistance. Small-molecule inhibitors (those ending in "-inib") are novel in that they are able to cross the cell membrane to affect the intracellular domain of cell-surface receptors and also block the activation of various downstream signaling pathways intracellularly; while this potentially increases their breadth of inhibition, it may also lead to more "off-target" adverse side effects. HDACIs (AR-42) have a novel mechanism by which they can indirectly dephosphorylate (deactivate) AKT through its interaction with protein phosphatase 1 (PP1).

chapter, we will review current candidate drugs for the treatment of VS in the NF2 patient.

83.2 Design of Medical Therapy Trials for Vestibular Schwannoma

The ideal drug for NF2 patients would be one that (1) permanently shrinks or eradicates the tumor as opposed to simply halting its growth temporarily; (2) will allow the patient to halt loss or potentially reverse sensorineural hearing loss from tumor involvement; (3) is effective for treating both VS and meningiomas, since these frequently co-exist; (4) is safe in both adults and children, particularly since many NF2 patients are diagnosed during adolescence; and (5) has minimal side effects and is easily administered.

To date, several preclinical and clinical studies have made progress toward these goals. These studies have focused on NF2 patients with progressive or symptomatic VS; however, testing in sporadic VS has also showed efficacy, likely because both forms of VS share similar pathobiology of merlin deficiency. In fact, approximately 90% of sporadic VSs have somatic *NF2* mutations. Currently, the major benchmarks to evaluate drug efficacy include (1) hearing outcomes as measured by speech discrimination (word recognition) scores and (2) radiographic outcomes based on changes in tumor volume.[3] While the ideal drug would permanently eradicate the tumor, quality of life may be improved by preserving hearing or avoiding surgery, even if only temporarily. Therefore, other clinically meaningful endpoints in the NF2 population have recently gained more attention, including "progression-free survival" and "time to disease progression," as delaying disease progression would be highly desirable in the NF2 population.[4]

83.3 Targeting Angiogenesis

Vascular endothelial growth factor (VEGF) has been demonstrated to be overexpressed in both VS and surrounding endothelial cells.[5] Therefore, targeting the tumor's blood supply with angiogenesis inhibitors presents one therapeutic approach in the medical treatment of VS.

83.3.1 Bevacizumab

Bevacizumab (Avastin, Roche), a humanized anti-VEGF-A monoclonal antibody that is FDA approved for use in various cancers, was one of the first medical therapies used for treatment of NF2-associated VS (▶ Table 83.1). In retrospective studies, bevacizumab has resulted in improved hearing and radiographic tumor shrinkage in about 50% of patients with progressive VS (defined as improvement in word recognition score above the 95% critical difference and ≥ 20% volume reduction).[6,7,8] A recent multicenter, phase 2 clinical trial (NCT01207687) of 14 patients with NF2 found a confirmed hearing response in 36% of patients (which was sustained ≥ 3 months) and radiographic response in 43% of patients, thereby confirming the efficacy and safety of bevacizumab in this subset of people with NF2 and progressive, symptomatic VSs.[9]

It is hypothesized that bevacizumab's effects on reducing tumor volume is secondary to decreasing vascular permeability and decreasing outgrowth of new vessels, as opposed to having a direct antiproliferative effect.[23] Unfortunately, tumor regrowth has been noted upon discontinuation of the drug, which may occur shortly after 6 months or longer following discontinuation of the drug; as a result, prolonged treatment may be necessary in order to sustain clinical benefit.[24] This can be challenging clinically given the relatively high incidence of long-term toxicities of bevacizumab, namely hypertension (58%) and proteinuria (62%).[25] In addition, bevacizumab impairs wound healing.[3] This is of particular concern for NF2 patient who are often afflicted with other tumors concurrently, which may require surgery.[3] Another ongoing clinical trial (NCT01767792) studying bevacizumab for children and young adults with hearing loss resulting from an NF2-associated VS will further investigate and expand upon the findings from this study.

83.3.2 Potential Future Therapies Targeting Angiogenesis

Given the initial success of previous studies with bevacizumab in NF2 patients, other methods of targeting VEGF have been explored. Recombinant human **endostatin**, formed by proteolytic cleavage of collagen XVIII, may impede the formation of blood vessels by inhibiting the migration of vascular endothelial cells through its interaction in multiple intracellular pathways.[26] A phase 2 clinical trial (NCT02104323) is ongoing in Beijing Tiantan Hospital using endostatin in patients with NF2-related tumors. **Axitinib** (Inlyta, Pfizer), a selective tyrosine kinases inhibitor (TKI) that is primarily active against VEGF receptors-1, -2, -3, is another promising antiangiogenic small molecule currently being tested in a phase 2 clinical trial for NF2 patients with progressive VS (NCT02129647).[27] Lastly, **PTC299** (PTC Therapeutics; South Plainfield, NJ) is a small molecule that inhibits VEGF at the posttranscriptional level, binding to the 5′- and 3′-untranslated regions of VEGF mRNA, thereby limiting its production.[28] A clinical trial was previously underway but is currently suspended according to clinicaltrials.gov.

83.4 Epidermal Growth Factor Family of Tyrosine Kinase Receptors

In NF2, dysfunction or loss of the merlin protein results in abnormal activation of epidermal growth factor family (EGFR) receptor tyrosine kinases (RTKs), specifically EGFR/ErbB1, ErbB2, and ErbB3, leading to increased cell proliferation and resistance to cell death.[11,29,30,31] Drugs targeting the EGFR/ErbB2 pathway have been tested in robust preclinical trials and have been shown to reduce schwannoma cell proliferation.[11,30]

83.4.1 Erlotinib

Erlotinib (Tarceva, Genentech) is an oral EGFR-selective RTK inhibitor approved by the FDA for treatment of non-small cell lung cancer and pancreatic cancer. In a study comparing the

Table 83.1 Molecular-targeted drug therapy candidates for NF2-related VS

Drug	Target	Outcomes[a]	Status (ClinicalTrials.gov identifier)
Candidate drugs with clinical outcomes			
Bevacizumab	VEGF mAB	57% hearing improved, 53% tumor shrinkage (retrospective).[6] 36% confirmed hearing response, 57% any hearing improvement, 43% tumor shrinkage (phase 2 trial)[9]	Phase 2 trials completed (NCT01207687) and ongoing (NCT01767792)
Lapatinib	EGFR and ErbB2	30.8% hearing improved, 23.5% tumor shrinkage[10]; (+) preclinical efficacy[11]	Phase 2 trial completed (NCT00973739) Phase 0 trial ongoing (NCT00863122)
Erlotinib	EGFR	No volumetric or audiological response[12]; (+) preclinical efficacy[13]	No active clinical trials
Everolimus	mTORC1	No volumetric or audiological response[14] but study limited by small number of patients, many of who had failed previous medical therapy; (+) preclinical efficacy[4]	Phase 2 trials completed (NCT01490476, NCT01419639) and ongoing (NCT01345136) Phase 0 trial ongoing (NCT01880749)
Aspirin	COX enzyme; IkB kinase	A significant inverse association was found among aspirin users and spontaneous VS growth (OR: 0.50)[15]	No active clinical trials
Candidate drugs showing preclinical efficacy			
Nilotinib	PDGFR, c-KIT, bcr-abl	(+) preclinical efficacy[16,17]	Phase 2 trial ongoing (NCT01201538)
AR-42	HDACI	(+) preclinical efficacy[18,19]	Phase 0 trial ongoing (NCT02282917)
AR-12	PDK-1	(+) preclinical efficacy[20]	No active clinical trials
Sorafenib	PDGFR, c-Raf, VEGFR-2, -3	(+) preclinical efficacy[21]	No active clinical trials
Selumetinib	MEK1/2	(+) preclinical efficacy[17,22]	No active clinical trials
Other novel candidate drugs			
Axitinib	VEGFR-1/2/3	No preclinical studies in VS	Phase 2 trial ongoing (NCT02129647)
Endostatin	VEGF, TNF-α	No preclinical studies in VS	Phase 2 trial ongoing (NCT02104323)
PTC299	VEGF mRNA	No preclinical studies in VS	Phase 2 trial ongoing (NCT00911248)

[a]Direct comparisons of outcomes between studies are limited by the variable definitions used for hearing improvement and volumetric tumor response between studies.

efficacy of erlotinib to trastuzumab (a monoclonal antibody against ErbB) *in vivo* using VS xenografts, both drugs significantly reduced the growth of VS xenografts; however, only erlotinib (but not trastuzumab) resulted in increased VS cell death.[13] Unfortunately, a retrospective clinical series studying erlotinib in 11 patients with NF2 and progressive VS did not achieve a formal radiographic response, although 3 patients (27%) demonstrated prolonged stable disease or slowing of their tumor growth rate, suggesting cytostatic effects of the drug.[12] Interestingly, five of these patients went on to be treated with bevacizumab and four demonstrated either a radiographic or hearing response, suggesting bevacizumab may be more effective in treating VS in these patients.[7]

83.4.2 Lapatinib

Lapatinib (Tykerb, GlaxoSmithKline) is a small molecule RTK inhibitor that is orally active and reversibly inhibits EGFR as well as ErbB2,[32] blocking phosphorylation and activation of ERK1/2 and AKT in EGFR and/or ErbB2-expressing tumor cell lines and animal xenografts.[33,34,35] Lapatinib can have cytostatic or cytotoxic antitumor effects depending on cell type.[35] Based on strong preclinical evidence of lapatinib's efficacy in schwannoma models,[11,33,34,35] a phase 2 clinical trial (NCT00973739) of lapatinib in adults and children with NF2-related tumors was performed.[10] The investigators reported a volumetric and audiological response rate of 23.5 and 30.8%, respectively, which was superior to the results of the retrospective review of 10 patients treated with erlotinib.[12] However, the duration of the response was brief, and patients who demonstrated a response subsequently had tumor regrowth. Moreover, these results were inferior to those obtained in the retrospective series of patients treated with bevacizumab, where a 70% of patients achieved a volumetric response (when defined as ≥ 15% volume reduction) and 57.1% had significant hearing improvement. In addition, patients treated with lapatinib did not show regression of coexisting meningiomas, as these tumors continued to progress with many of the patients during the study.[10] A phase 0 trial (NCT00863122) studying lapatinib's ability to access the tumor and bind to the target site is ongoing.

83.5 The MAPK (Raf/MEK/ERK) Pathway

The MAPK or Raf/MEK/ERK pathway is a key convergence point for multiple upstream signals and is affected by growth factor receptors such as platelet-derived growth factor receptor (PDGFR) and ErbB2.[21,36,37] Preclinical studies have demonstrated overexpression of PDGFR in NF2-deficient cells, resulting in sustained activation of the ERK1/2 and AKT pathways which ultimately lead to increased cell proliferation and tumor growth.[21,38,39]

83.5.1 Nilotinib

Nilotinib (Tasigna, Novartis Pharmaceuticals) is a second-generation, small-molecule RTK inhibitor that targets PDGFR and also targets intracellular players including c-KIT and the BCR-ABL oncoprotein.[16] Nilotinib has successfully inhibited tumor growth in preclinical models[16,17] and prolonged use induced apoptosis, which suggests that its cytotoxic effects may be able to reduce tumor size.[16] Currently, a phase 2 study of nilotinib for growing VS is underway in Canada (NCT01201538).

83.5.2 Sorafenib

Sorafenib (Nexavar, Bayer Pharmaceuticals) is an RTK inhibitor of PDGFR, VEGFR-2/-3, and c-Raf that has inhibited proliferation of schwannoma cells in preclinical studies, presumably through both receptor downregulation and antiangiogenic mechanisms.[21] Unfortunately, sorafenib is associated with severe side effects, which is not ideal as long-term therapy is often required to treat a slow-growing tumor like VS.

83.5.3 Selumetinib

Selumetinib (AZD6244, AstraZeneca) is a novel agent that selectively inhibits MEK1/2, one of the only known catalytic substrates of Raf kinases,[40] and a known convergence point for multiple cascades toward ERK1/2 activation and cell proliferation. Selumetinib completely inhibited PDGF-DD-mediated ERK1/2 activation and cell proliferation in human primary schwannoma cells,[22] and demonstrated greater inhibition when combined with nilotinib suggesting potential use for combination therapy.[17] Currently, there are no clinical trials investigating selumetinib in VS treatment.

83.6 The PI3K/AKT Pathway

The PI3-kinase/AKT pathway, a critical growth-regulating signaling cascade, has also been shown to be aberrantly activated in immunohistochemical studies of VS.[18,41,42]

83.6.1 AR-42

AR-42 (OSU-HDAC42; ARNO Therapeutics, Parsippany, NJ) is part of a new class of antitumor drugs known as histone deacetylase inhibitors (HDACIs). HDACIs act via multiple cell-signaling pathways to induce cell cycle arrest or cause apoptosis, thereby inhibiting tumor growth (▶ Fig. 83.3). AR-42 has been shown to inhibit the growth of schwannoma xenografts and meningioma cells at doses that correlate with AKT inactivation.[18,19] This feature is particularly beneficial for NF2 patients who often develop these tumors synchronously.[19] A phase 0 trial of AR-42 including NF2 patients with progressive VS and meningiomas is ongoing (NCT02282917).

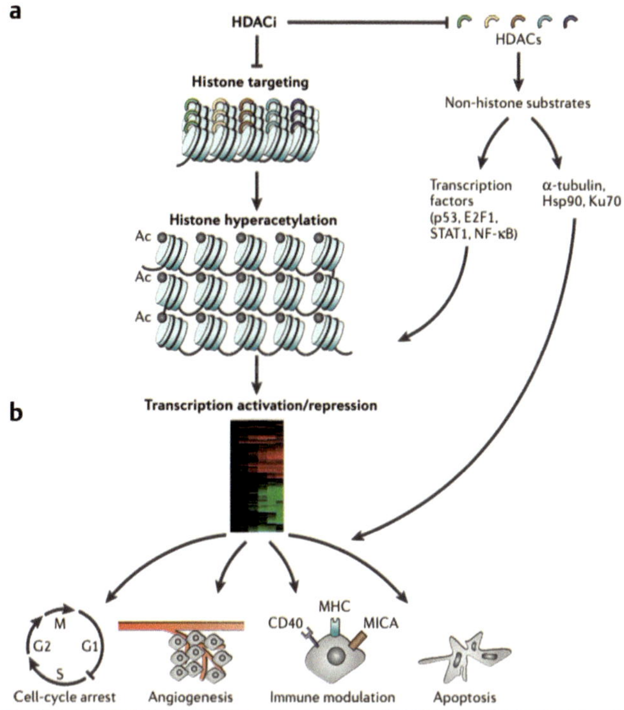

Fig. 83.3 Mechanisms of histone deacetylase inhibitors (HDACIs). **(a)** HDACIs inhibit the deacetylation of histones, permitting the chromatin scaffolding to assume a more relaxed, open conformation, which promotes gene transcription. These epigenetic modifications in gene expression result in upregulation of proapoptotic genes and downregulation of survival genes, which effectively lowers the apoptotic threshold of tumor cells. **(b)** In addition, HDACIs are able to interact with nonhistone proteins to induce cell-cycle arrest, modulate the PI3K/AKT or MEK/ERK signaling pathway, suppress angiogenesis through decreased expression of VEGF, and enhance a tumor cell's antigenicity through upregulating certain surface receptors. (Reprinted with permission from Nature Publishing Group: Nature Reviews Drug Discovery, Anticancer activities of histone deacetylase inhibitors. Bolden JE, Peart MJ, Johnstone RW. 2006 Sep; 5(9):769-84).

83.6.2 AR-12

AR-12 (OSU-03012; ARNO Therapeutics, Parsippany, NJ) is a novel phosphoinositide-dependent kinase-1 (PDK1) inhibitor that is derived from the cyclooxygenase-2 (COX-2) inhibitor Celebrex.[20] PDK1 is a key upstream kinase that phosphorylates and activates AKT, resulting in tumor growth, and blocking PDK-1 inhibition leading to decreased tumor growth *in vivo* that correlated with reduced AKT phosphorylation.[20] There are no clinical trials investigating AR-12 in VS treatment currently.

83.7 The mTOR Pathway

Merlin is a negative regulator of mammalian target of rapamycin complex 1 (mTORC1), and loss of merlin as occurs in NF2 results in activation of mTORC1 and the development of NF2-related tumors.[43,44] Since merlin may directly regulate mTOR activity, independent of AKT or MAPK activation,[45] a separate inhibitor of mTORC1 may need to suppress cell growth.

83.7.1 Everolimus (Rapamycin Analog)

Everolimus (Afinitor, RAD001; Novartis) is an oral inhibitor of mTORC1 and is FDA approved for advanced renal cell carcinoma and other tumors. Preclinical studies have shown that inhibition of mTORC1 may delay growth but does not completely suppress tumorigenesis of merlin-deficient cells.[4,44,45] There is also evidence that the mTORC1 inhibition also inhibits VEGF,[46] thereby reducing tumor angiogenesis, which has been previously shown to be an effective form of treatment.[7] Two phase 2 clinical trials (NCT01419639, NCT01490476) using everolimus in NF2 patients with progressive VS failed to show any clinically significant tumor shrinkage.[14,47] Importantly, Goutagny et al observed that everolimus has the potential to stabilize or delay tumor growth which may be of value for NF2 patients, but "rebound" growth occurred with cessation of the drug.[47] The drug is generally well tolerated with mild toxicities being reported, and the safety of everolimus in children has been studied.[48] A phase 0 trial (NCT01880749) and another phase 2 trial (NCT01345136) are ongoing to study the effects of everolimus on NF2-related VS and meningioma.

83.8 Targeting Mediators of Inflammation

Cyclooxygenase-2 (COX-2) and its downstream products including prostaglandin E2 have been shown to be aberrantly expressed in human VS and their activity correlates with VS cell proliferation rate.[49,50] In addition, nuclear factor kappa B (NF-kB), a transcription factor that orchestrates the immunogenic response of over 300 downstream genes and influences the growth, proliferation, and survival of cells, is overexpressed in human VS samples.[51]

83.8.1 Aspirin

Aspirin irreversibly inactivates the COX enzyme and is also a known inhibitor of NF-kB activation through its blockade of I kappa B kinase.[52,53] In a retrospective series, aspirin use was inversely associated with VS growth rate,[15] and it appears to have cytostatic effects *in vitro*, decreasing the growth rate of primary VS cultures by half.[15,49] Given its low toxicity profile, the use of aspirin to control VS growth may serve as a very attractive therapeutic option, especially given the other benefits of daily aspirin use such as reducing the risk of cardiovascular disease and certain cancers.[54,55,56] Future trials of COX-2 selective inhibitors such as celecoxib against VS are planned and may show similar efficacy but without the adverse effects of chronic use of general COX inhibitors, such as gastrointestinal bleed or ulceration.[57]

83.9 Future Research

Drug development for NF2-related VS is in its infancy and further multicenter, prospective trials are required before any definitive conclusions can be made. Advances in bioinformatics are leading to a better understanding of the functional relationships between differentially expressed genes and the molecular players of dysregulated pathways. High-throughput screening of compound libraries with phenotypic assays is serving as an efficient, nonbiased, empirical technique for researchers to quickly conduct millions of chemical, genetic, or pharmacological tests to aid in the drug discovery and target identification process. The use of genetically engineered mouse models to test rationally designed drug candidates prior to validating them in clinical trials is useful and important, particularly in NF2 where there is a limited patient population. Future discoveries will hopefully reveal chemoprevention strategies, whereby NF2 patients can safely take a drug that prevents or halts tumor growth before becoming symptomatic. With the development of increasingly novel molecular-targeted therapies, a surge of preclinical and clinical trials is sure to follow in the coming years ahead.

References

[1] Evans DG, Huson SM, Donnai D, et al. A clinical study of type 2 neurofibromatosis. Q J Med. 1992; 84(304):603–618

[2] Ogawa K, Kanzaki J, Ogawa S, Yamamoto M, Ikeda S, Shiobara R. The growth rate of acoustic neuromas. Acta Otolaryngol Suppl. 1991; 487:157–163

[3] Blakeley JO, Evans DG, Adler J, et al. Consensus recommendations for current treatments and accelerating clinical trials for patients with neurofibromatosis type 2. Am J Med Genet A. 2012; 158A(1):24–41

[4] Giovannini M, Bonne NX, Vitte J, et al. mTORC1 inhibition delays growth of neurofibromatosis type 2 schwannoma. Neuro-oncol. 2014; 16(4):493–504

[5] Cayé-Thomasen P, Baandrup L, Jacobsen GK, Thomsen J, Stangerup SE. Immunohistochemical demonstration of vascular endothelial growth factor in vestibular schwannomas correlates to tumor growth rate. Laryngoscope. 2003; 113(12):2129–2134

[6] Plotkin SR, Merker VL, Halpin C, et al. Bevacizumab for progressive vestibular schwannoma in neurofibromatosis type 2: a retrospective review of 31 patients. Otol Neurotol. 2012; 33(6):1046–1052

[7] Plotkin SR, Stemmer-Rachamimov AO, Barker FG, II, et al. Hearing improvement after bevacizumab in patients with neurofibromatosis type 2. N Engl J Med. 2009; 361(4):358–367

[8] Mautner VF, Nguyen R, Kutta H, et al. Bevacizumab induces regression of vestibular schwannomas in patients with neurofibromatosis type 2. Neuro-oncol. 2010; 12(1):14–18

[9] Blakeley JO, Ye X, Duda DG, et al. Efficacy and biomarker study of bevacizumab for hearing loss resulting from neurofibromatosis type 2-associated vestibular schwannomas. J Clin Oncol. 2016; 34(14):1669–1675

[10] Karajannis MA, Legault G, Hagiwara M, et al. Phase II trial of lapatinib in adult and pediatric patients with neurofibromatosis type 2 and progressive vestibular schwannomas. Neuro-oncol. 2012; 14(9):1163–1170

[11] Ammoun S, Cunliffe CH, Allen JC, et al. ErbB/HER receptor activation and preclinical efficacy of lapatinib in vestibular schwannoma. Neuro-oncol. 2010; 12(8):834–843

[12] Plotkin SR, Halpin C, McKenna MJ, Loeffler JS, Batchelor TT, Barker FG, II. Erlotinib for progressive vestibular schwannoma in neurofibromatosis 2 patients. Otol Neurotol. 2010; 31(7):1135–1143

[13] Clark JJ, Provenzano M, Diggelmann HR, Xu N, Hansen SS, Hansen MR. The ErbB inhibitors trastuzumab and erlotinib inhibit growth of vestibular schwannoma xenografts in nude mice: a preliminary study. Otol Neurotol. 2008; 29(6):846–853

[14] Karajannis MA, Legault G, Hagiwara M, et al. Phase II study of everolimus in children and adults with neurofibromatosis type 2 and progressive vestibular schwannomas. Neuro-oncol. 2014; 16(2):292–297

[15] Kandathil CK, Dilwali S, Wu CC, et al. Aspirin intake correlates with halted growth of sporadic vestibular schwannoma in vivo. Otol Neurotol. 2014; 35 (2):353–357
[16] Sabha N, Au K, Agnihotri S, et al. Investigation of the in vitro therapeutic efficacy of nilotinib in immortalized human NF2-null vestibular schwannoma cells. PLoS One. 2012; 7(6):e39412
[17] Ammoun S, Schmid MC, Triner J, Manley P, Hanemann CO. Nilotinib alone or in combination with selumetinib is a drug candidate for neurofibromatosis type 2. Neuro-oncol. 2011; 13(7):759–766
[18] Bush ML, Oblinger J, Brendel V, et al. AR42, a novel histone deacetylase inhibitor, as a potential therapy for vestibular schwannomas and meningiomas. Neuro-oncol. 2011; 13(9):983–999
[19] Jacob A, Oblinger J, Bush ML, et al. Preclinical validation of AR42, a novel histone deacetylase inhibitor, as treatment for vestibular schwannomas. Laryngoscope. 2012; 122(1):174–189
[20] Lee TX, Packer MD, Huang J, et al. Growth inhibitory and anti-tumour activities of OSU-03012, a novel PDK-1 inhibitor, on vestibular schwannoma and malignant schwannoma cells. Eur J Cancer. 2009; 45 (9):1709–1720
[21] Ammoun S, Flaiz C, Ristic N, Schuldt J, Hanemann CO. Dissecting and targeting the growth factor-dependent and growth factor-independent extracellular signal-regulated kinase pathway in human schwannoma. Cancer Res. 2008; 68(13):5236–5245
[22] Ammoun S, Ristic N, Matthies C, Hilton DA, Hanemann CO. Targeting ERK1/2 activation and proliferation in human primary schwannoma cells with MEK1/2 inhibitor AZD6244. Neurobiol Dis. 2010; 37(1):141–146
[23] Miller LE, Miller VM. Safety and effectiveness of microvascular decompression for treatment of hemifacial spasm: a systematic review. Br J Neurosurg. 2012; 26(4):438–444
[24] Mautner VF, Nguyen R, Knecht R, Bokemeyer C. Radiographic regression of vestibular schwannomas induced by bevacizumab treatment: sustain under continuous drug application and rebound after drug discontinuation. Ann Oncol. 2010; 21(11):2294–2295
[25] Slusarz KM, Merker VL, Muzikansky A, Francis SA, Plotkin SR. Long-term toxicity of bevacizumab therapy in neurofibromatosis 2 patients. Cancer Chemother Pharmacol. 2014; 73(6):1197–1204
[26] O'Reilly MS, Boehm T, Shing Y, et al. Endostatin: an endogenous inhibitor of angiogenesis and tumor growth. Cell. 1997; 88(2):277–285
[27] van Geel RM, Beijnen JH, Schellens JH. Concise drug review: pazopanib and axitinib. Oncologist. 2012; 17(8):1081–1089
[28] Knight D, Tiersten A, Miao H, et al. PTC299, a novel regulator of tumor VEGF expression, is well tolerated and achieves target plasma concentrations: dose-ranging results of a phase 1b study in women with metastatic breast cancer. Cancer Res. 2009; 69(24):853s–854s
[29] Lallemand D, Manent J, Couvelard A, et al. Merlin regulates transmembrane receptor accumulation and signaling at the plasma membrane in primary mouse Schwann cells and in human schwannomas. Oncogene. 2009; 28(6): 854–865
[30] Curto M, Cole BK, Lallemand D, Liu CH, McClatchey AI. Contact-dependent inhibition of EGFR signaling by Nf2/Merlin. J Cell Biol. 2007; 177(5):893–903
[31] Hansen MR, Linthicum FH, Jr. Expression of neuregulin and activation of erbB receptors in vestibular schwannomas: possible autocrine loop stimulation. Otol Neurotol. 2004; 25(2):155–159
[32] Montemurro F, Valabrega G, Aglietta M. Lapatinib: a dual inhibitor of EGFR and HER2 tyrosine kinase activity. Expert Opin Biol Ther. 2007; 7(2):257–268
[33] Xia W, Mullin RJ, Keith BR, et al. Anti-tumor activity of GW572016: a dual tyrosine kinase inhibitor blocks EGF activation of EGFR/erbB2 and downstream Erk1/2 and AKT pathways. Oncogene. 2002; 21(41):6255–6263
[34] Rusnak DW, Affleck K, Cockerill SG, et al. The characterization of novel, dual ErbB-2/EGFR, tyrosine kinase inhibitors: potential therapy for cancer. Cancer Res. 2001; 61(19):7196–7203
[35] Rusnak DW, Lackey K, Affleck K, et al. The effects of the novel, reversible epidermal growth factor receptor/ErbB-2 tyrosine kinase inhibitor, GW2016, on the growth of human normal and tumor-derived cell lines in vitro and in vivo. Mol Cancer Ther. 2001; 1(2):85–94
[36] Hansen MR, Roehm PC, Chatterjee P, Green SH. Constitutive neuregulin-1/ ErbB signaling contributes to human vestibular schwannoma proliferation. Glia. 2006; 53(6):593–600
[37] Yee KL, Weaver VM, Hammer DA. Integrin-mediated signalling through the MAP-kinase pathway. IET Syst Biol. 2008; 2(1):8–15
[38] Fraenzer JT, Pan H, Minimo L, Jr, Smith GM, Knauer D, Hung G. Overexpression of the NF2 gene inhibits schwannoma cell proliferation through promoting PDGFR degradation. Int J Oncol. 2003; 23(6):1493–1500
[39] Morrison H, Sperka T, Manent J, Giovannini M, Ponta H, Herrlich P. Merlin/ neurofibromatosis type 2 suppresses growth by inhibiting the activation of Ras and Rac. Cancer Res. 2007; 67(2):520–527
[40] Roberts PJ, Der CJ. Targeting the Raf-MEK-ERK mitogen-activated protein kinase cascade for the treatment of cancer. Oncogene. 2007; 26(22): 3291–3310
[41] Jacob A, Lee TX, Neff BA, Miller S, Welling B, Chang LS. Phosphatidylinositol 3-kinase/AKT pathway activation in human vestibular schwannoma. Otol Neurotol. 2008; 29(1):58–68
[42] Hilton DA, Ristic N, Hanemann CO. Activation of ERK, AKT and JNK signalling pathways in human schwannomas in situ. Histopathology. 2009; 55(6):744–749
[43] James MF, Stivison E, Beauchamp R, et al. Regulation of mTOR complex 2 signaling in neurofibromatosis 2-deficient target cell types. Mol Cancer Res. 2012; 10(5):649–659
[44] López-Lago MA, Okada T, Murillo MM, Socci N, Giancotti FG. Loss of the tumor suppressor gene NF2, encoding merlin, constitutively activates integrin-dependent mTORC1 signaling. Mol Cell Biol. 2009; 29(15):4235–4249
[45] James MF, Han S, Polizzano C, et al. NF2/merlin is a novel negative regulator of mTOR complex 1, and activation of mTORC1 is associated with meningioma and schwannoma growth. Mol Cell Biol. 2009; 29(15):4250–4261
[46] Lane HA, Wood JM, McSheehy PM, et al. mTOR inhibitor RAD001 (everolimus) has antiangiogenic/vascular properties distinct from a VEGFR tyrosine kinase inhibitor. Clin Cancer Res. 2009; 15(5):1612–1622
[47] Goutagny S, Raymond E, Esposito-Farese M, et al. Phase II study of mTORC1 inhibition by everolimus in neurofibromatosis type 2 patients with growing vestibular schwannomas. J Neurooncol. 2015; 122(2):313–320
[48] Fouladi M, Laningham F, Wu J, et al. Phase I study of everolimus in pediatric patients with refractory solid tumors. J Clin Oncol. 2007; 25(30):4806–4812
[49] Dilwali S, Kao SY, Fujita T, Landegger LD, Stankovic KM. Nonsteroidal anti-inflammatory medications are cytostatic against human vestibular schwannomas. Transl Res. 2015; 166(1):1–11
[50] Hong B, Krusche CA, Schwabe K, et al. Cyclooxygenase-2 supports tumor proliferation in vestibular schwannomas. Neurosurgery. 2011; 68(4): 1112–1117
[51] Dilwali S, Briët MC, Kao SY, et al. Preclinical validation of anti-nuclear factor-kappa B therapy to inhibit human vestibular schwannoma growth. Mol Oncol. 2015; 9(7):1359–1370
[52] Muller DN, Heissmeyer V, Dechend R, et al. Aspirin inhibits NF-kappaB and protects from angiotensin II-induced organ damage. FASEB J. 2001; 15(10): 1822–1824
[53] Kopp E, Ghosh S. Inhibition of NF-kappa B by sodium salicylate and aspirin. Science. 1994; 265(5174):956–959
[54] Chan AT, Ogino S, Fuchs CS. Aspirin use and survival after diagnosis of colorectal cancer. JAMA. 2009; 302(6):649–658
[55] Terry MB, Gammon MD, Zhang FF, et al. Association of frequency and duration of aspirin use and hormone receptor status with breast cancer risk. JAMA. 2004; 291(20):2433–2440
[56] Thorat MA, Cuzick J. Role of aspirin in cancer prevention. Curr Oncol Rep. 2013; 15(6):533–540
[57] Sobolewski C, Cerella C, Dicato M, Ghibelli L, Diederich M. The role of cyclooxygenase-2 in cell proliferation and cell death in human malignancies. Int J Cell Biol. 2010; 2010:215158

84 Auditory Rehabilitation in Neurofibromatosis Type 2

Daniel S. Roberts, Steven R. Otto, Marc S. Schwartz, and Eric P. Wilkinson

84.1 Introduction

Owing to the presence of bilateral vestibular schwannomas (VS) in neurofibromatosis type 2 (NF2), patients are often left completely deafened by either the natural course of the disease or by the necessity for therapeutic intervention.[1] Management of bilateral VS in patients with NF2 is highly individualized and hearing preservation or rehabilitation remains a prioritized goal for management. The development of the auditory brainstem implant (ABI) and auditory midbrain implant (AMI) provides a means of bypassing a diseased or absent cochlea and auditory nerve to directly stimulate the central auditory pathway in order to provide sound perception to a patient with profound hearing loss. Cochlear implantation (CI) may also provide benefit for a select group of patients with an anatomically intact cochlear nerve but nonserviceable hearing. This chapter discusses the clinical and surgical aspects of ABI, AMI, and CI in patients with NF2. Audiometric outcomes for each modality are reviewed.

84.2 History and Devices

84.2.1 Auditory Brainstem Implant

Drs. William Hitselberger and William House performed the first ABI in 1979 by placing a ball-type electrode onto the surface of the cochlear nucleus.[2,3] U.S. Food and Drug Administration (FDA) approval was obtained in 2000 for the multichannel ABI manufactured by Cochlear Limited (Sydney, Australia). ABIs have also been produced by other implant manufacturers including Med-El, which are currently not approved in the United States.

A penetrating electrode ABI was subsequently developed in an effort to improve the precision and selectivity of brainstem auditory neuron stimulation with the goal of improving speech recognition (▶ Fig. 84.1A). A hybrid ABI array consisting of a version of the present surface electrode and a 10-electrode penetrating array was studied in an FDA clinical trial of 10 patients. While this device resulted in increased selectivity and lowered charge requirements in the usable penetrating electrodes, the device did not provide improved speech discrimination.[4] As of 2017, all commercially available devices do not utilize penetrating electrodes.

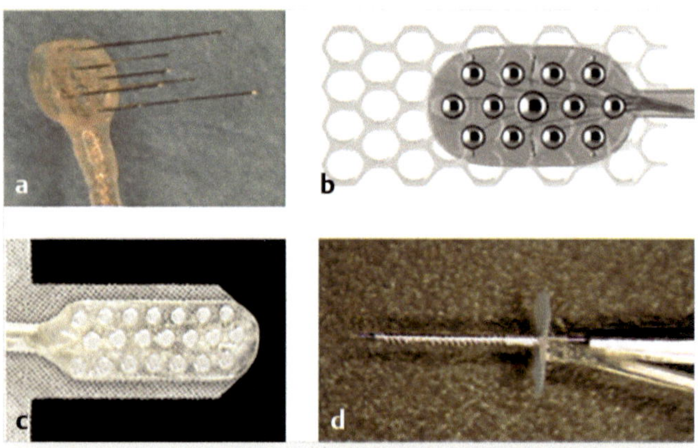

Fig. 84.1 Auditory brainstem implant (ABI) and auditory midbrain implant (AMI) electrode arrays. **(a)** Penetrating auditory brainstem implant array. **(b)** Cochlear ABI 541 21-electrode surface array. **(c)** Med-El Synchrony ABI 12-electrode surface array with a Dacron backing (cartoon). **(c)** AMI array.

The production of the Cochlear Nucleus 24 ABI was discontinued in 2015, and the replacement Cochlear Device, ABI 541, was not approved by the FDA until 2016 (▶ Fig. 84.1B). During this time, both Cochlear and Med-El devices were implanted under the auspices of "Compassionate Use" approval by the FDA in the United States on an individual, case-by-case basis.[5] FDA approval was granted in June 2016 for the ABI 541. The Med-El device continues to be implanted in the United States through an open clinical trial (ClinicalTrials.gov ID: NCT01736267). Approximately 1,300 patients have been implanted worldwide to date (▶ Fig. 84.1c).

84.2.2 Auditory Midbrain Implant

The inferior colliculus (ICC) is a desirable target for an AMI auditory prosthesis because the central nucleus of the ICC is a loci of convergence for ascending auditory pathways and is readily accessible during surgery.[6,7] Currently, two AMI options include the use of a surface electrode using the Med-El ABI array and a penetrating array utilizing a Cochlear Corporation deep brain stimulation (DBS) array (▶ Fig. 84.1D).[6,8]

84.2.3 Cochlear Implantation

The prospect of performing a CI in NF2 patients was first proposed by Cueva et al after successfully performing promontory stimulation in patients with deafness after VS resection.[9] The benefits of this approach were first realized in a single NF2 patient who received a CI after resection of VS where the cochlear nerve was spared.[10]

84.3 Patient Selection

84.3.1 Auditory Brainstem Implant

This device was originally designed for NF2 patients with bilateral VSs. FDA criteria includes bilateral eight-nerve tumors, age 12 years or older, psychological suitability, willingness to comply with the follow-up protocol, and realistic expectations. Several reports suggest positive outcomes in adults and children for the treatment of deafness resulting from traumatic transection or avulsion of the cochlear nerve, cochlear ossification after meningitis, and congenital cochlear aplasia or cochlear nerve deficiency. These topics will not be reviewed further in this chapter, but the following references are available for the interested reader.[11,12,13,14]

At the House Clinic, our NF2 protocol allows implantation at the time of first- or second-side VS removal or in patients whose tumors have previously been removed. Implantation during removal of the first tumor allows the patient to gain experience with the device with the goal of possible enhanced performance if the patient loses all hearing. Suitable candidates are patients undergoing translabyrinthine or retrosigmoid VS removal who have (1) nonaidable hearing or an only hearing ear with a symptomatic tumor or (2) serviceable hearing in the contralateral ear but a contralateral tumor of sufficient size to indicate that hearing will potentially be lost. Implantation on the first side gives the patient two chances at obtaining an optimally functioning system should the procedure in the first side not be successful, which may occur in up to 8% of cases.

84.3.2 Auditory Midbrain Implant

Damage to the brainstem region, either due to the tumor or during tumor removal, may make placement of an ABI impossible or ineffective. In these rare cases, AMI may be advantageous to bypass this damaged region to provide the best opportunity for auditory rehabilitation. AMI placement remains an area of active investigation and is only being performed in a research setting.[6]

84.3.3 Cochlear Implantation

Cochlear implantation is traditionally used in patients without retrocochlear disease because a lesion involving of the cochlear nerve or proximal could render the procedure ineffective. However, recent data suggest benefit for properly selected patients with NF2. CIs are advocated for cases of nonserviceable hearing with intracochlear and intralabyrinthine schwannomas.[15] Further indications include stable VSs with an anatomically intact cochlear nerve after surgical resection, radiosurgery, or during the course of conservative observation. The cochlear nerve is presumed to be intact in all patients with conservatively managed tumors or those who have received radiation treatment. Patient candidacy for CI after microsurgical resection may be more difficult, particularly if details regarding the original surgery are not well described. In such cases, electrical promontory stimulation testing may be beneficial.[16] Ideal postoperative candidates are those with smaller tumors who underwent attempted hearing preservation surgery, but lost serviceable hearing as a result of presumed vascular compromise. However, even patients who underwent translabyrinthine surgery may benefit from CI if the cochlear nerve was preserved. In these cases, use of a spacer or immediate implantation is recommended given the concern for cochlear ossification following translabyrinthine drilling. In an English consensus statement protocol evaluating the candidacy for ABI or CI in NF2, CI is considered to be the most efficacious modality for hearing rehabilitation in patients who have been treated with radiation or who have two stable VSs.[17]

84.4 Surgical Procedure

84.4.1 Auditory Brainstem Implant

During tumor dissection, care is taken to avoid trauma or injury to the area of the brainstem adjacent to the root entry zone of the vestibulocochlear nerve. The anatomical target for the ABI is the ventral cochlear nucleus, which is the main relay for cochlear nerve input and the ascending auditory pathway. The ventral cochlear nucleus lies within the lateral recess of the fourth ventricle. The surgical approach for tumor removal in ABI cases at the House Clinic has been exclusively via translabyrinthine craniotomy; however, other centers offer the retrosigmoid approach with success.[11,18] The retrosigmoid approach is particularly beneficial in cases where the sigmoid sinus is located extremely anteriorly or in pediatric cases. Electrodes are placed for recording electrically evoked auditory brainstem responses (EABRs) and for monitoring cranial nerves VII and IX/X. The choroid plexus marks the entrance to the lateral recess (foramen of Luschka), and the taenia choroidea obliquely traverses the roof of the lateral recess, marking the surface of the ventral cochlear nucleus. The ninth cranial nerve can also be used as a reference point for the lateral recess. After identifying the foramen of Luschka, microinstruments are used to insert the electrode array into the lateral recess with the electrodes facing superiorly (see Chapter 30).

The technique of electrode placement is dependent on the device that is utilized. The Med-El Synchrony device first uses a four-channel ABI placing electrode as a test electrode that is inserted into the lateral recess of the fourth ventricle to generate EABRs from the cochlear nucleus. Measurements are repeated until adequate EABR tracings are obtained for all electrode combinations. The placing electrode is then removed, and the active implant is then placed using EABR data to assist with positioning. A final EABR recording using the active electrode array is then performed confirming correct placement. For the Cochlear ABI 541 device, EABR is performed after placement of the active ABI, confirming placement at the cochlear nucleus. Repositioning is performed as needed with the active ABI device. Both electrode arrays are secured by a small piece of Teflon felt packed into the meatus of the lateral recess.

The cortical bone posterior to the mastoid is flattened, and a trough is drilled to accommodate the receiver/stimulator electrode similar to CI. The receiver/stimulator is placed into a circular area of bony cortex posterosuperior to the mastoid defect created by an otologic drill. A tie-down technique or tight periosteal pocket is used to secure the device. The magnet from the receiver-stimulator is removed to allow high-quality surveillance magnetic resonance imaging (MRI). Abdominal fat is used to obliterate the mastoid defect followed by a three-layered closure.

84.4.2 Auditory Midbrain Implant

Resection of VS followed by AMI placement utilizes a suboccipital craniotomy. Following resection of the VS, the cerebellum is retracted inferiorly to provide exposure to the ICC.[6] Arachnoid is dissected to expose the midbrain and the ICC is visualized. The AMI is inserted into the ICC with the tonotopic orientation of the ICC. Landmarks for insertion include the rostral border of the ICC with the superior colliculus, caudal ICC edge corresponding to the exit point of the trochlear nerve, and the midline between both ICCs.[19] Insertion requires an angle of 40 degrees relative to the sagittal plane.

84.4.3 Cochlear Implantation

Standard cochlear implant arrays and techniques are utilized for cases of implantation in patients with NF2. Carlson et al advocated consideration of an electrode with a stylet in cases of intracochlear schwannomas with late deployment to overcome possible resistance that may be encountered due to the presence of intracochlear tumor.[15]

84.5 Outcomes

84.5.1 Auditory Brainstem Implant

The goal of ABI is to provide the patient with some degree of environmental sound awareness, word recognition, and also improved communication in conjunction with lipreading. A minority of patients may also obtain some open-set speech understanding. Preoperatively, specific effort should be made to inform patients of these limitations and to help form realistic hearing expectations.

Over 310 patients with NF2 have been implanted with the Nucleus multichannel ABI system at the House Clinic between 1992 and 2017. With notable exceptions, ABI performance generally has not reached the high levels typically seen with CIs. Eighty percent of the patients are device users, and 92% have received auditory sensations from their ABIs. The majority of patients recognize a high percentage of environmental sounds, and the ability of speech understanding is enhanced an average of 35% when ABI sound is combined with lipreading. This enhancement has reached as high as 75% in some individuals. Although improvements are generally greatest during the first year, many patients have continued to improve even after 10 years of use. All patients have used the SPEAK (spectral maxima) speech processing strategy.[20]

At our center, approximately 25% of ABI users have achieved some open-set speech discrimination defined as at least 20% correct without lipreading cues on the CUNY Sentence Test.[21,22] Ten patients at the House Clinic have scored 65% or better, and three patients have scored 82% or better on this test. ▸ Table 84.1 shows outcomes from the House Ear Institute and from other centers.

Recent reports notably illustrate the successful ABI outcomes among NF2 patients with as high as a 37% rate of open speech perception at 1 year and 41% at 2 years after activation.[33,34] An inverse relationship between deafness duration and open speech perception was noted among these patients. These outcomes have reportedly improved upon data from the United States and factors accounting for these improved outcomes are not well understood and an area of active investigation.[37] Hypothetically, differences in surgical technique may account for improved outcomes. The retrosigmoid approach in the semi-sitting position with a Med-EL ABI device (not FDA approved in the United States) is primarily utilized by European centers. The semi-sitting position may facilitate brain relaxation and bloodless dissection. Positioning may improve hemostasis and health of the neural tissue in the auditory brainstem nucleus. The semi-sitting position does increase the risk of air embolism. A second untested hypothesis is that device differences may also account for differential outcomes. The Med-El device has enhanced cable flexibility and a smaller surface array profile, possibly aiding placement. The Med-El device also has a four-channel test electrode that allows EABR confirmation prior to opening the ABI device packaging and subsequent implantation. Other possible ABI hearing outcome prognostic factors include a history of Gamma Knife radiosurgery (GKRS) for VS which is associated with a higher rate of no hearing benefit (~30 vs. 9%). However, there are many examples of patients with large VS at our center, or a history of GKRS, who have experienced great benefit from their ABIs.

84.5.2 Auditory Midbrain Implant

Stimulation of the ICC is an active area of research with a small number of patients implanted.[6] The AMI was safe and provided auditory sensations, aided with lipreading, sound awareness, and some speech perception in a five-patient clinical trial from 2006 to 2008.[19] However, AMI has not yet demonstrated the outcomes comparable to the highest ABI performers, with no

Table 84.1 Auditory brainstem implant outcomes in neurofibromatosis type 2

First author	Year	*N*	Daily users	Open-set sentence recognition	No auditory response
Laszig[23]	1995	9	4 (42%)	0 (0%)	1 (11%)
Lenarz[24]	2002	13	13 (93%)	0 (%)	1/13 (8%)
Vincent[25]	2002	14	12 (85%)	3 (21%)	1 (7%)
Nevison[26]	2002	26	23 (88%)	2 (8%)	1 (4%)
Otto[27]	2002	61	55 (90%)	5%	6 (9%)
Kanowitz[28]	2004	18	11 (61%)	0 (0%)	1 (6%)
Sanna[29]	2006	20	18 (90%)	8 (42%)	NR
Grayeli[30]	2008	23	16 (70%)	8 (34%)	5 (22%)
Schwartz[31]	2003	230	NR	5%	15%
Maini[32]	2009	10	7 (70%)	5%	1 (10%)
Sanna[29]	2012	24	19 (79%)	4 (17%)	4 (17%)
Matthies[33]	2013	32	27 (84%)	37%	3 (9%)
Matthies[34]	2014	18	16 (88%)	41%	2 (11%)
Thong[35]	2016	8	3 (38%)	1 (13%)	2 (25%)
Ramsden[36]	2016	49	29 (59%)	5 (10%)	4 (8%)
Average			74%	14%	12%

Source: Used with permission from Sanna M, Di Lella F, Guida M, Merkus P. Auditory brainstem implants in NF2 patients: results and review of the literature. Otol Neurotol. 2012; 33(2):154 -164.[29]

Table 84.2 Cochlear implantation outcomes in neurofibromatosis type 2

First author	Year	N	Daily users	Open-set sentence recognition	No auditory response
Tono[41]	1996	1	NR	1 (100%)	0 (0%)
Graham[42]	1999	1	1 (100%)	1 (100%)	0 (0%)
Ahsan[43]	2003	1	NR	1 (100%)	0 (0%)
Nölle[44]	2003	1	NR	1 (100%)	0 (0%)
Arístegui[45]	2005	1	NR	1 (100%)	0 (0%)
Lustig[46]	2006	7	7 (100%)	6 (86%)	0 (0%)
Neff[39]	2007	5	NR	4 (80%)	0 (0%)
Vincenti[40]	2008	4	3 (75%)	3 (75%)	1 (25%)
Tran Ba Huy[47]	2009	3	NR	3 (100%)	0 (0%)
Trotter[48]	2010	3	3 (100%)	3 (100%)	0 (0%)
Roehm[49]	2011	6	5 (83%)	3 (50%)	1 (17%)
Carlson[38]	2012	10	9 (90%)	6 (60%)	1 (10%)
Sanna[29]	2012	5	5 (100%)	4 (80%)	0 (0%)
Lloyd[50]	2014	6	4 (67%)	4 (67%)	1 (17%)
Carlson[15]	2016	7	6 (86%)	5 (71%)	1 (28%)
Average			89%	85%	6.5%

patient achieving open-set sentence recognition. Despite these limitations, device and surgical modifications are an area of active investigation with further clinical trials planned.[19]

84.5.3 Cochlear Implantation

Cochlear implantation is a successful modality for hearing rehabilitation in properly selected cases and a high rate of open-set speech discrimination can be expected (▶ Table 84.2). While large series are not present in the literature, CI appears to be successful in most cases where a cochlear nerve is present, despite a prior history of stereotactic radiosurgery (SRS) or microsurgical resection. In a systematic review of all cases of CI in NF2 reported in the literature, open-set speech recognition was found in 65% of patients who had surgery, in 80% of those receiving SRS, and in 100% of patients who were observed.[38] Patients who had a duration of deafness of less than 10 years were statistically more likely to achieve open-set speech recognition. Time between surgery or SRS and CI, surgical approach, or tumor size had no influence on rates of open-set speech recognition.[39,40]

Several aspects of management merit discussion. Our experience suggests that cases amenable to CI are uncommon, with the preponderance of cases eventually leading to a lack of cochlear nerve continuity, because VS associated with NF2 are more adherent to neurovascular structures, possibly due to a more invasive histopathology.[51] Some cases of CI in the context of NF2 demonstrate variable results and the duration of CI use may be limited by further tumor growth or treatments. Patients should be apprised of this possibility, preoperatively. There are also several unanswered clinical dilemmas. Should surgical management include a strategy to preserve cochlear nerve continuity at the cost of gross total resection in effort to allow for CI? Should a greater number of NF2 patients be managed with SRS to allow for successful CI? These questions merit further analysis and must be balanced with the propensity for many NF2 VSs to require additional tumor treatment or revision surgery. Also, 5-year rates of successful NF2 tumor growth rate control for SRS are 66 to 85% which are historically lower than control rates for sporadic VS.[52] Certainly, the preponderance of evidence supports the use of CI in cases of nonserviceable hearing with an intact cochlear nerve, and a nongrowing tumor either before or after SRS or surgery.

84.6 Complications

For ABI, and possibly AMI, a notable complication is cerebrospinal fluid (CSF) leak which typically manifests with pseudomeningocele formation, or less likely incisional or nasal CSF leaks. ABI or AMI electrodes may serve as a pathway for CSF egress. Meticulous dural closure, adequate mastoid packing with fat, and plugging of the eustachian tube are critical. Despite these methods, ABI recipients are more likely to experience CSF leak compared to patients undergoing translabyrinthine resection of VS alone. Lumbar subarachnoid CSF drain and surgical exploration for persistent leakage are the main management techniques. CI in NF2 patients typically proceeds with the standard risks associated with CI surgery, with increased theoretical risk of CSF leak if performed concomitantly with or after craniotomy.

84.7 Tinnitus Suppression

Emerging data suggest that tinnitus suppression may be mediated by the use of an ABI in NF2 patients.[53] In a study of NF2 patient with tinnitus, ABI reduced tinnitus levels measured on a tinnitus visual analog scale (▶ Fig. 84.2, ▶ Fig. 84.3). Tinnitus levels were immediately reduced on ABI activation and after 1 hour of use, and suppression did not continue after the device was turned off. These studies not only provide additional information and guidance on counseling prospective ABI patients but also suggest that the cochlear nucleus may be a putative target for tinnitus suppression in patients with idiopathic tinnitus.

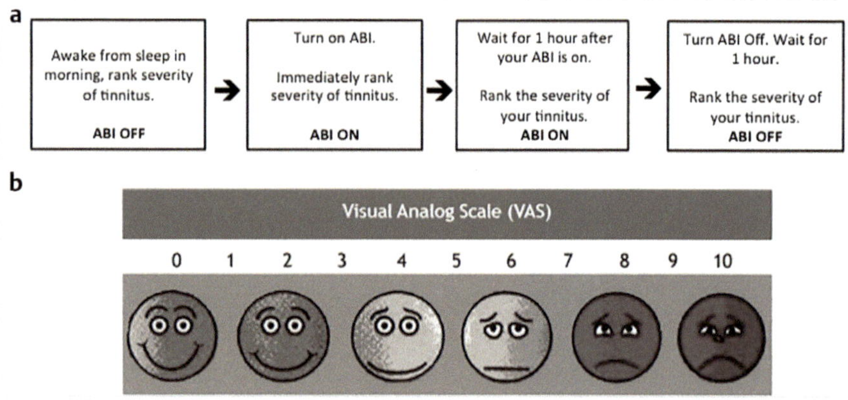

Fig. 84.2 Modulation of tinnitus levels with an auditory brainstem implant (ABI). **(a)** Patients were asked to rank tinnitus levels in four conditions with the ABI on or off according to the diagram. **(b)** Visual analog scale used to score tinnitus levels.

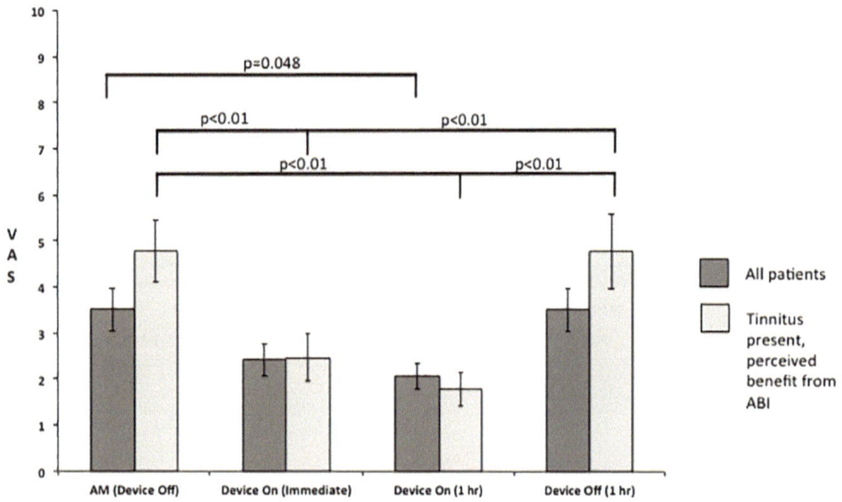

Fig. 84.3 Quantification of tinnitus levels. Data are mean visual analog scale scores ± SEM. *Dark bars* are all patients responded ($n = 33$). *Light bars* are for patients who believed the auditory brainstem implant reduced tinnitus loudness subjectively ($n = 16$). (Adapted from Roberts et al.[53])

84.8 Conclusion

When hearing preservation is not an option for patients with NF2, auditory rehabilitation may be accomplished by ABI or CI. ABI can safely and reliably produce useful auditory sensations by selective activation of the cochlear nucleus. Speech perception performance varies but typically does not reach high levels of open-set speech recognition in the majority of patients. In combination with lipreading cues, ABI has proven to be highly beneficial for the majority of recipients. CI in NF2 patients may more predictively provide the prospect of open-set sentence recognition in properly selected candidates. Further improvements in AMI may hold the prospect for a viable alternative to ABI in cases in which the brainstem has been damaged by tumor growth or treatment.

References

[1] Riccardi VM. Neurofibromatosis. Neurol Clin. 1987; 5(3):337–349
[2] Edgerton BJ, House WF, Hitselberger W. Hearing by cochlear nucleus stimulation in humans. Ann Otol Rhinol Laryngol Suppl. 1982; 91(2, Pt 3):117–124
[3] Hitselberger WE, House WF, Edgerton BJ, Whitaker S. Cochlear nucleus implants. Otolaryngol Head Neck Surg. 1984; 92(1):52–54
[4] Otto SR, Shannon RV, Wilkinson EP, et al. Audiologic outcomes with the penetrating electrode auditory brainstem implant. Otol Neurotol. 2008; 29 (8):1147–1154
[5] Roberts DS, Slattery WH, Chen BS, Otto SR, Schwartz MS, Lekovic GP. 'Compassionate use' protocol for auditory brainstem implantation in neurofibromatosis type 2: early House Ear Institute experience. Cochlear Implants Int. 2017; 18(1):57–62
[6] Lim HH, Lenarz M, Lenarz T. Auditory midbrain implant: a review. Trends Amplif. 2009; 13(3):149–180
[7] Casseday JH, Fremouw T, Covey E. The inferior colliculus: a hub for the central auditory system. In: Oertel D, Fay RR, Popper AN, eds. Springer Handbook of Auditory Research: Integrative Functions in the Mammalian Auditory Pathway, Vol. 15. New York: Springer-Verlag; 2002:238–318
[8] Colletti V, Shannon R, Carner M, et al. The first successful case of hearing produced by electrical stimulation of the human midbrain. Otol Neurotol. 2007; 28(1):39–43
[9] Cueva RA, Thedinger BA, Harris JP, Glasscock ME, III. Electrical promontory stimulation in patients with intact cochlear nerve and anacusis following acoustic neuroma surgery. Laryngoscope. 1992; 102(11):1220–1224
[10] Hoffman RA, Kohan D, Cohen NL. Cochlear implants in the management of bilateral acoustic neuromas. Am J Otol. 1992; 13(6):525–528
[11] Colletti V, Sacchetto L, Giarbini N, Fiorino F, Carner M. Retrosigmoid approach for auditory brainstem implant. J Laryngol Otol Suppl. 2000(27):37–40
[12] Colletti V, Carner M, Miorelli V, Guida M, Colletti L, Fiorino F. Auditory brainstem implant (ABI): new frontiers in adults and children. Otolaryngol Head Neck Surg. 2005; 133(1):126–138
[13] Colletti V, Shannon RV. Open set speech perception with auditory brainstem implant? Laryngoscope. 2005; 115(11):1974–1978
[14] Wilkinson EP, Eisenberg LS, Krieger MD, et al. Los Angeles Pediatric ABI Team. Initial results of a safety and feasibility study of auditory brainstem implantation in congenitally deaf children. Otol Neurotol. 2017; 38(2):212–220
[15] Carlson ML, Neff BA, Sladen DP, Link MJ, Driscoll CL. cochlear implantation in patients with intracochlear and intralabyrinthine schwannomas. Otol Neurotol. 2016; 37(6):647–653

[16] Temple RH, Axon PR, Ramsden RT, Keles N, Deger K, Yücel E. Auditory rehabilitation in neurofibromatosis type 2: a case for cochlear implantation. J Laryngol Otol. 1999; 113(2):161–163
[17] Tysome JR, Axon PR, Donnelly NP, et al. English consensus protocol evaluating candidacy for auditory brainstem and cochlear implantation in neurofibromatosis type 2. Otol Neurotol. 2013; 34(9):1743–1747
[18] Puram SV, Herrmann B, Barker FG, II, Lee DJ. Retrosigmoid craniotomy for auditory brainstem implantation in adult patients with neurofibromatosis type 2. J Neurol Surg B Skull Base. 2015; 76(6):440–450
[19] Lim HH, Lenarz T. Auditory midbrain implant: research and development towards a second clinical trial. Hear Res. 2015; 322:212–223
[20] McDermott HJ, McKay CM, Vandali AE. A new portable sound processor for the University of Melbourne/Nucleus Limited multielectrode cochlear implant. J Acoust Soc Am. 1992; 91(6):3367–3371
[21] Brackmann DE, Hitselberger WE, Nelson RA, et al. Auditory brainstem implant: I. Issues in surgical implantation. Otolaryngol Head Neck Surg. 1993; 108(6):624–633
[22] Shannon RV, Fayad J, Moore J, et al. Auditory brainstem implant: II. Postsurgical issues and performance. Otolaryngol Head Neck Surg. 1993; 108(6):634–642
[23] Laszig R, Sollmann WP, Marangos N. The restoration of hearing in neurofibromatosis type 2. J Laryngol Otol. 1995; 109(5):385–389
[24] Lenarz M, Matthies C, Lesinski-Schiedat A, et al. Auditory brainstem implant part II: subjective assessment of functional outcome. Otol Neurotol. 2002; 23 (5):694–697
[25] Vincent C, Zini C, Gandolfi A, et al. Results of the MXM Digisonic auditory brainstem implant clinical trials in Europe. Otol Neurotol. 2002; 23(1):56–60
[26] Nevison B, Laszig R, Sollmann WP, et al. Results from a European clinical investigation of the Nucleus multichannel auditory brainstem implant. Ear Hear. 2002; 23(3):170–183
[27] Otto SR, Brackmann DE, Hitselberger WE, Shannon RV, Kuchta J. Multichannel auditory brainstem implant: update on performance in 61 patients. J Neurosurg. 2002; 96(6):1063–1071
[28] Kanowitz SJ, Shapiro WH, Golfinos JG, Cohen NL, Roland JT, Jr. Auditory brainstem implantation in patients with neurofibromatosis type 2. Laryngoscope. 2004; 114(12):2135–2146
[29] Sanna M, Di Lella F, Guida M, Merkus P. Auditory brainstem implants in NF2 patients: results and review of the literature. Otol Neurotol. 2012; 33(2):154–164
[30] Grayeli AB, Kalamarides M, Bouccara D, Ambert-Dahan E, Sterkers O. Auditory brainstem implant in neurofibromatosis type 2 and non-neurofibromatosis type 2 patients. Otol Neurotol. 2008; 29(8):1140–1146
[31] Schwartz MS, Otto SR, Brackmann DE, Hitselberger WE, Shannon RV. Use of a multichannel auditory brainstem implant for neurofibromatosis type 2. Stereotact Funct Neurosurg. 2003; 81(1–4):110–114
[32] Maini S, Cohen MA, Hollow R, Briggs R. Update on long-term results with auditory brainstem implants in NF2 patients. Cochlear Implants Int. 2009; 10 Suppl 1:33–37
[33] Matthies C, Brill S, Kaga K, et al. Auditory brainstem implantation improves speech recognition in neurofibromatosis type II patients. ORL J Otorhinolaryngol Relat Spec. 2013; 75(5):282–295
[34] Matthies C, Brill S, Varallyay C, et al. Auditory brainstem implants in neurofibromatosis Type 2: is open speech perception feasible? J Neurosurg. 2014; 120(2):546–558
[35] Thong JF, Sung JK, Wong TK, Tong MC. Auditory brainstem implantation in Chinese patients with neurofibromatosis type II: the Hong Kong experience. Otol Neurotol. 2016; 37(7):956–962
[36] Ramsden RT, Freeman SR, Lloyd SK, et al. Manchester Neurofibromatosis Type 2 Service. Auditory brainstem implantation in neurofibromatosis type 2: experience from the Manchester Programme. Otol Neurotol. 2016; 37(9): 1267–1274
[37] Schwartz MS. Auditory brainstem implants in neurofibromatosis Type 2. J Neurosurg. 2014; 121(3):760–761
[38] Carlson ML, Breen JT, Driscoll CL, et al. Cochlear implantation in patients with neurofibromatosis type 2: variables affecting auditory performance. Otol Neurotol. 2012; 33(5):853–862
[39] Neff BA, Wiet RM, Lasak JM, et al. Cochlear implantation in the neurofibromatosis type 2 patient: long-term follow-up. Laryngoscope. 2007; 117(6):1069–1072
[40] Vincenti V, Pasanisi E, Guida M, Di Trapani G, Sanna M. Hearing rehabilitation in neurofibromatosis type 2 patients: cochlear versus auditory brainstem implantation. Audiol Neurootol. 2008; 13(4):273–280
[41] Tono T, Ushisako Y, Morimitsu T. Cochlear implantation in an intralabyrinthine acoustic neuroma patient after resection of an intracanalicular tumour. J Laryngol Otol. 1996; 110(6):570–573
[42] Graham J, Lynch C, Weber B, Stollwerck L, Wei J, Brookes G. The magnetless Clarion cochlear implant in a patient with neurofibromatosis 2. J Laryngol Otol. 1999; 113(5):458–463
[43] Ahsan S, Telischi F, Hodges A, Balkany T. Cochlear implantation concurrent with translabyrinthine acoustic neuroma resection. Laryngoscope. 2003; 113 (3):472–474
[44] Nölle C, Todt I, Basta D, Unterberg A, Mautner VF, Ernst A. Cochlear implantation after acoustic tumour resection in neurofibromatosis type 2: impact of intra- and postoperative neural response telemetry monitoring. ORL J Otorhinolaryngol Relat Spec. 2003; 65(4):230–234
[45] Arístegui M, Denia A. Simultaneous cochlear implantation and translabyrinthine removal of vestibular schwannoma in an only hearing ear: report of two cases (neurofibromatosis type 2 and unilateral vestibular schwannoma). Otol Neurotol. 2005; 26(2):205–210
[46] Lustig LR, Yeagle J, Driscoll CL, Blevins N, Francis H, Niparko JK. Cochlear implantation in patients with neurofibromatosis type 2 and bilateral vestibular schwannoma. Otol Neurotol. 2006; 27(4):512–518
[47] Tran Ba Huy P, Kania R, Frachet B, Poncet C, Legac MS. Auditory rehabilitation with cochlear implantation in patients with neurofibromatosis type 2. Acta Otolaryngol. 2009; 129(9):971–975
[48] Trotter MI, Briggs RJ. Cochlear implantation in neurofibromatosis type 2 after radiation therapy. Otol Neurotol. 2010; 31(2):216–219
[49] Roehm PC, Mallen-St Clair J, Jethanamest D, et al. Auditory rehabilitation of patients with neurofibromatosis Type 2 by using cochlear implants. J Neurosurg. 2011; 115(4):827–834
[50] Lloyd SK, Glynn FJ, Rutherford SA, et al. Ipsilateral cochlear implantation after cochlear nerve preserving vestibular schwannoma surgery in patients with neurofibromatosis type 2. Otol Neurotol. 2014; 35(1):43–51
[51] Linthicum FH, Jr, Brackmann DE. Bilateral acoustic tumors. A diagnostic and surgical challenge. Arch Otolaryngol. 1980; 106(12):729–733
[52] Mallory GW, Pollock BE, Foote RL, Carlson ML, Driscoll CL, Link MJ. Stereotactic radiosurgery for neurofibromatosis 2-associated vestibular schwannomas: toward dose optimization for tumor control and functional outcomes. Neurosurgery. 2014; 74(3):292–300, discussion 300–301
[53] Roberts DS, Otto S, Chen B, et al. Tinnitus suppression after auditory brainstem implantation in patients with neurofibromatosis type-2. Otol Neurotol. 2017; 38(1):118–122

Index

Note: Page numbers set **bold** or *italic* indicate headings or figures, respectively.

D

E

I

J

L

S

V

W

X